KV-014-037

Progress in Pain Research and Management
Volume 16

Proceedings of the 9th World Congress on Pain

Mission Statement of IASP Press®

The International Association for the Study of Pain (IASP) is a nonprofit, interdisciplinary organization devoted to understanding the mechanisms of pain and improving the care of patients with pain through research, education, and communication. The organization includes scientists and health care professionals dedicated to these goals. The IASP sponsors scientific meetings and publishes newsletters, technical bulletins, the journal *Pain,* and books.

The goal of IASP Press is to provide the IASP membership with timely, high-quality, attractive, low-cost publications relevant to the problem of pain. These publications are also intended to appeal to a wider audience of scientists and clinicians interested in the problem of pain.

Previous volumes in the series Progress in Pain Research and Management

Pharmacological Approaches to the Treatment of Chronic Pain: New Concepts and Critical Issues, edited by Howard L. Fields and John C. Liebeskind

Proceedings of the 7th World Congress on Pain, edited by Gerald F. Gebhart, Donna L. Hammond, and Troels S. Jensen

Touch, Temperature, and Pain in Health and Disease: Mechanisms and Assessments, edited by Jörgen Boivie, Per Hansson, and Ulf Lindblom

Temporomandibular Disorders and Related Pain Conditions, edited by Barry J. Sessle, Patricia S. Bryant, and Raymond A. Dionne

Visceral Pain, edited by Gerald F. Gebhart

Reflex Sympathetic Dystrophy: A Reappraisal, edited by Wilfrid Jänig and Michael Stanton-Hicks

Pain Treatment Centers at a Crossroads: A Practical and Conceptual Reappraisal, edited by Mitchell J.M. Cohen and James N. Campbell

Proceedings of the 8th World Congress on Pain, edited by Troels S. Jensen, Judith A. Turner, and Zsuzsanna Wiesenfeld-Hallin

Molecular Neurobiology of Pain, edited by David Borsook

Measurement of Pain in Infants and Children, edited by G. Allen Finley and Patrick J. McGrath

Sickle Cell Pain, by Samir K. Ballas

Assessment and Treatment of Cancer Pain, edited by Richard Payne, Richard B. Patt, and C. Stratton Hill.

Chronic and Recurrent Pain in Children and Adolescents, edited by Patrick J. McGrath and G. Allen Finley

Opioid Sensitivity of Chronic Noncancer Pain, edited by E. Kalso, H.J. McQuay, and Z. Wiesenfeld-Hallin

Psychological Mechanisms of Pain and Analgesia, by Donald D. Price

Progress in Pain Research and Management
Volume 16

Proceedings of the 9th World Congress on Pain

Editors

Marshall Devor, PhD

Department of Cell and Animal Biology,
Institute of Life Sciences,
Hebrew University of Jerusalem, Jerusalem, Israel

Michael C. Rowbotham, MD

Department of Clinical Neurology and Anesthesia
and UCSF Pain Clinical Research Center,
University of California, San Francisco,
California, USA

Zsuzsanna Wiesenfeld-Hallin, PhD

Department of Medical Laboratory Sciences and Technology,
Section of Clinical Neurophysiology,
Karolinska Institute, Huddinge, Sweden

IASP PRESS® • SEATTLE

Timely topics in pain research and treatment have been selected for publication, but the information provided and opinions expressed have not involved any verification of the findings, conclusions, and opinions by IASP®. Thus, opinions expressed in *Proceedings of the 9th World Congress on Pain* do not necessarily reflect those of IASP or of the Officers and Councillors.

No responsibility is assumed by IASP for any injury and/or damage to persons or property as a matter of product liability, negligence, or from any use of any methods, products, instruction, or ideas contained in the material herein. Because of the rapid advances in the medical sciences, the publisher recommends that there should be independent verification of diagnoses and drug dosages.

Library of Congress Cataloging-in-Publication Data

World Congress on Pain (9th: 1999: Vienna, Austria)
Proceedings of the 9th World Congress on Pain / editors, Marshall Devor, Michael C. Rowbotham, Zsuzsanna Wiesenfeld-Hallin.
p. ; cm. -- (Progress in pain research and management ; v. 16)
Includes bibliographical references and index.
ISBN 0-931092-31-0 (alk. paper)
1. Pain--Congresses. I. Title: Proceedings of the Ninth World Congress on Pain. II. Devor, Marshall. III. Rowbotham, Michael C. IV. Wiesenfeld-Hallin, Z. V. Title. VI. Series.
[DNLM: 1. Pain--Congresses. WL 704 W927p 2000]
RB127.W675 1999
616'.0472--dc21

00-023918

Published by:

IASP Press
International Association for the Study of Pain
909 NE 43rd St., Suite 306
Seattle, WA 98105 USA
Fax: 206-547-1703
www.halcyon.com/iasp

Printed in the United States of America

Contents

Contributing Authors

The 9th IASP World Congress on Pain and this congress proceedings volume are dedicated to our teacher and colleague, Professor Patrick D. Wall

Preface

The field of pain science and medicine is in a phase of extraordinary effervescence, creativity, and rapid growth, with new discoveries and insights appearing at a remarkable pace. This enthusiasm was dramatically reflected in the 9th World Congress on Pain, held in Vienna, Austria, August 22–27, 1999. The congress attracted a record number of pain professionals (nearly 6000) and provided an exciting forum for scientific discourse, with substantial media coverage and other opportunities for increasing public awareness. In preparing this proceedings volume, the editors have attempted to capture the dynamism that characterized the Vienna congress.

Under the theme, "Pain: from Molecule to Mind," the congress featured a full day of refresher courses, 19 plenary and special lectures, 90 workshops on topics in basic and clinical science, and more than 1700 poster presentations. In this volume, chapters written by the plenary and special lecturers place the reader at the cutting edge of the field on topics with which all pain professionals should have at least a passing familiarity. "Mini-reviews" present material related to various topical workshops. The remaining chapters provide a varied and eclectic selection of particularly novel and informative offerings from among the poster presentations in Vienna. Some of the poster-based chapters present new findings in areas of specialized pain research. Others will appeal to a broader audience. For example, if you have ever wondered on a hot summer's day why cold soda or beer produces that almost painful tingle as it runs down your throat, you will find the answer in Chapter 21. Overall, the proceedings volume constitutes an up-to-date handbook touching on virtually every aspect of pain science and medicine at the dawn of the 21st century. (Contents of the refresher courses are available in a separate volume: *Pain 1999—An Updated Review,* edited by M. Max; Seattle: IASP Press, 1999.)

Editing this book has given us an opportunity to reflect on some of the major themes that characterize our field at present. For example, there is a growing interest in neural mechanisms—a desire to understand the detailed workings of the biological machine that detects and responds to noxious stimuli. The pharmacology of analgesic drugs has always been of central importance, but now drug actions are increasingly being explored at the level of the molecule, its receptor(s), and the cellular processes that are triggered following receptor binding. Most would agree that the star molecule in Vienna was the Na^+ channel, but many others also played leading roles.

Scientists are also aggressively pursuing neural mechanisms at the systems level, largely thanks to a set of new and clinically relevant animal models of chronic pain states. The force of experimental evidence in this area is shattering many of our most cherished and deeply held beliefs. For example, most authorities are now convinced that pain is *not* the exclusive domain of C and Aδ nociceptors. Many chapters in this volume discuss pain ("allodynia") evoked by light-touch activation of low-threshold, fast-conducting, heavily myelinated Aβ afferent fibers. And let there be no mistake: this "Aβ pain" is not a rare peculiarity of odd clinical states. Rather, it is a common feature of mundane, everyday painful events such as burns, bruises, infections, and perhaps even migraine (see Chapters 12 and 55).

New areas of discourse have begun to penetrate and influence our thinking about pain. The Vienna congress was the first to spotlight the newly emerging area of "pain genetics." The identification of pain susceptibility genes may well lead to more powerful and selective analgesic agents in the future. But even in the near term such research offers potential benefits, notably the hope that those who experience pain more intensely than the norm may finally be freed of social stigma born of the erroneous assumption that such people are simply "complainers."

Some congress delegates stated that the striking advances in pain science seemed to overshadow the relatively slow progress in the clinical management of pain patients. As the outgoing IASP president, Jean-Marie Besson, pointed out, movement from the laboratory to the clinic is often agonizingly slow. Yet at the congress we celebrated the recent introduction into everyday use of an entirely new family of powerful and safer analgesic agents, the COX-2 inhibitors (see Chapter 74), and the continued success of another relatively new drug family, the migraine-relieving triptans.

Perhaps the most important new trend in clinical research evident in Vienna is the spirit of rationalism that is rapidly entering pain medicine. In the past, we have based our actions too much on historical authority and wishful thinking. In the future, pain medicine must be based on solid evidence. This volume highlights methods for obtaining and interpreting such evidence, including new approaches that permit quantitative comparisons among competing therapeutic agents (see Chapter 73). This new emphasis on "evidence-based medicine" should not be construed as an attack on alternative or nonconventional methods—very often we do not know the biological mechanism of treatments that are effective. But we do need evidence of efficacy. In the words of Kurt Vonnegut: "Science is magic that works." But one word of caution: Those who are the first to adopt evidence-based methods must take care not to alienate those who are still mulling over the meaning of this trend. Medical wisdom accumulated over years of practical clinical experience has undeniable value and should not be disdained.

Most participants in the Vienna congress, and the editors of this volume, fully acknowledge that pain cannot be understood simply as a set of molecular interactions, a state relieved by analgesic drugs or procedures. Pain is a sensory and emotional experience; it always occurs within the context of a person's life. Pain is powerfully modulated, for better or worse, by our beliefs and expectations and by the empathy and involvement of those around us. Richard Gracely eloquently points out in Chapter 99 that even in this watershed year 2000, the practical relief of pain remains in considerable part an art.

Finally, the editors wish to pay homage to our friend and mentor, Professor Patrick D. Wall, to whom the Vienna congress and this book are dedicated. Probably more than any other single living person, Pat Wall has put the puzzle of pain on the intellectual map. It is the combination of scientific and clinical progress that will give pain medicine the visibility and social impact it needs and deserves. Although fundamentally a basic scientist, Pat has always insisted on the importance of keeping the pain patient at the center of our focus. The average citizen needs to recognize that there is no excuse for severe pain—it simply should not be tolerated. In time we will look back on Vienna from the perspective of future world congresses on pain. Who knows which highlights of this book will by then have proved to be evanescent sparks, and which enduring themes that moved the field forward? But one thing can be predicted with confidence: the care and well-being of the pain patient will remain the central focus of all of our efforts.

MARSHALL DEVOR
MICHAEL C. ROWBOTHAM
ZSUZSANNA WIESENFELD-HALLIN

Acknowledgments

The editors of this volume and the officers and members of the Council of the International Association for the Study of Pain express their appreciation to the many individuals whose efforts were so important to the success of the 9th World Congress on Pain and of this book.

We first thank our colleagues on the Scientific Program Committee, Jean-Marie Besson, Sandra R. Chaplan, Michael J. Cousins, Andy Dray, Richard H. Gracely, Troels S. Jensen, Louisa E. Jones, Wade S. Kingery, Martin Koltzenburg, Sharon A. Lamb, Paolo Marchettini, Mitchell Max, Patricia McGrath, Henry McQuay, Jeffrey Mogil, Miklos Rethelyi, M. Omar Tawfik, Masaya Tohyama, Horacio Vanegas, Peter Wessely, and Clifford J. Woolf, upon whom the editorial group depended for the outline planning of the scientific program, which was so well received.

We thank Peter Wessely, chair of the Local Arrangements Committee in Vienna, and his colleagues Günther Lanner, Rudolf F. Morawetz, and Hans G. Kress. Special thanks are due to the Congress Secretariat in Vienna, ICOS Congress Organisation Service, and to their meeting coordinator, Silke Ortmann, who took great care in overseeing registration and all the on-site details. We are grateful for their hard work on our behalf. We also thank the staff at the Austria Center Vienna for their attentive care to our meeting. We extend special gratitude to Louisa Jones, IASP Executive Officer, for her invaluable efforts in organizing the Congress. Thanks also to all IASP staff members, especially Marilyn Carlson, Marleda di Pierri, Kathleen Havers, Karen Lauderback, Roberta Scholz, and Heather Spiess, whose hard work before and during the congress was an important contribution to the overall success of the meeting.

The editors express appreciation to the staff of the publications department of IASP and IASP Press, Elizabeth Endres, Sandra Marvinney, Dale Schmidt, and Roberta Scholz for their dedicated work in preparing this book for publication.

On behalf of the Council and members of IASP, the editors acknowledge and express their special appreciation for the financial support given to the 9th World Congress on Pain and related IASP programs by:

Allergan (UK)
ASTA Medica AG (Germany)
Boots Healthcare International (UK)
Endo Pharmaceuticals Inc. (USA)
Grünenthal GmbH (Germany)
Janssen Pharmaceutica (Belgium)
Medtronic, Inc. (USA, France)
Menarini International (Italy)
Neurex Corporation (USA)
Novartis (UK)
Parke-Davis (USA)
Pfizer Pharmaceuticals (USA)
The Procter & Gamble Company (USA)
Purdue Pharma L.P. (USA)
UPSA Laboratoires, a Bristol-Myers Squibb Company (France)
UPSA Pain Institute (France)

Proceedings of the 9th World Congress on Pain, Progress in Pain Research and Management, Vol. 16, edited by M. Devor, M.C. Rowbotham, and Z. Wiesenfeld-Hallin, IASP Press, Seattle, © 2000.

1

President's Address to the 9th World Congress on Pain: Basic Researchers and Clinicians Must Unite in the Fight against Pain

Jean-Marie Besson

Laboratory of Physiopharmacology of the Nervous System, INSERM; and Laboratory of Physiopharmacology of Pain, Ecole Pratique des Hautes Etudes, Paris, France

The International Association for the Study of Pain celebrated its 25th anniversary in 1998. In this chapter, I wish to draw several general conclusions about events along the long road that we have taken since the meeting in Issaquah in May 1973, at which the inspiration of J.J. Bonica led to the establishment of our association in 1973 and its incorporation in 1974. Not many of the participants in this 9th World Congress took part in that meeting in Issaquah, but the 5800 participants at this congress conclusively demonstrate the vitality of our association.

The booklet published to mark the 25th anniversary of IASP beautifully illustrates the philosophy and organization of our association. This booklet, tracing the maturation of IASP over the years, is a credit to the competence of our staff, led in such an excellent manner by Louisa Jones, our executive officer. That several of our officers and councillors also hold positions of responsibility in other national and international societies bears witness to the professionalism and rigorous approach of our members, whom we count among the great riches of our association. The future of IASP depends to a great extent on maintaining these standards.

From the financial perspective, IASP is prudently and efficiently managed. Thanks to the generous support of the contributing members and others who supported specific IASP programs and projects, IASP is completely independent financially. The journal *Pain* now provides income for the association. IASP was able to allocate $100,000 to help persons from developing and currency-restricted countries and trainees from developed countries attend the congress in Vienna.

I must also remind you that over the past 4 years the membership fees have not changed, and they will remain unchanged in the year 2000. This is remarkable, considering that among the benefits of membership are 15 issues of *Pain* (about 2000 pages this year, including the special issue in honor of Dr. P.D. Wall), the *IASP Newsletter, Pain Clinical Updates,* and other material. Additional good news is that IASP Press is doing very well and publishing high-quality and very inexpensive books.

We do, of course, recognize and regret the fact that our fees are too high for many of our colleagues in developing countries and in countries with currency restrictions. We have discussed this issue at council meetings since IASP's inception. For various reasons—financial, technical, and scientific—this problem has proved practically impossible to resolve.

As a practical solution, I would like to suggest that our members, regardless of nationality, personally contact companies (pharmaceutical and others) and ask them to consider paying the membership dues for a certain number of persons in countries with these difficulties. Some may say that I am living in a fantasy world, but I think this approach would be of great help to many members. I understand the concept that "business is business," but support in the form that I suggest would be ethically more acceptable than providing financial backing, often excessive, to particular individuals for foreign travel that is not always justified professionally. Health systems around the world are on the brink of crisis. The type of assistance I am suggesting would significantly advance good relations between industry and health professionals involved in the control of pain. I hope that this message is taken up by representatives of the pharmaceutical industry and other readers. This suggestion becomes even more valid given that the treatment of pain worldwide remains inadequate. Disparity among nations, religions, and age groups, socioeconomic and cultural difficulties, and inadequacies in the teaching of this subject are additional problems.

Although financial considerations sometimes forestall improvements in the care of patients with acute and chronic pain, pressure exerted by organizations (notably IASP and its national chapters), health professionals, patients, and a few rare politicians has forced governments to take greater responsibility. It is comforting to note that general practitioners in numerous countries are increasingly treating both acute and chronic pain. The consequence is an increase in the number of specialists involved in pain treatment and in the number of pain treatment centers. I am well aware that many members of IASP have selflessly put society's interests ahead of their own, and are playing a major role in our fight against pain. I thank them for their efforts.

We need to improve the functioning of IASP in a number of areas, including education and communication. I may appear to be stating the obvious, but the practical aspects are far from straightforward in an international organization with members from more than 90 countries. I have somewhat neglected some of these issues, but I am sure that our new president, Barry Sessle, an expert in the field of education, will give new impetus to our association in this regard.

Concerning communication, I would like to remind members and chapters that we encourage them to contact IASP's various committees and task forces. Members rarely do so, and I do not know why. Is it a lack of interest among our members or perhaps the relatively passive nature of some of our committees? I favor another explanation: after 25 years of existence, IASP is a highly structured organization, functional and efficient.

To improve the relations between IASP headquarters and national chapters, the Council has taken the following steps:

1) The president will appoint a liaison to facilitate relationships between regional organizations of IASP chapters and other multinational bodies.

2) Chapter presidents will receive Council and Executive Committee minutes after approval.

3) Chapters will receive a form for submitting an annual report, along with a copy of the previous year's report (if appropriate) and an example of a completed return.

4) IASP will encourage chapters to submit grant proposals for the translation into other languages of IASP's written materials. Such proposals will be renewed as appropriate.

5) Current educational material will be assessed. A strategy to implement the dissemination of information to the widest possible audience will be introduced.

6) The implementation group will consider the production of fact sheets that are brief, practical, and suitable for translation.

7) The secretary will be writing to chapter presidents to clarify the use of the IASP logo when advertising chapter and regional meetings.

8) Chapters are reminded that it is highly desirable that all chapter officers be members of IASP.

9) Council agrees to develop a program to support IASP visiting professors for chapter meetings as permitted by practical considerations.

These proposals lead me to mention the activity of various committees, task forces, and special interest groups. The standards of some have been very satisfactory, whereas others have unfortunately been quiet. I am personally very keen on the creation of guidelines for the editors of the special interest group (SIG) newsletters. Certain problems have arisen, and we must emphasize that these newsletters should not consist of personal viewpoints but must reflect discussions of the group members.

I wish to discuss in more detail the membership growth of IASP. Membership initially grew quickly after 1973, and then the rate of increase slackened. However, IASP welcomed about 500 new members between 1993 and 1996 and almost 800 between 1996 and 1999. The membership currently exceeds 7000. I am aware that some of you feel that this figure is not sufficient, considering the membership counts of the national pain societies. Our association, which encompasses many specialist fields and medical disciplines and counts as members various health professionals and basic scientists, has an open-door policy but has never had the goal of recruiting new members at all costs.

As our name implies, the aim of IASP is to encourage research on pain mechanisms and pain syndromes by bringing together highly competent and motivated people. Over the course of the past 25 years the composition of our membership has changed a great deal. At the 1973 meeting that mandated the creation of IASP, there were roughly equal numbers of clinicians and basic scientists. This is no longer the case: clinicians now form the majority. This can only be good news for patients, especially if we also consider that the absolute number of basic researchers is increasing rapidly. It is always gratifying to meet new young investigators during our congresses.

The encouragement of direct links between basic scientists and clinicians is one of the unique features of IASP. This must be maintained at all costs because it is a major factor in the quality of our meetings and of our diverse publications. Some clinicians have reproached us by saying that the science of pain is too complicated. I fully understand this viewpoint. However, I must say that this complexity is found not only in the pain area but in many fields of medicine, and is a feature of the neurosciences in general. The excellent scientific program and refresher courses in Vienna, organized by Marshall Devor and Mitchell Max, helped inform us all of developments in many important areas in basic and clinical pain research.

Although we have been through periods where understanding the relations among the different pieces of the puzzle of pain has been facilitated by important discoveries from the fundamental sciences, I nevertheless sense a degree of disillusionment among certain clinicians. This disappointment could be due in part to the fact that few original therapeutic agents have been produced for clinical use in recent years. We must remember that the production of new medicines is the goal and responsibility of the pharmaceutical industry, guided by the discoveries of scientists investigating basic mechanisms. We wish them every success in their search for new therapeutic agents.

Experimental researchers are well aware of the complexity and the difficulty of applying their discoveries, but they are themselves confronted by both methodological difficulties and the complexities of the nervous system itself (a jungle of neurochemical and anatomical connections from the periphery to the brain, with multiple receptors and subtypes of receptors). I sympathize with readers who are clinicians and find themselves confused by the descriptions of multiple substances involved in the circuitry of pain.

I will briefly consider a few of the problems arising in fundamental research. Our knowledge of the neurobiology of pain continues to grow, with discoveries in electrophysiology and molecular biology offering glimpses of potential therapeutic breakthroughs. However, I believe that the gaps between the clinical and basic sciences are widening. To put it simply, basic research is fascinating and flourishes in the public eye. However, too often it takes a naive approach to the difficult issues that confront clinicians providing therapy for certain types of pain. With few exceptions, clinicians have only "old molecules" available for treating pain. Providing clinicians with "new molecules" is difficult and takes a long time. For example, the opioid receptors were formally identified in 1973, but we are still awaiting the development of an opioid with the efficacy of morphine but without its side effects. The best research groups in molecular biology have spent 20 years in the race to clone the three main receptors: μ, δ, and κ. Many questions are still unresolved.

The relevance of the major behavioral models of clinical pain states has been widely debated. In most cases, stimuli are applied to healthy animals not afflicted by disorders that commonly occur in pain patients, such as hyperalgesia (extreme sensitivity to painful stimuli), allodynia (pain in response to a non-noxious stimulus), and hyperesthesia (abnormal sensitivity to a sensory stimulus). Some of these tests depend on spinal mechanisms, whereas others involve supraspinal structures. Some tests have good sensitivity for a particular class of analgesics, but other tests frequently produce false-positive results. In addition, many behavioral experiments use only one nociceptive test, and the exact method of its application can vary from investigator to investigator, making comparisons uncertain. Thus, controversy surrounds the pharmacology of pain. Laboratory and behavioral models are limited because they do not fully mimic chronic pain states in humans. Chronic pain differs substantially from acute pain with respect to persistence and adaptive changes such as neuroplasticity, which has been described at various levels of the nervous system. Such limitations have led to the development of more appropriate models of chronic pain in the last 15 years. These models include inflammatory pain and neuropathic pain.

Although they are not perfect, the development of such experimental models is essential, not only for the testing of new analgesics, but also for gaining a better understanding of the neural mechanisms underlying pain syndromes that are difficult to manage clinically. However, behavioral tests are limited and can be remarkably difficult to administer. Clinicians need to realize, for example, how hard it can be for a researcher to quantify allodynia by approaching an awake, freely moving rat or mouse with a calibrated von Frey hair.

Other difficulties encountered in the development of safe analgesics arise from the complexity of the nervous system. Some transmitters and receptors that may be involved in the transmission or modulation of pain are widely distributed throughout the nervous system, especially in the case of peptides and excitatory or inhibitory amino acids. Most of these neuroactive substances are involved in multiple physiological functions, thus agents developed to target these systems could produce widespread side effects. Additional difficulties result from the multiplicity of receptors and the colocalization of more than one neurotransmitter in a single neuron. Nevertheless, advances in the biological prediction of the structure of macromolecules will allow the three-dimensional structure of receptors to be elucidated. This, in turn, should ultimately lead to the development of agonists and antagonists with great specificity and fewer side effects, such as sodium channel blockers or adrenergic α_2-receptor ligands.

Various genetic approaches have been used to study pain processes, including the recent production of transgenic mice. Although there is no doubt that the deletion of receptors, channels, and transmitters by genetic manipulations produces a powerful tool for the dissection of the roles of these molecules in complex neuronal systems, the results of genetic approaches need to be interpreted with caution. Large-scale pharmacological research is needed to bring new drugs on line.

In the peripheral nervous system, a myriad of substances of neuronal or non-neuronal origin modulate the activity of nociceptors, and various interactions can occur between these mediators. Key immediate questions relevant to both the clinician and the pharmacologist are the following: Could the modulation of only one of these substances be sufficient to alter the level of pain in the periphery? Could there be a magic bullet with peripheral actions only? The latter option is unlikely, based on current pharmacological information. Only an in-depth analysis of the physiopathology of the different syndromes originating from peripheral processes can guide a clinician in prescribing the most effective substance. An alternative approach that seems more likely to be useful would be to produce an analgesic with mixed peripheral effects that acts on different receptor types, or perhaps to move toward a systematic analysis of the effects of administration of several agents.

The same questions arise at the spinal level, where numerous chemicals are implicated in the transmission and modulation of pain messages. Is it realistic to expect the development of a single magic bullet, or should we be thinking in terms of molecules with dual pharmacological actions or the use of a combination of drugs (multimodal analgesia) to elicit synergistic or additive actions of the combination? We have many examples of this approach, such as the association of morphine with agonists at the adrenergic α_2-receptor, or with antagonists at the cholecystokinin and the NMDA receptors. This type of approach has the potential dual advantages of improved effects and fewer side effects through use of lower doses of each agent. These examples are only a few of the many combinations that might enhance the usefulness of morphine. Although this approach is less spectacular than the magic bullet, it could be more beneficial to the patient and could be used as a general principle in this research.

I only have space here for these brief reflections on certain aspects of the pharmacology of the periphery and the spinal cord, and cannot describe the far greater complexity that arises when nociceptive messages arrive in the brain. Basic studies have described multiple ascending pathways; the spinothalamic tract is hardly the only route! We eagerly await clinical application of results that have recently been obtained with PET scans and fMRI.

The complexity of pain must not discourage us—we must face the problems with determination. On the other hand, I hope that scientists engaged in research will take a more realistic approach to their results so that clinicians are not misled into believing that many useful treatments for pain are just around the corner. Finally, I have two major wishes. One is that clinicians faced with the complexities of the nervous system take steps toward improving their understanding of basic science. The other is that basic scientists incorporate clinical aspects of pain when they plan their experimental studies. Furthermore, it is important for scientists to avoid "neuroscience show biz" and avoid giving false hopes either to cl-inicians or to patients and their families. Let us pull together for the benefit of IASP and our fight against pain.

Correspondence to: Jean-Marie Besson, DSc, INSERM, Unité 161, 2 rue d'Alésia, Paris, 75014, France. Tel: 33-1-4589-3662; Fax: 33-1-4588-1304; email: besson@broca.inserm.fr.

Proceedings of the 9th World Congress on Pain, Progress in Pain Research and Management, Vol. 16, edited by M. Devor, M.C. Rowbotham, and Z. Wiesenfeld-Hallin, IASP Press, Seattle, © 2000.

2

Incoming President's Address: Looking Back, Looking Ahead

Barry J. Sessle

Faculty of Dentistry, University of Toronto, Toronto, Ontario, Canada

It is a great pleasure to have the opportunity to write this chapter as the incoming president of the International Association for the Study of Pain (IASP). It is both an honor and a privilege to serve the association for the next three years, and to help steer it into the next century. IASP has grown in leaps and bounds since it was established just over 25 years ago under the visionary and dedicated leadership of John Bonica. I wish to recognize the remarkable contributions that all eight presidents have made to our association since its inception, especially the outstanding leadership that Dr. Jean-Marie Besson has given to IASP over the past three years. Along with the hard-working members of IASP Council and the various committees and task forces of IASP, Dr. Besson has helped ensure the continued growth and progress of the association and its influence worldwide on pain research and management. He and indeed all members of IASP have been extremely well served by the talented central office staff in Seattle under the very capable leadership of our executive officer, Louisa Jones. I also recognize Professor Marshall Devor and his Scientific Program Committee and Professor Peter Wessely and members of the Local Arrangements Committee for helping to make the recent world congress in Vienna a huge success. Regrettably, our enjoyment of the many positive aspects of the congress was partly offset by the earthquake disaster in Turkey that occurred just before the start of the congress, which limited the participation of many of our Turkish colleagues. I am pleased to note that in addition to the donations offered by individual congress participants at the IASP booth, IASP has provided a significant donation for Turkish disaster relief.

I join a line of IASP presidents whose diversity reflects the international character of our membership and accords well with the multidisciplinary nature not only of IASP but also of the study and management of pain. Our previous eight presidents have been from Australia, Canada, continental Europe, Great Britain, and the USA, and have come from the fields of anesthesiology, neurology, neuroscience, neurosurgery, and psychology. Being a native of Australia and a resident now of Canada, I reflect the geographic diversity of IASP. Furthermore, although my own research interests in pain primarily relate to my training and expertise as a neuroscientist, I am a dentist, the first dentist to assume the IASP presidency. Dentists are commonly associated with pain and pain relief, so who better to lead an association dedicated to improved pain research and management! Some of the most common pains in the body occur in the orofacial region, namely several types of toothaches and headaches. This region is a very common or selective site of chronic pain (e.g., temporomandibular disorders) and certain excruciatingly painful conditions (e.g., trigeminal neuralgia), but the etiology and pathogenesis and even the classification of many of these pain conditions are still unclear, partly because of the limited research focus on this field (Dubner et al. 1978; Woda and Pionchon 1999; Sessle 2000). One goal of my presidency will be to raise the consciousness of IASP members about the orofacial pain field and to enhance the visibility of IASP among my colleagues in dentistry. One step in this direction has been the formulation at the recent world congress of a provisional special interest group in orofacial pain.

During my 30 years or so in the fields of orofacial pain and sensorimotor research, I have witnessed the remarkable growth both of IASP and of our knowledge of pain processes and management. The last 30 years have seen the discovery of several endogenous neurochemicals and intrinsic pathways in the brain, and we have learned about their influences on nociceptive transmission and pain behavior. We have seen improvements in the pharmacological, surgical, and behavioral management of pain, and recognized the importance of biopsychosocial factors in pain expression and behavior. We have developed concepts and insights about peripheral and central sensitization, and recognized the neuroplasticity of pain processes, finding that these central processes and associated circuits are not "hard-wired," but that, in line with the gate-control theory of pain espoused by Melzack and Wall (1965) 35 years ago, they can be modulated by a number of factors. We have also witnessed the rapidly expanding fields of brain imaging and molecular and gene biology and their applicability to the pain field. These are just a few of the many areas where significant advances have been made in understanding and controlling pain during this period.

These advances in knowledge have not taken place in isolation, but in large part they reflect the tremendous parallel growth in the fields of neuroscience and molecular biology. We in the pain field have certainly benefited from the increased research focus on the brain over the past 30 years, but another major factor has been IASP itself. Through its primary mandate to foster pain research and management, it has helped fuel these many advances; surely it is not a coincidence that its progress has paralleled that of pain research, neuroscience, and molecular biology. As we enter the new millennium and a new era for IASP and the sciences, I believe that there is merit in taking stock of IASP, in noting its achievements over the 25 years of its existence, and in identifying the challenges that lie ahead for the association in the early years of the next century. I will examine how IASP has fared relative to its stated purposes, and use this "self-study" to outline my other goals for the next three years as president.

The association has 10 stated purposes that are outlined in its Articles of Incorporation and Bylaws (see Table I). I will concentrate on the first three, which in my view are the most important purposes, while the remaining seven are additional purposes to help achieve them.

Table I
IASP Purposes

A. To foster and encourage research of pain mechanisms and pain syndromes and to help improve the management of patients with acute and chronic pain by bringing together basic scientists, physicians, and other health professionals of various disciplines and backgrounds who have an interest in pain research and management.

B. To promote education and training in the field of pain.

C. To promote and facilitate the dissemination of new information in the field of pain, including sponsorship of a journal, *Pain*.

D. To promote and sponsor a triennial World Congress of the Association, and such other meetings as may be useful or desirable for the advancement of the purposes of the association.

E. To encourage the formation of national associations for the study and treatment of pain.

F. To encourage the adoption of a uniform classification, nomenclature, and definition regarding pain and pain syndromes.

G. To encourage the development of a national and international data bank and to encourage the development of a uniform records system with respect to information relating to pain mechanisms, syndromes, and management.

H. To inform the general public of the results and implications of current research in the area.

I. To advise international, national, and regional agencies on standards relating to the use of drugs, appliances, and other procedures in the therapy of pain.

J. To engage in such other activities as may be incidental to or in furtherance of the aforementioned purposes.

1) To foster and encourage research of pain mechanisms and pain syndromes and to help improve the management of patients with acute and chronic pain by bringing together basic scientists, physicians, and other health professionals of various disciplines and backgrounds who have an interest in pain research and management. As Dr. Besson mentioned in his president's address, encouraging pain research and improving pain management are very vital functions of IASP. Several yardsticks can be applied to determine how IASP has performed in this area. The association serves as the most prestigious organizational focus for those interested in pain research and management, and as a result the membership has grown phenomenally over this time (Fig. 1). The world's pain scientists and clinicians gather at IASP's World Congress on Pain, a blue ribbon event which has also grown. Membership stood at just over 1000 at the 1st World Congress on Pain held in Florence in 1975, which had fewer than 1000 participants representing 75 disciplines, and included around 250 free communications and plenary or workshop lectures. The multidisciplinary nature of our membership and of the congress participants was retained at the 9th World Congress, but our association has grown almost sevenfold to 7000 members, the number of participants has increased to almost 6000, and the number of presentations has grown to almost 1900 (Fig. 2). In bringing together pain scientists and clinicians from a wide variety of disciplines to its congress, IASP has addressed not only purpose A but also purpose D (Table I). Indeed, the quality of the congresses has been uniformly outstanding, and very informative and high-quality books have resulted from all of them. IASP has also encouraged many other meetings that have helped advance

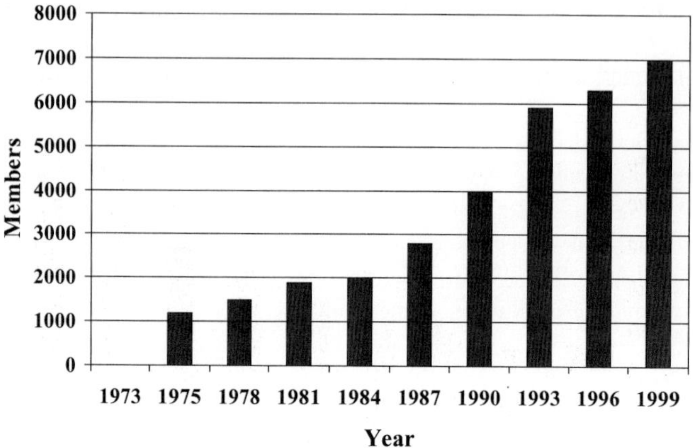

Fig. 1. Growth in IASP membership.

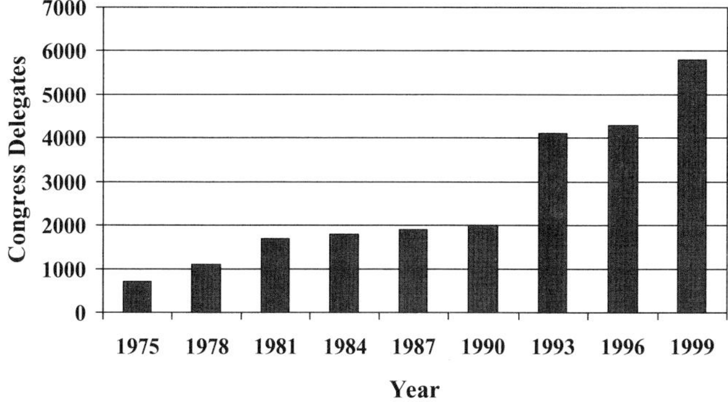

Fig. 2. Growth in number of participants at IASP world congresses on pain.

the objectives of the association. The challenge for the next congress in San Diego is to be even more successful by these various yardsticks than the exceptional congress in Vienna!

The number of IASP chapters has also grown 10-fold over this period (Fig. 3). In fostering the formation of IASP chapters that bring together members from different disciplines, both purposes A and E (Table I) are being addressed. At present 94 countries are represented in IASP. As noted in more detail below, a particular challenge for IASP is to foster chapter growth in regions with limited fiscal and infrastructure support.

The multidisciplinary nature of IASP and the broad perspectives that it helps bring to bear on various aspects of pain are also evidenced in the growth of the special interest groups (SIGs) in the space of just 10 years; there are currently nine active SIGs (Table II), and I anticipate that three others will receive provisional status in the very near future from IASP Council.

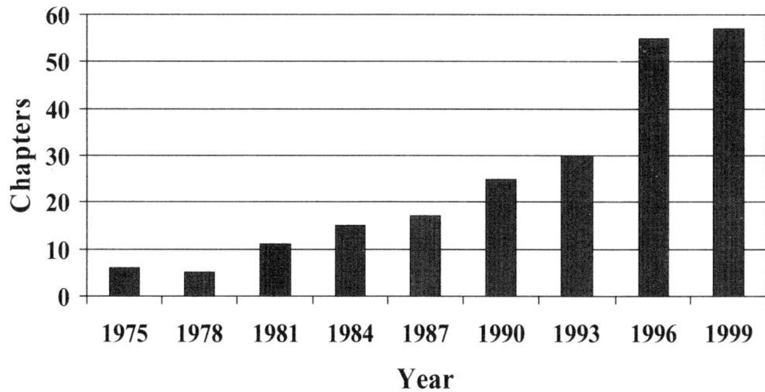

Fig. 3. Growth in number of IASP chapters.

Table II
Current IASP Special Interest Groups

Pain in Childhood (1989)
Pain and the Sympathetic Nervous System (1990)
Clinical/Legal Issues in Pain (1994)
Systematic Reviews in Pain Relief (1996)
Rheumatic Pain (1996)
Placebo (1997)
Sex, Gender, and Pain (1997)
Pain of Urogenital Origin (1998)
Refractory Angina (1999)

IASP also has taken an active leadership role in fostering research into pain mechanisms and management, not only by providing new knowledge through such vehicles as its world congresses and its publications, but also by recognizing outstanding research achievements through its research awards and by establishing last year a series of annual research symposia. Additional approaches, which have addressed purposes F and G (Table I) as well as A, have been the development of a manual and database for treatment center records and data retrieval, and the archiving of material related to IASP and to pain in general. A notable achievement in this area has been the recent establishment of the John C. Liebeskind History of Pain Collection at the University of California at Los Angeles, dedicated last year to the memory of IASP President-Elect John Liebeskind, a friend and colleague of many of us who tragically passed away before he could assume the IASP presidency. The association must continue to foster the development of these valuable resources. In addition, through the efforts of Professor Harold Merskey and other members, IASP has established landmark guidelines on the classification and description of pain conditions. This is not to say that IASP can rest on its laurels; rather it should continue to foster other ways of looking at pain classification, as exemplified in one of the workshop sessions at the recent world congress, "A Mechanisms-Based Pain Classification Scheme," organized by Ronald Dubner.

The association has tried to provide support and encouragement for developing countries and others in which currency restrictions, funding, or infrastructure may not be conducive to fostering pain research and management. It has also tried to work with the World Health Organization and other nongovernmental organizations in these countries, but as Dr. Besson has recently pointed out (Besson 1999), such liaisons have had limited success. IASP has taken other initiatives such as funding the participation of members from some of these countries in the congress or encouraging IASP members to "adopt a member" by supporting his or her dues payment. I believe IASP should continue to make concerted efforts along these lines, but should also broaden its international activities to include providing financial support to selected young investigators and young clinician-scientists in the pain field. Support from IASP, perhaps subsidized by industrial partners, could enable talented young researchers and clinicians in developing or currency-restricted countries to travel and learn from more established colleagues in their own geographic region or beyond. IASP could also support visits by pain experts to help educate researchers and clinicians in such regions. Because of the fiscal and infrastructure limitations in many of these countries, I see little value in trying to encourage extensive research development there. The focus, at least for the short term, should be on enhancing pain education and pain management approaches. IASP could also make itself more visible in these regions, for example by having the president or one of the executive committee members of IASP attend an annual meeting of each chapter at least once every six years. Such a visit would provide an opportunity for formal or informal presentations at other venues in the region so as to disseminate, first hand, information on the principles and activities of IASP and to encourage the efforts of local IASP members.

The development of broad multidisciplinary approaches to pain research and management at the local level is another direction that IASP should encourage. As I noted earlier, one of the successes of IASP has been its ability to bring together at its triennial congress large numbers of pain researchers and clinicians from a broad spectrum of disciplines, and to introduce multidisciplinary perspectives in its many publications. This philosophy has been adopted at several academic and clinical institutions around the world that have created multidisciplinary pain centers. However, most of these have focused on management, and many are dominated by one or two disciplines and offer a limited number of diagnostic or therapeutic approaches. Indeed, these centers have come under a lot of self-study and critical appraisal in recent years. All too often we also see excellent pain researchers or clinicians working in relative isolation. I believe that one of the next leaps forward in understanding and managing pain will come from an even greater emphasis on multidisciplinary and team approaches. Recognizing that research and treatment approaches should go hand in hand, the University of Toronto recently established the Center for the Study of Pain with the goal of fostering multidisciplinary pain research, management, and education. I hope that others will also adopt this approach, so that the seminal issues and challenges facing the pain field can be addressed more expeditiously. For example, we know that the nervous system can undergo neuroplastic changes in chronic or persistent pain, but how are the neural connections "rewired"? What are the underlying molecular mechanisms? We also know that inhibitory neural control mechanisms in the brain can be recruited by painful experiences, but why are they not always sufficient to control the development of chronic pain? To what extent are genetic factors involved in the expression of pain? What are the relationships between pain and gender, and what is the neural substrate underlying the high predominance of females in many chronic pain states? What is the neural substrate that causes some persons to seek care and not others, and what psychological factors and societal influences promote these behaviors? These are just some of the questions for our field in the future—challenges that require an integrated, cohesive, and multidisciplinary attack. IASP could provide greater advocacy for such an approach, particularly in countries and centers that have the critical mass of disciplines to meet these challenges.

2) To promote education and training in the field of pain. Some of the activities of IASP related to research and management have also addressed this mandate on education, and others include the triennial congresses and other IASP-sponsored meetings and refresher courses, IASP Press books, the journal *Pain,* other IASP publications, and SIGs. The IASP also maintains a file of training opportunities on pain on the IASP Web site. These activities are all extremely valuable from an educational point of view. Another initiative has been, through the work of the IASP Education Committee members and others, the development of the pain curricula, an activity in which many of us have participated from the mid 1980s to the present (Table III). The Education Committee is to be complimented for this effort; it has accomplished one of its primary purposes in establishing course syllabi for various professional groups and in disseminating information on pain education. Nonetheless, I have to wonder about the impact of these curricular guidelines on pain education in the health sciences and allied fields. Have they been used to guide and implement pain curricula in most of the institutions with which our members are affiliated? And has IASP fully addressed its objective of promoting excellence in pain teaching and training? I doubt if the answer to these questions is a resounding yes, and I believe that IASP

Table III
IASP Pain Curricula (1988–1998)

Medicine
Dentistry
Pharmacy
Nursing
Occupational and Physical Therapy
Psychology

could put more effort into ensuring that it is effectively promoting pain education and training. The association and its members must ensure that IASP pain curricula and principles are adopted and given sufficient visibility and content time in educational programs. If we intend to enhance the understanding of pain and improve its management, I suggest that we start at one of the front lines, i.e., the education of students in the health sciences and allied programs. One of the principal goals of my presidency will be to rejuvenate the educational mandate of IASP to ensure that these objectives are met.

3) To promote and facilitate the dissemination of new information in the field of pain, including sponsorship of a journal, Pain. The association has made great strides in disseminating new knowledge, principally through several avenues already mentioned above: its journal *Pain,* congresses, satellite meetings, IASP publications and guidelines, and more recently books published by the IASP Press, started just six years ago. The Committee on Publications and members of the IASP Executive Committee have made significant progress in meeting this objective, and Professor Howard Fields as Editor-in-Chief of IASP Press has done a fine job in overseeing the publications of several high-quality texts. Particular mention must also be made of Professors Patrick Wall and Ronald Dubner, whose editorship of *Pain* has been exemplary. The journal has the most rigorous peer review, highest standards, and highest level of citation compared to any other journal in the field. Professor Wall was the founding editor of *Pain* and has served as an editor-in-chief for 25 years. He is stepping down from this role at the end of the year, and we all owe him a great debt of gratitude in ensuring that the flagship journal of the association has become the flagship journal of the field. His departure leaves the editorship of the journal in the very capable hands of Professor Dubner.

Purposes H, I, and J (Table I) are also relevant to the dissemination of new information. The IASP has played a leadership role in advocating several pain management strategies (e.g., use of narcotic analgesics) and in establishing standards and ethical guidelines for pain research in human and experimental animals, pain treatment facilities, etc. The association has a Committee on Public Information and Education, and a number of media contacts and public information resources have been developed so as to lay the groundwork for a communication network. The Web page of IASP, the development of which is overseen by a task force, is up and running, and offers considerable scope for wider use. During my presidency, I intend that the association should encourage further development of the Web site as an information resource, and that through the IASP Committee on Public Information and Education it should identify and implement other approaches that will better inform the public and health professionals. These approaches should include more extensive use of material already developed at the local chapter level. Indeed, there are many opportunities to enhance communication and interaction with IASP chapters, and I will endeavor to put in place a mechanism for enhanced liaisons among the chapters.

I wish to conclude this chapter by again recognizing and thanking Dr. Besson for the leadership he has given to our association over the past three years, and by affirming that I look forward to working effectively with my colleagues on the new slate of IASP officers and councillors. May we all benefit from another successful three years that will culminate in the 10th World Congress on Pain in San Diego in August, 2002!

REFERENCES

Besson J-M. President's message. *IASP Newsletter* 1999 (Spring).

Dubner R, Sessle BJ, Storey AT (Eds). *The Neural Basis of Oral and Facial Function*. New York: Plenum Press, 1978, p 483.

Melzack R, Wall PD. Pain mechanisms: a new theory. *Science* 1965; 150:971–978.

Sessle BJ. Acute and chronic craniofacial pain: brainstem mechanisms of nociceptive transmission and neuroplasticity, and their clinical correlates. *Crit Rev Oral Biol Med* 2000; 11:57–91.

Woda A, Pionchon P. A unified concept of idiopathic orofacial pain: clinical features. *J Orofac Pain* 1999; 13:172–184.

Correspondence to: Barry J. Sessle, BDS, MDS, PhD, FRSC, Faculty of Dentistry, University of Toronto, 124 Edward Street, Toronto, Ontario, Canada M5G 1G6. Tel: (416) 979-4910; Fax: (416) 979-4937; email: barry.sessle@utoronto.ca.

Proceedings of the 9th World Congress on Pain,
Progress in Pain Research and Management,
Vol. 16, edited by M. Devor, M.C. Rowbotham, and
Z. Wiesenfeld-Hallin, IASP Press, Seattle, © 2000.

3

Pain in Context: The Intellectual Roots of Pain Research and Therapy[1]

Patrick D. Wall

Sensory Functions Group, King's College, Guy's Campus, London, United Kingdom

This chapter summarizes the theory of a hard-wired, line-labeled, modality-dedicated pain mechanism as a preface to rejecting it. Reasons are given as to why this theory persists despite its sterility. Facts observed in the clinic and in the laboratory require the recognition of an integrated, distributed dynamic series of pain mechanisms. Before the cognitive identification of pain, preceding processes such as attention and orientation must occur. I propose that pain itself is best seen as a need state in which the brain analyzes the input in terms of what action would be appropriate. To achieve this, the brain involves parts of both the classical sensory and motor systems and represents the pain state in distributed structures in a temporal and spatial pattern that differs among individuals.

Few invitations are more likely to generate a deadly combination of pomposity and pretentiousness than a request to write on intellectual roots. It is not a contemporary subject. To ask a modern neuroscientist working on pain problems to explain the intellectual roots of a recent experiment is to provoke puzzlement. For most scientists, it is still true that pain is provoked by injury, and the duty of the scientist is to collect data that would permit a break in the link between the injury and the pain. Perl (1998) writes:

> Most people accept that the sensations of vision, hearing, taste and vibration are subserved by dedicated neural pathways in which the physical stimulus is transduced by specialised sensory cells and processed by certain neurons and regions of the central nervous system that are dominated by their particular sensory input. Is this also true of pain?

---

[1] Mini-review based on a congress workshop.

Despite all that has happened in the past 50 years, most would answer "yes" to the question and would label the nociceptor as the specialized cell. I will show that they are fundamentally wrong, since they confuse sensory categories and place vision in the same category as pain. Twenty of my good friends and colleagues have honored me by writing of their latest work in a special issue of the journal *Pain* (Dubner 1999). Careful reading of these brilliant papers shows that some remain ambiguous on this question. I have tried to show that pain is an attribute assigned by the brain as a quality. I think at least three reasons can explain the persistence of the simplistic view of a hard-wired pain mechanism.

PERSISTENCE OF A SIMPLISTIC VIEW OF PAIN MECHANISMS

GENERALIZATION FROM THRESHOLD MEASURES

Perl (1998) chooses vibration as the only other somatic sensation to compare with pain. This conclusion derives from the undoubted results of Mountcastle et al. (1967), and we need to examine the data precisely. Trained subjects were required to be alert for vibration in a plate on the skin and announce when they first detected it. The subjects' ability to detect low-frequency vibration precisely matched the ability of axons attached to Meissner corpuscles to respond to a low-frequency vibration. If the trial was to detect high-frequency vibration, the subjects' detection abilities exactly followed those of axons attached to Pacinian corpuscles. The overall psychophysical tuning curve from low to high frequencies could be superimposed on the tuning curves of the two types of receptor. This is the basis for the general statement that our threshold ability to detect vibration depends on two dedicated pathways. How could it be otherwise? The subject has been trained to announce the arrival of any nerve impulses, and the stimulus has been designed to excite only one type of receptor. The subject has been turned into a one-bit detection machine. These experiments could only show a dedicated receptor by virtue of the experimental design. Similarly, some properties of retinal rods can be measured by asking trained, dark-adapted subjects whether they detect light when a few photons are absorbed in the retina (Hecht et al. 1942). A rat with all whiskers but one shaved off will jump a gap in the dark if he can feel the far side of the gap with his one whisker. It would be foolhardy indeed to generalize from these carefully designed minimal inputs and responses to explain the whole of normal vision or somatic sensation.

Psychophysical experiments with normal subjects designed to detect pain thresholds are a travesty compared to the designed genuine simplicity of the experiments just described on vibration threshold detection. The subjects' task is not to detect a single stimulus or sensation but to detect a transition from one sensation to another. They have been repeatedly exposed to the stimulus and coached to respond in an expected way. They have learned that this particular sensation is not associated with impending damage. Training is continued until consistency is ensured and anxiety is eliminated. Even then, comparison of results of apparently identical experiments performed at different laboratories reveals a huge variation (Sternbach and Tursky 1975).

THE RELATION OF NOCICEPTOR ACTIVITY TO PAIN SENSATIONS

This key topic has obviously attracted great attention (reviewed in Raja et al. 1999). Some studies have attempted to relate the firing of nociceptors in undamaged tissue to perceived pain. The greatest enthusiasts for the specificity of pain-related nociceptive firing are clearly unable to explain hyperalgesia or allodynia by excitation of nociceptors, and therefore limit themselves to undamaged tissue and a sensation they bizarrely label as "normal" or "physiological" pain. Even with carefully designed experiments, more exceptions exist than examples to support any claim that pain thresholds and nociceptor thresholds coincide. Nociceptors must reach a discharge frequency above 0.5 Hz before pain occurs (van Hees 1976; Bromm and Treede 1984). Painful pressure stimuli must produce a much higher firing rate for painful responses than do temperature stimuli (van Hees and Gybels 1981). (I was of course delighted by these results because they fulfill a prediction of the gate control theory.) Prolonged, steadily painful heat stimuli evoke quite different time courses of response in A and C mechanical-heat nociceptors (Meyer and Campbell 1981). The increase in pain as temperature rises fails to match the rate of firing of nociceptors (Yarnitsky et al. 1992). And so on. It is difficult to maintain a relation between the level of perceived pain and of nociceptor firing in undamaged tissue.

Any such attempt collapses completely in the areas of frank damage and in surrounding areas of secondary hyperalgesia. While Lewis (1942) tried to incorporate primary and secondary areas in a single mechanism involving only peripheral nerves, the idea was abandoned by Hardy et al. (1948), who recognized the role of central mechanisms in addition to peripheral ones. The idea was taken up by the clinicians Livingstone (1943) and Noordenbos (1959). The change in the origin of pain clearly involving inputs from normal low-threshold afferents has been studied in detail by many, including LaMotte et al. (1991) and Treede et al. (1992). When damage has occurred, many types of afferent neurons, including nociceptors, can trigger pain. If we are now to enter a period where pains are named by the mechanisms that produce them (Woolf and Decosterd 1999), then the commonly used term "nociceptive pain" will disappear because it is rarely justified.

A GENERAL ATMOSPHERE FAVORING A SIMPLISTIC ANSWER

We must try to explain why the general attitude to pain mechanisms has remained in the doldrums for the past 50 years while genuinely revolutionary attitudes have appeared in theories of olfaction, audition, and vision. Three discoveries of the fifties completely changed studies of vision: (1) Kuffler (1953) showed that the receptive fields of retinal ganglion cells were complex and were formed by convergence; (2) Lettvin showed event detectors in the frog optic nerve; and (3) Hubel and Wiesel showed shape detectors in the cortex. These discoveries led to the present sophisticated state of visual physiology and psychology with the complete dismissal of modality-labeled cells. Yet, despite the massive evidence for convergence, plasticity, and feedback and "feed forward", the common attitude about pain mechanisms describes pathways moving in one direction from periphery to cortex with pain-labeled fibers, cells, pathways, and centers. How could that be?

The revolutionary shift of attitude in vision and audition has had no practical impact on clinical practice, so scientists were free to explore the challenges of a brain containing multiple systems acting in a unified way, as exemplified by the last three chapters in Mountcastle's (1998) book on the cerebral cortex. In contrast, those working on pain mechanisms rightly focused on the practical search for effective therapy and were anxious to help, influence, and educate clinicians. If we examine contemporary textbooks and research reports by those concerned with practice, particularly anesthetists and pharmacologists, we see that basic pain mechanisms are still represented as unidirectional pathways running from injury to pain. Even the old gate control diagram, which incorporates convergence and feedback, is "dumbed down" to represent nothing but a gain control. The legitimate, insistent demands of patients in misery do not permit the luxury of fantasy speculation.

For practical reasons, basic science concentrates on the periphery rather than venturing into the deep morass of the central nervous system. A survey of the abstracts at this conference (IASP 1999) shows the periphery as a major attack point. We must be impressed by the spectacular and elegant cell biology that has revealed the nature of inflammation (Levine and Reichling 1999) and of the neurotrophins (McMahon and Bennett 1999).

Similarly, the observations we began 30 years ago now reveal an extraordinary plasticity of the entire length of peripheral nerves in the presence of damage (Devor and Selzer 1999).

We must also recognize the existence of a medical-industrial complex that influences the direction of research and development with a major financial input that far exceeds government and charity contributions to basic and practical studies of pain. There is nothing sinister about the goals of this industry, which is forced by its own overt rules to concentrate on and accelerate the solution of best guesses. In practice, that means attempting to optimize existing therapies or to perform powerful molecular analysis of the most clearly defined target in the periphery. It is highly unlikely that such organizations would spend time on the possibility that the brain is anything but a passive recipient of messages from the periphery.

SPINAL CORD CELLS

It has become standard practice to divide cells in the dorsal horn that receive primary afferents into four categories; low-threshold, nociceptor-specific, wide-dynamic-range, and proprioceptive. In the vast majority of papers in the past 20 years, cells are given one or other of these labels. In 1953, Kuffler showed that retinal ganglion cells responded to an organized convergence of inputs with contrasting effects from different parts of the retina. Intensive studies of the retina since then have revealed the anatomy, physiology, and pharmacology of this convergence. We have shown the elaborate nature of convergence from different parts of the receptive field for dorsal horn lamina V cells (Hillman and Wall 1969). I am unaware of serious subsequent attempts to analyze this convergence, given that it was more convenient to consider cells as simple excitatory convergence points from specified types of afferents that would permit a single label. I suspect an intellectual block against tackling the much more difficult task of describing the nature of inhibitory and excitatory convergences. This is surprising in view of the obvious relevance of convergence mechanisms to such phenomena as referred pain, secondary hyperalgesia and allodynia, and above all the induced central hyperexcitabilities. The latter have been wonderfully explored by Mendell and especially by Woolf (Doubell et al. 1999). The existence of hidden silent convergences has been revealed. For example, a nociceptive-specific cell in lamina I is converted into a wide-dynamic-range cell by the arrival in the vicinity of a brief volley of impulses in unmyelinated afferents from muscle (Cook et al. 1987). At any one moment, the entire structure is in a single state that can change fundamentally as a consequence of neuronal activity and of slowly changing chemistry. This dynamic state needs to be appreciated as such and not oversimplified as a fixed state with rare alternative options.

We now know that the response of single units depends on (1) the convergent activity of different types of afferent, (2) the past history of afferent barrages of nerve impulses and of transported chemicals, and (3) tonic and phasic effects of descending impulses. From the time of Sherrington (Sherrington and Sowton 1915) it was recognized that the spinal reflex circuits in a decerebrate animal were dominated by the proprioceptive input, while a spinal animal responded preferably to cutaneous inputs. This was shown on a single cell where the receptive field was entirely proprioceptive in the decerebrate state, but if descending impulses were cold blocked, the cell became responsive only to a cutaneous input in the spinal state (Wall 1967). The Fields group (Fields and Basbaum 1999) has shown how phasic descending volleys give permission to cord cells to respond to a cutaneous input. Most dramatically, the Dubner group (Dubner et al. 1981) has shown that single cells in a trained monkey respond to temperature changes on the skin, and again the same cell responds equally well to an alerting signal that the stimulus would occur in the future.

There are two ways of achieving stability: structural and dynamic. It is surely time for a paradigm shift in our way of thinking about even a small group of cells such as the dorsal horn. The classical way was structural: function was assigned only by the anatomical origin of the input and the anatomical destination of the output. Dynamic stability is achieved in a quite different way. We can take the analogy of a plane flying a steady course on autopilot. The autopilot has precisely defined inputs from a variety of sensors and has equally simple outputs to the engines and control surfaces. However, within the apparatus, it is fatuous to assign a single function to any one component because they are all in a dynamic looped interaction. The whole ensemble has a stable function, but the components play a subtle, variable role in achieving the overall single function. It is now crucial that we shift our way of thinking about neuronal assemblies from the classical structural state to the dynamic, interconnected form.

I admit to having played a passive role as editor of the journal *Pain* in allowing without complaint a persistent confusion between structural and dynamic descriptions. One such error of passivity began in 1969 when I declined to join my friends Melzack and Casey in their 1969 paper. Melzack had analyzed words used by people in pain; their classification of these words led to the enormously useful and influential McGill Pain Questionnaire. One group of words, such as sharp and burning, were called "sensory-discriminative." They describe the person's belief in the quality, intensity, and location of a past stimulus event. Another group of words, such as frightening and sickening, were called "affective." They describe how the person is reacting now to the past event. So far, so good; but now began a hopeless confusion of categories. The two categories of words were labeled as separate, independent dimensions. This is a highly dangerous step, with an air of physical separation and no consideration of the attributes or serial consequences of words. Melzack and Casey swallowed the bait and reverted to the very Cartesian solution that I thought we had demolished (Melzack and Wall 1965). They assigned separate input pathways for the two categories. The sensory-discriminative sensation was attributed to the action of cells that gave rise to the lateral neo-spinothalamic-primary sensory cortex system. The affective sensation was assigned to cells of origin of the medial-paleo-spino-thalamic-limbic system. In the 30 years since this proposal we have gained considerable new knowledge of the effect of lesions, of local recording, and of images, so we might have expected some support for the dual-input theory, but I have yet to see it. Nevertheless, some of the most respected and productive workers in the field (Treede et al. 1999) seem to accept the idea as established fact. I and others (Fields 1999) prefer to analyze the multitude of painful responses as the outcome of integrated dynamic systems that provide a clear, stable analysis of consequences of an overall situation.

THE STABILITY OF PAIN MECHANISMS

A diagnostic characteristic to differentiate hard-wired from dynamic interactive systems is their response to injury. This applies to frank lesions and to pharmacological blockade as well as genetic knockouts. Hard-wired systems progressively decrease their performance with progressive block, while dynamic systems often appear immune to substantial loss. Pain famously demonstrates its stability. Dose-response curves of morphine analgesia have a step function with large variations between individuals, as would be expected of dynamic control mechanisms. When hard-wired circuits are progressively damaged, a simple progressive decrease in function takes place. Faulty dynamic loop circuits may oscillate, as occurs in several pain states with sudden phasic attacks, or they may shift to a set stable abnormal input-output function. Noordenbos and I (1981) encountered an extreme example of stable abnormal pain mechanisms in a series of patients with partial median nerve injuries and intractable pain in the hand. They had been observed in careful detail for more than 6 months and had failed to respond to a series of therapies. In desperation, we asked neurosurgeons to excise the entire area of partially damaged median nerve and to span the gap with multiple sural nerve grafts. The immediate effect was, of course, a completely anesthetic and paralyzed median hand that was pain free. Over a period of months, all patients experienced successful regeneration and a return of hand sensitivity. Unfortunately, there was also a detailed reconstruction of the precise areas of hypersensitivity suffered by patients before their operations. The original lesion had been a partial section of the nerve, while the surgical lesion was a complete section with widespread excision. Clearly, the origin of the pain state had migrated centrally from the site of injury and had established itself in a stable state that recreated the spatial distribution and degree of the abnormal sensitivity.

The phenomenon of stability of pain mechanisms despite lesions has plagued surgical attempts to cure pain. Section of dorsal roots (Dubuisson 1999) or central lesions (Gybels and Sweet 1989) demonstrate a remarkably consistent effect. Initial results are highly satisfactory, but wherever the lesion, they are followed by a recurrence of pain, with a mixture of deafferentation and provoked pains. The most common operation is the open anterolateral cordotomy, which cuts 50% of all the ascending and descending fibers on one side. The lesion produced by percutaneous cordotomy is variable in size and location but is just as effective as open surgery. The operation is fully justified in cancer patients with intractable pain with a few weeks to live, but after that the analgesia fades and is often replaced by an even more unpleasant pain. The failure of cordotomy to cure chronic pain has prompted a century of attempts to locate the single final pathway by making lesions in the midbrain, thalamus, and cortex. Lesions of the medial lemniscus were rapidly abandoned when the recurrence of pain was discovered to be rapid and violent. Widely targeted single and multiple lesions have been tried and abandoned. Lesions in structures such as the pulvinar, which are not on a classical pain pathway, produce the same sequence of analgesia followed by recurrence. Clearly, the brain tissue capable of producing a pain state is widely distributed, but it is not adequate to conclude that pain is provoked by a number of parallel, redundant, hard-wired circuits. If that were true, each lesion would limit the maximal level of pain perceived. Since that is not true, we are faced with a distributed mechanism whose stability is characteristic of dynamic feed-forward and feedback mechanisms capable of producing a standard output consequence despite the loss of individual components.

Some clinicians conclude that any patient who fails to report pain characteristic of a hard-wired system is guilty of faulty thinking. Proponents of this rigid view have to work hard on censoring what the patients say. Their selective quotation of the literature would be hilarious if it were not taken so seriously. The beginning of their hard-line approach is Brown-Séquard's

(1857) demonstration that hemisection of the cord produces contralateral analgesia. In 1892, Sir Frederick Mott produced contradictory findings with ipsilateral changes. In 1894, Brown-Séquard, then aged 77, wrote in agreement with Mott:

> Fifteen years ago, I began to revise my previous opinion that sensation from one side of the body was transmitted to the perception centre by way of the opposite side of the spinal cord. The research method based on the notion that those functions which disappear after destruction of central structures are the functions of the lesioned structures is essentially vicious. Against that conclusion, it is enough to say that the loss of function could just as well be caused by inhibition or excitation at a distance of those nervous structures which are actually responsible for the function.

The neurological establishment completely ignored Mott's results and Brown-Séquard's second thoughts. Eighty years later, Denny-Brown (1979) confirmed Mott's and Brown-Séquard's new results in detail. It is too much to hope that the hard-liners would change their simplistic views, even when three of the most distinguished neurologists of the century differed with their hard-wired scheme. Another beloved "fact" of the single-line fanatics is the rigid fixture dermatome despite repeated demonstrations of the extreme plasticity of dermatomal boundaries (Kirk and Denny-Brown 1970; Denny-Brown et al. 1973). Referred pain was an embarrassment to doctors of the hard-wired view, especially when it was shown that the area to which the pain was referred became tender and responded to local anesthesia (Lewis 1942). Lewis and Kellgren (1939) provided some sense of order to referred pain by showing that the evident convergence must occur in the same segment, given that referred pain occupied the same dermatome as the initiating stimulus. Even this observation could not be repeated when Hockaday and Whitty (1967) repeated the experiments on subjects who had not been to medical school and did not know about dermatomes. These subjects reported pain in definite but differing areas, but not in dermatomal arrangements; when the stimulus was repeated, the subjects again responded with reports of pain in the same distant area. It is evident that even the most basic observations fail to support the proponents of the hard-wired, rigid structural systems. We do not need to recruit the detailed modern results on plasticity of function to favor a dynamic distributed model of pain mechanisms. To explore that we need to consider the brain and the whole creature beyond the input.

BEYOND THE SPINAL CORD

I have pointed out that many of the best neuroscientists wisely stick to the periphery. They in turn can accuse me of concentrating on the spinal cord. Clearly we must assign a function to more rostral structures if we are to propose a plausible pain mechanism. I have already given reasons to doubt the existence of a hard-wired, line-labeled, modality-specific mechanism. If that is accepted, the following types of experiment are likely to be sterile: (1) the location of cells responding to intense peripheral stimuli; (2) the effect of lesions; and (3) the assignment of single-output functions to single subdivisions, i.e., movement, affect, autonomic responses, endocrine responses, and others. Even the effects of local stimulation, while of potential therapeutic interest, do not define the nature of the mechanism. If, as I propose, the mechanism is a distributed dynamic loop process, the experiments that would reveal such a mechanism are far more complex, but they are becoming possible. Such experiments involve simultaneous recording at multiple sites in order to define temporal-spatial patterns. That does not mean that it is necessary to scan the entire brain with continuous analysis. Simple observation shows a sequence of processes preceding the final mature, cognitive description of a single pain.

ATTENTION

I have written elsewhere (Wall 1999) that a series of processes must have occurred before pain is perceived. They include vigilance, alerting, orientation, and attention. They are neither trivial nor simple. In a continuous precognitive process the entire available sensory input is being scanned to assign biological significance. This process continues not only during quiet rest periods but most impressively during skilled motor action. Highly skilled sportsmen and musicians consistently report their best performance while their attention is switched off. Even in tests where the subject is in trained expectation to recognize the consequences of a stimulus, there is a delay of 1–200 ms during which preparatory settings of the sensory system occur. An example is the firing of first-order sensory cells timed to the warning stimulus that signals that the stimulus to be discriminated is about to be applied (Dubner et al. 1981). We know almost nothing about the mechanism by which sensory inputs initially switch our attention.

The earliest and still the most surprising result of brain imaging positron emission tomography (PET) scans of subjects in pain was the appearance of activity in the anterior cingulate cortex reviewed by Ingvar (1999). Some still label this structure as a "pain area." However, this area lights up whenever the subject is involved in an attention shift for whatever reason (Hsieh et al. 1995). Activation also occurs when the subject imagines an event. Furthermore, my earliest work (Fulton et al. 1949; Wall and Davis 1951) showed this area to be the posterior part of a continuous strip of cortex that ran from anterior cingulate to supraorbital cortex to medial temporal lobe to anterior insula. Activity in the latter is also apparent when people are in pain, as is activity in the intermediate areas.

The switching of attention is a necessary event that precedes the awareness of sensation. When attention is locked onto events that have a higher biological priority than response to injury, the paradoxical phenomenon of painless injury occurs. The oldest pain therapy is distraction or counterirritation, in which the attention is captured by some event other than the cause of pain. We may therefore predict the detection of neural processes related to attention that precede the cognitive awareness of pain but involve an analysis of the same sensory input, which is eventually assigned a pain label. PET scans have poor temporal resolution, but the newer scanning methods, including functional magnetic resonance imaging (fMRI), have potentially good temporal resolution. Therefore we may expect data on signals of the time and location of crucial events that precede the process of cognitive classification. A paradox of attention is that it permits only one analysis at a time.

THE ENGRAM OF PAIN

The most classical and unquestioned model of the brain is that it consists of three parts: the sensory brain, the premotor-associative planning brain, and the motor brain. This separation of the brain into three major areas that sequentially communicate with each other may be another of those intellectual traps we have set ourselves. The most persistent of these traps is the Cartesian plan in which there is first a relatively mechanical sensory mechanism that feeds into a separate cognitive, mental perceptive structure. I have given reasons to doubt this dualistic separation (Wall 1999). If we are to seek a distributed dynamic mechanism that signals the perception of pain, we need a hypothesis of where and how to look. It is possible that the engram we seek is incorporated in some subtle synchronous pattern of activity (Abeles 1991; Singer 1998). Even if that were true, it may be that the significant area is marked by a general increase of activity that should be detectable with the present imaging methods. These areas show remarkably widespread zones of activity (Ingvar 1999). I have already suggested that some of the surprising areas such as the anterior cingulate cortex, supra-orbital cortex, anterior insula, and posterior parietal cortex might be associated with activity that precedes perception and is associated with attention and orientation. Of the classical primary and secondary somatosensory association areas, activity detected in these areas is not convincingly associated with the perception of pain. Even activity in the sensory thalamus fails to correlate with perceived pain in patients with chronic neuropathic pain (Iadarola et al. 1995; Ingvar 1999). However, many reports locate activity in structures classically assigned a motor function. These include the motor cortex itself and the basal ganglia, including the putamen and globus pallidus, and the cerebellum. Activity in these classical motor areas is reported in subjects who are in pain but show no signs of motor activity. This observation raises the question of the validity of excluding these areas from models of sensory processing. Therefore, let us explore the possibility that the brain analyzes its sensory input in terms of the possible action that would be appropriate to the event that triggered the whole process. There is no suggestion that actual movement occurs, only that the brain is scanning possible responses that would abolish the input. In this way, pain would join sensations such as hunger, thirst, and itch, which are best defined as needs that signify the next most probable action. If pain is perceived in terms of probable actions, it would occur only in relation to a single solution at one time and would correlate with a single target of attention, which is a strange and unexpected characteristic of attention and pain. The placebo, the most paradoxical feature of pain, would then become an action rather than a stimulus. Expectation and training lead the subject to the "knowledge" that the action of taking a placebo leads to relief.

Classical thinking would strongly predict the discovery of a definable pattern of brain activity, an engram, in all normal people in pain. Such a pattern would provide objective evidence for a common coded representation of pain, free from the subjective inconsistencies produced by what the subject thought about the pain. The issue is crucial to any concept of the nature of sensation. Locke (1975) wondered what would happen "if, by the different structure of our organs, it were so ordered that the same object should produce in several men's minds different ideas at the same time."

Locke doubts this variation between individuals. Wittgenstein (1958) writes: "The assumption would thus be possible—though unverifiable—that one section of mankind has one sensation of red and another section another." He was so disturbed by this possibility that he did not discuss further the nature of private sensation. The question now is whether Wittgenstein's "assumption" has become verifiable through imaging.

It was not possible in the earlier PET studies to localize activity in individuals because the signal strength was too weak and it was necessary to pool results from 8 to 12 subjects. An exception was Vogt et al. (1996), who showed variable locations of activity in the cingulate gyrus among subjects. Paulson et al. (1998) reported marked quantitative differences between groups of men and of women subjected to painful hot stimuli. Fortunately, the development of fMRI greatly increased temporal and spatial resolution and signal strength to a level where individuals can be examined. Davis et al. (1998) investigated 12 trained subjects stimulated with hot or cold or tactile stimuli. They focused on four areas; thalamus, S-2 sensory cortex, insula, and basal ganglia. When all 12 subjects were pooled, activity was observed in all four areas, as had been reported previously. However, no person has the same pattern of activity as any other person. Similar results were reported at this congress with fMRI studies and with other types of localized activity recording. These results are a major nightmare for the classical neuroscientist, and many will therefore dismiss or ignore them. Clinical psychologists, however, have repeatedly reported profound variability among individuals. This variation goes far beyond the relation of the size of the stimulus to the intensity of the pain. Individuals show a wide variety of tactics in responding to identical stimuli. These tactics amount to a variety of sensory postures that could be represented in the brain as differing motor plans. It is therefore possible that there is not just a single engram for pain but that a family of distributed brain activities is associated with unpleasantness, which we group together as pain by social linguistic convention.

REFERENCES

Abeles M. *Corticonics*. Cambridge: Cambridge University Press, 1991.

Bromm B, Treede R-D. Nerve fibre discharges, cerebral potentials and sensations. *Human Neurobiol* 1984; 3:33–40.

Brown-Séquard E. *Experimental Researches Applied to Physiology and Pathology*. New York: Ballière, 1857.

Brown-Séquard E. Remarque à propos des recherches du Dr F W Mott. *Arch Physiol Norm Pathol* 1894; 6:195–198.

Cook AJ, Woolf CJ, Wall PD, McMahon SB. Dynamic receptive field plasticity. *Nature* 1987; 325:151–153.

Davis KD, Kwan CL, Crawley AP, Mikulis DJ. Functional MRI study of thalamic and cortical activations. *J Neurophysiol* 1998; 80:1533–1546.

Denny-Brown D. The enigma of crossed sensory loss. In: Bonica JJ, et al. (Eds). *Advances in Pain Research and Therapy*, Vol. 3. New York: Raven Press, 1979, pp 889–895.

Denny-Brown D, Kirk EJ, Yanagisawa N. The tract of Lissauer in relation to sensory transmission. *J Comp Neurol* 1973; 151:175–200.

Devor M, Selzer Z. Pathophysiology of damaged nerve. In: Wall PD, Melzack R (Eds). *Textbook of Pain,* 4th ed. Edinburgh: Churchill Livingstone, 1999.

Doubell TP, Mannion RJ, Woolf CJ. The dorsal horn. In: Wall PD, Melzack R (Eds). *Textbook of Pain,* 4th ed. Edinburgh: Churchill Livingstone, 1999.

Dubner R (Ed). A tribute to Patrick D Wall. *Pain* 1999; (Suppl 6).

Dubner R, Hoffman DS, Hayes RL. Task related responses. *J Neurophysiol* 1981; 46:444–464.

Dubuisson D. Root and ganglion surgery. In: Wall PD, Melzack R (Eds). *Textbook of Pain,* 4th ed. Edinburgh: Churchill Livingstone, 1999.

Fields HL, Basbaum AI. Central nervous mechanisms of pain modulation. In: Wall PD, Melzack R (Eds). *Textbook of Pain,* 4th ed. Edinburgh: Churchill Livingstone, 1999.

Fulton JF, Pribram KH, Stevenson JAF, Wall PD. Interrelations between orbital gyrus, insula, temporal tip and anterior cingulate. *Trans Am Neurol Assoc* 1949; 21:175–179.

Gybels JM, Sweet WH. *Neurosurgical Treatment of Persistent Pain.* Basel: Karger, 1989.

Hardy JD, Wolff HG, Goodell H. *Pain Sensations and Reactions.* New York: Williams & Wilkins, 1948.

Hecht S. Visual mechanisms. *J Gen Physiol* 1942; 25:819–840.

Hillman P, Wall PD. Inhibitory and excitatory factors controlling lamina V cells. *Exp Brain Res* 1969; 9:284–306.

Hockaday JM, Whitty CWM. Patterns of referred pain in normal subjects. *Brain* 1967; 90:481–496.

Hsieh JC, Belfrage M, Stone-Elander S, Hansson P, Ingvar M. Central representation of chronic ongoing pain. *Pain* 1995; 63:225–236.

Iadarola MJ, Max MB, Berman KF, et al. Unilateral decrease of thalamic activity. *Pain* 1995; 63:55–64.

IASP. *Abstracts: 9th World Congress on Pain.* Seattle: IASP Press, 1999.

Ingvar M, Hsieh JC. The image of pain. In: Wall PD, Melzack R (Eds). *Textbook of Pain,* 4th ed. Edinburgh: Churchill Livingstone, 1999.

Kirk EJ, Denny-Brown D. Functional variation in dermatomes. *J Comp Neurol* 1970; 138:307–320.

Kuffler SW. Discharge patterns and functional organisation of mammalian retina. *J Neurophysiol* 1953; 16:37–67.

LaMotte RH, Shain CN, Simone D A, Tsai E-FP. Neurogenic hyperalgesia. *J Neurophysiol* 1991; 66:190–211.

Levine JD, Reichling DB. Peripheral mechanisms of inflammatory pain. In: Wall PD, Melzack R (Eds). *Textbook of Pain,* 4th ed. Edinburgh: Churchill Livingstone, 1999.

Lewis T. *Pain.* New York: Macmillan, 1942.

Lewis T, Kellgren JH. Observations relating to referred pain. *Clin Sci* 1939; 4:47–71.

Livingstone EK. *Pain Mechanisms. A Physiological Interpretation of Causalgia.* New York: Macmillan, 1943.

Locke J. An essay concerning human understanding. In: Niddital P (Ed*). Collected Works.* Oxford: Clarendon Press, 1975, p 1690.

McMahon SB, Bennett DLH. Trophic factors and pain. In: Wall PD, Melzack R (Eds). *Textbook of Pain,* 4th ed. Edinburgh: Churchill Livingstone, 1999.

Melzack R, Casey KL. Sensory, motivational and central control determinants of pain. In: Kenshalo DR (Ed). *The Skin Senses.* Springfield: Thomas, 1968, pp 423–439.

Melzack R, Wall PD. Pain mechanisms: a new theory. *Science* 1965; 150:971–979.

Meyer RA, Campbell JN. Myelinated nociceptive afferents account for the hyperalgesia that follows a burn. *Science* 1981; 213:1527–1529.

Mott FW. Results of hemisection of the spinal cord in monkeys. *Philos Trans R Soc* 1892; 83:1–59.

Mountcastle VB. *Perceptual Neuroscience: The Cerebral Cortex.* Cambridge: Harvard University Press, 1998.

Mountcastle VB, Talbot WH, Darian-Smith I, Kornhuber HH. A neural base for the sense of flutter vibration. *Science* 1967; 155:597–600.

Noordenbos W. *Pain*. Amsterdam: Elsevier, 1959.
Noordenbos W, Wall PD. Implications of the failure of nerve resection and graft to cure chronic pain produced by nerve lesions. *J Neurol Neurosurg Psychiatry* 1981; 44:1068–1073.
Paulson PE, Minoshima S, Morrow TJ, Casey KL. Gender differences in pain perception. *Pain* 1998; 76:223–230.
Perl ER. Getting a line on pain: is it mediated by dedicated pathways. *Nat Neurosci* 1998; 1:177–178.
Raja SN, Meyer RA, Ringkamp M, Campbell JN. Peripheral neural mechanisms of nociception. In: Wall PD, Melzack R (Eds). *Textbook of Pain*, 4th ed. Edinburgh: Churchill Livingstone, 1999.
Sherrington CS, Sowton SCM. Observations on reflex responses to break shocks. *J Physiol* 1915; 49:331–343.
Singer W. Consciousness and the structure of neural representation. *Philos Trans R Soc Lond B Biol Sci* 1998; 353:1829–1840.
Sternbach RA, Tursky B. On the psychophysical power function in electric shock. *Psychosom Sci* 1975; 1:217–218.
Treede R-D, Meyer RA, Raja SM, Campbell JN. Mechanisms of cutaneous hyperalgesia. *Prog Neurobiol* 1992; 38:397–421.
Treede R-D, Kenshalo DR, Gracely RH, Jones AKP. The cortical representation of pain. *Pain* 1999; 79:105–111.
van Hees J. Human C-fibre input during painful and non-painful skin stimulation. In: Bonica JJ, Albe-Fessard DG (Eds). *Advances in Pain Research and Therapy*, Vol. 1. New York: Raven Press, 1976, pp 35–40.
van Hees J, Gybels JC. C nociceptor activity during painful and non-painful stimulation. *J Neurol Neurosurg Psychiatry* 1981; 44:600–607.
Vogt BA, Derbyshire S, Jones AK. Pain processing in four regions of human cingulate cortex localized with co-registered PET and MR imaging. *Eur J Neurosci* 1996; 8:1461–1473.
Wall PD. *Pain the Science of Suffering*. London: Wiedenfeld & Nicholson, 1999.
Wall PD. The laminar organization of the dorsal horn and effects of descending impulses. *J Physiol* 1967; 188:403–423.
Wall PD, Davis GD. Three cerebral cortical systems affecting autonomic function. *J Neurophysiol* 1951; 14:507–518.
Woolf CJ, Decosterd I. Implications of recent advances in the understanding of pain pathophysiology. *Pain* 1999; (Suppl 6):141–148.
Wittgenstein L. *Philosophical Investigations*. Oxford: Blackwell, 1958.
Yarnitsky D, Simone DA, Dotson RM, Cline MA, Ochoa JL. Single C nociceptor responses and psychophysical parameters of evoked pain. *J Physiol* 1992; 450:581–592.

Correspondence to: Patrick D. Wall, DM, FRS, Sensory Functions Group, King's College, Guy's Campus, Hodgkin Building, London SE1 1UK, United Kingdom. Tel/Fax: 44-(0)20-7435-9139; email: p.wall@umds.ac.uk.

Proceedings of the 9th World Congress on Pain,
Progress in Pain Research and Management,
Vol. 16, edited by M. Devor, M.C. Rowbotham, and
Z. Wiesenfeld-Hallin, IASP Press, Seattle, © 2000.

4

Influencing Cancer Pain Management: Medical Writing in the Second Half of the 20th Century

Christina Faull

St Mary's Hospice and University Hospital Birmingham NHS Trust, Birmingham, United Kingdom

When physicians in the early 20th century began to find ways to influence the course of illness, the focus of clinical care became the disease process. The hope (and expectation) was to cure. The health service and medical training in the United Kingdom were sculpted from the belief that diseases could be cured. However, in the same year that the National Health Service was founded, the medical curriculum committee of the British Medical Association warned:

> In the last fifty years the necessary division of medical practice into specialities has encouraged 'piece-meal' medicine, especially in hospital practice, where very often no one is interested in the patient as a person. Interest in the impersonal scientific aspect of medicine is being allowed to overshadow the human and the individual problems. (Medical Curriculum Committee of the British Medical Association 1948)

Patrick Wall has described the ubiquitous nihilistic regard for pain: "Symptoms were placed on one side as sign posts along a highway which was being driven toward the intended destination. Therapy directed at the sign posts was denigrated and dismissed as merely symptomatic." (Wall 1986).

During the 1950s, parallel but synergistic moves developed against this professional disregard for pain and for the appropriate care of patients with terminal cancer. John Bonica published *The Management of Pain* (Bonica 1953), and Cicely Saunders first aired her vision for what was to become the Hospice movement (Saunders 1958). Alongside these efforts, but remarkably separate until the formation of the International Association for the

Study of Pain, was a growing interest in the neurophysiology and pharmacology of pain. The identification of opioid receptors (Pert and Snyder 1973) and the subsequent discovery of the endogenous ligands for the receptors (Hughes et al. 1975) were seminal events in the mid-1970s, as attested by the large numbers of citations of these publications, over 1000 and 2000, respectively.

This chapter explores qualitative and quantitative changes in medical writing about cancer pain in the second half of the 20th century in generalist medical journals and undergraduate textbooks. Specific attention is given to the influence of the discovery of the endogenous opioids and their receptors.

CANCER, PAIN, AND ENDOGENOUS OPIOIDS IN MEDICAL JOURNALS

Articles focusing on cancer-related pain published in the *British Medical Journal* (*BMJ*), *Lancet,* or *New England Journal of Medicine* (*NEJM*) have increased from 0.01% of all articles in the period 1966–1970 to 0.09% in the period 1991–1995 (Table I). The absolute number of articles, however, particularly those containing original research, remains very low. During 1966–1995 the *Lancet* published 45 articles on cancer-related pain, the

Table I
Number of publications concerning cancer and pain in generalist medical journals (percentage of all published articles is shown in parentheses)

Journal	Topic	1966–1970	1971–1975	1976–1980	1981–1985	1986–1990	1991–1995
BMJ	Pain	79 (0.9)	91 (0.9)	143 (1.2)	109 (1.2)	102 (1.2)	161 (1.4)
	Cancer	494 (5.6)	735 (7.2)	825 (6.7)	632 (7.0)	686 (8.0)	738 (6.6)
	Cancer and pain	0 (0)	1 (0.01)	0 (0)	4 (0.04)	6 (0.07)	4 (0.04)
Lancet	Pain	43 (0.5)	93 (0.7)	165 (1.2)	155 (1.3)	149 (1.2)	176 (1.3)
	Cancer	629 (7.1)	1363 (9.9)	1450 (10.8)	1377 (11.4)	1336 (10.4)	1434 (10.6)
	Cancer and pain	3 (0.03)	5 (0.04)	2 (0.01)	5 (0.04)	15 (0.12)	15 (0.11)
NEJM	Pain	11 (0.2)	21 (0.3)	32 (0.5)	36 (0.6)	22 (0.4)	75 (1.2)
	Cancer	353 (7.3)	590 (9.2)	822 (12.3)	754 (12.8)	613 (12.1)	923 (14.3)
	Cancer and pain	0 (0)	3 (0.05)	3 (0.04)	7 (0.12)	1 (0.02)	9 (0.14)

Note: BMJ = British Medical Journal; NEJM = New England Journal of Medicine.

NEJM 23 articles, and the *BMJ* only 15 articles. Interest in the subject appeared to peak in the United States in the early 1980s and in the United Kingdom in the late 1980s.

These generalist journals appear to have provided a vehicle for debate through correspondence rather than publishing original pain research (Table II). They featured a high proportion of articles of "expert opinion." In 30 years, they presented only 14 publications of original research to a generalist readership.

The MEDLINE database of medical literature identifies 14,987 indexed entries between 1966 and 1998 that focus on endogenous or exogenous opioid peptides; of these, 380 (2.5%) also focus on malignancy and 683 (4.6%) on pain. In this period, only 22 articles relating to pain in malignancy focus on the endogenous opioids: 2 reviews, 2 reports of research in animals, and 18 of research in humans, the first of which was in 1980.

MEDICAL TEACHING THROUGH UNDERGRADUATE TEXTBOOKS

The Principles and Practice of Medicine: A Textbook for Student Doctors, first published in 1952 as a summary of Stanley Davidson's lecture notes for Scottish medical students, has become a standard undergraduate text in the United Kingdom and other countries. It is now in its 17th edition. The first edition briefly described the symptom of pain and its diagnostic value in the section, "Diseases of the Digestive System." Pain was attributed to cancer, but with little clear advice on therapy: "As in the management of other carcinomatous patients, analgesics should be given in sufficient amounts to control pain. For suitable diet see Appendix 1" (Davidson 1952). There were no indexed entries to opium, narcotics, or morphine. This superficial approach to pain has continued until very recent years:

Table II
The type of published articles in the *NEJM*, *BMJ*, and *Lancet* concerning cancer-related pain

Article Type	1966–1970	1971–1975	1976–1980	1981–1985	1986–1990	1991–1995
Editorial	0	1	0	2	2	2
Review	0	0	0	10	3	3
Original research	1	0	2	4	2	5
Case report	0	2	0	0	4	0
Letter	2	6	3	9	11	17
Education guidelines	0	0	0	0	0	1
All articles	3	9	5	16	22	28

> Pain due to invasion of the chest wall by malignant tumour, if not relieved by radiotherapy, usually demands a powerful analgesic such as pethidine or morphine given by injection. In advanced cases these drugs may be ineffective and neurosurgical measures may be required for the relief of intractable pain." (Grant et al. 1977)

> Morphine and diamorphine play an essential role in the management of severe chronic pain, but these substances are all too often prescribed in sub-optimal ways. Two common mistakes are the over cautious prescription for fear of inducing addiction, and prescribing "cocktails" containing substances such as cocaine and chlorpromazine. Addiction is irrelevant in the management of severe pain in advanced malignancy. (Smyth 1995)

The endogenous opioid system, first mentioned in the late 1980s, has found a place only within endocrinology.

Harrison's *Principles of Internal Medicine* was first published in the United States in 1950. In contrast to Davidson's textbook, 70 pages were devoted to discussion of pain, but largely as a presenting symptom of disease. The management of pain was related to treatment of the disease, for example in discussing the pain of the cauda equina syndrome: "Here, as in spinal cord tumours, treatment, other than surgical removal, is of no avail." (Harrison et al. 1950, p. 69). The 1553-page text contained 2½ pages on the detailed management of intoxication by morphine and related alkaloids. In contrast, the management of the pain of advanced cancer of the stomach is discussed thus:

> Sedatives, analgesics, hypnotics and narcotics should be used freely and wisely. The diagnosis should not be disclosed to the patient. Not even the most mentally rugged can maintain hope in the knowledge of an inoperable cancer. A stable, responsible member of the family, however, should be informed. (Harrison et al. 1950, p. 1171)

The author conveys the deep fear of the use of opioids that presumably was widely held: "Some physicians believe that he should learn to endure pain, with the hope that it may lessen rather than be put on narcotics with the impression that it is hopeless and he might just as well be an addict" (Dock 1950). This fear persisted for over 30 years: "Intractable pain due to incurable disease such as metastatic carcinoma is one of the most difficult of therapeutic problems. As a rule, one resorts to narcotic drugs because of their strong analgesic action, and habituation is accepted as the lesser of two evils" (Harrison et al. 1966; Wintrobe et al. 1974). "Narcotic analgesics are the mainstay of therapy in malignant disease. Pain relief can be achieved in over 95% of patients, but narcotic use must be balanced against the undesirable side effects of sedation, constipation, tolerance, physical dependence and addiction" (Adams and Martin 1983).

The endogenous opioids are discussed with excitement but realism in 1980: "It is impossible to predict which areas of clinical medicine will reap the fruits of these remarkable peptides. Perhaps the most likely will be the field of psychiatry." "It seems unlikely that the development of analogs of opioid peptides will lead to the production of analgesics with non-addictive properties. However, drugs may be developed with a different spectrum of activity compared with the presently known analgesic narcotics" (Unger and Ipp 1980). In more recent years the discussion of endogenous opioids is mostly related to endocrinology.

CONCLUSIONS

The number of published articles in generalist journals concerning cancer-related pain has increased almost 10-fold in the past 30 years, but remains very low. Publication of original research is rare, and the nonspecialist doctor thus has little exposure to this subject. The discovery of the opiate receptor and the endogenous opioid peptides has had no influence on the generalist literature and has led to very few publications of pain research in humans.

Teaching about pain has progressed slowly in the second half of the century, from consideration solely as a clue to a diagnosis, to discussion of the phenomena of pain and of the specifics of pain relief and the use of opioids. The reluctance to use morphine for fear of addiction has been long lived. Entries in the indexes have been dominated by addiction, intoxication, and other negative images of morphine. The discovery of the opioid receptors is briefly alluded to as leading to an increased understanding of pain. These discoveries have had little influence on medical writing specifically about cancer pain, but their influence is greater in the field of endocrinology.

ACKNOWLEDGMENTS

This work was supported by a Wellcome Trust Research Fellowship in the History of Medicine.

REFERENCES

Adams RD, Martin JB. In: Petersdorf RG, Adams RD, Braunwald E, et al. (Eds). *Harrison's Principles of Internal Medicine,* 10th ed. New York: McGraw-Hill, 1983, p 14.

Bonica JJ (Ed). *Management of Pain: With Special Emphasis on the Use of Analgesic Block in Diagnosis, Prognosis, and Therapy.* Philadelphia: Lea & Febiger, 1953.

Davidson LSP (Ed). *The Principles and Practice of Medicine: Notes for Scottish Medical Students.* Edinburgh: Churchill Livingstone, 1952, pp 608.

Dock W. Principles of neoplasia. In: Harrison TR, Resnick WR, Wintrobe MM, Thorn GW, Beeson PB (Eds). *Principles of Internal Medicine.* New York: McGraw-Hill, 1950, pp 290.

Grant IWB, Horrie NW, McHardy GJR. Diseases of the respiratory system. In: Macleod J (Ed). *Davidson's Principles and Practice of Medicine: Notes for Scottish Medical Students,* 12th ed. Edinburgh: Churchill Livingstone, 1977, p 268.

Harrison TR, Resnick WR, Wintrobe MM, Thorn GW, Beeson PB (Eds). *Principles of Internal Medicine.* New York: McGraw-Hill, 1950.

Harrison TR, Adams RD, Bennett IL, et al. (Eds). *Principles of Internal Medicine,* 5th ed. New York: McGraw-Hill, 1966, p 17.

Hughes J, Smith TW, Kosterlitz HW, et al. Identification of two related pentapeptides from the brain with potent agonist activity. *Nature* 1975; 258:577–579.

Medical Curriculum Committee of the British Medical Association. *The Training of a Doctor.* London: Butterworths Medical Publications, 1948, p 52.

Pert CB, Snyder SH. The opiate receptor: demonstration in nervous tissue. *Science* 1973; 179:1011.

Saunders C. Dying of cancer. *St. Thomas's Hospital Gazette* 1958; 56:37–47.

Smyth JF. Oncology. In: Edwards CRW, Bouchier IAD, Haslett C, Chilvers ER (Eds). *Davidson's Principles and Practice of Medicine: A Textbook for Students and Doctors,* 17th ed. Edinburgh: Churchill Livingstone, 1995, p 861.

Unger RH, Ipp E. In: Isselbacher KJ, Adams RD, Braunwald E, Petersdorf RG, Wilson JD (Eds). *Harrison's Principles of Internal Medicine,* 9th ed. New York: McGraw-Hill, 1980, pp 1665–1666.

Wall PD. 25 volumes of Pain. *Pain* 1986; 25:1–2.

Wintrobe MM, Thorn GW, Adams RD, et al. (Eds). *Harrison's Principles of Internal Medicine,* 7th ed. New York: McGraw-Hill, 1974, pp 18.

Correspondence to: Christina Faull, MBBS, MD, FRCP, Consultant in Palliative Medicine, 3rd Floor, Nuffield House, Queen Elizabeth Hospital, Edgbaston, Birmingham B15 2TH, United Kingdom. Tel: 44-121-472-1311; Fax: 44-121-472-4159; email: faull@moseley104.freeserve.co.uk.

Proceedings of the 9th World Congress on Pain,
Progress in Pain Research and Management,
Vol. 16, edited by M. Devor, M.C. Rowbotham, and
Z. Wiesenfeld-Hallin, IASP Press, Seattle, © 2000.

5

A Web-Based Multidisciplinary Course in Pain Management

Stephen Loftus, Isobel Taylor, Ross Harris,
and Michael Cousins

*Pain Management and Research Centre, Royal North Shore Hospital,
St. Leonards, Sydney, New South Wales, Australia*

The graduate diploma/master's degree in Pain Management from the University of Sydney, initially offered in 1996 as a residential program, was the first of its kind in the world. Students attend six intensive teaching weekends each year, for 2 years, to qualify for the graduate diploma; a dissertation completed in a third year qualifies candidates for the master's degree. The course has always been heavily oversubscribed, and students are willing to travel great distances to attend weekend intensives. To meet the demand for higher training in this growing field, the degree is now available not only as a residential course, but is open to pain professionals worldwide in a Web-based format.

Two strong themes underlie the treatment philosophy of the Pain Management and Research Centre: a multidisciplinary approach to assessment and treatment and an evidence-based approach to clinical practice. These themes are reflected in the course subject matter, the orientation of teaching staff, and the recruitment of students from a wide spectrum of professions. Students may include doctors, dentists, nurses, physiotherapists, and clinical psychologists; any health care professional involved in pain management who supports a multidisciplinary approach should feel at home in the program.

EDUCATIONAL TECHNOLOGIES

The distance course exploits several educational technologies. The main point of contact is a secure World Wide Web site, which uses a proprietary course management system, TopClass, produced by WBT Systems, Inc. Access is by user name and password.

Students are organized into small tutorial groups, and all are also enrolled in an "Open Forum." Discussions are organized in a manner that allows multi-threading, so that users can quickly and easily see messages grouped into themes. Study guides offering an overview of various topics are provided in Adobe Acrobat's PDF format. These can be read or printed direct from the Web site or downloaded to students' machines, to be read offline or printed. The PDF format allows platform independence.

Study guides are supplemented by several online, interactive quizzes and computer-aided learning programs. In addition, a folio of readings on each subject is mailed out each semester and comprises key journal papers and book chapters considered core material for mastery of a specified subject. In addition, students receive videotapes that include interviews with experts in the pain management field (for example Professor Patrick Wall) and demonstrations of clinical procedures.

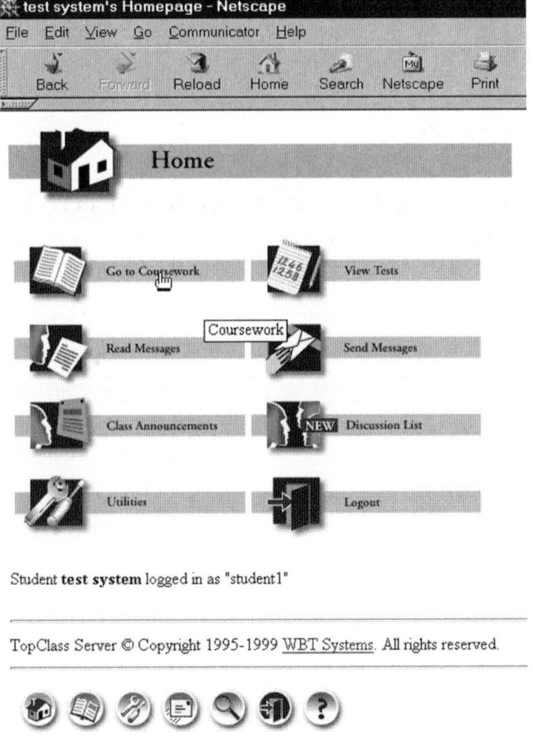

Fig. 1. Distance education home page. Each user has a home page generated by the course management system.

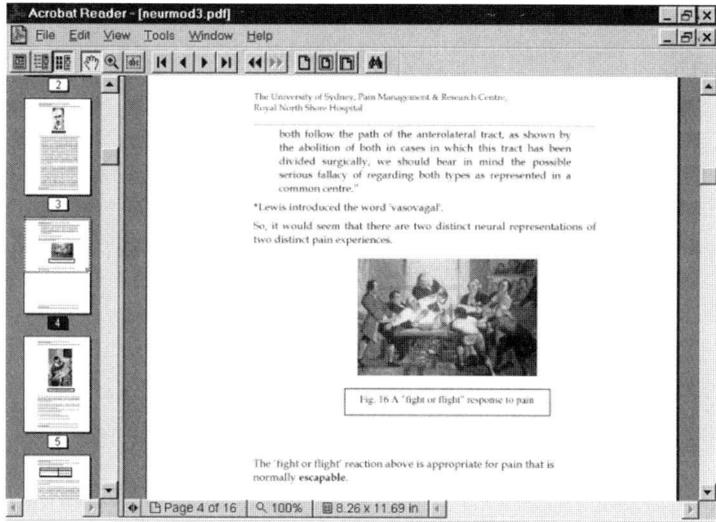

Fig. 2. The subject study guide. Displays a sample from a study guide that is provided online, but can be downloaded to be read or printed offline. Reading from the computer allows users to access features such as the thumbnail sketches of each page (on the left). This permits rapid and easy navigation within the document.

STUDENT LEARNING

Distance education is based on one of two models: the remote classroom and the correspondence course (Daniel 1996). An example of the remote classroom is Australia's School of the Air, which for many years has provided education by radio to children in sparsely occupied regions. More

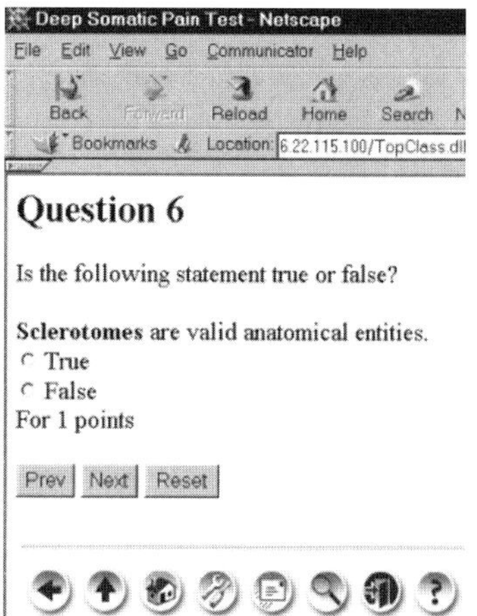

Fig. 3. Interactive online quizzes, shown here, and tutorials supplement the readings and aid formative self-assessment.

recent examples of this model include audioconferencing and videoconferencing. These technologies have their strengths, but can be criticized for shrinking distance only, as users must be connected in real time. The correspondence course model forms the basis for most Web-based systems and can effectively shrink both time and distance. Communication is asynchronous, meaning that users can log on and communicate when it is convenient to them. This flexibility enables busy clinicians in different time zones and continents to communicate easily.

Computer-mediated communication (CMC) or computer conferencing is relatively new, but has already been enthusiastically adopted by many institutions around the world (Kaye 1989). It has numerous benefits for student learning (Bates 1995). It can encourage academic discourse: participants in a face-to-face discussion must respond to each other in real time, whereas the asynchronous nature of CMC allows students to compose and edit responses in a more considered manner, which can enhance the quality of contributions. Students who are more reflective are not marginalized by the more impulsive members of a group, but can take a full and active part. Students from four continents are enrolled in the course; our experience reflects that of other institutions (Riel 1993) in that CMC "raises cross-cultural awareness and brings into the learning process different perspectives from different cultures."

CMC helps to overcome social isolation, a notorious fault in traditional correspondence courses using the postal system. Regular communication with staff and other students enables participants to support each other; this benefit is proving to be one of the greatest strengths of the CMC facility. Many students seek help from colleagues and faculty in managing problem pain cases. With their multidisciplinary backgrounds, staff and fellow students have considerable clinical experience and expertise in solving problem cases submitted by students. Tutors take on the role of mentors and facilitators rather than teachers, and students can also initiate interactions, allowing for a student-centered approach to learning.

THE FUTURE

Distance education, which arose soon after the appearance of a reliable postal system in the 19th century, long remained a fringe activity because of the limitations of the technology. Now, with recent technological advances, distance education is coming of age as one of the most rapidly growing areas of educational activity.

We are continuing to explore ways to exploit the potential of the technology to enhance the educational experience of our students. A patient simulator is under development, to be distributed on CD-ROM, which will allow students to enhance their clinical skills through role-playing the assessment and treatment planning of a patient in a multidisciplinary center. How can we structure online tutorials and train our tutors to ensure continuing support and a high level of interaction and academic discourse? We are committed to using the World Wide Web to explore these and other questions about effective postgraduate medical education.

There are also wider issues to face (Farrington 1997). Distance education is now becoming an important concept in mainstream education (McIsaac and Gunarwardena 1996). Soon most universities will be in a position to offer courses worldwide and will have the option of competing or collaborating with each other. We at the Pain Management and Research Centre are interested in collaborating with other institutions that wish to become involved in this phenomenon that is transforming higher education, and has been summarized as follows:

> Education today must, like any enterprise, be a bold or dangerous undertaking, preparing people for a changing world rather than one of permanence. The enterprising college or university must understand that its mission is not so much to teach as it is to create a culture—driven by technology—in which students, faculty and staff are continuously learning. (Heterick 1994)

SUMMARY

The Pain Management and Research Centre at the University of Sydney's Royal North Shore Hospital has pioneered multidisciplinary postgraduate education in pain management. This course, making use of modern educational technology, is now available throughout the world. Further information can be obtained from our Web page in the section on postgraduate degrees at http://www.painmgmt.usyd.edu.au/, or by contacting the first author at sloftus@doh.health.nsw.gov.au.

REFERENCES

Bates AW. Computer-mediated communication. In: *Technology, Open Learning and Distance Education*. London: Routledge, 1995, pp 202–208.

Daniel J. The essentials of distance education. In: *Mega-Universities and Knowledge Media—Technology Strategies for Higher Education*. London: Kogan Page, 1996, pp 46–66.

Farrington G. Higher education in the Information Age. In: *The Learning Revolution: The Challenge of Information Technology in the Academy*. Boston: Anker, 1997, pp 54–74.

Heterick RC Jr. Technological change and higher education policy. *AGB Priorities* 1; 1994, Spring.

Kaye A. Computer mediated communication and distance education. In: Mason R, Kaye A. (Eds). *Mindweave: Communication, Computers, and Distance Education*. Oxford and New York: Pergamon Press, 1989, pp 2–21.

McIsaac MS, Gunarwardena CM. Distance education. In: Jonassen D (Ed). *A Handbook of Research in Educational Communications and Technology: A Project of the Association for Educational Communications and Technology*. New York: Macmillan, 1996, pp 403–438.

Riel M. Global education through Learning Circles. In: Harasim L (Ed). *Global Networks: Computers and International Communication*. Cambridge, MA: MIT Press, 1993, pp 221–236.

Correspondence to: Stephen Loftus, Pain Management and Research Centre, Royal North Shore Hospital, St. Leonards, NSW 2065, Australia. Tel: 61-(0)2-9926-7387; Fax: 61-(0)2-9926-6548; email: sloftus@doh.health.nsw.gov.au.

Proceedings of the 9th World Congress on Pain,
Progress in Pain Research and Management,
Vol. 16, edited by M. Devor, M.C. Rowbotham, and
Z. Wiesenfeld-Hallin, IASP Press, Seattle, © 2000.

6

The Primary Nociceptor: Special Functions, Special Receptors

John N. Wood,[a] Armen N. Akopian,[a] Paolo Cesare,[a] Yanning Ding,[a] Rey Garcia,[a] Mark Heath,[b] Anastasia Liapi,[a] Misbah Malik-Hall,[a] Mohammed Nassar,[a] Kenji Okuse,[a] Samantha Ravenall,[a] Oro Rufian,[a] Veronika Souslova,[a] and Madhu Sukumaran[a]

[a]*Biology Department, University College, London, United Kingdom;*
[b]*Department of Anesthesiology, Columbia University, New York, New York, USA*

Specialized sensory neurons that respond to tissue damage (nociceptors) have long been a focus of interest for biologists interested in pain perception (Wood and Perl 1999). The detection of noxious chemical, thermal, and mechanical stimuli seems to be mediated by receptors on these cells, and there has been much debate about the role of chemical mediators in these processes. Biochemical and electrophysiological studies of the consequences of applying noxious thermal mechanical and chemical stimuli to sensory neurons have suggested that the thresholds of activation of specific receptors on sensory neurons mirror pain thresholds detected psychophysically (Cesare and McNaughton 1996), providing support for the view that blocking nociceptor activation may be the focus of choice for developing new analgesic drugs. The past few years have seen dramatic increases in our understanding of nociceptors, as technical advances in molecular genetics and cellular physiology have been applied to the study of nociceptor function. We now have a good idea of some of the developmental regulatory pathways that lead to the acquisition of a nociceptor phenotype, and of the molecular mechanisms that underlie nociceptor activation and sensitization. This knowledge is likely to prove valuable for the development of new types of analgesic drugs. In this chapter we focus on receptors and channels that are expressed specifically by nociceptors. Genes expressed only by particular cell types are likely to play a specialized functional role. The hunt for sensory-neuron-specific genes has involved a variety of difference and homology cloning methods that have resulted in the identification of sensory-neuron-specific channels and receptors that may play important roles in nociception.

CLONING STRATEGIES

The receptors and channels expressed by nociceptors can be cloned in various ways. cDNA libraries made from mRNA expressed in dorsal root ganglia (DRG) can be depleted of broadly expressed transcripts by subtractive hybridization with RNA isolated from other tissues. The basis of this technique is to complex cDNA from sensory neurons with RNA from a variety of other tissues that has been coupled to biotin. The common transcripts present in all tissues can be solvent extracted after addition of streptavidin, and a tiny amount of cDNA-encoding transcripts only present in the tissue of interest are left to be amplified using the polymerase chain reaction (PCR) and cloned (Sive and St John 1988; Akopian and Wood 1995). More recently, differential screening of single-cell libraries has become a feasible and productive method, which has been exploited to identify pheromone receptors (Dulac and Axel 1995). A substantial number of DRG-specific clones have been identified using differential screening. These include the voltage-gated sodium channel SNS (also called PN3) and the adenosine triphosphate (ATP)-gated cation channel P2X3 (Chen et al. 1995; Akopian et al. 1996).

Another approach relies upon expression-cloning to identify transcripts that encode a functional protein that can be detected by functional assays in eukaryotic expression systems. This approach has been used to identify serotonin receptors by means of electrophysiological screens in *Xenopus* oocytes (Julius et al. 1988). Calcium imaging of transfected cells has more recently been used to identify the capsaicin receptor VR1 (Caterina et al. 1997), and homology cloning has identified other capsaicin-like clones (Caterina et al. 1999).

SENSORY NEURON ATP-GATED ION CHANNELS

An ATP-gated cation channel named P2X3 was first identified in a DRG difference library (Chen at al. 1995). Injection of ATP in human blister bases can evoke pain (Bleehan and Keele 1977), a finding consistent with a direct action of ATP on nociceptive sensory neurons. This explanation for the pain-inducing actions of ATP is supported by electrophysiological studies that have shown that many DRG sensory neurons respond to ATP with elevated intracellular free calcium concentrations, or with depolarizing responses (Buell et al. 1996). These effects are probably mediated by the P2X class of ATP-gated ion channels, which are all expressed by DRG neurons. Such receptors comprise a family of glycosylated proteins of apparent molecular mass of about 60 kDa, which have intracellular N- and C-terminal domains, two-membrane-spanning hydrophobic domains, the second of which lines the channel pore, and a large extracellular domain. The subunits are encoded by different genes, although alternatively spliced transcripts of particular subtypes also occur. The channels are 35–50% identical at the amino acid level and are permeable to both monovalent and divalent cations. These channels show some similarities with amiloride-sensitive sodium channel subunits and with *Caenorhabditis elegans degenerins,* but have a distinct pattern of expression of conserved cysteine residues, in the predicted extracellular domain of the proteins. Seven different P2X receptors have been cloned and expressed in *Xenopus* oocytes, and their distribution has been analyzed by in situ hybridization. Six known P2X-subtype mRNA transcripts are expressed in sensory neurons of the dorsal root, nodose, and trigeminal ganglia (Buell et al. 1996). However, only one subtype, P2X3, is expressed selectively in small-diameter sensory neurons that generally subserve a nociceptive function. An electrophysiological analysis of the properties of the expressed P2X3 channel showed many similarities with rat sensory neurons in culture (Chen et al. 1995). The channel rapidly desensitized, and was activated by ATP congeners with the same rank order of potency as that described for sensory neurons in culture (at low concentrations, 2-methyl-thio ATP >> ATP > αβ-methylene ATP > γ-thio ATP > 2′deoxy ATP > cytidine triphosphate [CTP] > adenosine disphosphate [ADP] >> uridine triphosphate [UTP] βγ-methylene ATP > guanidine triphosphate [GTP]). Indirect evidence for heteromultimeric channels in sensory neurons has been provided by co-expression studies of distinct P2X subunits in *Xenopus* oocytes. Some nodose ganglion cells desensitize slowly in response to αβ-methylene ATP (Khakh et al. 1995). However, the oocyte-expressed P2X3 receptor desensitizes rapidly. If P2X2 (first identified in PC12 cells) is co-expressed with P2X3 in oocytes, a slowly desensitizing form of the receptor is generated (Lewis et al. 1995). This evidence is consistent with other data, but does not prove that heteromultimeric receptors exist in sensory neurons. Structural studies using cross-linking reagents suggest that monomeric receptors exist as trimers, unlike other known classes of ion channels. Recent evidence suggests that P2X3 is expressed predominantly by c-ret-positive sensory neurons sensitive to glial-derived neurotrophic factor (GDNF), which comprise a subset of the nociceptor population. Developmental analysis has shown that P2X3 transcripts are expressed as early as the period of sensory neurogenesis (E11.5 in the rat, where E = embryonic day). In the E12.5 rat, P2X3 transcripts are found in somatovisceral primary sensory neurons, including neurons of trigeminal, facial, petrosal, nodose, and dorsal root ganglia, but not in other kinds of primary sensory neurons, such as olfactory epithelia, retina, and trigeminal mesencephalic nuclei.

Evidence of a role for P2X3 in nociception comes from physiological studies of conscious rats following subplantar injection of ATP and the ultrapotent congener αβ-methylene ATP, which shows some selectivity for P2X3. Hindpaw lifting and licking occurred in animals given subplantar injections of αβ-methylene ATP. Nociceptive behaviors were dose-related, while desensitization with a subplantar injection of capsaicin abolished all pain-related behavior in animals subsequently injected with αβ-methylene ATP (Bland-Ward and Humphrey 1997).

A specific role of P2X3 in nociception is thus an interesting possibility, given its selective expression pattern on nociceptive neurons. Non-desensitizing P2X receptors seem to be present on dorsal horn neurons, and probably correspond to P2X2, P2X4, and P2X6 receptor subtypes. Recent studies on spinal cord splices confirm that ATP applied to DRG neuron spinal cord co-cultures stimulates glutamate release (Gu and MacDermott 1997). Interestingly, an expression-cloned mechanoreceptor that corresponds to a P2Y1 receptor was recently reported. The authors found that tissue distortion caused by mechanical stimulation could also activate P2X3 through the release of ATP from distended cells, suggesting a possible role for P2X3 in mechanical, as well as chemotransduction (Nakamura and Strittmatter 1996).

The hypothesis that P2X3 receptors have a specialized role in nociception is supported by the observation that P2X3-immunostaining and ATP-induced inward current indeed appear in fluorescence-traced nociceptors of rat tooth pulp (Cook et al. 1997). In the absence of specific inhibitors for P2X subtypes, the generation of null mutants for P2X receptors is a route to defining their function. P2X1, 2, 3, and 4 null mutants are now available, and an analysis of their responses to noxious stimuli is under way. Preliminary studies suggest that all the ATP-evoked fast desensitizing responses of primary sensory neurons in culture are lost in P2X3 null mutant mice (Cesare et al. 2000).

SENSORY NEURON PROTON-GATED CHANNELS

Proton-gated channels associated with sensory neurons are of particular interest because low pH is an important component in the induction of inflammatory pain (Vyklicky et al. 1998). An unusual nondesensitizing proton-gated calcium current has been described in sensory neurons in culture, and it has been suggested that a related channel could be the capsaicin receptor (Bevan and Geppetti 1994). Support for this view is increasing, as the cloned capsaicin receptor VR1 is activated at low pH. Recently, a new set of cation-selective (predominantly sodium) ion channels gated by protons has been described in sensory neurons that may contribute to such currents (Waldmann and Lazdunski 1998). A proton-gated cation channel named ASIC (acid-sensing ion channel) that is expressed throughout the nervous system was the first channel to be identified (Waldmann et al. 1997a). The ASIC channels also comprise a two-transmembrane subunit with some topological similarities to the P2X receptors, but with distinct primary sequences that place them in the family of amiloride-sensitive epithelial sodium channels (ENaC). The family has expanded to include the MDEG (mammalian degenerin) channels, renamed ASIC2a and 2b, and a related clone expressed in DRG sensory neurons named DRASIC or ASIC-3 (Garcia-Anoveros et al. 1997). Interestingly, all the ASIC clones have highly conserved extracellular cysteine residues, suggesting that, as with the P2X class of receptors, the overall topology of the extracellular domain is similar within this particular class of receptor. Recent studies have provided compelling evidence that the members of the ENaC family are tetramers, when heterologously expressed, in contrast to the trimeric P2X receptors (Coscoy et al. 1998).

Using homology cloning techniques, the ASIC homologue (DRASIC) was found in sensory-neurons (Waldmann et al. 1997b). DRASIC is predominantly expressed in sensory neurons, but some evidence indicates that it is expressed in spinal cord and other central nervous system (CNS) locations at lower levels (Chen et al. 1998). In addition, two splice variants of an additional channel named MDEG (mammalian degenerin) have been identified (Lingueglia et al. 1997). MDEG1 is a functional proton-gated ion channel, but MDEG2 is a splice variant that does not function except as a heteromultimer with ASIC or DRASIC. Interestingly, the properties of DRASIC/MDEG2 heteromultimers are distinct from DRASIC, with altered kinetics and ionic permeabilities, which provides strong evidence that members of the ENaC family may form heteromultimers, presumably of four subunits in total (Coscoy et al. 1998). MDEG1 and 2 are also known as ASIC2a and ASIC2b. Only ASIC2b is found in sensory neurons (Chen et al. 1998).

Homology cloning has recently identified an ASIC-related clone with distinct 5´ and 3´ untranslated regions (UTRs) named ASIC-α and a splice variant with a unique 5´ region and the same C terminal and 3´ UTR as

ASIC-α, named ASIC-β. ASIC-β has a unique 172-amino-acid N-terminal region with a putative first-transmembrane domain that is homologous to the DRASIC channel sequence (Chen et al. 1998). A single ASIC-α 3.2-kilobase transcript is expressed in sensory neurons and other tissues. A similar sized transcript is expressed by ASIC-β in DRG alone, and is present only in a subset of small-diameter sensory neurons. The functional properties of ASIC-β are subtly different to those of other members of this family. Unlike ASIC-α, both DRASIC and ASIC-β show fast and slow components of proton-evoked channel opening. However, the slow response of ASIC-β is less marked than that of DRASIC, and is unaffected by the application of amiloride, which blocks the fast component in both channels, but potentiates the slow component in DRASIC. Like ASIC-α, ASIC-β discriminates poorly between cations, since the reversal potential for the pH-gated current in ASIC-β-expressing COS cells was some 50 mV more negative than would be expected for a "pure" sodium conductance (+22 mV versus calculated sodium reversal potential of +73 mV). ASIC-β shows some calcium permeability, since increasing extracellular calcium enhances the size of currents, whilst ASIC-α is markedly inhibited, even with physiological levels of extracellular calcium. Interestingly, in sensory neurons in culture, proton-evoked ion fluxes are calcium permeable (Bevan and Geppetti 1994), which implies that either the capsaicin-gated cation channel or a novel combination of ASIC subunits mediate proton-evoked fluxes. Identification of sensory-neuron-specific channels that alone or in combination account for a long-lasting component of proton-evoked cation flux provides another potential new route to the development of novel anti-inflammatory analgesic drugs.

The possibility that some of the proton-gated channels may participate in mechanosensitive ion channel complexes should also be considered. There is clear evidence that C fibers can be activated mechanically, which suggests that receptors are present on the sensory neurons themselves. Of the mechanosensitive channels defined by genetic studies of *C. elegans* and *Drosophila melanogaster,* all seem to fall into the class of two-transmembrane receptors exemplified by the ENaC/degenerin family. Expression cloning of rat mechanoreceptors in *Xenopus* oocytes suggests that ATP released through mechanical distortion may activate the P2Y1 receptor present on large-diameter sensory neurons, whilst more active mechanical distortion causes activation of the P2X3 receptor (also a two-transmembrane ion channel, see above) (Nakamura and Strittmatter 1996). Several mechanisms for mechanosensation may thus exist. Two novel *Drosophila* DEG/ENaC proteins, Pickpocket (PPK) and Ripped Pocket (RPK), appear to be ion channel subunits. Expression of RPK generated multimeric Na^+ channels that were dominantly activated by a mutation associated with neurodegeneration. Amiloride and gadolinium, which block mechanosensation in vivo, inhibited RPK channels. Although PPK did not form channels on its own, it associated with and reduced the current generated by a related human brain Na^+ channel. The vertebrate homologues of these channels are thus candidates for mechanoreception (Wood and Perl 1999).

HEAT-OPERATED AND CAPSAICIN-GATED CHANNELS

Noxious heat causes an inward current in a subset of nociceptive neurons with a threshold of activation of about 42°C (Cesare and McNaughton 1996). Recent studies suggest that this effect is mediated through a cation-selective ion channel that is also gated by capsaicin, the pungent ingredient of red peppers (Caterina et al. 1997).

Capsaicin causes depolarization of sensory neurons, increases in intracellular calcium, and release of neuropeptides such as calcitonin gene-related peptide (CGRP). The depolarization is caused by capsaicin-induced inward currents carried mainly by Ca^{2+} and Na^+ ions mediated by opening of a nonspecific cation channel. There are two widely used capsaicin antagonists. Capsazepine is a close analogue of capsaicin and is a competitive antagonist (Bevan et al. 1992), and ruthenium red is a noncompetitive antagonist (Dray et al. 1990; Amman and Maggi 1991; Bevan et al. 1992).

A functional vanilloid (capsaicin) receptor (VR1) activated both by capsaicin and noxious heat (46°C) has recently been cloned by the Julius laboratory (Caterina et al. 1997). The investigators used a rat DRG cDNA library in a shuttle vector to isolate and sib-select pools of clones that conferred a capsaicin response; they then used the calcium-sensitive Fura-2 dye to measure increases in intracellular calcium in HEK293 (human embryonic kidney) cells transfected with defined pools of cDNA clones. The functional receptor resembles members of the "TRP" (transient receptor potential) family of proteins in terms of topological organization. TRP proteins are six-transmembrane monomers, first identified in *Drosophila* mutants that showed deficits in photoreception. VR1 has the characteristic N-terminal ankyrin repeats. Considerable sequence similarity is also apparent in, but is limited to, the sixth-transmembrane domain. Its flanking sequences and the loop between transmembrane domains 5 and 6 are believed to form part of the presumptive pore region.

Several lines of evidence have established that some TRP genes provide the molecular basis for the phenomenon known as capacitative calcium entry (CCE). CCE is loosely defined as the influx of Ca^{2+} from the extracellular space following inositol 1,4,5-triphosphate-induced mobilization of internal stores (Putney 1986). As such, it has also been referred to as store-operated calcium entry. This mode of calcium influx appears to be ubiquitous, having been observed in most cells examined. Expression of the *Drosophila* TRP gene (*Dtrp*) in Sf9 (Vaca et al. 1994) and 293T cells (Xu et al. 1997) causes the appearance of novel membrane currents that show modest selectivity for Ca^{2+} and are sensitive to store depletion. In contrast, the *Drosophila* TRP-like gene (*Dtrpl*) forms a rather nonselective, constitutively active cation channel when heterologously expressed (Hu et al. 1994). To date, six mammalian TRP genes have been cloned and sequenced, either through initial searches of expressed sequence tag databases using the *Dtrp* amino acid sequence as the query sequence; or through degenerate reverse transcription-polymerase reaction (RT-PCR) using primers designed from the highly conserved regions (transmembrane domains 5 and 6) of *Dtrp* and *Dtrpl*. *Dtrp1* (Wes et al. 1995; Zhu et al. 1995), *Dtrp3* (Zhu et al. 1996), *Dtrp4* (Philipp et al. 1996), and *Dtrp6* (Boulay et al. 1997) have been sequenced in their full length, and partial sequences have also been reported for *Dtrp2* (possibly a pseudogene) and *Dtrp5* (Zhu et al. 1996). Functional expression of the available full-length clones in mammalian cells enhances CCE (Birnbaumer 1996; Philipp et al. 1996; Zhu et al. 1996; Boulay et al. 1997), whereas expression of TRP cDNA fragments in antisense orientation interferes with endogenous CCE (Birnbaumer 1996; Zhu et al. 1996), providing a direct connection between TRP proteins and store-operated calcium entry. Like *Drosophila* TRP, bovine *trp4* appears to be fairly selective for Ca^{2+} and sensitive to store depletion when expressed in HEK293 cells (Philipp et al. 1996). Human *TRP1*, when expressed in CHO (Chinese hamster ovary) cells, is also activated by store depletion, but the channel formed is fairly nonselective (Zitt et al. 1996). *Trp3* and *trp6* have also been functionally expressed; they form nonselective cation channels insensitive to store depletion (Zhu et al. 1998; Boulay et al. 1997). Homomeric and/or heteromultimeric interactions between the different TRP proteins may help explain the functional heterogeneity of store-operated conductances observed in various cell types.

The capsaicin receptor VR1 also probably exists in a multimeric form (Hill coefficient of 2 for capsaicin), as a cation-selective ion channel with a preference for calcium, but it does not appear to play any role in CCE. Whether VR1 can heteromultimerize with other TRP proteins or further VR1-like receptors is unknown, but there is certainly strong evidence for an additional VR1-like receptor present in mast cells. Biro et al. (1998) have characterized a calcium-45 uptake response in these cells, but interestingly, in contrast to sensory neurons, capsaicin does not kill mast cells, and does not even induce their degranulation.

The existence of other VR1-like receptors and the large number of TRP family members raises the possibility that members of this channel family may be gated by ligands other than noxious heat. It is already clear that TRP channels play a critical role in phototransduction in *Drosophila,* and evidence that bradykinin, a hyperalgesic mediator, can gate *trp3* via activation of heterotrimeric G_q proteins has been obtained in a heterologous expression system. Studies by the Bargmann group in *C. elegans* (Colbert et al. 1997, Bargmann et al. 1998) suggest that TRP channels also play a role in mechanosensory transduction. Homology cloning and expression studies of VR1 in combination with other TRP channels, and of their regulation by G-protein-coupled receptors, should provide interesting evidence not only about mechanisms of nociception, but also on the normal gating mechanisms of TRP channels.

A possible endogenous ligand for vanilloid receptors that has been the subject of much debate is low pH. Bevan and Geppetti (1994) have used electrophysiological studies to show that protons may gate the capsaicin channel, and studies with VR1 clones confirm that protons potentiate the actions of capsaicin and may activate the channel directly. These observations are particularly intriguing in the context of studies on soups of inflammatory mediators carried out by the Reeh laboratory. They have found that an inward current is evoked by bradykinin, prostaglandin E_2, and serotonin in sensory neurons at low pH, but not at physiological pH (Vyklicky et al. 1998). As the current is blocked by 10 μM Capsezapine, it is possible that the vanilloid receptor/ion channel is responsible for the inward current.

An additional vanilloid receptor, broadly expressed in DRG neurons, T cells, and various other tissues, named VR-L, has also recently been homology cloned and may be activated by very high temperatures (Caterina et al. 1999). A further member of the family is present in silico (i.e., in DNA databases). The creation and analysis of knock-out mice for these channels should prove illuminating.

SENSORY-NEURON-SPECIFIC SODIUM CHANNELS

The functional voltage-gated sodium channels (VGSCs) present in both the peripheral and central nervous systems comprise a large membrane-spanning α subunit of 260 kDa, which comprises four repeated domains of six transmembrane segments. In addition, there are associated regulatory subunits—a β_1 subunit of 36 kDa and a covalently associated β_2 subunit of 33 kDa (Isom and Catterall 1996). Indirect evidence indicates that several β_2 subunits exist. The α-subunit mRNAs can direct the translation of functional channels, while the accessory β_1 and β_2 subunits enhance functional channel expression in *Xenopus* oocytes and regulate the kinetic properties of expressed channels. In addition, the β_2 subunit may play a role in anchoring the protein at particular locations within the cell (Isom and Catterall 1996).

The functional VGSC α subunit SNS (Akopian et al. 1996), which was homology cloned and named PN3 by Sangameswaran et al. (1996), is particularly interesting because it corresponds to an unusual type of sodium channel that is present in small-diameter sensory neurons and is resistant to the puffer fish poison, tetrodotoxin (TTX). Mounting evidence suggests that this TTX-resistant (TTX-r) sodium channel plays a unique role in the transmission of nociceptive information to the spinal cord. For example, peripherally applied TTX failed to affect bradykinin-dependent release of CGRP or the C-fiber-mediated depolarization of dorsal horn cells (Jeftinija 1994). However, a more prevalent view is that in most nerves, essentially all electrically evoked depolarizations leading to both A- and C-fiber-mediated action potential propagation are TTX sensitive, and thus the role of SNS may be to regulate the threshold of activation of small-diameter sensory neurons.

The sodium channel transcripts present in DRG have been explored by Northern blots and PCR (Table I). The neuronal forms type I and II are present, while the embryonic type III reappears after axotomy. Both SNS and the TTX-s channel PN1 are present at high levels in peripheral neurons. PN1, type I, NaCh6, and type II TTX-s transcripts occur in descending order of abundance. The atypical sodium channel NaG is expressed predominantly by Schwann cells, but is also found in sensory neurons. Only the small-diameter, sensory-neuron-specific SNS subunit is exclusively present in small-diameter sensory neurons, however. This pattern of distribution has been

Table I
Sodium channels in dorsal root ganglia

Name	Gene	Chromosome		Functional?
Type I	*SCN1a*	2	X03638	Yes
Type II	*SCN2a*	2	X03639	Yes
Type IIa				Yes
Type III	*SCN3a*	2	Y00766	Yes
SM1	*SCN4a*	11	JN0007	Absent
SM2	*SCN5a*	9	A33996	Absent
NaCh6	*SCN8a*	15	U59966	Yes
PN1, HneNa	*SCN9a*	2	X82835	Yes
SNS/PN3	*SCN10a*	9	X92184	Yes
NaN/SNS2	*SCN11a*	9	AF059030	Yes
NaG/SCL11	*SCN7a*	?	Y09164	?

demonstrated by in situ hybridization and RT-PCR examination of a range of tissues. In addition, the destruction of small-diameter sensory neurons by capsaicin (which acts predominantly on nociceptors) leads to loss of the SNS transcript (Akopian et al. 1996). These observations, combined with its resistance to TTX block (IC_{50} [inhibitory concentration] = 60 μM) support the view that SNS underlies the TTX-insensitive (TTX-i) currents observed in C fibers and small-diameter neurons. The molecular basis for the TTX insensitivity exhibited by SNS has recently been addressed by site-directed mutagenesis experiments. A critical residue in the pore of the channel of TTX-sensitive (TTX-s) VGSCs that is normally hydrophobic is transformed to a serine in SNS. When this single amino acid position is altered to phenylalanine, the sensitivity to TTX is dramatically increased (IC_{50} = 2 nM) (Sivilotti et al. 1997). These studies confirm earlier ideas about the TTX-binding site in sodium channel atria based on mutagenesis studies of the cardiac sodium channel.

Gold et al. (1996) and England et al. (1996) have demonstrated the functional modulation of TTX-i VGSC activity in sensory neurons by inflammatory mediators that are known to lower pain thresholds. Prostaglandin E_2, adenosine, and serotonin all increased the magnitude of sodium current, shifted its conductance-voltage relation in a hyperpolarizing direction, and increased the rates of activation and inactivation of sodium channels in small-diameter sensory neurons in culture. Such data suggest that TTX-i sodium currents play an important role in regulating pain thresholds.

Although SNS does not appear to be completely dependent upon nerve growth factor (NGF) for expression, both the transcript and the protein are upregulated and an unusual, and apparently nonfunctional, splice variant appears on addition of NGF to sensory neurons in culture (Okuse et al. 1997). In addition, a soluble factor released by Schwann cells, which may well be NGF, seems to be involved in the upregulation of SNS expression (Dib-Hajj et al. 1998). Given the restricted expression of the high-affinity NGF receptor trkA on the neuronal subpopulation that is principally concerned with nociception, NGF regulation of sodium channels, particularly of SNS, may play a role in regulating inflammatory pain thresholds. Interestingly, IB4-positive, GDNF-sensitive small-diameter sensory neurons also express SNS; this finding raises the possibility that other factors such as GDNF may regulate SNS expression in this class of nociceptor. In contrast to the upregulation of TTX-r currents and of SNS transcripts with inflammatory mediators, various manipulations that lead to neuropathic pain (ligature-induced and diabetic neuropathies) have downregulated SNS expression. This finding suggests that SNS may play a more significant role in inflammatory rather than neuropathic pain states.

The recently described anti-hyperalgesic agent BW2040W92 (Trezise et al. 1998) appears to be a use-dependent blocker of TTX-r activity in sensory neurons, and some of its antihyperalgesic actions may be ascribed to SNS block, although the compound also acts on TTX-s channels. These observations provide further indirect support for a role for SNS in setting pain thresholds. The unique low-affinity TTX-binding site in the SNS channel atrium has been partially defined, and substituted guanidines specifically directed against SNS could thus provide an additional approach to selective channel block. A direct approach to determine the functional significance of SNS is to ablate the expression of the channel in a null mutant mouse and measure the behavioral and electrophysiological consequences. Studies of such mice demonstrate that all TTX-r activity found in sensory neurons in culture is encoded by SNS (Akopian et al. 1999). The behavioral correlates of a loss of SNS expression are of major interest in terms of nociceptive processing. To obtain meaningful data, behavioral analysis depends upon careful manipulation of genetic backgrounds by repeated backcrosses to produce congenic strains, as well as the assessment of any compensatory developmental changes that may occur in *sns* null mutants. The loss of SNS seems to lead to a compensatory upregulation of expression of the TTX-s channel PN1, with lower thresholds of electrical excitation of C fibers in null mutants. There are nonetheless major deficits in pain pathways in such mice, which emphasize the important role on SNS in nociception (Akopian et al. 1999).

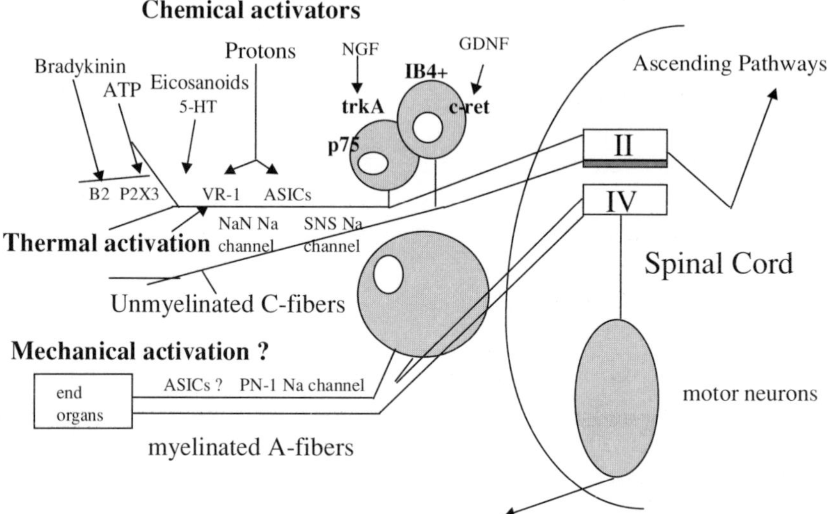

Fig. 1. Sensory-neuron-specific receptors and channels.

Recently a new sodium channel transcript named NaN has been identified in small-diameter sensory neurons (Dib-Hajj et al. 1998; Tate et al. 1998). The channel contains the appropriate sodium selectivity filters and voltage sensor motifs, although it has three less positively charged residues in its S4 domains than does SNS. Interestingly, the channel expresses a serine residue at the same position of the TTX-binding site as does SNS, suggesting that the channel is likely to be TTX-r. There is evidence, however, that the transcript encodes a functional channel, although analysis of SNS null mutants (which have no sensory neuron TTX-r currents) argues against a functional role as a TTX-i sodium channel for NaN.

WIDELY-EXPRESSED RECEPTORS PRESENT IN NOCICEPTORS

Several receptors that have been characterized at the molecular level, such as prostanoid and serotonin receptors, appear to play a functional role in nociception, as well as being broadly expressed elsewhere. The prostacyclin receptor seems to be particularly important in the induction of hyperalgesia, as the null mutant does not exhibit acetic-acid-induced writhing behavior. Binding and pharmacological studies have also identified a number of serotonin (5-HT) receptor subtypes on sensory neurons, including 5HT-1A, 5HT-1D, 5HT-2, and 5HT-3. The 5HT-3 receptor (previously classified as a β_5 nicotinic receptor subunit) is the only directly gated cation channel present, and is found on about 40% of DRG neurons grown in tissue culture. It is known to form a heteromeric cation channel. Unmyelinated C fibers seem to respond particularly well to 5-HT. Apart from these direct actions mediated through the 5HT-3 receptor, the action of other chemical or mechanical activators of sensory neurons are enhanced by 5-HT acting through other receptor subtypes. Glutamate receptors, nicotinic and muscarinic receptors, and bradykinin B2 receptors also occur on nociceptive sensory neurons (Wood and Docherty 1997). Interestingly, an epibatidine-related compound (ABT-594) has potent analgesic activity, and appears to act on nociceptor presynaptic nicotinic receptors in the spinal cord. The generation of tissue-specific knockouts for these globally expressed receptors would be valuable in helping to clarify their role in nociception and pain induction. One way to do this is to create mice that express the bacterial recombinase Cre in DRG neurons alone. The site-specific DNA recombinase Cre mediates the recombination of two repeated target sites (loxP) to a single loxP site, with concomitant excision of the DNA segment flanked by the loxP sites. Gene excision can be achieved by mating two different animals, one carrying a target gene flanked by loxP sites and one carrying a Cre transgene (Kuhn et al. 1995).

FUTURE PROSPECTS

Difference, expression, and homology cloning have led to the identification of several selectively expressed ion channels and receptors that may prove to be useful analgesic drug targets. A better understanding of the regulatory sequences that specify sensory-neuron-specific gene expression may also be useful in designing screens for modulators that alter channel expression rather than function. Tissue-specific gene ablation using the Cre-lox system will also allow us to examine the contribution of broadly expressed genes to nociceptive pathways. Taken together, these various approaches demonstrate that the application of molecular genetics to the study of sensory neurobiology has been valuable and informative, and should lead to useful treatments for pain disorders that result from aberrant nociceptor activity.

REFERENCES

Akopian AN, Wood JN. Peripheral nervous system-specific genes identified by subtractive cDNA cloning. *J Biol Chem* 1995; 270:21264–21270.

Akopian AN, Sivilotti L, Wood JN. A tetrodotoxin-resistant sodium channel expressed by C-fibre associated sensory neurons. *Nature* 1996; 379:257–262.

Akopian AN, Souslova V, England S, et al. The tetrodotoxin-resistant sodium channel SNS plays a specialised role in pain pathways. *Nat Neurosci* 1999; 2:541–548.

Amman R, Maggi CA. Ruthenium red as a capsaicin antagonist. *Life Sci* 1991; 49:849–856.

Bargmann CI, Kaplan JM. Signal transduction in the *Caenorhabditis elegans* nervous system. *Annu Rev Neurosci* 1998; 21:279–308.

Bevan S, Geppetti P. Protons: small stimulants of capsaicin-sensitive nerves. *Trends Neurosci* 1994; 17:509–512.

Bevan S, Hothi S, Hughes G. Capsazepine: a competitive antagonist of the sensory neuron excitant capsaicin. *Br J Pharmacol* 1992; 107:544–552.

Biro T, Maurer M, Modarres S, et al. Characterization of functional vanilloid receptors expressed by mast cells. *Blood* 1998; 91:1332–1340.

Birnbaumer L, Zhu X, Jiang M, et al. On the molecular basis and regulation of cellular capacitative calcium entry: roles for Trp proteins. *Proc Natl Acad Sci USA* 1996; 93:15195–15202.

Bland-Ward PA, Humphrey P. Acute nociception mediated by hindpaw P2X receptor activation in the rat. *Br J Pharmacol* 1997; 122(2):365–371.

Bleehen T, Keele CA. Observations on the algogenic actions of adenosine compounds on the human blister base preparation. *Pain* 1977; 4:367–377.

Boulay G, Zhu X, Peyton M, et al. Cloning and expression of a novel mammalian homolog of *Drosophila* transient receptor potential (Trp) involved in calcium entry secondary to activation of receptors coupled by the Gq class of G protein. *J Biol Chem* 1997; 272:29672–29680.

Buell G, Collo G, Rassendren F. P2X receptors: an emerging channel family. *Eur J Neurosci* 1996; 8:2221–2228.

Caterina MJ, Schumacher MA, Tominaga M, et al. The capsaicin receptor: a heat-activated ion channel in the pain pathway. *Nature* 1997; 389:816–824.

Caterina MJ, Rosen TA, Tominaga M, Brake AJ, Julius D. A capsaicin-receptor homologue with a high threshold for noxious heat. *Nature* 1999; 398(6726):436–441.

Cesare P, McNaughton PA. Novel heat-activated current in nociceptive neurons and its sensitization by bradykinin. *Proc Natl Acad Sci USA* 1996; 24,93(26):15435–15439.

Cesare P, Souslova V, Akopian A, Rufian O, Wood JN. Fast-inactivating responses to ATP are lost in DRG neurons from P2X3 knock-out mice. *J Physiol* 2000; in press.

Chen C-C, Akopian AN, Sivilotti L, et al. A P2X purinoceptor expressed by a subset of sensory neurons. *Nature* 1995; 377:428–431.

Chen C-C, England S, Akopian AN, Wood JN. A sensory neuron specific proton-gated cation channel. *Proc Natl Acad Sci USA* 1998; 18,95(17):10240–10245.

Colbert HA, Smith TL, Bargmann CI. OSM-9, a novel protein with structural similarity to channels, is required for olfaction, mechanosensation, and olfactory adaptation in *Caenorhabditis elegans*. *J Neurosci* 1997; 17(21):8259–8269.

Cook SP, Vulchanova L, Hargreaves KM, Elde R, McCleskey EW. Distinct ATP receptors on pain-sensing and stretch-sensing neurons. *Nature* 1997; 387:505–508.

Coscoy S, Lingueglia E, Lazdunski M, Barbry P. The Phe-Met-Arg-Phe-amide-activated sodium channel is a tetramer. *J Biol Chem* 1998; 273(14):8317–8322.

Dib-Hajj SD, Tyrrell L, Black JA, Waxman SG. NaN, a novel voltage-gated Na channel, is expressed preferentially in peripheral sensory neurons and down-regulated after axotomy. *Proc Natl Acad Sci USA* 1998; 95(15):8963–8968.

Dray A, Forbes CA, Burgess G. Ruthenium red blocks the capsaicin-induced increases in intracellular calcium and activation of membrane currents in sensory neurons as well as the activation of peripheral nociceptors in vitro. *Neurosci Lett* 1990; 110:52–59.

Dulac C, Axel R. A novel family of genes encoding putative pheromone receptors in mammals. *Cell* 1995; 83(2):195–206.

Elliott-AA, Elliott-JR. Characterization of TTX-sensitive and TTX-resistant sodium currents in small cells from adult rat dorsal root ganglia. *J Physiol (Lond)* 1993; 463:39–56.

England S, Bevan S, Docherty RJ. PGE2 modulates the tetrodotoxin-resistant sodium current in neonatal rat DRG neurones via the cAMP-protein kinase A cascade. *J Physiol* 1996; 495.2:429–440.

Garcia-Anoveros J, Derfler B, Neville-Golden J, Hyman BT, Corey DP. BNaC1 and BNaC2 constitute a new family of human neuronal sodium channels related to degenerins and epithelial sodium channels. *Proc Natl Acad Sci* 1997; 94:1459–1464.

Gold MS, Reichling DB, Shuster MJ, Levine JD. Hyperalgesic agents increase a tetrodotoxin-resistant Na current in nociceptors. *Proc Natl Acad Sci* 1996; 93:1108–1112.

Gu JG, MacDermott AB. Activation of ATP P2X receptors elicits glutamate release from sensory neuron synapses. *Nature* 1997; 389(6652):749–753.

Hu Y, Vaca L, Zhu X. Appearance of a novel Ca^{+2}-influx pathway in Sf9 insect cells following expression of the transient receptor potential-like (trpl) protein of *Drosophila*. *Biochem Biophys Res Commun* 1994; 132:346–354.

Hurst RS, Zhu X, Boulay G, Birnbaumer L, Stefani E. Ionic currents underlying HTRP3 mediated agonist-dependent Ca^{2+} influx in stably transfected HEK293 cells. *FEBS Lett* 1998; 422(3):333–338.

Isom LL, Catterall WA. Na^{+} channel subunits and Ig domains. *Nature* 1996; 383:307.

Jeftinija S. Bradykinin excites tetrodotoxin-resistant primary afferent fibres. *Brain Res* 1994; 665:69–76.

Julius D, MacDermott AB, Axel R, Jessell TM. Molecular characterization of a functional cDNA encoding the serotonin 1c receptor. *Science* 1998; 241:558–564.

Khakh BS, Humphrey PP, Surprenant A. Electrophysiological properties of P2X-purinoceptors in rat superior cervical, nodose and guinea-pig coeliac neurones. *J Physiol* 1995; 484:385–395.

Kuhn R, Schwenk F, Aguet M, Rajewsky K. Inducible gene targeting in mice. *Science* 1995; 269(5229):1427–1429.

Lewis C, Neidhart S, Holy C, et al. Heteropolymerization of P2X receptor subunits can account for ATP-induced current in sensory neurons. *Nature* 1995; 377:432–435.

Lingueglia E, de Weille JR, Bassilana F. A modulatory subunit of acid sensing ion channels in brain and dorsal root ganglion cells. *J Biol Chem* 1997; 272:29778–29783.

Nakamura F, Strittmatter SM. P2Y1 purinergic receptors in sensory neurons: contribution to touch-induced impulse generation. *Proc Natl Acad Sci USA* 1996; 93:10465–10470.

Okuse K, Akopian AN, Sivilotti L, Dolphin AC, Wood JN. Sensory neuron voltage-gated sodium channels and nociception. In: Borsook D (Ed). *Molecular Neurobiology of Pain*, Progress in Pain Research and Management, Vol. 9. Seattle: IASP Press, 1997, pp 239–257.

Philipp S, Cacalie A, Freichel M, et al. A mammalian capacitative calcium entry channel homologous to *Drosophila* TRP and TRPL. *EMBO J* 1996; 15:6166–6171.

Putney JW Jr. A model for receptor-regulated calcium entry. *Cell Calcium* 1986; 7:1–12.

Sangameswaran L, Delgado SG, Fish LM, et al. Structure and function of a novel voltage-gated TTX-resistant sodium channel specific to sensory neurons. *J Biol Chem* 1996; 271:5953–5956.

Sinkins WG, Hu Y, Kunze DL, Schilling WP. Activation of recombinant trp by thapsigargin in Sf9 insect cells. *Am J Physiol* 1994; 266:C1501–C1505.

Sive HL, St. John T. A simple subtractive hybridisation technique employing photoactivatable biotin and phenol extraction. *Nucl Acids Res* 1988; 16:10937.

Sivilotti L, Okuse K, Akopian AN, Moss S, Wood JN. A single serine residue confers TTX insensitivity on the rat SNS sodium channel. *FEBS Lett* 1997; 409:49–52.

Tate S, Benn S, Hick C, Trezise D, et al. Two sodium channels contribute to the TTX-R sodium current in primary sensory neurons. *Nat Neurosci* 1998; 1(8):653–655.

Trezise DJ, John VH, Xie X.M. Voltage- and use-dependent inhibition of Na^+ channels in rat sensory neurones by 4030W92, a new antihyperalgesic agent. *Br J Pharmacol* 1998; 124(5):953–963.

Vaca L, Sinkins WG, Hu Y, Kunze DL, Schilling WP. Activation of recombinant trp by thapsigargin in Sf9 insect cells. *Am J Physiol* 1994; Nov, 267(5 Pt 1):C1501–C1505.

Vyklicky L, Knotkova-Urbancova H, Vitaskova Z, et al. Inflammatory mediators at acidic pH activate capsaicin receptors in cultured sensory neurons from newborn rats. *J Neurophysiol* 1998; Feb, 79(2):670–676.

Waldmann R, Lazdunski M. H(+)-gated cation channels: neuronal acid sensors in the NaC/DEG family of ion channels. *Curr Opin Neurobiol* 1998; 8(3):418–424.

Waldmann R, Champigny G, Bassilana F, Heurteaux C, Lazdunski M. A proton-gated cation channel involved in acid-sensing. *Nature* 1997a; 386:173–177.

Waldmann R, Basilana F, de Weille J, et al. Molecular cloning of a non-inactivating proton-gated Na^+ channel specific for sensory neurons. *J Biol Chem* 1997b; 272:20975–20978.

Wes PD, Chevesich J, Jeromin A, et al. TRPC1, a human homolog of a *Drosophila* store-operated channel. *Proc Natl Acad Sci USA* 1995; 92:9652–9659.

Winter J, Forbes CA, Sternberg J, Lindsay RM. Nerve growth factor (NGF) regulates adult rat cultured dorsal root ganglion neuron responses to capsaicin. *Neuron* 1988; 1:973–981.

Wood JN, Docherty R. Chemical activators of sensory neurons. *Annu Rev Physiol* 1997; 59:457–482.

Wood JN, Perl ER. Pain. *Curr Opin Genet Dev* 1999; 9:328–332.

Xu X-Z S, Li H-S, Guggino WB, Montell C. Coassembly of TRP and TRPL produces a distinct store-operated conductance. *Cell* 1997; 89:1155–1164.

Zhu X, Chu PB, Peyton M, Birnbaumer L. Molecular cloning of a widely expressed human homologue for the *Drosophila* trp gene. *FEBS Lett* 1995; 373:193–198.

Zhu X, Jiang M, Peyton M. trp, a novel mammalian gene family essential for agonist-activated capacitative Ca^{+2} entry. *Cell* 1996; 85:661–671.

Zhu X, Jiang M, Birnbaumer L. Receptor-activated Ca^{+2} influx via human trp3 stably expressed in human embryonic kidney (HEK) 293 cells. *J Biol Chem* 1998; 273:133–142, 1189–1196.

Correspondence to: John N. Wood, DSc, Biology Department, University College, London, WC1E 6BT, United Kingdom. Tel: 44-171-380-7800; Fax: 44-171-380-7800; email: j.wood@ucl.ac.uk.

Proceedings of the 9th World Congress on Pain,
Progress in Pain Research and Management,
Vol. 16, edited by M. Devor, M.C. Rowbotham, and
Z. Wiesenfeld-Hallin, IASP Press, Seattle, © 2000.

7

ATP (P2X) Receptors and Pain[1]

G. Burnstock,[a] S.B. McMahon,[b] P.P.A. Humphrey,[c] and S.G. Hamilton[b]

[a]Autonomic Neuroscience Institute, Royal Free and University College Medical School, London; [b]Department of Physiology, King's College London, and St. Thomas's Hospital Medical School, London; [c]Glaxo Institute of Applied Pharmacology, and Department of Pharmacology, University of Cambridge, Cambridge, United Kingdom

This chapter begins with a brief overview of the history and current status of purinergic signaling in general, discusses the early hints of the involvement of purine nucleotides and nucleosides in nociception, and then focuses on the current evidence offered by various pain models.

PURINERGIC SIGNALING

EARLY HISTORY

The early studies of Drury and Szent-Györgyi (1929) demonstrated the potent extracellular actions of adenosine triphosphate (ATP). Holton (1959) presented the first hint of a transmitter role for ATP in the nervous system by demonstrating release of ATP during antidromic stimulation of sensory nerves. Then, in 1970, it was proposed that nonadrenergic, noncholinergic (NANC) nerves supplying the gut and bladder used ATP as a motor neurotransmitter (Burnstock et al. 1970, 1972). In an early pharmacological review, Burnstock (1972) introduced the term "purinergic" and presented the first evidence for purinergic transmission in a wide variety of systems.

[1] Mini-review based on a congress workshop.

CURRENT STATUS OF RECEPTORS FOR PURINES AND PYRIMIDINES

Implicit in the concept of purinergic neurotransmission is the existence of postjunctional purinergic receptors (Burnstock 1976). A brief history of the development of the purinoceptor nomenclature follows. In 1978, Burnstock proposed a basis for distinguishing two types of purinoceptor, identified as P1 and P2 (for adenosine and ADP/ATP, respectively), but a basis for distinguishing two types of P2 receptor (P2X and P2Y) was not formulated until 1985 (Burnstock and Kennedy 1985). A year later, Gordon (1986) tentatively named two further P2 purinoceptor subtypes, namely a P2T receptor selective for ADP on platelets and a P2Z receptor on macrophages. Further subtypes followed, perhaps the most important being the P2U receptor, which could recognize pyrimidines such as UTP as well as ATP (O'Connor et al. 1991). Based on studies of transduction mechanisms (Dubyak 1991) and the cloning of the P2Y purinoceptor (Lustig et al. 1993; Webb et al. 1993) and later the P2X purinoceptor (Brake et al. 1994; Valera et al. 1994), Abbracchio and Burnstock (1994) proposed that purinoceptors belong to two major families: a P2X family of ligand-gated ion channel receptors and a P2Y family of G-protein-coupled receptors. This nomenclature has been widely adopted, and seven P2X subtypes and about eight P2Y receptor subtypes are now recognized (Ralevic and Burnstock 1998).

PURINERGIC SIGNALING AND PAIN

EARLY HINTS OF INVOLVEMENT OF ATP AND ADENOSINE IN PAIN

Bleehen and Keele (1977) described the algogenic actions of adenine compounds on the human skin; later, ATP was implicated in migraine (Burnstock 1981, 1989). Several papers described ATP as a central synaptic mediator for subpopulations of primary afferent fibers (Fyffe and Perl 1984; Salter and Henry 1985; Sawynok and Sweeney 1989; Li and Perl 1995).

CLONING OF THE P2X3 RECEPTOR AND ITS DISTRIBUTION ON NOCICEPTIVE SENSORY NEURONS

The amino acid sequence of a distinct P2X receptor subtype (P2X3) has been described (Chen et al. 1995; Lewis et al. 1995). This receptor is present in a subset of dorsal root ganglion (DRG) sensory neurons that express peripherin, a cytoskeletal protein associated with small-diameter sensory neurons, a high proportion of which are nociceptive. This suggested that ATP might play an important role in nociceptor activation (Burnstock and Wood 1996).

A molecular mechanism for the pain-inducing actions of ATP has been suggested by studies of rat sensory neurons in culture. Electrophysiological analysis has shown that between 40% and 96% of DRG sensory neurons in culture respond to ATP by increasing intracellular free calcium concentrations or by depolarizing (Bouvier et al. 1991; Robertson et al. 1996; Rae et al. 1998). P2X1–6 mRNA transcripts are expressed in sensory neurons of DRG, nodose, and trigeminal ganglia (North 1996). However, only one subtype, P2X3, is expressed selectively in cell populations enriched in nociceptors, as judged by in situ hybridization analysis with markers for small-diameter neurons. This finding demonstrates that other P2X receptors probably account for the depolarizing actions of ATP on large-diameter neurons. The level of expression of mRNA detected in small-diameter sensory neurons by in situ and Northern blots suggests relatively greater amounts of P2X3 compared to other P2X subunits, such as P2X2.

An electrophysiological analysis of the properties of the expressed P2X3 channel showed many similarities with currents in rat sensory neurons in culture (Robertson et al. 1996). The channel rapidly desensitized, and was activated by ATP congeners with the same rank order of potency as that described for sensory neurons in culture (at low concentrations, 2-methylthioATP >> ATP > α,β-methylene ATP > γ-thioATP > CTP > ADP >> UTP ≈ β,γ-methylene ATP > GTP) (Chen et al. 1995). In addition, the channel is blocked by suramin, a general antagonist of P2X purinoceptors (with the exception of P2X4 and P2X6). However, it is not clear whether P2X3 exists as a homomultimer or a heteromultimer with P2X2 in sensory neurons in vivo. A recent study of rat nodose ganglion neurons that used 2′,3′-*O*-trinitrophenyl ATP (TNP-ATP) as a selective P2X antagonist concluded that some neurons used homomeric P2X2 receptors, whereas others used heteromeric P2X2/3 receptors (Thomas et al. 1998; Virginio et al. 1998a,b). Evidence indicates that the capsaicin-sensitive, small DRG neurons of the rat express mainly the homomeric P2X3 subunit, while capsaicin-insensitive, medium-sized neurons express the heteromultimeric P2X2/3 receptor (Ueno et al. 1999).

Indirect evidence for heteromultimeric channels in sensory neurons has been provided by co-expression of P2X subunits in *Xenopus* oocytes. Some nodose ganglion neurons desensitize slowly in response to α,β-methylene ATP (α,β-meATP), but P2X3 shows a rapid desensitization in oocytes. However, co-expression of P2X2 and P2X3 produces a channel that has a slowly desensitizing response (Lewis et al. 1995). This confirms that heteromultimeric P2X2/3 channels formed that may account for some slowly desensitizing responses in subsets of sensory neurons.

It seems likely, as discussed above, that P2X3 receptors form heteromultimeric combinations with P2X2 receptors. Thus, while P2X3 receptors are not sensitive to pH, recombinant P2X2 receptors are strongly pH-sensitive (King et al. 1996; Wildman et al. 1999). Acid pH augments the excitatory actions of ATP on dissociated mammalian sensory neurons (Li et al. 1996). Therefore, the sensitivity to nociceptive P2 receptors is likely to be enhanced in inflammatory conditions with slow acidosis. In contrast, physiological concentrations of extracellular Mg^{2+} inhibit ATP-activated current in rat nodose ganglion cells (Li et al. 1997). A more recent study of dissociated DRG neurons from 1- to 4-day-old rats showed that the relative actions of various ATP analogues and, in particular, the very low activity of β,γ-methylene-L-ATP confirmed the presence of P2X3 receptors (Rae et al. 1998). Synergistic interactions between ATP and other known nociceptive agents on sensory terminals in the periphery have been proposed (Green et al. 1991; Hu and Li 1996; Wildman et al. 1997).

Immunohistochemical studies of P2X3 receptors on sensory ganglia have been carried out at both the light microscope (Vulchanova et al. 1996, 1997, 1998; Bradbury et al. 1998; Xiang et al. 1998; Bo et al. 1999) and electron microscope level (Llewellyn-Smith and Burnstock 1998). They show that the P2X3 receptors are predominantly located on the nonpeptidergic subpopulation of small nociceptive neurons that label with the lectin IB4. In trigeminal ganglia, P2X3-receptor immunoreactivity occurs in both small and large nerve cell bodies and their processes. P2X3 receptors are expressed in approximately equal numbers of sensory neurons projecting to the skin and viscera, but in few of those innervating skeletal muscle. The central projections of P2X3-labeled nerves in the DRG are located in inner lamina II of the dorsal horn of the spinal cord. For the labeled nerve profiles in lamina II, P2X3 receptors were located largely in terminals with the ultrastructural characteristics of sensory afferent terminals, which suggests that ATP is released onto primary afferent terminals, thereby modulating sensory input coming from the periphery. In the nucleus solitarius, P2X3-receptor-positive boutons synapse on dendrites and cell bodies and have complex synaptic relationships with other axon terminals and dendrites. Peripheral projections of nociceptive neurons in the skin, tongue, and tooth pulp are immunopositive for P2X3 receptors. After sciatic nerve axotomy, P2X3-receptor expression dropped by more than 50% in L4/L5 DRG. Glial-cell-derived neurotrophic factor (GDNF), delivered intrathecally, completely reversed axotomy-induced downregulation of the P2X3 receptor (Bradbury et al. 1998). In contrast, the P2X3 receptor was transiently upregulated and anterogradely transported in trigeminal primary sensory nerves after nerve injury (Eriksson et al. 1998).

NOCICEPTIVE ACTIONS OF ATP

Animal studies

In vivo studies of the functional consequences of P2X receptor activation of peripheral neurons in animal models are beginning to appear. Behavioral indices of acute nociception were monitored in the conscious rat following subplantar injection of ATP and α,β-meATP into the hindpaw (Bland-Ward and Humphrey 1997). Signs of overt nociception, i.e., hindpaw lifting and licking, were apparent following injection of α,β-meATP; these effects were dose related and were inhibited by selective desensitization of the P2X3 receptor.

Parallel electrophysiological studies examined the activity of single nociceptors in response to ATP analogues applied directly to the peripheral receptive field (Fig. 1) (Hamilton et al. 1999). Among all C-fiber nociceptors recorded, 49% responded either to ATP or to α,β-meATP. Interestingly, most (76%) C-mechanoheat units (polymodal nociceptors) responded to a P2X agonist, whereas significantly fewer C-mechanonociceptors (27%) responded to the same chemical stimuli. The proportion of Aδ nociceptors responding to a P2X agonist was similar to that of C-mechanonociceptors (24%). Low-threshold Aδ-fiber mechanonocieceptors and down-hair afferents did not respond to either ATP or α,β-meATP. These results directly demonstrate that ATP can selectively activate cutaneous nociceptors and further suggest that the P2X3 receptor plays a major role in nociceptive responses to ATP.

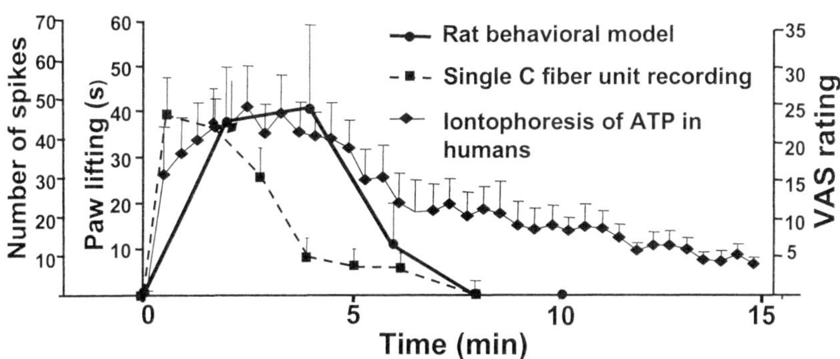

Fig. 1. The time course of the response to ATP analogues in three different models: rat nocifensive behavior following intraplantar injection of 50 nmol of α,β-meATP (n = 10), iontophoresis of ATP in human subjects (n = 6), and single C-fiber unit recordings from a rat in vitro skin nerve preparation (n = 7). The method of quantifying the response to ATP analogues is indicated in the y-axis: paw lifting in 2-minute bins was measured in the rat behavioral model, the average number of spikes in 1-minute bins was calculated for the single-unit recordings, and the human subjects rated their pain according to the VAS every 20 seconds. It is apparent that the response to ATP analogues remains constant regardless of the methodology.

ATP can also excite nociceptors in other tissues. Dowd et al. (1998) applied ATP and α,β-meATP to the peripheral terminals of primary afferent articular nociceptors in rat knee joints and recorded neural activity from the medial articular nerve in rats anesthetized with pentobarbitone. Rapid, short-lasting excitations of a subpopulation of C and Aδ nociceptive afferents were evoked that were antagonized by pyridoxalphosphate-6-azophenyl-2′,4′-disulfonic acid (PPADS). This effect was still evident in unilateral arthritic joints, which suggests that ATP, found in the synovial fluid of patients with arthritis, may be implicated in the associated pain (Ryan et al. 1991; Dowd et al. 1998).

The nociceptive effects of ATP also have been examined in several animal models of experimental inflammation. Carrageenan-induced inflammation of the rat hindpaw greatly enhanced and prolonged the response to α,β-meATP (Fig. 2): a dose of 50 nmol of α,β-meATP induced 311.6 ± 35.2 seconds of nocifensive paw-lifting compared to 81.8 ± 22.1 seconds in naive animals (mean ± SEM). Furthermore, the threshold dose required to elicit a nocifensive response was reduced more than 100-fold, to micromolar concentrations, in inflamed skin (Hamilton et al. 1999). In other experiments, the inflammation produced by UV irradiation has been studied (Hamilton et al. 1999). At a dose of UVB irradiation capable of producing significant thermal hyperalgesia, the paw-lifting response to injected ATP and α,β-meATP was significantly augmented 6 and 24 hours following irradiation. The effect of α,β-meATP was also potentiated in the presence of PGE_2. Co-administration resulted in almost double the expected paw-lifting response. The nociceptive actions of ATP analogues are therefore markedly augmented

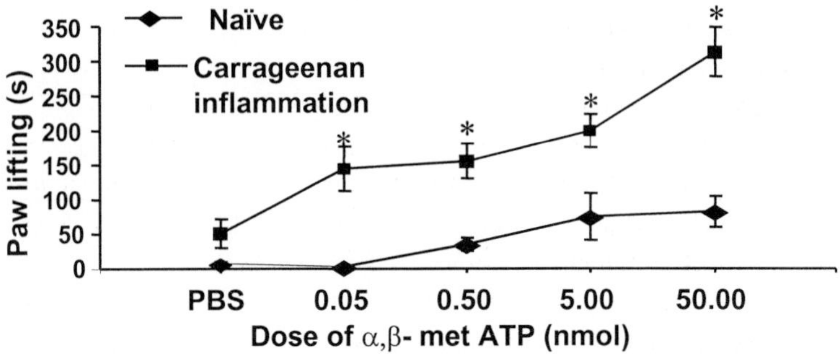

Fig. 2. Nocifensive behavior induced by intraplantar injections of α,β-meATP or vehicle (50 μL) into a hindpaw inflamed with carrageenan (50 μL of 0.25% solution) 2 hours previously (n = 5 rats per group). The total hindpaw-lifting time in the 10-minute period following intraplantar injection is plotted. The increases seen in carrageenan-inflamed skin are significant ($P < 0.05$, ANOVA). Asterisks indicate significant differences between inflamed and normal animals ($P < 0.05$, Dunnett's post hoc test).

in the presence of inflammation or inflammatory mediators, with a time course that makes altered nociceptor gene expression (e.g., upregulation of receptors) an unlikely explanation. These data suggest that endogenous levels of ATP are more likely to reach levels capable of exciting nociceptors in inflamed as opposed to normal skin.

The studies described above do not reveal the role of endogenous ATP in nociception. However, such a role is reported in experiments using the formalin test in the rat hindpaw. Following intradermal formalin injections, two distinct nocifensive components are elicited: an initial phase that reflects direct sensory nerve activation, and a later phase that may reflect an inflammatory component (see Tjølsen et al. 1992). The P2 antagonists, suramin, Evans blue, trypan blue, and reactive blue 2, produced antinociception in this model when applied intrathecally (Driessen et al. 1994). Sawynok and Reid (1997) conducted related experiments that suggested a peripheral contribution from ATP. Another study used the formalin and writhing tests in adult male albino mice. Systemically administered ATP and ADP, which rapidly degrade to adenosine, caused a reduction in the number of writhes and the time of licking the formalin-injected paw (Mello et al. 1996). However, P1 but not P2 antagonists reversed these reactions, prompting the conclusion that adenosine mediates the antinociceptive effects of adenosine nucleotides.

Human studies

Only two published studies address the effects of ATP on human pain-signaling systems. Bleehen and Keele (1977) applied ATP to blister bases raised in human volunteers, and Coutts et al. (1981) injected ATP intradermally. These studies report conflicting information about the threshold dose required to elicit a pain response. In the Coutts et al. study, pain was elicited only with doses of about 250 nmol or more of ATP (extrapolated from their data), whereas Bleehen and Keele found doses of 0.2–0.6 nmol effective. These studies provide limited information about the magnitude of the pain produced by ATP, the duration of response, the desensitization and recovery of response, and the potential changes in inflamed skin.

We recently used a non-invasive method of iontophoresis to deliver ATP to the volar forearm skin of healthy volunteers while subjects rated the magnitude of the evoked pain on a visual analogue scale (VAS) (Hamilton et al. 2000). ATP consistently produced a modest burning pain but no other sensation. The pain began within 20 seconds after commencing ATP delivery, and with continuing iontophoresis was maintained for several minutes (Fig. 1). Persistent iontophoresis of ATP led to desensitization within 12 minutes, and recovery was almost complete 1 hour later. The average pain rating for ATP increased with increasing current. With use of 0.8 mA iontophoretic current, subjects reported pain averaging 27.7 ± 2.8 on a scale ranging from 0 to 100. The pain produced by ATP was dependent on capsaicin-sensitive sensory neurons as it was virtually abolished in skin treated repeatedly with topical capsaicin. Conversely, the pain-producing effects of ATP were greatly potentiated in several models of hyperalgesia. Thus, with acute capsaicin treatment when subjects exhibited touch-evoked hyperalgesia but no persisting pain, the average pain rating increased threefold during ATP iontophoresis. Moreover, ATP iontophoresed onto skin 24 hours after UV irradiation (to create sunburn) resulted in double the pain rating compared with the same procedure in normal skin (Fig. 3).

ORIGIN OF ATP INVOLVED IN PAIN INITIATION

ATP released from different cell types may be implicated in the initiation of pain by acting on nociceptive purinoceptors on sensory nerve terminals (Burnstock 1996, 1999). In complex regional pain syndrome (CRPS), type II (causalgia), type I (reflex sympathetic dystrophy), and other syndromes involving "sympathetically maintained pain" there appears to be sympathetic hyperinnervation (or hyperactivity), although the precise mechanisms involved are much debated (McMahon 1994). Burnstock (1996) proposed that in these pathological conditions, the ATP that is released from sympathetic nerves as a cotransmitter with noradrenaline and neuropeptide Y (Burnstock 1990a) acts on purinergic nociceptive receptors on sensory nerve endings to contribute to the initiation of pain. Consistent with this

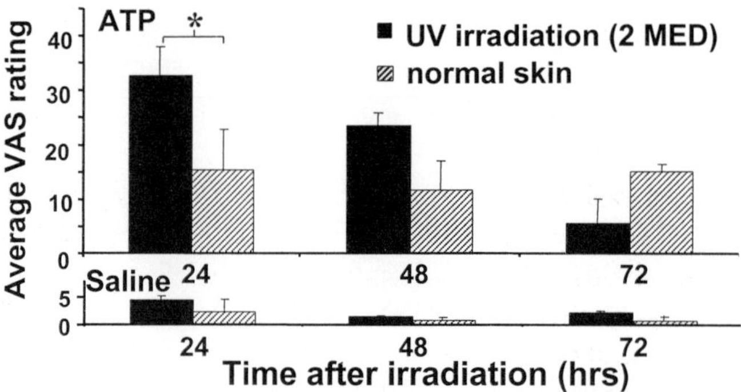

Fig. 3. Average VAS rating elicited by ATP (top) and saline (bottom) at 24, 48, and 72 hours in human skin treated with a dose of 2 MED of UV irradiation. The potentiation of the pain response to ATP is significant at 24 hours ($P < 0.05$, paired t test); the trend continues at 48 hours, but the effect is lost at 72 hours. The pain elicited by saline is unaffected by UV irradiation.

hypothesis are reports (e.g., Yasuda 1994) that surgical sympathectomy, sympathetic ganglion blockers, and guanethidine (which prevents release of sympathetic cotransmitters) are more effective in preventing pain in these conditions than are adrenoceptor antagonists or reserpine (which depletes noradrenaline, but not ATP, from sympathetic nerve terminals).

Sympathetic nerve activity also appears to be involved with other painful conditions, including the inflammation associated with arthritis (Levine et al. 1987). As ATP induces prostaglandin synthesis (and prostaglandins are known to be mediators of inflammation), ATP may play a further, indirect role as a sympathetic cotransmitter in the generation of pain (Burnstock 1996). Merkel cells, which contain high levels of ATP, are closely associated with sensory nerve endings in the skin (Malinovsky and Pac 1985) and may be another source of ATP involved in the maintenance of pain in CRPS-I.

Vascular pain—including angina, ischemic muscle pain, migraine, lumbar pain, and pelvic pain in women—appears to occur during the reactive hyperemic phase that follows local vasospasm. Burnstock (1981) proposed that ATP may play a role in mediating these effects in migraine. During reactive hyperemia, large amounts of ATP are released from vascular endothelial cells that act on endothelial P2Y receptors, resulting in the release of nitric oxide and vasodilatation (Burnstock 1990b). Burnstock (1996) proposed that in the microcirculation, ATP diffuses from the endothelial cells to activate nociceptive endings of sensory nerve fibers in the adventitia. A central role for adenosine also has been considered in relation to anginal pain (see Sylvén 1993). ATP released from platelets during aggregation, which increases in migraine, may also contribute to the initiation of pain via nociceptive purinoceptors. Consistent with this hypothesis is the recent report that nociception from blood vessels is independent of the sympathetic nervous system under physiological conditions in humans (Kindgen-Milles and Holthusen 1997).

Tumor cells are known to contain exceptionally high levels of ATP (Maehara et al. 1987). When the tumor reaches a size that leads to breakage of cells during abrasive movements, the ATP released may act on nociceptive endings of sensory nerves in the vicinity to produce the sensation of pain (Burnstock 1996). ATP released from damaged muscle following major accidents or surgery also could be involved in local pain and in pain associated with traumatic shock (Trams et al. 1980).

A new hypothesis (Burnstock 1999) proposes that in tubes (including the ureter, salivary duct, bile duct, vagina, and intestine) and sacs (including the urinary bladder, gall bladder, and lung), nociceptive mechanosensory transduction occurs where distension releases ATP from the epithelial cells lining these organs, which then activate P2X2/3 receptors on subepithelial sensory nerve plexuses to relay messages to pain centers of the central nervous system. Supporting evidence for this concept comes from studies of the rat bladder where ATP was released from the urothelial cells by hydrostatic pressure changes (Ferguson et al. 1997) and from studies in which nerve discharges were produced in pelvic nerve afferent from the bladder during slow distension and infusion of α,β-meATP; these discharges were antagonized by suramin (Morrison et al. 1998). New in vivo electrophysiological evidence for the presence of P2X receptors on mesenteric afferent nerve endings might suggest that ATP is involved in the perception of abdominal discomfort and pain that occurs in functional bowel disorders (Kirkup et al. 1999).

DISCUSSION

Now that the molecular structure of the nociceptor-associated P2X3 receptor has been identified, the search for selective antagonists at the P2X3 receptor can be pursued. When identified, such antagonists could then be tested both on both recombinant receptors expressed in oocytes or transfected cells and in vivo models of the different types of pain. P2X3 receptors are clearly not the only receptors involved in pain, so a synergism with receptors for other agents that modulate pain (such as bradykinin, histamine, and 5-hydroxytryptamine) should be explored. In addition to our review of the action of ATP on receptors on sensory nerve terminals, other reports indicate that ATP acts on dorsal horn neurons in the spinal cord after being released from a subpopulation of small primary afferent nerves involved in pain pathways (see Sawynok 1997). The future identification of a selective adenosine A1-receptor agonist to attenuate pain at the spinal cord level and of an A2 antagonist at the peripheral sensory terminal level are also of obvious clinical interest (see Segerdahl and Sollevi 1998).

Some intriguing parallels need to be explored further regarding capsaicin-gated channels and P2X nociceptive receptors, including the mechanism of desensitization through calcineurin action (King et al. 1997), the pronounced pH dependence of channel gating, the distribution and expression of capsaicin sensitivity at the P2X3 receptor, and the ion selectivity of the channel (see Krylova 1997). Interactions with the recently identified acid sensory ion channel localized on small primary afferent neurons (Olson et al. 1998) also will be of great interest.

ACKNOWLEDGMENTS

We gratefully acknowledge the support of Roche Bioscience, Palo Alto (G. Burnstock and S.B. McMahon), and of the Wellcome Trust (G. Burnstock) and the British Heart Foundation (G. Burnstock). S.G. Hamilton is in receipt of a research grant from the Special Trustees of St. Thomas' Hospital, London.

REFERENCES

Abbracchio M, Burnstock G. Purinoceptors: are there families of P_{2X} and P_{2Y} purinoceptors? *Pharmacol Ther* 1994; 64:445–475.

Bland-Ward PA, Humphrey PPA. Acute nociception mediate by hindpaw P2X receptor activation in the rat. *Br J Pharmacol* 1997; 122:365–371.

Bleehen T, Keele CA. Observations on the algogenic actions of adenosine compounds on human blister base preparation. *Pain* 1977; 3:367–377.

Bo X, Alavi A, Xiang Z, et al. Localization of $P2X_2$ and $P2X_3$ receptor immunoreactive nerves in rat taste buds. *Neuroreport* 1999; 10:11107–1111.

Bouvier MM, Evans ML, Benham CD. Calcium influx induced by stimulation of ATP receptors on neurons cultured from rat dorsal root ganglia. *Eur J Neurosci* 1991; 3:285–291.

Bradbury EJ, Burnstock G, McMahon SB. The expression of $P2X_3$ purinoceptors in sensory neurons: effects of axotomy and glial-derived neurotrophic factor. *Mol Cell Neurosci* 1998; 12:256–268.

Brake AJ, Wagenbach MJ, Julius D. New structural motif for ligand-gated ion channels defined by an inotropic ATP receptor. *Nature* 1994; 371:519–523.

Burnstock G. Purinergic nerves. *Pharmacol Rev* 1972; 24:509–581.

Burnstock G. Purinergic receptors. *J Theor Biol* 1976; 62:491–503.

Burnstock G. A basis for distinguishing two types of purinergic receptor. In: Straub RW, Bolis L (Eds). *Cell Membrane Receptors for Drugs and Hormones: A Multidisciplinary Approach*. New York: Raven Press, 1978, pp 107–118.

Burnstock G. Pathophysiology of migraine: a new hypothesis. *Lancet* 1981; i:1397–1399.

Burnstock G. The role of adenosine triphosphate in migraine. *Biomed Pharmacother* 1989; 43:727–736.

Burnstock G. Co-transmission. The Fifth Heymans Lecture. Ghent, February 17, 1990. *Arch Int Pharmacodyn Ther* 1990a; 304:7–33.

Burnstock G. Local mechanisms of blood flow control by perivascular nerves and endothelium. *J Hypertens* 1990b; 8 (Suppl 7):S95–S106.

Burnstock G. A unifying purinergic hypothesis for the initiation of pain. *Lancet* 1996; 347:1604–1605.

Burnstock G. Release of vasoactive substances from endothelial cells by shear stress and purinergic mechanosensory transduction. *J Anat* 1999; 194:335–342.

Burnstock G, Kennedy C. Is there a basis for distinguishing two types of P_2-purinoceptor? *Gen Pharmacol* 1985; 16:433–440.

Burnstock G, Wood JN. Purinergic receptors: their role in nociception and primary afferent neurotransmission. *Curr Opin Neurobiol* 1996; 6:526–532.

Burnstock G, Campbell G, Satchell D, Smythe A. Evidence that adenosine triphosphate or a related nucleotide is the transmitter substance released by non-adrenergic inhibitory nerves in the gut. *Br J Pharmacol* 1970; 40:668–688.

Burnstock G, Dumsday B, Smythe A. Atropine resistant excitation of the urinary bladder: the possibility of transmission via nerves releasing a purine nucleotide. *Br J Pharmacol* 1972; 44:451–461.

Chen C-C, Akopian AN, Sivilotti L, et al. A P2X purinoceptor expressed by a subset of sensory neurons. *Nature* 1995; 377:428–431.

Coutts AA, Jorizzo JL, Eady RAJ, Greaves MW, Burnstock G. Adenosine triphosphate-evoked vascular changes in human skin: mechanism of action. *Eur J Pharmacol* 1981; 76:391–401.

Dowd E, McQueen DS, Chessell IP, Humphrey PPA. P2X receptor-mediated excitation of nociceptive afferents in the normal and arthritic rat knee joint. *Br J Pharmacol* 1998; 125:341–346.

Driessen B, Reimann W, Selve N, Friderichs E, Bültmann R. Antinociceptive effect of intrathecally administered P_2-purinoceptor antagonists in rats. *Brain Res* 1994; 666:182–188.

Drury AN, Szent-Györgyi A. The physiological activity of adenine compounds with special reference to their action upon the mammalian heart. *J Physiol* 1929; 68:213–237.

Dubyak GR. Signal transduction by P_2-purinergic receptors for extracellular ATP. *Am J Respir Cell Mol Biol* 1991; 4:295–300.

Eriksson J, Bongenhielm U, Kidd E, Matthews B, Fried K. Distribution of $P2X_3$ receptors in the rat trigeminal ganglion after inferior alveolar nerve injury. *Neurosci Lett* 1998; 254:37–40.

Ferguson DR, Kennedy I, Burton TJ. ATP is released from rabbit urinary bladder epithelial cells by hydrostatic pressure changes—a possible sensory mechanism? *J Physiol* 1997; 505:503–511.

Fyffe REW, Perl ER. Is ATP a central synaptic mediator for certain primary afferent fibres from mammalian skin? *Proc Natl Acad Sci USA* 1984; 81:6890–6893.

Gordon JL. Extracellular ATP: effects, sources and fate. *Biochem J* 1986; 233:309–319.

Green PG, Basbaum AI, Helms C, Levine JD. Purinergic regulation of bradykinin-induced plasma extravasation and adjuvant-induced arthritis in the rat. *Proc Natl Acad Sci USA* 1991; 88:4162–4165.

Hamilton SG, Wade A, McMahon SB. The effects of inflammatory mediators on nociceptive behaviour induced by ATP analogues in the rat. *Br J Pharmacol* 1999; 126:326–332.

Hamilton SG, Warburton J, Bhattachajee A, Ward J, McMahon SB. ATP in human skin elicits a dose related pain response which is potentiated under conditions of hyperalgesia. *Brain* 2000; in press.

Holton P. The liberation of adenosine triphosphate on antidromic stimulation of sensory nerves. *J Physiol* 1959; 145:494–504.

Hu HZ, Li ZW. Substance P potentiates ATP-activated currents in rat primary sensory neurons. *Brain Res* 1996; 739:163–168.

Kindgen-Milles D, Holthusen H. Nociception from blood vessels is independent of the sympathetic nervous system under physiological conditions in humans. *Eur J Pharmacol* 1997; 328:41–44.

King BF, Ziganshina LE, Pintor J, Burnstock G. Full sensitivity of $P2X_2$ purinoceptor to ATP revealed by changing extracellular pH. *Br J Pharmacol* 1996; 117:1371–1373.

King B, Chen C, Akopian AN, Burnstock G, Wood JN. A role for calcineurin in the desensitization of the $P2X_3$ receptor. *Neuroreport* 1997; 8:1099–1102.

Kirkup AJ, Booth CL, Chessell IP, Humphrey PPA, Grundy D. Excitatory effect of P2X receptor activation on mesenteric afferent nerves in the anaesthetised rat. *J Physiol* 1999; 520:551–563.

Krylova O, Chen CC, Akopian A, et al. Ligand-gated ion channels of sensory neurons: from purines to peppers. *Biochem Soc Trans* 1997; 25:842–844.

Levine JD, Goetzl EJ, Basbaum AI. Contribution of the nervous system to the pathophysiology of rheumatoid arthritis and other poly arthrites. *Pathol Chronic Inflamm Arthr* 1987; 13:369–383.

Lewis C, Neidhart S, Holy C, North RA, Surprenant A. Coexpression of $P2X_2$ and $P2X_3$ receptor subunits can account for ATP-gated currents in sensory neurons. *Nature* 1995; 377:432–435.

Li C, Peoples RW, Weight FF. Acid pH augments excitatory action of ATP on a dissociated mammalian sensory neuron. *Neuroreport* 1996; 7:2151–2154.

Li C, Peoples RW, Weight FF. Mg^{2+} inhibition of ATP-activated current in rat nodose ganglion neurons: evidence that Mg^{2+} decreases the agonist affinity of the receptor. *J Neurophysiol* 1997; 77:3391–3395.

Li J, Perl ER. ATP modulation of synaptic transmission in the spinal substantia gelatinosa. *J Neurosci* 1995; 15:3357–3365.

Llewellyn-Smith IJ, Burnstock G. Ultrastructural localization of $P2X_3$ receptors in rat sensory neurons. *Neuroreport* 1998; 9:2245–2250.

Lustig KD, Shiau AK, Brake AJ, Julius D. Expression cloning of an ATP receptor from mouse neuroblastoma cells *Proc Natl Acad Sci USA* 1993; 90:5113–5117.

Maehara Y, Kusumoto H, Anai H, Kusumoto T, Sugimachi K. Human tumor tissues have higher ATP contents than normal tissues. *Clin Chim Acta* 1987; 169:341–343.

Malinovsky L, Pac L. Is the Merkel cell a secondary sensory cell? (A contribution to the classification of Merkel cell neurite complexes). *Z Mikroskop Anat Forsch* 1985; 99:119–128.

McMahon SB. Mechanisms of cutaneous, deep and visceral pain. In: Wall PD, Melzack R (Eds). *Textbook of Pain*. London: Churchill Livingstone, 1994; 129–151.

Mello CF, Begnini J, De La Vega DD, et al. Antinociceptive effect of purine nucleotides. *Braz J Med Biol Res* 1996; 29:1379–1387.

Morrison JFB, Namasivayam S, Eardley I. ATP may be a natural modulator of the sensitivity of bladder mechanoreceptors during slow distension [Abstract]. *Proceedings of the 1st International Consultation on Incontinence,* 1998, p 84.

North RA. P2X purinoceptor plethora. In: Burnstock G (Guest Ed). *Purinergic Neurotransmission Seminars in the Neurosciences,* Vol. 8. Cambridge: Academic Press, 1996, pp 187–195.

O'Connor SE, Dainty IA, Leff P. Further subclassification of ATP receptors based on agonist studies. *Trends Pharmacol Sci* 1991; 12:137–141.

Olson TH, Riedl MS, Vulchanova L, Ortiz-Gonzalez XR, Elde R. An acid sensing ion channel (ASIC) localizes to small primary afferent neurons in rats. *Neuroreport* 1998; 9:1109–1113.

Rae MG, Rowan EG, Kennedy C. Pharmacological properties of $P2X_3$-receptors present in neurones of the rat dorsal root ganglia. *Br J Pharmacol* 1998; 124:176–180.

Ralevic V, Burnstock G. Receptors for purines and pyrimidines. *Pharmacol Rev* 1998; 50:413–492.

Robertson SJ, Rae MG, Rowan EG, Kennedy C. Characterization of a P2X-purinoceptor in cultured neurones of the rat dorsal root ganglia. *Br J Pharmacol* 1996; 118:951–956.

Ryan LM, Rachow JW, McCarty DJ. Synovial fluid ATP: a potential substrate for the production of inorganic pyrophosphate. *J Rheumatol* 1991; 18:716–720.

Salter MW, Henry JL. Effects of adenosine 5´-monophosphate and adenosine 5´-triphosphate on functionally identified units in the cat spinal dorsal horn. Evidence for a differential effect of adenosine 5´-triphosphate on nociceptive vs non-nociceptive units. *Neuroscience* 1985; 15:815–825.

Sawynok J. Purines and nociception. In: Jacobson KA, Jarvis MF (Eds). *Purinergic Approaches in Experimental Therapeutics*. New York: Wiley-Liss, 1997, pp 495–513.

Sawynok J, Reid A. Peripheral adenosine 5´-triphosphate enhances nociception in the formalin test via activation of a purinergic P_{2X} receptor. *Eur J Pharmacol* 1997; 330:115–121.

Sawynok J, Sweeney MI. The role of purines in nociception. *Neuroscience* 1989; 32:557–569.

Segerdahl M, Sollevi A. Adenosine and pain relief: a clinical overview. *Drug Dev Res* 1998; 45:151–158.

Sylvén C. Mechanisms of pain in angina pectoris—a critical review of the adenosine hypothesis. *Cardiovasc Drug Ther* 1993; 7:745–759.

Thomas S, Virginio C, North RA, Surprenant A. The antagonist trinitrophenyl-ATP reveals co-existence of distinct P2X receptor channels in rat nodose neurones. *J Physiol* 1998; 509:411–417.

Tjølsen A, Berge O-G, Hunskaar S, Rosland JH, Hole K. The formalin test: an evaluation of the method. *Pain* 1992; 51:5–17.

Trams EJ, Kauffman H, Burnstock G. A proposal for the role of ecto-enzymes and adenylates in traumatic shock. *J Theor Biol* 1980; 87:609–621.

Ueno S, Tsuda M, Iwanaga T, Inoue K. Cell type-specific ATP-activated responses in rat dorsal root ganglion neurons. *Br J Pharmacol* 1999; 126:429–436.

Valera S, Hussy N, Evans RJ, et al. A new class of ligand-gated ion channel defined by P_{2X} receptor for extra-cellular ATP. *Nature* 1994; 371:516–519.

Virginio C, North RA, Surprenant A. Calcium permeability and block at homomeric and heteromeric $P2X_2$ and $P2X_3$ receptors, and P2X receptors in rat nodose neurones. *J Physiol* 1998a; 510:27–35.

Virginio C, Robertson G, Surprenant A, North RA. Trinitrophenyl-substituted nucleotides are potent antagonists selective for $P2X_1$, $P2X_3$ and heteromeric $P2X_{2/3}$ receptors. *Mol Pharmacol* 1998b; 53:969–973.

Vulchanova L, Arvidsson U, Riedl M, et al. Differential distribution of two ATP-gated channels (P2X receptors) determined by imunocytochemistry. *Proc Natl Acad Sci USA* 1996; 93:8063–8067.

Vulchanova L, Arvidsson U, Riedl M, et al. Imunocytochemical study of the $P2X_2$ and $P2X_3$ receptor subunits in rat and monkey sensory neurons and their central terminals. *Neuropharmacology* 1997; 36:1229–1242.

Vulchanova L, Riedl M, Shuster SJ, et al. $P2X_3$ is expressed by DRG neurons that terminate in inner lamina II. *Eur J Neurosci* 1998; 10:3470–3478.

Webb TE, Simon J, Krishek BJ, et al. Cloning and functional expression of a brain G-protein coupled ATP receptor. *FEBS Lett* 1993; 324:219–225.

Wildman SS, King BF, Burnstock G. Potentiation of ATP-responses at a recombinant $P2X_2$ receptor by neurotransmitters and related substances. *Br J Pharmacol* 1997; 120:221–224.

Wildman SS, King BF, Burnstock G. Modulatory activity of extracellular H^+ and Zn^{2+} on ATP responses at $rP2X_1$ and $rP2X_3$ receptors. *Br J Pharmacol* 1999; 128:486–492.

Xiang Z, Bo X, Burnstock G. Localization of ATP-gated P2X receptor immunoreactivity in rat sensory and sympathetic ganglia. *Neurosci Lett* 1998; 256:105–108.

Yasuda JM. Guanethidine for reflex sympathetic dystrophy. *Ann Pharmacother* 1994; 28:338–341.

Correspondence to: G. Burnstock, PhD, DSc, FAA, MRCP(Hon), FRCS(Hon), FMedSci FRS, Autonomic Neuroscience Institute, Royal Free and University College Medical School, University College London, Rowland Hill Street, London NW3 2PF, United Kingdom. Tel: 44-171-830-2948; Fax: 44-171-830-2949; email: g.burnstock@ucl.ac.uk.

Proceedings of the 9th World Congress on Pain,
Progress in Pain Research and Management,
Vol. 16, edited by M. Devor, M.C. Rowbotham, and
Z. Wiesenfeld-Hallin, IASP Press, Seattle, © 2000.

8

Sodium Channels as Molecular Targets in Pain

Theodore R. Cummins, Sulayman D. Dib-Hajj,
Joel A. Black, and Stephen G. Waxman

Department of Neurology and PVA/EPVA Neuroscience Research Center, Yale Medical School, New Haven, Connecticut; and Rehabilitation Research Center, VA Connecticut, West Haven, Connecticut, USA

EXPRESSION OF SODIUM CHANNELS IN DRG NEURONS

The pain pathway begins with primary sensory neurons of the dorsal root ganglia (DRG) and trigeminal nerve. Injuries can result in chronic pain by triggering abnormal spontaneous burst activity in these neurons (Ochoa and Torebjörk 1980; Scadding 1981; Nordin et al. 1984; Devor 1994). Sodium channels within primary sensory neurons are likely to be involved in generating the abnormal action potential activity associated with pain. Thus these channels might be expected to present useful molecular targets for the treatment of pain, and experimental and clinical observations have in fact demonstrated partial efficacy of sodium channel blockers in both experimental models and clinical cases of neuropathic pain (Chabal et al. 1989; Devor et al. 1992; Omana-Zapata et al. 1997; Rizzo 1997).

The molecular revolution in neurobiology over the past decade has shown that at least eight distinct sodium channels, encoded by different genes, are expressed within the nervous system. These channels, which have different distributions and different physiological signatures, are expressed in a regionally and temporally specific manner. We have recently demonstrated (Black et al. 1996) that DRG neurons express at least six presumptive sodium channels, some of which are specific to sensory neurons. Moreover, injury to primary sensory neurons triggers the deployment of a new and different repertoire of sodium channels, and can contribute to hyperexcitability of these cells through a process of abnormal channel expression that includes the downregulation of some sodium channel genes and the upregulation of other, previously silent sodium channel genes. This chapter discusses the expression of sodium channels in DRG neurons, the changes in expression of sodium channel genes that occur in DRG neurons following injury, and the contributions of these changes in sodium channel expression to hyperexcitability of these cells.

HYPEREXCITABILITY OF PRIMARY SENSORY NEURONS FOLLOWING INJURY

A hint that sodium channel expression might change in injured neurons was provided by early electrophysiological studies (Eccles et al. 1958; Kuno and Llinas 1970), which demonstrated changes in excitability of spinal motor neurons following injury of their axons, suggesting increased sodium channel expression over the cell body and the dendrites. Similar changes were subsequently observed following axonal transection of sensory neurons (Gurtu and Smith 1988). Immunocytochemical observations have more recently demonstrated abnormal sodium channel accumulations at the tips of injured axons (Devor et al. 1989; England et al. 1994). Biophysical and electrophysiological studies indicate that abnormal increases in sodium conductance can lead to inappropriate, repetitive action potential activity (see, e.g., Waxman and Brill 1978; Matzner and Devor 1992, 1994; Zhang et al. 1997).

MULTIPLE SODIUM CHANNELS IN PRIMARY SENSORY NEURONS

Nearly a dozen molecularly distinct voltage-gated sodium channels are known to be encoded by different genes within mammals. At least eight of these sodium channel genes are expressed in the nervous system. Thus, in trying to understand the molecular basis of pain, it is important to know what type(s) of sodium channels are expressed in primary sensory neurons, and what types of channels produce inappropriate sensory neuron discharge associated with pain.

DRG neurons exhibit multiple, distinct sodium currents with different voltage dependence and different kinetic and pharmacological properties (Kostyuk et al. 1981; Caffrey et al. 1992; Roy and Narahashi 1992; Elliott and Elliott 1993). These cells are now known to express at least six presumptive sodium channel transcripts (Black et al. 1996). The α-I and Na6 channels (which are also expressed at high levels by other neuronal cell types within the central nervous system [CNS]) produce tetrodotoxin-sensitive (TTX-s) sodium currents, and are expressed at high levels in DRG neurons. In addition, DRG neurons express four distinct putative sodium channel transcripts that are not expressed at significant levels in other neuronal cell types: (1) PN1/hNE is expressed preferentially in DRG neurons (Toledo-Aral et al. 1997); this channel produces a fast, transient TTX-s sodium current in response to sudden depolarizations, and a slowly inactivating current in response to slow depolarizations close to resting membrane potential (Cummins et al. 1998). (2) SNS/PN3, expressed preferentially in small DRG and trigeminal neurons, encodes a slowly inactivating TTX-resistant (TTX-r) sodium current (Akopian et al. 1996; Sangameswaran et al. 1996). (3) NaN, expressed preferentially in small DRG and trigeminal neurons, exhibits an amino acid sequence, which although only 47% similar to SNS/PN3, predicts that it encodes a TTX-r sodium channel (Dib-Hajj et al. 1998a); patch-clamp studies on mouse (Cummins et al. 1999) and human (Dib-Hajj et al. 1996b) DRG neurons indicate that NaN ecodes a persistent TTX-r sodium channel whose activity probably contributes to setting resting potential and excitability. (4) NaG, another putative sodium channel, was initially cloned from an astrocyte library and at first was considered to be glial specific (Gautron et al. 1992), but it is also preferentially expressed at high levels within DRG neurons (Black et al. 1996) and at lower levels within other neurons of neural crest origin (Felts et al. 1997). Because NaG mRNA is also present in the lung, pituitary, and bladder and encodes relatively few positively charged amino acid residues in the putative voltage sensor region, some investigators have expressed doubt as to whether NaG functions as a voltage-dependent sodium channel (Akopian et al. 1997).

The preferential expression, within small DRG neurons, of SNS/PN3 and NaN provides a molecular correlate for the observation (Kostyuk et al. 1981; Roy and Narahashi 1992; Elliott and Elliott 1993; Rizzo et al. 1995a; Rush et al. 1998; Scholz et al. 1998) that these cells express multiple sodium currents, including TTX-r currents. Physiological experiments have shown that TTX-r sodium channels play a role in action potential conduction within nociceptive sensory neurons and their axons (Jeftinija 1994; Quasthoff et al. 1995; Brock et al. 1998).

SODIUM CHANNEL GENE EXPRESSION CHANGES IN DRG NEURONS FOLLOWING AXONAL INJURY

Knowing that DRG neurons express multiple sodium channels, we asked whether there is a switch in the type of channels produced in these cells following axonal injury. Our early observations (Waxman et al. 1994) demonstrated a significant upregulation of expression of the previously silent α-III sodium channel gene in DRG neurons following axotomy within the sciatic nerve. We also demonstrated a downregulation of the SNS/PN3 gene that can persist for as long as 210 days following axotomy (Dib-Hajj et al. 1996) and a downregulation of the NaN gene (Dib-Hajj et al. 1998a). These changes in sodium channel gene expression are illustrated in Fig. 1.

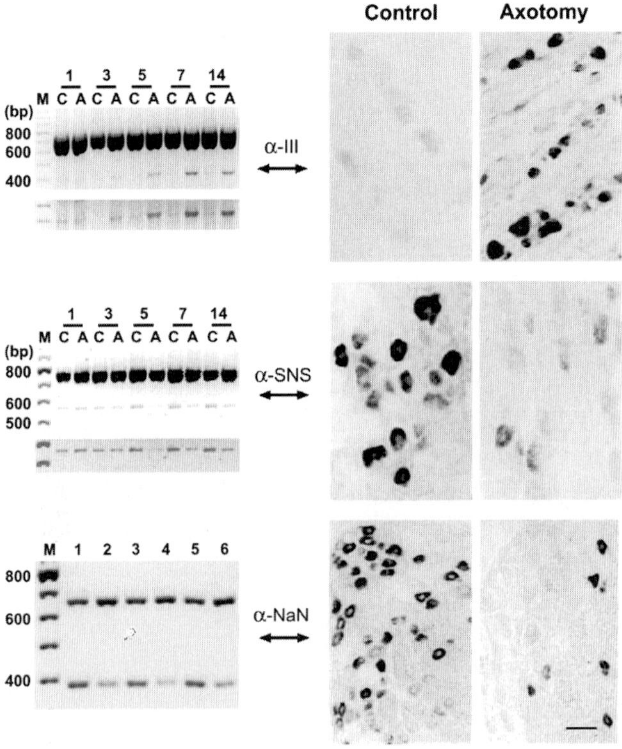

Fig. 1. Expression of mRNA is upregulated for sodium channel α-III (upper) and downregulated for SNS (middle) and NaN (lower panel) in DRG neurons following transection of their axons within the sciatic nerve. Micrographs (at right) show in situ hybridizations in control DRG and 5–7 days post-axotomy. Gels (at left) show products of co-amplification of α-III (upper left) and SNS (middle left) together with β-actin transcripts in control and axotomized DRG (days post-axotomy indicated above gels), with computer-enhanced images of amplification products shown below gels. Co-amplification of NaN (392 base pairs [bp]) and glyceraldehyde-3-phosphate dehydrogenase (GAPDH) (606 bp) (lower left) shows decreased expression of NaN mRNA at 7 days post-axotomy (lanes 2, 4, 6) compared to controls (lanes 1, 3, 5). Upper and middle panels were modified from Dib-Hajj et al (1996) and lower panels from Dib-Hajj et al (1998a), with permission.

Because expression of the SNS/PN3 and NaN sodium channel genes is downregulated in DRG neurons following axonal transection, we expected that TTX-r sodium currents would be reduced in these cells following axotomy. Our patch-clamp studies demonstrated that, indeed, there is a significant attenuation of TTX-r sodium currents in medium-sized cutaneous afferent DRG neurons following axonal transection within the sciatic nerve (Rizzo et al. 1995b). We observed a similar downregulation of TTX-r sodium currents in small DRG neurons that persisted for at least 60 days after axotomy (Cummins and Waxman 1997), consistent with the long-lasting changes in gene expression that we observed in these cells (Dib-Hajj et al. 1996). Both slowly inactivating TTX-r sodium currents (Fig. 2) and low-voltage-activated (LVA) persistent TTX-r sodium currents (Fig. 3) were decreased by axotomy (Cummins and Waxman 1997). In addition, we observed a significant switch in the properties of the TTX-s sodium currents, including the emergence of a rapidly repriming current (i.e., a current that recovers rapidly from inactivation) in these cells following axotomy (Cummins and Waxman 1997). Cummins and Waxman (1997) suggested

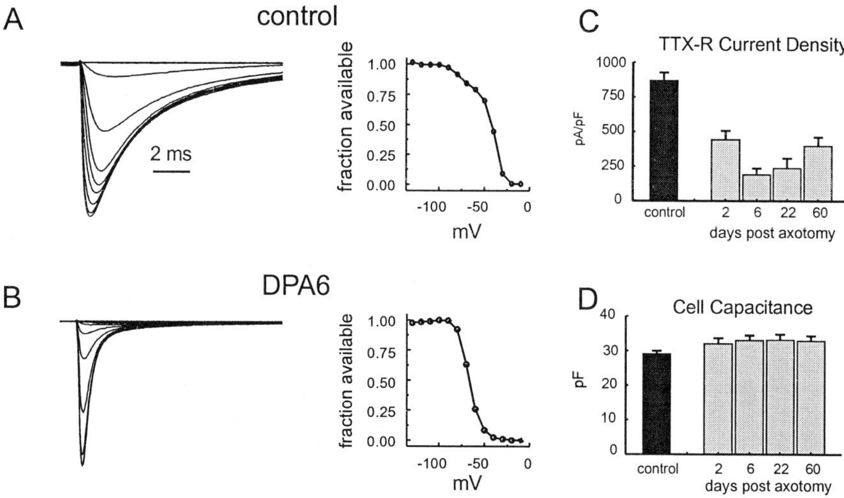

Fig. 2. TTX-resistant (TTX-r) sodium currents in small DRG neurons are downregulated following axotomy within the sciatic nerve. Whole-cell patch clamp recordings from (A, left) representative control and (B, left) DPA6 (6 days post-axotomy) DRG neurons show that the TTX-r, slowly inactivating component of sodium current is attenuated following axotomy. Steady-state inactivation curves (A, B; right side) show loss of a component characteristic of TTX-r currents. (C) Attenuation of TTX-r current persists for at least 60 days post-axotomy. (D) Cell capacitance, which provides a measure of cell size, does not change significantly following axotomy. Modified from Cummins and Waxman (1997), with permission.

that the expression of the type III sodium channel underlies the emergence of the rapidly repriming sodium current in axotomized DRG neurons. Similar changes in sodium currents and sodium channel mRNA levels have also been observed in the DRG neurons of rats that exhibited hyperalgesia following chronic constriction of the sciatic nerve (Dib-Hajj et al. 1999a).

Several mechanisms might cause these changes to contribute to spontaneous activity, or to activity at inappropriately high frequencies in DRG neurons, following injury to their axons. Increased sodium conductance due to increased numbers of channels will tend to lower the threshold for generation of action potentials (Matzner and Devor 1992). Overlap between steady-state activation and inactivation curves, together with the relatively weak voltage dependence of TTX-r sodium channels, suggests that co-expression of abnormal combinations of several types of channels could allow subthreshold oscillations in voltage, supported by TTX-r channels, to cross-activate other sodium channels, thereby triggering spontaneous action potential activity (Rizzo et al. 1996). As a result of the rapid repriming of the TTX-s sodium current in DRG neurons following axotomy, the refractory period is reduced in injured neurons and they should sustain higher firing frequencies (Cummins and Waxman 1997). If persistent currents participate

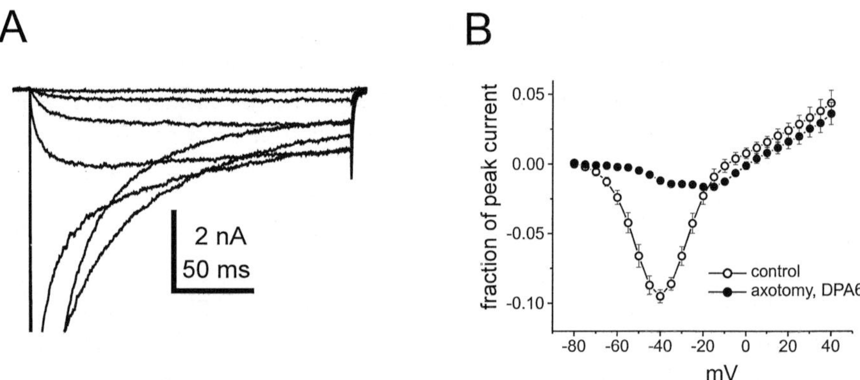

Fig. 3. Axotomy decreases persistent currents in small neurons. (A) Family of currents recorded from a control small DRG neuron. Current was elicited by test potentials from –75 to –25 in 10-mV steps. The peak current in this cell was 47 nA. (B) Relationship between current and voltage for the persistent current in small DRG neurons. Cells were held at –100 mV and increased in steps from –80 to 40 mV. The average current was normalized to the maximum peak current for each cell and is plotted against the test voltage. Data are shown for control (n = 11) and axotomized (n = 14) neurons. The persistent current was measured using test depolarizations of 200 ms for control neurons and 40 ms for axotomized neurons. Modified from Cummins and Waxman (1997), with permission.

in setting the resting potential, as demonstrated in optic nerve axons (Stys et al. 1993), reduction of LVA persistent TTX-r sodium currents following injury to the axons of DRG neurons could produce a hyperpolarizing shift in resting membrane potential that, by relieving resting inactivation, might increase the availability of TTX-s sodium current for electrogenesis (Cummins and Waxman 1997).

NEUROTROPHINS MODULATE SODIUM CHANNEL EXPRESSION IN NORMAL AND INJURED DRG NEURONS

Early experiments in vitro demonstrated that nerve growth factor (NGF) can affect sodium channel expression in DRG neurons (Aguayo and White 1992; Zur et al. 1995). One possibility was that peripheral axotomy caused changes in sodium channel gene expression in DRG neurons, at least in part, as a result of interruption of access to a peripheral supply of NGF. Using an in vitro model that mimics axotomy, Black et al. (1997) observed that NGF, delivered directly to DRG cell bodies, downregulates α-III mRNA and maintains high levels of SNS/PN3 mRNA expression in small DRG neurons. Extending these observations to an in vivo model, Dib-Hajj et al. (1998b) studied small DRG neurons following axotomy, and demonstrated that administration of exogenous NGF to the proximal transected nerve stump results in a partial rescue of SNS/PN3 mRNA levels and of TTX-r sodium current in small DRG neurons (Fig. 4). These results indicate that at least some of the changes in sodium channel expression in DRG neurons following axotomy of the sciatic nerve are due to loss of access to peripheral pools of neurotrophic factors.

Sodium channel expression in DRG neurons may reflect combined effects of multiple neurotrophic factors. Brain-derived neurotrophic factor (BDNF) does not alter the expression of sodium currents in DRG neurons, although it has significant effects on the expression of GABA-receptor-mediated currents in these cells (Oyelese et al. 1997). Glial-derived neurotrophic factor (GDNF) modulates the expression of NaN and of TTX-r sodium currents in a subpopulation of small DRG neurons that express the ret receptor (Fjell et al. 1999). Changes in the expression of several neurotrophins and in the accessibility of peripheral pools of neurotrophins may contribute to abnormal expression of sodium channels in injured DRG neurons.

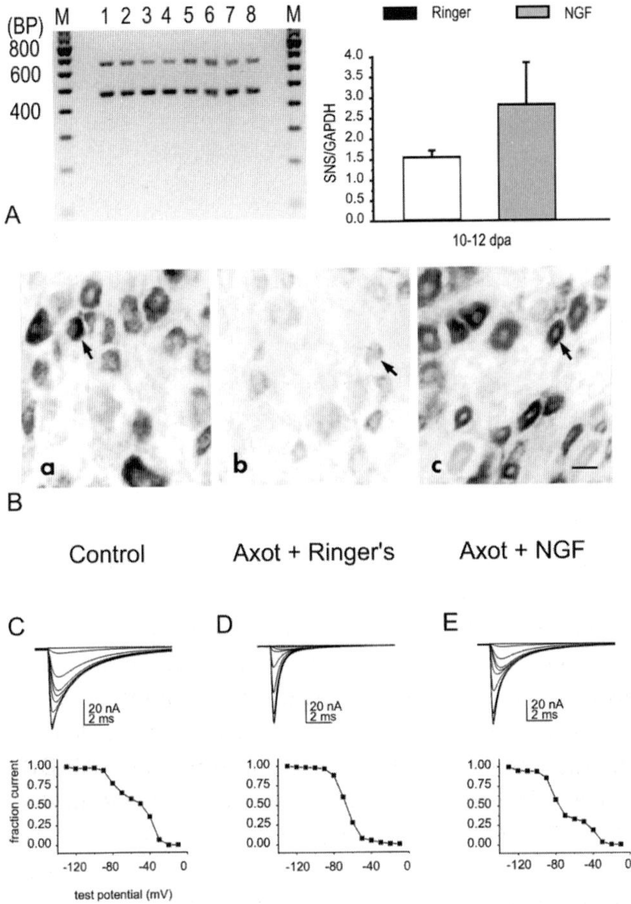

Fig. 4. SNS mRNA and TTX-r sodium currents are partially rescued in axotomized DRG neurons following delivery of nerve growth factor (NGF) to the proximal nerve stump. (A) Gel showing co-amplification of SNS (979 bp) and GAPDH (666 bp) products in Ringer-treated axotomized DRG (lanes 1, 2, 5, 6) and NGF-treated axotomized DRG (lanes 3, 4, 7, 8). The graph shows the increase in SNS amplification product in NGF-treated DRG. (B) In situ hybridization shows downregulation of SNS mRNA in DRG following axotomy (axotomy + Ringers) compared to control, and shows the partial rescue of SNS mRNA by NGF. (C, D, E) A partial rescue of slowly inactivating TTX-r sodium currents in axotomized DRG neurons following exposure to NGF. Representative patch-clamp recordings from (C) control, (D) Ringer-treated axotomized, and (E) NGF-treated axotomized neurons; corresponding steady-state inactivation curves are shown below the recordings. Modified from Dib-Hajj et al. (1998b), with permission.

SODIUM CHANNEL EXPRESSION CHANGES IN INFLAMMATORY PAIN MODELS

The evidence described above suggests that abnormal expression of sodium channels contributes to the pathophysiology of neuropathic pain. In addition, evidence implicates abnormal sodium channel expression in inflammatory pain. Inflammatory molecules, such as prostaglandins and serotonin, can modulate TTX-r sodium currents in DRG neurons (Gold et al. 1996), possibly acting via a cascade involving cyclic adenosine monophosphate (cAMP) and protein kinase A that affects one or more of the channel's phosphorylation sites (England et al. 1996). In addition to this modulation of pre-existing channels, recent studies have revealed changes in sodium channel gene expression in inflammatory models of pain. Our studies, carried out before our cloning of NaN, focused on SNS/PN3 because its expression was known to be especially dynamic. Because we had observed peak changes in SNS/PN3 mRNA 5 days following axotomy (Dib-Hajj et al. 1996), we studied sodium channel expression in DRG neurons in rats 4 days following injection of carrageenan into the hindpaw (Tanaka et al. 1998). Using in situ hybridization, we observed significantly increased SNS/PN3 mRNA expression in DRG neurons projecting to the inflamed limb, compared with DRG neurons from the contralateral side or naive (uninjected) controls (Fig. 5). Our patch-clamp recordings at 4 days post-injection demonstrated an increase in the amplitude of the TTX-r sodium current in small DRG neurons projecting to the inflamed limb (31.7 ± 3.3 nA) compared to the contralateral side (20.1 ± 2.1 nA) (Tanaka et al. 1998). The TTX-r current density (which provides a measure of the density of channels per unit area of membrane) was also significantly increased in the carrageenan-challenged DRG neurons.

Consistent with a contribution of altered sodium channel expression to the pathophysiology of inflammatory pain, Gould et al. (1998) reported an increase in sodium channel immunoreactivity in DRG neurons that persists for at least 2 months following injection of complete Freund's adjuvant into their projection field, and Tate et al (1998) reported an increase in NaN/SNS-2 mRNA 7 days following injection of complete Freund's adjuvant. The molecular trigger for these changes in sodium channel gene expression in these models of inflammatory pain is not known, but it may involve neurotrophins. NGF is normally produced in peripheral target cells including fibroblasts, Schwann cells, and keratinocytes; NGF production is stimulated in immune cells, and exposure to inflammatory agents such as carrageenan and Freund's adjuvant increases concentrations of NGF in various cell types (Weskamp and Otten 1987; Woolf et al. 1994). Thus inflammation may result in changes in neurotrophin levels within target tissues, which in turn trigger changes in the expression of sodium channels within primary sensory neurons.

SODIUM CHANNELS AS MOLECULAR TARGETS

Sodium channels contribute in several ways to the hyperexcitability of primary sensory neurons that can be associated with pain. Pre-existing sodium channels within the membrane and processes of DRG neurons participate in electrogenesis in these cells. Profound changes also occur in the molecular organization of injured DRG neurons, including changes in sodium channel gene expression such as the downregulation of some sodium channel subtypes and the upregulation of other, previously unexpressed, sodium channel subtypes.

We do not yet know whether secondary sensory neurons, postsynaptic to primary sensory cells, also exhibit altered expression of sodium channel genes in chronic pain states. A growing body of evidence demonstrates

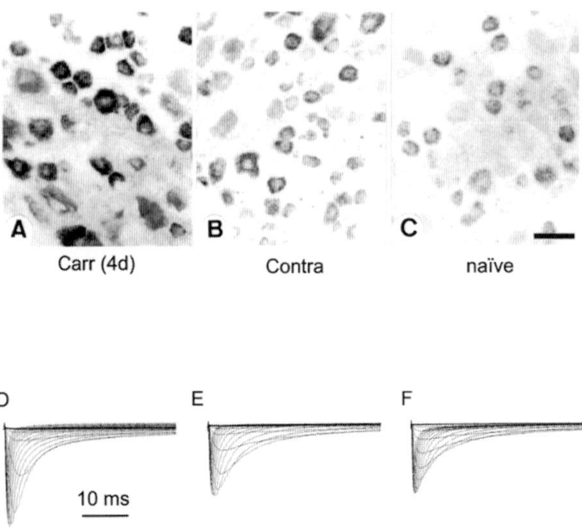

Fig. 5. SNS mRNA levels and TTX-r sodium currents are increased 4 days following injection of carrageenan into the projection fields of DRG neurons. Top: In situ hybridization showing SNS mRNA in (A) carrageenan-injected, (B) contralateral control, and (C) naive DRG cells. Patch-clamp recordings (D, E, F) reveal no change in voltage dependence of activation or steady-state inactivation of TTX-r sodium currents following carrageenan injection, but demonstrate an increase in TTX-r current amplitude (D) and density. Modified from Tanaka et al. (1998), with permission.

activity-related regulation of sodium channel expression in uninjured central neurons. Deafferentation of the olfactory bulb via surgical transection of the olfactory nerve in neonatal rats downregulates α-II sodium channel mRNA expression of tufted and mitral cells (Sashihara et al. 1996). This change is not due to denervation per se, but appears to result from a change in the level of incoming synaptic activity, since similar changes occur following cauterization of the naris, which abolishes access to olfactory stimuli without denervating the olfactory bulb (Sashihara et al. 1997). Sodium channel expression is also a dynamic process within some types of neurons in the nervous system of intact adult rats. Within the supraoptic nucleus of the hypothalamus, the α-II and Na6 sodium channel transcripts are upregulated and sodium currents increase in response to physiological changes in the osmotic milieu (Tanaka et al. 1999). Thus, physical injury is not a prerequisite for resetting the pattern of sodium channel expression within neurons. In view of the dynamic nature of sodium channel expression in intact neurons, it seems reasonable to ask whether there are changes in sodium channel expression in uninjured neurons, located centrally along the pain pathway, in chronic pain states.

We still need to delineate the precise contribution of each sodium channel subtype in the physiology of electrogenesis within primary sensory neurons and in the pathophysiology of hyperexcitability associated with pain, and we must assess the effects of selective blockade of each channel subtype in these cells. DRG and trigeminal neurons express several presumptive sodium channel genes (SNS/PN3, NaN, PN1, and NaG) in a preferential manner, at levels much higher than in other neuronal cell types. Selective pharmacological manipulation may thus be possible for primary sensory neurons in general, or nociceptive neurons in particular. Molecular and functional studies on ion channels and in vivo studies in pain models promise to reveal, in the relatively near future, whether selective sodium channel blockade will emerge as a viable strategy for the treatment of pain.

SUMMARY

Hyperexcitability and increased baseline sensitivity of primary sensory neurons following nerve injury can lead to abnormal burst activity associated with pain, and thus the molecules underlying these events represent important therapeutic targets. Early investigations on motor neurons demonstrated that, following axonal injury, neurons can display altered excitability consistent with increased sodium channel expression. Moreover, abnormal accumulations of sodium channels have been observed at the tips of injured axons. Our laboratory has used molecular, electrophysiological, and pharmacological techniques to discover what types of sodium channels contribute to the hyperexcitability of primary sensory neurons following injury. We have demonstrated the expression of multiple sodium channels, with distinct physiological properties, within small DRG neurons, which include nociceptive cells. Several sodium channels that are preferentially expressed within DRG and trigeminal neurons have now been cloned and sequenced. Following injury to the axons of DRG neurons, sodium channel expression in these cells changes dramatically, with downregulation of the SNS/PN3 and NaN sodium channel genes and upregulation of the previously silent type III sodium channel gene. These alterations in sodium channel expression can produce electrophysiological changes in DRG neurons that cause them to fire spontaneously or at inappropriately high frequencies. Changes in sodium channel gene expression also occur in experimental models of inflammatory pain. Sodium channels thus may provide important molecular targets in the search for new, more effective drugs for the treatment of pain.

ACKNOWLEDGMENTS

This work has been supported in part by grants from the National Multiple Sclerosis Society and the Paralyzed Veterans of America/Eastern Paralyzed Veterans Association, and by the Medical Research Service and Rehabilitation Research Service, Department of Veterans Affairs.

REFERENCES

Aguayo LG, White G. Effects of nerve growth factor on TTX- and capsaicin-sensitivity in adult rat sensory neurons. *Brain Res* 1992; 570:61–67.

Akopian AN, Sivilotti L, Wood JN. A tetrodotoxin-resistant voltage-gated sodium channel expressed by sensory neurons. *Nature* 1996; 379:257–262.

Akopian AN, Souslova V, Sivilotti L, Wood JN. Structure and distribution of a broadly expressed atypical sodium channel. *FEBS Lett* 1997; 400:183–187.

Black JA, Dib-Hajj S, McNabola K, Jeste S, et al. Spinal sensory neurons express multiple sodium channel α-subunit mRNAs. *Mol Brain Res* 1996; 43:117–132.

Black JA, Langworthy K, Hinson A.W, Dib-Hajj SD, Waxman SG. NGF has opposing effects on Na^+ channel III and SNS gene expression in spinal sensory neurons. *Neuroreport* 1997; 8:2331–2335.

Brock JA, McLachlan EM, Belmonte C. Tetrodotoxin-resistant impulses in single nociceptor nerve terminals in guinea-pig corneas. *J Physiol* 1998; 512:211–217.

Caffrey JM, Eng DL, Black JA, Waxman SG, Kocsis JD. Three types of sodium channels in adult rat dorsal root ganglion neurons. *Brain Res* 1992; 592:283–297.

Chabal C, Russell LC, Burchiel KJ. The effect of intravenous lidocaine, tocainide, and mexiletine on spontaneously active fibers originating in rat sciatic neuromas. *Pain* 1989; 38:333–338.

Cummins TR, Waxman SG. Downregulation of tetrodotoxin-resistant sodium currents and upregulation of a rapidly repriming tetrodotoxin-sensitive sodium current in small spinal sensory neurons after nerve injury. *J Neurosci* 1997; 17:3503–3514.

Cummins TR, Howe JR, Waxman SG. Slow closed-state inactivation: a novel mechanism underlying ramp currents in cells expressing the hNE/PN1 sodium channel. *J Neurosci* 1998; 18:9607–9619.

Cummins TR, Dib-Hajj S, Black JA, et al. Novel persistent tetrodotoxin-resistant sodium current in SNS-null and wild-type small primary sensory neurons. *J Neurosci* 1999; 19:RC43 (1–6).

Devor M. The pathophysiology of damaged peripheral nerves. In: Wall PD, Melzack R (Eds). *Textbook of Pain,* 2nd ed. Edinburgh: Churchill Livingstone, 1994, pp 79–101.

Devor M, Keller CH, Deerinck TJ, Ellisman MH. Na^+ channel accumulation on axolemma of afferent endings in nerve end neuromas in *Apteronotus. Neurosci Lett* 1989; 102:149–154.

Devor M, Wall PD, Catalan N. Systemic lidocaine silences ectopic neuroma and DRG discharge without blocking nerve conduction. *Pain* 1992; 48:261–268.

Dib-Hajj S, Black JA, Felts P, Waxman SG. Down-regulation of transcripts for Na channel α-SNS in spinal sensory neurons following axotomy. *Proc Natl Acad Sci USA* 1996; 93:14950–14954.

Dib-Hajj SD, Tyrrell L, Black JA, Waxman SG. NaN, a novel voltage-gated Na channel, is expressed preferentially in peripheral sensory neurons and down-regulated after axotomy. *Proc Natl Acad Sci USA* 1998a; 95:8963–8969.

Dib-Hajj SD, Black JA, Cummins TR, et al. Rescue of α-SNS sodium channel expression in small dorsal root ganglion neurons after axotomy by nerve growth factor in vivo. *J Neurophysiol* 1998b; 79:2668–2678.

Dib-Hajj SD, Fjell J, Cummins TR, et al. Plasticity of sodium channel expression in DRG neurons in the chronic constriction injury model of neuropathic pain. *Pain* 1999a; in press.

Dib-Hajj SD, Tyrrell L, Cummins TR, et al. Two tetrodotoxin-resistant sodium channels in human dorsal root ganglian neurons. *FEBS Lett* 1996; 462:117–121.

Eccles JC, Libet B, Young RR. The behavior of chromatolysed motoneurons studied by intracellular recording. *J Physiol (Lond)* 1958; 143:11–40.

Elliott AA, Elliott JR. Characterization of TTX-sensitive and TTX-resistant sodium currents in small cells from adult rat dorsal root ganglia. *J Physiol (Lond)* 1993; 463:39–56.

England JD, Gamboni F, Ferguson MA, Levinson SR. Sodium channels accumulate at the tips of injured axons. *Muscle Nerve* 1994; 17:593–598.

England S, Bevan S, Docherty RJ. PGE_2 modulates the tetrodotoxin-resistant sodium current in neonatal rat dorsal root ganglion neurones via the cyclic AMP-protein kinase A cascade. *J Physiol (Lond)* 1996; 495:429–440.

Felts PA, Black JA, Dib-Hajj SD, Waxman SG. NaG: A sodium channel-like mRNA shared by Schwann cells and other neural crest derivatives. *Glia* 1997; 21:269–277.

Fjell J, Cummins TR, Dib-Hajj SD, et al. Differential role of GDNF and NGF in the maintenance of two TTX-resistant sodium channels in adult DRG neurons. *Mol Brain Res* 1999; 67:267–282.

Gautron S, Dos Santos G, Pinto-Henrique D, et al. The glial voltage-gated sodium channel: cell- and tissue-specific mRNA expression. *Proc Natl Acad Sci USA* 1992; 89:7272–7276.

Gold MS, Reichling DB, Shuster MJ, Levine JD. Hyperalgesic agents increase a tetrodotoxin-resistant Na^+ current in nociceptors. *Proc Natl Acad Sci USA* 1996; 93:1108–1112.

Gould HJ III, England JD, Liu ZP, Levinson SR. Rapid sodium channel augmentation in response to inflammation induced by complete Freund's adjuvant. *Brain Res* 1998; 802:69–74.

Gurtu S, Smith PA. Electrophysiological characteristics of hamster dorsal root ganglion cells and their response to axotomy. *J Neurophysiol* 1988; 59:408–423.

Jeftinija S. The role of tetrodotoxin-resistant sodium channels of small primary afferent fibers. *Brain Res* 1994; 639:125–134.

Kostyuk PG, Veselovsky NS, Tsyandryenko AY. Ionic currents in the somatic membrane of rat dorsal root ganglion neurons. I. Sodium currents. *Neuroscience* 1981; 6:2423–2430.

Kuno M, Llinas R. Enhancement of synaptic transmission by dendritic potentials in chromatolysed motoneurons of the cat. *J Physiol (Lond)* 1970; 210:807–821.

Matzner O, Devor M. Na^+ conductance and the threshold for repetitive neuronal firing. *Brain Res* 1992; 597:92–98.

Matzner O, Devor M. Hyperexcitability at sites of nerve injury depends on voltage-sensitive Na^+ channels *J Neurophysiol* 1994; 72:349–359.

Nordin M, Nystrom B, Wallin U, Hagbarth K-E. Ectopic sensory discharges and paresthesiae in patients with disorders of peripheral nerves, dorsal roots and dorsal columns. *Pain* 1984; 20:231–245.

Ochoa J, Torebjörk HE. Paresthesiae from ectopic impulse generation in human sensory nerves. *Brain* 1980; 103:835–854.

Omana-Zapata I, Khabbaz MA, Hunter JC, Bley KR. QX-314 inhibits ectopic nerve activity associated with neuropathic pain. *Brain Res* 1997; 771:228–237.

Oyelese AA, Rizzo MA, Waxman SG, Kocsis JD. Differential effects of NGF and BDNF on axotomy-induced changes in $GABA_A$-receptor-mediated conductance and sodium currents in cutaneous afferent neurons. *J Neurophysiol* 1997; 78:31–42.

Quasthoff S, Grosskreutz J, Schroder JM, Schneider U, Grafe P. Calcium potentials and tetrodotoxin-resistant sodium potentials in unmyelinated C fibres of biopsied human sural nerve. *Neuroscience* 1995; 69:955–965.

Rizzo MA. Successful treatment of painful traumatic mononeuropathy with carbamazepine: insights into a possible molecular pain mechanism. *J Neurol Sci* 1997; 152:103–106.

Rizzo MA, Kocsis JD, Waxman SG. Slow sodium conductances of dorsal root ganglion neurons: intraneuronal homogeneity and interneuronal heterogeneity. *J Neurophysiol* 1995a; 72:2796–2816.

Rizzo MA, Kocsis JD, Waxman SG. Selective loss of slow and enhancement of fast Na^+ currents in cutaneous afferent dorsal root ganglion neurones following axotomy. *Neurobiol Dis* 1995b; 2:87–96.

Rizzo MA, Kocsis JD, Waxman SG. Mechanisms of paresthesiae, dysesthesiae, and hyperesthesiae: Role of Na^+ channel heterogeneity. *Eur Neurol* 1996; 36:3–12.

Roy ML, Narahashi T. Differential properties of tetrodotoxin-sensitive and tetrodotoxin-resistant sodium channels in rat dorsal root ganglion neurons. *J Neurosci* 1992; 12:2104–2111.

Rush AM, Brau ME, Elliott AA, Elliott JR. Electrophysiological properties of sodium current subtypes in small cells from adult rat dorsal root ganglia. *J Physiol* 1998; 511:771–789.

Sangameswaran L, Delgado SG, Fish LM, et al. Structure and function of a novel voltage-gated, tetrodotoxin-resistant sodium channel specific to sensory neurons. *J Biol Chem* 1996; 271:5953–5956.

Sashihara S, Greer CA, Oh Y, Waxman SG. Cell specific differential expression of Na^+ channel β1 subunit mRNA in the olfactory system during postnatal development and following denervation. *J Neurosci* 1996; 16:702–714.

Sashihara S, Waxman SG, Greer CA. Down-regulation of Na^+ channel mRNA following sensory deprivation of tufted cells in the neonatal rat olfactory bulb. *Neuroreport* 1997; 8:1289–1293.

Scadding JW. Development of ongoing activity, mechanosensitivity, and adrenalin sensitivity in severed peripheral nerve axons. *Exper Neurol* 1981; 73:345–364.

Scholz A, Appel N, Vogel W. Two types of TTX-resistant and one TTX-sensitive Na^+ channel in rat dorsal root ganglion neurons and their blockade by halothane. *Eur J Neurosci* 1998; 10:2547–2556.

Stys PK, Ransom BR, Waxman SG. Non-inactivating, TTX-sensitive Na^+ conductance in rat optic nerve axons. *Proc Natl Acad Sci USA* 1993; 90:6976–6980.

Tanaka M, Cummins TR, Ishikawa K, et al. SNS Na^+ channel expression increases in dorsal root ganglion neurons in the carrageenan inflammatory pain model. *Neuroreport* 1998; 9:967–972.

Tanaka M, Cummins TR, Ishikawa K, et al. Molecular and functional remodeling of electrogenic membrane of hypothalamic neurons in response to changes in their input. *Proc Natl Acad Sci USA* 1999; 96:1088–1093.

Tate S, Benn S, Hick C, et al. Two sodium channels contribute to the TTX-R sodium current in primary sensory neurons. *Nat Neurosci* 1998; 1:653–655.

Toledo-Aral JJ, Moss BL, He Z-J, et al. Identification of PN1, a predominant voltage-dependent sodium channel expressed principally in peripheral neurons. *Proc Natl Acad Sci USA* 1997; 94:1527–1532.

Waxman SG, Brill MH. Conduction through demyelinated plaques in multiple sclerosis: computer simulations of facilitation by short internodes. *J Neurol Neurosurg Psychiat* 1978; 41:408–417.

Waxman SG, Kocsis JK, Black JA. Type III sodium channel mRNA is expressed in embryonic but not adult spinal sensory neurons, and is reexpressed following axotomy. *J Neurophysiol* 1994; 72:466–471.

Weskamp G, Otten U. An enzyme-linked immunoassay for nerve growth factor (NGF): a tool for studying regulatory mechanisms involved in NGF production in brain and in peripheral tissues. *J Neurochem* 1987; 48:1779–1786.

Woolf CJ, Safieh-Garabedian B, Ma Q-P, Crilly P, Winters J. Nerve growth factor contributes to the generation of inflammatory sensory hypersensitivity. *Neuroscience* 1994; 62:327–331.

Zhang J-M, Donnelly DF, Song X-J, LaMotte RH. Axotomy increases the excitability of dorsal root ganglion cells with unmyelinated axons. *J Neurophysiol* 1997; 78:2790–2794.

Zur KB, Oh Y, Waxman SG, Black JA. Differential up-regulation of sodium channel α- and β-subunit mRNAs in cultured embryonic DRG neurons following exposure to NGF. *Mol Brain Res* 1995; 30:97–103.

Correspondence to: Stephen G. Waxman, MD, PhD, Department of Neurology, LCI 707, Yale Medical School, 333 Cedar Street, New Haven, CT 06510, USA. Tel: 203-785-6351; Fax: 203-785-7826; email: stephen.waxman@yale.edu.

Proceedings of the 9th World Congress on Pain, Progress in Pain Research and Management, Vol. 16, edited by M. Devor, M.C. Rowbotham, and Z. Wiesenfeld-Hallin, IASP Press, Seattle, © 2000.

9

Ectopic Discharge in Primary Sensory Neurons Depends on Intrinsic Membrane Potential Oscillations

Ron Amir,[a] Martin Michaelis,[b] and Marshall Devor[a]

[a]Department of Cell and Animal Biology, Institute of Life Sciences, Hebrew University of Jerusalem, Jerusalem, Israel; [b]Physiology Institute, Christian-Albrechts University, Kiel, Germany

The abnormal discharge that develops at ectopic sites in some injured sensory neurons is an important generator of neuropathic paresthesias and pain (reviewed by Devor and Seltzer 1999). Ectopic discharge directly evokes persistent paresthesias and pain, and in addition may trigger and maintain "central sensitization," a hyperexcitability state of the central nervous system (CNS) in which normally non-noxious input carried on large myelinated Aβ touch afferents is felt as painful ("allodynia"; Woolf 1983; Campbell et al. 1988). Both persistent pain and allodynia are eliminated by preventing ectopic discharge from gaining access to the CNS (e.g., Gracely et al. 1992; Sheen and Chung 1993).

It is generally presumed that ectopic neuropathic discharge results from the classical (Hodgkin-Huxley) repetitive firing process whereby a sustained depolarization repeatedly draws the membrane potential toward threshold. We now report evidence that the discharge in fact results from a quite different process related to the presence of subthreshold membrane potential oscillations in a subpopulation of primary sensory neurons in the dorsal root ganglion (DRG) (for more details see Amir et al. 1999).

METHODS

Immature (22–88 g) and adult (165–530 g) male and female rats of the Wistar-derived Sabra strain were deeply anesthetized (Nembutal, >60 mg/kg i.p.) and killed. We excised DRG L4 and L5 with the dorsal root (DR) and a variable length of the spinal/sciatic nerve attached. In some adult animals the sciatic nerve was tightly ligated and cut just distal to the ligature 2–15 days prior to excision. All work adhered to national, university, and International Association for the Study of Pain (IASP) guidelines for the humane care and use of laboratory animals.

We made intracellular recordings from DRG neurons using sharp micropipettes in current clamp mode and applying electrical stimuli to the nerve. The evoked compound action potential, monitored on the dorsal root, served as an indicator of spike propagation through the ganglion. DRG neurons were categorized by axon conduction velocity (CV) and the shape of the intracellularly recorded spike (Amir and Devor 1996; Villiere and McLachlan 1996). Briefly, we took the axon to be myelinated (A-neuron) if CV > 1 m/s. Cells with CV ≤ 1 m/s were designated as having nonmyelinated axons (C-neurons). Values are presented as mean ± SD.

RESULTS

When first penetrated, most DRG neurons in young rats had a stable resting potential. A minority (9/73 A-neurons), however, exhibited periodic, sinusoidal membrane potential oscillations, with a mean frequency of 96 ± 18 Hz. The small amplitude of the oscillations at resting membrane potential (1.4 ± 0.6 mV peak-to-peak) and their high frequency may explain why they have not been reported previously despite the abundant attention DRG cells have attracted.

We routinely shifted the membrane potential in the depolarizing direction by intracellular current injection. With this search protocol the number of A-neurons with oscillations more than doubled from that seen at resting potential (9/73 vs. 20/73, $P < 0.05$). In addition, oscillations were revealed in three of 12 C-neurons, none of which had oscillations at rest. Fourier analysis showed that each neuron with oscillations had a single frequency peak, the cell's "dominant oscillation frequency." The oscillation amplitude gradually increased to a peak as the cell was depolarized, and the dominant frequency also rose (Fig. 1). With further depolarization, however, oscillation frequency continued to increase, but the amplitude declined until oscillations were no longer discernible. It was thus possible to define a "best oscillation frequency" at which the oscillation amplitude was maximal. Peak oscillation amplitude usually fell within the range of 3–6 mV. Best frequency for A-neurons averaged 118 ± 26 Hz ($n = 20$) and for C-neurons 11.7 ± 2.9 Hz ($n = 3$).

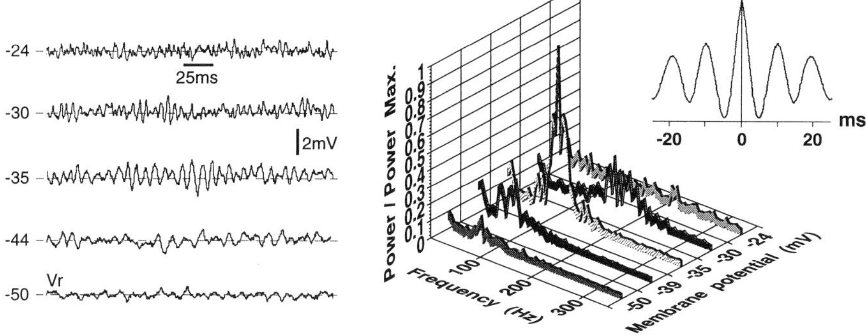

Fig. 1. Membrane potential oscillations recorded from a DRG A-neuron. Oscillation amplitude increased when the cell was depolarized from rest (Vr), and subsequently decreased with still deeper depolarization (left). The Fourier analysis (FFT) profile in this cell illustrates oscillation amplitude (power) peak (103 Hz) at –35 mV (right). Power scale was normalized relative to the maximal power recorded at –35 mV. The inset shows the autocorrelogram at –35 mV. Reprinted from Amir et al. (1999).

We also looked at neurons in DRGs taken from adult rats. Both A- and C-neurons in adults showed sinusoidal oscillations similar to those seen in young animals. The prevalence of A-neurons with subthreshold oscillations was higher in immature than in adult rats (27% vs. 11%, $P < 0.01$). In C-neurons, it was slightly higher in adults, although the difference was not statistically significant. In all cases, the amplitude, frequency, and prevalence of the oscillations were dependent on membrane potential, much as in immature animals.

In DRGs from both immature and adult rats repetitive spike discharge was rare at resting membrane potential (4/205 neurons). However, on injection of depolarizing current, either by a step function or a slow ramp, a significant proportion of the cells began to discharge repetitively (24/205 neurons, X^2, $P < 0.001$). Depolarization promoted spiking in two ways: it increased oscillation amplitude and it brought the neuron closer to spike threshold. In each case action potentials emerged from the depolarizing phase of oscillatory sinusoid, which indicates a causal relation between the oscillations and spiking (Fig. 2). In contrast, neurons that did not show subthreshold oscillations never fired repetitively, either spontaneously or on ramp depolarization (0/165 neurons vs. 24/205, $P < 0.0001$).

Two patterns of repetitive discharge were observed in neurons with oscillatory capability: slow/irregular (0.5–4 impulses/second) and bursting. In neurons that fired irregularly, single spikes occurred when individual oscillations reached threshold. In bursting cells, individual oscillations that

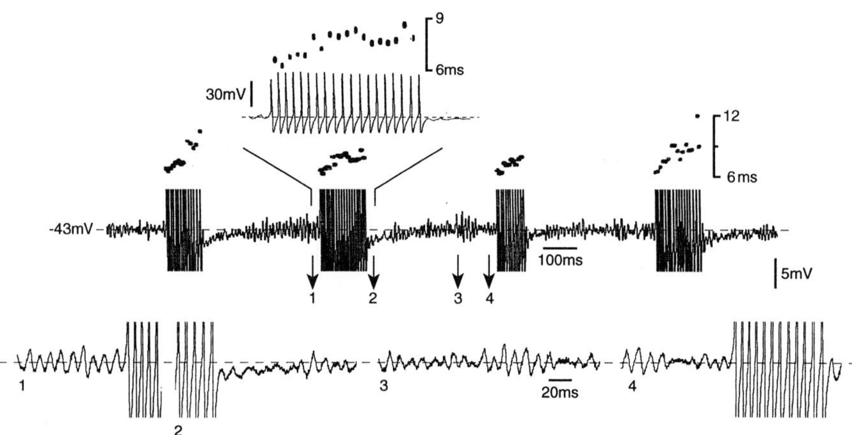

Fig. 2. Bursting discharge in a DRG A-neuron from an immature rat. Spikes are truncated except in the inset at top, which shows one of the bursts on a faster time base. Segments of the record at time points 1–4 are shown below on a still faster time base to illustrate the triggering of spike bursts by membrane potential oscillations. Reprinted from Amir et al. (1999).

reached threshold triggered a burst of spikes (interspike interval 4–15 ms). The burst was terminated by a burst-induced hyperpolarizing shift of the membrane potential (Amir and Devor 1997, Fig. 2). Both the bursting and the slow/irregular ectopic discharge pattern have been described previously in DRG neurons in vivo (Wall and Devor 1983).

We next investigated the effect of sciatic nerve cut and ligation on membrane potential oscillations and on the ectopic spike discharge that they trigger. This form of injury induces both persistent pain in the area of denervation and allodynia in the adjacent partially denervated territory (e.g., Wall et al. 1979; Markus et al. 1984; Kingery and Vallin 1989). We found that nerve injury induced a significant increase in the prevalence of DRG neurons with subthreshold oscillations, at least in A-neurons. The proportion of A-neurons with oscillations increased from 11% (10/95) to 30% (16/54, $P < 0.005$). In C-neurons the proportion increased from 28% (7/25) to 44% (18/41, $P > 0.2$). Consequent to the increased incidence of oscillations, the incidence of repetitive spike discharge also significantly increased ($P < 0.005$ for the total population).

A voltage- and tetrodotoxin (TTX)-sensitive Na^+ conductance(s) appears to contribute to the resonance characteristic responsible for subthreshold membrane potential oscillations in both A- and C-fiber DRG neurons as oscillations were eliminated by (partial) substitution of Na^+ with choline in the perfusion solution, or bath application of TTX or lidocaine (Fig. 3).

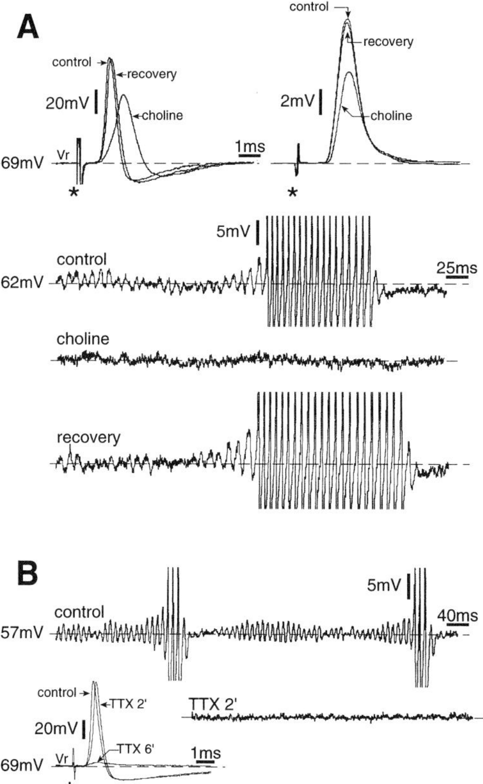

Fig. 3. Subthreshold membrane potential oscillations, and resulting spike bursting, depend on voltage-sensitive Na^+ conductance. (A) Subthreshold oscillations triggered a spike burst in an A-neuron (control). Replacing NaCl in the bath solution with choline chloride, thus reducing the bath Na^+ concentration from 151 mM to 27 mM., abolished the oscillations and the resulting spikes. Washout of the choline and return to the control bath solution restored both the oscillations and bursting (recovery). All three traces recorded at –62 mV. Upper traces show (left) the intracellularly recorded spike before, during, and after choline application (at resting potential [Vr] = –69 mV), and (right) the simultaneously recorded DR compound action potential. Both spike and compound action potential persisted, if with a reduced amplitude, when oscillations and ectopic spiking were eliminated. Propagation distance from the sciatic nerve stimulation site was 37 mm to the cell soma, and 50 mm to the compound action potential recording electrode. (B) In this A-neuron, DRG depolarization from rest (Vr = –69 mV) yielded subthreshold oscillations that triggered spike bursting (control trace, spikes truncated). Bath application of 1 μM TTX abolished the oscillations and spikes within 2 minutes (TTX 2´). Spike propagation in response to nerve stimulation at a distance of 7 mm persisted at this time, although it failed 4 minutes later (TTX 6´). Reprinted from Amir et al. (1999).

Once eliminated, oscillations could not be restored by further depolarization, but they generally reappeared following washout of the blocker (Fig. 3). Bath-applied Co^{2+} (5 mM), a wide-spectrum Ca^{2+} channel blocker, was not effective at blocking the oscillations. Suppression of oscillations with Na^+ substitution, TTX, or lidocaine always suppressed repetitive firing (Fig. 3). Interestingly, oscillations and consequent firing were consistently blocked at times when propagation of spikes evoked by axonal stimulation persisted (Fig. 3). For example, with high concentrations of lidocaine (0.4–40 mM) spike propagation was blocked along with the oscillations, but with low concentrations (4 μM) oscillations were eliminated while spike propagation persisted (4/4 A-neurons). Ectopic firing in vivo is also suppressed by local anesthetic concentrations insufficient to block axon conduction (e.g., Devor et al. 1992).

DISCUSSION

Our data indicate that repetitive firing in primary sensory neurons depends on the presence of intrinsic resonance properties that give rise to subthreshold oscillations of the membrane potential. One or more TTX and lidocaine-sensitive Na^+ channels play a central role in the generation of the oscillations, and hence the resulting ectopic discharge and neuropathic pain. We recorded from afferent neuron somata in the DRG. However, because the behavior of the DRG soma is often mirrored, at least in part, in the behavior of the axon shaft and end, it is likely that ectopic discharge generated at sites of nerve injury, such as neuromas and areas of demyelination (Kapoor et al. 1997), is also subserved by TTX-sensitive Na^+ channel-dependent membrane potential oscillations.

DRG neurons rarely fire at resting membrane potential and the DRG is essentially devoid of synaptic input, so what could induce depolarization and trigger ectopic discharge and pain in vivo? In fact, several nonsynaptic processes are able to depolarize sensory neurons. These include mechanical stress (e.g., during movement or straight-leg lifting; Nordin et al. 1984), cell-cell cross-depolarization (Amir and Devor 1996, 2000), and sympathetic efferent activity (Petersen et al. 1996). All these conditions increase ectopic firing in vivo and exacerbate neuropathic pain (Devor and Seltzer 1999). Oscillatory behavior in DRG neurons can be thought of as a "motor" ready to be engaged when the "clutch" of a slow-onset physiological depolarization is released.

Together, these considerations add to the growing body of evidence that injury-triggered processes that regulate the expression and vectorial transport of Na^+ channels are a major factor in the emergence of electrical hyperexcitability and ectopic firing in injured primary afferent neurons, and hence in the development of neuropathic pain (Devor and Seltzer 1999). The oscillatory behavior of primary afferent neurons, and the regulatory processes that control it, provide new targets for development of novel drugs to treat many devastating and often intractable chronic pain states.

ACKNOWLEDGMENTS

This work was supported by the U.S.-Israel Binational Science Foundation (BSF), the German-Israel Foundation for Research and Development (GIF), and the Leopold, Norman and Sara Yisraeli Memorial Fund. Martin Michaelis receives a Heisenberg fellowship from the Deutsche Forschungsgemeinschaft.

REFERENCES

Amir R, Devor M. Chemically mediated cross-excitation in rat dorsal root ganglia. *J Neurosci* 1996; 16:4733–4741.

Amir R, Devor M. Spike-evoked suppression and burst patterning in dorsal root ganglion neurons. *J Physiol (Lond)* 1997; 501:183–196.

Amir R, Devor M. Functional cross-excitation between afferent A- and C-neurons in dorsal root ganglia. *Neuroscience* 2000; 95:189–195.

Amir R, Michaelis M, Devor M. Membrane potential oscillations in dorsal root ganglion neurons: role in normal electrogenesis and in neuropathic pain. *J Neurosci* 1999; 19:8589–8596.

Campbell JN, Raja SN, Meyer RA, MacKinnon SE. Myelinated afferents signal the hyperalgesia associated with nerve injury. *Pain* 1988; 32:89–94.

Devor M, Seltzer Z. Pathophysiology of damaged nerves in relation to chronic pain. In: Wall PD, Melzack R (Eds). *Textbook of Pain,* 4th ed. London: Churchill Livingstone, 1999, pp 129–164.

Devor M, Wall PD, Catalan N. Systemic lidocaine silences ectopic neuroma and DRG discharge without blocking nerve conduction. *Pain* 1992; 48:261–268.

Gracely RH, Lynch SA, Bennett GJ. Painful neuropathy: altered central processing maintained dynamically by peripheral input. *Pain* 1992; 51:175–194.

Kapoor R, Li Y-G, Smith KJ. Slow sodium-dependent potential oscillations contribute to ectopic firing in mammalian demyelinated axons. *Brain* 1997; 120:647–652.

Kingery WS, Vallin JA. The development of chronic mechanical hyperalgesia, autotomy and collateral sprouting following sciatic nerve section in rat. *Pain* 1989; 38:321–332.

Markus H, Pomerantz B, Krushelnychy D. Spread of saphenous somatotopic projection map in spinal cord and hypersensitivity of the foot after chronic sciatic denervation in adult rat. *Brain Res* 1984; 296:27–39.

Nordin M, Nystrom B, Wallin U, Hagbarth K-E. Ectopic sensory discharges and paresthesiae in patients with disorders of peripheral nerves, dorsal roots and dorsal columns. *Pain* 1984; 20:231–245.

Petersen M, Zhang J, Zhang J-M, LaMotte RH. Abnormal spontaneous activity and responses to norepinephrine in dissociated dorsal root ganglion cells after chronic nerve constriction. *Pain* 1996; 67:391–397.

Sheen K, Chung JM. Signs of neuropathic pain depend on signals from injured fibers in a rat model. *Brain Res* 1993; 610:62–68.

Villiere V, McLachlan EM. Electrophysiological properties of neurons in intact rat dorsal root ganglia classified by conduction velocity and action potential duration. *J Neurophysiol* 1996; 76:1924–1941.

Wall PD, Devor M. Sensory afferent impulses originate from dorsal root ganglia as well as from the periphery in normal and nerve-injured rats. *Pain* 1983; 17:321–339.

Wall PD, Devor M, Inbal R, et al. Autotomy following peripheral nerve lesions: experimental anaesthesia dolorosa. *Pain* 1979; 7:103–113.

Woolf CJ. Evidence for a central component of post-injury pain hypersensitivity. *Nature* 1983; 306:686–688.

Correspondence to: Ron Amir, BPT, PhD, Department of Cell and Animal Biology, Institute of Life Sciences, Hebrew University of Jerusalem, Jerusalem 91904, Israel. Tel: 972 (2) 6585916; Fax: 972 (2) 6520261; email: ronamir@pob.huji.ac.il.

Proceedings of the 9th World Congress on Pain,
Progress in Pain Research and Management,
Vol. 16, edited by M. Devor, M.C. Rowbotham, and
Z. Wiesenfeld-Hallin, IASP Press, Seattle, © 2000.

10

Spontaneous Action Potential Discharge in Cultured Dorsal Root Ganglion Neurons from Patients with Neuropathic Pain

Thomas K. Baumann[a,b] and Melissa E. Martenson[a]

[a]*Department of Neurological Surgery and* [b]*Department of Physiology and Pharmacology, Oregon Health Sciences University, Portland, Oregon, USA*

Neurophysiological studies in animals with various types of peripheral nerve injury have demonstrated that nerve injury causes ectopic action potential discharge in primary afferent neurons. Such ectopic action potential activity in dorsal root ganglion (DRG) neurons is believed to cause allodynia and hyperalgesia. Following experimental nerve injury, action potentials emanate not only from the neuroma at the site of injury, but also from the DRG (Wall and Devor 1983; Burchiel 1984; Devor et al. 1992; Kajander et al. 1992). However, it is not known whether the somata of DRG neurons generate spontaneous action potential discharge in patients with neuropathic pain. Our study examined the incidence of action potential discharge in the somata of DRG neurons obtained from patients treated by ganglionectomy for chronic intractable pain. We show that a large percentage of the cell bodies of DRG neurons from patients with neuropathic pain fire action potentials spontaneously and that a large proportion of the spontaneously active neurons respond to capsaicin. Furthermore, we also observed that 300 nM tetrodotoxin (TTX) did not block spontaneous action potential discharge by the somata of human DRG neurons. We have reported some of our results as abstracts (Baumann et al. 1993, 1994).

MATERIALS AND METHODS

We obtained adult human cervical, thoracic, and lumbar DRG neurons from 20 patients (11 women, 9 men, age 38–72 years) treated surgically (by ganglionectomy) for chronic intractable pain (Table I). Specimens from four patients (HC, HD, HE, and HT, Table I) were included in a previous study on the responses of cultured human DRG neurons to capsaicin and protons (Baumann et al. 1996). The experiments were approved by the institutional review board.

Table I
Patient history and percentage of dorsal root ganglion (DRG) neurons with spontaneous activity (SA)

Sex	Age	Pain Diagnosis	DRG	Neurons (n)	SA (%)	Culture Code
F	49	Post-thoracotomy pain, intercostal neuralgia	Rt T6–T9	15	20	HC
F	54	Intercostal neuralgia	Lt T6–T8	24	8	HD
F	55	Neurofibromatosis, scoliosis, cervical kyphosis	Lt T2–T4	15	40	HE
M	55	Right occipital neuralgia and multiple sclerosis	Rt C3	24	17	HG
F	38	Long history of post-thoracotomy pain	Rt T5–T7	21	29	HI*
M	59	Left post-thoracotomy painful neuralgia	Lt T2–T5	20	35	HJ
M	57	Left occipital neuralgia	Lt C2-C3	25	20	HK
M	41	Occipital neuralgia	Lt C3	17	24	HN
F	48	Post-thoracotomy pain with possible neuroma formation	Rt T6–T8	19	21	HO
M	42	Right T12 neuralgia post transurethral stone resection by laser	Rt T11, T12, L1	38	53	HP
M	56	Left occipital neuralgia	Lt C2	9	22	HQ
M	55	Intractable pain due to metastatic lung carcinoma	Lt T2–T6	19	21	HR
M	72	17-year history of left occipital and retro-auricular pain	Lt C2–C3	15	27	HS
M	47	Chronic pain due to failed back surgery syndrome	T9–T11	20	5	HT
F	49	Pain following resection of a schwannoma	Rt C3–C5	24	25	HU
F	44	Chronic bilateral occipital headache pain after vehicle accident	Bilat C2	1	0	HY
F	38	10-year history of trigeminal neuralgia and multiple sclerosis	Lt C3	3	0	HZ
F	41	Long history of post-thoracotomy pain	Rt T8–T9	22	5	HAA*
F	40	Stump pain resulting from a work-related crush injury	Rt T2	19	32	HAB
F	51	Postmastectomy pain syndrome; intercostal brachial neuralgia	Bilat T2–T5	46	22	HAG
F	39	Intractable pain, intercostal neuralgia	Rt T7–T9	15	7	HAI

Note: Rt = right; Lt = left; Bilat = bilateral; * same patient, but different ganglionectomies; n = number of neurons tested per culture.

Cell culture. Immediately following surgical excision, we immersed the DRG in cold, balanced salt solution with nutrients (BSS; see below for composition) and transported them to the laboratory for processing. The method for dissociation and primary culture was in all aspects identical to that used previously (Baumann et al. 1996), except for longer duration of enzymatic digestion (4.5 hours on average, with a maximum of 7.5 hours). Baumann (1999) describes the procedure in detail. Briefly, the contents of the connective tissue capsule were extirpated, minced, and dissociated enzymatically (with a mixture of 0.1% trypsin, 0.1% collagenase, and 0.01% DNase, w/v). The progress of tissue dissociation was monitored microscopically and the duration of exposure to enzymes adjusted accordingly. Dissociated cells were collected in a solution containing 0.2% soybean trypsin inhibitor, 0.1% bovine serum albumin, and 10% fetal calf serum, washed several times by centrifugation and suspended in a growth medium (L-15/air, Gibco) with added supplements of mouse 7S nerve growth factor and horse serum. Cells were subsequently seeded on polylysine-coated glass coverslips. The cultures were maintained in a humidified air incubator (36°C). One half of the growth medium was replaced with fresh medium every 2–3 days.

Measurement of soma diameter. We used phase-contrast optics (IM inverted microscope, Zeiss) to observe neurons subjected to electrophysiological recording and a calibrated ocular reticle to measure the size of the soma. Most somata were ellipsoid; we calculated the average diameter along the major and minor axes.

Electrophysiology. Recordings were made from 411 cultured DRG neurons at room temperature (approximately 21°C). To make tight-seal, whole-cell recordings we used thick-wall borosilicate glass electrodes (Sutter Instrument Co.) and a patch-clamp amplifier (3900/3911A, Dagan) interfaced to a computer running commercially available software (pClamp, versions 5.1.1. and 6.0.3, Axon Instruments). Recording pipettes typically had resistances of 4 MΩ. We used the main amplifier circuitry to compensate for series resistance and the whole-cell plug-in module (3911A, Dagan) to neutralize membrane capacitance and resistance.

We determined the presence or absence of spontaneous action potential discharge from the presence or absence of action currents upon first breaking the patch membrane and establishing the whole-cell recording (before compensating for access resistance, membrane capacitance, and membrane resistance). During this time the pipette tip potential was held near –60 mV. Subsequently, we applied compensation and measured responses to capsaicin in either current-clamp (by recording action potential discharge with zero holding current applied) or voltage-clamp recording mode (by recording membrane current while the membrane voltage was switched between

–60 and –70 mV every 2.05 seconds so that we could also monitor membrane conductance). The effect of TTX on spontaneous action potential discharge was examined under current clamp recording conditions.

Composition and application of solutions. Recording solutions made from distilled, deionized water were passed through filters of 0.2 μm pore size (Millipore). Patch electrodes were filled with a solution composed of 160 mM KCl, 7.4 mM EGTA (ethylene glycol-bis (β-aminoethyl ether) N, N, N´, N´-tetraacetic acid), and 9.1 mM HEPES (N-[2-hydroxyethyl] piperazine-N´-[2-ethanesulfonic acid]) (pH adjusted to 7.2 with 1 N KOH). The external balanced salt solution (BSS) had the following composition (in millimoles per liter): NaCl 137.7, KCl 5.0, $CaCl_2$ 1.0, $MgSO_4$ 1.2, H_3PO_4 2.0, D,L-alanine 5.0, glucose 5.5, HEPES 32.0 (pH adjusted to 7.35 with 1 N NaOH). Capsaicin-containing physiological solutions (1 and 10 μM) were prepared by dissolving, respectively, 9.2 and 92 μL of 5.45 mM capsaicin stock solution in 50 mL BSS. Lower concentrations of capsaicin (30, 100, and 300 nM) were made using 9.2 μL of 0.181, 0.545, or 1.69 mM capsaicin stock solution, respectively. To make the stock solutions, we dissolved capsaicin (Fluka) in 98% ethanol.

All solutions were supplied by gravity via a glass pipe placed approximately 100 μm from the neuron under study (flow rate ca. 0.4 mL/min). The volume of fluid in the recording chamber (0.6 mL) was kept constant by a remote suction device, and the input to the glass pipe was switched manually by operating a six-way valve. Capsaicin stimuli were applied for 1 minute, and TTX was applied for 30 seconds. We excluded the possibility of inadvertent desensitization or sensitization of neurons from previous application of chemical stimuli by studying only one neuron per coverslip and rinsing the recording chamber with BSS between recordings.

Data analysis. We retrieved current-clamp recording traces stored by the computer, counted the action potentials, and divided by elapsed recording time to determine mean discharge rate. Classification of neurons as capsaicin responders or nonresponders was based upon visual inspection of voltage-clamp responses recorded at slow speed (1 cm/min) on the chart recorder. Neurons that displayed unambiguous, stimulus-related currents ≥20 pA were classified as responders (Baumann et al. 1996). We used Clampfit software (pClamp, Axon Instruments) to determine stimulus-evoked current amplitudes. We calculated net current amplitude by subtracting the baseline holding current (measured 4 seconds prior to stimulus application) from the maximum sustained inward current registered during the 1-minute stimulus application. All descriptive statistics are reported as means and standard deviations.

RESULTS

We tested 411 adult human DRG neurons after 1–90 days in culture (12 ± 12 days). The sample included small to medium-size (Dyck et al. 1993) neurons (diameter 46 ± 10 μm, range 19–74 μm, n = 389). Most cultures (19/21) contained neurons that had spontaneous action potential discharge in the absence of any intentional stimulus (96/411 neurons). Among the active cultures, as many as 53% (23 ± 12%) of the neurons had background discharge. Table I reports the incidence of spontaneous activity, by patient and culture.

Many of the spontaneously active neurons responded to capsaicin (50/60 neurons tested with ≥ 30 nM capsaicin in either current- or voltage-clamp mode). Spontaneously active cells tested with capsaicin, irrespective of concentration, ranged in size from 29 to 74 μm. The largest human DRG neuron studied (74 μm mean diameter) was both spontaneously active and capsaicin-sensitive (100 μm). Most voltage-clamped, spontaneously active neurons responded to capsaicin with an inward current (Table II). As observed previously (Baumann et al. 1996), the amplitude of the capsaicin-evoked current increased with the concentration of capsaicin applied.

Spontaneously active neurons displayed either regular (not illustrated) or irregular discharge (Fig. 1). Discharge rates ranged from 0.03 to 13.9 impulses/second with 14/37 neurons displaying a rate ≥1 impulse/second. The soma diameter of spontaneously active neurons (46 ± 9 μm) did not differ significantly from that of quiescent neurons (46 ± 10 μm). Similarly, time in culture of spontaneously active neurons (13 ± 11 days in vitro) did not differ significantly from that of cells lacking spontaneous discharge (11 ± 12 days in vitro). Spontaneous discharge, tested in five capsaicin-responsive neurons (all from culture HAG, see Table I), was resistant to a moderate concentration (300 nM) of TTX (Fig. 1).

Table II
Response of spontaneously active human DRG neurons to capsaicin

Capsaicin	30 nM	100 nM	1 μM	10 μM
No. neurons tested	6	33	7	2
Responders	4	24	7	2
Nonresponders	2	9	0	0
Whole-cell current (pA)	–20 to –148	–39 to >–3702*	–504 to >–10,000*	–441 to >–9165*

* Current saturated the amplifier.

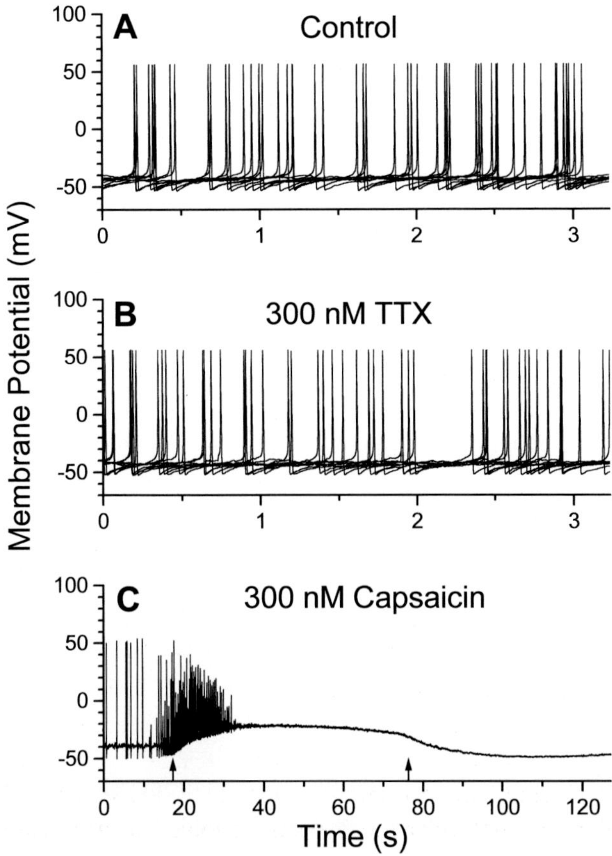

Fig. 1. Spontaneous action potential discharge and capsaicin response of a cultured human DRG neuron. (A) Relatively irregular background discharge, average frequency 1.5 impulses/second. (B) Lack of an effect of 300 nM tetrodotoxin on spontaneous discharge of this neuron. Superimposed traces in both A and B represent 10 contiguous sweeps. (C) Depolarization and action potential discharge evoked by a 1-minute application (between arrows) of 300 nM capsaicin (current-clamp recording, no holding current applied to the recording electrode in A–C). Background action potential discharge was silenced after capsaicin despite return of membrane potential from depolarization. Some action potentials do not display full amplitude because the computer program could only store 16,384 points/sweep, which led to undersampling. The same neuron is shown in all three panels, recorded after 3 days in culture.

DISCUSSION

Our study shows for the first time that many somata of DRG neurons from patients with neuropathic pain fire action potentials spontaneously. Spontaneous action potential discharge occurred in a substantial proportion of the somata. Most of the spontaneously active neurons were excited by capsaicin and thus could be regarded as nociceptive (Baumann et al. 1991; Gold 1996).

Notably, 300 nM TTX did not affect the discharge frequency of spontaneously active human DRG neurons, and all five neurons tested with TTX were subsequently excited by capsaicin. If this preliminary finding proves to be typical of spontaneously active human DRG neurons, it would suggest that TTX-sensitive sodium conductances are not responsible for driving the spontaneous discharge in capsaicin-sensitive nociceptive human DRG neurons.

Given the lack of control human DRG neurons from patients without intractable pain, we cannot discount the possibility that the incidence of spontaneous activity would have been no different had we been able to obtain such controls. Aspects of the culturing process that could have caused a high incidence of spontaneous activity include the prolonged exposure to enzymes, which is required to dissociate adult human DRG neurons, and the chronic axotomy, which is inherent in the dissociation and culturing process. However, studies using cultured DRG neurons from rats with nerve injury reported a similarly high incidence of spontaneously active neurons (approximately 20%), but found a negligible (essentially 0%) incidence of spontaneous action potential discharge for DRG neurons from rats without prior nerve injury (Petersen et al. 1996; Study and Kral 1996).

While not conclusive, the results of our study strongly suggest that abnormal spontaneous activity of the somata of nociceptive DRG neurons may be a source of pain in patients with nerve injury. If future experiments confirm these findings, the cell culture approach could be applied to examine the cellular and molecular mechanisms involved in neuropathic pain in humans.

ACKNOWLEDGMENTS

Supported in part by a PHS grant R01 NS37149, a grant from the American Cancer Society (Oregon Chapter), and a grant from the National Headache Foundation (to T.K. Baumann). We thank Dr. Kim J. Burchiel for providing the human tissue and Drs. Susan L. Ingram and Joseph H. Arguelles for participating in some experiments.

REFERENCES

Baumann TK. Human spinal sensory ganglia. In: Haynes LW (Ed). *The Neuron in Tissue Culture*, IBRO Handbook Series. New York: John Wiley and Sons, 1999, pp 398–406.

Baumann TK, Simone DA, Shain C, LaMotte RH. Neurogenic hyperalgesia: the search for the primary cutaneous afferent fibers that contribute to capsaicin-induced pain and hyperalgesia. *J Neurophysiol* 1991; 66:212–227.

Baumann TK, Burchiel KJ, Ingram SL, Martenson ME. Patch clamp recordings from cultured adult human dorsal root ganglion neurons. *Proceedings of the American Association of Neurological Surgeons 61st Annual Meeting* [abstract]. 1993, p 432.

Baumann TK, Burchiel KJ, Martenson ME, Ingram SL. Chemo- and mechanosensitivity of adult human DRG neurons. *Proceedings of the American Pain Society 13th Annual Meeting* [abstract]. 1994, p A-139.

Baumann TK, Burchiel KJ, Ingram SL, Martenson ME. Responses of adult human dorsal root ganglion neurons in culture to capsaicin and low pH. *Pain* 1996; 65:31–38.

Burchiel KJ. Effects of electrical and mechanical stimulation on two foci of spontaneous activity which develop in primary afferent neurons after peripheral axotomy. *Pain* 1984; 18:249–265.

Devor M, Wall PD, Catalan N. Systemic lidocaine silences ectopic neuroma and DRG discharge without blocking nerve conduction. *Pain* 1992; 48:261–268.

Gold MS. Co-expression of nociceptor properties in dorsal root ganglion neurons from the adult rat *in vitro*. *Neuroscience* 1996; 71:265–275.

Kajander KC, Wakisaka S, Bennett GJ. Spontaneous discharge originates in the dorsal root ganglion at the onset of a painful peripheral neuropathy in the rat. *Neurosci Lett* 1992; 138:225–228.

Petersen M, Zhang J, Zhang JM, LaMotte RH. Abnormal spontaneous activity and responses to norepinephrine in dissociated dorsal root ganglion cells after chronic nerve constriction. *Pain* 1996; 67:391–397.

Study RE, Kral MG. Spontaneous action potential activity in isolated dorsal root ganglion neurons from rats with a painful neuropathy. *Pain* 1996; 65:235–242.

Wall PD, Devor M. Sensory afferent impulses originate from dorsal root ganglia as well as from the periphery in normal and nerve injured rats. *Pain* 1983; 17:321–339.

Correspondence to: Thomas K. Baumann, PhD, Department of Neurological Surgery, L472, Oregon Health Sciences University, Portland, OR 97201, USA. Tel: 503-494-4985; Fax: 503-494-7161; email: baumannt@ohsu.edu.

Proceedings of the 9th World Congress on Pain,
Progress in Pain Research and Management,
Vol. 16, edited by M. Devor, M.C. Rowbotham, and
Z. Wiesenfeld-Hallin, IASP Press, Seattle, © 2000.

11

Action of the Hyperpolarization-Activated Current Blocker ZD7288 in Dorsal Root Ganglion Neurons Classified by Conduction Velocity

Junichi Yagi,[a,b] Naoki Hirai,[a] and Rhyuji Sumino[b]

[a]Department of Physiology, Kyorin University School of Medicine, Tokyo, Japan; [b]Department of Physiology, Nihon University School of Dentistry, Tokyo, Japan

A hyperpolarization-activated current has been found in a variety of neurons, including dorsal root ganglion (DRG) neurons and cardiac pacemaker myocytes, and is generally termed the I_h or H-current in neurons and I_f in cardiac cells (Yanagihara and Irisawa 1980; Mayer and Westbrook 1983; DiFrancesco et al. 1986; McCormick and Pape 1990; Scroggs et al. 1994; Villière and McLachlan 1996). Under voltage clamp conditions, I_h is evoked by a hyperpolarizing voltage step as a slowly activating inward cation (Na^+ and K^+) current. Since I_h is active at a membrane potential more negative than approximately –50 mV and does not inactivate, the partial activation of I_h at the resting level of excitable cells is thought to participate in determining the resting membrane potential. I_h is also called the "pacemaker current" because it is assumed to produce the pacemaker depolarization during generation of oscillatory activity and to play a role in accelerating the firing frequency. Therefore, modulation of I_h by neurotransmitters, intracellular second messengers, or certain chemical agents could affect cell excitability.

In rat DRG neurons I_h is observed in most medium and large cells, but infrequently in the smallest cells (Scroggs et al. 1994). In view of the properties of I_h, it might be expected that I_h would contribute to facilitating the ectopic spontaneous discharges of DRG neurons that develop after injury to a peripheral nerve. Our study evaluated the effects of ZD7288 (Zeneca

Pharmaceuticals), a bradycardiac agent known as the I_h blocker (BoSmith et al. 1993; Maccaferri and McBain 1996; Gasparini and DiFrancesco 1997; Lüthi et al. 1998), on I_h and neuronal excitability in rat DRG neurons. More specifically, we wished to investigate the possibility that the ZD7288-induced inhibition of I_h might decrease the discharge frequency of abnormally active DRG neurons and produce antinociceptive effects.

MATERIALS AND METHODS

Whole-cell patch-clamp recordings from adult rat DRG neurons were made using isolated whole ganglia with their sciatic nerves attached. The aim of this novel approach was to classify the DRG neurons according to axonal conduction velocity.

SURGICAL AND CELL PREPARATION

Adult female rats (Sprague Dawley, 6–14 weeks old) were anesthetized deeply with sodium pentobarbital (80 mg/kg) injected intraperitoneally. Bilateral L4 and L5 DRGs along with the sciatic nerves were excised and placed immediately in oxygenated artificial cerebrospinal fluid (ACSF) comprising: 125 mM NaCl, 3.8 mM KCl, 2.0 mM $CaCl_2$, 1.0 mM $MgCl_2$, 1.2 mM KH_2PO_4, 26 mM $NaHCO_3$, 10 mM D-glucose (pH = 7.4). The preparations were digested with collagenase (1 mg/mL, Wako) for 30 minutes at room temperature (24°–27°C), after which the epineurium around each was removed as carefully as possible. Each ganglion was placed on the bottom of a recording chamber on the stage of an upright microscope (Nikon, E600FN) fitted with Nomarski optics. The ganglion was then superfused with ACSF equilibrated with 95% O_2 and 5% CO_2. The sciatic nerve was drawn out of the chamber into an adjacent narrow trough where it was laid over two pairs of bipolar stimulating electrodes with cathodes 10 mm apart. The tissue and continuous satellite cells overlying the somata were loosened by focal application of collagenase (10 mg/mL, Wako) and thermolysine (100 U/mL, Sigma) through a pipette for 10–30 minutes at room temperature (Yagi and Sumino 1998).

In some experiments designed to study the effects of ZD7288 on spontaneous activity of DRG neurons, the preparations were obtained from rats that previously had sciatic nerve transection near the sciatic notch under anesthesia with pentobarbital (50 mg/kg).

ELECTROPHYSIOLOGICAL TECHNIQUES

Patch pipettes were made by pulling borosilicate thin-walled glass capillaries (GC150T-10, Clark Electromedical). The standard internal solution comprised: 147 mM KCl, 5 mM NaCl, 0.1 mM $CaCl_2$, 2 mM $MgCl_2$, 1.0 mM EGTA, 5 mM HEPES, 2 mM Na_2ATP, and 0.2 mM Na_3GTP. The pH of the solution was adjusted to 7.2 with KOH. The pipette filled with this internal solution had a resistance of 1.4–2.4 MΩ. A continuous satellite cell around the target DRG neuron was ruptured by applying positive pressure through the patch pipette. Negative pressure was then immediately applied to form a gigaohm seal (>5 GΩ) (Yagi and Sumino 1998). Voltage- and current-clamp experiments were carried out using an Axopatch 200B patch-clamp amplifier (Axon Instruments) at room temperature (24°–27°C). The DRG neurons were classified, according to axonal conduction velocity, as Aα/β (>10 m/s), Aδ (2–7 m/s), and C-type (<1 m/s).

RESULTS

MAGNITUDES OF I_h IN DRG NEURONS OF DIFFERENT TYPES

The current densities of peak I_h were estimated in DRG neurons classified according to their axonal conduction velocity. Fig. 1 shows representative recordings of the somatic action potential and I_h in Aα/β and C-type DRG neurons. Under voltage-clamp conditions, the inward currents evoked by a hyperpolarizing voltage step in DRG neurons consisted of two current components: an instantaneous inward current (I_{inst}) and a slowly activating inward current (I_h). We observed I_h in all 29 Aα/β, all 3 Aδ, and 9 of 14 C-type DRG neurons, and while the amplitudes of I_h were obviously large in Aα/β-type cells, they were small in Aδ and C-type cells. The magnitudes of peak I_h evoked by a 400-ms voltage step to –120 mV from –50 mV were normalized to cell membrane capacitance for each DRG neuron to estimate the values per unit area of the cell membrane. The normalized magnitude of I_h tended to be proportional to the conduction velocity, and averaged 93.2 ± 7.2 (SE) pA/pF (n = 29), 22.2 ± 3.1 pA/pF (n = 3), and 4.2 ± 0.9 pA/pF (n = 9) in Aα/β-, Aδ-, and C-type DRG neurons, respectively. The current density of I_h was significantly larger in Aα/β-type DRG neurons than in Aδ- and C-type DRG neurons (one-way factorial ANOVA test, $P < 0.001$).

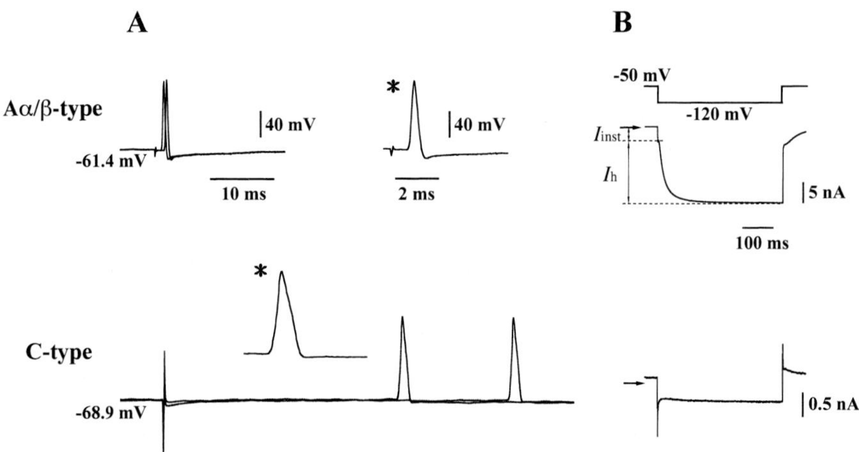

Fig. 1. Representative examples of somatic action potential and hyperpolarization-activated current (I_h) in Aα/β- and C-type dorsal root ganglion (DRG) neurons. (A) Somatic action potentials evoked by stimulating the sciatic nerve trunk with two pairs of bipolar stimulating electrodes. The conduction velocities were 25.4 m/s and 0.59 m/s in the Aα/β- and C-type, respectively. Insets (*) show the action potential shapes on an expanded time scale. (B) Whole-cell currents of the DRG neurons in panel A recorded under voltage-clamp conditions in response to a 400-ms step (upper trace) to –120 mV from –50 mV. The inward currents consisted of an instantaneous inward current (I_{inst}) and a slowly activating inward current (I_h). While the amplitude of I_h was large in the Aα/β-type, it was small in the C-type cell. The arrows indicate the zero-current level.

BLOCKADE OF I_h BY ZD7288

In voltage-clamp mode, the effects of ZD7288 on I_{inst} and I_h evoked by hyperpolarization were investigated. As shown in Fig. 2, about 1 minute after the start of ZD7288 (40 μM) perfusion, the amplitude of I_h started to decline slowly, and by 4 minutes was fully blocked. It did not recover even after the preparation had been perfused with ACSF free of ZD7288 for 1 hour. In contrast, ZD7288 seemed to have little influence on I_{inst}. I_{inst} includes a leak current (I_{leak}) carried largely by potassium ions or an inward rectifier potassium current (I_{ir}) (Scroggs et al. 1994). We thus can conclude that ZD7288 selectively blocks I_h, but has little, if any, influence on I_{leak} and I_{ir}.

A concentration–response curve was generated for ZD7288 (data not shown), and 40 μM ZD7288 was found to evoke almost saturated responses. In the presence of 40 μM ZD7288, I_h was inhibited by 97.2 ± 0.7% (SE) (n = 11) and 100 ± 0.0% (n = 3) in Aα/β and C-type DRG neurons, respectively. Curve fitting by the Hill equation yielded values of 1.2 μM for the half-maximal effective concentration and 1.1 for the Hill coefficient (n = 13).

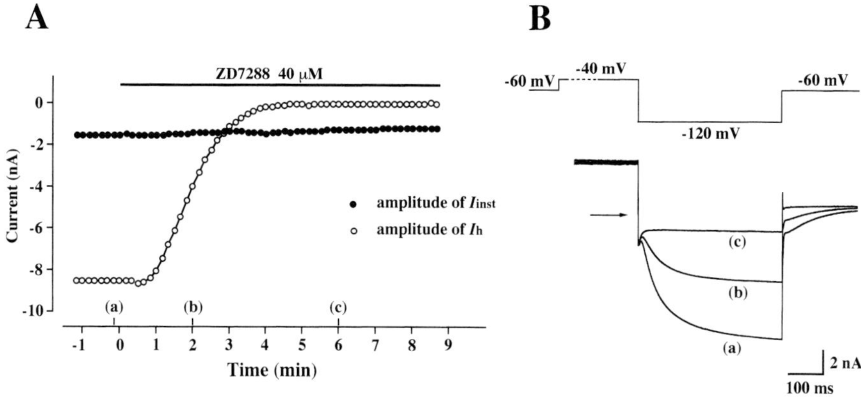

Fig. 2. Time course of the amplitudes of I_h and I_{inst} during ZD7288 application. In voltage-clamp mode, whole-cell currents of an Aα/β-type (conduction velocity = 31.5 m/s) DRG neuron were recorded in response to a twin pulse protocol comprising a 500-ms depolarizing prepulse to –40 mV from a holding potential of –60 mV, which was applied to block I_h activated tonically at the holding level, followed by a 400-ms test pulse to –120 mV. The twin pulses were delivered every 10 s before and during application of 40 μM ZD7288. I_{inst} amplitude was measured at 7 ms after initiation of the test pulse to avoid the minimized capacitative transient, and I_h amplitude was determined by subtracting the I_{inst} amplitude from that of the total peak current. (A) Plots of I_{inst} (filled circles) and I_h (open circles) amplitudes versus time. ZD7288 was applied by superfusion during the period indicated by the horizontal bar. Application of ZD7288 resulted in nearly complete blockade of I_h with little influence on I_{inst}. (B) Twin pulse protocol (upper trace) and representative examples of raw current traces (lower traces) recorded at times a, b, and c labeled in panel A. The arrows indicate the zero-current level.

EFFECTS OF ZD7288 ON DRG NEURONAL EXCITABILITY

We then investigated the influence of ZD7288 on DRG neuronal excitability in current-clamp mode. All of 5 Aα/β- and all 4 C-type DRG neurons that possessed I_h responded to 40 μM ZD7288 with hyperpolarization (>2 mV) with mean (± SE) values of 6.7 ± 1.9 mV (n = 5) and 4.7 ± 1.0 mV (n = 4), respectively. In addition, in intact Aα/β-type cells, ZD7288 prevented the repetitive action potentials elicited by injecting a depolarizing current pulse and also blocked time-dependent rectification produced by injecting a hyperpolarizing current pulse (Fig. 3A).

Next, we tested the effects of ZD7288 on spontaneous firing activity in injured Aα/β-type DRG neurons. An injured Aα/β-type DRG neuron illustrated in Fig. 3B displayed membrane potential oscillations and spontaneous discharge under conditions of positive direct current (DC) injection. ZD7288 reduced the firing frequency under conditions where the membrane potential was held constant by DC. While ZD7288 did not modify the action potential wave form in the depolarization and repolarization phase, it reduced the depolarizing influence during afterhyperpolarization (AHP).

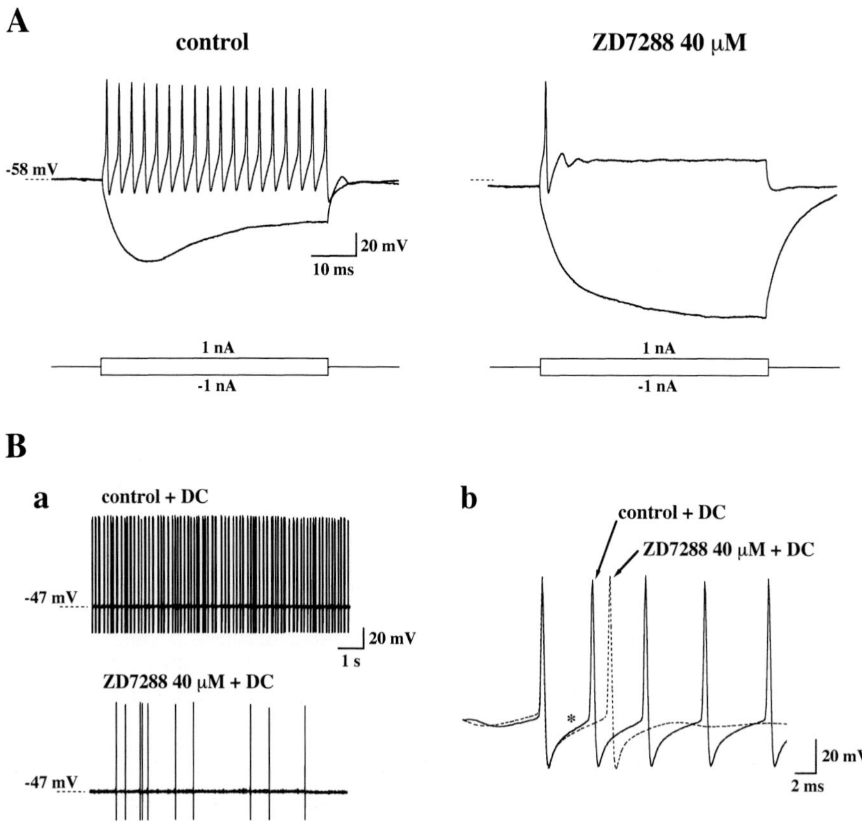

Fig. 3. Effects of ZD7288 on DRG neuronal excitability. (A) Current-clamp recordings of an intact Aα/β-type (conduction velocity = 23.6 m/s) DRG neuron. The resting potential before drug application was –58.0 mV (indicated by the dotted lines). Application of 40 μM ZD7288 induced a 4.0-mV hyperpolarization of the resting membrane potential. ZD7288 prevented the repetitive action potentials elicited by injection of a 50-ms depolarizing current pulse and also blocked time-dependent rectification produced by injection of a hyperpolarizing current pulse. (B) Current-clamp recordings of an Aα/β-type (conduction velocity = 31.5 m/s) DRG neuron obtained from a rat that had sciatic nerve transection 5 days previously. This neuron was quiescent at the original membrane potential of –61.4 mV. When the membrane potential was depolarized to be more positive than –52 mV by direct current (DC), this cell exhibited spontaneous firing activity. (a) Spontaneous discharges before (control) and during application of 40 μM ZD7288. The membrane potential was held at –47 mV (dotted line) by manually controlling the DC. Before drug application, a high-frequency bursting discharge pattern with irregular interburst intervals was observed (mean over a 10-s period: 46.3 Hz). ZD7288 reduced the firing frequency (mean: 3.2 Hz). In (b), two bursting discharges recorded in the control (continuous line) and in the presence of ZD7288 (dotted line) in (a) were superimposed and shown over an expanded scale. Note that ZD7288 led to a reduction of the depolarizing influence (*) during the after hyperpolarization, resulting in delayed initiation of the second action potential.

DISCUSSION

ZD7288 blocked I_h selectively in rat DRG neurons. In current-clamp experiments, ZD7288 induced hyperpolarization of the membrane and reduced the frequency of repetitive action potentials evoked by a depolarizing current pulse. The actions of ZD7288 on rat DRG neurons reported here are similar to those described for other cells (BoSmith et al. 1993; Maccaferri and McBain 1996; Gasparini and DiFrancesco 1997; Lüthi et al. 1998). Since I_h is activated partially at a membrane potential of around –60 mV, which is close to the resting membrane potential of DRG neurons, it has been assumed that I_h contributes to the resting membrane potential (Mayer and Westbrook 1983; Scroggs et al. 1994; Yagi and Sumino 1998). The resting potential is determined by the counterbalancing actions of some ionic conductances. The partial activation of I_h at the resting level will play a role in positively shifting the membrane potential toward the reversal potential of I_h (–30 to –40 mV). It follows from this view that inhibition of I_h by ZD7288 would lead to a small hyperpolarization. In addition, I_h is expected to contribute to shaping an AHP. I_h activated by membrane hyperpolarization during the AHP might exert a depolarizing influence, even if the amount of the activated I_h is small, resulting in acceleration of repetitive action potentials. This action is supported by the finding that ZD7288 decreased the slope of the depolarizing influence during the AHPs even after compensation for the ZD7288-induced hyperpolarization (Fig. 3B). Hence, it could be concluded that I_h is involved in the excitability of DRG neurons and is able to elevate the firing frequency.

After injury to a peripheral nerve, a proportion of the DRG neurons develop spontaneous discharges (Wall and Devor 1983; Burchiel 1984; Petersen et al. 1996; Study and Kral 1996) with Aα/β-type DRG neurons in particular discharging spontaneously at 10–50 Hz (Kajander and Bennett 1992). This ability to produce such a high discharge frequency might be partially caused by Aα/β-type cells possessing a high density of I_h channels. In contrast, Aδ- and C-type DRG neurons have a low density of I_h channels. However, it is still likely that I_h participates to some extent in determining the neuronal excitability even in Aδ- and C-type neurons, because conductance of other ions that counteracts the action of I_h near the resting level is also low in these neurons. In fact, some of the tested C-type DRG neurons responded to ZD7288 with hyperpolarization.

Although the question of the functional roles of I_h in DRG neurons is still open, our results indicate that I_h may be associated with the "frequency code" for receptor potential in peripheral terminals of primary sensory neurons. However, we would also like to highlight another action of I_h—that is,

I_h could be associated with ectopic spontaneous activity in DRG neurons. It is well known that after a nerve is injured, DRG neurons discharge spontaneously, causing abnormal pain. It is possible that I_h participates in facilitating the firing discharges in such spontaneously active DRG neurons. Recently, we observed that ZD7288-induced inhibition of I_h reduced the spontaneous activity in nerve-injured Aα/β-DRG neurons (Fig. 3B). We suggest that local application of ZD7288 to injured sensory neurons might produce antinociceptive effects by inhibiting I_h. In addition, the action of ZD7288 could have the advantage of not completely blocking the cell excitability, so the cell retains the capacity to conduct impulses. From this study it appears that ZD7288 may be useful for the clinical treatment of neuropathic pain.

ACKNOWLEDGMENTS

We thank Zeneca Pharmaceuticals (Macclesfield, UK) for kindly supplying the ZD7288. This work was supported by a Grant-in-Aid for Scientific Research (11780595) from the Japanese Ministry of Education, Science and Culture, a Research Project Grant from Kyorin University, and the Sato Foundation of Nihon University.

REFERENCES

BoSmith RE, Briggs I, Sturgess NC. Inhibitory actions of ZENECA ZD7288 on whole-cell hyperpolarization activated inward current (I_f) in guinea-pig dissociated sinoatrial node cells. *Br J Pharmacol* 1993; 110:343–349.

Burchiel KJ. Spontaneous impulse generation in normal and denervated dorsal root ganglia: sensitivity to alpha-adrenergic stimulation and hypoxia. *Exp Neurol* 1984; 85:257–272.

DiFrancesco D, Ferroni A, Mazzanti M, Tromba C. Properties of the hyperpolarizing-activated current (i_f) in cells isolated from the rabbit sino-atrial node. *J Physiol (Lond)* 1986; 377:61–88.

Gasparini S, DiFrancesco D. Action of the hyperpolarization-activated current (I_h) blocker ZD 7288 in hippocampal CA1 neurons. *Pflügers Arch* 1997; 435:99–106.

Kajander KC, Bennett GJ. Onset of a painful peripheral neuropathy in rat: a partial and differential deafferentation and spontaneous discharge in A beta and A delta primary afferent neurons. *J Neurophysiol* 1992; 68:734–744.

Lüthi A, Bal T, McCormick DA. Periodicity of thalamic spindle waves is abolished by ZD7288, a blocker of I_h. *J Neurophysiol* 1998; 79:3284–3289.

Maccaferri G, McBain CJ. The hyperpolarization-activated current (I_h) and its contribution to pacemaker activity in rat CA1 hippocampal stratum oriens-alveus interneurones. *J Physiol (Lond)* 1996; 497:119–130.

Mayer ML, Westbrook GL. A voltage-clamp analysis of inward (anomalous) rectification in mouse spinal sensory ganglion neurons. *J Physiol (Lond)* 1983; 340:19–45.

McCormick DA, Pape HC. Properties of a hyperpolarization-activated cation current and its role in rhythmic oscillation in thalamic relay neurons. *J Physiol (Lond)* 1990; 431:291–318.

Petersen M, Zhang J, Zhang JM, LaMotte RH. Abnormal spontaneous activity and responses to norepinephrine in dissociated dorsal root ganglion cells after chronic nerve constriction. *Pain* 1996; 67:391–397.

Scroggs RS, Todorovic SM, Anderson EG, Fox AP. Variation in I_H, I_{IR}, and I_{LEAK} between acutely isolated adult rat dorsal root ganglion neurons of different size. *J Neurophysiol* 1994; 71:271–279.

Study RE, Kral MG. Spontaneous action potential activity in isolated dorsal root ganglion neurons from rats with a painful neuropathy. *Pain* 1996; 65:235–242.

Villière V, McLachlan EM. Electrophysiological properties of neurons in intact rat dorsal root ganglia classified by conduction velocity and action potential duration. *J Neurophysiol* 1996; 76:1924–1941.

Wall PD, Devor M. Sensory afferent impulses originate from dorsal root ganglia as well as from the periphery in normal and nerve injured rats. *Pain* 1983; 17:321–339.

Yagi J, Sumino R. Inhibition of a hyperpolarization-activated current by clonidine in rat dorsal root ganglion neurons. *J Neurophysiol* 1998; 80:1094–1104.

Yanagihara K, Irisawa H. Inward current activated during hyperpolarization in the rabbit sinoatrial node cell. *Pflügers Arch* 1980; 385:11–19.

Correspondence to: Junichi Yagi, DDS, PhD, Department of Physiology, Kyorin University School of Medicine, 6-20-2 Shinkawa, Mitaka-shi, Tokyo 181-8611, Japan. Tel: 81-422-47-5511 (ext. 3445); Fax: 81-422-44-1816; email: jun-y@po.iijnet.or.jp.

Proceedings of the 9th World Congress on Pain,
Progress in Pain Research and Management,
Vol. 16, edited by M. Devor, M.C. Rowbotham, and
Z. Wiesenfeld-Hallin, IASP Press, Seattle, © 2000.

12

Altered Excitability of Large-Diameter Cutaneous Afferents following Nerve Injury: Consequences for Chronic Pain[1]

Jeffery D. Kocsis[a,b] and Marshall Devor[c]

[a]Department of Neurology, PVA/EPVA Neuroscience and Regeneration Research Center, Yale University School of Medicine, New Haven, Connecticut, USA; [b]Rehabilitation Research and Development Center, Department of Veterans Affairs Medical Center, West Haven, Connecticut, USA; [c]Department of Cell and Animal Biology, Institute of Life Sciences, Hebrew University of Jerusalem, Jerusalem, Israel

Disease or trauma affecting peripheral nerves often results in the development of chronic, frequently intractable pain. The clinical importance of these "neuropathic" pain syndromes provides a strong incentive for understanding the underlying physiological mechanisms. There is a general consensus that both peripheral (PNS) and central (CNS) nervous system processes play a role in these syndromes. Normally, pain is experienced when signals reach the brain as a result of impulse activity in peripheral nociceptors, nonmyelinated C fibers, or lightly myelinated Aδ fibers. For this reason, discussions of pain mechanisms almost always focus on nociceptors. However, there is now good evidence that activity in non-nociceptive, fast-conducting, thickly myelinated Aβ touch afferents may evoke pain in the event of inflammation or after nerve injury (e.g., Campbell et al. 1988; Price et al. 1989, 1992; Koltzenburg et al. 1992, 1994; Torebjörk et al. 1992, 1995; Lindblom 1994; Rowbotham and Fields 1996). Allodynia (pain from normally nonpainful stimuli) in these cases is believed to result from abnormal central processing of low-threshold tactile inputs by CNS mechanisms collectively termed "central sensitization" (Hardy et al. 1952; Devor et al. 1991; Woolf 1991; Baba et al. 1999). For example, elevated background

---

[1] Mini-review based on a congress workshop.

activity may partially depolarize spinal convergent neurons, rendering them more responsive to otherwise nonpainful tactile signals. Peptides released by active nociceptors may enable normally blocked glutamate-sensitive NMDA (N-methyl D-aspartate) receptors and amplify postsynaptic effects of low-threshold glutaminergic afferent inputs. Finally, recent work suggests that Aβ fibers, which normally terminate in dorsal horn lamina III, may sprout after nerve injury, form new synapses in the substantia gelatinosa, and hence activate pain-signaling spinal neurons (Shortland and Woolf 1993; Kohama et al. 1999).

The ability of Aβ activity to evoke pain means that under conditions of central sensitization, changes in the excitability of large-diameter myelinated axons and their cell bodies may play a crucial role in the pathogenesis of chronic pain sensation. Moreover, an emerging body of evidence suggests that in the event of nerve injury, Aβ afferents themselves might be able to trigger and maintain central sensitization (e.g., Ma and Woolf 1996; Mannion et al. 1999; Michael et al. 1999; Liu et al. 2000). Thus, Aβ afferents may contribute to neuropathic pain in several ways (Devor and Seltzer 1999): (1) They are the active element in cutaneous tactile allodynia (in the presence of central sensitization); (2) spontaneous ectopic discharge of Aβ afferents contributes to ongoing pain (in the presence of central sensitization); (3) ectopic mechanosensitivity of Aβ afferents at sites of nerve injury and associated dorsal root ganglia (DRGs) contributes to pain on movement and deep palpation (in the presence of central sensitization); and (4) Aβ activity may contribute to central sensitization itself. In light of the potential importance of altered activity in Aβ touch afferents to the pathophysiology of chronic pain, this chapter will summarize some of the electrophysiological and biophysical changes that may occur in these neurons following nerve injury.

ECTOPIC REPETITIVE FIRING OF INJURED PERIPHERAL AXONS

Important early observations indicated that the axons of injured nerves fire abnormally to produce spontaneous impulse activity, ectopic mechanosensitivity, and abnormal responses to adrenaline and other chemical agonists (Fig. 1A; Kirk 1974; Wall and Gutnick 1974; Govrin-Lippmann and Devor 1978; reviewed by Devor and Seltzer 1999). While the prevalence of axons that show ectopic activity after nerve injury can be determined with some accuracy (Fig. 1B), information about the types of afferents that preferentially generate ectopic firing is much more difficult to obtain. Axotomy disconnects the peripheral receptor ending from the proximal preserved axon,

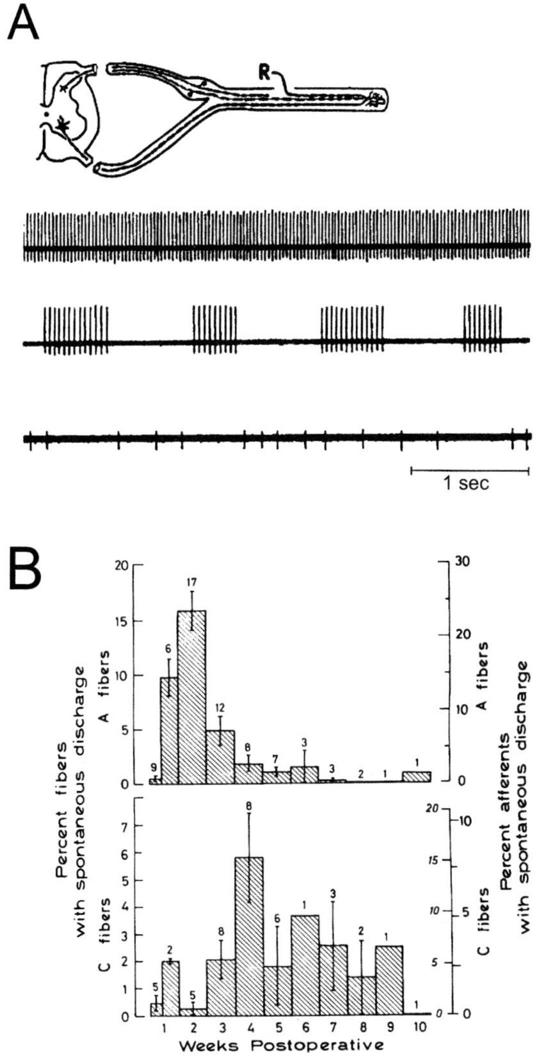

Fig. 1. Spontaneous ectopic discharge generated in a chronic sciatic nerve end neuroma in vivo. (A) Sketch of the teased-fiber recording method, with examples of typical spontaneous firing patterns obtained in experiments using adult rats. The top two traces illustrate tonic and interrupted (bursty) autorhythmic firing in fast-conducting afferent A fibers. The bottom trace illustrates the slow, irregular firing pattern typical of neuroma C fibers. (B) Prevalence of spontaneous ectopic discharge in afferent A and C fibers in rat neuromas as a function of time following sciatic nerve section. The left scale refers to all axons sampled; the right scale refers to afferent fibers only (see Devor and Seltzer 1999).

so receptor typing cannot be accomplished directly. Nonetheless, some information can be obtained from conduction velocity and threshold measurements, by comparing recordings from dorsal (sensory) versus ventral (motor) roots, and from study of cutaneous versus muscle nerves (Devor and Seltzer 1999).

Such studies indicate that the great bulk of spontaneous ectopic activity is generated in sensory, rather than motor fibers. Aβ and Aδ afferents are represented roughly according to their numbers in the nerve, with activity very prominent during the first 2 weeks postinjury and then subsiding. C fibers are under-represented in the ectopic barrage at short postinjury times and are over-represented in chronic preparations (Fig. 1B). With regard to receptor type, slowly adapting afferents, particularly muscle and joint proprioceptors, appear to make up the bulk of the spontaneous A-fiber discharge in mixed nerves. Cutaneous afferents show mechanosensitivity, but relatively little spontaneous activity (Johnson and Munson 1991; Proske et al. 1995; Tal and Devor 1998; Michaelis et al. 2000). These observations suggest that neuroma endbulbs and sprouts develop the same types of sensitivities that the terminal region of the neuron had before the nerve injury (Devor et al. 1990; Koschorke et al. 1991; Michaelis et al. 1995). This speculation is attractive because the transduction properties of an afferent are mostly determined by the types of transducer, receptor, and channel proteins produced in the cell soma and transported down to the sensory axon end.

Regardless of the type of nerve injury, ectopic firing in A afferents is usually rhythmic. That is, the interval between adjacent impulses within a train is highly regular, typically falling within the range of 35–65 ms. This translates to an instantaneous discharge rate in the range of 15–30 Hz, frequencies that correspond to a substantial sensory stimulus (Fig. 1A). In about a third of neuroma A afferents, spontaneous rhythmic discharge is interrupted by silent pauses resulting in a "bursty," on-off firing pattern ("interrupted autorhythmicity"). Most C fibers, and the remaining A fibers, fire in a slow, irregular pattern (0.1–10 Hz).

Investigators report considerable variability in ectopic afferent firing from one experiment to the next. Following clues based on animal-to-animal variation in neuropathic pain behavior, we examined neuromas of different rat strains. Inbred Lewis rats, a strain that expresses very low levels of autotomy, show much less ectopic neuroma activity than do Wistar-derived Sabra strain rats, which have much higher levels of autotomy (Devor et al. 1982; also see Hao and Wiesenfeld-Hallin 1994). Moreover, first-generation offspring of Sabra × Lewis parents, in whom autotomy is low, revealed low levels of activity resembling the Lewis parent. These observations and others suggest that susceptibility to neuropathic sensory abnormalities is related to ectopic hyperexcitability, and may be in part heritable (Devor and Raber 1990; Mogil et al. 1999). This conclusion, which has obvious implications for the gross variability of neuropathic symptoms in human patient populations, focuses attention on genes that code for the proteins responsible for neuronal excitability. While precise mechanisms of ectopic hyperexcitability after nerve injury are not yet clear, much work indicates the involvement of important injury-induced changes in the organization of ion channel proteins.

For technical reasons most research on injury-induced changes in the organization of ion channels is carried out on sensory neurons that have been excised from animals with prior nerve injury, and that are maintained under in vitro conditions. In the absence of the peripheral sensory ending, identifying such neurons as cutaneous versus muscle afferents, for example, is not trivial. Some cues are available, such as cell size. However, while the functional class of DRG neurons does bear some relationship to cell size, size alone is not a reliable predictor of function (Harper and Lawson 1985a,b). Recent studies have used retrograde marking techniques as an alternative way of distinguishing cutaneous from muscle afferents after cell dissociation. Specifically, DRG neurons that contain a retrograde tracer that had been injected into the skin are unequivocally marked as cutaneous afferents. Using this approach, we have shown striking differences among different cell types in action potential waveform, Na^+ and K^+ channel organization, and $GABA_A$ receptor properties, as described below. In addition, we have shown that after nerve ligation and neuroma formation, cutaneous afferents undergo distinct changes in their electrophysiological properties, changes that differ from muscle afferents. Some of these changes are mediated by neurotrophins, including nerve growth factor (NGF) and brain-derived neurotropic factor (BDNF).

SODIUM CHANNEL DYSREGULATION IN INJURED LARGE CUTANEOUS AFFERENT NEURONS

The Na^+ channel is the main ion channel responsible for the ionic currents that underlie the generation of action potentials. Much work over the past several years points to a diversity of Na^+ channel subtypes, and indicates that different types of primary afferent neurons employ different combinations of these channels. Moreover, nerve injury has differential effects on different neuronal types, partly by virtue of their differential effects on the various Na^+ channels. For example, it has been known for a long time that small C-neurons have tetrodotoxin-sensitive (TTX-s) and TTX-resistant

(TTX-r) sodium currents (Kostyuk et al. 1981; Roy and Narahashi 1992; Elliot and Elliot 1993). More recent studies have demonstrated that larger DRG neurons, those that give rise to myelinated axons, also have kinetically and pharmacologically diverse sodium currents (Caffrey et al. 1993; Honmou et al. 1994; Rizzo et al. 1995; Oyelese et al. 1997).

Early studies on axons indicated that following the blockade of potassium currents, sensory axons generate a delayed depolarization that is calcium-independent (Kocsis et al. 1983, 1986). This sensory neuron-specific delayed depolarization fits the criterion of being generated by a kinetically slow sodium current distinct from the faster current responsible for the action potential (Kocsis et al. 1983; Honmou et al. 1994). Fig. 2 shows intra-axonal recordings from a biopsied human sural nerve after application of the potassium channel blocker 4-aminopyridine (4-AP). Note the emergence of the delayed depolarization following the action potential (arrow), which gives rise to additional spikes. Delayed depolarization is important because it increases the number of impulses generated, favors repetitive firing, and triggers spike bursts. Paired pulse experiments (Fig. 2B) indicate that the delayed depolarization is followed by a prolonged refractory period. Subsequent studies revealed that the delayed depolarization is not present in muscle afferents or motor neurons, that it is unique to large myelinated cutaneous afferents and their cell bodies, and that it is generated by a kinetically distinct slow Na^+ current (Honmou et al. 1994; Oyelese et al. 1997).

Following nerve injury (sciatic nerve ligation), the slow sodium current decreases as assayed in whole-cell patch clamp recordings made from the cell bodies of large cutaneous afferent DRG neurons (Rizzo et al. 1995). Likewise, the delayed depolarization observed in cutaneous afferents is reduced by nerve ligation and neuroma formation (Sakai et al. 1998). This finding indicates that the axons as well as the cell bodies of large cutaneous afferents downregulate the kinetically slow sodium current after axotomy. In addition, both large cutaneous A-afferents and small cutaneous C-afferents

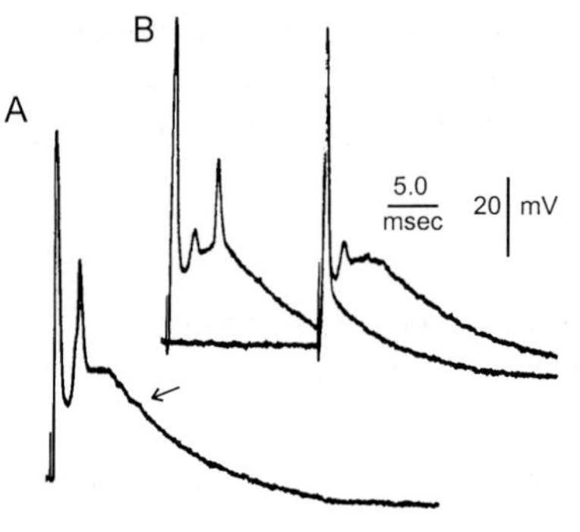

Fig. 2. Recordings obtained from human sural nerve in vitro. (A) Intra-axonal recording in the presence of 4-AP. Note the delayed depolarization and burst activity (arrow). (B) The delayed depolarization has a greater refractory period than the initial spike. Traces show responses to a single stimulus pulse (delivered 15 ms after the beginning of the sweep) that evoked a spike with a delayed depolarization, and to two pulses separated by 15 ms. Note that in the two-pulse experiment, an action potential is evoked by the second pulse, but no delayed depolarization is evoked. Modified from Kocsis (1986).

show accelerated repriming of their fast TTX-s Na^+ current after nerve injury (Cummins and Waxman 1997; Everill et al. 1999b). An important functional consequence of the reduced slow TTX-r current, and the accelerated repriming of the TTX-s current, is that injured cutaneous afferents become prone to generating more prolonged and higher frequency discharges. Correspondingly, their refractory period is reduced (Sakai et al. 1998).

Molecular analysis of the expression of different types of Na^+ channels largely accords with the observed changes of membrane currents. For example, the type III sodium channel is upregulated following nerve injury. In contrast, the PN3/SNS and the NaN/SNS2 Na^+ channel subtypes are downregulated (Waxman et al. 1994; Cummins and Waxman 1997; Oaklander and Belzberg 1997; Novakovic et al. 1998; Dib-Hajj et al. 1998b). Given that the PN3/SNS channel is thought to contribute significantly to the TTX-r kinetically slow current, the downregulation of this Na^+ channel isoform is consistent with the biophysical observations on Na^+ currents noted above.

In addition to up- and downregulation in the synthesis of various Na^+ channel transcripts, evidence indicates that nerve injury brings about abnormal spatial distribution of Na^+ channels along the axonal trajectory, and that this effect contributes to abnormal impulse activity. For example, Na^+ channels accumulate in excess numbers in the axonal membrane at neuroma endbulbs, in patches of demyelination, and in aborted and regenerating sprouts (Lombet et al. 1985; Devor et al. 1989, 1994; England et al. 1996; Novakovic et al. 1998). Interestingly, the PN3/SNS channel subtype accumulates at neuroma endings even though its synthesis in the cell body is reduced (Novakovic et al. 1998). Na^+ channel accumulation renders the injured axons electrically hyperexcitable so they become an ectopic source of afferent impulse discharge (Devor et al. 1994b; Matzner and Devor 1994). Although the evidence is still fragmentary, it is likely that other channels types, and transducer and receptor molecules, likewise accumulate at sites of nerve injury. This accumulation is expected to contribute to the abnormal mechanosensitivity, thermosensitivity, and chemosensitivity that frequently characterize ectopic pacemaker sites (Devor and Seltzer 1999). Correspondingly, partial axoplasmic transport block reduces spontaneous firing and mechanosensitivity in neuromas (Devor and Govrin-Lippmann 1983; Koschorke et al. 1994).

SUBTHRESHOLD MEMBRANE POTENTIAL OSCILLATIONS UNDERLIE REPETITIVE AFFERENT DISCHARGE

We have recently shown that spontaneous repetitive firing in large-diameter DRG neurons does not result from the classical (Hodgkin-Huxley) repetitive firing process whereby a sustained (generator) depolarization repeatedly draws the membrane potential to spike threshold. Rather, the discharge is due to intrinsic subthreshold oscillations in the afferent neuron's membrane potential (Amir et al. 1999). Spiking occurs when individual oscillation sinusoids reach threshold (Fig. 3). Nearly all DRG neurons with subthreshold oscillations fire repetitively either at rest or when they are depolarized. In contrast, neurons without subthreshold oscillations fail to fire repetitively at any membrane potential. The delayed depolarization noted above, which facilitates bursting discharge, is closely associated with the oscillatory process; both processes are dependent of Na^+ currents (Sakai et al. 1998; Amir et al. 1999). Interestingly, nerve injury greatly enhances oscillatory behavior, both by increasing the prevalence of cells that show oscillations and by revealing oscillations at membrane potentials closer to the cell's resting membrane potential. The enhanced oscillatory behavior increases ectopic spike discharge and its sensory consequences.

POTASSIUM CHANNEL REORGANIZATION IN INJURED NEURONS

Potassium currents also have an important role in the regulation of neuronal excitability. For example, computer simulations predict that a reduction in K^+ channel density after nerve injury could contribute to sensory neuron hyperexcitability (Devor et al. 1994b). Indeed, the application of pharmacological K^+ channel antagonists to sites of ectopic afferent discharge facilitates ectopic firing, and injection of such agents into nerve-end neuromas in humans provokes intense pain (Devor et al. 1983; Chabal et al. 1989). Characterization of K^+ currents in axotomized DRG cutaneous afferents is thus important for understanding the mechanisms of neuronal hyperexcitability.

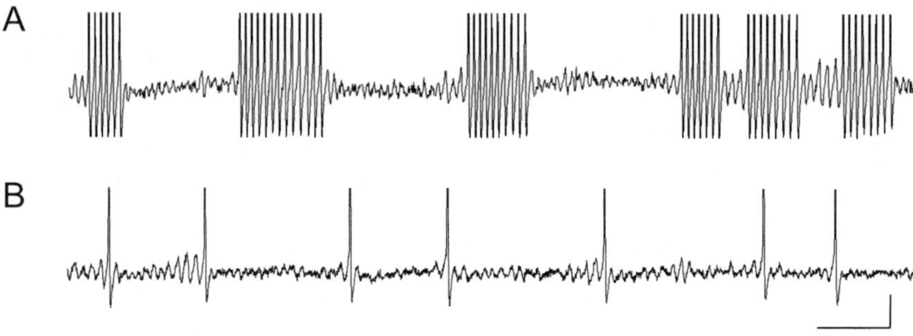

Fig. 3. Samples of (A) bursty and (B) irregular ongoing discharge, recorded intracellularly from axotomized DRG A-neurons in vitro. In each case spikes (or spike bursts) are triggered by subthreshold membrane potential oscillations. Calibration: 100 ms/10 mV.

Gold (1996) characterized several transient K^+ currents previously unidentified in adult rat DRG neurons. However, he focused on small-diameter nociceptive neurons, not the larger low-threshold mechanoreceptor-type neurons that we are considering here. In a recent study (Everill et al. 1998), we demonstrated that large cutaneous neurons express three distinct classes of K^+ current: a dominant sustained K-current (I_K), a fast inactivating A-current (I_A), and a more slowly inactivating D-current (I_D). Foehring and Surmeier (1993) have proposed that the D-current is not associated with a distinct K^+ channel, but rather is in effect a residue of several transient K^+ currents other than I_A. The D-current differs from the A-current in its slower inactivation rate, different voltage dependence of steady-state properties, and enhanced sensitivity to dendrotoxin (DTx) and mast cell degranulating peptides (for review see Castle et al. 1989).

Nerve ligation is followed by a large and selective reduction in I_K and I_A in axotomized cutaneous afferent neurons (Everill and Kocsis 1999a); these currents are reduced by about 50% (Fig. 4). Fig. 4A,B shows the overall K^+ current profiles for control and injured large cutaneous afferent DRG neurons. Note the large reduction in sustained K^+ current after injury. Isolation of transient currents also indicates a reduction in I_A. The size of the neurons studied suggested they give rise to myelinated Aβ fibers, and hence are functionally involved in tactile sensation of the skin. This large reduction in the K^+ current most likely contributes to the injury-induced increase in excitability in these neurons by reducing the ability of the neuron to hyperpolarize.

NEUROTROPHINS PROTECT NEURONS FROM INJURY-INDUCED CHANGES IN SODIUM AND POTASSIUM CHANNEL EXPRESSION

When applied to the cut ends of axotomized neurons, NGF reduces the loss of the slow Na^+ current (Oyelese et al. 1997) as shown in Fig. 5. Quantification using reverse transcription polymerase chain reaction (RT-PCR) also indicates a protective effect of NGF on the injury-induced decline in the expression of the PN3/SNS Na^+ channel subtype (Fig. 6; Dib-Hajj et al. 1998a). Dib-Hajj et al. (1998a) recently reported that the accelerated repriming of TTX-s Na^+ current in axotomized DRG neurons is also prevented by NGF application. In contrast, NGF had no effect on nerve injury-induced changes in $GABA_A$ currents in cutaneous afferent DRG neurons. Rather, the change in $GABA_A$ current was reduced by application to the nerve of BDNF (Oyelese et al. 1997). These effects of NGF and BDNF are specific to cutaneous afferent neurons and are not seen in muscle afferents.

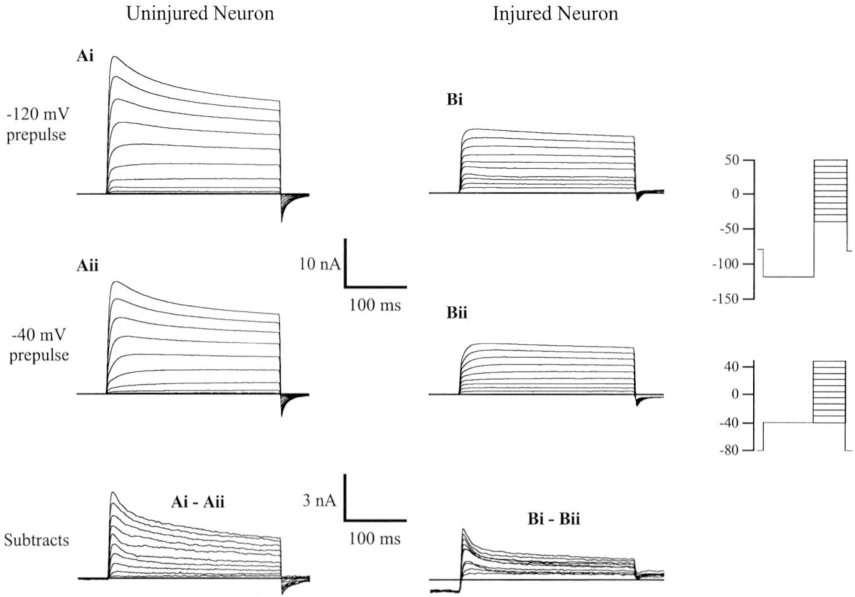

Fig. 4. Comparison of uninjured with injured neurons showing that axotomy triggers a decrease in neuronal K^+ conductance. Representative waveforms of depolarization-activated K^+ currents in (left) control (uninjured) and (right) injured cutaneous afferent DRG neurons (48 μm in diameter) recorded in control solutions. Waveforms in panels (Ai) and (Bi) were initiated using a prepulse of –120 mV. In (Aii) and (Bii) the prepulse was –40 mV (both of 500 ms). The prepulse protocol was followed by a series of test pulses rising from –40 mV to +50 mV in 10-mV steps of 300 ms (right). The subtractions in the bottom traces (Ai – Aii, Bi – Bii) reveal transient A- and D-type currents. The peak K and A currents of injured neurons are seen to be reduced by about 50% in both prepulse conditions. Modified from Everill and Kocsis (1999).

NGF also modulates nerve injury-induced changes in K^+ current (Sharma et al. 1993; Everill and Kocsis 1999b). As noted above, I_K and I_A currents in adult DRG neurons are reduced by about half after axotomy. NGF supplied to the cut nerve end maintains these currents at levels similar to those recorded in cells that were not axotomized. In the intact animal, appropriate levels of neurotrophins are provided to sensory neurons by the peripheral tissues that they innervate (e.g., skin or muscle). Following axotomy, this supply is interrupted. It is interesting that nerve crush does not result in the same degree of reduction of K^+ currents as do nerve cut and ligation; following nerve crush we find no reduction in I_A and only a small reduction in I_K (Everill and Kocsis 1999a). The nerve crush procedure results in transection of the axons, but they rapidly begin to regenerate back to the periphery and to reestablish functional connections (Devor and Govrin-Lippmann 1979; Kenney and Kocsis 1998). It is known that Schwann cells, macrophages, and

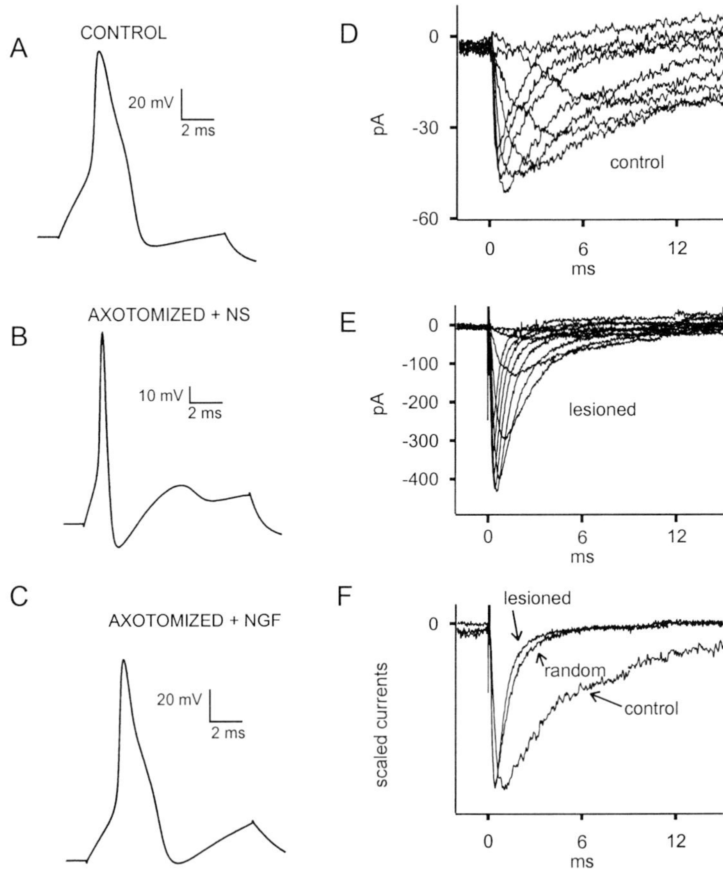

Fig. 5. NGF provides protection from effects of axotomy. (A–C) Action potentials were induced by depolarizing current pulse in control neurons (A), and in axotomized neurons after treatment with normal solution (B), or NGF (C). (D) Na^+ currents recorded from a 3-μm diameter somatic membrane bleb excised from a control (nonaxotomized) 48-μm-diameter identified cutaneous afferent DRG neuron. The membrane was held at –100 mV, conditioned at –140 mV for 100 ms, then depolarized in the range of –50 to +30 mV in steps of 10 mV. (E) The same protocol was applied to an 8-μm diameter bleb excised from a previously axotomized cutaneous afferent DRG neuron. Note that in both (D) and (E), each trace represents the mean of four records. The increased noise in (D) is indicative of the lower number of Na^+ channels recorded from. In (F), records obtained from the blebs in (D) and (E) at +10 mV test potential are scaled and superimposed with the record from a bleb excised from an unlabeled (hence non-cutaneous) DRG neuron randomly selected from a culture prepared under the same conditions. The control neuron reveals slower activation and inactivation kinetics, and the inactivation phase reveals an inflection, suggesting two underlying Na^+ channel populations with different kinetics. In the lesioned neuron (E), the kinetically slow currents are much reduced. Modified from Oyelese et al. (1998) and Rizzo et al. (1995).

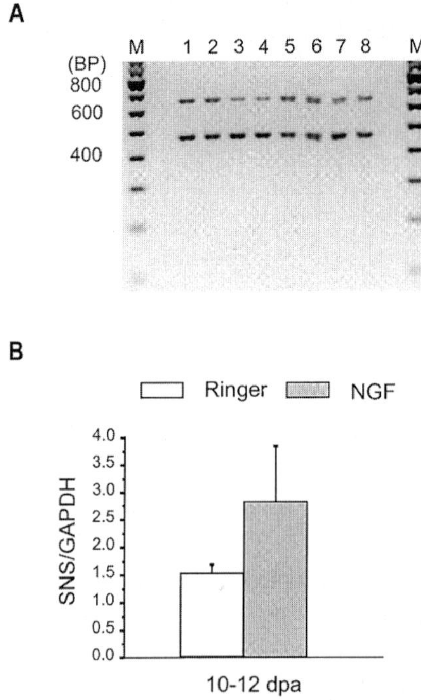

Fig. 6. Reverse transcription-polymerase chain reaction (RT-PCR) quantification of the SNS Na^+ channel from axotomized DRG neurons treated with Ringer or NGF. (A) Representative gel analysis of the coamplified (SNS) and glyceraldehyde-3-phosphate dehydrogenase (GAPDH) products. Column "M" denotes 100-base pair standard (Pharmacia). Lanes 1, 2, 5, and 6: PCR products from two independent amplifications of cDNA from Ringer-treated axotomized DRG. Lanes 3, 4, 7, and 8: PCR products from two independent amplifications of cDNA from NGF-treated axotomized DRG. Gel image was digitized using GelBase 7500 system (UVP) and printed on a Fargo Primera Pro laser color printer (Fargo Electronics) in black-and-white dye sublimation mode. (B) Mean levels of SNS amplification products normalized to GAPDH in eight independent amplifications of cDNA templates from Ringer- and NGF-treated DRG. Data were extracted from gel analysis of PCR products as shown in panel (A). Error bars represent standard deviations. Modified from Dib-Hajj et al. (1998).

fibroblasts in the distal degenerating nerve segment begin to express NGF and BDNF (Heumann et al. 1987; Taniuchi et al. 1988). The regenerating sprouts that enter the distal zone can access these neurotrophins, which thus provide sustained trophic support for the neuron and maintain the ongoing regulation of K^+ current.

The role of NGF, BDNF, and other neurotrophins in the regulation of membrane channel expression and neuronal excitability stresses the multiple and complexly interacting changes set into play by nerve injury. For example, while nerve section cuts the normal supply of NGF from the skin, it also increases the synthesis and supply of neurotrophins in the distal nerve stump, and indeed in the DRG itself (e.g., Sebert and Shooter 1993; Michael et al. 1999). Axotomy also changes the responsiveness of DRG neurons to neurotrophins by regulating the synthesis of their high-affinity tyrosine kinase receptors (e.g., Sebert and Shooter 1993; Shen et al. 1999). Finally, recent evidence suggests that some neurotrophins may act directly as (fast) neurotransmitters, in additional to filling a trophic role (Kafitz et al. 1999).

CONCLUSIONS

Discussions of pain associated with changes in the excitability of primary afferent neurons usually focus exclusively on nociceptors. However, the phenomenon of central sensitization demands a radical change in this outlook. It is now well documented that in the area of "secondary hyperalgesia" surrounding focal lesions and sites of irritation, tactile allodynia (particularly to phasic brushing-type stimuli) is signaled by activity in low-threshold Aβ mechanoreceptors (references in the Introduction). The most widely held explanation of this "Aβ pain" is that nociceptor activity originating in the area of the lesion triggers and maintains a state of central sensitization that amplifies the sensory effects of Aβ touch input, rendering it painful. An unavoidable extension of this line of reasoning is that Aβ activity originating in the area of injury itself, i.e., the area of "primary hyperalgesia," is also rendered painful by central sensitization. Thus, a substantial fraction of the tactile pain and tenderness felt during everyday injuries such as minor burns, bruises, and abrasions must originate in Aβ touch afferents rather than in sensitized nociceptors.

This conclusion also extends to neuropathic pain, where evidence is strong that tactile allodynia is signaled by intact Aβ afferents that are rendered pain-provoking by central sensitization triggered and maintained by ectopic firing of injured afferents (e.g., Price et al. 1989, 1992; Gracely et al. 1992; Kajander et al. 1992; Sheen and Chung 1993; Koltzenburg et al. 1994; Torebjörk et al. 1995; Rowbotham and Fields 1996; Devor and Seltzer 1999; Liu et al. 2000). By the same token, spontaneous discharge in injured Aβ afferents must contribute to spontaneous pain in neuropathy, and ectopic mechanosensitivity of injured Aβ afferents must contribute to pain on movement and on deep palpation. Therefore, our report of the nerve-injury-evoked changes in membrane ionic currents that underlie hyperexcitability in large cutaneous afferents has direct implications for the pathophysiology of neuropathic pain.

ACKNOWLEDGMENTS

We gratefully acknowledge the support of the United States–Israel Binational Science Foundation, the Medical Research Service of the Department of Veterans Affairs, and the National Institutes of Health (NS 10174).

REFERENCES

Amir R, Michaelis M, Devor M. Membrane potential oscillations in dorsal root ganglion neurons: role in normal electrogenesis and in neuropathic pain. *J Neurosci* 1999; 19:8589–8596.

Baba H, Doubell TP, Woolf CF. Peripheral inflammation facilitates Aβ fiber-mediated synaptic input to the substantia gelatinosa of the adult rat spinal cord. *J Neurosci* 1999; 19:859–867.

Caffrey JM, Eng DL, Black JA, Waxman SG, Kocsis JD. Three types of sodium channels in adult rat dorsal root ganglion neurons. *Brain Res* 1993; 592:283–287.

Campbell JN, Raja SN, Meyer RA, Mackinnon SE. Myelinated afferents signal the hyperalgesia associated with nerve injury. *Pain* 1988; 32:89–94.

Castle NA, Haylett DG, Jenkinson DH. Toxins in the characterization of potassium channels. *Trends Neurosci* 1989; 12:59–65.

Chabal C, Jacobson L, Burchiel KJ. Pain responses to perineuronal injection of normal saline, gallamine, and lidocaine in humans. *Pain* 1989; 36:321–325

Cummins TR, Waxman SG. Downregulation of tetrodotoxin-resistant sodium currents and upregulation of a rapidly repriming tetrodotoxin-sensitive sodium current in small spinal sensory neurons after nerve injury. *J Neurosci* 1997; 17:3503–3514.

Devor M. Potassium channels moderate ectopic excitability of nerve-end neuromas in rats. *Neurosci Lett* 1983; 40:181–186.

Devor M, Govrin-Lippmann R. Selective regeneration of sensory fibers following nerve crush injury. *Exp Neurol* 1979; 63:243–254.

Devor M, Govrin-Lippmann R. Axoplasmic transport block reduces ectopic impulse generation in injured peripheral nerves. *Pain* 1983; 16:73–86.

Devor M, Raber P. Heritability of symptoms in an experimental model of neuropathic pain. *Pain* 1990; 42:51–67.

Devor M, Seltzer Z. Pathophysiology of damaged nerves in relation to chronic pain. In: Wall PD, Melzack R (Eds). *Textbook of Pain,* 4th ed. London: Churchill Livingstone, 1999, pp 129–164.

Devor M, Wall PD. Cross excitation among dorsal root ganglion neurons in nerve injured and intact rats. *J Neurophysiol* 1990; 64:1733–1746.

Devor M, Inbal R, Govrin-Lippmann R. Genetic factors in the development of chronic pain. In: Lieblich L (Ed). *Genetics of the Brain.* Amsterdam: Elsevier, 1982.

Devor M, Keller CH, Deerinck T, Levinson SR, Ellisman MH. Na^+ channel accumulation on axolemma of afferents in nerve end neuromas in *Apteronotus*. *Neurosci Lett* 1989; 102:149–154.

Devor M, Keller CH, Ellisman MH. Spontaneous discharge of afferents in a neuroma reflects original receptor tuning. *Brain Res* 1990; 517:245–250.

Devor M, Basbaum AI, Bennett GJ, et al. Group report: mechanisms of neuropathic pain following peripheral injury. In: Basbaum AI, Besson J-M (Eds). *Toward a New Pharmacotherapy of Pain.* Chichester: Wiley, 1991, pp 417–440.

Devor M, Jänig W, Michaelis M. Modulation of activity in dorsal root ganglion (DRG) neurons by sympathetic activation in nerve-injured rats. *J Neurophysiol* 1994a; 71:38–47.

Devor M, Lomazov P, Matzer O. Na^+ channel accumulation in injured axons as a substrate for neuropathic pain. In: Boivie J, Hansson P, Lindblom U (Eds). *Touch, Temperature and Pain in Health and Disease: Mechanisms and Assessments,* Progress in Pain Research and Management, Vol. 3. Seattle: IASP Press, 1994b, pp 207–230.

Dib-Hajj SD, Black JA, Cummins TR, et al. Rescue of α-SNS sodium channel expression in small dorsal root ganglion neurons after axotomy by nerve growth factor in vivo. *J Neurophysiol* 1998a, 79:2668–2676.

Dib-Hajj SD, Tyrrell L, Black JA, Waxman SG. NaN, a novel voltage-gated Na^+ channel preferentially in peripheral sensory neurons and down-regulated after axotomy. *Proc Natl Acad Sci USA* 1998b; 95:8963–8968.

Elliott AA, Elliott JR. Characterization of TTX-sensitive and TTX-resistant sodium currents in small cells from adult rat dorsal root ganglia. *J Physiol (Lond)* 1993; 463:39–56.

England JD, Happel LT, Kline DG. et al. Sodium channel accumulation in humans with painful neuromas. *Neurology* 1996; 47, 272-276.

Everill B, Kocsis JD. Reduction in potassium currents in identified cutaneous afferent DRG neurons after axotomy. *J Neurophysiol* 1999a; 82:700–708.

Everill B, Kocsis JD. Effects of nerve growth factor on potassium conductance after nerve injury in adult cutaneous afferent dorsal root ganglion neurons. *Soc Neurosci Abstracts* 1999b; 24:1332.

Everill B, Rizzo MA, Kocsis JD. Morphologically identified cutaneous afferent DRG neurons express three different potassium currents in varying proportions. *J Neurophysiol* 1998; 79:1814–1824.

Foehring RC, Surmeier DJ. Voltage-gated potassium currents in acutely dissociated rat cortical neurons. *J Neurophysiol* 1993; 70:51–63.

Gold M, Shuster MJ, Levine JD. Characterization of six voltage-gated K^+ currents in adult rat sensory neurons. *J Neurophysiol* 1996; 75:2629–2646.

Govrin-Lippmann R, Devor M. Ongoing activity in severed nerves: source and variation with time. *Brain Res* 1978; 159:406–410.

Gracely RH, Lynch SA, Bennett GJ. Painful neuropathy: altered central processing , maintained dynamically by peripheral input. *Pain* 1992; 51: 175–194.

Hao J-X, Wiesenfeld-Hallin Z. Variability in the occurrence of ongoing discharges in primary afferents originating in the neuroma after peripheral nerve section in different strains of rats. *Neurosci Lett* 1994; 169:119–121.

Hardy JD, Wolf HG, Goodell H. *Pain Sensations and Reactions.* New York: William and Wilkins, 1952.

Harper AA, Lawson SN. Conduction velocity is related to morphological cell type in rat dorsal root ganglion neurons. *J Physiol (Lond)* 1985a; 359:31–46.

Harper AA, Lawson SN. Electrical properties of dorsal root ganglion neurons with different peripheral nerve conduction velocities. *J Physiol (Lond)* 1985b; 359:47–63.

Heumann R, Korsching S, Bandtlow C, Thoenen H. Changes of nerve growth factor synthesis in non-neuronal cells in response to sciatic nerve transection. *J Cell Biol* 1987: 104:1623–1631

Honmou O, Utzschneider DA, Rizzo MA, et al. Delayed depolarization and slow sodium currents in cutaneous afferents. *J Neurophysiol* 1994; 71:1627–1637.

Johnson RD, Munson JB. Regenerating sprouts of axotomized cat muscle afferents express characteristic firing patterns to mechanical stimulation. *J Neurophysiol* 1991; 66:2155–2158.

Kafitz KW, Rose CR, Thoenen H, Konnerth A. Neurotrophin-evoked rapid excitation through TrkB receptors. *Nature* 1999; 410:918-921.

Kajander KC, Wakisaka S, Bennett GJ. Spontaneous discharge originates in the dorsal root ganglion at the onset of a painful peripheral neuropathy in the rat. *Neurosci Lett* 1992; 138:225–228.

Kenney AM, Kocsis JD. Peripheral axotomy induces long-term c-jun amino-terminal kinase-1 activation and activator protein-1 binding activity by c-Jun and JunD in adult rat dorsal root ganglia *in vivo*. *J Neurosci* 1998; 18:1318–1328.

Kirk E. Impulses in dorsal spinal nerve rootlets in cats and rabbits arising from dorsal root ganglia isolated from the periphery. *J Comp Neurol* 1974; 2:165–176.

Kocsis JD. Functional characteristics of potassium channel of normal and pathological mammalian axons. In: Ritchie JM, Keynes RD, Bolls L (Eds). *Ion Channels in Neural Membranes.* New York: Alan R Liss, 1986, pp 123–144.

Kocsis JD, Ruiz JA, Waxman SG. Maturation of mammalian myelinated fibers: changes in action-potential characteristics following 4-aminopyridine application. *J Neurophysiol* 1983; 50:449–463.

Kohama I, Kocsis JD. Changes in synaptic transmission of rat dorsal horn neurons after demyelination or C-fiber ablation to the sciatic nerve. *Soc Neurosci Abstracts* 1999; 25:1671.

Koltzenburg M, Lundberg LER, Torebjörk HE. Dynamic and static components of mechanical hyperalgesia in human hairy skin. *Pain* 1992; 51:207–219.

Koltzenburg M, Torebjörk HE, Wahren LK. Nociceptor modulated central sensitization causes mechanical hyperalgesia in acute chemogenic and chronic neuropathic pain. *Brain* 1994; 117:579–591.

Koschorke GM, Meyer RA, Tillman DB, Campbell JD. Ectopic excitability of injured nerves in monkey: entrained responses to vibratory stimuli. *J Neurophysiol* 1991; 65:693–701.

Koschorke GM, Meyer RA, Campbell JN. Cellular components necessary for mechanoelectrical transduction are conveyed to primary afferent terminals by fast axonal transport. *Brain Res* 1994; 641:99–104.

Kostyuk PG, Veselovsky NS, Tsyndrenko AY. Ionic currents in the somatic membrane of rat dorsal root ganglion neurons. I. Sodium currents. *Neuroscience* 1981; 6:2423–2430.

Lindblom U. Analysis of abnormal touch, pain and temperature sensation in patients. In: Boivie J, Hanson P, Lindblom U (Eds). *Touch, Temperature, and Pain in Health and Disease: Mechanisms and Assessments,* Progress in Pain Research and Management, Vol. 3. Seattle: IASP Press, 1994, pp 63–84.

Liu C-N, Wall PD, Ben-Dor E, et al. Tactile allodynia in the absence of C-fiber activation: altered firing properties of DRG neurons following spinal nerve injury. *Pain* 2000; in press.

Lombet A, Laduron P, Mourre C, Jacomet Y, Lazdunski M. Axonal transport of the voltage-dependent Na^+ channel protein identified by its tetrodotoxin binding site in rat sciatic nerves. *Brain Res* 1985; 345:153–158.

Ma Q-P, Woolf CJ. Progressive tactile hypersensitivity: an inflammation-induced incremental increase in the excitability of the spinal cord. *Pain* 1996; 67:97–106.

Mannion RJ, Costigan M, Decosterd I, et al. Neurotrophins: peripherally and centrally acting modulators of tactile stimulus-induced inflammatory pain hypersensitivity. *Proc Natl Acad Sci USA* 1999; 96:9385–9390.

Matzner O, Devor M. Hyperexcitability at sites of nerve injury depends on voltage -sensitive Na^+ channels. *J Neurophysiol* 1994; 72:349–357.

Michael GJ, Averill S, Shortland PJ, Yan Q, Priestley JV. Axotomy results in major changes in BDNF expression by dorsal root ganglion cells: BDNF expression in large trkB and trkC cells, in pericellular baskets, and in projections to deep dorsal horn and dorsal column nuclei. *Eur J Neurosci* 1999; 11:3539–3551.

Michaelis M, Blenk K-H, Jänig W, Vogel C. Development of spontaneous activity and mechanosensitivity in axotomized afferent nerve fibers during the first hours after nerve transection in rats. *J Neurophysiol* 1995; 74:1020–1027.

Michaelis M, Liu X-G, Jänig W. Muscle afferents but not skin afferents develop ongoing discharges of dorsal root ganglion origin following peripheral nerve lesion. *J Neurosci* 2000; in press.

Mogil JS, Wilson SG, Bon K, et al. Heritability of nociception I: Responses of 11 inbred mouse strains on 12 measures of nociception. *Pain* 1999; 80:67–82.

Novakovic SD, Tzoumaka E, McGivern JC. Distribution of the tetrodotoxin-resistant sodium channel PN3 in rat sensory neurons in normal and neuropathic conditions. *J Neurosci* 1998; 18:2174–2187.

Oaklander AL, Belzberg A. Unilateral nerve injury down-regulates mRNA for Na^+ channel SCN10A bilaterally in rat dorsal root ganglion. *Mol Brain Res* 1997; 52:162–165.

Oyelese AA, Rizzo MA Waxman SG, Kocsis JD. Differential effects of NGF and BDNF on axotomy-induced changes in $GABA_A$ receptor-mediated conductances and sodium currents in cutaneous afferent neurons. *J Neurophysiol* 1997; 78:31–41.

Price DD, Bennett GJ, Rafii A. Psychophysical observations on patients with neuropathic pain relieved by sympathetic block. *Pain* 1989; 36:273–288.

Price DD, Long S, Huitt C. Sensory testing of pathophysiological mechanisms of pain in patients with reflex sympathetic dystrophy. *Pain* 1992; 49:163–173.

Proske U, Iggo A, Luff AR. Mechanical sensitivity of regenerating myelinated skin and muscle afferents in the cat. *Exp Brain Res* 1995; 104:89–98.

Rizzo MA, Kocsis JD, Waxman SG. Selective loss of slow and enhancement of fast Na^+ currents in cutaneous afferent dorsal root ganglion neurons following axotomy. *Neurobiol Dis* 1995; 2:87–96.

Rowbotham MC, Fields HL. The relation of pain, allodynia and thermal sensation in post-herpetic neuralgia. Brain 1996; 119:347–354

Roy ML, Narahashi T. Differential properties of tetrodotoxin-sensitive sodium channels in rat dorsal root ganglion neurons. *J Neurosci* 1992; 12:2104–2111.

Sakai J, Honmou O, Kocsis JD, Hashi K. The delayed depolarization in rat cutaneous afferent axons is reduced following nerve transection and ligation, but not crush: implications for injury-induced axonal Na^+ channel reorganization. *Muscle Nerve* 1998; 21:1040–1047.

Sebert ME, Shooter EM. Expression of mRNA for neurotrophic factors and their receptors in the rat dorsal root ganglion and sciatic nerve following nerve injury. *J Neurosci Res* 1993; 36:357–367.

Sharma N, D'Arcangelo G, Kleinklaus A, Halegoua S, Trimmer JS. Nerve growth factor regulates the abundance and distribution of K^+ channels in PC12 Cells. *J Cell Biol* 1993; 123:1835–1843.

Sheen K, Chung JM. Signs of neuropathic pain depend on signals from injured fibers in a rat model. *Brain Res* 1993; 610:62–68.

Shen H, Chung JM, Coggeshall RE, Chung K. Changes in trkA expression in the dorsal root ganglion after peripheral nerve injury. *Exp Brain Res* 1999; 127:141–146.

Shortland P, Wolf CJ. Chronic peripheral nerve section results in a rearrangement of the central axonal arborizations of axotomized A beta primary afferent neurons in the rat spinal cord. *J Comp Neurol* 1993; 330:65–82.

Strong PN. Potassium channel toxins. *Pharmacol Ther* 1990; 46;137–162.

Tal M, Devor M. Myelinated afferent types that become spontaneously active following transection of a mixed nerve. *Soc Neurosci Abstracts* 1998; in press.

Taniuchi, M, Clark HB, Schweitzer JB, Johnson EM. Expression of nerve growth factor receptors by Schwann cells of axotomized peripheral nerves: ultrastructure location, suppression by axonal contact and binding properties. *J Neurosci* 1988; 8:664–681.

Torebjörk HE, Lundberg LER, LaMotte RH. Central changes in processing of mechanoreceptive input in capsaicin-induced secondary hyperalgesia in humans. *J Physiol (Lond)* 1992; 448:765–780.

Torebjörk E, Wahren LK, Wallin G, Hallin R, Koltzenberg M. Noradrenaline-evoked pain in neuralgia. *Pain* 1995; 63:11–20.

Wall PD, Gutnick M. Ongoing activity in peripheral nerves: the physiology and pharmacology of impulses originating from a neuroma. *Exp Neurol* 1974; 43:580–593.

Waxman SG, Kocsis JD, Black JA. Type III sodium channel mRNA is expressed in embryonic but not in adult spinal sensory neurons, and is reexpressed following axotomy. *J Neurophysiol* 1994; 72:466–470.

Woolf CJ. Excitability changes in central neurons following peripheral damage, In: Willis WD Jr (Ed). *Hyperalgesia in Allodynia.* New York: Raven Press, 1991, pp 221–243.

Correspondence to: Jeffery D. Kocsis, PhD, Yale University School of Medicine, Neuroscience Research Center (127A), Department of Veterans Affairs Medical Center, West Haven, CT 06516, USA. Tel: 203-937-3802; Fax: 203-937-3801; email: jeffery.kocsis@yale.edu.

Proceedings of the 9th World Congress on Pain,
Progress in Pain Research and Management,
Vol. 16, edited by M. Devor, M.C. Rowbotham, and
Z. Wiesenfeld-Hallin, IASP Press, Seattle, © 2000.

13

The Role of Neighboring Intact Dorsal Root Ganglion Neurons in a Rat Neuropathic Pain Model

Tetsuo Fukuoka, Atsushi Tokunaga, Eiji Kondo, and Koichi Noguchi

Department of Anatomy and Neuroscience, Hyogo College of Medicine, Hyogo, Japan

Unilateral L5 spinal nerve (SpN) ligation (L5 SpNL) causes mechano- and thermo-allodynia in the ipsilateral plantar hindpaw in rats (Kim and Chung 1992). In this model, the natural stimuli applied to the ipsilateral plantar foot surface must be transferred through the neighboring intact SpNs, mainly through the L4 SpN, because the plantar surface of the rat hindpaw is innervated by the L3–L5 spinal segments (Takahashi et al. 1994) and the L5 SpN distal to the ligation site retains no functional contact with spinal cord.

We have studied functional changes in gene expression in the ipsilateral L4 dorsal root ganglion (DRG) in this model. In previous studies, we demonstrated that calcitonin gene-related peptide (CGRP) mRNA and preprotachykinin (PPT) mRNA increased in the ipsilateral L4 DRG neurons 7 and 14 days after L5 SpNL, respectively (Fukuoka et al. 1998a,b). In this study, we further examined the time course of the upregulation of these neuropeptides, quantified nerve growth factor (NGF) content using enzyme-linked immunosorbent assay (ELISA), and measured NGF mRNA expression using Northern blot analysis and in situ hybridization histochemistry (ISHH) in L4 DRG, L4 SpNs, and sciatic nerves (ScNs) in this model. In addition, we investigated the change in vanilloid receptor subtype 1 (VR1) mRNA expression in L4 DRG and co-expression of trkA mRNA with PPT, CGRP, and VR1 mRNAs in L4 DRG using ISHH.

MATERIALS AND METHODS

Animal model and behavioral tests. All animal experiments conformed to the regulations of the Hyogo College of Medicine Committee on Animal Research and were carried out in accordance with the guidelines of the National Institutes of Health on animal care. A total of 65 male Sprague-Dawley rats weighing 170–200 g were used. Under adequate anesthesia with sodium pentobarbital, the left L5 SpN was isolated and tightly ligated with 5-0 silk thread. The right L5 SpN was also isolated but left without ligation. Mechanical and heat allodynia of the plantar surface of hindpaws were tested using von Frey filaments (2.13 and 72.2 mN) and the plantar test (7370, Ugo Basile).

Collection of tissue samples. All animals were deeply anesthetized and killed by decapitation at the postoperative days (PODs) described below. In all experiments, naive animals were used for control.

For ISHH, on the 1st, 3rd, 5th, 7th, 14th, and 28th POD, L4 DRG were dissected out and rapidly frozen in powdered dry ice; 16-μm sections were then cut using a cryostat at –18°C. The sections from the ipsilateral and contralateral L4 DRG of each rat were thaw-mounted onto the same vectabond (Vector)-coated slides, and stored at –80°C until use. For ISHH of serial sections, L4 DRG were collected on the 14th POD and 6-μm sections were cut as described above.

For ELISA, L4 DRG, L4 SpNs, and ScNs were collected on the 4th, 7th, and 14th PODs. To ensure detectable NGF protein, we included tissues from 3–4 rats in each sample. For Northern blot analysis, L4 DRG, L4 SpNs, and ScNs were collected on the 14th POD. To ensure sufficient total RNA, each sample contained tissues from 4–5 rats.

Analysis. We used oligonucleotide probes recognizing mRNA for CGRP, PPT, VR1, trkA, and NGF. Previous reports confirmed the specificity of the probes used in this study. Our protocol for ISHH of freshly cut sections has been described in detail (Fukuoka et al. 1998b).

We used a computerized image analysis system (NIH Image version 1.61) to measure the density of silver grains over selected tissue profiles, and calculated signal/noise (S/N) ratio for each cell in each tissue as previously described (Fukuoka et al. 1998b). The S/N ratio of an individual neuron and its cross-sectional area were plotted as shown in Figs. 1 and 2. Based on these scattergrams, neurons with a grain density of five-fold the background level or higher were considered positively labeled for mRNAs for PPT and CGRP. Neurons with a grain density of double the background level or higher were considered positively labeled for VR1.

The percentage of positively labeled DRG neurons is expressed throughout as mean ± SEM. Pairwise comparisons (*t* test) allowed us to determine

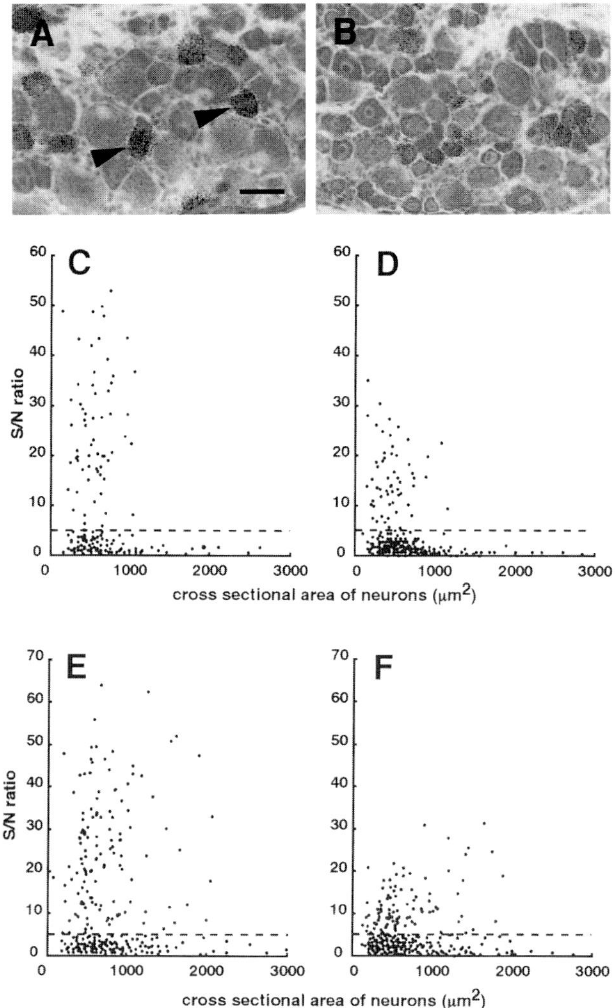

Fig. 1. Effect of L5 spinal nerve ligation on PPT and CGRP mRNA expression in L4 DRG neurons. Rats received unilateral L5 spinal nerve ligation 14 days before sacrifice. Bright-field photomicrographs showing in situ hybridization products for PPT mRNA (A,B) are shown. In the ipsilateral L4 DRG (A), several neurons were intensely labeled (arrow heads) compared to the contralateral L4 DRG (B). Scale bar = 50 μm. Scatterplot diagrams of PPT mRNA (C,D) and CGRP mRNA (E,F) expression in the ipsilateral (C,E) and contralateral (D,F) L4 DRG from one representative rat are shown. Individual cell profiles are plotted according to the cross-sectional area (μm^2; along the x-axis) and signal/noise (S/N) ratio (along the y-axis). The dashed lines indicate the border between the non- and weakly labeled neurons (S/N ratio = 5). A subpopulation of small (<600 μm^2) and medium-sized (600–1200 μm^2) neurons increased in S/N ratio for both mRNAs in the ipsilateral side compared to the contralateral side.

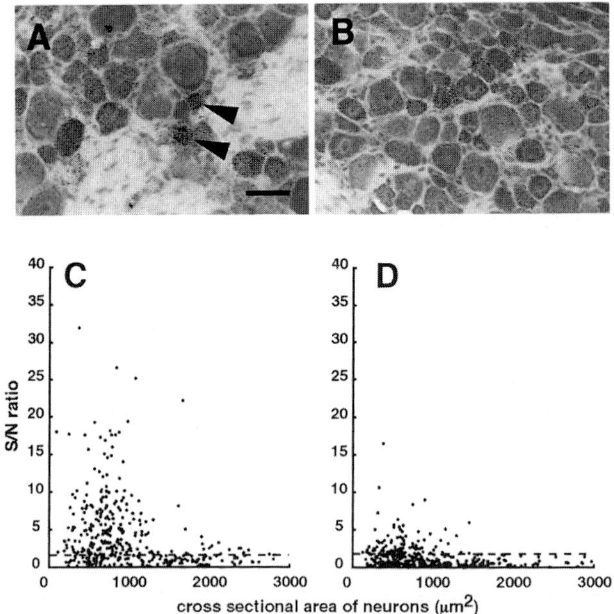

Fig. 2. Effect of L5 spinal nerve ligation on VR1 mRNA expression in L4 DRG neurons. Rats received unilateral L5 spinal nerve ligation 14 days before sacrifice. Bright-field photomicrographs showing in situ hybridization products for VR1 mRNA (A,B) are shown. In the ipsilateral L4 DRG (A), several neurons were intensely labeled (arrow heads) compared to the contralateral L4 DRG (B). Scale bar = 50 μm. Scatterplot diagrams of VR1 mRNA expression in the ipsilateral (C) and contralateral (D) L4 DRG from one representative rat are shown. Individual cell profiles are plotted according to the cross-sectional area (μm^2; along the *x*-axis) and signal/noise (S/N) ratio (along the *y*-axis). The dashed lines indicate the border between the non-labeled and weakly labeled neurons (S/N ratio = 2). A subpopulation of small ($<600\ \mu m^2$) and medium-sized (600–1200 μm^2) neurons increased in S/N ratio in the ipsilateral compared to the contralateral side.

the differences of values between ipsilateral and contralateral DRG. Neurons co-expressing trkA with PPT, CGRP, and VR1 mRNAs were counted using camera lucida. Data are expressed as mean percentage ± SEM.

We measured β-NGF content with a two-site ELISA immunoassay based on a protocol provided by Boehringer Mannheim. The first antibody was a monoclonal anti-mouse β-NGF antibody (clone 27/21, Boehringer Mannheim) and the second was the same antibody conjugated with β-galactosidase. Recombinant rat β-NGF (R&D Systems, Inc.) was used to obtain a standard curve. The ipsilateral/contralateral ratio of the NGF content (picograms) per wet mass (milligrams) of the samples was calculated and expressed as mean ± SEM.

For Northern blot analysis, total cellular RNA was purified from the samples using ISOGEN (Nippon Gene). Twenty micrograms of total RNA was electrophoresed in a 1% agarose gel containing 2% formaldehyde, and transferred to a nitrocellulose filter (Hybond-N+). An oligonucleotide probe recognizing NGF mRNA was labeled with α-[^{32}P]-dATP (NEN) and terminal deoxynucleotidyl transferase (Amersham), which gave a specific activity of approximately 5–10 × 10^9 cpm/μg. The filters were hybridized overnight at 42°C, washed at high stringency (1 × SSC, 0.1% SDS, 55°C), and exposed to Kodak BioMax films at –80°C.

RESULTS

Following unilateral L5 spinal nerve ligation, most of the rats developed mechanical and heat allodynia as reported in our previous study (Fukuoka et al. 1998b).

From the 1st to the 7th POD, there was no significant difference in PPT mRNA expression between ipsilateral and contralateral L4 DRG. As shown in Fig. 1A,B, some neurons intensely labeled for PPT mRNA were observed on the 14th POD in the ipsilateral L4 DRG as compared to the contralateral side. This upregulation was also observed on the 28th POD (data not shown). Cross-sectional area S/N ratio distributions of the L4 DRG from a typical rat established that the increase in signal intensity was exclusively seen in a subpopulation of small (<600 μm^2) to medium-sized (600–1200 μm^2) neurons (Fig. 1C,D). The mean percentages of non-labeled neurons (S/N ratio < 5) were significantly decreased (58.2 ± 2.0% vs. 72. 5 ± 2.0%, $P < 0.01$), while moderately (20 ≤ S/N ratio < 40) and intensely (40 ≤ S/N ratio) labeled neurons were significantly increased in the ipsilateral L4 DRG compared to the contralateral DRG (19.3 ± 2.3% vs. 4.3 ± 1.5%, $P < 0.001$ and 4.6 ± 0.8% vs. 0%, $P < 0.001$, respectively).

Our previous study (Fukuoka et al. 1998b) reported the increase in CGRP mRNA expression in the ipsilateral L4 DRG 7 days after L5 spinal nerve ligation. We also observed this increase in this study and continued at least until the 28th POD (data not shown). Most of the intensely (40 ≤ S/N ratio) labeled neurons were small to medium-sized (Fig. 1E,F). On the 14th POD, the mean percentage of intensely labeled neurons was significantly increased in the ipsilateral L4 DRG compared to the contralateral side (15.8 ± 2.2% vs. 3.9 ± 2.0%, $P < 0.01$). No significant difference was seen in the non-labeled (S/N ratio < 5), weakly labeled (5 ≤ S/N ratio < 20), or moderately labeled (20 ≤ S/N ratio < 40) neurons between the ipsilateral and contralateral sides.

At the L4 level, some neurons intensely labeled for VR1 mRNA were observed on the ipsilateral side on the 14th POD (Fig. 2A). This increase was also observed on the 28th POD (data not shown). Cross-sectional area

S/N ratio distributions of the L4 DRG from a typical rat are shown in Fig. 2C,D. A subpopulation of small and medium-sized neurons in the ipsilateral L4 DRG increased the signal intensity as compared to the contralateral L4 DRG. The mean percentages of non-labeled neurons (S/N ratio < 2) were significantly decreased (53.5 ± 3.2% vs. 74.0 ± 4.8%, $P < 0.01$), while moderately (5 ≤ S/N ratio < 10) and intensely (10 ≤ S/N ratio) labeled neurons were significantly increased in the ipsilateral L4 DRG compared to the contralateral DRG (16.0 ± 2.1% vs. 5.5 ± 1.8%, $P < 0.01$; and 6.1 ± 1.4% vs. 1.3 ± 0.7%, $P < 0.05$, respectively).

Most of the PPT and CGRP mRNA-expressing neurons of the ipsilateral L4 DRG co-expressed trkA mRNA (84.0 ± 1.7%, and 91.8 ± 2.1%, respectively). However, only 36.5 ± 2.9% of VR1 mRNA-expressing neurons of the DRG were labeled for trkA mRNA.

NGF content in the ipsilateral L4 DRG increased with time and reached a significantly greater value than did that in the contralateral L4 DRG on the 14th POD (ELISA; Fig. 3A). NGF content in the ipsilateral L4 SpN slightly increased as compared to the contralateral side from the 4th through 14th POD (Fig. 3C). NGF content in the ipsilateral ScN significantly increased at the 4th POD and returned to around normal value after the 7th POD (Fig. 3E).

Neither in the L4 DRG (data not shown) nor in the L4 SpN (Fig. 3D) could NGF mRNA be detected by Northern blot analysis on the 14th POD. However, NGF mRNA clearly increased in the ipsilateral ScN as compared to the contralateral side at the same time point (Fig. 3F). We further confirmed the lack of expression of NGF mRNA in the ipsilateral L4 DRG using ISHH (Fig. 3B).

DISCUSSION

Our previous studies demonstrated increases in expression of PPT and CGRP mRNAs in the ipsilateral L4 DRG following L5 SpNL (Fukuoka et al. 1998a,b). In the current study, we confirmed these increases and for the first

---

Fig. 3. Change in NGF content and NGF mRNA in L4 DRG, L4 spinal nerve (SpN), and sciatic nerve (ScN) after L5 spinal nerve ligation. NGF content was measured by ELISA and expressed as ipsilateral/contralateral (ipsi./contra.) ratio (mean ± SEM of four independent experiments). The ratio increased with time in L4 DRG (A) and reached statistical significance on the 14th postoperative day (POD). The ratio increased slightly in SpN (C). However, the ratio in ScN (E) increased at the 4th POD but returned to around 1 at the 7th POD. Asterisks (*) denote $P < 0.05$. Northern blot analysis was used to examine NGF mRNA expressions in L4 DRG (data not shown), L4 SpN (D) and ScN (F) at the 14th POD, and ISHH was also used for L4 DRG (B). NGF mRNA was upregulated only in the ipsilateral ScN. ⟶

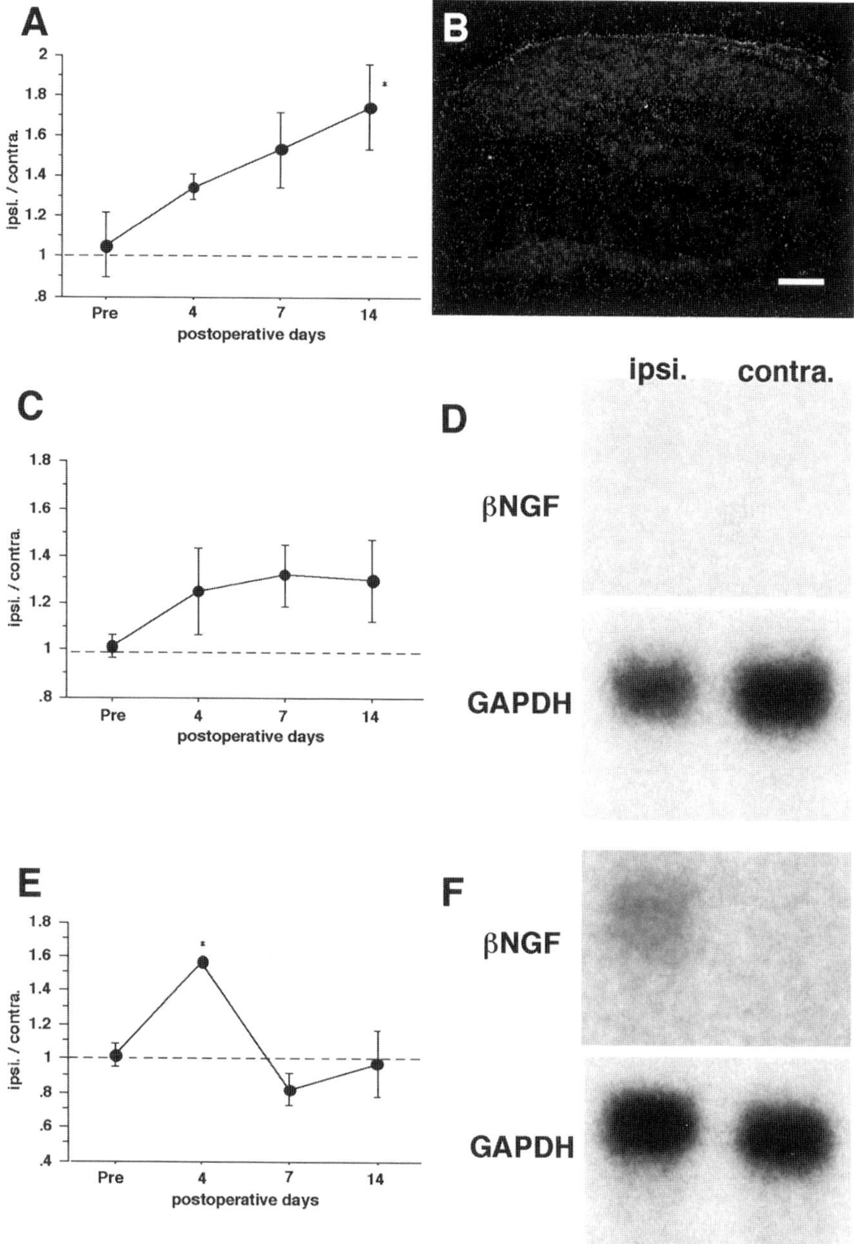
A
2
1.8
1.6
1.4
1.2
1
.8
ipsi. / contra.
Pre
4
7
14
postoperative days
B
C
1.8
1.6
1.4
1.2
1
.8
ipsi. / contra.
Pre
4
7
14
postoperative days
D
ipsi.
contra.
βNGF
GAPDH
E
1.8
1.6
1.4
1.2
1
.8
.6
.4
ipsi. / contra.
Pre
4
7
14
postoperative days
F
βNGF
GAPDH

time demonstrated an increase in VR1 mRNA in the ipsilateral L4 DRG in this neuropathic pain model. Substance P and CGRP are important neuromodulators for sensory transmission in the dorsal horn. These neuropeptides are co-released from the primary afferent terminals by natural and electrical stimuli (Morton and Hutchison 1990). They directly activate dorsal horn neurons (Miletic and Tan 1988; Ryu et al. 1988), potentiate the excitatory effects of noxious stimulation and of each other on dorsal horn neurons (Wiesenfeld-Hallin et al. 1984; Woolf and Wiesenfeld-Hallin 1985, 1986), and increase the release of glutamate into spinal slice perfusate (Kangrga et al. 1990). Therefore, the increases in these neuropeptides in the ipsilateral L4 DRG could facilitate sensory transmission through the L4 spinal segment.

The regulatory effects of various neurotrophic factors on peptide expression in DRG have been examined (for review, see Hökfelt et al. 1997). At present, NGF is the leading candidate to upregulate and maintain the expression of SP or CGRP in adult rat DRG neurons in various conditions (Kessler and Black 1980; Otten et al. 1980; Goedert et al. 1981; Lindsay and Harmar 1989; Diemel et al. 1994; Sango et al. 1994). This conclusion is also supported by our observation in this study that a high proportion of PPT mRNA- and CGRP mRNA-expressing neurons in the ipsilateral L4 DRG co-express trkA mRNA (also see Averill et al. 1995; Bennett et al. 1996; Kashiba et al. 1996). Therefore, we quantified the NGF content in the L4 DRG and its peripheral nerves. As expected, NGF content increased with time in the ipsilateral L4 DRG compared to the contralateral side (Fig. 3A). It also slightly increased in the ipsilateral L4 SpN (Fig. 3C); however, the increase in the ipsilateral ScN, distal to the ligation site, was transient and returned to control values on the 7th POD (Fig. 3E).

Where is the NGF synthesized? Examination detected NGF mRNA in these tissues only in the ipsilateral ScN on the 14th POD (Fig. 3F), when the NGF content was significantly increased in the ipsilateral L4 DRG and the contents in bilateral ScNs had already returned to equal. NGF mRNA could not be detected in the ipsilateral L4 DRG by ISHH. These data strongly suggest that NGF is synthesized in the ipsilateral ScN, perhaps in the L5 SpN distal to the ligation site, and then diffuses to the neighboring fibers including the L4 SpN, is retrogradely transported through it, and influences the gene expression in L4 DRG.

VR1 is the first cloned capsaicin receptor. This receptor is a nonselective cation channel gated by capsaicin and noxious heat and is expressed by a subpopulation of DRG small cells with unmyelinated or thinly myelinated fibers, including polymodal nociceptors and heat-sensitive fibers (Holzer 1991). Therefore, this receptor is a candidate heat transducer in primary afferents and may play an important role in thermal hyperalgesia in this neuropathic pain model. In this study, we demonstrated the upregulation of VR1 mRNA in a subpopulation in the ipsilateral L4 DRG. NGF increases the sensitivity of DRG neurons to capsaicin (Winter et al. 1988). However, only about one-third of the VR1 mRNA-expressing neurons co-expressed trkA mRNA. The remaining two-thirds should be included in another subclass of DRG small neurons that are characterized by binding with isolectin B4 and sensitivity to glial cell line-derived neurotrophic factor (GDNF) (Bennett et al. 1998; Snider and McMahon 1998). It has not yet been confirmed whether GDNF regulates the expression of VR1 mRNA in DRG neurons. The detailed neurochemical characterization of the VR1 mRNA-expressing neurons and quantification of GDNF in the ipsilateral L4 DRG in this model are necessary to address the mechanism of upregulation of VR1.

ACKNOWLEDGMENTS

We gratefully acknowledge technical assistance from Masako Tatsumi and Yuko Doi. This study was supported by the Science Research Promotion Fund of the Japan Private School Promotion Foundation, and by Grants-in-Aid for Science Research from the Japanese Ministry of Education, Science and Culture.

REFERENCES

Averill S, McMahon SB, Clary DO, et al. Immunocytochemical localization of trkA receptors in chemically identified subgroups of adult rat sensory neurons. *Eur J Neurosci* 1995; 7:1484–1494.

Bennett DL, Dmietrieva N, Priestley JV, et al. trkA, CGRP and IB4 expression in retrogradely labelled cutaneous and visceral primary sensory neurones in the rat. *Neurosci Lett* 1996; 206:33–36.

Bennett DL, Michael GJ, Ramachandran N, et al. A distinct subgroup of small DRG cells express GDNF receptor components and GDNF is protective for these neurons after nerve injury. *J Neurosci* 1998; 18:3059–3072.

Diemel LT, Brewster WJ, Fernyhough P, et al. Expression of neuropeptides in experimental diabetes; effects of treatment with nerve growth factor or brain-derived neurotrophic factor. *Brain Res Mol Brain Res* 1994; 21:171–175.

Fukuoka T, Miki K, Tokunaga A, et al. Up-regulation of calcitonin gene-related peptide and preprotachykinin mRNA in L4 dorsal root ganglion neurons following L5 spinal nerve ligation; a rat neuropathic pain model. *Neurosci Abstr* 1998a; 24:1392

Fukuoka T, Tokunaga A, Kondo E, et al. Change in mRNAs for neuropeptides and the GABA(A) receptor in dorsal root ganglion neurons in a rat experimental neuropathic pain model. *Pain* 1998b; 78:13–26.

Goedert M, Stoeckel K, Otten U. Biological importance of the retrograde axonal transport of nerve growth factor in sensory neurons. *Proc Natl Acad Sci USA* 1981; 78:5895–5898.

Hökfelt T, Zhang X, Xu Z-Q, et al. Phenotype regulation in dorsal root ganglion neurons after nerve injury: focus on peptides and their receptors. In: Borsook D (Ed). *Molecular Neurobiology of Pain,* Progress in Pain Research and Management, Vol. 9. Seattle: IASP Press, 1997, pp 115–143.

Holzer P. Capsaicin: cellular targets, mechanisms of action, and selectivity for thin sensory neurons. *Pharmacol Rev* 1991; 43:143–201.

Kangrga I, Larew JSA, Randic M. The effects of substance P and calcitonin gene-related peptide on the efflux of endogenous glutamate and aspartate from the rat spinal dorsal horn in vitro. *Neurosci Lett* 1990; 108:155–160.

Kashiba H, Ueda Y, Senba E. Coexpression of preprotachykinin-A, alpha-calcitonin gene-related peptide, somatostatin, and neurotrophin receptor family messenger RNAs in rat dorsal root ganglion neurons. *Neuroscience* 1996; 70:179–189.

Kessler JA, Black IB. Nerve growth factor stimulates the development of substance P in sensory ganglia. *Proc Natl Acad Sci USA* 1980; 77:649–652.

Kim SH, Chung JM. An experimental model for peripheral neuropathy produced by segmental spinal nerve ligation in the rat. *Pain* 1992; 50:355–363.

Lindsay RM, Harmar AJ. Nerve growth factor regulates expression of neuropeptide genes in adult sensory neurons. *Nature* 1989; 337:362–364.

Miletic V, Tan H. Iontophoretic application of calcitonin gene-related peptide produces a slow and prolonged excitation of neurons in the cat lumbar dorsal horn. *Brain Res* 1988; 446:169–172.

Morton CR and Hutchison WD. Morphine does not reduce the intraspinal release of calcitonin gene-related peptide in the cat. *Neurosci Lett* 1990; 117:319–324.

Otten U, Goedert M, Mayer N, et al. Requirement of nerve growth factor for development of substance P containing sensory neurones. *Nature (Lond)* 1980; 287:158–159.

Ryu PD, Gerber G, Murase K, et al. Actions of calcitonin gene-related peptide on rat spinal dorsal horn neurons. *Brain Res* 1988; 441:357–361.

Sango K, Verdes JM, Hikawa N, et al. Nerve growth factor (NGF) restores depletions of calcitonin gene-related peptide and substance P in sensory neurons from diabetic mice in vitro. *J Neurol Sci* 1994; 126:1–5.

Snider WD, McMahon SB. Tackling pain at the source: new ideas about nociceptors. *Neuron* 1998; 20:629–632.

Takahashi Y, Nakajima Y, Sakamoto T. Dermatome mapping in the hindlimb by electrical stimulation of the spinal nerves. *Neurosci Lett* 1994; 168:85–88.

Wiesenfeld-Hallin Z, Hökfelt T, Lundberg JM, et al. Immunoreactive calcitonin gene-related peptide and substance P coexist in sensory neurons to the spinal cord and interact in spinal behavioral responses of the rat. *Neurosci Lett* 1984; 52:199–204.

Winter J, Forbes CA, Sternberg J, et al. Nerve growth factor (NGF) regulates adult rat cultured dorsal root ganglion neuron responses to the excitotoxin capsaicin. *Neuron* 1988; 1:973–981.

Woolf CJ, Wiesenfeld-Hallin Z. Substance P and calcitonin gene-related peptide produce synergistic excitability changes in the spinal cord. *Neurosci Lett Suppl* 1985; 22:S239.

Woolf CJ, Wiesenfeld-Hallin Z. Substance P and calcitonin gene-related peptide synergistically modulate the gain of the nociceptive flexor withdrawal reflex in the rat. *Neurosci Lett* 1986; 66:226–230.

Correspondence to: Tetsuo Fukuoka, MD, PhD, Department of Anatomy and Neuroscience, Hyogo College of Medicine, 1-1 Mukogawa-cho, Nishinomiya, Hyogo, 663-8501, Japan. Tel: 81-798-45-6416; Fax: 81-798-45-6417; email: tfukuoka@hyo-med.ac.jp.

Proceedings of the 9th World Congress on Pain,
Progress in Pain Research and Management,
Vol. 16, edited by M. Devor, M.C. Rowbotham, and
Z. Wiesenfeld-Hallin, IASP Press, Seattle, © 2000.

14

The Molecular Biology of Mu Opioid Analgesia

Gavril W. Pasternak

The Cotzias Laboratory of Neuro-Oncology, Memorial Sloan-Kettering Cancer Center, New York, New York, USA

Opioid analgesics have long been the mainstay in the management of pain. While several clinically important drugs act through kappa (κ) receptors, most clinical opioids work through mu (μ), or morphine, receptors. Yet, subtle differences in the pharmacology of these analgesics have raised questions about their optimal use. Some patients respond better to one opioid than another, both for analgesia and side effects, particularly nausea and vomiting. Indeed, patients incapacitated by adverse effects from one agent may tolerate another without problem. Unfortunately, it is almost impossible to predict which drug will be superior for an individual patient.

Clinicians also have observed incomplete cross-tolerance among many μ analgesics, even though they all act through μ-opioid receptors. Switching tolerant patients to a different analgesic typically restores significant analgesic sensitivity, an observation that has led some clinicians to consider opioid rotation to enhance analgesic effectiveness. Why should drugs acting through the same receptor show subtle, but clinically important, differences? Recent advances at the molecular level of opioid receptor pharmacology have provided new insights into these areas. This chapter will review the pharmacological and molecular biological evidence for multiple subtypes of μ-opioid receptors and their implications in opioid pharmacology.

OPIOID SYSTEMS IN THE BRAIN

The primary function of sensory nervous systems is to interpret stimuli from the outside world. However, the simultaneous presentation of all sensory input would be chaotic. Sensory input must be "filtered" to permit the brain to focus its attention upon specific sensory stimuli. Pain is an excellent example. The perception of pain can vary dramatically, depending upon the situation in which the nociceptive input occurs. While trivial insults can sometimes be perceived as very painful, in other circumstances people report little pain despite severe injuries. This was documented in an early study comparing the analgesic requirements of wounded soldiers during World War II to those of civilians undergoing elective surgery (Beecher 1946). Despite their more extensive wounds, the soldiers required far less analgesic medication, demonstrating that the stress of life-threatening situations can affect the ability of individuals to tolerate pain.

We now understand that sensitivity to pain is modulated by the endogenous opioid system, among others (Pasternak 1993; Reisine and Pasternak 1996). This system is composed of several distinct families of opioid peptides and their receptors. The endogenous opioid peptides include the enkephalins, the dynorphins, the endomorphins, and β-endorphin. These agents act through opioid receptors, which have provided the most effective targets for the development of strong analgesics. Three major families of opioid receptors were initially proposed, based upon a wide variety of pharmacological approaches: μ, κ, and δ. While most opioids interact with several different opioid receptors, a number of highly selective agents have been developed that have been useful in defining the pharmacology of these receptor classes. Morphine and most clinical opioid analgesics (Fig. 1) act through μ-opioid receptors. The κ_1 opioid receptors, defined by their high affinity for the endogenous opioid peptide dynorphin A and for several highly selective synthetic opiates, have a number of problematic side effects, including psychotomimetic activity, dysphoria, and a profound diuresis. While δ drugs may prove to be important in the future, few nonpeptides are available for study. Thus, the μ-opioid analgesics will remain the mainstay in the control of pain for the near future.

MU RECEPTOR PHARMACOLOGY

Mu analgesics are potent, effective analgesics. However, μ-opioid receptors also mediate various other actions, including respiratory depression, sedation, and constipation (Reisine and Pasternak 1996). Within the μ-receptor family, evidence has been mounting for multiple subtypes. Although clinical observations, such as incomplete cross-tolerance, have provided strong evidence for different μ-analgesic mechanisms, animal studies have permitted more detailed investigations in the attempt to define multiple μ-opioid receptors.

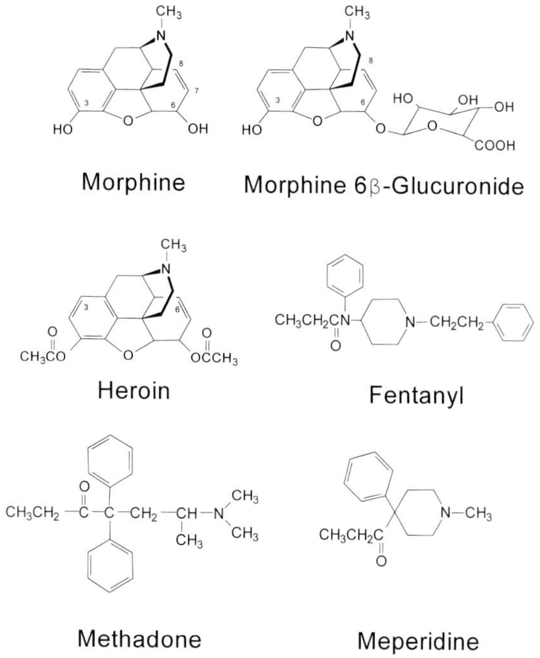

Morphine Morphine 6β-Glucuronide

Heroin Fentanyl

Methadone Meperidine

Fig. 1. Diagram showing wide variety of structures of μ-opioid analgesics.

In many areas of pharmacology, selective antagonists have long been used to define receptors. In the opioid field, naloxone was the first opioid antagonist; it has been often used to define actions as opioid or nonopioid. More selective antagonists are now available that can distinguish among the various classes (Pasternak 1993). For example, β-funaltrexamine selectively antagonizes μ-opioid receptors (Ward et al. 1982), while naltrindole selectively blocks δ-opioid sites (Abdelhamid et al. 1991) and nor-binaltorphimine acts against κ_1-opioid receptors (Portoghese et al. 1987). Other agents have been described that can further differentiate subtypes of receptors. The first two antagonists, naloxonazine and naloxazone, suggested subtypes of μ receptors (Pasternak et al. 1980a,b; Hahn and Pasternak 1982; Hahn et al. 1982). Since then, 3-*O*-methylnaltrexone has implied a third μ receptor (Brown et al. 1997), while several other agents have suggested subtypes of δ receptors (Jiang et al. 1990, 1991; Mattia et al. 1991; Sofuoglu et al. 1992; Chakrabarti et al. 1993).

Soon after the initial descriptions of opioid binding (Pert and Snyder 1973; Simon et al. 1973; Terenius 1973), we observed a novel site of very high affinity (Pasternak and Snyder 1975), which we termed μ_1 to distinguish it from the morphine-selective μ_2 site (Wolozin and Pasternak 1981). Naloxonazine and naloxazone selectively blocked the very high affinity binding component both in vitro and in vivo (Pasternak et al. 1980a,b; Hahn and Pasternak 1982), suggesting that they might be μ_1-selective antagonists and thus could define the pharmacological actions of the μ-opioid binding sites. When given to rats or mice, the two antagonists blocked the analgesic actions of morphine given systematically or supraspinally, without significantly affecting morphine's respiratory depression or inhibition of gastrointestinal transit (Pasternak 1982; Hahn and Pasternak 1982; Ling et al. 1983, 1984, 1985, 1986; Bodnar et al. 1988; Heyman et al. 1988; Paul and Pasternak 1988; Paul et al. 1989b). Additional studies examined other μ effects, dividing them into naloxonazine-sensitive (μ_1) or insensitive (μ_2) actions (Pasternak 1993).

More recently, great interest has centered upon morphine-6β-glucuronide (M6G) (Fig. 1), a very potent morphine metabolite. Although M6G was first demonstrated to be an active metabolite in the early 1970s (Shimomura et al. 1971; Yoshimura et al. 1973), its true importance was not appreciated until much later. Systemically, M6G is twice as potent as morphine in animal models (Pasternak et al. 1987; Paul et al. 1989a) and in humans (Hand et al. 1987; Osborne et al. 1988; Tiseo et al. 1995). When administered centrally in rodents to bypass the blood–brain barrier, M6G is over 100-fold more potent then morphine. Yet, M6G is less potent than morphine in receptor-binding assays. This disparity between its pharmacological potency and its binding affinity for the traditional μ-opioid receptor suggested that M6G may act through a different receptor than does morphine.

Cross-tolerance is commonly used to establish a common mechanism of action for different drugs. Morphine and codeine, for example, show cross-tolerance. However, mice tolerant to morphine retained their analgesic sensitivity toward M6G (Rossi et al. 1996). In addition, the morphine-tolerant mice responded normally to a number of other μ opioids, including heroin and its active metabolite 6-acetylmorphine, etonitazine, and fentanyl. Thus, this animal model recapitulates the clinical observations of incomplete cross-tolerance noted above, in which patients regain analgesic sensitivity when switched from one μ analgesic to another.

Genetic factors also play significant roles in analgesic sensitivity. Various strains of mice show differing sensitivities to various classes of opioid analgesics. One mouse strain has provided a valuable model system. The inbred CXBK strain has long been known to be insensitive to morphine given either systemically or supraspinally (Baron et al. 1975; Reith et al. 1981; Moskowitz and Goodman 1985; Vaught et al. 1988; Pick et al. 1993; Connelly et al. 1994; Mogil et al. 1996; Chang et al. 1998). However, CXBK mice respond normally to M6G, heroin, and 6-acetylmorphine, consistent with the suggestion of a distinct M6G receptor (Rossi et al. 1996). The concept of a unique M6G receptor was furthered strengthened by the observation that 3-*O*-methylnaltrexone can selectively block M6G, heroin, and 6-acetylmorphine analgesia at doses that are ineffectual against morphine (Brown et al. 1997). 3-*O*-Methylnaltrexone also antagonizes self-administered heroin, raising the possibility that the self-rewarding properties of heroin may involve the M6G receptor (Walker et al. 1999).

THE MOLECULAR BIOLOGY OF MU OPIOID RECEPTORS

Opiates act through receptors on the outside of the neurons. Opioid receptors are members of the large G-protein receptor family, which includes hundreds of different receptors for a wide variety of neurotransmitters and hormones (Lefkowitz 1993, 1996; Knapp et al. 1995). Despite their wide diversity of ligands, all G-protein receptors share several important characteristics. Structurally, they all contain seven transmembrane regions, with the amino terminus outside the cell and the carboxy terminus inside. Functionally, they all interact with heterotrimeric G proteins, which in turn can influence a number of transduction systems.

Opioid receptor genes have been cloned that encode a μ-opioid receptor (MOR-1) (Chen et al. 1993; Wang et al. 1993), a δ-opioid receptor (DOR-1) (Evans et al. 1992; Kieffer et al. 1992), or a κ_1-opioid receptor (KOR-1) (Chen et al. 1993; Li et al. 1993; Reisine and Bell 1993; Yasuda et al. 1993). A fourth member of the opioid receptor family also has been cloned (Bunzow et al. 1994; Fukuda et al. 1994; Keith Jr et al. 1994; Mollereau et al. 1994; Pan et al. 1994, 1995). This receptor, termed "opioid-receptor-like" (ORL1), is quite unusual. Its endogenous ligand is orphanin FQ (Reinscheid et al. 1995), also known as nociceptin (OFQ/N) (Meunier et al. 1995). While its homology to the classical opioid receptors is quite high, none of the traditional opioids label ORL1 with high affinity; its ligand, OFQ/N, shows very poor affinity for the classical opioid receptors.

In the original descriptions, MOR-1 was reported to contain four exons that spanned over 50 kilobases (kb) in the genome (Chen et al. 1993; Wang et al. 1993). Genes contain both exons and introns. The exons are the sequences that are kept within the mRNA, which in turn is translated into the protein (Fig. 2). The sequences between exons, termed introns, are spliced out and eliminated from the mature mRNA. Exon 1 encodes the first transmembrane region, while exons 2 and 3 each encode three additional transmembrane regions, for a total of seven (Fig. 3). The fourth exon encodes a short peptide sequence at the tip of the intracellular tail. When expressed in cell lines, MOR-1 binds opiate ligands with the selectivity and affinity simi-

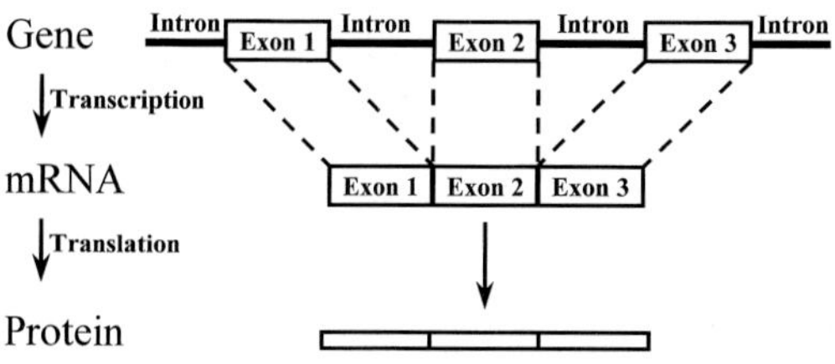

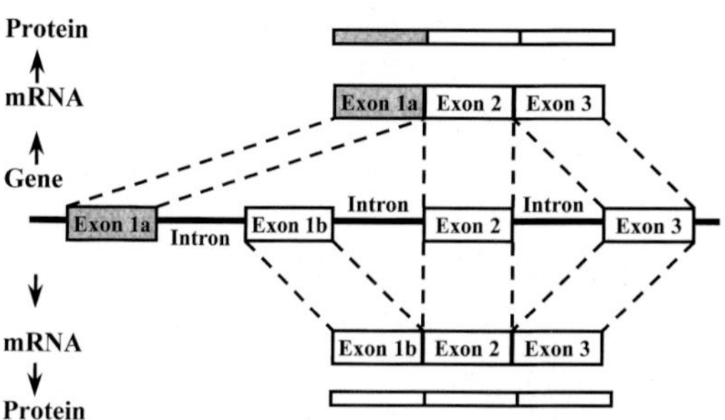

Fig. 2. Schematic of intron-exon splicing. (A) Simple intron-exon splicing; The gene contains regions that comprise mRNA, termed exons, and regions that do not, termed introns. Many mRNAs are composed of a series of different exons that are linked together. The introns between the exons are spliced out and are not present in the mature mRNA. (B) Alternative splicing: In one form of alternative splicing, the gene may have several exons from which one can be incorporated into the protein. This is denoted in this figure. The final protein can have either exon 1a or exon 1b. However, alternative splicing also can be quite complex, inserting and/or deleting multiple different exons.

lar to that previously demonstrated in brain tissue for μ-opioid receptors (Chen et al. 1993; Wang et al. 1993). Mu ligands, such as morphine, have high affinity, whereas selective δ and κ drugs are virtually inactive.

Although the cloned receptor clearly fell within the μ-opioid receptor family, was this receptor responsible for mediating morphine analgesia? Correlating individual proteins with behavior can be difficult. There are two major approaches. Antisense approaches target the mRNA and provide a transient and limited decrease in the protein. Alternatively, the gene itself can be disrupted, as in knockout mice. The first such indication that MOR-1 was involved with morphine analgesia came from antisense studies (Rossi et al. 1994). In this approach, short oligodeoxynucleotide sequences are designed that are complementary to regions of the mRNA and therefore bind to form a duplex, which destabilizes the mRNA and leads to a downregulation in mRNA levels and a corresponding reduction in receptor levels (Crooke 1993; Stein and Cheng 1993). One advantage of antisense approaches is that they can be carried out quickly and easily. Furthermore, antisense probes can be targeted anywhere along the mRNA, provided the oligodeoxynucleotide probe is designed appropriately. This technique permits the exploration of the role of splice variants in the actions being investigated.

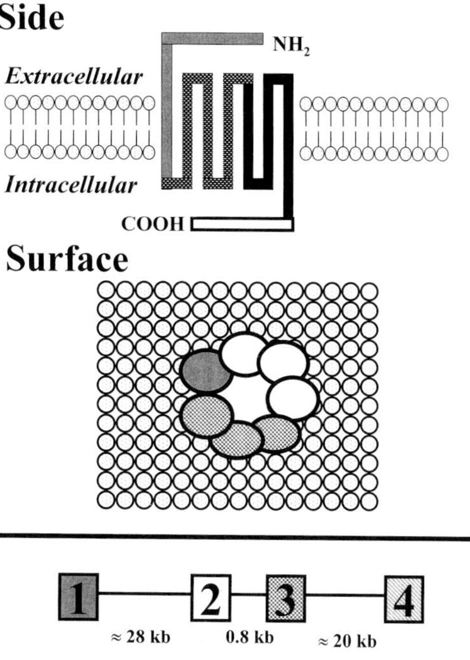

Fig. 3. Schematic of initial MOR-1 gene. The original gene contained four exons which that approximately 50 kilobases (kb). The receptor is a traditional G-protein-coupled receptor. The first exon encodes the extracellular amino terminus and the first-transmembrane (TM) region. The second exon encodes the next three TM regions and their corresponding intracellular loops. Exon 3 encodes the last three TM regions, while exon 4 supplies the amino acids at the tip of the COOH-terminus.

However, antisense approaches are not applicable for all systems. Studying the opioid system has the advantage that the regions of interest are mostly periventricular, which ensures that the probes have access to the regions responsible for the behaviors being monitored. Furthermore, modest shifts of the opioid analgesic dose-response curves are relatively straightforward to detect. This is important because antisense treatments typically reduce opioid receptor binding and mRNA levels by only 30–50%. Antisense approaches require a number of controls. First, it is necessary to establish the specificity of the sequence and ensure that the actions are not simply due to nonspecific effects. The specificity of the antisense oligodeoxynucleotide sequence is very strict. For example, mismatch probes that switch the sequence of four bases of the 20 in the antisense typically are inactive. This strict specificity of the sequence also means that probes usually are restricted to single species. It is reassuring to see more than one antisense probe targeting the protein of interest, and helpful to document a decrease in both mRNA and protein levels.

Soon after the initial cloning of MOR-1 from the rat, we designed an antisense probe that targeted the first exon of MOR-1 and examined its actions on morphine analgesia after microinjection into the periaqueductal gray of the rat (Rossi et al. 1994). The antisense dramatically lowered the morphine response, implying that MOR-1 did encode the receptor responsible for morphine analgesia.

Antisense approaches can be used to target sites anywhere along an mRNA, an approach we termed antisense mapping (Standifer et al. 1994; Rossi et al. 1995, 1997). Three different antisense probes targeting the first exon of MOR-1 all blocked morphine analgesia (Rossi et al. 1995). However, these three probes were without effect against M6G analgesia. Conversely, probes targeting exons 2 and 3, which effectively blocked M6G analgesia, were inactive against morphine. Thus, antisense mapping studies underscored important differences in the receptor mechanisms of morphine and M6G analgesia at the molecular level. Furthermore, these results implied that both the morphine and the M6G receptor were related to, but distinct from, the initial MOR-1 clone, although all seemed to be generated from the MOR-1 gene. Together, these observations raised the possibility that the receptors may represent splice variants of the MOR-1 gene.

Knockout approaches offer an alternative method by which to explore the functional significance of proteins. Unlike antisense, the protein being targeted in the knockout model is absent throughout development, which raises the concern that the animal may develop compensatory systems to take over the functions normally associated with the targeted protein. Recent studies have also observed another potential problem when individual exons in the gene are disrupted. Disrupting an exon may or may not completely eliminate all products of the gene. In genes that undergo alternative splicing, variants that normally do not contain the targeted exon may still be expressed, as was recently reported with a knockout of the neuronal nitric oxide synthase gene (Brenman et al. 1996).

The first MOR-1 knockout, an insertional disruption at exon 2, was insensitive to all μ opioids tested, including both morphine and M6G (Matthes et al. 1996; Kieffer 1999). Morphine analgesia also was lost in all knockout mice in which either exon 1 or exons 2 and 3 together were targeted (Sora et al. 1997; Loh et al. 1998; Schuller et al. 1999). However, one exon 1 knockout mouse remained sensitive to M6G and heroin (Schuller et al. 1999), although the potency of these drugs was slightly diminished in the experimental mouse compared to wild-type controls. A different exon 1 knockout mouse did not respond to either morphine or M6G (Kitanaka et al. 1998). The reasons for this difference are not entirely clear, but it is interesting that the promoter region of the gene was deleted in the exon 1 knockout mouse that was insensitive to all opioids, unlike the M6G-sensitive exon 1 knockout mouse, where the promoter region was left intact. Additional studies indicate that the M6G-sensitive exon 1 knockout mice still express MOR-1 gene transcripts containing exons 2 and 3, as determined by reverse transcription polymerase chain reaction (RT-PCR), while immunohistochemical studies have revealed persistent expression of epitopes associated with some recently described MOR-1 splice variants in the knockout mice, as discussed below. Thus, M6G-sensitive exon 1 knockout mice still demonstrate expression of MOR-1 gene products. Together, these findings support the concept that distinct receptors mediate morphine and M6G analgesia.

Pharmacological studies had implied the existence of multiple μ-opioid receptors, a concept supported by the antisense and knockout approaches. However, evidence from many laboratories had described a single gene. The antisense mapping studies described above led us to believe that there would be additional alternatively spliced variants of MOR-1. In alternative splicing, a gene can have more than one possible exon to place in the mRNA, resulting in multiple unique proteins from a single gene (Fig. 2B). Prior efforts had identified two MOR-1 splice variants. MOR-1A was a minor variant lacking exon 4 (Bare et al. 1994), while MOR-1B contained a new exon (exon 5) in place of the original exon 4 (Zimprich et al. 1995) (Fig. 4A). Overall, these variants differed only slightly from MOR-1 at the intracellular COOH terminus (Fig. 4B) and both displayed a traditional μ-opioid-binding selectivity profile. The regional distribution of MOR-1B differed from MOR-1, which suggests region-specific processing and expression (Zimprich et al. 1995). We recently isolated five more exons within the MOR-1 gene (Fig. 4A) (Pan et al. 1999). With these exons, we demonstrated that the MOR-1 gene was over 250 kb long, about fivefold longer than the original estimate. These additional five exons combine to yield four new splice variants (Fig. 4B). When expressed in cells, all the variants retain high affinity for morphine and morphine-like drugs and can be considered members of the μ-receptor family (Pan et al. 1999). There are some differences in binding, but they are subtle and are most evident with the endogenous opioid peptides.

The regional distribution of the μ receptors also differs at the level of the mRNA, as shown by using RT-PCR and immunohistochemical assays (Abbadie et al. 1999; Pan et al. 1999). The differences in the distribution of MOR-1C and MOR-1 are dramatic. MOR-1-like immunoreactivity (MOR-1-LI) is present in clusters within the striatum, a pattern first described for μ receptors using autoradiographic approaches (Atweh and Kuhar 1977a,b,c; Goodman and Pasternak 1985). Yet, there is no MOR-1C-like immunoreactivity (MOR-1C-LI) within the striatum. Rather, MOR-1C-LI is high in the lateral septum, a region with little MOR-1-LI. MOR-1D-LI also has a distinct regional distribution. Although some regions contain all three types of receptor, including regions of the dorsal horn of the spinal cord associated with pain processing, confocal microscopy suggests that the receptors are not typically colocalized to the same neurons.

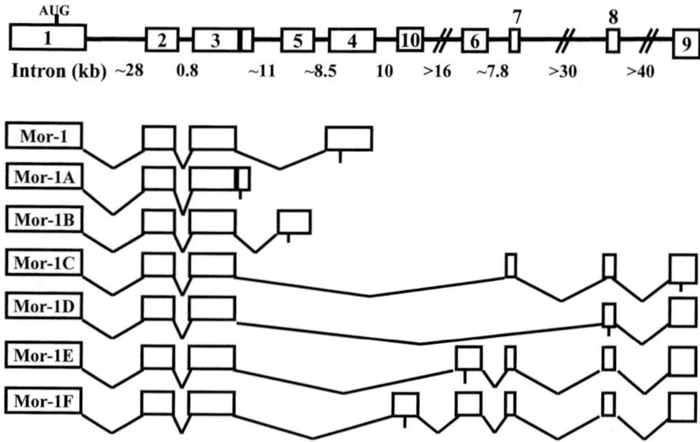

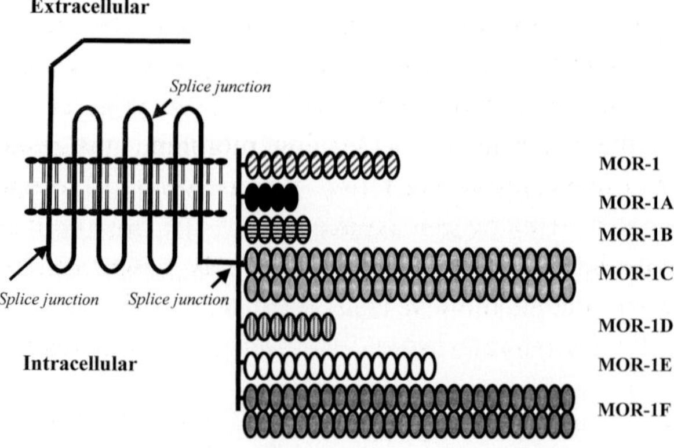

Fig. 4. Schematic of current MOR-1 gene. (A) Nucleotide structure: Exons are noted as boxes and are numbered according to their discovery. Intron distances between exons are noted as kilobases (kb). In the variants, the termination codons are indicated by a small line on the bottom of the exon box. Although some variants share coding exons, none share an amino acid sequence due to frame shifts. (B) Amino acid structure: All the variants result in changes in the amino acid sequences in the terminal portion of the COOH terminus of the receptor. The number of amino acids for each variant is indicated. Note that the amino acid sequences encoded by the various variants are all unique.

These variants also appear to be functionally relevant. Antisense mapping studies demonstrate that probes targeting exons 6, 7, 8, or 9 all down-regulate morphine analgesia, but not M6G analgesia (Pan et al. 1999). Since MOR-1E is the only variant containing exon 6, MOR-1E clearly is involved in morphine analgesia. However, the roles of MOR-1C and MOR-1D cannot be easily ascertained from these studies because the exons contained within these variants are also contained in MOR-1E. The antisense probes targeting exons 7, 8, and 9 may be decreasing morphine analgesia by downregulating MOR-1C or MOR-1D. Alternatively, they also might reflect activity only at MOR-1E. In additional studies, an antisense probe targeting exon 10, which is contained only within MOR-1F, shows only a modest effect against morphine analgesia, suggesting that it may play a small role in morphine's analgesic actions. However, the evidence implies that a number of MOR-1 variants are involved with morphine actions.

CONCLUSIONS

Morphine analgesia is becoming increasingly complex. The early pharmacological studies implied three subdivisions of μ receptors, but cloning studies now have identified at least seven MOR-1 splice variants encoding μ-opioid receptors. Many questions remain regarding the mechanisms of μ analgesics. Although the evidence suggests a distinct M6G receptor at both the pharmacological and molecular level, this receptor has not yet been isolated. Even the mechanisms underlying morphine analgesia are uncertain. However, it does appear that more than one μ-opioid receptor mediates morphine analgesia. If many μ-receptor variants are important in producing analgesia, incomplete cross-tolerance may simply reflect differences in selectivity of drugs among these receptors (Fig. 5). Tolerance would be expected only at the receptors being activated. If a new μ analgesic activated a

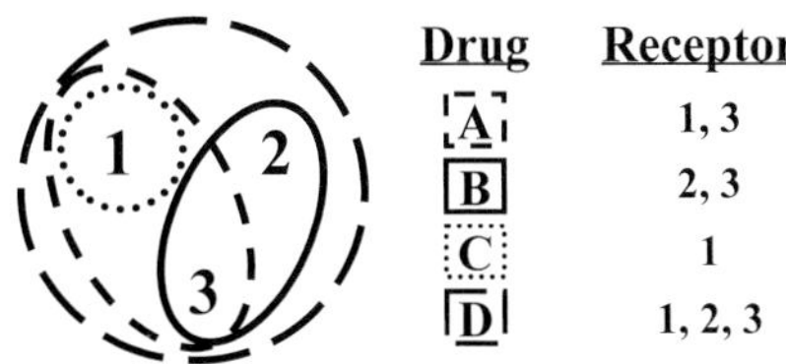

Fig. 5. Schematic of a hypothetical approach to incomplete cross-tolerance. The receptor selectivity of each drug is indicated by the receptors included within its circle. Thus, Drug A activates receptors 1 and 3; Drug B receptors 2 and 3; Drug C receptor 1; and Drug D receptors 1, 2, and 3. Drugs presumably would induce tolerance to the receptors that they activate.

Cross Tolerance

Challenge Drug	If tolerant to A	B	C	D
A	-	Slight	Slight	Yes
B	Slight	-	No	Yes
C	Yes	No	-	Yes
D	Slight	Slight	Slight	-

subtype not made tolerant previously, only limited cross-tolerance would be expected. Although intriguing, however, this hypothesis has still not been adequately tested experimentally.

The identification of these additional μ-receptor variants also offers interesting opportunities in future drug development. Will certain subtypes of μ-opioid receptors mediate problematic side effects, such as respiratory depression, sedation, and constipation, as suggested by the studies with naloxonazine? Will it be possible to design either agonists or antagonists that interact with only one μ-receptor subtype? It seems likely that further μ-receptor variants will be uncovered, emphasizing the ever-increasing complexity of the μ-receptor system and potential new targets in the search for safe, effective analgesics lacking side effects.

ACKNOWLEDGMENTS

I would like to thank the National Institute on Drug Abuse and the National Cancer Institute for their support of much of the work described in this chapter.

REFERENCES

Abbadie C, Pan Y-X, Pasternak GW. Distribution in rat brain of a new mu opioid receptor splice variant MOR1C: evidence for region specific-specific processing. *Mol Pharmacol* 1999; 56:396–403.

Abdelhamid EE, Sultana M, Portoghese PS, Takemori AE. Selective blockage of delta opioid receptors prevents the development of morphine tolerance and dependence in mice. *J Pharmacol Exp Ther* 1991; 258:299–303.

Atweh SF, Kuhar MJ. Autoradiographic localization of opiate receptors in rat brain. I. Spinal cord and lower medulla. *Brain Res* 1977b; 124:53–67.

Atweh SF, Kuhar MJ. Autoradiographic localization of opiate receptors in rat brain. II. The brain stem. *Brain Res* 1977c; 129:1–12.

Atweh SF, Kuhar MJ. Autoradiographic localization of opiate receptors in rat brain. III. The telencephalon. *Brain Res* 1977a; 134:393–405.

Bare LA, Mansson E, Yang D. Expression of two variants of the human μ opioid receptor mRNA in SK-N-SH cells and human brain. *FEBS Lett* 1994; 354:213–216.

Baron A, Shuster L, Elefterhiou BE, Bailey DW. Opiate receptors in mice: genetic differences. *Life Sci* 1975; 17:633–640.

Beecher HK. Pain in men wounded in battle. *Ann Surgery* 1946; 123:96–105.

Bodnar RJ, Williams CW, Pasternak GW. Role of mu_1 opiate receptors in supraspinal opiate analgesia: a microinjection study. *Brain Res* 1988; 447:45–52.

Brenman JE, Chao DS, Gee SH, et al. Interaction of nitric oxide synthase with the postsynaptic density protein PSD-95 and α1-syntrophin mediated by PDZ domains. *Cell* 1996; 84:757–767.

Brown GP, Yang K, King MA, et al. 3-Methoxynaltrexone, a selective heroin/morphine-6β-glucuronide antagonist. *FEBS Lett* 1997; 412:35–38.

Bunzow JR, Saez C, Mortrud M, et al. Molecular cloning and tissue distribution of a putative member of the rat opioid receptor gene family that is not a μ, δ or kappa opioid receptor type. *FEBS Lett* 1994; 347:284–288.

Chakrabarti S, Sultana M, Portoghese PS, Takemori AE. Differential antagonism by naltrindole-5'-isothiocyanate on [^{3}H]DSLET and [^{3}H]DPDPE binding to striatal slices of mice. *Life Sci* 1993; 53:1761–1765.

Chang A, Emmel DW, Rossi GC, Pasternak GW. Methadone analgesia in morphine-insensitive CXBK mice. *Eur J Pharmacol* 1998; 351:189–191.

Chen Y, Mestek A, Liu J, Yu L. Molecular cloning of a rat kappa opioid receptor reveals sequence similarities to the μ and δ opioid receptors. *Biochem J* 1993; 295:625–628.

Connelly CD, Martinez RP, Schupsky JJ, Porreca F, Raffa RB. Etonitazene-induced antinociception in μ_1 opioid receptor deficient CXBK mice: Evidence for a role for μ_2 receptors in supraspinal antinociception. *Life Sci* 1994; 54:369–374.

Crooke ST. Progress toward oligonucleotide therapeutics: pharmacodynamic properties. *FASEB J* 1993; 7:533–539.

Evans CJ, Keith DE Jr, Morrison H, Magendzo K, Edwards RH. Cloning of a delta opioid receptor by functional expression. *Science* 1992; 258:1952–1955.

Fukuda K, Kato S, Mori K, et al. cDNA cloning and regional distribution of a novel member of the opioid receptor family. *FEBS Lett* 1994; 343:42–46.

Goodman RR, Pasternak GW. Visualization of mu_1 opiate receptors in rat brain using a computerized autoradiographic subtraction technique. *Proc Natl Acad Sci USA* 1985; 82:6667–6671.

Hahn EF, Pasternak GW. Naloxonazine, a potent, long-acting inhibitor of opiate binding sites. *Life Sci* 1982; 31:1385–1388.

Hahn EF, Carroll-Buatti M, Pasternak GW. Irreversible opiate agonists and antagonists: the 14-hydroxydihydromorphinone azines. *J Neurosci* 1982; 2:572–576.

Hand CW, Blunnie WP, Claffey LP, et al. Potential analgesic contribution from morphine-6-glucuronide in CSF. *Lancet* 1987; 1207–1208.

Heyman JS, Williams CL, Burks TF, Mosberg HI, Porreca F. Dissociation of opioid antinociception and central gastrointestinal propulsion in the mouse: studies with naloxonazine. *J Pharmacol Exp Ther* 1988; 245:238–243.

Jiang Q, Mosberg HI, Porreca F. Antinociceptive effects of [D-ala^2] deltorphin II, a highly selective δ agonist *in vivo*. *Life Sci* 1990; 47:PL43–PL47.

Jiang Q, Takemori AE, Sultana M, et al. Differential antagonism of opiate delta antinociception by [D-Ala^2,Cys^6]enkephalin and naltrindole-5'-iosothiocyanate: evidence for subtypes. *J Pharmacol Exp Ther* 1991; 257:1069–1075.

Keith D Jr, Maung T, Anton B, Evans C. Isolation of cDNA clones homologous to opioid receptors. *Regul Pept* 1994; 54:143–144.

Kieffer BL. Opioids: first lessons from knockout mice. *Trends Pharmacol Sci* 1999; 20:19–26.

Kieffer BL, Befort K, Gaveriaux-Ruff C, Hirth CG. The δ-opioid receptor: isolation of a cDNA by expression cloning and pharmacological characterization. *Proc Natl Acad Sci USA* 1992; 89:12048–12052.

Kitanaka N, Sora I, Kinsey S, Zeng ZZ, Uhl GR. No heroin or morphine 6β-glucuronide analgesia in μ-opioid receptor knockout mice. *Eur J Pharmacol* 1998; 355:R1–R3.

Knapp RJ, Malatynska E, Collins N, et al. Molecular biology and pharmacology of cloned opioid receptors. *FASEB J* 1995; 9:516–525.

Lefkowitz RJ. G protein-coupled receptor kinases. *Cell* 1993; 74:409–412.

Lefkowitz RJ. G protein-coupled receptors and receptor kinases: from molecular biology to potential therapeutic applications. *Bio Technology* 1996; 14:283–286.

Li S, Zhu J, Chen C, et al. Molecular cloning and expression of a rat kappa opioid receptor. *Biochem J* 1993; 295:629–633.

Ling GSF, Spiegel K, Nishimura S, Pasternak GW. Dissociation of morphine's analgesic and respiratory depressant actions. *Eur J Pharmacol* 1983; 86:487–488.

Ling GSF, MacLeod JM, Lee S, Lockhart SH, Pasternak GW. Separation of morphine analgesia from physical dependence. *Science* 1984; 226:462–464.

Ling GSF, Spiegel K, Lockhart SH, Pasternak GW. Separation of opioid analgesia from respiratory depression: evidence for different receptor mechanisms. *J Pharmacol Exp Ther* 1985; 232:149–155.

Ling GSF, Simantov R, Clark JA, Pasternak GW. Naloxonazine actions in vivo. *Eur J Pharmacol* 1986; 129:33–38.

Loh HH, Liu HC, Cavalli A, et al. μ Opioid receptor knockout in mice: effects on ligand-induced analgesia and morphine lethality. *Mol Brain Res* 1998; 54:321–326.

Matthes HWD, Maldonado R, Simonin F, et al. Loss of morphine-induced analgesia, reward effect and withdrawal symptoms in mice lacking the μ-opioid-receptor gene. *Nature* 1996; 383:819–823.

Mattia A, Vanderah T, Mosberg HI, Porreca F. Lack of antinociceptive cross tolerance between [D-Pen^2,D-Pen^5]enkephalin and [D-Ala^2]deltorphin II in mice: evidence for delta receptor subtypes. *J Pharmacol Exp Ther* 1991; 258:583–587.

Meunier JC, Mollereau C, Toll L, et al. Isolation and structure of the endogenous agonist of the opioid receptor like ORL_1 receptor. *Nature* 1995; 377:532–535.

Mogil JS, Kest B, Sadowski B, Belknap JK. Differential genetic mediation of sensitivity to morphine in genetic models of opiate antinociception: Influence of nociceptive assay. *J Pharmacol Exp Ther* 1996; 276:532–544.

Mollereau C, Parmentier M, Mailleux P, et al. ORL-1, a novel member of the opioid family: cloning, functional expression and localization. *FEBS Lett* 1994; 341:33–38.

Moskowitz AS, Goodman RR. Autoradiographic analysis of mu_1, mu_2, and delta opioid binding in the central nervous system of C57BL/6BY and CXBK (opioid receptor-deficient) mice. *Brain Res* 1985; 360:108–116.

Osborne R, Joel S, Trew D, Slevin M. Analgesic activity of morphine-6-glucuronide. *Lancet* 1988; 828–828.

Pan Y-X, Cheng J, Xu J, Pasternak GW. Cloning, expression and classification of a $kappa_3$-related opioid receptor using antisense oligodeoxynucleotides. *Regul Pept* 1994; 54:217–218.

Pan Y-X, Cheng J, Xu J, et al. Cloning and functional characterization through antisense mapping of a $kappa_3$-related opioid receptor. *Mol Pharmacol* 1995; 47:1180–1188.

Pan YX, Xu J, Bolan EA, et al. Identification and characterization of three new alternatively spliced mu opioid receptor isoforms. *Mol Pharmacol* 1999; 56:396–403.

Pasternak GW. Pharmacological mechanisms of opioid analgesics. *Clin Neuropharmacol* 1993; 16:1–18.

Pasternak GW, Snyder SH. Identification of a novel high affinity opiate receptor binding in rat brain. *Nature* 1975; 253:563–565.

Pasternak GW, Bodnar RJ, Clark JA, Inturrisi CE. Morphine-6-glucuronide, a potent mu agonist. *Life Sci* 1987; 41:2845–2849.

Pasternak GW, Childers SR, Snyder SH. Opiate analgesia: evidence for mediation by a subpopulation of opiate receptors. *Science* 1980a; 208:514–516.

Pasternak GW, Childers SR, Snyder SH. Naloxazone, long-acting opiate antagonist: effects in intact animals and on opiate receptor binding in vitro. *J Pharmacol Exp Ther* 1980b; 214:455–462.

Paul D, Pasternak GW. Differential blockade by naloxonazine of two μ opiate actions: analgesia and inhibition of gastrointestinal transit. *Eur J Pharmacol* 1988; 149:403–404.

Paul D, Standifer KM, Inturrisi CE, Pasternak GW. Pharmacological characterization of morphine-6β-glucuronide, a very potent morphine metabolite. *J Pharmacol Exp Ther* 1989a; 251:477–483.

Paul D, Bodnar RJ, Gistrak MA, Pasternak GW. Different μ receptor subtypes mediate spinal and supraspinal analgesia in mice. *Eur J Pharmacol* 1989b; 129:307–314.

Pert CB, Snyder SH. Opiate receptor: demonstration in nervous tissue. *Science* 1973; 179:1011–1014.

Pick CG, Nejat R, Pasternak GW. Independent expression of two pharmacologically distinct supraspinal mu analgesic systems in genetically different mouse strains. *J Pharmacol Exp Ther* 1993; 2265:166–171.

Portoghese PS, Lipkowski AW, Takemori AE. Binaltorphimine and nor-binaltorphimine, potent and selective κ-opioid receptor agonists. *Life Sci* 1987; 40:1287–1292.

Reinscheid RK, Nothacker HP, Bourson A, et al. Orphanin FQ: a neuropeptide that activates an opioidlike G protein-coupled receptor. *Science* 1995; 270:792–794.

Reisine T, Bell GI. Molecular biology of opioid receptors. *Trends Neurosci* 1993; 16:506–510.

Reisine T, Pasternak GW. Opioid analgesics and antagonists. In: Hardman JG, Limbird LE (Eds). *Goodman & Gilman's: The Pharmacological Basis of Therapeutics.* McGraw-Hill, 1996, pp 521–556.

Reith MEA, Sershen H, Vadasz C, Lajtha A. Strain differences in opiate receptors in mouse brain. *Eur J Pharmacol* 1981; 74:377–380.

Rossi GC, Pan Y-X, Cheng J, Pasternak GW. Blockade of morphine analgesia by an antisense oligodeoxynucleotide against the mu receptor. *Life Sci* 1994; 54:PL375–379.

Rossi GC, Pan Y-X, Brown GP, Pasternak GW. Antisense mapping the MOR1 opioid receptor: Evidence for alternative splicing and a novel morphine-6β-glucuronide receptor. *FEBS Lett* 1995; 369:192–196.

Rossi GC, Brown GP, Leventhal L, Yang K, Pasternak GW. Novel receptor mechanisms for heroin and morphine-6β-glucuronide analgesia. *Neurosci Lett* 1996; 216:1–4.

Rossi GC, Leventhal L, Pan YX, et al. Antisense mapping of MOR1 in the rat: distinguishing between morphine and morphine-6β-glucuronide antinociception. *J Pharmacol Exp Ther* 1997; 281:109–114.

Schuller AG, King MA, Zhang J, et al. Retention of heroin and morphine-6 beta-glucuronide analgesia in a new line of mice lacking exon 1 of MOR1. *Nat Neurosci* 1999; 2:151–156.

Shimomura K, Kamata O, Ueki S, et al. Analgesic effect of morphine glucuronides. *Tohoku J Exp Med* 1971; 105:45–52.

Simon EJ, Hiller JM, Edelman I. Stereospecific binding of the potent narcotic analgesic [^{3}H]Etorphine to rat-brain homogenate. *Proc Natl Acad Sci USA* 1973; 70:1947–1949.

Sofuoglu M, Portoghese PS, Takemori AE. 7-benzylidenenaltrexone (BNTX): A selective δ_1 opioid receptor antagonist in the mouse spinal cord. *Life Sci* 1992; 52:769–775.

Sora I, Takahashi N, Funada M, et al. Opiate receptor knockout mice define μ receptor roles in endogenous nociceptive responses and morphine-induced analgesia. *Proc Natl Acad Sci USA* 1997; 94:1544–1549.

Standifer KM, Chien C-C, Wahlestedt C, Brown GP, Pasternak GW. Selective loss of δ opioid analgesia and binding by antisense oligodeoxynucleotides to a δ opioid receptor. *Neuron* 1994; 12:805–810.

Stein CA, Cheng Y-C. Antisense oligonucleotides as therapeutic agents—is the bullet really magical? *Science* 1993; 261:1004–1012.

Terenius L. Stereospecific interaction between narcotic analgesics and a synaptic plasma membrane fraction of rat cerebral cortex. *Acta Pharmacol Toxicol* 1973; 32.

Tiseo PJ, Thaler HT, Lapin J, et al. Morphine-6-glucuronide concentrations and opioid-related side effects: a survey in cancer patients. *Pain* 1995; 61:47–54.

Vaught JL, Mathiasen JHR, Raffa RB. Examination of the involvement of supraspinal and spinal mu and delta opioid receptors in analgesia using the mu receptor deficient CXBK mouse. *J Pharmacol Exp Ther* 1988; 245:12–16.

Walker JR, King M, Izzo E, Koob GF, Pasternak GW. Antagonism of heroin and morphine self-administration in rats by the morphine-6β-glucuronide antagonist 3-0-methylnaltrexone. *Eur J Pharmacol* 1999; in press.

Wang JB, Imai Y, Eppler CM, et al. μ Opiate receptor: cDNA cloning and expression. *Proc Natl Acad Sci USA* 1993; 90:10,230–10,234.

Ward SJ, Portoghese PS, Takemori AE. Pharmacological characterization in vivo of the novel opiate, β-funaltrexamine. *J Pharmacol Exp Ther* 1982; 220:494–498.

Wolozin BL, Pasternak GW. Classification of multiple morphine and enkephalin binding sites in the central nervous system. *Proc Natl Acad Sci USA* 1981; 78:6181–6185.

Yasuda K, Raynor K, Kong H, et al. Cloning and functional comparison of kappa and δ opioid receptors from mouse brain. *Proc Natl Acad Sci USA* 1993; 90:6736–6740.

Yoshimura H, Ida S, Oguri K, Tsukamoto H. Biochemical basis for analgesic activity of morphine-6β-glucuronide. I: Penetration of morphine-6β-glucuronide in the brain of rats. *Biochem Pharmacol* 1973; 22:1423–1430.

Zimprich A, Simon T, Hollt V. Cloning and expression of an isoform of the rat μ opioid receptor (rMOR 1B) which differs in agonist induced desensitization from rMOR-1. *FEBS Lett* 1995; 359:142–146.

Correspondence to: Gavril W. Pasternak, MD, PhD, Department of Neurology, Memorial Sloan-Kettering Cancer Center, 1275 York Avenue, New York, NY 10021, USA. Tel: 212-639-7046; Fax: 212-794-4332; email: pasterng@mskmail.mskcc.org.

Proceedings of the 9th World Congress on Pain,
Progress in Pain Research and Management,
Vol. 16, edited by M. Devor, M.C. Rowbotham, and
Z. Wiesenfeld-Hallin, IASP Press, Seattle, © 2000.

15

Approaches to the Study of Altered Gene Expression in Pain[1]

Katia Befort and Michael Costigan

Neural Plasticity Research Group, Department of Anesthesia and Critical Care, Massachusetts General Hospital and Harvard Medical School, Charlestown, Massachusetts, USA

Molecular control within the cell can occur at several stages. The first major rate-limiting step is transcription, the conversion of the DNA genetic blueprint into the RNA message en route to protein production. The pattern of messenger RNA (mRNA) expression is therefore the molecular determinant of a cell's functional potential. Studies of altered gene expression are essentially concerned with changes in mRNA levels. Messenger RNAs are very unstable molecules, however, reflecting the fact that they represent a transient communication point within the cell. To analyze mRNA levels it is necessary to convert this unstable molecule into a more permanent facsimile. An enzyme called reverse transcriptase is used to produce a complementary DNA (cDNA) copy of the mRNA, and the cDNA molecules are used as a tool to identify changes in gene expression. However, changes in mRNA levels are not the only way a cell exercises molecular control of its function: translational (the conversion of mRNA into protein) and post-translational changes (protein modification by phosphorylation, for example) are equally important (Woolf and Costigan 1999).

Several methods have been developed over the last decade to isolate genes, know and unknown, that are important in various cellular processes. Methods of looking at altered gene expression include differential display, expressed sequence tags (ESTs), serial analysis of gene expression (SAGE), various subtractive cloning techniques, gene grids, and microarrays (Table I). For homology cloning, methods include degenerate polymerase chain reaction (PCR) and in silico cloning. This chapter aims to critically evaluate

---

[1] Mini-review based on a congress workshop.

Table I

Summary of different techniques to isolate novel regulated genes

Method	RNA Requirement	Sequencing Needs	Each Way Analysis	Multiple Sample Analysis	Advantages and Disadvantages
Differential display	10–100 ng poly-A RNA	Medium	Yes	Very simple	Relatively easy to set up, low cost. Prone to false positives. Often pulls out 3´UTR sequence.
EST	1–5 μg poly-A RNA	High	Yes	Very expensive	Relatively easy, but high cost. Sequencer required. Large amounts of sequencing are required for adequate depth, thus most studies are likely to identify only highly regulated genes.
SAGE	1–5 μg poly-A RNA	High	Yes	Difficult	Medium cost. Very high relative output. Technically demanding. Sequencer and software required.
Microarray chips	>1 μg poly-A RNA	Low	Yes	Expensive but simple	Expensive; usually company driven. Practical processing not routine.
Commercial gene grids	>1 μg poly-A RNA	Low	Yes	Fairly expensive but simple	Fairly expensive. Relatively low number of genes analyzed; only obvious candidates. Technically very simple.
Subtractive hybridization	10–100 ng poly-A RNA	Medium	No	Simple	Low cost. High relative output for small operation. Technically demanding. Often pulls out 3´UTR sequence.

Note: See Table II for explanation of abbreviations..

Table II
Abbreviations and definitions

Abbreviation or Term	Definition
cDNA	Complementary DNA (a DNA copy of the less stable mRNA)
DD-PCR	Differential display PCR (an expression profiling method)
Degenerate PCR	PCR using protein sequence to produce the oligonucleotide primers
Driver	The control population in subtractive hybridization
EST	Expressed sequence tag (random sequencing of clones from a cDNA library)
Grid	A collection of genes, represented by cDNAs, arranged on a nylon membrane
In silico	With the aid of a computer
Microarray	A collection of genes, represented by oligonucleotides, arranged on a silica chip
mRNA	Messenger RNA (the genes expressed within a cell type)
Oligonucleotide	Short sequence of single-stranded DNA
PCR	Polymerase chain reaction
RDA	Representational difference analysis (a cDNA subtraction method)
SAGE	Serial analysis of gene expression (an expression profiling method)
Tester	The treated population in subtractive hybridization

these techniques; where possible, we provide examples of studies that have used these methods with regard to isolating genes that are involved in pain signaling or in responses to peripheral nerve damage.

DIFFERENTIAL DISPLAY

First introduced by Liang and Pardee in 1992 (Liang et al. 1994, 1995; Liang and Pardee 1995, 1997) and adapted to a slightly different protocol by McClelland and colleagues (McClelland et al. 1993, 1995; McClelland and Welsh 1994), the differential display method uses a PCR-based protocol to produce a molecular "bar code" of a cDNA sample. If all the reaction conditions are kept constant between a control and a treated cDNA population, then it is proposed that any differences in the fingerprint are the result of differentially regulated genes (for reviews see Livesey and Hunt 1996; Matz and Lukyanov 1998).

Protocols differ slightly, but differential display PCR (DD-PCR) is essentially performed as follows. Messenger RNA is purified from total RNA and reverse transcribed with a poly-d(T) primer to produce first-strand cDNA. This is amplified using both an arbitrary primer and the reverse transcription primer. The arbitrary primers, usually 10 bases long, can prime on multiple transcripts to produce a number of different-sized bands, which represent different genes. An effective molecular bar code of the genes present in the mRNA sample can then be produced on a gel; differences in the bar code represent differentially regulated genes (Fig. 1).

This method is very popular because it is inexpensive and relatively simple to perform. Differential display PCR (DD-PCR) requires only small amounts of RNA, and can reliably produce cDNA with as little as 50 ng of total RNA. One of the major advantages of this method is that multiple samples can be run simultaneously, so that a whole treatment time course can be run on the same gel and the gene expression profile monitored.

Differential display is, however, prone to a high false-positive rate, due to the fact that PCR is an amplification process; thus, the minutest of differences in the starting material can lead to huge differences in the final molecular fingerprint (Debouck 1995). It is essential, therefore, to control against this by amplifying independent samples for each cDNA sample and by being very careful to standardize all of the preparation conditions among samples. Another disadvantage of DD-PCR is that the molecular bar codes produced in each PCR reaction contain bands that represent only a very few genes, around 50–100 genes in one reaction. To analyze the sample in detail, many reactions must be performed, each with a different arbitrary primer. Kits are available from various companies to perform DD-PCR. Despite its disadvantages, this method probably represents the best option for nonmolecular laboratories hoping to start down the road of gene discovery.

Differential display has been used to isolate genes regulated in response to axotomy of the sciatic nerve (Livesey et al. 1997), many of which may play key roles in regenerative mechanisms (Livesey and Hunt 1998).

EXPRESSED SEQUENCE TAG SEQUENCING

Expressed sequence tags or ESTs were first introduced in 1991 (Adams et al. 1991). With this method, whole cDNA libraries are produced for a control and a treated population separately, and these libraries are then sequenced. With the aid of an automated sequencer, many randomly picked individual cDNA clones can be sequenced in a relatively short time. This method is fairly simple to perform, but requires at least two cDNA libraries and the dedicated use of an automated sequencer—resources not available to most laboratories. With this method, the greater the number of individual

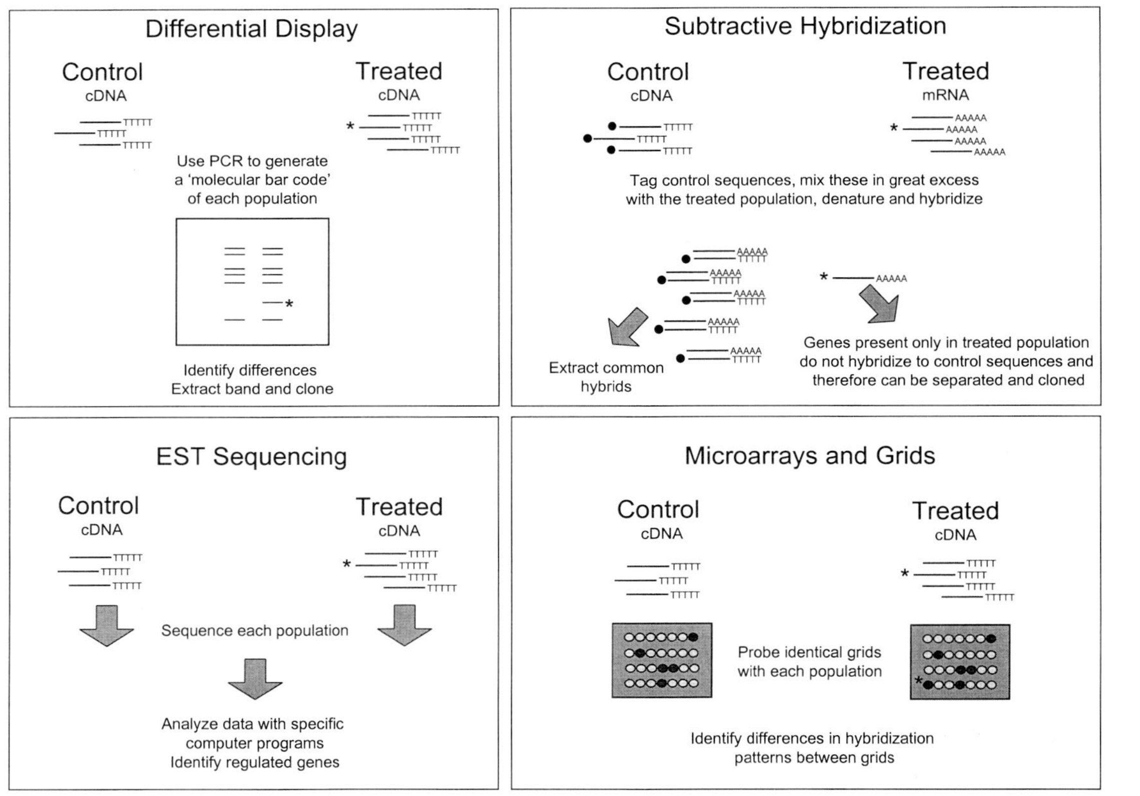

Fig.1. Methods used to isolate differentially regulated genes.

clones sequenced from each library, the more meaningful are the results; meaningful results require at least 3000 sequences per library (Lee et al. 1995).

Several biotechnology companies are involved in enormous cDNA library sequencing projects. The sequences that are obtained are placed in databases that can be compared using sophisticated bioinformatic software packages that can detect genes that are expressed in only one of the populations and identify genes that are up- or downregulated. These sequence databases thus represent a very valuable resource for profiling gene expression, and even make it possible to clone genes in silico without the need for any bench work. In silico cloning begins when a new gene is published, for example, for an ion channel or a receptor. This sequence is then fed into the database, and homology searches are performed for ESTs that may represent a new unknown family member. Once an interesting EST is identified, the cDNA database is searched, and in a method analogous to conventional cloning from cDNA libraries, new ESTs with homology to the original sequence are used to walk along the gene sequence (Fig. 2). Once the gene has been assembled within the computer, PCR or conventional cloning techniques are used to isolate a "wet" copy, which can then be expressed and the function of the protein analyzed.

With respect to cloning of genes related to pain, homology searches for ESTs were used to isolate VRL1, a family member of the capsaicin receptor VR1, which has been postulated to act as the transduction protein for the high-threshold Aδ heat receptor (Caterina et al. 1999).

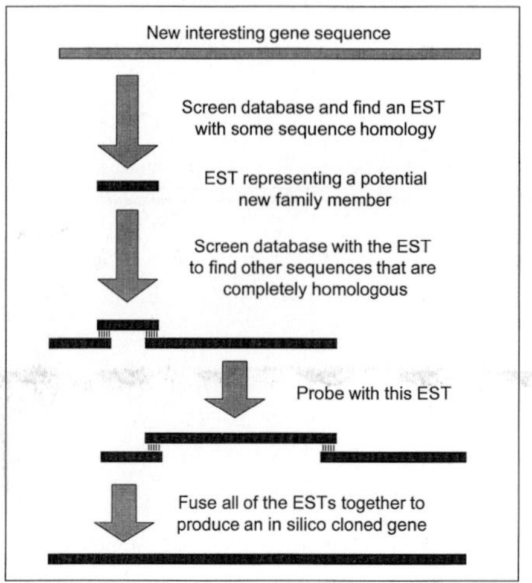

Fig. 2. Method of cloning genes in silico.

SERIAL ANALYSIS OF GENE EXPRESSION

The serial analysis of gene expression (SAGE) technique is a method that constructs two gene databases in a similar way to that described above for EST analysis (Velculescu et al. 1995; Adams 1996). SAGE, however, avoids the practical problem inherent in EST analysis (which requires the production of massive data sets) by giving every gene a short code, allowing the expression profile of far larger sets of genes to be assembled.

In a complex process, described in detail elsewhere (Adams 1996), libraries are created containing very short sequence tags, nine base pairs in length. Theoretically, nine base pairs are sufficient to distinguish between every gene in the pool; a tag is produced for every gene present, and every gene is given its own nine-digit code. The tags are then ligated to one another to produce concatemers, or linked mixtures, of 20 or more gene codes, which are then cloned and sequenced. A profile of gene expression in a given RNA sample can then be derived using the relative number of each gene code present. If two RNA samples are subjected to SAGE analysis, the gene expression databases can be compared, and up- and downregulated gene codes can be identified. Once a tag of interest is found, it can be decoded by a standard database search to determine the identity of the gene from which it arose. If the gene is unknown, the nine-mer can be incorporated into a PCR primer to isolate a longer clone.

These very short ESTs offer an unparalleled ability to perform high-throughput screening of the expression profile of an RNA sample, as every sequenced clone represents 20 or more genes as opposed to just one in standard EST analysis. Where a sample set may consist of 3000 individual genes when sequenced by conventional EST analysis, SAGE allows tens of thousands of genes to be sequenced per sample. The greater the depth of the expression profile, the more likely is the identification of all the relevant changes in mRNA levels. On a more negative front, SAGE is a very complex technique that requires a high level of competence in molecular biology and a great deal of automated sequencing. SAGE does, however, offer the opportunity for single laboratories to comprehensively profile the expression of genes in given RNA samples, and the method has produced some impressive results. In one study, 7000 individual genes were identified; only 14 of these genes (0.19%) were upregulated in a colorectal carcinoma cell line in response to p53-induced apoptosis. Strikingly, many of these genes were predicted to encode proteins that could generate or respond to oxidative stress (Polyak et al. 1997). To our knowledge, no studies using SAGE have been directed toward pain research.

SUBTRACTIVE HYBRIDIZATION

Subtractive hybridization (SH) was developed in the late 1980s to produce subtracted cDNA libraries. However, this method was inapplicable for studying many biological events because of the vast amounts of poly-A mRNA required (around 5–10 μg). The development of PCR as a tool for amplification has meant that SH can now be applied to biological events where mRNA is a limited resource. Many different subtraction protocols have been developed, including suppression subtractive hybridization (Diatchenko et al. 1999), representational difference analysis (Hubank and Schatz 1999), and various more conventional PCR-based subtraction techniques (Sagerstrom et al. 1997; Mannion et al. 2000). Each method differs in the molecular steps involved, but the aim of each is the same—to isolate sequences present in a treated (tester) mRNA sample but not in the control (driver) mRNA sample. Two mRNA samples are generated corresponding to the tester and driver populations, and the treated mRNA pool is reverse transcribed to produce a cDNA population. The control mRNA population is chemically linked to a molecule that allows it to be recognized later. A large quantity of chemically tagged control mRNA is mixed with the treated cDNA population, and the mixture is denatured and allowed to hybridize. Because of the stoichiometry of the reaction, sequences common to the control and treated populations hybridize as heteromeric molecules, and only sequences unique to the treated population remain as single-stranded cDNA (Fig. 1). The chemical tag present on the control molecules is then used to subtract out common hybrid molecules from the mixture, leaving only genes present in the treated population. Genes present only in the treated population can then be amplified by PCR, cloned, and sequenced.

Although conceptually simple, this method contains several complex molecular steps. For a molecular laboratory, however, it is an inexpensive and very effective method of cloning differentially regulated genes. One of the major disadvantages of most SH protocols is that the subtraction product often contains a proportion of clones that are not regulated but remain in the pool; however, reaction conditions can be modified to reduce this background (Wang and Brown 1991). It is often advisable to perform a further screening phase to lower the number of false positives encountered (Dulac and Axel 1995; Sagerstrom et al. 1997). Another disadvantage of SH is that each reaction only isolates genes regulated in one direction, so that two separate reactions must be performed, whereas many of the other available methods simultaneously identify up- and downregulated genes.

Gene expression in primary sensory neurons has been analyzed by subtractive hybridization. One such method was used to isolate genes expressed only in dorsal root ganglia (DRG) (Akopian and Wood 1995), such as the sensory-neuron-specific sodium channel (SNS) (Akopian et al. 1996). We have used a similar protocol to isolate genes that are up- and downregulated following axotomy of the sciatic nerve (Mannion et al. 2000). One of the genes thus isolated, the heat shock protein HSP27, is upregulated 10-fold within DRG neurons after nerve injury (Costigan et al. 1998). We have subsequently shown that this molecule is an intrinsic survival factor that may protect DRG neurons following peripheral nerve damage (Lewis et al. 1999).

MICROARRAYS AND GENE GRIDS

Another approach to obtaining novel genes that are differentially regulated between two samples is to perform a differential screen of pre-plated gene libraries. This protocol relies on the duplicate production of a library or grid of known genes spotted onto nylon or another material (Marshall and Hodgson 1998; Ramsay 1998). As these duplicate gene grids are ostensibly identical, if one is probed with a labeled control cDNA population probe and the other with the treated cDNA population, then any differences in the hybridization events that occur should identify differentially regulated genes (Fig. 1).

Certain pharmaceutical companies are now producing high-density arrays of oligonucleotides, which are generated on silica microchips (Schena 1996; Marshall and Hodgson 1998; Ramsay 1998). The sequence of each oligonucleotide is specific to an individual gene, and multiple oligonucleotides are produced for each gene. The RNA populations are then labeled to produce two complex probes, and each probe is hybridized with separate oligonucleotide microarrays. The gene chips are then scanned to look for specific genes, which display an altered expression profile. Because multiple copies of each gene are present, these copies can be checked to ensure that they show the same change in expression.

This novel method has a number of distinct advantages, the most important being that it does not involve the initial cloning step that would be necessary for cDNA library; only the gene sequences are required. Several complete genome sequencing projects are nearing completion, so in theory at least, the expression levels of every gene within a particular organism could be assayed by this method. Microarrays also facilitate investigation of gene families and splice variants, as well as polymorphic allele analysis of genetic traits. The major disadvantage with this technology is the expense, which restricts access to biotechnology or pharmaceutical companies. The potential strengths of these techniques are obvious, particularly once the human genome project is completed, and while some concerns have been raised over the sensitivity of these techniques, recent results are encouraging (Iyer et al. 1999).

A cheaper alternative to gene chips, available commercially from a number of different suppliers, are gene grids. Similar to microarrays, these are matrices of different genes (Trenkle et al. 1999). The differences are that the genes are represented not by oligonucleotides but by cDNAs, and that the clones are spotted onto standard nylon mesh as opposed to silica. Any investigator could purchase these arrays; however, they are fairly expensive when the software programs designed for the analysis of these gene grids are included. Also, the number of genes represented in the arrays is low, usually measured in the hundreds. The major advantages of gene grids are that very little practical knowledge is required and that results can be obtained in a very short time.

DEGENERATE PCR

Degenerate polymerase chain reaction can be used to discover new gene family members by exploiting homologous sequences. Such groups include ion channels, which are likely to play a major role in the molecular mechanisms of nociception (Woolf and Costigan 1999). Most gene families have conserved areas of protein sequences that represent features important to the function of these molecules, e.g., the membrane-spanning domains of receptor families. Sequence alignment can readily identify these areas within a family, and the sequences can then be used to produce degenerate PCR primers. PCR is used to amplify a product that will contain all of the known family members and, it is hoped, some new species. This PCR product can be used to screen a cDNA library to obtain larger novel clones. We have applied degenerate primer screening to a DRG cDNA library with the aim of cloning novel sodium channels. Primers were designed for conserved sequences within the 3′ coding region of the rat brain II, heart, skeletal muscle, and glial voltage-gated sodium channels. These primers were used to amplify a sodium channel panspecific probe from rat genomic DNA. A rat cDNA library was then used to assemble a novel sensory-neuron-specific, full-length sodium channel, SNS2 (Tate et al. 1998). The expression profile and electrophysiology of this channel suggests that it has an important role in the conduction of nociceptive input from the periphery (Tate et al. 1998). Other investigators have used degenerate PCR to isolate further new and exciting molecular targets, such as the neurotrophic factor persephin (Milbrandt et al. 1998) and the ion channel ASIC-β (Chen et al. 1998).

CONCLUSIONS

The techniques detailed above serve only to isolate a gene of interest. Following this first stage, the gene's differential expression must be confirmed. The gold standards for this are northern blotting, RNase protection, and in situ hybridization. If the gene of interest is expressed at medium to high levels, the best method for relative quantification is northern blotting, whereas if the gene is expressed at low levels then RNase protection should be used. Although these two methods are commonly employed to study changes in the levels of particular mRNAs, they offer no information on the cellular localization of the mRNA, which in a heterogeneous population of cells, such as a DRG, may be neurons, Schwann cells, or fibroblasts. In situ hybridization allows localization and comparative quantification of transcripts at a cellular level.

Molecular biological techniques offer a powerful approach for identifying the mechanisms that operate to produce pain. The full potential of these techniques, however, can only be realized when they are combined with nonmolecular techniques that allow us to study the function of identified genes. Cloning novel genes expressed in the pain somatosensory system is only the beginning. The formidable task ahead is to devise a strategy for identifying the physiological or pathophysiological role of these genes. Once this is in place, we will truly be on the way to understanding the molecular basis of pain.

REFERENCES

Adams MD. Serial analysis of gene expression: ESTs get smaller. *Bioessays* 1996; 18:261–262.

Adams MD, Kelley JM, Gocayne JD, et al. Complementary DNA sequencing: expressed sequence tags and human genome project. *Science* 1991; 252:1651–1656.

Akopian AN, Wood JN. Peripheral nervous system-specific genes identified by subtractive cDNA cloning. *J Biol Chem* 1995; 270:21264–21270.

Akopian AN, Sivilotti L, Wood JN. A tetrodotoxin-resistant voltage-gated sodium channel expressed by sensory neurons. *Nature* 1996; 379:257–262.

Caterina MJ, Rosen TA, Tominaga M, Brake AJ, Julius D. A capsaicin-receptor homologue with a high threshold for noxious heat. *Nature* 1999; 398:436–441.

Chen CC, England S, Akopian AN, Wood JN. A sensory neuron-specific proton-gated ion channel. *Proc Natl Acad Sci USA* 1998; 95:10240–10245.

Costigan M, Mannion RJ, Kendall G, et al. Heat Shock Protein 27: developmental regulation and expression after peripheral nerve injury. *J Neurosci* 1998; 18:5891–5900.

Debouck C. Differential display or differential dismay? *Curr Opin Biotechnol* 1995; 6:597–599.

Diatchenko L, Lukyanov S, Lau Y-FC, Siebert PD. Suppression subtractive hybridization: a versatile method for identifying differentially expressed genes. *Methods Enzymol* 1999; 303:369–380.

Dulac C, Axel R. A novel family of genes encoding putative pheromone receptors in mammals. *Cell* 1995; 83:195–206.

Hubank M, Schatz DG. cDNA representational difference analysis: a sensitive and flexible method for identification of differentially expressed genes. *Methods Enzymol* 1999; 303:325–349.

Iyer VR, Eisen MB, Ross DT, et al. The transcriptional program in the response of human fibroblasts to serum. *Science* 1999; 283:83–87.

Lee NH, Weinstock KG, Kirkness EF, et al. Comparative expressed-sequencing analysis of differential gene expression profiles in PC-12 cells before and after nerve growth factor treatment. *Proc Natl Acad Sci USA* 1995; 92:8303–8307.

Lewis SE, Mannion RJ, White FA, et al. A role for HSP27 in sensory neuron survival. *J Neurosci* 1999; 19:8945–8953.

Liang P, Pardee AB. Recent advances in differential display. *Curr Opin Immunol* 1995; 7:274–280.

Liang P, Pardee AB. Differential display. A general protocol. *Methods Mol Biol* 1997; 85:3–11.

Liang P, Zhu W, Zhang X, et al. Differential display using one-base anchored oligo-dT primers. *Nucleic Acids Res* 1994; 22:5763–5764.

Liang P, Bauer D, Averboukh L, et al. Analysis of altered gene expression by differential display. *Methods Enzymol* 1995; 254:304–321.

Livesey F, Hunt SP. Identifying changes in gene expression in the nervous system: mRNA differential display. *Trends Neurosci* 1996; 19:84–88.

Livesey F, Hunt SP. Differential display cloning of genes induced in regenerating neurons. *Methods* 1998; 16:386–395.

Livesey F, O'Brien J, Li M, et al. A Schwann cell mitogen accompanying regeneration of motor neurons. *Nature* 1997; 390:614–618.

Mannion RJ, Costigan M, Woolf CJ. Molecular approaches to the study of pain. In: Wood JN (Ed). *Molecular Basis of Pain Induction.* New York: Wiley-Liss, 2000, pp 87–111.

Marshall A, Hodgson J. DNA chips: an array of possibilities. *Nat Biotechnol* 1998; 16:27–31.

Matz MV, Lukyanov SA. Different strategies of differential display: areas of application. *Nucleic Acids Res* 1998; 26:5537–5543.

McClelland M, Welsh J. RNA fingerprinting by arbitrarily primed PCR. *PCR Methods* (1994) Appl 4:S66–S81.

McClelland M, Chada K, Welsh J, Ralph D. Arbitrary primed PCR fingerprinting of RNA applied to mapping differentially expressed genes. *EXS* 1993; 67:103–115.

McClelland M, Matheiu-Daude F, Welsh J. RNA fingerprinting and differential display using arbitrarily primed PCR. *Trends Genet* 1995; 11:242–246.

Milbrandt J, de Sauvage FJ, Fahrner TJ, et al. Persephin, a novel neurotrophic factor related to GDNF and neurturin. *Neuron* 1998; 20:245–253.

Polyak K, Xia Y, Zwieler JL, Kinzler KW, Vogelstein B. A model for p53-induced apoptosis. *Nature* 1997; 389:300–305.

Ramsay G. DNA chips: state-of-the-art. *Nat Biotechnol* 1998; 16:40–44.

Sagerstrom CG, Sun BI, Sive HL. Subtractive cloning: past, present, and future. *Annu Rev Biochem* 1997: 66:751–783.

Schena M. Genome analysis with gene expression microarrays. *Bioessays* 1996; 18:427–431.

Tate S, Benn S, Hick C, et al. Two sodium channels contribute to the TTX-R sodium current in primary sensory neurons. *Nat Neurosci* 1998; 1:653–655.

Trenkle T, Mathieu-Daude F, Welsh J, McClelland M. Reduced complexity probes for DNA arrays. *Methods Enzymol* 1999; 303:381–392.

Velculescu VE, Zhang L, Vogelstein B, Kinzler KW. Serial analysis of gene expression. *Science* 1995; 270:484–487.

Wang Z, Brown DD. A gene expression screen. *Proc Natl Acad Sci USA* 1991; 88:11505–11509.

Woolf CJ, Costigan M. Transcriptional and posttranslational plasticity and the generation of inflammatory pain. *Proc Natl Acad Sci USA* 1999; 96:7723–7730.

Correspondence to: Michael Costigan, Neural Plasticity Research Group, Dept of Anesthesia and Critical Care, Massachusetts General Hospital and Harvard Medical School, 149 13th Street, Room 4309, Charlestown, MA 02129, USA. Tel: 617-724-3614; Fax: 617-724-3632; email: costigan@helix.mgh.harvard.edu.

Proceedings of the 9th World Congress on Pain,
Progress in Pain Research and Management,
Vol. 16, edited by M. Devor, M.C. Rowbotham, and
Z. Wiesenfeld-Hallin, IASP Press, Seattle, © 2000.

16

Neurotrophic Factor Effects on Pain-Signaling Systems[1]

Tim J. Boucher, Bradley J. Kerr, Matt S. Ramer, S.W.N. Thompson, and Stephen B. McMahon

Neuroscience Research Centre, King's College London, London, United Kingdom

The last decade has seen considerable growth in our knowledge of neurotrophic factors in general and their effects on pain-signaling systems in particular. It is now clear that various factors act on this system in a variety of ways and at multiple sites. This chapter will focus principally on three factors: nerve growth factor (NGF), brain-derived neurotrophic factor (BDNF), and glial cell line-derived neurotrophic factor (GDNF). We concentrate on these factors because adult cutaneous nociceptors fall into two minimally overlapping groups expressing receptors for NGF and GDNF, respectively. Moreover, nociceptors in one of these groups—those sensitive to NGF—constitutively express BDNF, which may be released from central terminals to act as a spinal neuromodulator of nociceptive transmission. In Fig. 1 we summarize the properties of these two groups of nociceptors and illustrate how they are distinct from each other and from the large-diameter, mechanoreceptive sensory neurons that have large myelinated axons. In the sections below we consider the role played by each of these trophic factors.

NERVE GROWTH FACTOR

NGF AND NOCICEPTOR DEVELOPMENT

The prototypical neurotrophic molecule NGF was initially characterized by its ability to promote sensory and sympathetic axon outgrowth. In intact

[1] Mini-review based on a congress workshop.

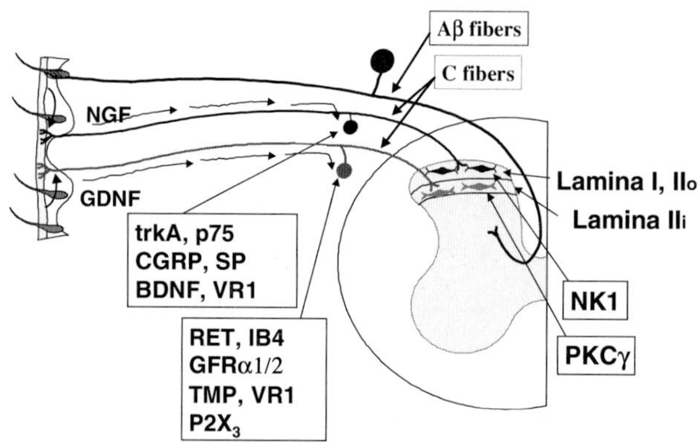

Fig. 1. Peripheral and central target fields of primary sensory neurons. The trophic factor dependence and biochemical properties of the two major classes of cutaneous nociceptors (C fibers) are shown. TrkA-expressing neurons represent roughly 40% of dorsal root ganglion (DRG) neurons, while the IB4 population comprises approximately 30%. Most of the remaining 30% of neurons are myelinated Aβ fibers, which predominantly transduce innocuous mechanical information. BDNF = brain-derived neurotrophic factor; CGRP = calcitonin gene-related peptide; GDNF = glial-derived neurotrophic factor; GFR = GDNF family receptor; NGF = nerve growth factor; PKCγ = protein kinase C (gamma); SP = substance P; TMP = thiamine monophosphatase.

adult animals, NGF is produced in minute quantities in peripheral tissues and is retrogradely transported to afferent somata within axons expressing the NGF-specific tyrosine kinase receptor trkA. There it maintains the neurochemical and electrophysiological phenotype of small-diameter dorsal root ganglia (DRG) neurons (Fitzgerald et al. 1985; Verge et al. 1995). The development of all small-diameter DRG neurons depends on NGF, as exemplified by the sensory neuronal deficit in transgenic mice that lack trkA (Smeyne et al. 1994), and by the faulty phenotypic development of high-threshold cutaneous mechanoreceptors in rats treated with NGF antiserum during development. During the first three postnatal weeks of life, about half the small-diameter neurons downregulate trkA so that in adulthood only about 40% of DRG neurons remain NGF-responsive. During late prenatal development and the first postnatal week, the population of small-diameter afferents that lose their trkA begin to express receptor components for GDNF (Molliver et al. 1997). The sensitivity of these neurons to GDNF is maintained into adulthood (Bennett et al. 1998), as discussed below.

NGF IN INFLAMMATION

Inflammation is a complex cellular and biochemical response to tissue injury or the presence of foreign substances. Pain produced by inflammation is primarily due to the chemical sensitivity of primary afferent nociceptive endings, but important morphological and neurochemical changes in sensory neurons have also been described. While drastic modifications in central processing also occur, this chapter focuses on plasticity of primary sensory neurons.

NGF is a well-studied mediator of inflammatory pain (Lewin et al. 1993). Injections of NGF or other agents that induce the local expression of NGF, such as complete Freund's adjuvant or carrageenan, increase sensitivity to thermal and mechanical stimulation, and these behaviors can be ameliorated by systemically or locally administered NGF antiserum or NGF-sequestering molecules (Woolf et al. 1994; McMahon et al. 1995). NGF can increase the expression of a sensory neuron-specific sodium channel (PN1), possibly leading to increased excitability, and NGF can regulate current through the capsaicin receptor-channel complex and expression of the capsaicin (VR1) receptor itself (Tominaga et al. 1998). Peptides induced by NGF in inflammation include the nociceptive neuropeptides substance P (SP) and calcitonin gene-related peptide (CGRP). These may be released centrally to increase the excitability of dorsal horn neurons, or peripherally to exacerbate inflammation neurogenically. In addition to these molecular and neurochemical changes, NGF upregulation in inflammation may also induce the peripheral sprouting of trkA-expressing sensory and sympathetic axons.

Indirect actions of NGF on nociceptor function may be mediated through mast cells (Woolf et al. 1996), as they express trkA and degranulate in the presence of NGF to release a host of sensitizing mediators. Various types of leukocytes also respond to NGF: eosinophils and neutrophils accumulate in the skin at the site of NGF injections and may be responsible for leukotriene-mediated nociceptor sensitization.

NGF AND NEUROPATHIC PAIN

While the role of NGF in inflammatory pain is well understood, its possible involvement in "neuropathic" pain is less clear. Following peripheral nerve injury, Wallerian degeneration occurs in the severed distal stump and Schwann cells, macrophages, and other cell types such as fibroblasts upregulate growth factors and cytokines. Of these substances, the best-studied is NGF. Interleukin-1β released by the invading macrophages stimulates the production and release of NGF from Schwann cells and fibroblasts (Heumann et al. 1987). Expression of the p75 neurotrophin receptor also increases in glial cells in degenerating nerve.

The expression of both trkA and p75 decreases in axotomized DRG neurons, and the retrograde transport of NGF to sensory perikarya is decreased. The lack of peripherally derived NGF contributes to many of the cell body changes following axotomy. However, NGF mRNA is modestly upregulated in DRG following nerve injury (Zhou et al. 1999), and p75 expression increases in satellite cells surrounding axotomized DRG neurons, which suggests possible compensation, at least in part, for the loss of target-derived NGF.

Animal models of neuropathic pain most often involve incomplete lesions to peripheral nerves, such as a chronic constriction injury (CCI) to the sciatic nerve. Induced by loosely tying the sciatic nerve with chromic gut ligatures, CCI results in the slow edematous axotomy of predominantly large-diameter myelinated axons. The result is that a sciatic nerve connection to the periphery is spared, and the remaining (mainly small unmyelinated) axons reside for a time in a peripheral nerve environment in which Wallerian degeneration is occurring. This degeneration seems crucial to the development of abnormal cutaneous sensitivity that follows CCI, and it has been suggested that contact between spared axons and the trophically enriched environment of the distal stump is particularly important in the development of CCI-induced pain. Indeed, treatment with NGF antiserum can attenuate pain associated with CCI (Herzberg et al. 1997). Conversely, some data suggest that NGF itself might be used therapeutically to relieve some of the pain-related abnormalities associated with nerve damage (Ren et al. 1995).

NGF AND MORPHOLOGICAL CHANGES OF PRIMARY AFFERENTS FOLLOWING NERVE INJURY

Following sciatic nerve lesions, spared nociceptive axons sprout into the denervated cutaneous sciatic territory. This sprouting may be a result of increased levels of NGF in the denervated skin, as it can be inhibited by anti-NGF treatment. Skin innervated by these collateral sprouts is hyperalgesic to mechanical stimulation.

We have known for some time that the central terminals of primary afferents can sprout in the dorsal horn under appropriate conditions. A possible explanation for touch-evoked allodynia that often accompanies nerve lesions is Woolf et al.'s (1992) finding that mechanoreceptive or proprioceptive Aβ myelinated primary afferent axons, which normally terminate in the deeper lamina of the spinal cord dorsal horn, send new projections to superficial laminae following nerve injury. A recent study demonstrated that this reorganization can be prevented by intrathecally delivered exogenous NGF or GDNF (Bennett et al. 1998), which suggests that it may be mediated by atrophic changes in C fibers. Interestingly, in this case it is the lack of NGF mediating the morphological changes putatively involved in neuropathic pain, rather than an excess, that seems to be associated with the peripheral sprouting described earlier.

NGF, SYMPATHETIC SPROUTING, AND NEUROPATHIC PAIN

In the intact state, little or no interaction occurs between sympathetic efferent fibers and primary afferent axons in the periphery, yet following either inflammation or nerve injury, pain often relies to a certain extent on the sympathetic nervous system. Sympathetic-sensory coupling may occur in the skin, damaged nerve trunk, or DRG (where sympathetic axons sprout to surround sensory neurons), and provides a putative anatomical substrate for sympathetically maintained pain (reviewed in Jänig et al. 1996). NGF is a likely chemical mediator of the sprouting phenomenon, as exogenous NGF induces sympathetic sprouting into the DRG in uninjured animals, and NGF antisera reduce sympathetic sprouting and abnormal pain behavior in rats following nerve injury (reviewed in Ramer et al. 1999).

NGF AND CHANGES IN AFFERENT NEUROCHEMISTRY FOLLOWING NERVE INJURY

Given that peptidergic transmitters are important in modulating nociceptive neurotransmission in the spinal cord, several studies have focused on nerve injury-induced changes in neuropeptide expression in DRG neurons and their central processes. Of particular interest are SP, the primary nociceptive peptide in intact animals, and galanin, which can act as an excitatory or inhibitory modulator of pain transmission (Hökfelt et al. 1994). Complete sciatic nerve transection is associated with a decrease in SP expression in the DRG and a dramatic upregulation of galanin. NGF applied to the distal stump of transected nerves can attenuate the reduction of SP following axotomy. In contrast to its stimulating effects on SP expression, NGF partially suppresses the upregulation of galanin (presumably in trkA-expressing neurons) when applied to a cut nerve. These and other NGF effects are summarized in Fig. 2.

BRAIN-DERIVED NEUROTROPHIC FACTOR

Brain-derived neurotrophic factor (BDNF) was the second member of the neurotrophin family to be characterized. Recent examination of BDNF or trkB (the high-affinity receptor for BDNF) knock-out mice showed a pronounced loss of placode-derived sensory neurons (Klein et al. 1993). However, for spinal sensory neurons (that is those with their cell bodies in the DRG), very limited, if any, cell death occurs in these knock-outs. In these animals, however, BDNF appears to be crucial in regulating the mechanosensitivity of slowly adapting mechanoreceptors (Carroll et al. 1998).

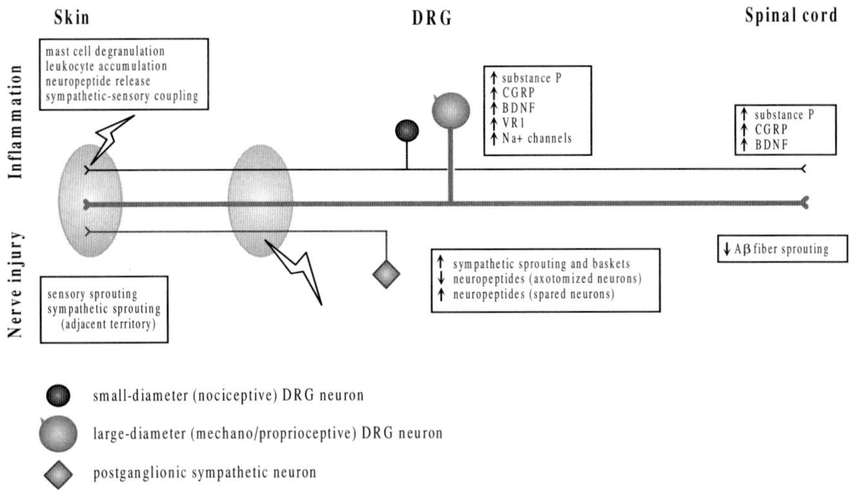

Fig. 2. Peripheral actions of NGF in inflammation and nerve injury. In inflammatory states (skin/joint inflammation), peripherally produced NGF causes mast cell degranulation and leukocyte infiltration, which may result in sensitization of nociceptors. Nociceptive neuropeptides, BDNF, and sodium channels are upregulated in DRG neurons, and transport of SP, CGRP, and BDNF to the spinal cord increases and may contribute to central sensitization. Following nerve injury, there is an NGF-dependent sprouting of both sensory and sympathetic axons into denervated skin from adjacent, uninjured territory. In the DRG, while some peptides are downregulated in axotomized neurons in response to a loss of target-derived NGF, others are upregulated in spared neurons in response to decreased competition for NGF in partially denervated targets. Sympathetic axons sprout in the DRG in response to locally produced NGF. In the spinal cord, exogenous NGF (or GDNF) can prevent Aβ terminal reorganization.

Along with these peripheral trophic and maintenance roles, strong evidence is now emerging that BDNF may function centrally, within the spinal cord, to modulate nociceptive sensory signaling.

BDNF EXPRESSION IN SPINAL CORD AND DRG

BDNF, like other neurotrophins, is retrogradely transported by sensory neurons in the DRG. However, BDNF shows an unusual property in that it is constitutively expressed by a small number of primary sensory neurons (Michael et al. 1997). Cells expressing BDNF mRNA and protein are small in diameter and co-localize with the neuropeptide CGRP and the high-affinity NGF-receptor trkA. These cells are likely to be nociceptors with unmyelinated or thinly myelinated axons. BDNF is anterogradely transported to the dorsal horn and packaged into dense core vesicles. Furthermore, trkB-receptor expression is abundant in the dorsal horn of the spinal cord.

Levels of BDNF protein and mRNA are regulated by NGF: exogenous NGF can upregulate both BDNF mRNA and protein within the cell bodies of primary sensory neurons and their terminal fields in the spinal cord (Michael et al. 1997). A recent study has shown that inflammation, which is known to elevate levels of NGF peripherally (see McMahon et al. 1995), can also induce an upregulation of BDNF protein in the DRG (Mannion et al. 1999). These authors report that the inflammation-induced upregulation of BDNF is accompanied by a novel expression of BDNF in large-diameter DRG cells. Another recent study reported that BDNF expression can be induced in large-diameter, trkB- and trkC-positive sensory neurons in response to nerve injury (Michael et al. 1999). Furthermore, the axotomy induced upregulation of BDNF in these large-diameter primary afferents is reflected centrally by an increased expression of BDNF within deeper laminae in the dorsal horn, the site of central terminations for large-diameter fibers. Electron microscopy revealed that these novel BDNF-expressing axons within the deeper laminae possess varicosities that may represent sites of synaptic contact with adjoining dendrites.

Thus, both inflammation and axotomy can upregulate levels of BDNF expression. However, in the former case, the increase appears to occur predominantly in small (nociceptive) neurons, while in the latter it is seen in large (presumably mechanoreceptive) neurons. BDNF is packaged in dense core vesicles, so it is likely to be released with activity from the afferent terminals. Clear evidence points to altered connectivity between sensory and dorsal horn neurons following both inflammation and nerve injury. As we review below, BDNF appears to be a promising candidate molecule contributing to such changes.

BDNF AS A NEUROMODULATOR: ELECTROPHYSIOLOGICAL EVIDENCE

Although evidence supports the activity-dependent secretion of neurotrophins from hippocampal slices (Blochl and Thoenen 1995), no evidence yet confirms that BDNF is released within the spinal cord following afferent fiber activation. The localization of BDNF and its injury-associated regulation detailed above, however, are consistent with a possible neuromodulatory role for this neurotrophin. Recent data obtained from experiments examining BDNF actions on hippocampal activity has shown that BDNF can rapidly and specifically enhance phosphorylation of the post-synaptic N-methyl-D-aspartic acid (NMDA) receptor (Levine et al. 1998). These experiments have also shown that BDNF can potentiate NMDA responses via a three-fold increase in NMDA-receptor open time. Furthermore, it has recently been established that BDNF can directly depolarize neurons in a manner similar to other classical excitatory neurotransmitters such as glutamate (Kafitz et al. 1999).

We have recently used an in vitro hemisected spinal cord preparation from juvenile rats to examine the effects of BDNF on spinal excitability and its effects on NMDA responses at the spinal level (Kerr et al. 1999). This preparation is used to monitor alterations in synaptic excitability. Reflex responses to C-fiber inputs may be recorded from the ventral root, which appear as prolonged ventral root potentials (VRPs). These extracellularly recorded potentials are a good measure of spinal excitability. Alternatively, hemisected spinal cord preparations can be briefly superfused with experimental agents such as NMDA and the resulting short-duration depolarizing responses can be recorded from the ventral roots. In these experiments we have shown that pretreatment of spinal cords with BDNF can potentiate NMDA-induced depolarizations. In addition, we also found that superfusion of the spinal cord with BDNF can specifically enhance the C-fiber-evoked component of the prolonged VRP, thus indicating an overall increase in spinal reflex excitability. Delivery of a trkB-IgG fusion protein, which sequesters and effectively antagonizes BDNF, had no effect on the evoked VRPs of naive preparations. However, animals pretreated 24 hours previously with NGF to upregulate levels of BDNF in nociceptor terminals, showed a modest enhancement of the C-fiber component of the reflex. In these NGF-pretreated preparations, superfusion with trkB-IgG produced a sustained and significant depression of the C-fiber-evoked component.

BDNF AS A NEUROMODULATOR: BEHAVIORAL EVIDENCE

To date, most of the work on effects of BDNF on synaptic transmission has used isolated preparations in vitro. Recent experiments have examined the effects of BDNF antagonism on nociceptive behavioral responses in vivo. BDNF appears to have no role in acute noxious signaling in a naive state; the administration of trkB-IgG does not alter the basal sensitivity to noxious thermal or mechanical stimuli (Mannion et al. 1999). Similarly, intrathecal administration of trkB-IgG had no effect on the behavioral responses to injection of dilute formalin. However, when rats were pretreated with NGF for 24 hours, intrathecal trkB-IgG effectively antagonized the second, prolonged phase of behavioral responses to formalin injection. The second phase of the formalin response has a centrally mediated component that is NMDA dependent. Additionally, the thermal hyperalgesia induced by carrageenan inflammation is reduced by intrathecal trkB-IgG (Fig. 3) (Kerr et al. 1999).

These results strongly suggest that upregulation of BDNF is a major

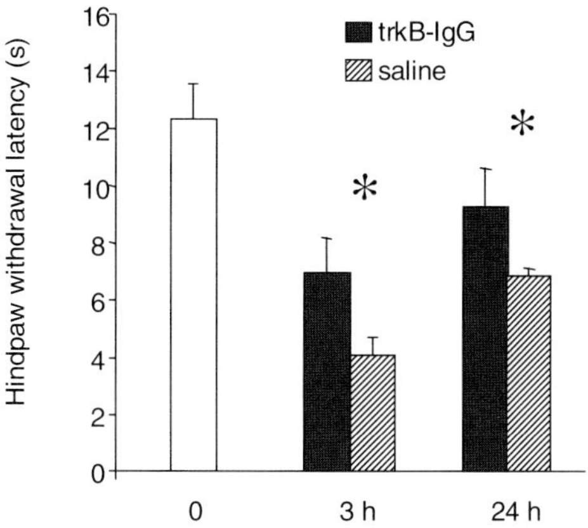

Fig. 3. The effect of intrathecal trkB-IgG (10 μL; 0.16 mg/mL + 10 μL flush) or saline vehicle (20 μL) upon hindpaw thermal withdrawal latencies following intraplantar injection of carrageenan (50 μL, 2%). Latency for hindpaw withdrawal from a noxious thermal stimulus was measured 3 and 24 hours following intraplantar injection. Compounds were administered 30 minutes prior to each testing point. TrkB-IgG significantly ameliorated thermal hyperalgesia at both time points. Asterisks (*) denote significant difference between saline- and trkB-IgG-treated animals ($P < 0.05$, two-way, repeated-measures ANOVA).

contributor to the central mechanism of NGF- and inflammation-induced hyperalgesia. In addition, the evidence suggests that BDNF targets NMDA receptors to facilitate central sensitization. Central sensitization is believed to underlie some aspects of altered sensibility found in chronic pain states. Thus, current data are consistent with the idea that BDNF may be a key mediator of central sensitization within the spinal cord via an interaction at the NMDA-receptor site.

THE GDNF FAMILY OF NEUROTROPHIC FACTORS

Glial cell line-derived neurotrophic factor (GDNF) is the prototypical member of a small family of trophic factors that are distant members of the TGFβ superfamily. GDNF was originally described on the basis of its ability to promote the survival of embryonic midbrain dopaminergic neurons in vitro (Lin et al. 1993). Analysis of GDNF-deficient mice has shown that, in addition to playing a critical role in the development of the enteric nervous system, GDNF is also essential for the development of a subpopulation of sensory neurons in the DRG (Moore et al. 1996). To date, three other members of the GDNF family have been identified: neurturin (NTN), persephin (PSP), and artemin (ART). While GDNF, NTN, and ART promote the survival of sympathetic (superior cervical ganglion) and sensory (trigeminal, nodose, and DRG) neurons in culture, PSP does not have any survival-promoting effects on these populations. It is clear, however, that three of the four members of this family have trophic effects on sensory neurons.

RECEPTORS FOR THE GDNF FAMILY

The GDNF family of neurotrophic factors signal via a receptor complex consisting of a transmembrane tyrosine kinase signal-transducing domain (RET), and one of four GPI-linked receptors, which act as ligand-binding domains (GFRα1–4). It is thought that GDNF, NTN, ART, and PSP bind preferentially to GFRα1, α2, α3, and α4, respectively, and these complexes all signal through phosphorylation of the shared RET component. However, significant cross-talk occurs between ligands and the GFRα receptors; for example either GFRα1 or GFRα2 in conjunction with RET can mediate GDNF or NTN signaling. However, in vivo interactions are generally fairly specific, with GDNF activating mainly GFRα1, and NTN predominantly using GFRα2 (Rosenthal 1999).

EXPRESSION OF GDNF RECEPTOR COMPONENTS IN THE DRG

Cells sensitive to GDNF will normally express either GFRα1 or α2 and RET. Analysis of mRNA distribution has shown that approximately 60% of DRG cells express message for RET, while 40% and 30% express GFRα1 and α2, respectively (Molliver et al. 1997; Bennett et al. 1998). RET and GFRα1 are expressed in subpopulations of both large- and small-diameter cells, while GFRα2 is expressed almost exclusively in small cells.

As shown in Fig. 1, adult DRG cells can be divided into three broad groups. Studies combining in situ hybridization with these chemically defined subpopulations have found a high level of expression of GDNF receptor components in the nonpeptidergic IB4-binding cells. Almost all IB4-binding cells express RET mRNA and protein, and most of these cells also express the ligand-binding domains GFRα1 or GFRα2. In contrast, few of the peptidergic/trkA-expressing cells have GDNF receptor components. This pattern of receptor component expression thus suggests that one-half of C fibers are responsive to NGF, while the other half respond to GDNF. A subgroup of the large myelinated fibers also expresses RET and GFRα1, and thus is likely to be sensitive to GDNF.

Peripheral nerve injury induces a variety of changes in the expression of GDNF receptor components. Two weeks after sciatic nerve axotomy the proportion of DRG cells that express RET and GFRα1 increases dramatically (to 75% and 65%, respectively), so that virtually all large-diameter DRG cells express these receptor components. A significant number of small cells still fail to express these components, which probably represent the trkA subpopulation of C fibers. Conversely, the expression of message for GFRα2 is downregulated following axotomy (to 12% of sciatic afferents). These changes in receptor expression imply that the proportion of cells that are sensitive to GDNF may change after axotomy, with more of the large myelinated neurons responding to this trophic factor. The downregulation of GFRα2 suggests that injured sensory neurons are less sensitive to NTN.

NEUROPROTECTIVE EFFECTS OF GDNF

Sciatic nerve axotomy induces a series of reactive changes in both DRG cells and their primary afferent terminals. These include a downregulation of markers for both populations of C fibers, such as CGRP, SP, and IB4 binding, or thiamine monophosphatase expression. Continuous intrathecal delivery of NGF, GDNF, or vehicle (1.2 or 12 μg/day, via an osmotic minipump), concomitant with axotomy, have differential and complementary effects on the expression of these markers within the DRG and dorsal horn. NGF completely prevents the downregulation of CGRP, but has no effect on the proportion of IB4-binding cells. Conversely, GDNF has no effect on CGRP expression, but almost completely prevents the downregulation of IB4 binding in both DRG and dorsal horn, in a dose-dependent fashion. The differential and specific effects on these two subpopulations suggest that they have distinct trophic requirements. Further evidence comes from the effects of NGF and GDNF on another axotomy-induced phenomenon, namely the slowing in axonal conduction velocity.

Axotomy leads to a pan-neuronal decrease in the expression of structural proteins (such as neurofilament), which reduces axonal caliber, and thus leads to a slowing in conduction velocity. Treatment with either NGF or GDNF partially (and significantly) reverses this slowing, consistent with each of these trophic factors acting on separate subpopulations of C fibers. Treating animals with a mixture of GDNF and NGF restores conduction velocity even further (to a level not significantly different from normal), which indicates a rescue in both populations of C fibers (Bennett et al. 1998).

Intra-axonal and bulk labeling methods have shown that after axotomy, large myelinated fibers sprout into the superficial laminae, an area that normally receives input from unmyelinated C fibers. We have found that intrathecal treatment with NGF or GDNF prevents the myelinated fiber sprouting seen after axotomy, presumably by preventing atrophic changes in C-fiber terminals. It is not clear why "rescuing" either of the C-fiber subpopulations

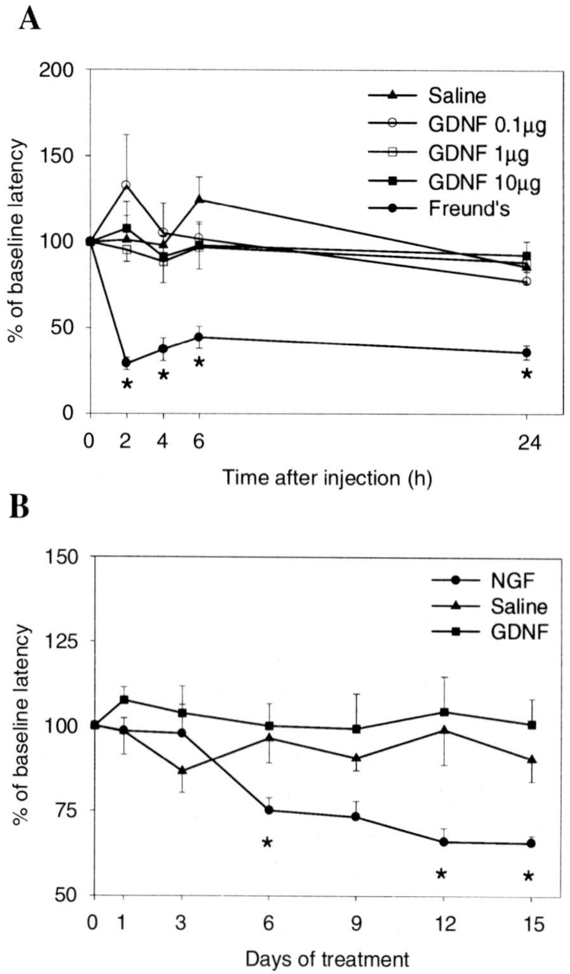

Fig. 4. Intraplantar injections of GDNF do not induce any change in thermal threshold (50 μL; 0.1, 1, or 10 μg). Complete Freund's adjuvant (50 μL) induces a rapid and persisting thermal hyperalgesia. Asterisks (*) denote significant difference from saline controls ($P < 0.01$, two-way repeated-measures ANOVA, Tukey post hoc test). In contrast to NGF, continuous intrathecal infusion of GDNF does not induce thermal hyperalgesia in otherwise normal animals. Trophic factors were delivered via an osmotic mini-pump over a 2-week period (12 μg/day).

prevents this sprouting. However these findings indicate that these trophic factors may be of use in the treatment of peripheral neuropathies.

We have further investigated this possibility by using a model of peripheral nerve injury that is accompanied by quantifiable measures of neuropathy. Unilateral ligation of about one-third to one-half of the sciatic nerve results in thermal and mechanical hyperalgesia in the ipsilateral paw. Preliminary data from our laboratory suggest that the infusion of GDNF (as above) can largely prevent the development of this neuropathy, although the mechanisms are unknown.

THE ROLE OF ENDOGENOUS GDNF

Considerable evidence reveals that NGF plays an important role in inflammatory pain and the regulation of nociceptors (see above). However much less is known about the role of GDNF in these processes. We have found that, in contrast to NGF, chronic intrathecal GDNF does not affect thresholds to noxious thermal stimulation. Intraplantar injections of GDNF also do not affect thermal thresholds (Fig. 4).

Although it has no acute sensitizing effects, GDNF may play a tonic modulatory role in nociceptive processing; a recent in vitro study has shown that GDNF increases thermal sensitivity and TTX-resistant sodium current in IB4-binding neurons (Stucky and Lewin 1999). Work by Holstege and coworkers has shown that GDNF protein is present in primary afferent terminals and appears to be transported anterogradely from the DRG (Holstege et al. 1998). Interestingly, and apparently in a similar fashion to BDNF (see above), GDNF is present in the terminal fields of trkA-expressing DRG neurons, and acute intrathecal administration of GDNF induces dorsal horn *c-fos*. These findings indicate the possibility that GDNF may have both neuromodulatory and trophic effects, although current knowledge is fragmentary.

CONCLUSIONS

The last five years have seen a considerable expansion in our knowledge of the actions of trophic factors on pain-signaling systems. The expansion relates both to the range of effective factors and the sites at which they act. The early studies focused on the pro-nociceptive effects of NGF, and particularly its role as a peripheral mediator of some aspects of inflammatory pain. As we review in this chapter, this molecule is also implicated in some aspects of neuropathic pain, notably in neurochemical and morphological changes in both sensory and sympathetic neurons. It has also become clear that a substantial proportion of nociceptors are sensitive not to NGF but to GDNF. While exogenous GDNF appears to lack the pro-nociceptive effects so apparent with NGF, this protein has potent neuroprotective actions on nociceptors and is a powerful regulator of gene expression in those cells. Finally, an emerging body of evidence suggests that another factor, BDNF, may play an important role as a neuromodulator of spinal nociceptive processing. The expression of this molecule by nociceptors is regulated by peripheral inflammation and nerve injury.

The study of the effects of neurotrophic factors is likely to increase our understanding of both the development of pain-signaling systems and their plasticity in the mature animal. It is also possible that these studies will provide the rationale for the development of novel analgesic strategies.

ACKNOWLEDGMENTS

The work of the authors described in this chapter is supported by the Wellcome Trust and the Medical Research Councils of Great Britain and Canada. Special thanks to Viv Cheah for all assistance, and Elizabeth Bradbury and Dave Bennett for comments on the manuscript.

REFERENCES

Bennett DLH, Michael GJ, Ramachandran N, et al. A distinct subgroup of small DRG cells express GDNF receptor components and GDNF is protective for these neurons after nerve injury. *J Neurosci* 1998; 18:3059–3072.

Blochl A, Thoenen H. Characterization of nerve growth factor (NGF) release from hippocampal neurons: evidence for a constitutive and an unconventional sodium-dependent regulated pathway. *Eur J Neurosci* 1995; 7:1220–1228.

Carroll P, Lewin GR, Koltzenburg M, Toyka KV, Thoenen H. A role for BDNF in mechanosensation. *Nat Neurosci* 1998; 1(1):42–46.

Fitzgerald M, Wall PD, Goedert M, Emson PC. Nerve growth factor counteracts the neurophysiological and neurochemical effects of chronic nerve section. *Brain Res* 1985; 332:131–141.

Herzberg U, Eliav E, Dorsey JM, Gracely RH, Kopin IJ. NGF involvement in pain induced by chronic constriction injury of the rat sciatic nerve. *Neuroreport* 1997; 8:1613–1618.

Heumann R, Korsching S, Bandtlow C, Thoenen H. Changes of nerve growth factor synthesis in non-neuronal cells in response to sciatic nerve transection. *J Cell Biol* 1987; 104:1623–1631.

Hökfelt T, Zhang X, Wiesenfeld-Hallin Z. Messenger plasticity in primary sensory neurons following axotomy and its functional implications. *Trends Neurosci* 1994; 17:22–30.

Holstege JC, Jongen JL, Kennis JH, van Rooyen-Boot AA, Vecht CJ. Immunocytochemical localization of GDNF in primary afferents of the lumbar dorsal horn. *Neuroreport* 1998; 9:2893–2897.

Jänig W, Levine JD, Michaelis M. Interactions of sympathetic and primary afferent neurons following nerve injury and tissue trauma. *Prog Brain Res* 1996; 113:161–183.

Kafitz KW, Rose CR, Thoenen H, Konnerth A. Neurotrophin-evoked rapid excitation through TrkB receptors. *Nature* 1999; 401:918–921.

Kerr BJ, Bradbury EJ, Bennett DLH, et al. Brain-derived neurotrophic factor modulates nociceptive sensory inputs and NMDA-evoked responses in the rat spinal cord. *J Neurosci* 1999; 19(12):5138–5148.

Klein R, Smeyne RJ, Wurst W, et. al. Targeted disruption of the trkB neurotrophin receptor gene results in nervous system lesions and neuronal death. *Cell* 1993; 75:113–122.

Levine ES, Crozier RA, Black IB, Plummer MR. BDNF modulates hippocampal synaptic transmission by increasing NMDA receptor activity. *Proc Natl Acad Sci USA* 1998; 95:10235–10238.

Lewin GR, Ritter AM, Mendell LM. Nerve growth factor-induced hyperalgesia in the neonatal and adult rat. *J Neurosci* 1993; 13:2136–2148.

Lin LF, Doherty DH, Lile JD, Bektesh S, Collins F. GDNF: a glial cell line-derived neurotrophic factor for midbrain dopaminergic neurons. *Science* 1993; 260:1130–1132.

Mannion RJ, Costigan M, Decosterd I, et al. Neurotrophins: peripherally and centrally acting modulators of tactile stimulus-induced inflammatory pain hypersensitivity. *Proc Natl Acad Sci USA* 1999; 96:9385–9390.

McMahon SB, Bennett DLH, Priestley JV, Shelton DB. The biological effects of endogenous nerve growth factor on adult sensory neurons revealed by trkA-IgG fusion molecule. *Nat Med* 1995; 1:774–780.

Michael GJ, Averill S, Nitkunan A, et al. Nerve growth factor treatment increases brain-derived neurotrophic factor selectively in trka-expressing dorsal root ganglion cells and their central terminations within the spinal cord. *J Neurosci* 1997; 17(21):8476–8490.

Michael GJ, Averill S, Shortland PJ, Yan Q, Priestley JV. Axotomy results in major changes in BDNF expression by dorsal root ganglion cells: BDNF expression in large trkB and trkC cells, in pericellular baskets, and in projections to deep dorsal horn and dorsal column nuclei. *Eur J Neurosci* 1999; 11:1–13.

Molliver DC, Wright DE, Leitner ML, et al. IB4-binding DRG neurons switch from NGF to GDNF dependence in early postnatal life. *Neuron* 1997; 19:849–861.

Moore MW, Klein RD, Farinas I, et al. Renal and neuronal abnormalities in mice lacking GDNF. *Nature* 1996; 382:76–79.

Ramer MS, Thompson SWN, McMahon SB. Causes and consequences of sympathetic basket formation in dorsal root ganglia. *Pain* 1999; (Suppl)6:S111–S120.

Ren K, Thomas DA, Dubner R. Nerve growth factor alleviates a painful peripheral neuropathy in rats. *Brain Res* 1995; 699:286–292.

Rosenthal A. The GDNF protein family: gene ablation studies reveal what they really do and how. *Neuron* 1999; 22:201–202.

Smeyne RJ, Klein R, Schnapp A, et al. Severe sensory and sympathetic neuropathies in mice carrying a disrupted trk/NGF receptor gene. *Nature* 1994; 368:246–249.

Stucky CL, Lewin GR. Isolectin B(4)-positive and -negative nociceptors are functionally distinct. *J Neurosci* 1999; 19:6497–6505.

Tominaga M, Caterina MJ, Malmberg AB, et al. The cloned capsaicin receptor integrates multiple pain-producing stimuli. *Neuron* 1998; 21:531–543.

Verge VMK, Richardson PM, Wiesenfeld-Hallin Z, Hökfelt T. Differential influence of nerve growth factor on neuropeptide expression in vivo: a novel role in peptide suppression in adult sensory neurons. *J Neurosci* 1995; 15(3):2081–2096.

Woolf CJ, Shortland P, Coggeshall RE. Peripheral nerve injury triggers central sprouting of myelinated afferents. *Nature* 1992; 355:75–78.

Woolf CJ, Safiehgarabedian B, Ma QP, Crilly P, Winter J. Nerve growth factor contributes to the generation of inflammatory sensory hypersensitivity. *Neuroscience* 1994; 62:327–331.

Woolf CJ, Ma QP, Allchorne A, Poole S. Peripheral cell types contributing to the hyperalgesic action of nerve growth factor in inflammation. *J Neurosci* 1996; 16:2716–2723.

Zhou XF, Deng YS, Chie E, et al. Satellite cell-derived nerve growth factor and neurotrophin-3 are involved in noradrenergic sprouting in the dorsal root ganglia following peripheral nerve injury in the rat. *Eur J Neurosci* 1999; 11:1711–1722.

Correspondence to: T.J. Boucher, MSc, Neuroscience Research Centre, King's College London, St Thomas Campus, Lambeth Palace Road, London SE1 7EH, United Kingdom. Tel: 44(0) 171-928-9292 ext. 2241; Fax: 44(0) 171-928-0729; email: timothy.boucher@kcl.ac.uk.

Proceedings of the 9th World Congress on Pain,
Progress in Pain Research and Management,
Vol. 16, edited by M. Devor, M.C. Rowbotham, and
Z. Wiesenfeld-Hallin, IASP Press, Seattle, © 2000.

17

Phosphorylation of ERK and CREB in Nociceptive Neurons after Noxious Stimulation

Ru-Rong Ji, Gary J. Brenner, Raymond Schmoll,
Hiroshi Baba, and Clifford J. Woolf

Neural Plasticity Research Group, Department of Anesthesia and Critical Care, Massachusetts General Hospital and Harvard Medical School, Boston, Massachusetts, USA

ERK/MAPK CASCADE

The mitogen-activated protein kinase (MAPK) cascade is a major signaling system by which cells transduce extracellular stimuli into intracellular responses. MAPK is a family of serine/threonine kinases, which are activated by phosphorylation on threonine and tyrosine (Seger and Krebs 1995). The extracellular signal-regulated kinases (ERKs) ERK1 and ERK2 are the most intensively studied members of the MAPK family. The discovery of two other MAPK subtypes, the *c-Jun* N-terminal kinase/stress-activated protein kinase (JNK/SAPK) and p38 MAPK, adds complexity within the family. MAPKs have been classically studied as regulators of cell proliferation and differentiation. In particular, MAPKs have been identified as primary effectors of growth factor receptor signaling, a cascade that involves activation of Ras, Raf, and MEK (MAPK and ERK kinase), and regulates cell proliferation and differentiation (Seger and Krebs 1995). However, the pattern of MAPK cascade is not restricted to growth factor signaling. ERK is widely expressed in postmitotic neurons in the mammalian nervous system. It is localized primarily in neuronal cell bodies and dendrites (Fiore et al. 1993). ERK is activated by stimulation of N-methyl-D-aspartate (NMDA) receptors (Bading and Greenberg 1991), and depolarization/calcium influx (Rosen et al. 1994). Light and the circadian rhythm regulate ERK activation in the suprachiasmatic nuclei (Obrietan et al. 1998), and ERK is phosphorylated in the hippocampus by long-term potentiation (LTP; English and Sweatt 1996). ERK phosphorylation is required, moreover, for LTP and associative long-term memory in mammals (English and Sweatt 1997; Atkins et al. 1998; Impey et al. 1998). Thus, ERK phosphorylation is both a marker of and contributor to activity-dependent synaptic plasticity.

CREB PHOSPHORYLATION

The cAMP response element binding protein (CREB) is a transcriptional factor that has been implicated in the transcriptional regulation of many genes. For example, CREB-mediated *c-fos* expression has been well characterized (Ginty 1997). CREB constitutively binds with high affinity to the cAMP response element (CRE) and phosphorylation of CREB at serine 133 is required for CREB-mediated transcription (Gonzalez and Montminy 1989; Ginty 1997). CREB-mediated signaling has been implicated in memory formation (Bourtchuladze et al. 1994; Yin et al. 1994) and morphological plasticity of dendritic spines (Murphy and Segal 1997). Interestingly, all the major signaling pathways converge on CREB activation. For example, CREB is phosphorylated by calcium/calmodulin-dependent protein kinase II and IV (CaMKII/CaMKIV), protein kinase A and C (PKA, PKC) (Bito et al. 1996, Ginty 1997), and especially by ERK via CREB kinase ribosomal S-6 kinase 2 (RSK2) (Xing et al. 1996; Impey et al. 1998). CRE sites have been identified in those genes, such as *c-fos,* zif 268, dynorphin, enkephalin, galanin, neurokinin-1 (NK-1), brain-derived neurotrophic factor (BDNF), and vasoactive intestinal peptide (VIP), which are regulated in dorsal horn or dorsal root ganglia (DRG) by tissue injury and inflammation (Dubner and Ruda 1992; Ji et al. 1995; Ji and Rupp 1997; Woolf and Costigan 1999) or nerve injury (Hökfelt et al. 1994) and may contribute to inflammatory pain and neuropathic pain, respectively. Thus, CREB may be an important transcriptional factor in the dorsal horn and DRG that regulates expression of genes that mediate pain.

ACTIVITY-DEPENDENT NEURONAL PLASTICITY AFTER NOXIOUS STIMULATION

Activation of high-threshold C-fiber primary sensory neurons by peripheral noxious stimuli has two effects. It leads first to an immediate sensation of pain as a consequence of the transfer of the input from the periphery through nociceptive pathways in the central nervous system (CNS) to the cortex. In addition, it leads to an increase in the responsiveness of neurons in the dorsal horn of the spinal cord that outlasts the initiating stimulus for tens of minutes. This activity-dependent regulation of neuronal excitability, known as central sensitization (Woolf 1983), plays a major role in the heightened pain sensitivity that follows injury or intense noxious stimuli. After tissue damage/inflammation, increase in basal sensitivity occurs not only within the site of inflammation (primary hyperalgesia), but also in the neighboring noninflamed tissue (secondary hyperalgesia). These changes can result from peripheral sensitization (alteration of sensitivity of nociceptors) or central sensitization. Central sensitization also plays an important role in neuropathic pain (Woolf and Mannion 1999). The mechanisms responsible for C-fiber-induced, activity-dependent plasticity in DRG and the spinal cord may result from both post-translational modification such as phosphorylation of membrane-bound receptors, especially the NMDA receptor, and transcriptional regulation producing a potentiated system (Woolf and Costigan 1999). To explore the post-translational and transcriptional roles of ERK and CREB, we investigated ERK and CREB activation in nociceptive neurons in the DRG and spinal dorsal horn.

ERK ACTIVATION IN NOCICEPTIVE NEURONS

Experiments were approved by the animal use committee at Massachusetts General Hospital. Adult male Sprague-Dawley rats (200–250 g) were anesthetized with sodium pentobarbital anesthesia (60 mg/kg, i.p.). Capsaicin (25 μL, 75 μg, dissolved in 10% Tween 80), a pungent ingredient in chili pepper and an activator of C-fiber nociceptors, was injected into the plantar surface of the left hindpaw. After appropriate survival times, the rats were perfused and processed for immunohistochemistry as described previously (Ji et al. 1994, 1999). Briefly, transverse spinal cord sections (30 μm) were cut and blocked with 1% goat serum in 0.3% triton for 1 hour at room temperature, and then incubated over night at 4°C with monoclonal primary antibody for pERK1/2 (1:200, New England BioLabs), and polyclonal primary antibody for PKCγ (1:2000, Santa Cruz).

In normal nonstimulated lumbar spinal cord (L4–L5), pERK levels are very low. However, 2 minutes after an intraplantar capsaicin injection, pERK immunoreactivity (ir) was detected within many neurons of the most superficial layers (laminae I and IIo) of the ipsilateral dorsal horn of the spinal cord (Fig. 1a, 1b). No staining was evoked contralateral to the capsaicin injection. The pERK label was located in the medial half of the dorsal horn in the L4 and L5 lumbar segments, topographically corresponding with inputs from the hindlimb (Ji et al. 1999). Double immunofluorescence staining

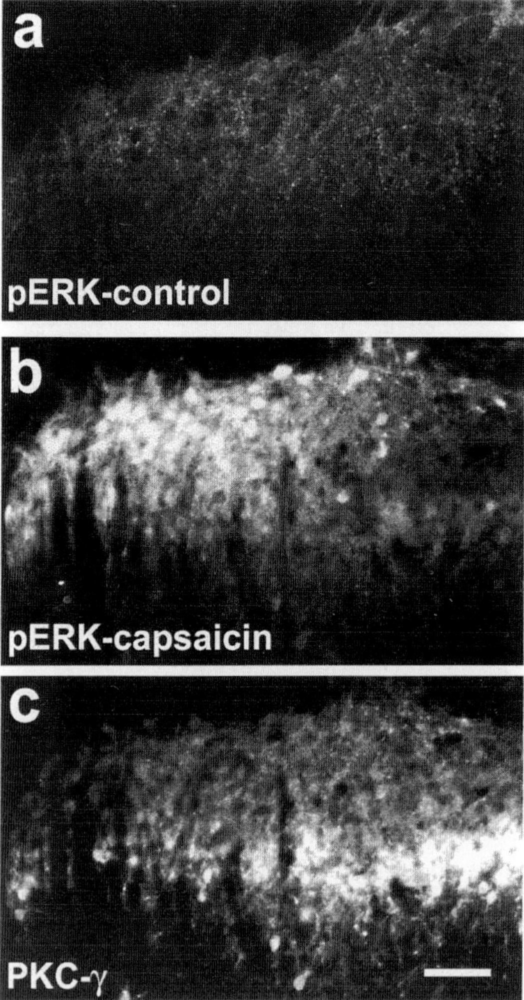

Fig. 1. Immunofluorescence images showing pERK (a,b) and PKCγ (c) immunoreactivity (ir) in the medial part of the superficial spinal dorsal horn (L5). pERK-ir is very low in normal control rats (a); 2 minutes after intraplantar capsaicin, pERK-ir is induced in the medial lamina I and IIo of the ipsilateral dorsal horn (b), but is not colocalized with PKCγ in lamina IIi (c). Scale bar 50 μm.

indicated that pERK did not overlap with PKCγ (Fig. 1b,c), which is predominantly localized in lamina IIi (Malmberg et al. 1997). pERK is also induced in small DRG neurons immediately after capsaicin injection. It can also be induced by a KCl-produced depolarization (Ji and Woolf 1999).

CREB PHOSPHORYLATION IN NOCICEPTIVE NEURONS

To examine an activity-dependent activation of CREB, we electrically stimulated the sciatic nerve at C-fiber strength (5 mA, 500 μs, 10 Hz) in halothane-anesthetized rats for 30 minutes, waited for 2, 4, and 6 hours, and sacrificed the rats under terminal anesthesia. The L4–L5 DRG from control and electrically stimulated rats were immediately dissected and processed with Western blot analysis as described before (Ji and Rupp 1997; Ji et al. 1998). Briefly, the samples were homogenized with a hand-held pellet pestle in boiling lysis buffer and separated on SDS-PAGE gel and transferred to PVDF filters. The filters were incubated overnight at 4°C with polyclonal anti-pCREB antibody (1:3000, Upstate Biotech). The blots were visualized in enhanced chemiluminescence (ECL) solution and exposed onto X-ray films, and then stripped and reprobed with anti-CREB antibody (1:2000, New England Biolabs). The results shown in Fig. 2 indicate that C-fiber stimulation induces an obvious increase in pCREB levels, as compared to the control (Fig. 2, upper panel). The total CREB protein levels are stable (Fig. 2, lower panel). The increased pCREB-ir was found in the nuclei of small DRG neurons after formalin (Ji and Rupp 1997) or capsaicin stimulation (Ji and Woolf 1999). As compared to pERK, pCREB has a higher basal level in the dorsal horn. Intraplantar injection of formalin produced a bilateral increase in pCREB levels, not only in the superficial dorsal horn (laminae I–II), but also in the deep dorsal horn (laminae III–VI), and this induction is partially NMDA-receptor-dependent (Ji and Rupp 1997). The bilateral CREB phosphorylation has been confirmed in another study that used the complete Freund's adjuvant (CFA) model (Messersmith et al. 1998). An

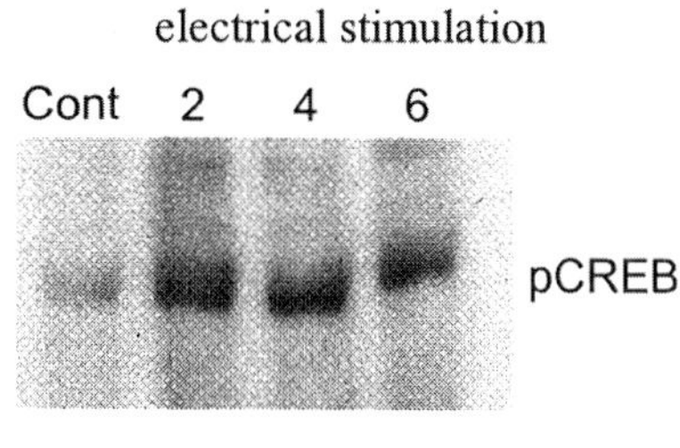

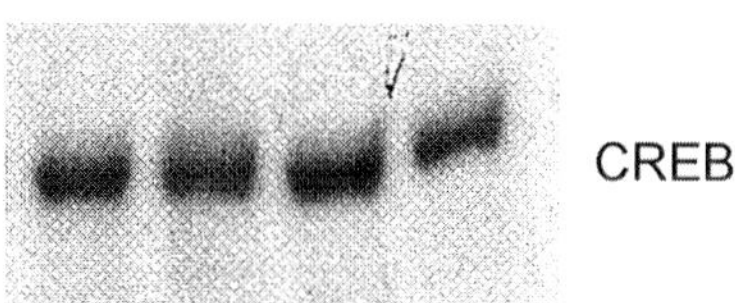

Fig. 2. Western blot analysis obtained from control (Cont) and electrically stimulated DRG (L4, L5) indicating an increased pCREB levels after electrical stimulation. Bottom panel shows the total level of CREB protein from the same blot. The sciatic nerve was stimulated at C-fiber strength (5 mA, 500 μs, 10 Hz) in halothane-anesthetized rats for 30 minutes.

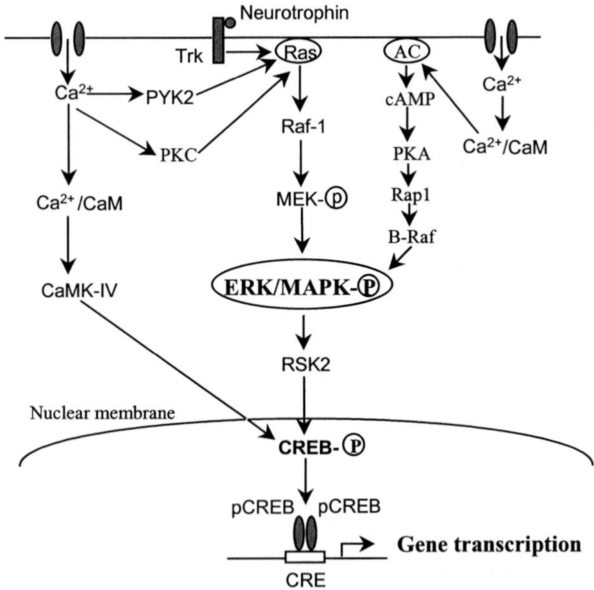

Fig. 3. Schematic diagram indicating putative signal transduction pathways in nociceptive neurons. In the most well-studied pathway, neurotrophin receptor activates the small guanosine triphosphate (GTP)-binding protein Ras. Recruitment of Raf-1 to the plasma membrane by Ras leads to its activation. Stimulation of the NMDA receptor, other voltage-gated calcium channels, and metabotropic receptors results in calcium influx or release from intracellular stores, which in turn activates several calcium-dependent kinases, such as PKC, adenylate cyclase (AC), and tyrosine kinase PYK2. The activation of these kinases activates the MAPK cascade, leading to ERK phosphorylation. The capability of cAMP to stimulate ERK is linked with a Ras homologue Rap-1, and Raf isoform B-Raf. In the nucleus CREB is phosphorylated on Serine 133 by RSK2, which is activated by ERK. CREB is also phosphorylated by a calcium/calmodulin-dependent kinase IV (CaMK-IV), which is present in small DRG neurons (Ji et al. 1996). The phosphorylated CREB then binds to CRE sites on the promotor regions of DNA and initiates gene transcription.

increased level of pCREB in the dorsal horn is also induced by capsaicin (Wu et al. 1999).

CONCLUDING REMARKS

Noxious stimulation leads to an activation both of the MAP kinase ERK and the transcription factor CREB in neurons of the dorsal horn and dorsal root ganglia. The MAP kinase cascade is likely to be a major signaling pathway in nociceptive neurons. As shown in Fig. 3, ERK is downstream to both PKA and PKC, and a variety of neuromodulatory neurotransmitter receptors couple to ERK activation via these two cascades. The convergence on final common effectors has an implication: the failure of one pathway may be compensated by others. We have shown that ERK activation is required for the second-phase nociceptive response to formalin (Ji et al. 1999). Due to the short onset of the formalin response, ERK activation must contribute to changes in dorsal horn neuronal properties by nontranscriptional means, presumably as a result of directly or indirectly phosphorylating kinases, key receptors, and ion channels, modifying membrane excitability. However, CREB phosphorylation in nociceptive neurons, possibly via ERK activation after noxious stimulation, may regulate the CRE-mediated transcription and contribute to the establishment of long-term pain.

ACKNOWLEDGMENT

This research is funded by NIH NS 38253-01 (C.J. Woolf) and Human Frontier Science Program RG73/96 (C.J. Woolf).

REFERENCES

Atkins CM, Selcher JC, Petraitis JJ, Trzaskos JM, Sweatt JD. The MAPK cascade is required for mammalian associative learning. *Nat Neurosci* 1998; 1:602–609.

Bading H. Greenberg ME. Stimulation of protein tyrosine phosphorylation by NMDA receptor activation. *Science* 1991; 253:912–914.

Bito H, Deisseroth K, Tsien RW. CREB phosphorylation and dephosphorylation: a Ca^{2+}- and stimulus duration-dependent switch for hippocampal gene expression. *Cell* 1996; 87:1203–1214.

Bourtchuladze R, Frenguelli B, Blendy J, et al. Deficient long-term memory in mouse with a targeted mutation of the cAMP-response element-binding protein. *Cell* 1994; 79:59–68.

Dubner R, Ruda MA. Activity-dependent neuronal plasticity following tissue injury and inflammation. *Trends Neurosci* 1992; 15:96–103.

English JD, Sweatt JD. Activation of p42 mitogen-activated protein kinase in hippocampal long term potentiation. *J Biol Chem* 1996; 271:24329–24332.

English JD, Sweatt JD. A requirement for the mitogen-activated protein kinase cascade in hippocampal long term potentiation. *J Biol Chem* 1997; 272:19103–19106.

Fiore RS, Bayer VE, Pelech SL, et al. p42 mitogen-activated protein kinase in brain: prominent localization in neuronal cell bodies and dendrites. *Neuroscience* 1993; 55:463–472.

Ginty DD. Calcium regulation of gene expression: isn't that spatial? *Neuron* 1997; 18:183–186.

Gonzalez GA, Montminy MR. Cyclic AMP stimulates somatostatin gene transcription by phosphorylation of CREB at serine 133. *Cell* 1989; 59:675–680.

Hökfelt T, Zhang X, Wiesenfeld-Hallin Z. Messenger plasticity in primary sensory neurons following axotomy and its functional implications. *Trends Neurosci* 1994; 17:22–30.

Impey S, Obrietan K, Wong ST, et al. Cross talk between Erk and PKA is required for Ca^{2+} stimulation of CREB-dependent transcription and Erk nuclear translocation. *Neuron* 1998; 21:869–883.

Ji RR, Rupp F. Phosphorylation of transcription factor CREB in rat spinal cord after formalin-induced hyperalgesia: relationship to c-fos induction. *J Neurosci* 1997; 17:1776–1785.

Ji RR, Woolf CJ. Activity-dependent activation of CREB and MAPK in dorsal root ganglia and spinal cord. *Abstracts: 9th World Congress on Pain.* Seattle: IASP Press, 1999, p 5.

Ji RR, Zhang X, Zhang Q, et al. Central and peripheral expression of galanin in response to inflammation. *Neuroscience* 1995; 68:563–576.

Ji RR, Shi TJ, Xu ZQ, et al. Calcium^{2+}/calmodulin-dependent protein kinase type IV in dorsal root ganglion: colocalization with peptides, axonal transport and effect of axotomy. *Brain Res* 1996; 721:167–173.

Ji RR, Bose CM, Lesuisse L, et al. Specific agrin isoforms induce cAMP response element binding protein phosphorylation in hippocampal neurons. *J Neurosci* 1998; 18:9695–8702.

Ji RR, Baba H, Brenner JG, Woolf CJ. Nociceptive-specific activation of ERK in spinal neurons contributes to pain hypersensitivity. *Nat Neurosci* 1999; 2:1114–1119.

Malmberg AB, Chen C, Susumu T. Basbaum AI. Preserved acute pain and reduced neuropathic pain in mice lacking PKC gamma. *Science* 1997; 278:279–283.

Messersmith DJ, Kim DJ, Iadarola MJ. Transcription factor regulation of prodynorphin gene expression following rat hindpaw inflammation. *Mol Brain Res* 1998; 53:260–269.

Murphy D, Segal M. Morphological plascticity of dendritic spines in central neurons is mediated by activation of cAMP response element binding protein. *Proc Natl Acad Sci USA* 1997; 94:1482–1487.

Obrietan K, Impey S, Storm DR. Light and circadian rhythmicity regulate MAP kinase activation in the suprachiasmatic nuclei. *Nat Neurosci* 1998; 1:693–700.

Rosen LB, Ginty DD, Weber MJ, Greenberg ME. Membrane depolarization and calcium influx stimulate MEK and MAP kinase via activation of Ras. *Neuron* 1994; 12:1207–1221.

Seger R, Krebs EG. The MAPK signaling cascade. *FASEB J* 1995; 9:726–735.

Woolf CJ. Evidence for a central component of post-injury pain hypersensitivity. *Nature* 1983; 306:686–688.

Woolf CJ, Costigan M. Transcriptional and post-translational plascticity and the generation of inflammatory pain. *Proc Natl Acad Sci USA* 1999; 96:7723–7730.

Woolf CJ, Mannion RJ. Neuropathic pain: the relationship between aetiology, symptoms, mechanisms and management. *Lancet* 1999; 353:1959–1964.

Wu J, Fang L, Lin Q, Willis WD. Involvement of cAMP-responsive element-binding protein (CREB) in central sensitization following intradermal capsaicin injection. *Abstracts: 9th World Congress on Pain.* Seattle: IASP Press, 1999, p 5.

Xing J, Ginty DD, Greenberg ME. Coupling of the RAS-MAPK pathway to gene activation by RSK2, a growth factor-regulated CREB kinase. *Science* 1996; 273:959–963.

Yin JCP, Wallach JS, Del Vecchio M, et al. Induction of a dominant negative CREB transgene specifically blocks long-term memory in *Drosophila. Cell* 1994; 79:49–58.

Correspondence to: Ru-Rong Ji, PhD, Neural Plasticity Research Group, Department of Anesthesia and Critical Care, Massachusetts General Hospital, Harvard Medical School, 149 13th Street, Room 4309, Charlestown, MA 02129, USA. Tel: 617-724 3302; Fax: 617-724 3632; email: ji@helix.mgh.harvard.edu.

Proceedings of the 9th World Congress on Pain, Progress in Pain Research and Management, Vol. 16, edited by M. Devor, M.C. Rowbotham, and Z. Wiesenfeld-Hallin, IASP Press, Seattle, © 2000.

18

Subpopulations of Human C Nociceptors and Their Sensory Correlates[1]

Erik Torebjörk

Department of Neuroscience, Clinical Neurophysiology, University Hospital, Uppsala, Sweden

MICRONEUROGRAPHY

In 1968, Vallbo and Hagbarth published a technique of microneurography that allowed recordings from individual large myelinated fibers in intact nerves in awake human subjects. The recording electrodes are thin sharp microelectrodes that are inserted manually through the skin into the nerve to be explored. In the following year, R.G. Hallin and I discovered that such microelectrodes allow detection of multifiber discharges in unmyelinated C fibers, and even single-unit recordings from individual afferent nociceptive or efferent sympathetic C axons. We were anxious to publish our results, so we sent the papers to the local journal, *Acta Societatis Medicorum Upsaliensis,* where they appeared in 1970 (Hallin and Torebjörk 1970a,b; Torebjörk and Hallin 1970). Our findings were confirmed and expanded by van Hees and Gybels in 1972.

In 1973, John Bonica invited Dr. Hallin and myself to participate in the International Symposium on Pain held May 21–26 at the Providence Heights Conference Center, Issaquah (near Seattle), Washington. Participants decided to found the International Association for the Study of Pain. In a paper presented at that meeting, we showed activity-dependent slowing of conduction velocity in C fibers, which can be used to discriminate between electrically activated afferent and sympathetic C fibers (Hallin and Torebjörk 1973; Torebjörk and Hallin 1973).

For a long time, recordings from human C nociceptors were heavily biased toward detection of polymodal (Bessou and Perl 1969) or C mechano-

[1] John J. Bonica distinguished lecture.

heat (CMH) units (Campbell et al. 1989) because we used mechanical scratching of the skin to search for the long-latency C-fiber response and the typical afterdischarges of polymodal nociceptors to such stimuli. In collaboration with R.H. LaMotte and his group at Yale University, we showed that the stimulus-response pattern of these units to heating more or less (but not entirely) paralleled pain magnitude ratings (Torebjörk et al. 1984), that their dynamic responsiveness corresponded to subjective detection of small increments of heat stimuli (Robinson et al. 1983), and that peripheral sensitization of these units could contribute to primary hyperalgesia to heat after a mild heat injury to the skin (Torebjörk et al. 1984).

The combined techniques of microneurographic recording and electrical intraneural microstimulation (Torebjörk and Ochoa 1980) provided evidence that allodynia to stroking of the skin in the area of secondary hyperalgesia after intradermal capsaicin injection was due not to peripheral sensitization of CMH nociceptors (LaMotte et al. 1992), but rather to C-fiber-induced central sensitization, by which a normal input from Aβ mechanoreceptors could give rise to unpleasant sensations (Torebjörk et al. 1992).

Changing the search strategy from mechanical scratching to transcutaneous electrical stimuli (Meyer and Campbell 1988), we used a pointed probe to detect the cutaneous innervation territories of C fibers without introducing mechanical bias. Once the innervation territory of a C unit was found, two needles were inserted 5 mm apart at that spot, and intracutaneous electrical stimulation was performed at a low, monotonous frequency (0.25 Hz) for the rest of the experiment. After a while the C-fiber responses would stabilize at latencies characteristic for each unit in a multifiber recording (Torebjörk and Hallin 1974). Activation of a C fiber by additional natural or electrical stimuli would result in a transient, activity-dependent slowing of impulse conduction, seen as a transient increase in latency of the responses to the monotonous electrical stimulation. In this way C units were shown to be afferent by their responsiveness to mechanical, thermal, or chemical stimuli. In addition, sympathetic fibers could be classified by their activation related to sympathetic reflexes caused, for instance, by arousing stimuli (Hallin and Torebjörk 1974). A single extra impulse can be reliably detected with this "marking" technique (Schmelz et al. 1995). All of the experiments described were performed by recording from the peroneal nerve at knee level, and a distance of 20–50 cm was typical between the recording and stimulation sites. This means that small differences in conduction velocities caused latency separation of multiple C fibers recorded in one intraneural site. Furthermore, the marking method never caused any ambiguity as to which unit responded to a particular stimulus, even if two or more units had adjacent or even overlapping innervation territories. This powerful method is very useful for classifying of C nociceptors of different types, for mapping the extensions of their innervation territories, for determining their thresholds, for estimating suprathreshold responses, and for studying ongoing activity (Torebjörk 1974; Schmidt et al. 1995; Olausson 1998).

MECHANOSENSITIVE AND MECHANOINSENSITIVE C FIBERS

In a long-term collaboration with H.O. Handwerker and his group in Erlangen, we have detected novel types of C nociceptors in human skin (Schmidt et al. 1995). In addition to the CMH nociceptors responsive to mechanical and heat stimuli, there are CM nociceptors responsive to mechanical stimuli but not to heat, and mechanoinsensitive C nociceptors that respond to heating (CH) or are insensitive to heating (CMiHi). However, following chemical inflammation of the skin by topical application of mustard oil or capsaicin, even the "sleeping" (CMiHi) nociceptors can become responsive to mechanical stimuli and to heat, proving that they were afferents (Schmidt et al. 1995) and might contribute to primary hyperalgesia to tonic pressure and heat in an inflamed area (Torebjörk et al. 1996). In the following section I will describe some distinctly different features of the mechanoresponsive CMH and CM units versus the mechanoinsensitive CH and CMiHi units, suggesting that they may be involved in different aspects of nociception.

C-mechanoresponsive units have fairly low mechanical thresholds, always below 750 mN, with a median around 30 mN (Schmidt et al. 1995). C-mechanoinsensitive units have thresholds considerably greater than 750 mN, and many of them do not even respond to needle insertion in their electroreceptive fields (Weidner et al. 1999; Schmelz et al., in press). During firm (12 N) tonic pressure for 2 minutes, the mechanosensitive units gave an immediate phasic response, but fatigued fairly quickly. By contrast, the insensitive units did not respond at the beginning of the stimulus, but started firing after 30 seconds or so; their response increased during the firm pressure in parallel with the increasing pain (Schmelz et al. 1997b). Mechanoresponsive units had fairly small innervation territories, about 2 cm^2 on the leg and 1 cm^2 on the foot (Schmidt et al. 1997). C-mechanoinsensitive units had much larger innervation territories, as mapped by electrical stimulation on the skin. Such electroreceptive fields were of the order of 6 cm^2, both on the leg and the foot (Schmidt et al. 1998). Taken together, these data suggest that C-mechanoresponsive units may play a role in the detection and the fairly precise C-fiber-mediated localization of noxious stimuli applied to the skin (Jørum et al. 1989; Koltzenburg et al. 1993), but they cannot account for the increasing pain during prolonged pressure. By contrast, the mechanoinsensitive units cannot detect the onset of a noxious mechanical stimulus, and their large innervation territories are not suited for very precise spatial discrimination of noxious stimuli. But they are likely to contribute to the increasing pain during sustained pressure, perhaps because they respond to algogenic substances released by the stimulus.

C-mechanoresponsive units have fairly low electrical thresholds on transcutaneous stimulation (less than 15 mA, mean around 2 mA, tested with a 30 mm^2 electrolytic probe), whereas the mechanoinsensitive units have much higher thresholds (more than 35 mA, often exceeding the tolerance limit of 50–80 mA) (Weidner et al. 1999). This finding opened up the possibility of stimulating C units differentially to study their contributions to the axon reflex flare. Electrical stimulation at a strength sufficient for activation of all mechanoresponsive C units in the vicinity of the probe caused no axon reflex flare as tested with a Laser Doppler Scanner, whereas stimulation at a strength that also activated the insensitive units caused a pronounced, large flare (author's unpublished observations). This result is consistent with the large innervation territories of the insensitive units and suggests that they play an important role in neurogenic inflammation, in line with findings in the skin of the pig (Lynn et al. 1996).

The responsiveness to intracutaneous capsaicin injection (20 μL, 0.1%) also differed among types of C unit. Mechanoresponsive units responded to insertion of the needle in the skin and gave an immediate, short-lasting discharge during injection, but were silent and desensitized at the injection site thereafter. By contrast, the insensitive units did not respond immediately to insertion of the needle, but responded with a delay of about 20 seconds. They were spontaneously active for several minutes after the injection (some of them for 20 minutes or more) during the entire period of ongoing pain and concomitant secondary allodynia to touch (Schmelz et al., in press). In addition, they became responsive to heating and pressure at the injection site, but not in the surrounding area. Thus, the mechanoinsensitive C nociceptors are likely candidates for mediating the ongoing burning pain following capsaicin injection, and may play an important role in maintaining central sensitization that manifests itself as allodynia to touch from normal Aβ-mechanoreceptor input (Torebjörk et al. 1992). We have no evidence that any type of C nociceptor becomes sensitized in the area of secondary hyperalgesia well outside the injured site (LaMotte et al 1992; Schmelz et al. 1996, in press), as has sometimes been suggested (Serra et al. 1995, 1998).

ITCH

CMH units have significantly higher conduction velocities (mean 0.95 m/s) (Schmidt et al. 1995; Olausson 1998) than do C-mechanoinsensitive units (mean 0.8 m/s) (Schmidt et al. 1995). Among the CH and CMiHi units, a subpopulation was discovered that had low conduction velocities (mean 0.5 m/s) and were sensitive to histamine iontophoresis. The discharge profiles of these units mirrored the magnitude and duration of histamine-evoked itch; these units are thus likely candidates for mediating itch (Schmelz et al. 1997a). On repetitive low-frequency stimulation at 1/8, 1/4, and 1/2 Hz, the activity-dependent slowing of impulse conduction was much greater in the mechanoinsensitive versus the sensitive units (Weidner et al. 1999). Activity-dependent slowing of conduction reportedly differentiates between nociceptive and cold-specific C fibers in rats (Thalhammer et al. 1994; Gee et al. 1996) and in humans (Serra et al. 1999), but to our knowledge Weidner et al.'s results represent the first time that differentiation has been observed between different types of C-nociceptive fibers. Statistical analysis revealed that this differentiation cannot be explained simply by differences in conduction velocities. Instead, the data suggest that mechanoresponsive and mechanoinsensitive C nociceptors have different membrane characteristics (Weidner et al. 1999). These data are interesting from a methodological point of view because the pronounced slowing allows a quick identification of "sleeping" and "itch" C units in a multifiber recording. Even more fascinating is the possibility that different types of human C-nociceptive fibers may have different ionic channels. Evidence in favor of this hypothesis would introduce the prospect of pharmacological agents targeted against fibers involved in inflammation, itching, and central sensitization, without affecting normal pain sensation. Preliminary evidence in this direction comes from recent experiments showing that systemically applied lidocaine in low concentrations inhibits mechanical hyperalgesia to tonic pressure, histamine-induced itch, axon reflex flare, and capsaicin-induced hyperalgesia to punctate and touch-evoked stimuli, but leaves acute heat and mechanical pain thresholds intact (Koppert et al. 1998, 1999).

CONCLUSIONS

Human skin contains several types of C nociceptors with distinctly different properties. The mechanoresponsive units may be involved in detection and localization of very acute noxious events. The CMH units have the capacity to detect small increments in heat on a painful background, and they give graded responses to painful heat stimuli. The finding that CMH and CM units are sensitized to heat following a mild burn injury or inflammation in the skin suggests that they contribute to primary heat hyperalgesia in the injured region.

The mechanoinsensitive C nociceptors are less suited for the detection and localization of initial noxious events, but they can become spontaneously active for long periods of time following chemical irritation or inflammation. Their sensitization may contribute to primary hyperalgesia to heat and to tonic pressure in the injured region. In addition, their ongoing discharges may contribute to central sensitization involved in secondary hyperalgesia outside the injured area. They are responsible for the axon reflex flare and are likely to be engaged in neurogenic inflammation.

A subpopulation of the mechanoinsensitive units appears to have a unique sensitivity to histamine. Their discharge profiles mirror the magnitude and duration of histamine-evoked itch. These CH and CMiHi units are candidates for mediating itch.

An important finding is the very different degree of activity-dependent slowing of impulse conduction for mechanoresponsive versus mechanoinsensitive C fibers, which suggests that they may have different membrane channels.

ACKNOWLEDGMENTS

This work was supported by the Swedish Medical Research Council Project 5206, the Max Planck Research Award for International Cooperation (E. Torebjörk), and the Deutsche Forschungsgemeinshaft (SFB 353). All experiments were approved by the local ethics committees, and all subjects gave their written informed consent according to the Declaration of Helsinki.

REFERENCES

Bessou P, Perl ER. Responses of cutaneous sensory units with unmyelinated fibers to noxious stimuli. *J Neurophysiol* 1969; 32:1025–1043.

Campbell JN, Raja SN, Cohen RH, et al. Peripheral neural mechanisms of nociception. In: Wall PD, Melzack R (Eds). *Textbook of Pain*. London: Churchill Livingstone, 1989, pp 22–45.

Gee MD, Lynn B, Cotsell B. Activity-dependent slowing of conduction velocity provides a method for identifying different functional classes of C-fibre in the rat saphenous nerve. *Neuroscience* 1996; 73:667–675.

Hallin RG, Torebjörk HE. C-fibre components in electrically evoked compound potentials recorded from human median nerve fascicles in situ. *Acta Soc Med Upsal* 1970a; 75:77–80.

Hallin RG, Torebjörk HE. Afferent and efferent C-units recorded from human skin nerves in situ. *Acta Soc Med Upsal* 1970b; 75:277–281.

Hallin RG, Torebjörk HE. Activity in unmyelinated nerve fibers in man. In: Bonica JJ (Ed). *International Symposium on Pain,* Advances in Neurology, Vol. 4. New York: Raven Press, 1973, pp 19–27.

Hallin RG, Torebjörk HE. Methods to differentiate electrically induced afferent and sympathetic C unit responses in human cutaneous nerves. *Acta Physiol Scand* 1974; 92:318–331.

van Hees J, Gybels JM. Pain related to single afferent C fibers from human skin. *Brain Res* 1972; 48:397–400.

Jørum E, Lundberg LER, Torebjörk HE. Peripheral projections of nociceptive unmyelinated axons in the human peroneal nerve. *J Physiol (Lond)* 1989; 416:291–301.

Koltzenburg M, Handwerker HO, Torebjörk HE. The ability of humans to localize noxious stimuli. *Neurosci Lett* 1993; 150:219–222.

Koppert W, Zeck S, Sittl R, et al. Low-dose lidocaine suppresses experimentally induced hyperalgesia in humans. *Anesthesiology* 1998; 89:1345–1353.

Koppert W, Sittl R, Zeck S, Ostermeier N, Schmelz M. Peripheral and spinal mechanisms of systemic lidocaine in human pain models. *Abstracts: 9th World Congress on Pain.* Seattle: IASP Press, 1999, pp 293–294.

LaMotte RH, Lundberg LER, Torebjörk HE. Pain, hyperalgesia and activity in nociceptive C units in humans after intradermal injection of capsaicin. *J Physiol (Lond)* 1992; 448:749–764.

Lynn B, Schutterle S, Pierau FK. The vasodilator component of neurogenic inflammation is caused by a special subclass of heat-sensitive nociceptors in the skin of the pig. *J Physiol (Lond)* 1996; 494:587–593.

Meyer RA, Campbell JN. A novel electrophysiological technique for locating cutaneous nociceptive and chemospecific receptors. *Brain Res* 1988; 561:252–261.

Olausson B. Recordings of polymodal single C-fiber nociceptive afferents following mechanical and argon-laser heat stimulation of human skin. *Exp Brain Res* 1998; 122:44–54.

Robinson CJ, Torebjörk HE, LaMotte RH. Psychophysical detection and pain ratings of incremental thermal stimuli. A comparison with nociceptor responses in humans. *Brain Res* 1983; 274:87–106.

Schmelz M, Forster C, Schmidt R, et al. Delayed responses to electrical stimuli reflect C-fibre responsiveness in human microneurography. *Exp Brain Res* 1995; 104:331–336.

Schmelz M, Schmidt R, Ringkamp M, et al. Limitation of sensitization to injured parts of receptive fields in human skin C-nociceptors. *Exp Brain Res* 1996; 109:141–147.

Schmelz M, Schmidt R, Bickel A, Handwerker HO, Torebjörk HE. Specific C-receptors for itch in human skin. *J Neurosci* 1997a; 17:8002–8008.

Schmelz M, Schmidt R, Bickel A, Handwerker HO, Torebjörk HE. Differential sensitivity of mechanosensitive and -insensitive C-fibers in human skin to tonic pressure and capsaicin. *Soc Neurosci Abstr* 1997b; 23:1004.

Schmelz M, Schmidt R, Bickel A, Handwerker HO, Torebjörk HE. Encoding of burning pain from capsaicin treated human skin in two categories of unmyelinated nerve fibres. *Brain*, in press.

Schmidt R, Schmelz M, Forster C, et al. Novel classes of responsive and unresponsive C nociceptors in human skin. *J Neurosci* 1995; 15:333–341.

Schmidt R, Schmelz M, Ringkamp M, Handwerker HO, Torebjörk HE. Innervation territories of mechanically activated C nociceptor units in human skin. *J Neurophysiol* 1997; 78:2641–2648.

Schmidt R, Schmelz M, Bickel A, et al. Innervation territories of mechanoinsensitive C nociceptor units in human skin. *Soc Neurosci Abstr* 1998; 24:383.

Serra J, Campero M, Ochoa J. Sensitization of silent C nociceptors in areas of secondary hyperalgesia (SH). *Neurology* 1995; 45:A365.

Serra J, Campero M, Ochoa J. Flare and hyperalgesia after intradermal capsaicin injection in human skin. *J Neurophysiol* 1998; 80:2801–2810.

Serra J, Campero M, Ochoa J, Bostock H. Activity-dependent slowing of conduction differentiates functional subtypes of C fibres innervating human skin. *J Physiol (Lond)* 1999; 515:799–811.

Thalhammer JG, Raymond SA, Popitz-Bergez FA, Strichartz GR. Modality-dependent modulation of conduction by impulse activity in functionally characterized single cutaneous afferents in the rat. *Somatosensory Motor Res* 1994; 11:242–257.

Torebjörk HE. Afferent C units responding to mechanical, thermal and chemical stimuli in human non-glabrous skin. *Acta Physiol Scand* 1974; 92:374–390.

Torebjörk HE, Hallin RG. C-fibre units recorded from human sensory nerve fascicles in situ. *Acta Soc Med Upsal* 1970; 75:81–84.

Torebjörk HE, Hallin RG. Excitation failure in thin nerve fibre structures and accompanying hypalgesia during repetitive electric skin stimulation. In: Bonica JJ (Ed). *International Symposium on Pain,* Advances in Neurology, Vol. 4. New York: Raven Press, 1973, pp 733–735.

Torebjörk HE, Hallin RG. Responses in human A and C fibres to repeated electrical intradermal stimulation. *J Neurol Neurosurg Psychiatry* 1974; 37:653–664.

Torebjörk HE, Ochoa JL. Specific sensations evoked by activity in single identified sensory units in man. *Acta Physiol Scand* 1980; 110:443–447.

Torebjörk HE, LaMotte RH, Robinson CJ. Peripheral neural correlates of the magnitude of cutaneous pain and hyperalgesia: simultaneous recordings in humans of sensory judgments of pain and evoked responses in nociceptors with C-fibers. *J Neurophysiol* 1984; 51:325–339.

Torebjörk HE, Lundberg LER, LaMotte RH. Central changes in processing of mechanoreceptive input in capsaicin–induced secondary hyperalgesia in humans. *J Physiol (Lond)* 1992; 448:765–780.

Torebjörk HE, Schmelz M, Handwerker HO. Functional properties of human cutaneous nociceptors and their role in pain and hyperalgesia. In: Belmonte C, Cervero F (Eds). *Neurobiology of Nociceptors*. Oxford: Oxford University Press, 1996, pp 349–369.

Vallbo ÅB, Hagbarth K-E. Activity from skin mechanoreceptors recorded percutaneously in awake human subjects. *Exp Neurol* 1968; 21:270–289.

Weidner C, Schmidt R, Schmelz M, et al. Functional attributes discriminating mechano-insensitive and mechano-responsive C-nociceptors in human skin. *J Neurosci* 1999; 19:10184–10190.

Correspondence to: Erik Torebjörk, MD, PhD, Department of Neuroscience, Clinical Neurophysiology, University Hospital, S-75185 Uppsala, Sweden. Tel: 46-18-663433; Fax: 46-18-556106; email: erik.torebjork@neurofys.uu.se.

Proceedings of the 9th World Congress on Pain,
Progress in Pain Research and Management,
Vol. 16, edited by M. Devor, M.C. Rowbotham, and
Z. Wiesenfeld-Hallin, IASP Press, Seattle, © 2000.

19

Sensory Functions of Epidermal Nerve Fibers in Humans

Donald A. Simone,[a] Nidal Khalili,[b]
Jill-Desiree Brederson,[a] Courtney Feder,[a]
Gwen Wendelschafer-Crabb,[b]
and William R. Kennedy[b]

Departments of [a]Psychiatry, and [b]Neurology, University of Minnesota, Minneapolis, Minnesota, USA

Recent studies using the pan-neuronal marker protein gene product 9.5 (PGP 9.5) have identified a network of epidermal nerve fibers (ENFs) that arise from the subepidermal neural plexus just below the basement membrane and extend to the very superficial epidermis (Wang et al. 1990; Kennedy and Wendelschafer-Crabb 1993). Clinical studies support the notion that ENFs possess a sensory function because they degenerate in a variety of neuropathic conditions associated with sensory deficits, including diabetic neuropathy (Kennedy et al. 1996) and small-fiber painful neuropathy (McCarthy et al. 1995; Holland et al. 1997; Herrmann et al. 1999; Periquet et al. 1999).

To evaluate sensory functions of ENFs, we determined whether topical application of capsaicin, a neurotoxin selective for small-diameter sensory fibers (Lynn 1990; Holzer 1991; Winter et al. 1995), would cause degeneration of ENFs, and whether loss of ENFs would produce detectable changes in cutaneous sensation.

METHODS

SUBJECTS AND PROCEDURES

Twelve healthy human subjects, eight male and four female (29–70 years of age), participated. None of the subjects was taking any medication. Subjects applied 0.075% capsaicin cream four times daily for 1 week to a 4 × 5 cm area of skin marked on the volar aspect of one forearm. The same area on the contralateral forearm served as the control site. Sensations of heat and mechanical pain were assessed during days 1–6 of capsaicin application, and once weekly for 5 weeks after the cessation of capsaicin treatment. The sensation of itch was determined following 3 days of capsaicin application for three subjects.

Skin biopsies were obtained from capsaicin-treated skin during 1–6 days of capsaicin application and once a week for 5 weeks following cessation of capsaicin, immediately following sensory testing. One biopsy was obtained from normal, control skin from each subject. Psychophysical measures of cutaneous sensation were obtained for all subjects, and skin biopsies were taken from five subjects. All procedures were performed with informed consent as approved by the Internal Review Board and the Human Subjects Committee of the University of Minnesota.

PSYCHOPHYSICAL MEASURES OF CUTANEOUS SENSATION

Sensations of heat pain, pricking pain, touch, and itch were assessed. Heat pain sensation was measured with a Peltier-type thermode with a contact area of 7.1 mm^2 (WR Medical Electronics Co., Stillwater, MN). The thermode was set at a temperature of 53°C, and was applied to the volar forearm at random locations within areas of control or capsaicin-treated skin. The stimulus was applied 5 times in treated and control skin, each for a duration of 5 seconds. Subjects judged the maximum magnitude of pain produced by each stimulus using a visual analogue scale (VAS; on a scale of 0–10).

The sensation of sharp, pricking pain was evoked by a sharp probe (50 μm diameter tip) attached to a calibrated nylon monofilament (95 mN bending force) applied to 10 randomly selected locations within control and capsaicin-treated skin, each for a duration of 2 seconds. Subjects reported whether they experienced sharp pain or only touch. The proportion of trials reported painful was determined.

Tactile detection threshold (mN) was determined with calibrated nylon von Frey monofilaments. Threshold was defined as the smallest force that was perceived at least 50% of the time.

The sensation of itch was produced by intradermal injection of 100 μg histamine in a volume of 10 μL. Histamine was injected into normal and capsaicin-treated skin. Subjects judged the magnitude of itch every 15 seconds for 10 minutes after injection (or until the itch sensation disappeared) using the method of magnitude estimation.

SKIN BIOPSIES AND IMMUNOHISTOCHEMISTRY

Skin biopsies were collected from the control and capsaicin sites in five subjects and processed as described previously (Kennedy et al. 1996). The biopsies were fixed in Zamboni's solution for 24 hours and cryoprotected with 20% sucrose in 0.1 M phosphate buffered saline until sectioned. Frozen sections (100 μm) were immunostained using antibodies to the pan-neuronal marker PGP 9.5, and to type IV collagen. Antibodies were visualized with cyanine 2, 3, or 5 fluorescent probes conjugated to appropriate secondary antibodies. Confocal images were acquired at 2-μm intervals throughout the depth of the specimen. Each image could be viewed individually, or the entire series could be projected into a single focused image, for counts of ENFs.

DATA ANALYSES

One-way ANOVA was used to compare the number of ENFs per millimeter length of epidermis in capsaicin-treated skin and normal skin at various times after capsaicin treatment. Two-way ANOVAs with repeated measures were used to assess differences over time between capsaicin-treated and untreated skin in the magnitude of heat pain, the proportion of mechanical stimuli perceived as painful, tactile threshold, and the magnitude and duration of itch. Post hoc comparisons were made using the Tukey procedure. $P < 0.05$ was considered significant. All data are represented as the mean (± 1 SEM).

RESULTS

MORPHOLOGY OF ENFS FOLLOWING CAPSAICIN TREATMENT

In normal, untreated skin, the epidermis and subepidermal neural plexus were richly innervated by nerve fibers, immunoreactive for PGP 9.5, that arose from the subepidermal plexus and projected up through the basement membrane to terminate in the superficial epidermis (Fig. 1). Capsaicin produced a dramatic loss of ENFs that was evident 24 hours after capsaicin treatment. Fig. 1 shows confocal images of skin biopsies from normal and capsaicin-treated skin at various times after treatment for a typical subject. The mean number of ENFs (per millimeter length of epidermis) for all subjects decreased by 76% at 24 hours after capsaicin treatment (Fig. 2), and by 91% 48 hours after treatment. ENFs were rarely observed at the end of 3 days of capsaicin application. There was no obvious alteration of fibers located in the subepidermal plexus or deeper in the dermis.

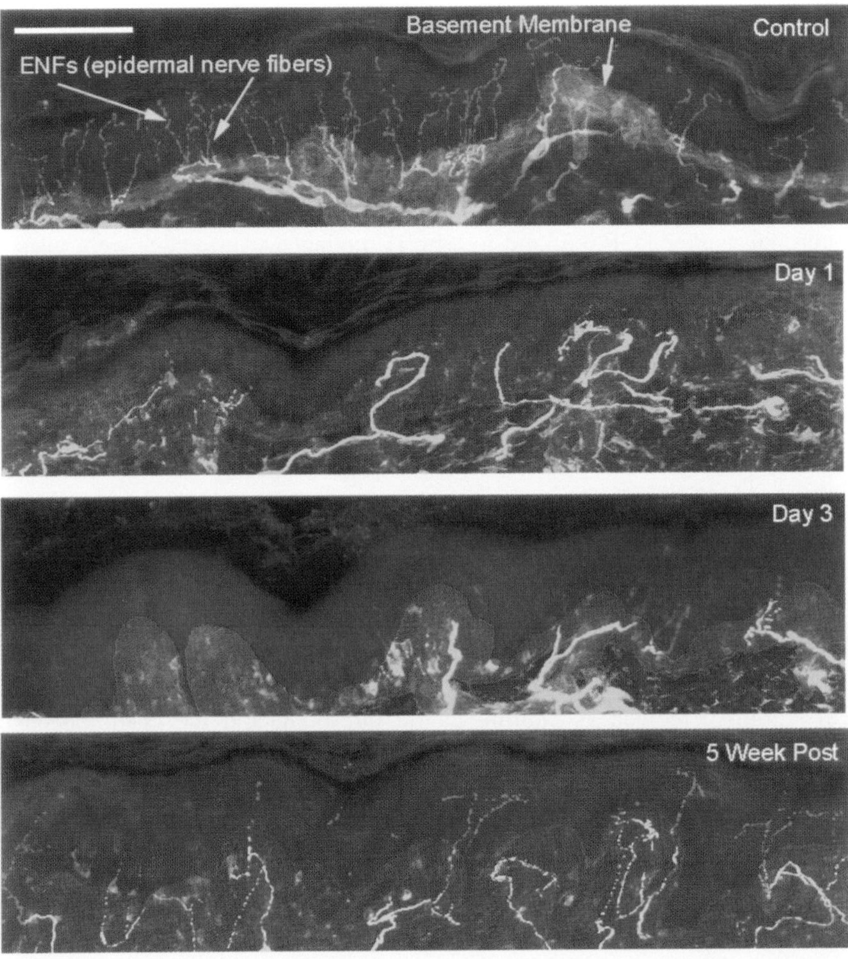

Fig. 1. Confocal images of skin biopsies from one subject showing epidermal nerve fibers (ENFs) in normal, control skin, following 1 and 3 days of capsaicin application, and at 5 weeks following capsaicin treatment. PGP 9.5 staining of nerve fibers appears yellow or green, and type IV collagen staining of the basement membrane and blood vessels appears red. Each is labeled in the top panel. The scale bar in the top panel = 100 μm and applies to all panels.

Reinnervation of the epidermis was gradual, and was evident at 2 weeks following cessation of capsaicin, with few ENFs having regenerated into the epidermis. A representative example of epidermal reinnervation is illustrated in Fig. 1. The mean number of ENFs per millimeter length of epidermis for all subjects at 1, 2, and 5 weeks following capsaicin treatment was 12%, 29%, and 52% of normal, respectively (Fig. 2).

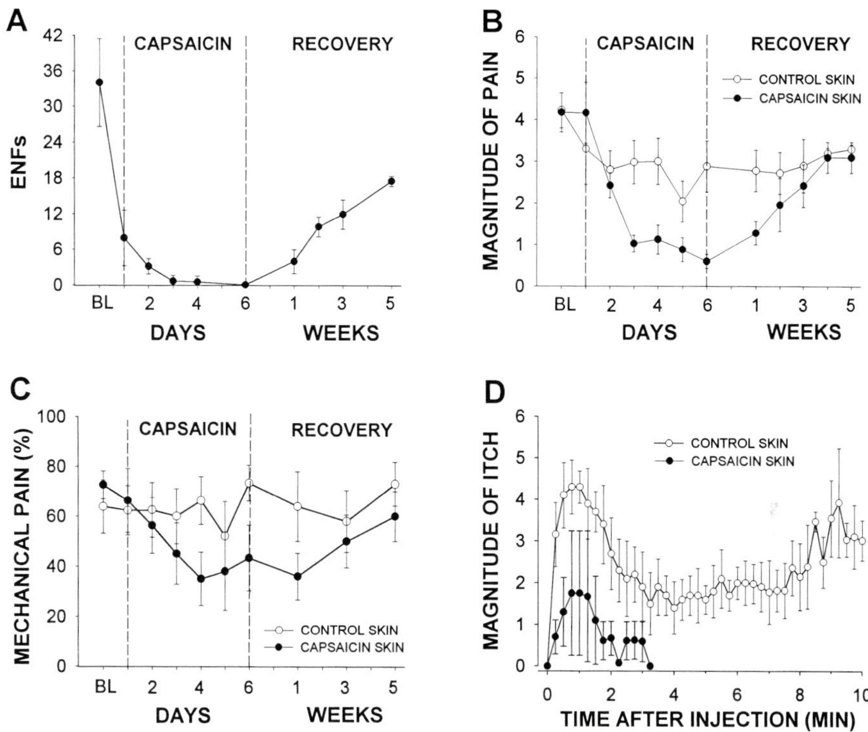

Fig. 2. Effect of capsaicin on ENFs and on pain and itch sensations. Measurements of ENFs, heat pain, and sharp mechanical pain were obtained at baseline (BL), during 1 week of capsaicin application, and for 5 weeks after capsaicin treatment (recovery). The sensation of itch was assessed following 3 days of capsaicin application. (A) Mean (± SEM) number of ENFs per millimeter length of epidermis; (B) mean (± SEM) magnitude of heat pain; (C) mean (± SEM) percentage of trials that the mechanical stimulus was perceived as painful; (D) mean (± SEM) normalized magnitude estimates of itch following injection of histamine (given at time "0").

EFFECT OF CAPSAICIN ON CUTANEOUS SENSATION

Capsaicin significantly decreased sensations of heat pain, sharp pain, and itch, without affecting tactile sensation. The magnitude of heat pain decreased by 47% following 2 days of capsaicin application (Fig. 2), and by 6 days, heat pain was barely detected. Detection of sharp pain sensation also decreased significantly (Fig. 2). Following 2 days of capsaicin application, the mean proportion of trials reported as painful decreased from 72.5% ± 5.6% to 56.3% ± 11.2%, and decreased further following continued capsaicin treatment.

The magnitude and duration of itch sensation decreased following 3 days of capsaicin application (Fig. 2). In untreated skin, itch persisted for over 10 minutes. However, in capsaicin-treated skin, the maximum magnitude of itch was approximately 50% of that reported in normal skin, and itch sensation lasted for only 3 minutes.

The restoration of pain sensation occurred gradually, beginning 2 weeks after cessation of capsaicin, and was consistent with the reappearance of ENFs. At 4–5 weeks following capsaicin treatment, the heat and pricking pain sensations did not different from control values. Itch sensation was not evaluated following discontinuation of capsaicin.

DISCUSSION

The results confirm and extend our previous findings that intradermal injection (Simone et al. 1998) or topical application (Nolano et al. 1999) of capsaicin produces loss of ENFs associated with a decrease in heat pain and mechanical (sharp) pain sensation. In our previous study using topical application of capsaicin, we first examined epidermal innervation 3 days following capsaicin application. In the present study we found a reduction in ENFs and heat and mechanical pain sensations as early as 24 hours following capsaicin treatment. This implies that the process of ENF degeneration may occur soon after capsaicin application, as suggested by Reilly et al. (1997). We also found that the sensation of itch diminished following capsaicin treatment. Together, our results suggest that at least a portion of ENFs are nociceptors and contribute to sensations of pain and itch.

Results of the present study also show that ENFs possess a remarkable regenerative capacity following discontinuation of capsaicin. Reinnervation was apparent 2 weeks following discontinuation of capsaicin and was consistent with the gradual return of pain sensation. The mechanisms underlying ENF regeneration are unclear, but may depend in part on trophic influences (Pincelli and Yarr 1997). Capsaicin may therefore be a useful tool to further elucidate the complex mechanisms of peripheral nerve regeneration and restoration of function.

ACKNOWLEDGMENTS

This work was supported by NIH grants NS31223 (D.A. Simone) and NS31397 (W.R. Kennedy), and by Toray Industries, Tokyo (W.R. Kennedy).

REFERENCES

Hermann DN, Griffin JW, Hauer P, Cornblath DR, McArthur JC. Intraepidermal nerve fiber density, sural nerve morphometry and electrodiagnosis in peripheral neuropathies. *Neurology* 1999; 53:1634–1640.

Holland NR, Stocks A, Hauer P, et al. Intraepidermal nerve fiber density in patients with painful sensory neuropathy. *Neurology* 1997; 48:708–711.

Holzer P. Capsaicin: cellular targets, mechanisms of action and selectivity for thin sensory neurons. *Pharmacol Rev* 1991; 43:143–201.

Kennedy WR, Wendelschafer-Crabb G. The innervation of human epidermis. *J Neurol Sci* 1993; 115:184–190.

Kennedy WR, Wendelschafer-Crabb G, Johnson T. Quantitation of epidermal nerves in diabetic neuropathy. *Neurology* 1996; 47:1042–1048.

Lynn B. Capsaicin: actions on nociceptive C-fibers and therapeutic potential. *Pain* 1990; 41:61–69.

McCarthy BG, Hsieh S-T, Stocks EA, et al. Cutaneous innervation in sensory neuropathies. *Neurology* 1995; 45:1848–1855.

Nolano M, Simone DA, Wendelschafer-Crabb, et al. Topical capsaicin in humans: parallel loss of epidermal nerve fibers and pain sensation. *Pain* 1999; 81:135–145.

Periquet MI, Novak V, Collins MP, et al. Painful sensory neuropathy: prospective evaluation of painful feet using electrodiagnosis and skin biopsy. *Neurology* 1999; 53:1641–1647.

Pincelli C, Yarr M. Nerve growth factor: its significance in cutaneous biology. *J Invest Dermatol Symp Proc* 1997; 2:31–36.

Reilly DM, Ferdinando D, Johnston C, et al. The epidermal nerve fiber network: characterization of nerve fibers in human skin by confocal microscopy and assessment of racial variations. *Br J Dermatol* 1997; 137:163–170.

Simone DA, Ochoa J. Early and late effect of prolonged topical capsaicin on cutaneous sensibility and neurogenic vasodilation in humans. *Pain* 1991; 47:285–294.

Simone DA, Nolano M, Wendelschafer-Crabb G, Kennedy WR. Intradermal injection of capsaicin in humans produces rapid degeneration and subsequent reinnervation of epidermal nerve fibers: correlation with sensory function. *J Neurosci* 1998; 18:8947–8959.

Wang L, Hilliges M, Jernberg T, Wiegleb-Edström D, Johansson O. Protein gene product 9.5-immunoreactive nerve fibres and cells in human skin. *Cell Tissue Res* 1990; 261:25–33.

Winter J, Bevan S, Campbell EA. Capsaicin and pain mechanisms. *Br J Anaesthesiol* 1995; 75:157–168.

Correspondence to: Donald A. Simone, PhD, Department of Psychiatry, University of Minnesota, 420 Delaware Street SE, Box 392, UMHC, Minneapolis, MN 55455, USA. Tel: 612-625-6464; Fax: 612-624-8935; email: simon003@tc.umn.edu.

Proceedings of the 9th World Congress on Pain,
Progress in Pain Research and Management,
Vol. 16, edited by M. Devor, M.C. Rowbotham, and
Z. Wiesenfeld-Hallin, IASP Press, Seattle, © 2000.

20

Secondary Hyperalgesia to Punctate Stimuli Is Mediated by A-Fiber Nociceptors

Ellen Jørum,[a] Torhild Warncke,[a] Esther A. Ziegler,[b] Walter Magerl,[b] Perry N. Fuchs,[c,d] Richard A. Meyer,[c] and Rolf-Detlef Treede[b]

[a]*Laboratory of Clinical Neurophysiology, Department of Neurology, The National Hospital, Oslo, Norway;* [b]*Institute of Physiology and Pathophysiology, Johannes Gutenberg University, Mainz, Germany;* [c]*Department of Neurosurgery, Johns Hopkins University, Baltimore, Maryland, USA;* [d]*Department of Psychology, University of Texas at Arlington, Arlington, Texas, USA*

Cutaneous injury elicits hyperalgesia to heat and mechanical stimuli at the site of the injury (primary hyperalgesia) and hyperalgesia to mechanical stimuli in an area surrounding the injury (secondary hyperalgesia) (Lewis 1936; Hardy et al. 1950; LaMotte et al. 1982, 1991; Raja et al. 1984). Primary hyperalgesia to heat stimuli is believed to be mediated by sensitization of nociceptive afferents (peripheral sensitization) (Meyer and Campbell 1981; LaMotte et al. 1982). Secondary hyperalgesia is the consequence of sensitization of spinal cord dorsal horn neurons by conditioning noxious input (Simone et al. 1991; Pertovaara 1998).

In the secondary zone, two main subtypes of mechanical hyperalgesia have been described after experimental skin injuries (LaMotte et al. 1991; Koltzenburg et al. 1992; Kilo et al. 1994): hyperalgesia to light touch elicited by tactile stimuli such as light stroking of the skin with cotton wool (also termed allodynia), and hyperalgesia to punctate stimuli elicited by pointed stimuli such as sharp needles or von Frey hairs. Although central sensitization subserves both types of mechanical hyperalgesia in the secondary zone (LaMotte et al. 1991), different neural mechanisms must be involved because the characteristics of the two forms of hyperalgesia differ. For example, in human experimental models, such as application of capsaicin or thermal injury, hyperalgesia to punctate stimuli is more easily induced, more frequent, longer lasting, and encompasses a larger area in comparison to hyperalgesia to light touch (LaMotte et al. 1991; Koltzenburg et al. 1992; Kilo et al. 1994; Warncke et al. 1997; Magerl et al. 1998). Secondary hyperalgesia to light touch is mediated by A-fiber, low-threshold mechanoreceptors (LTMs), which are normally responsible for touch sensations (Torebjörk et al. 1992). In contrast, punctate hyperalgesia may be mediated by nociceptive fibers (Treede and Cole 1993; Cervero et al. 1994; Kilo et al. 1994).

To determine whether Aδ or C-fiber nociceptors are responsible for secondary hyperalgesia to punctate stimuli, we performed two different experiments using differential nerve conduction blockade.

EXPERIMENT A

MATERIALS AND METHODS

Ten healthy, unmedicated volunteers (3 males, 7 females; age range 23–33 years, median age 26 years) took part in the study at the National Hospital in Oslo, Norway. Hyperalgesia was induced by a burn injury on the medial surface of the right or left calf. A 25 × 50 mm rectangular thermode (Thermotest, Somedic AB, Sweden) at 47°C was applied with a standardized pressure (8 kPa) for 7 minutes. This resulted in a first-degree burn injury with erythema without any visible edema or blister, which resolved within less than 24 hours. Immediately after the thermal injury, no spontaneous pain was experienced at the injured skin, and pain was only reported thereafter during mechanical or thermal stimulation.

Thresholds for sensations of heat, cold, heat pain, and cold pain were determined by a computerized Thermotest (Somedic AB, Sweden). Tactile thresholds were determined by hand-held nylon filaments (von Frey hair, 0.29–745.6 mN) (Stoelting) applied in an ascending and descending order of force. The area of secondary hyperalgesia to punctate stimuli was determined with a hand-held von Frey hair (83.7 mN). The borders of the hyperalgesic area were identified by stimulating along eight linear paths arranged radially around the site of thermal injury (Fig. 1). Stimulation along each path with a von Frey hair started well outside the hyperalgesic area where no sensation of pain was experienced, and progressed towards the site of thermal injury until the subject reported a definite change of perception

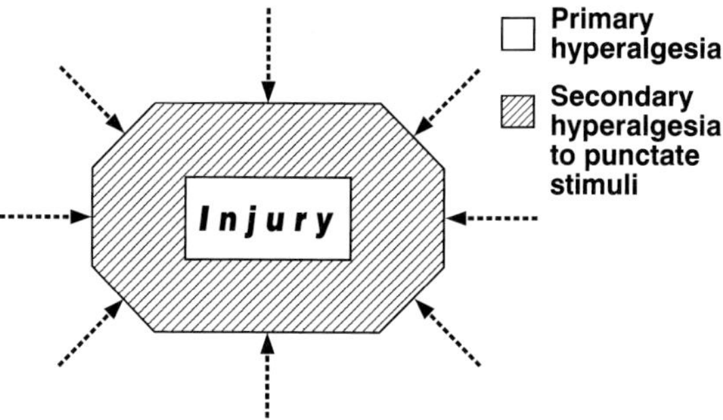

Fig. 1. Mapping of the area of secondary hyperalgesia (shaded area) following the burn injury (white rectangle). The borders of the hyperalgesic skin zone were identified by stimulating with a von Frey hair (83.7 mN force) along eight linear paths (broken lines) arranged radially around the site of thermal injury. Stimulation started from well outside the hyperalgesic area, and progressed toward the injury site until subjects experienced an abrupt increase in pain when the border of the hyperalgesic skin area was met (position of arrowheads).

from nonpainful touch to a burning or pricking pain. The presence of primary and secondary hyperalgesia was verified before ischemic nerve conduction blockade was induced by inflating a sphygmomanometer applied to the calf above the site of thermal injury to 200 mm Hg. The ischemic block was left until the sensation of touch (block of A-fiber LTMs) and cold (block of Aδ cold fibers) was eliminated distal to the block.

RESULTS

Following a burn injury, an area of punctate hyperalgesia was induced that was characterized by a decrease in mechanical pain threshold (Table I). A reduction of pain threshold to heat was found in the primary, but not secondary zone. Distal to the pressure cuff, the sensation of touch was lost after 40 ± 1 minutes (mean ± SEM), and the sensation of cold was lost after 38 ± 2 minutes of ischemic nerve block. In three subjects, the sensation of cold was lost before the sensation of touch. In the remaining seven subjects, the sensation of cold was lost simultaneously with the sensation of touch. After perception of touch and cold was lost, the hyperalgesia to punctate stimuli persisted unaltered in both primary and secondary zones. Most subjects described the sensation as different in quality: stimuli appeared less definite and less pricking, but in fact more unpleasant, with an unpleasant after-sensation that was not present before the ischemic block.

Table I
Mean sensory thresholds (± SEM) before thermal injury and 30 minutes after thermal injury (a first-degree burn)

	Primary Zone		Secondary Zone	
Sensory Threshold	Before	After	Before	After
Heat detection thresh. (°C)	35.9 ± 0.6	36.5 ± 0.6	35.7 ± 0.4	36.0 ± 0.5
Cold detection thresh. (°C)	29.8 ± 0.6	29.8 ± 0.6	31.3 ± 1.2	29.9 ± 0.3
Heat pain detection thresh. (°C)	44.5 ± 0.7	39.1 ± 0.8**	43.8 ± 0.8	43.7 ± 0.9
Cold pain detection thresh. (°C)	NA	NA	NA	NA
Tactile detection thresh. (mN)	8.7 ± 1.4	6.6 ± 1.3*	8.7 ± 1.4	7.2 ± 1.2
Mechanical pain thresh. (mN)	95.9 ± 5.0	44.5 ± 5.6**	95.9 ± 5.0	60.4 ± 6.7*
Skin temperature (°C)	31.9 ± 0.4	33.5 ± 0.4	31.7 ± 0.4	31.9 ± 0.4

Note: Primary zone = area of thermal injury; secondary zone = outside area of thermal injury. Area of hyperalgesia from thermal injury = 58.3 ± 4.1 cm^2. NA = not assessable. Significant differences: * $P < 0.05$, ** $P < 0.01$.

EXPERIMENT B

METHODS

Ten healthy subjects (3 males, 7 females; age 23–55 years, median age 27 years) took part in the study at the Johannes Gutenberg University in Mainz, Germany. Capsaicin (40 μg in 12.5 μL volume) was injected intradermally into the hairy skin on the dorsum of the left hand to induce secondary hyperalgesia. As a control, capsaicin was also injected intradermally into the hairy skin on the dorsum of the right hand. Pain perception to mechanical stimuli was tested by weight-loaded punctate mechanical probes (200 μm diameter, 35–407 mN force).

Differential nerve conduction blockade of myelinated nerve fibers of the radial nerve was performed in the left hand proximal to the wrist by pressing the superficial radial nerve to the radial bone with a 2.5-cm wide rubber band loaded with a 1.2-kg weight. Tests of A- and C-fiber sensory modalities were performed before, during, and after the nerve block for: (1) touch sensitivity to a 4-mN von Frey hair and compound sensory nerve action potential (SNAP) for large-diameter Aβ-fiber mechanoreceptors; (2) cold detection for small-diameter Aδ-fiber cold receptors; (3) fast reaction times to a 125-mN weighted pinprick (<500 ms, i.e., first pain) for A-fiber nociceptors; (4) innocuous heat (warm) detection for C-fiber warm receptors; and (5) slow reaction times to 125-mN pinprick (>500 ms, i.e., second pain) and capsaicin-evoked pain for C-fiber nociceptors (for details see Ziegler et al. 1999).

When these tests indicated that the ability to detect both touch and cold had largely disappeared, the autonomous zone of the superficial branch of the radial nerve was mapped (Fig. 2A). Pain perception to punctate stimuli was tested after conduction blockade of non-nociceptive and nociceptive A fibers was complete. Capsaicin was then injected intradermally, well inside the autonomous zone, and pain perception to punctate stimuli was tested

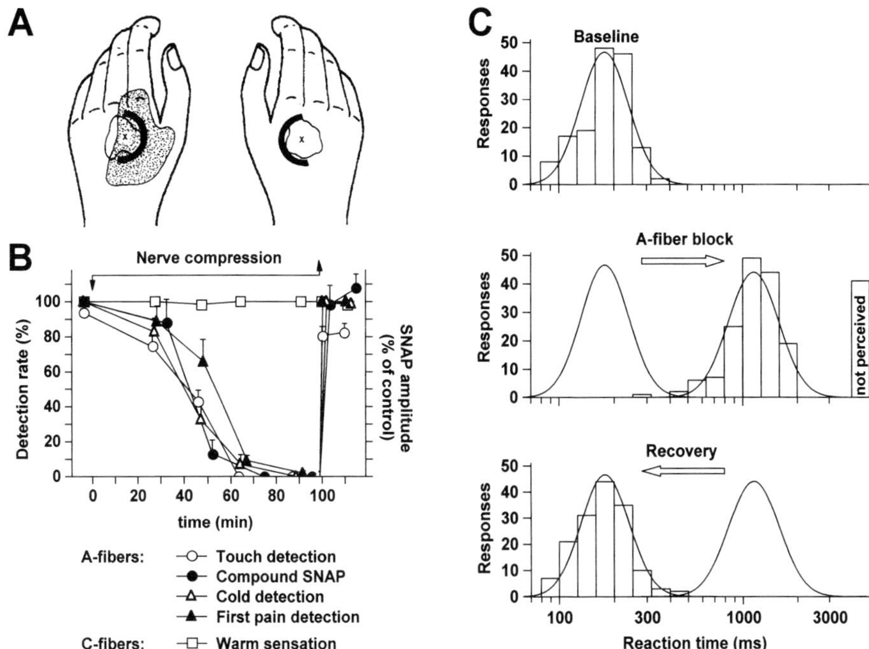

Fig. 2. Secondary hyperalgesia and A-fiber conduction blockade. (A) A-fiber conduction was blocked by pressure to the superficial radial nerve, resulting in a temporary block of A-fiber-mediated sensations within the autonomous zone of this nerve (stippled area). Capsaicin (40 µg) was intradermally injected within this area (marked by x), resulting in a flare (white area) and secondary hyperalgesia in adjacent skin. Secondary hyperalgesia was tested by 200-µm flat-tip probes at 15 mm distance (black semicircle) within the skin zone affected by the A-fiber blockade. (B) Loss of A-fiber-mediated perception by nerve compression. Note that Aδ-mediated first pain is blocked significantly later than are Aβ-fiber-mediated touch and sensory nerve action potential (SNAP) and Aδ-fiber-mediated cold perception. At approximately 90 minutes of pressure, all A-fiber-mediated perception is completely blocked, while C-fiber-mediated warmth perception is readily preserved. (C) Detailed analysis of first pain perception. Reaction times to touching the skin with a needle probe were on average 180 ms in normal skin (lognormal distribution). Under fully established A-fiber conduction blockade, approximately 80% of skin stimuli were still perceived, but reaction times were now in the range of C-fiber-mediated second pain (on average 1150 ms). Reaction times returned to normal within minutes after termination of nerve compression. Modified with permission from Ziegler et al. (1999).

again at 10 minutes after the injection. Sensory tests before and after capsaicin injection were used to verify that, in the time window of pain and hyperalgesia testing (60–90 minutes after block onset), A-fiber conduction blockade was complete, and that C-fiber function was still intact. The block was released at 96 ± 3 minutes.

RESULTS

The time course of conduction blockade was very similar for all non-nociceptive A-fiber functions: time to 50% decay of function was 42 ± 3 minutes for touch, 39 ± 4 minutes for cold, and 38 ± 4 minutes for SNAP. In contrast, 50% loss of first pain detection occurred significantly later at 57 ± 3 minutes ($P < 0.001$ vs. touch, cold and SNAP, Fig. 2B,C). For the sensory testing performed 65 ± 2 minutes after initiation of nerve compression, the reaction time to touching the skin with a sharp needle-tip increased dramatically, indicating a blockade of nociceptive and non-nociceptive A-fiber function at this stage. After 1 hour of nerve compression, pricking pain to the punctate stimuli of the left hand was strongly diminished to 25% of baseline values ($P < 0.001$). According to the shift in reaction times to pin-pricks, the remaining pain evoked by the punctate probes was mediated by C fibers.

Capsaicin injection caused an equally strong burning pain in both hands (right control hand: 84 ± 6%; left hand under A-fiber block: 89 ± 6% on a numerical rating scale). In the control hand, capsaicin elicited a robust and

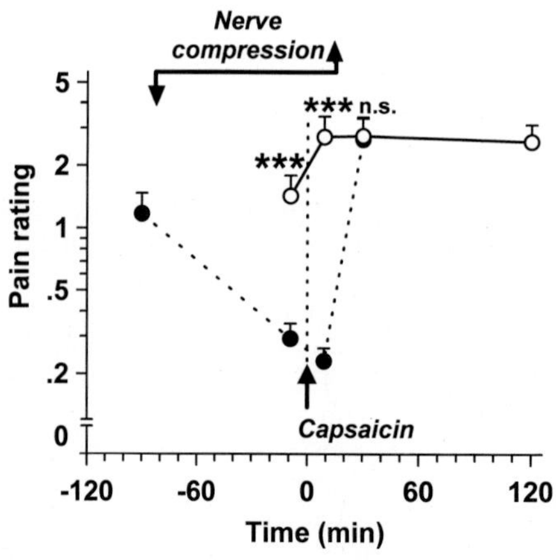

Fig. 3. Impact of A-fiber conduction blockade on perception of pricking pain and secondary hyperalgesia to punctate stimuli. Capsaicin injection (black arrow, vertical broken line at time = 0) in the control hand (open symbols) induced a highly significant increase of pain sensation in adjacent uninjured skin, which remained stable for at least 2 hours. Complete A-fiber conduction blockade of the left superficial radial nerve strongly reduced the magnitude of pricking pain in the left hand (closed symbols). Notably, the remaining (C-fiber-mediated) pain was not increased following the capsaicin injection (although the pain evoked by the capsaicin injection was similar to normal skin). However, the hyperalgesia became apparent when A-fiber conduction was re-established after removal of the nerve compression. Reprinted with permission from Ziegler et al. (1999).

long-lasting secondary hyperalgesia to punctate stimuli for at least 2 hours (Fig. 3). In contrast, pain ratings to the punctate stimuli at 10 minutes after the capsaicin injection to the left hand (80 minutes after induction of pressure block) decreased even further. However, when the A-fiber conduction blockade was released, secondary hyperalgesia to punctate stimuli was fully present and did not differ from the control hand ($P = 0.78$).

DISCUSSION

Secondary hyperalgesia is generally accepted to result from sensitization of nociceptive neurons in the dorsal horn of the spinal cord (Simone et al. 1991). Whereas secondary hyperalgesia to light touch is signaled by low-threshold mechanosensitive Aβ fibers, hyperalgesia to punctate stimuli derives from activation of nociceptive primary afferents.

Nerve fiber conduction blockades have traditionally been used to differentiate between A and C fibers, with loss of touch and cold perception as criteria for blocking conduction in A fibers (Sinclair 1967). However, this does not necessarily indicate complete conduction blockade of A-fiber nociceptors. Future experiments employing nerve blocks need to differentiate between non-nociceptive and nociceptive A-fiber function. Although cold fibers and A-fiber nociceptors have similar conduction velocities in the Aδ range, they differ substantially with respect to other properties, such as absolute and relative refractory periods (Raymond et al. 1990). Our experiments show that when perception of light touch and cold had disappeared distal to an ischemic nerve block (at around 40 minutes), punctate hyperalgesia remained present, suggesting apparent mediation through nonmyelinated C fibers. However, as shown in more detail in experiment B, explicit testing of A-fiber nociceptor function under pressure nerve block revealed that nociceptive A fibers are significantly more resistant to nerve block than are non-nociceptive mechanoreceptive and cold fibers. Notably, conduction blockade of non-nociceptive A fibers occurred in the same time-range (38–42 minutes) under pressure block as under ischemic block (40 minutes). In contrast, blockade of A-fiber nociceptors, as shown by conversion of fast (i.e., first pain) into slow (i.e., second pain) reaction times did not occur until 15–20 minutes later. In this critical time window, when detection of touch and cold were already lost, the hyperalgesia to punctate stimuli was still mediated by A-fiber nociceptors, as demonstrated by the presence of first pain reaction times. However, when conduction in nociceptive *and* non-nociceptive A-fiber subtypes was lost, with C-fibers still being unaffected, hyperalgesia to punctate stimuli was completely eliminated.

In conclusion, secondary hyperalgesia to punctate stimuli is signaled by A-fiber nociceptors. Secondary hyperalgesia is confined to mechanical stimuli, while hyperalgesia to heat is absent adjacent to an injury (as shown in experiment A and by Raja et al. 1984; LaMotte et al. 1991; Ali et al. 1996). Likewise, sensitization of spinal dorsal horn neurons is restricted to mechanical input (Simone et al. 1991; Pertovaara 1998), while noxious thermal input may even be transiently inhibited (Dougherty et al. 1998). Therefore, the relevant A-fiber nociceptors likely encompass only those subpopulations that are either heat-insensitive or have very high heat thresholds, i.e., high-threshold mechanoreceptive and type I mechano-heat-sensitive A-fiber nociceptors (Treede et al. 1998). The recent observation that punctate hyperalgesia persists in capsaicin-desensitized skin also supports this conclusion (Fuchs et al. 1999; Magerl et al. 1999).

REFERENCES

Ali Z, Meyer RA, Campbell JN. Secondary hyperalgesia to mechanical but not heat stimuli following a capsaicin injection in hairy skin. *Pain* 1996, 68:401–411.

Cervero F, Meyer RA, Campbell JN. A psychophysical study of secondary hyperalgesia: evidence for increased pain to input from nociceptors. *Pain* 1994; 58:21–28.

Dougherty PM, Willis WD, Lenz FA. Transient inhibition of responses to thermal stimuli of spinal sensory tract neurons in monkeys during sensitization by intradermal capsaicin. *Pain* 1998; 77:129–136.

Fuchs PN, Campbell JN, Meyer RA. Secondary hyperalgesia in capsaicin desensitized skin. *Pain* 1999, in press.

Hardy JD, Wolff G, Goodell H. Experimental evidence on the nature of cutaneous hyperalgesia. *J Clin Invest* 1950; 29:115–140.

Kilo S, Schmelz M, Koltzenburg M, Handwerker HO. Different patterns of hyperalgesia induced by experimental inflammation in human skin. *Brain* 1994; 117:385–396.

Koltzenburg M, Lundberg LER, Torebjörk HE. Dynamic and static components of mechanical hyperalgesia in human hairy skin. *Pain* 1992; 51:207–219.

LaMotte RH, Thalhammer JG, Torebjörk HE, Robinson CJ. Peripheral neural mechanisms of cutaneous hyperalgesia following mild injury by heat. *J Neurosci* 1982; 6:765–781.

LaMotte RH, Shain CN, Simone DA, Tsai EF. Neurogenic hyperalgesia: psychophysical studies of underlying mechanisms. *J Neurophysiol* 1991; 66:190–211.

LaMotte RH, Lundberg LER, Torebjörk HE. Pain, hyperalgesia and activity in nociceptive C units in humans after intradermal injection of capsaicin. *J Physiol* 1992; 448:749–764.

Lewis T. Experiments relating to cutaneous hyperalgesia and its spread through somatic nerves. *Clin Sci* 1936; 2:373–423.

Magerl W, Wilk SH, Treede R-D. Secondary hyperalgesia and perceptual wind-up following intradermal injection of capsaicin in humans. *Pain* 1998; 74:257–268.

Magerl W, Fuchs PN, Meyer RA, Treede R-D. Secondary hyperalgesia to punctate stimuli in humans is mediated by capsaicin-insensitive A-fiber nociceptors. Abstracts: 9th World Congress on Pain. Seattle: IASP Press, 1999, p 407.

Meyer RA, Campbell JN. Myelinated nociceptive afferents account for the hyperalgesia that follows a burn to the hand. *Science* 1981; 213:1527–1529.

Pertovaara A. A neuronal correlate of secondary hyperalgesia in the rat spinal dorsal horn is submodality selective and facilitated by supraspinal influence. *Exp Neurol* 1998; 149:193–202.

Raja SN, Campbell JN, Meyer RA. Evidence for different mechanisms of primary and secondary hyperalgesia following heat injury to the glabrous skin. *Brain* 1984; 107:1179–1188.

Raymond SA, Thalhammer JG, Popitz-Berger F, Strichartz GR. Changes in axonal impulse conduction correlate with sensory modality in primary afferent fibers in the rat. *Brain Res* 1990; 526:318–321.

Simone DA, Sorkin LS, Oh U, et al. Neurogenic hyperalgesia: central neural correlates in responses of spinothalamic tract neurons. *J Neurophysiol* 1991; 66:228–246.

Sinclair DC. *Cutaneous Sensation*. London: Oxford University Press, 1967.

Torebjörk HE, Lundberg LER, LaMotte RH. Central changes in processing of mechanoreceptive input in capsaicin-induced secondary hyperalgesia in humans. *J Physiol* 1992; 448:765–780.

Treede R-D, Cole J. Dissociated secondary hyperalgesia in a subject with a large-fiber sensory neuropathy. *Pain* 1993; 53:169–174.

Treede R-D, Meyer RA, Campbell JN. Myelinated mechanically insensitive afferents from monkey skin: heat response properties. *J Neurophysiol* 1998; 80:1082–1093.

Warncke T, Stubhaug A, Jørum E. Ketamine, an NMDA receptor antagonist, suppresses spatial and temporal properties of burn-induced secondary hyperalgesia in man: a double-blind, cross-over comparison with morphine and placebo. *Pain* 1997; 72:99–106.

Ziegler EA, Magerl W, Meyer RA, Treede R-D. Secondary hyperalgesia to punctate mechanical stimuli. Central sensitization to A-fibre nociceptor input. *Brain* 1999; 122:2245–2257.

Correspondence to: Walter Magerl, PhD, Institute of Physiology and Pathophysiology, Johannes Gutenberg University Mainz, Saarstr. 21, D-55099 Mainz, Germany. Tel: 49-6131-3925218; Fax: 49-6131-3925902; email: magerl@mail.uni-mainz.de.

Proceedings of the 9th World Congress on Pain, Progress in Pain Research and Management, Vol. 16, edited by M. Devor, M.C. Rowbotham, and Z. Wiesenfeld-Hallin, IASP Press, Seattle, © 2000.

21

The Tingling Sensation of Carbonated Drinks Is Mediated by a Carbonic Anhydrase-Dependent Excitation of Trigeminal Nociceptive Neurons

Christopher T. Simons,[a,b] Jean-Marc Dessirier,[a,b] Mirela Iodi Carstens,[a] Michael O'Mahony,[b] and E. Carstens[a]

[a]*Section of Neurobiology, Physiology and Behavior; and* [b]*Department of Food Science and Technology, University of California, Davis, Davis, California, USA*

The popularity of "fizzy" drinks has continued to increase since medieval times when Europeans consumed naturally carbonated water (*spiritus silvestris*) in an effort to combat the plague. Today, the soft drink industry boasts lucrative sales estimated in the billions of dollars annually in the United States (Anonymous 1997). The pungency elicited by carbonated beverages seems to contribute to their acceptance. Historically, this tingling sensation has been attributed to the activation of mechanoreceptors via bursting bubbles. However, when carbonated water is consumed under hyperbaric conditions, which prevent bubble formation, subjects still judged tingling, stinging, pricking, and throatburn qualities to be just as intense as those elicited by bubbling water under normal atmospheric pressure (S. McEvoy, personal communication). Furthermore, the oral pungency elicited by carbonated water is maintained for a prolonged period after expectoration (Green 1992). These observations are more consistent with a chemogenic mechanism, rather than a mechanical bursting action of bubbles, to induce the tingling sensation.

Carbon dioxide (CO_2), when applied to the nasal epithelium (Cain and Murphy 1980; Peppel and Anton 1993; Thürauf et al. 1993), the cornea (Chen et al. 1995), or subcutaneously (Steen et al. 1992), elicits activity in nociceptive afferents. The underlying mechanism is thought to involve the conversion of CO_2 to carbonic acid (H_2CO_3) in a reaction catalyzed by carbonic anhydrase. The H_2CO_3 dissociates, generating protons capable of activating peripheral chemonociceptors (Lingueglia et al. 1997; Waldmann et al. 1997a,b). In support of this mechanism, the carbonic anhydrase blocker, acetazolamide, inhibited CO_2-induced activity in nociceptive afferents of the rat lingual nerve (Komai and Bryant 1993) or skin (Steen et al. 1992) and in chorda tympani fibers (Komai et al. 1994). This mechanism may help explain the "champagne blues," a phenomenon reported anecdotally in mountaineers who, after taking acetazolamide (Diamox) for mountain sickness, stated that carbonated beverages had lost their tingling sensation and beer tasted like "dishwater" (Graber and Kelleher 1988).

We used psychophysical methods to test the hypothesis that carbonated water elicits a sensation that can be reduced by dorzolamide, a blocker of carbonic anhydrase. We further hypothesized that this sensation is mediated at least partly by CO_2-induced excitation of intraoral nociceptors that, in turn, project to the trigeminal subnucleus caudalis (Vc) to excite neurons in the somatotopically appropriate (dorsomedial) region (Carstens et al. 1995, 1998). To this end, we employed two additional complementary approaches, electrophysiological single-unit recording and *c-fos* immunohistochemistry, to determine if activation of Vc neurons in rats induced by lingual application of carbonated water is reduced by dorzolamide.

METHODS

Human psychophysical methods. A dorzolamide-saturated filter paper was placed on one side of the dorsal lingual surface of 21 subjects, and a control solution matched in bitterness and viscosity was applied to the opposite side in a counterbalanced design. After 5 minutes the filter papers were removed and subjects rinsed the mouth. Using a two–alternative, forced-choice procedure, we asked subjects to choose the side of the tongue perceived to have the strongest sensation when carbonated water was flowed bilaterally over the dorsal surface for 5 or 15 seconds. Additionally, each subject was asked to give intensity ratings for both sides of the tongue independently, using a scale from 0 (no carbonation sensation) to 10 (intense carbonation sensation). To control for the possibility that any effect of dorzolamide was specific to CO_2, we repeated the same procedure in a separate session but applied pentanoic acid (200 mM by filter paper) bilaterally to the tongue. Finally, to control for the possibility that dorzolamide did not affect lingual tactile sensitivity, subjects were asked to report whether they detected a weak tactile stimulus (von Frey filament applied randomly to the dorzolamide-treated side, the untreated side, or not at all, 10 times each), and whether they were sure or not sure. An R-index (O'Mahony 1992) was used to assess any difference in tactile sensitivity between the two sides of the tongue. A binomial analysis determined whether a significant majority of individuals chose the nontreated side as having a stronger carbonation- or acid-evoked sensation. We used Student's t test to compare mean intensity scores for the treated and untreated sides of the tongue. For all comparisons, $P < 0.05$ was considered to be significant.

Electrophysiological methods. In adult male Sprague-Dawley rats anesthetized with thiopental (80 mg/kg), the lower brainstem and upper cervical spinal cord were exposed for extracellular single-unit recording from neurons in superficial laminae of Vc that responded to ipsilateral noxious pinch and heat (54°C) stimuli and to carbonated water. After establishing that unit responses to repeated application of carbonated water from freshly opened bottles (delivered by constant flow at a rate of 0.1 mL/s for 30 seconds onto the anterior dorsal surface of the tongue) were consistent across trials, we applied dorzolamide (Merck; 22.3 mg/mL) topically (three applications of 0.1 mL at 5-minute intervals) to the tongue. The unit's response to carbonated water was retested 10 minutes following dorzolamide, and at approximately 10-minute intervals thereafter to test for recovery. Responses were quantified as the total number of impulses/30-second period before and after the onset of the carbonated water stimulus, and paired t test was used to compare mean neuronal responses before and after dorzolamide, with $P < 0.05$ considered to be significant.

Immunohistochemical methods. Adult male Sprague-Dawley rats anesthetized with sodium pentobarbital (65 mg/kg; i.p.) were assigned to one of the following groups: (1) carbonated water only (n = 6), applied to the dorsal anterior tongue (10 mL/minute for 10 minutes); (2) dorzolamide pretreatment (three 0.1-mL applications at 5-minute intervals) followed 10 minutes later by carbonated water (n = 11); (3) 0.9% NaCl control, delivered in the same manner as dorzolamide (n = 5); (4) flat (uncarbonated) water control, delivered in the same manner as carbonated water (n = 7); and (5) unstimulated anesthetized controls (n = 5) receiving no oral stimulation. Two hours following the onset of stimulation, rats were perfused with 4% paraformaldehyde. Brain stems were cut in 50-μm frozen sections and processed for *c-fos* immunohistochemistry (primary *c-fos* antibody [Arnel, 1:50,000] followed by secondary biotinylated goat-antirabbit antibody; avidin-biotin-complex reaction; visualization by Ni-diaminobenzidine reaction). Numbers of cell nuclei expressing FOS-like immunoreactivity (FLI) were counted in (1) the dorsomedial aspect of Vc, (2) the ventrolateral aspect of Vc, (3) the ventrolateral medulla, (4) the nucleus of the solitary tract (NTS) between the level of pyramidal decussation caudally and the area postrema rostrally, and (5) the area postrema. We compared cell counts in each region by using an unpaired *t* test, with $P < 0.05$ considered to be significant.

RESULTS

Psychophysical results. A significant majority of subjects reported a stronger sensation on the side of the tongue not receiving dorzolamide, and assigned significantly higher intensity ratings to that side, when carbonated water was flowed over the tongue for 5 seconds (Fig. 1A). However, when the carbonated water was flowed for 15 seconds, these differences disappeared (Fig. 1B). Dorzolamide pretreatment had no effect on the perceived intensity of irritation elicited by pentanoic acid (Fig. 1C). These data confirm the selectivity of the dorzolamide treatment. Finally, dorzolamide treatment had no significant effect on lingual tactile sensitivity as indicated by equivalent ($P = 0.44$) R-indices for the treated (72%) and untreated sides (71%) of the tongue.

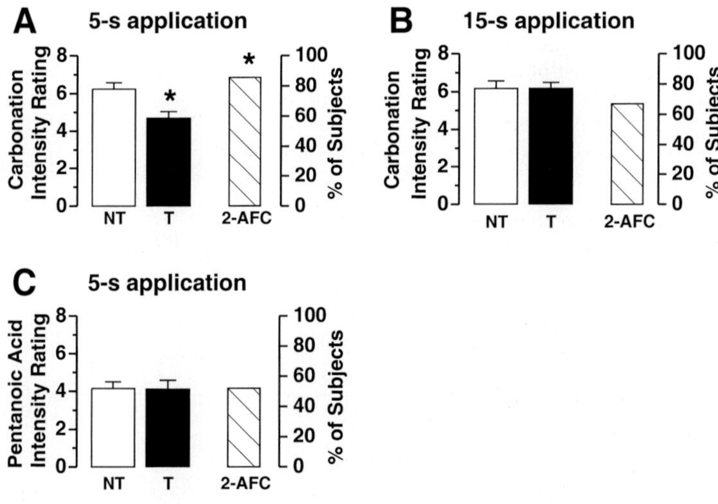

Fig. 1. Psychophysical results. (A) Bar graph (left) gives intensity ratings of carbonation for the nontreated (NT, open bar) and dorzolamide pretreated (T, filled bar) side of the tongue, respectively. Hatched bar (right) indicates proportion of subjects noting a stronger sensation on the nontreated side. Ratings were made 5 seconds after application of carbonated water to the tongue by continuous flow. Error bars indicate SEM. Asterisks indicate significant difference between groups (to left), and significant majority choosing nontreated side (to right). (B) Graph as in A for responses 15 seconds after application of carbonated water. (C) Graph as in A showing lack of effect of dorzolamide pretreatment on irritation evoked by pentanoic acid. Reproduced from Simons et al. (1999), by permission of the Society for Neuroscience.

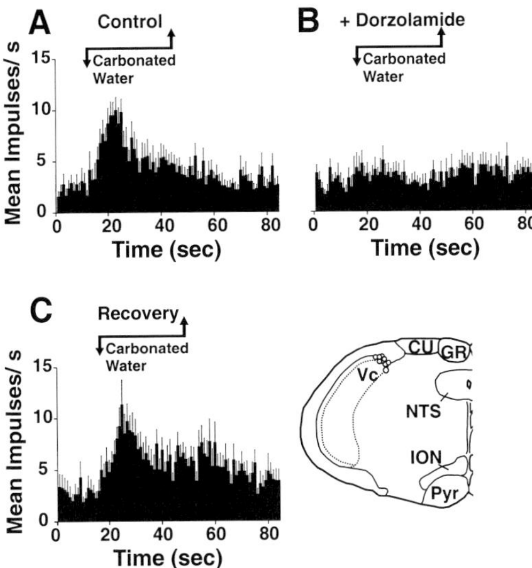

Fig. 2. Mean peristimulus-time histograms (bin width, 1 second) of 10 neurons to carbonated water applied for 30 seconds to the dorsal surface of the rat tongue, (A) prior to application of dorzolamide, (B) after dorzolamide, and (C) during recovery. Spontaneous activity not subtracted. Error bars indicate SEM. Inset shows histologically localized recording sites. Abbreviations as in Fig. 3. Reproduced from Simons et al. (1999), by permission of the Society for Neuroscience.

Electrophysiological results. Ten wide-dynamic-range-type Vc units responded to carbonated water; Fig. 2A shows an averaged peristimulus-time histogram (PSTH) of their response. Dorzolamide treatment significantly reduced the response to the carbonated water (Fig. 2B), with recovery to predorzolamide levels after approximately 40 minutes (Fig. 2C). The effect of dorzolamide appeared to be selective for carbonated water, in that responses to application of HCl (pH = 1) were not reduced following dorzolamide pretreatment in the units tested.

Immunohistochemical results. Carbonated water elicited significantly higher FLI in dorsomedial Vc compared to flat water, saline, or unstimulated control groups. Carbonated water also significantly elevated FLI in the ventrolateral Vc over saline and unstimulated control levels, and in NTS over unstimulated controls. An example of the brainstem distribution of FLI elicited by carbonated water is shown in Fig. 3A. For dorsomedial Vc, dorzolamide treatment significantly reduced FLI elicited by carbonated water (Fig. 3B). For comparison, Fig. 3C shows an example of the brainstem distribution of FLI following control application of flat water.

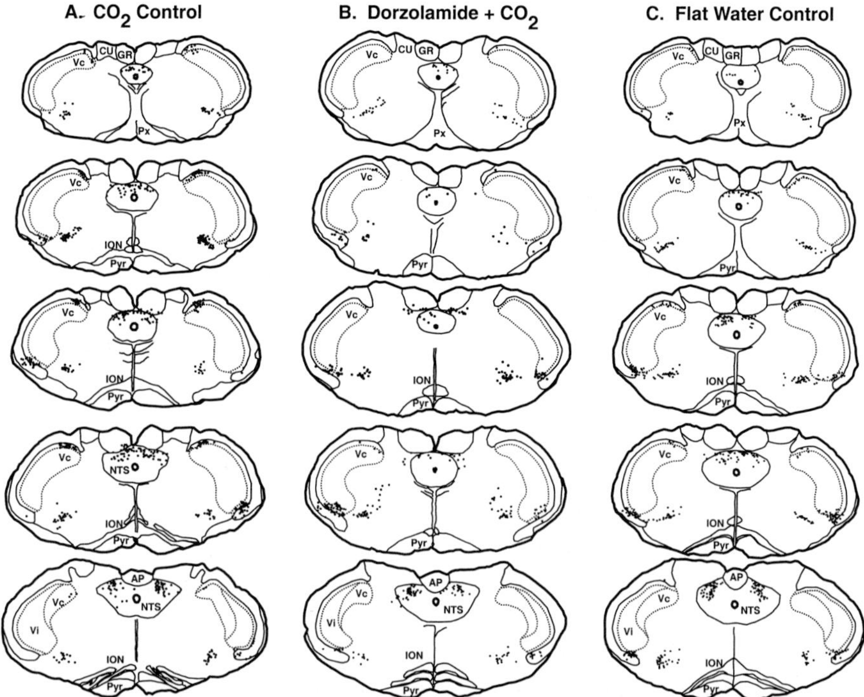

Fig. 3. Individual examples of brainstem distribution of FLI. (A) Carbonated water only. Sections are arranged from caudal (top) to rostral (bottom). Dots indicate FLI. (B) Dorzolamide followed by carbonated water. (C) Flat (uncarbonated) water control. Abbreviations: CU = cuneate nucleus; GR = nucleus gracilis; ION = inferior olivary nucleus; Pyr = pyramid; Vc = trigeminal nucleus caudalis; Vi = trigeminal nucleus interpolaris. Reproduced from Simons et al. (1999), by permission of the Society for Neuroscience.

DISCUSSION

These psychophysical results, showing that dorzolamide pretreatment significantly reduced the sensation elicited by carbonated water, are consistent with the idea that this tingling sensation has a largely chemogenic origin. This concept receives further support from the electrophysiological and neuroanatomical studies, which show that dorzolamide pretreatment significantly attenuated activation of neurons in Vc. Furthermore, the latter data are consistent with the hypothesis that carbonated drinks activate trigeminal nociceptive pathways. The Vc neurons that responded to carbonated water also responded to noxious mechanical and thermal stimuli in the present study; such neurons may thus participate in the transmission of nociceptive information from the oral cavity (see Carstens et al. 1998). Moreover, neurons in the same region of Vc exhibited increased FLI following application of carbonated water. Expression of FLI is thought to reflect strong activation of neurons (see Carstens et al. 1995). Previous studies have shown that lingual nerve and chorda tympani fibers respond to aqueous CO_2 solutions in a carbonic anhydrase-dependent manner (Komai and Bryant 1993; Komai et al. 1994). These findings, together with our data, support the notion that carbonated water is converted into carbonic acid to excite lingual nociceptive afferents which, in turn, project to Vc to excite nociceptive neurons that are presumably involved in signaling oral irritation.

The psychophysical data show that dorzolamide treatment selectively reduced the sensation elicited by carbonated water, but not that evoked by pentanoic acid, which has a lipophilicity comparable to that of CO_2. Moreover, tactile sensitivity was not compromised by dorzolamide. These data provide additional support for the idea that the sensation evoked by carbonated water is primarily of chemogenic origin and is not due to tactile stimulation of lingual mechanoreceptors by bursting bubbles. Of note, the effect of dorzolamide diminished when carbonated water was flowed over the tongue for 15 seconds (Fig. 1B). We speculate that CO_2, being highly lipophilic, may have penetrated more deeply into the lingual epithelium during the longer stimulus application to access tissue that the dorzolamide was unable to reach.

The mechanism by which H_2CO_3 excites nociceptive afferents is not known and cannot be directly assessed using the present methods. Localization of carbonic anhydrase both intracellularly (Wong et al. 1983) and extracellularly (Feldstein and Silverman 1984; Murakami and Sly 1987) suggests two possible, speculative mechanisms. One possibility is that CO_2 could traverse the plasma membrane of nociceptive endings and be converted to H_2CO_3 via intracellular carbonic anhydrase; dissociation of H_2CO_3 might then lead to intracellular acidification and cellular activation. Alternatively, CO_2 could be converted into H_2CO_3 extracellularly; proton activation of nociceptors could then occur via an acid-sensing ion channel (ASIC or DRASIC) in the membrane of nociceptor endings (Lingueglia et al. 1997; Waldmann et al. 1997b). Further studies are necessary to differentiate between these two possibilities.

ACKNOWLEDGMENTS

Supported by grants from the NIH (NS-35778) and the California Tobacco Disease-Related Research Program (6RT-0231).

REFERENCES

Anonymous. 1997 retail value of the carbonated soft drink business in the US only: $54.7 billion. *Beverage Digest,* 1997, February 20:1.

Cain WS, Murphy CL. Interaction between chemoreceptive modalities of odour and irritation. *Nature* 1980; 284(5753):255–257.

Carstens E, Saxe I, Ralph R. Brainstem neurons expressing c-Fos immunoreactivity following irritant chemical stimulation of the rat's tongue. *Neuroscience* 1995; 69(3):939–953.

Carstens E, Kuenzler N, Handwerker HO. Activation of neurons in rat trigeminal subnucleus caudalis by different irritant chemicals applied to oral or ocular mucosa. *J Neurophysiol* 1998; 80(2):465–492.

Chen X, Gallar J, Pozo MA, Baeza M, Belmonte C. CO_2 stimulation of the cornea: a comparison between human sensation and nerve activity in polymodal nociceptive afferents of the cat. *Eur J Neurosci* 1995; 7(6):1154–1163.

Feldstein JB, Silverman DN. Purification and characterization of carbonic anhydrase from the saliva of the rat. *J Biol Chem* 1984; 259(9):5447–5453.

Graber M, Kelleher S. Side effects of acetazolamide: the champagne blues. *Am J Med* 1988; 84(5):979–980.

Green BG. The effects of temperature and concentration on the perceived intensity and quality of carbonation. *Chem Senses* 1992; 17:435–450.

Komai M, Bryant BP. Acetazolamide specifically inhibits lingual trigeminal nerve responses to carbon dioxide. *Brain Res* 1993; 612(1–2):122–129.

Komai M, Bryant B, Takeda T, Suzuki H, Kimura S. The effect of topical treatment with a carbonic anhydrase inhibitor, MK-927, on the response of the chorda tympani nerve to carbonated water. In: Kurikara K, Suzuki N, Ogawa H (Eds). *Olfaction and Taste XI*. Tokyo: Springer-Verlag, 1994, p 92.

Lingueglia E, de Weille JR, Bassilana, et al. A modulatory subunit of acid sensing ion channels in brain and dorsal root ganglion cells. *J Biol Chem* 1997; 272(47):29778–29783.

Murakami H, Sly WS. Purification and characterization of human salivary carbonic anhydrase. *J Biol Chem* 1987; 262(3):1382–1388.

O'Mahony M. Understanding discrimination tests: a user friendly treatment of response bias, rating and ranking R-index tests and their relationship to signal detection. *J Sensory Studies* 1992; 7:1–47.

Peppel P, Anton F. Responses of rat medullary dorsal horn neurons following intranasal noxious chemical stimulation: effects of stimulus intensity, duration, and interstimulus interval. *J Neurophysiol* 1993; 70(6):2260–2275.

Simons CT, Dessirier J-M, Iodi Carstens M, O'Mahony M, Carstens E. Neurobiological and psychophysical mechanisms underlying the oral sensation produced by carbonated water. *J Neurosci* 1999; 19(18):8134–8144.

Steen KH, Reeh PW, Anton F, Handwerker HO. Protons selectively induce lasting excitation and sensitization to mechanical stimulation of nociceptors in rat skin, in vitro. *J Neurosci* 1992; 12(1):86–95.

Thürauf N, Hummel T, Kettenmann B, Kobal G. Nociceptive and reflexive responses recorded from the human nasal mucosa. *Brain Res* 1993; 629(2):293–299.

Waldmann R, Bassilana F, de Weille J, et al. Molecular cloning of a non-inactivating proton-gated Na^+ channel specific for sensory neurons. *J Biol Chem* 1997a; 272(34):20975–20978.

Waldmann R, Champigny G, Bassilana F, Heurteaux C, Lazdunski M. A proton-gated cation channel involved in acid-sensing. *Nature* 1997b; 386(6621):173–177.

Wong V, Barrett CP, Donati EJ, Eng LF, Guth L. Carbonic anhydrase activity in first-order sensory neurons of the rat. *J Histochem Cytochem* 1983; 31(2):293–300.

Correspondence to: Earl Carstens, PhD, Section of Neurobiology, Physiology, and Behavior, University of California, Davis, Davis, CA 95616, USA. Tel: 530-752-6640; Fax: 530-752-5582; email: eecarstens@ucdavis.edu.

Proceedings of the 9th World Congress on Pain, Progress in Pain Research and Management, Vol. 16, edited by M. Devor, M.C. Rowbotham, and Z. Wiesenfeld-Hallin, IASP Press, Seattle, © 2000.

22

Unidirectional Conduction Block at Branching Points of Human Nociceptive C Afferents: A Peripheral Mechanism for Pain Amplification

C. Weidner,[a] M. Schmelz,[a] R. Schmidt,[b] H.O. Handwerker,[a] and H.E. Torebjörk[b]

[a]*Department of Physiology and Experimental Pathophysiology, University of Erlangen-Nürnberg, Erlangen, Germany;* [b]*Department of Clinical Neurophysiology, University of Uppsala, Uppsala, Sweden*

Investigations of primary afferent nociceptors usually focus on characteristics of peripheral and spinal terminals or cell bodies. The axon, however, has mainly been regarded as a mere conductor of action potentials, and not involved directly in pain processing. Its contribution at best is indirect by providing the structural basis of the axon reflex flare. According to the widely accepted theory, action potentials originating from one terminal of an excited nociceptor invade all arborizations of this axon and propagate in a retrograde direction to depolarize the terminals and release vasodilatory neuropeptides (antidromic vasodilatation). Matching innervation territories of single C nociceptors and the flare reaction in humans confirmed this view. There is ample structural evidence for branching of unmyelinated axons in the skin (Reilly et al. 1997). Also, the frequent observation of discontinuous innervation territories of nociceptors consisting of several island-like innervated areas implies that branching is a regular phenomenon in nociceptors (Schmidt et al. 1997). In electrophysiological studies, distinct steps in response latency have been observed following electrical stimulation inside the receptive field. These discontinuous changes in response latency have been attributed to alternating activation of different terminal branches of a single parent axon. This phenomenon has been termed "branching" or "hobbing" (Peng et al. 1999) and has been described in animal

(Pierau et al. 1982) and human studies (Torebjörk and Hallin 1974). The distinct steps of response latency observed in the recordings reflect the difference in conduction time between different branches. A recent study that systematically investigated branching in Aδ fibers in monkey skin (Peng et al. 1999) found extensive branching with branching points located up to 10 cm proximal from the most distal part of the innervation territory.

According to the axon reflex theory, action potentials from the fastest daughter branch should invade all the other branches and lead to occlusion or resetting. Thus, maximum firing frequency of the parent axon would be limited to the maximum frequency of the fastest branch. However, this condition only holds true if the nerve impulses penetrate all the terminal arborizations. Evidence indicates that this is not the case for the central terminals of myelinated afferents in the dorsal column of rat. Presynaptic control of propagation probability in fine arborizations has been hypothesized to regulate the number of terminals activated by incoming action potentials. Thus, control of propagation probably represents a mechanism for pain processing in the spinal cord (Wall 1995). Signs of unidirectional conduction block at branching points in peripheral nerves have also been reported in rat sural nerve (McMahon and Wall 1987). This chapter presents data on the phenomenon of unidirectional block in the peripheral arborizations of primary afferent nociceptors in human skin and discusses its possible implications.

METHODS

Microneurographic methods have been described in detail elsewhere (Torebjörk 1974) and thus will be summarized only briefly in the following section.

Subjects. None of the young subjects participating in the microneurography experimental series suffered from any dermatological or neurological disease. All gave their written informed consent according to the guidelines of the local ethics committees.

C-fiber recordings. A microelectrode (0.2 mm diameter) was manually inserted into the peroneal nerve dorsolateral to the fibular head and a reference microelectrode was placed subcutaneously nearby. The uninsulated tip of the recording electrode was inserted in a cutaneous fascicle. Positioning of the electrode was guided by the characteristic noise of multifiber discharges evoked by gently stroking the skin in the expected innervation territory (lower leg or foot dorsum).

Transcutaneous electrical search stimuli. Single electrical pulses (0.2 ms, 30–50 mA from an insulated constant current stimulator, Digitimer DS7) were then applied from a pointed steel probe with a small contact surface (1 mm in diameter), which was moved on the skin until single C-unit responses were obtained, characterized by their stable, long latencies. When the skin innervation territory of a C fiber was found, two needle electrodes (0.2 mm shaft diameter) were inserted 5 mm apart in this territory for repetitive intracutaneous electrical stimulation (0.25 Hz, 0.2 ms, 10–150 V, from an insulated Grass S88 stimulator).

Conduction velocity measurements. The response latency to the first electrical shock after a rest period of at least 2 minutes was used to calculate the conduction velocities. The shortest distance between the stimulating needles in the skin and the recording electrode in the nerve was measured with an accuracy of 1 millimeter. Room temperature was kept constant at 22–24°C.

C-unit classification. Sympathetic C units were identified by their response to maneuvers known to elicit sympathetic sudomotor or vasoconstrictor reflexes in human skin nerves (Hallin and Torebjörk 1970, 1974; Hagbarth et al. 1972). Afferent C units were identified by their responses induced by stimulation of their innervation territories in the skin. Mechanical sensitivity was tested with von Frey hairs (Stoelting Co.). Units that responded to forces below 750 mN were classified as mechanoresponsive (Schmidt et al. 1995). Heat sensitivity was tested by elevating skin surface temperature from a baseline of 32°C to a maximum of 52°C at a rate of 1°C/4 s by radiant heat from a halogen bulb with a thermocouple feedback control mechanism (Beck et al. 1974). The subjects were asked to stop the heating at their tolerance limit.

Marking method. Responsiveness of the units under study was assessed by analyzing prolonged slowing of conduction velocity in a C fiber following activation (Fig. 1B) (Torebjörk and Hallin 1974). Pronounced slowing is characteristic for C fibers and probably due to prolonged changes of membrane properties after excitation. Even a single additional spike induced in a C fiber by a conditioning stimulus produces an increased delay of the subsequent electrically induced spike by about 1 ms (intracutaneous electrical stimulation at 4-s intervals). The length of the delay is strongly correlated to the number of additional spikes (Schmelz et al. 1995).

RESULTS

"Branching" and "hobbing." The schematic diagram in Fig. 1 shows the phenomena of "hobbing" and "marking." Hobbing (Fig. 1A) is characterized by distinct steps in response latency. A single unit is responding to

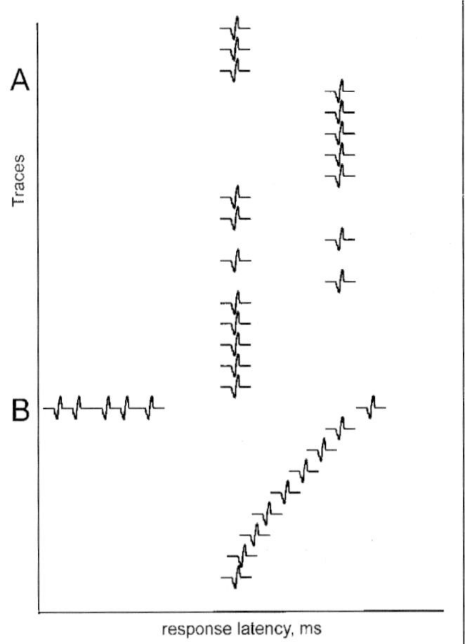

Fig. 1. Schemes of "branching" and "marking." (A) Responses of a single C nociceptor to repetitive electrical stimulation at 0.25 Hz are shown in successive traces from top to bottom. Response latencies alternate between two distinct values, which suggests the existence of two branches with different conduction velocity. Note that no activity-dependent slowing is observed during the alternating responses. (B) Activation at high frequency (five spikes shown) induced activity-dependent slowing of conduction velocity and a sudden shift in response latency. The decreased conduction velocity gradually recovers, typical for the "marking" phenomenon.

electrical stimuli with alternating conduction velocities. Identity of the spike shape and strict alternations are proof that a single unit is observed and not two units with different conduction velocities. Increase of stimulus intensity regularly leads to stepwise decrease of response latency indicating the activation of faster conducting branches. This response is not surprising, because we can expect that action potentials from newly recruited slower branches would collide with faster conducted ones. The "branching" phenomenon is not accompanied by "marking," which is shown in Fig. 1B.

Unidirectional block. The absence of "marking" during the "hobbing" shown in Fig. 1A proves that both branches were activated once with each stimulus, which implies that the spike reaching the branching point first invades the other branch antidromically. This sequence, however, does not always seem to hold true. Fig. 2 shows a specimen record in which single electrical pulses in the cutaneous receptive field induced two action potentials recorded at knee level. The shapes of the two action potentials were virtually identical (inset Fig. 2). In addition, each double response caused activity-dependent slowing in the unit under study and its absence was always followed by a recovery of conduction velocity. This observation indi-

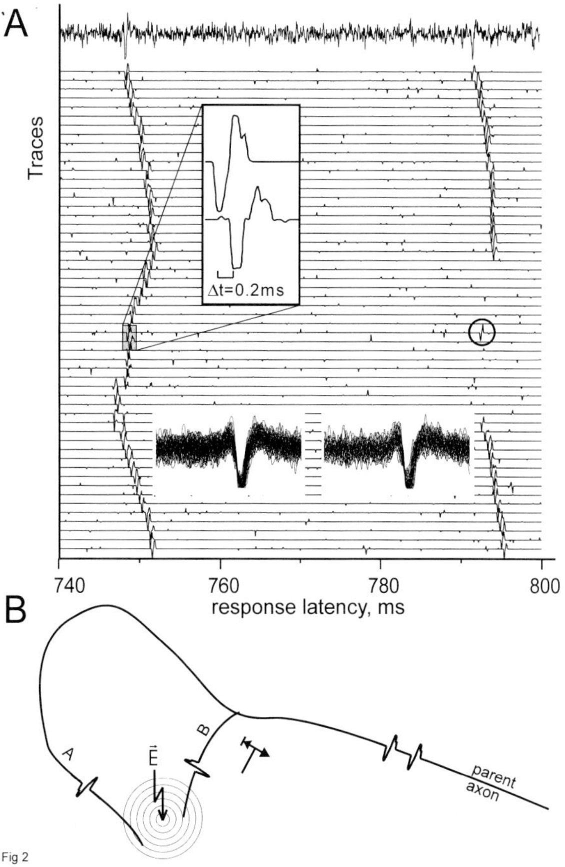

Fig. 2. Unidirectional block of a human mechanoinsensitive C unit: Responses of a single C nociceptor to repetitive electrical stimulation in the innervation territory at 0.25 Hz are shown in successive traces from top to bottom. In the first trace the unfiltered signal is shown while the successive traces passed a band pass filter. (A) Without changing the external stimulus parameters the depicted unit developed a double response pattern. In the period of double response, activity-dependent slowing of conduction velocity can be observed in both branches. Each trace showing a double response is followed by a slowing of the two branches (enlarged inset). Correspondingly, absence of the double response (middle traces in the raster) is followed by recovery of the faster branch in each trace. In the inset the action potentials of all first (left) and all second (right) responses during the unidirectional block are superposed to show their identical shape. (B) The scheme of a branched axon illustrates the proposed mechanism of the unidirectional block (see Discussion).

cates unidirectional blockade of antidromic conduction (see schematic diagram in Fig. 2B).

DISCUSSION

Ample anatomical and electrophysiological evidence points to branching in nociceptive nerve fibers. Abrupt changes between two response latencies to electrical stimulation inside the innervation territory of nociceptors (Fig. 1A) can be attributed to the excitation of two branches of the same nociceptive unit. Previous studies have convincingly shown that other explanations such as current spread are unlikely (Peng 1999). In line with these electrophysiological results, innervation territories of C nociceptors can extend to more than 7 cm (Schmelz et al. 1997), and innervation territories often consist of several distinct areas separated by noninnervated parts (Schmidt et al. 1997). Thus, the existence of branching in nociceptors is well established. However, the functional role of branching is less clear. According to the classical concept, an action potential initiated in one branch should be conducted along the complete axonal tree into the complete innervation territory. This assumption would predict that a single electrical stimulus in the innervation territory of a nociceptor should elicit a single response in the parent axon with a latency representing the conduction delay of the fastest activated branch. If the electrical stimulus also activates other branches, antidromic invasion would cause collisions of their action potentials. However, in this study we observed two action potentials of the same unit following a single electrical pulse applied to the innervation territory at the dorsum of the foot.

These double responses (Fig. 2A) could arise from the following conduction pattern: two branches (A,B) of the same axon are excited by a single stimulus. The action potential reaching the branching point first (B) is only centrally propagated. Antidromic conduction into the slower branch (A) is blocked unidirectionally. This block of conduction is crucial because otherwise the orthodromically conducted action potential in the slower branch would be abolished. When the action potential of the faster branch fails to invade the slower branch, the slower action potential can be conducted centrally if it arrives after the end of the refractory period at the branching point. Under this condition, two action potentials of the same unit can be recorded at knee level (Fig. 2A). Both share the parent axon as they progress centrally. Thus, during the unidirectional block the axon must conduct two action potentials instead of one. This additional activity induces activity-dependent slowing ("marking") (Torebjörk and Hallin 1974). Likewise, termination of a unidirectional block is followed by recovery of response latency. A unidirectional block in peripheral nociceptive axons induces two instead of one action potentials in the parent axon, thereby increasing the frequency of the discharge. It could thus compensate for the low maximum repetition rate of the thin terminal branches and increase the maximum frequency in the parent axon. Extensive terminal branching may thus not only increase the area of the innervation territory but also the probability of unidirectional blockade and thus the maximum firing frequency in the parent axon. In conclusion, the branching points of nociceptors in the periphery represent potential sites for modulation of pain processing. Thus, the traditional view of a strictly conductive role of the axonal tree, restricted to conduction of action potentials, is challenged.

ACKNOWLEDGMENTS

This work was supported by a Max Planck Price grant to H.E. Torebjörk, Deutsche Forschungsgemeinschaft Grant SFB 353, Swedish Medical Council Project 5206, and a grant to R. Schmidt from the Swedish Foundation for Brain Research.

REFERENCES

Beck PW, Handwerker HO, Zimmermann M. Nervous outflow from the cat's foot during noxious radiant heat stimulation. *Brain Res* 1974; 67:373–386.

Hagbarth KE, Hallin RG, Hongell A, et al. General characteristics of sympathetic activity in human skin nerves. *Acta Physiol Scand* 1972; 84:164–176.

Hallin RG, Torebjörk HE. Afferent and efferent C units recorded from human skin nerves in situ. A preliminary report. *Acta Soc Med Ups* 1970; 75:277–281.

Hallin RG, Torebjörk HE. Single unit sympathetic activity in human skin nerves during rest and various manoeuvres. *Acta Physiol Scand* 1974; 92:303–317.

McMahon SB, Wall PD. Physiological evidence for branching of peripheral unmyelinated sensory afferent fibers in the rat. *J Comp Neurol* 1987; 261:130–136.

Peng YB, Ringkamp M, Campbell JN, Meyer RA. Electrophysiological assessment of the cutaneous arborization of a-delta-fiber nociceptors. *J Neurophysiol* 1999; 82:1164–1177.

Pierau FK, Taylor DC, Abel W, Friedrich B. Dichotomizing peripheral fibres revealed by intracellular recording from rat sensory neurones. *Neurosci Lett* 1982; 31:123–128.

Reilly DM, Ferdinando D, Johnston C, et al. The epidermal nerve fibre network: characterization of nerve fibres in human skin by confocal microscopy and assessment of racial variations. *Br J Dermatol* 1997; 137:163–170.

Schmelz M, Forster C, Schmidt R, et al. Delayed responses to electrical stimuli reflect C-fiber responsiveness in human microneurography. *Exp Brain Res* 1995; 104:331–336.

Schmelz M, Schmidt R, Bickel A, et al. Specific C-receptors for itch in human skin. *J Neurosci* 1997; 17:8003–8008.

Schmidt R, Schmelz M, Forster C, et al. Novel classes of responsive and unresponsive C nociceptors in human skin. *J Neurosci* 1995; 15:333–341.

Schmidt R, Schmelz M, Ringkamp M, et al. Innervation territories of mechanically activated C nociceptor units in human skin. *J Neurophysiol* 1997; 78:2641–2648.

Torebjörk HE. Afferent C units responding to mechanical, thermal and chemical stimuli in human non-glabrous skin. *Acta Physiol Scand* 1974; 92:374–390.

Torebjörk HE, Hallin RG. Responses in human A and C fibres to repeated electrical intradermal stimulation. *J Neurol Neurosurg Psychiatry* 1974; 37:653–664.

Wall PD. Do nerve impulses penetrate terminal arborizations? A pre-presynaptic control mechanism. *Trends Neurosci* 1995; 18:99–103.

Correspondence to: Herman O. Handwerker, Dr. med., Department of Physiology and Experimental Pathophysiology, University of Erlangen/Nürnberg, Universitätsstr. 17, 91054 Erlangen, Germany. Fax: 91-31-85-224-00; email: handwerker@physiologie1.uni-erlangen.de.

Proceedings of the 9th World Congress on Pain,
Progress in Pain Research and Management,
Vol. 16, edited by M. Devor, M.C. Rowbotham, and
Z. Wiesenfeld-Hallin, IASP Press, Seattle, © 2000.

23

Mid-Axonal TNF Causes Allodynia and C-Nociceptor Activity: TNF-Induced Activity Is Blocked by Low-Dose Intravenous Lidocaine

Heidi Junger, Carmen M. Doom, and Linda S. Sorkin

Anesthesia Research Labs, University of California, San Diego, La Jolla, California, USA

Previous work from our laboratory indicates that tumor necrosis factor alpha (TNF) applied to the nerve trunk in anesthetized rats elicits ectopic activity in C and, to a lesser extent, Aδ nociceptive afferent fibers (Sorkin et al. 1997). As these experiments were designed to look at sequential doses and to construct a dose-response curve, we examined activity for only a brief period at each dose. To examine the physiological relevance of acute TNF application, our present study looked at pain behavior in awake rats following administration of TNF in the vicinity of the sciatic nerve. In addition, we examined the duration of the TNF-induced ectopic activity and its sensitivity to low-dose intravenous lidocaine.

METHODS

All experimental protocols were approved by the university animal care committee.

Behavior. Male Sprague-Dawley rats (300–325 g) were acclimated to the testing apparatus for at least 30 minutes. Mechanical withdrawal thresholds were measured using von Frey hairs with buckling forces of 0.4, 0.7, 1.2, 2.0, 3.6, 5.5, 8.5, and 15.1 g (Chaplan et al. 1994). Rats were then anesthetized with halothane and an incision made to expose the sciatic nerve, which was cleared of connective tissue. The exposed segment was mildly stretched to no more than 10% greater than its initial length because of the potential effect of stretch in increasing perineurial permeability (Abbott et al. 1997). A catheter was then tunneled subcutaneously from the back of the neck to the incision site. The caudal end was inserted through the muscle layer to the nerve. The muscle was loosely sutured and the incision closed. After recovery from anesthesia, any rat with signs of weakness or motor difficulties was killed. Several hours later, rats were again placed in the testing apparatus. Baseline measurements were taken every 15 minutes for 1 hour. At 60 minutes, rats were injected through the catheter with 90 μL TNF (0.9 or 7.7 ng) or saline, followed by 20 μL of sterile saline. Rats were then returned to the apparatus and tested every 15 minutes for 1 hour and every 30 minutes for the next 2 hours. To verify access of the injected substance to the nerve, 150 μL of 0.75% bupivacaine was given through the catheter at the end of the experiment. Loss of withdrawal to pinch was interpreted as a positive response and normal reflex withdrawal as negative. Animals with negative bupivacaine responses and TNF injections were treated as another control group based on the assumption that the injected drugs did not have access to the nerve.

To analyze data we used ANOVA followed by Bonferroni/Dunn's post hoc test for multiple comparisons. $P \leq 0.05$ was considered to be significant.

Electrophysiology. Rats (male Holtzman) used in electrophysiological experiments were anesthetized with pentobarbital sodium (50 mg/kg i.p.) and prepared for sural nerve recording as previously described (Puig and Sorkin 1996). Anesthesia was maintained by a pentobarbital/saline infusion. Briefly, we exposed the sural nerve and separated it from the sciatic under microscopic control. The foot was supported by a clay block to provide stability. We inserted a silver reference electrode between skin and underlying muscle and placed two silver hook stimulating electrodes under the sural nerve. Proximal to these electrodes, the nerve ran through a small slotted chamber that was sealed with petroleum jelly. The chamber was filled with 100 μL saline containing 0.1% bovine serum albumin (TNF vehicle). The portion of the nerve in the chamber was partially stripped. The sural stump was freed from peri- and epineuria and teased into small strands; an individual strand was then draped over a silver hook recording electrode. Search stimuli of 0.3 Hz and a duration of 0.5 ms were applied to the nerve trunk. The nerve strand was further dissected until activity from only a few units was activated. If conduction velocity of an individual spike was determined to be ≤ 1.5 m/s and the spike was clearly differentiated, basal activity was recorded (1401 plus, Spike2, CED). We then replaced vehicle in the chamber with TNF (2 pg/100 μL) and continued to record neural activity. The concentration of TNF used in the chamber was much lower than that used in the behavioral experiments. Optimal concentrations were defined experimentally; it is assumed that higher concentrations were required with epineurial injections due both to diffusion away from the nerve and to dilution of the remaining TNF with bodily fluids and the saline flush. In other C fibers, after TNF-induced activity, we administered a lidocaine infusion through a jugular catheter until ongoing activity stopped. The infusion was terminated and recording continued until activity resumed. Plasma lidocaine levels were determined at baseline and at the end of the infusion.

RESULTS

Behavior. Prior to injection, mean mechanical withdrawal threshold was 14.5 g ± 0.3 SEM for all groups. Epineurial injection of TNF at either dose was followed by a drop in withdrawal threshold that reached its nadir 45–60 minutes after injection (Fig. 1). The decrease was significant at 45–90 minutes for both doses of TNF, and threshold remained lower than in saline-injected animals for the remainder of the observation period. In a few animals, one or more small red spots appeared on the paw immediately following TNF injection. These red spots appeared to be much more sensitive to von Frey hair application than did the surrounding tissue. Animals

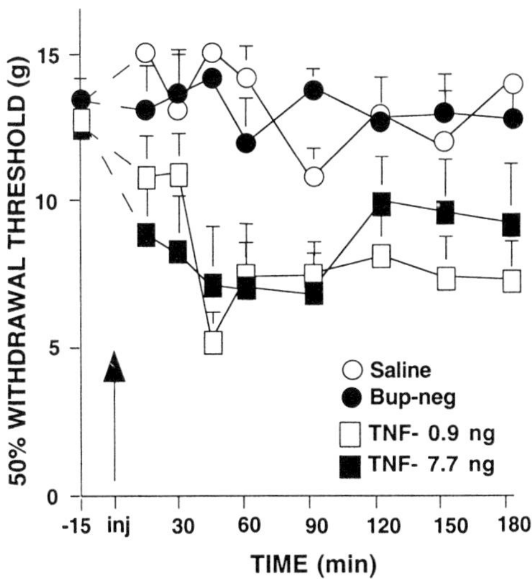

Fig. 1. Mean withdrawal thresholds for animals injected with TNF (0.9 ng, n = 12; 7.7 ng, n = 7), saline (n = 5), or animals injected with TNF that maintained their response to pinch after bupivacaine injection at the end of the experiment (Bup-neg, n = 8). The latter were placed in a separate control group. Time of injection is indicated by arrow.

that retained their response to pinch (bupivacaine negative) had no change in mechanical threshold following TNF injection, displayed a time course identical to saline-injected animals, and did not develop red spots on their paws.

Electrophysiology. In most animals exchange of vehicle for TNF solution in the chamber initiated ectopic activity in C fibers provided that mineral oil did not leak into the chamber and blood did not accumulate along the nerve. Latency varied from 1 to 40 minutes with a mean onset of 13.9 ± 3.1 minutes (n = 18). We attribute this variability to several factors including degree of nerve stripping, location of the axon within the nerve, and amount of nerve stretch during preparation. Once TNF initiated activity, fibers observed for the duration of the effect continued to fire for up to 2 hours or more. When activity was averaged over 100-second epochs, peak firing rate was 5.6 ± 1.0 Hz with a range of 0.5–14 Hz. Fig. 2 illustrates an example of gradual onset followed by sustained activity; this was the most prevalent pattern. About 20 minutes after TNF was added to the chamber, the C fiber started to fire slowly; the rate gradually increased over the next several minutes until it was roughly stable, firing at 2–3 Hz. Other patterns of activity involved periodic bursting. The most common was to see several low-frequency bursts (0.6–1 Hz) lasting less than 1 minute each and separated by 1-minute silent periods. Each set of bursts was separated by a longer silent period of up to 5 or 6 minutes. When activity was averaged over 1000-second epochs, firing rate was 0.03–0.05 Hz.

In nine animals, a lidocaine infusion via the jugular catheter was started when background activity reached 2–3 Hz (averaged in 100-second epochs). In eight of nine fibers, firing frequency began to decrease within minutes

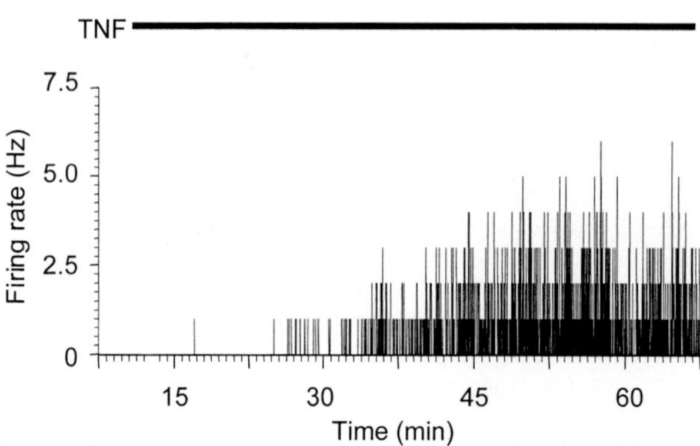

Fig. 2. Histogram indicating spikes fired by a C-nociceptive fiber. The fiber was silent until about 20 minutes after TNF solution was placed in the chamber. Solid line indicates duration of TNF in the chamber. Action potentials were collected in 100-ms bins.

and stopped completely within 5 minutes (Fig. 3). The infusion was terminated at this point and fiber activity resumed within 20–30 minutes. During the intervening silent period, activity could always be evoked mechanically from the receptive field or by electrical nerve stimulation. Plasma samples (preceded by a discarded fraction) were taken from an arterial line at baseline, after ectopic firing had ceased (just as the infusion pump was turned off). We used solid-phase extraction chromatography quantification by capillary gas chromatography with nitrogen-phosphorous detection to assay samples for lidocaine. Mean peak plasma lidocaine concentration was 1.67 ± 0.26 μg/mL. The range was 0.8–2.15 μg/mL. The example in Fig. 3 illustrates not only the resumption of firing after plasma lidocaine levels decreased, but also the even faster onset of the inhibition with the second administration.

DISCUSSION

Our data indicate that TNF applied to the sciatic nerve trunk results in an acute mechanical allodynia. This pain behavior is due to actions on elements within the nerve, i.e., nerve fibers, Schwann cells, or mast cells, as TNF injection into the surrounding tissue in the bupivacaine-negative animals was without effect. While Wagner and Myers (1996) showed that endoneurial injection of TNF resulted in pain behavior 1 day after treatment, our study demonstrates that epineurial TNF causes pain behavior within an

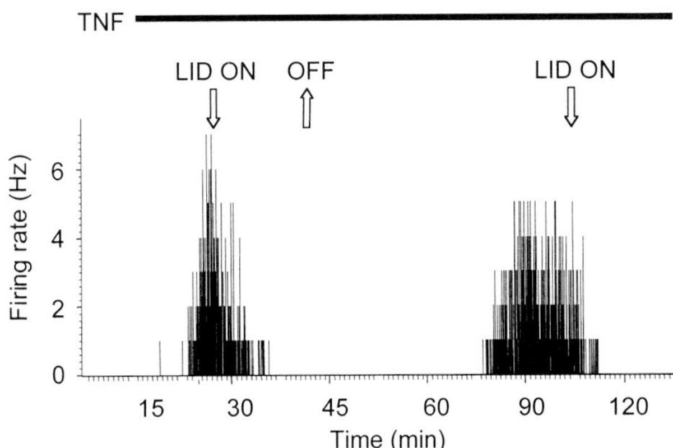

Fig. 3. This C fiber was silent until about 7 minutes after TNF solution was placed in the chamber. When mean activity reached 2–3 Hz, the lidocaine infusion started and continued until the fiber was silent. After 20 minutes, firing resumed and a repeated administration of lidocaine was effective. Solid line indicates duration of TNF in the chamber. Plasma lidocaine was 1.99 μg/mL just before the "off" upward arrow. Initial level was 0 μg/mL.

hour. Resolution of the allodynia in our study could be due to disappearance of the exogenous TNF in the whole animal. In parallel to the behavior, we repeated our earlier study (Sorkin et al. 1997) in a different nerve and confirmed that epineurial TNF can induce ectopic activity in C nociceptors. However, in recent experiments we have seen a smaller percentage of fibers responding to TNF exposure with ectopic activity. This neural activity is presumably responsible for the appearance of the pain behavior. As yet, the mechanism is unknown. Previously, we proposed that the TNF trimer inserted itself into the neural membrane and formed a nonspecific cation channel (Kagan et al. 1992) that provided the source of the depolarization. However, capsaicin-sensitive, isolated dorsal root ganglion cells do not develop background discharge following incubation with 10 ng/mL TNF (Nicol et al. 1997). Although our previous study demonstrated little to no activity at this concentration (Sorkin et al. 1997), the evidence is increasing that TNF-induced activity is receptor mediated. Hyperalgesia in an experimental neuropathy model is partially reduced by an epineurially injected neutralizing antibody to the TNF receptor 1 (Sommer et al. 1998). However, much of this effect could be indirect. TNF could degranulate endoneurial mast cells to release several potential algesic agents. Alternatively, subcutaneous TNF causes plasma extravasation in skin (Junger and Sorkin 2000) and likely has a similar effect on the endoneurial vasculature. Given the potent chemotactic actions of TNF, it is probable that infiltration of immune-competent cells increased vascular permeability.

Low plasma levels of lidocaine reversibly inhibited the TNF-associated ectopic discharge. The effective levels are within the range considered to be therapeutic for neuropathic pain. Thus, one result of TNF could be to activate Na^+ channels. Both prostaglandin E_2 (PGE_2) and serotonin can increase current through tetrodotoxin-resistant voltage-gated Na^+ channels (Gold et al. 1996). As serotonin is released from mast cells and plasma platelets and as many TNF effects are prostanoid mediated (Nicol et al. 1997), much of the neural activity could result from indirect actions of TNF.

In summary, TNF applied to the nerve trunk has an acute effect resulting in ectopic activity and allodynia. Longer term changes in behavior following nerve injury could be due in part to a continuing supply of endogenous TNF, synergy between TNF and other pro-inflammatory and injury-related mediators, or processes set into action by early exposure to TNF.

ACKNOWLEDGMENT

Supported by National Institutes of Health NS35630.

REFERENCES

Abbott NJ, Mitchell G, Ward KJ, Abdullah F, Smith IC. An electrophysiological method for measuring the potassium permeability of the nerve perineurium. *Brain Res* 1997; 776:204–213.

Chaplan SR, Bach FW, Pogrel JW, Chung JM, Yaksh TL. Quantitative assessment of tactile allodynia in the rat paw. *J Neurosci Meth* 1994; 53:55–63.

Gold MS, Reichling DB, Shuster MJ, Levine JD. Hyperalgesic agents increase a tetrodotoxin-resistant Na+ current in nociceptors. *Proc Natl Acad Sci USA* 1996; 93:1108–1112.

Junger H, Sorkin LS. Nociceptive and inflammatory effects of subcutaneous TNF-alpha. *Pain* 2000; 85:145–151.

Kagan BL, Baldwin RL, Munoz D, Wisnieski BJ. Formation of ion-permeable channels by tumor necrosis factor-α. *Science* 1992; 255:1427–1430.

Nicol GD, Lopshire JC, Pafford CM. Tumor necrosis factor enhances the capsaicin sensitivity of rat sensory neurons. *J Neurosci* 1997; 17:975–982.

Puig S, Sorkin LS. Formalin-evoked activity in identified primary afferent fibers: systemic lidocaine suppresses phase-2 activity. *Pain* 1996; 64:345–355.

Sommer C, Schmidt C, George A. Hyperalgesia in experimental neuropathy is dependent on the TNF receptor 1. *Exp Neurol* 1998; 151:138–142.

Sorkin LS, Xiao WH, Wagner R, Myers RR. Tumour necrosis factor-alpha induces ectopic activity in nociceptive primary afferent fibres. *Neuroscience* 1997; 81:255–262.

Wagner R, Myers RR. Endoneurial injection of TNF-alpha produces neuropathic pain behaviors. *Neuroreport* 1996; 7:2897–2901.

Correspondence to: Linda S. Sorkin, PhD, Anesthesia Research Labs, University of California, San Diego, 9500 Gilman Drive, La Jolla, CA 92093-0818, USA. Tel: 619-543-3498; Fax: 619-543-6070; email: lsorkin@ucsd.edu.

Proceedings of the 9th World Congress on Pain,
Progress in Pain Research and Management,
Vol. 16, edited by M. Devor, M.C. Rowbotham, and
Z. Wiesenfeld-Hallin, IASP Press, Seattle, © 2000.

24

Pain-Related Behavior in TNF-Receptor-Deficient Mice

Carola Vogel,[a] Thies Lindenlaub,[a] Gisa Tiegs,[b]
Klaus V. Toyka,[a] and Claudia Sommer[a]

[a]Department of Neurology, Julius-Maximilians-University, Würzburg, Germany; [b]Institute of Experimental and Clinical Pharmacology and Toxicology, University of Erlangen-Nürnberg, Erlangen, Germany

Tumor necrosis factor alpha (TNF) is an important mediator of inflammatory pain and also modulates hyperalgesia after peripheral nerve injury (Cunha et al. 1992; Sommer et al. 1998). TNF is rapidly upregulated in the endoneurium of injured nerves (George et al. 1999). Various methods of reducing TNF in the nerve have enabled us to reduce behavioral signs of hyperalgesia in animals with chronic constriction injury (CCI, Bennett and Xie 1988), a model of neuropathic pain. In particular, we reduced thermal hyperalgesia and mechanical allodynia by administering either drugs that reduce TNF synthesis (Sommer and Marziniak 1996) or a metalloproteinase inhibitor that prevents shedding of TNF from the cell membrane (Sommer et al. 1997), or by neutralizing antibodies to TNF and to the TNF receptors TNFR1 and TNFR2 (Sommer et al. 1998). Interestingly, blocking TNF and TNFR1 also decreased hyperalgesia, whereas blocking TNFR2 had no effect. We thus decided to investigate whether similar behavioral observations could be made in mice deficient in one or both of the TNF receptors.

MATERIALS AND METHODS

Animals and surgery. We obtained 36 female mice (B6 × 129) weighing 18–39 g (H. Bluethmann, Hoffmann La Roche). They included 12 wild-type mice, 9 lacking the TNF receptor 1 (TNFR1-/-, Rothe et al. 1993), 4 deficient in TNF receptor 2 (TNFR2-/-, Erickson et al. 1994), and 11 lacking both receptors (TNFR1/2-/-). The animals were housed on a light:dark cycle of 14:10 hours with standard rodent chow and water ad libitum. All experiments were approved by the Bavarian state authorities. We administered deep barbiturate anesthesia to 24 mice and performed a CCI of one sciatic nerve, by placing three ligatures (7-0 prolene) around the nerve at mid-thigh level and tying them until they just lightly touched the nerve and elicited a brief twitch in the limb. A sham operation was performed contralaterally.

Behavioral testing and paw temperature. Twelve mice were not operated and served as controls. The mice were supplied in two approximately equal groups several months apart. Therefore, we conducted behavioral tests separately on each group. Testing procedures for mechanical and cold stimuli and skin temperature were reproducibly established at the time of the second experiment. Therefore, the number of mice tested for mechanical and cold thresholds and for skin temperature was smaller than for heat thresholds.

Withdrawal thresholds to radiant heat were assessed using the device of Hargreaves (Hargreaves et al. 1988) purchased from Ugo Basile, as described previously (Sommer and Schäfers 1998). The withdrawal latency of the animals' hindpaw was recorded automatically. A significant decrease of the withdrawal latency after CCI compared to the baseline was defined as heat hyperalgesia. For innocuous mechanical stimulation of the animals' hindpaws, we used calibrated von Frey hairs with circular plain tips of 0.8 mm diameter made from nylon filaments. The force required to bend the hairs ranged from 0.2 mN to 53.9 mN. Mechanical testing was based on the up-and-down method of Dixon (1965) according to Chaplan et al. (1994), modified for mice (Sommer and Schäfers 1998). We recorded the 50% withdrawal threshold, i.e., force of the von Frey hair to which an animal reacts in 50% of the presentations. Cold stimulation of the animals' hindpaws followed the method of Choi et al. (1994), modified for mice. A drop of acetone from a polyethylene tube with a tip diameter of 0.8 mm was gently applied at the plantar aspect of the hindpaw. A drop of room temperature water from a similar tube served as a control. A response to acetone was defined as sharp withdrawal of the hindpaw lasting >1 second, and the time of hindpaw elevation was recorded with a digital stopwatch. We used a thermometer (GTH 1200) with an infrared sensor (Raynger IP, F. Greisinger; inner diameter of 0.4 cm) to assess skin temperature of the plantar surface of the animals' hindpaws. By this device skin temperature was measured with a resolution of 0.1°C and an accuracy of ± 0.5°C within the range of 22.0–39.0°C. Skin temperature was recorded if stable for at least 10 seconds.

Tissue processing and microscopy. Tissue was harvested on day 15 post CCI. Four-mm long sciatic nerve segments distal to the ligatures and the corresponding segments from the controls were deep-frozen. A 2-mm segment distal to the previous one was processed for plastic embedding, and 1-µm sections were stained with toluidine blue. Sections were viewed and photographed on an Axiophot 2 microscope (Zeiss).

Statistical analysis. We used SPSS (Version 9.0) for statistical analysis and present results as mean ± SD. To compare the data between groups, we used ANOVA (for normally distributed values) and Kruskal-Wallis (for non-parametric analysis, and for post hoc comparison we used Scheffé's procedure (parametric) and the Mann-Whitney test (nonparametric). A paired Student's *t* test and Wilcoxon test permitted comparison between two means in the same subject. A *P* value of < 0.05 indicates significance.

RESULTS

Baseline thresholds for heat, mechanical and acetone stimuli, and skin temperature. TNFR1-/- mice had significantly lower paw-withdrawal latencies to heat at baseline (3.6 ± 0.9 seconds) than did wild-type mice (6.9 ± 1.2 seconds), TNFR2-/- (8.1 ± 1.4 seconds), and TNFR1/2-/- mice (6.7 ± 0.9 seconds). In TNFR2-/- mice the paw withdrawal latency to heat was increased compared to TNFR1-/- ($P < 0.01$) and TNFR1/2-/- mice ($P < 0.05$, Fig. 1a). Mechanical 50% thresholds at baseline in TNFR1-/- mice (13.2 ± 5.1 mN) and to a lesser extent in TNFR1/2-/- mice (16.9 ± 9.8 mN) were lower than in wild-type mice (20.4 ± 10.9 mN). However, the differences were not significant (Fig. 1b). Similar results were obtained for the baseline paw elevation time to acetone, which was decreased in TNFR1-/- (1.5 ± 0.9 seconds) and—less markedly—in TNFR1/2-/- mice (1.9 ± 0.9 seconds) in comparison with wild-type mice (2.4 ± 0.7 seconds), again without reaching statistical significance (Fig. 1c). Baseline skin temperatures of the hindpaw were clearly reduced in TNFR1-/- (32.3 ± 1.2°C, $P < 0.01$) and slightly decreased in TNFR1/2-/- mice (34.2 ± 2.4°C, $P > 0.05$) compared to wild-type mice (35.9 ± 1.9°C, Fig. 1d).

Thresholds to heat, mechanical and cold stimuli, and morphometry after CCI. Skin temperature after CCI varied too greatly to permit a comparison between the groups. Postoperative data for TNFR2-/- mice are not available due to the small sample tested.

Heat hyperalgesia measured as a significant reduction in paw withdrawal latency was evident from the first day after CCI in wild-type and from day 3 in TNFR1/2-/- mice. Heat hyperalgesia was not observed in TNFR1-/- mice (Fig. 2a–c). Heat thresholds in wild-type mice were decreased from day 1 to day 14 postoperatively (p.o.) to values between 86.9 ± 11.9% and 60.8 ± 14.9%. In TNFR1/2-/- mice the withdrawal latencies to heat were

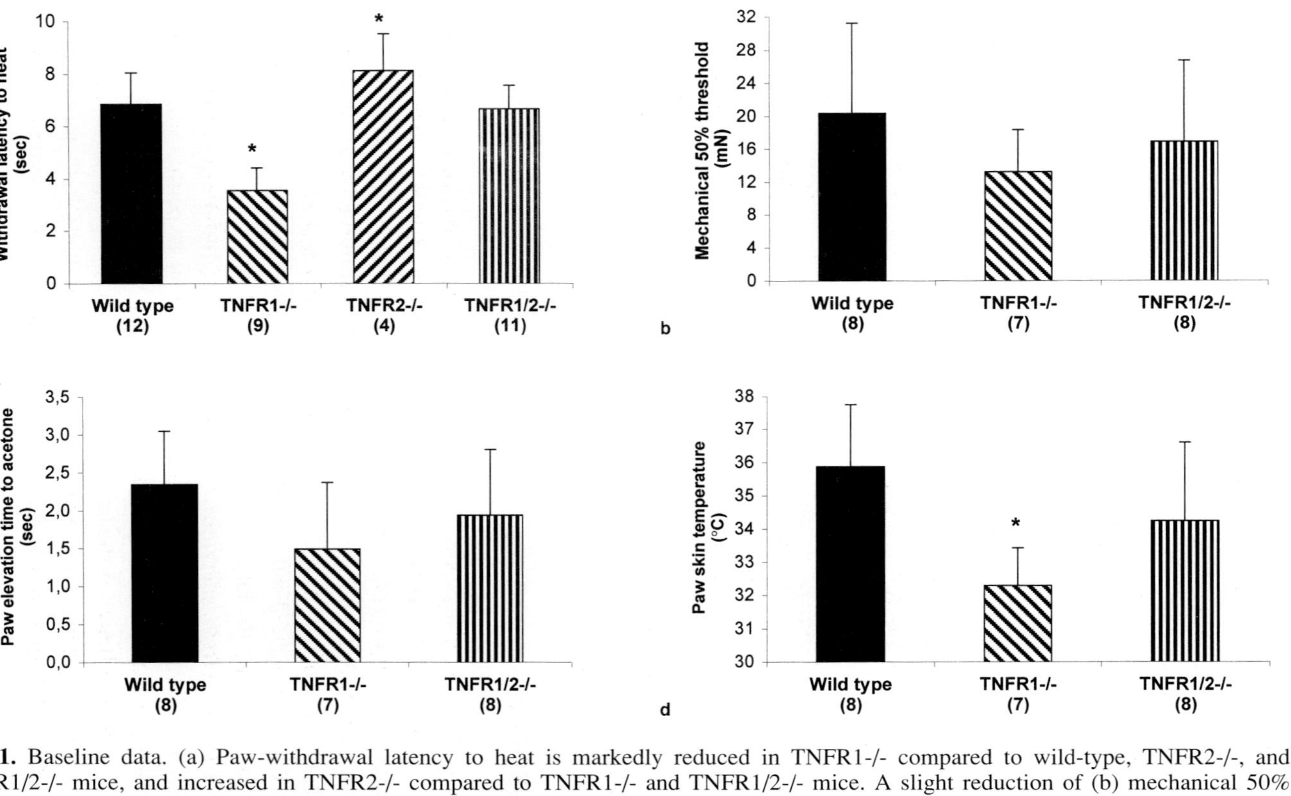

Fig. 1. Baseline data. (a) Paw-withdrawal latency to heat is markedly reduced in TNFR1-/- compared to wild-type, TNFR2-/-, and TNFR1/2-/- mice, and increased in TNFR2-/- compared to TNFR1-/- and TNFR1/2-/- mice. A slight reduction of (b) mechanical 50% thresholds and (c) paw elevation time to acetone in TNFR1-/- and TNFR1/2-/- mice lacked statistical significance. (d) Paw skin temperature is significantly reduced in TNFR1-/- mice. Data represent the mean (± SD) over two test days, pooled for the right and left hindpaw. Asterisks: $P < 0.05$. Numbers in parentheses show number of animals tested.

reduced from day 3 to day 9 p.o. with values between 75.1 ±25.1% and 89 ± 27.2% and returned to control levels on day 11. *Mechanical allodynia* was present in all groups tested within the first week after CCI (Fig. 2d–f). Mechanical thresholds decreased to a minimum of 3.1 ± 1.5 mN in wild-type mice and 1.3 ± 1 mN in TNFR1/2-/- mice on day 2 after CCI. In TNFR1-/- mice the reduction began on day 6 with a minimum of 2.9 ± 4 mN on day 10 p.o. *Cold allodynia* was evident from the second week but until day 14 p.o. we saw no obvious difference between the groups tested during the observation period. The paw elevation time to acetone increased from baseline values of 2.7 ± 0.2 seconds in wild-type mice, 1.5 ± 0.9 seconds in TNFR1-/-, and 2.1 ± 0.8 seconds in TNFR1/2-/- mice to a maximum of 9.1 ± 2.8 seconds in wild-type mice, 6.3 ± 3.7 seconds in TNFR1-/-, and 6.3 ± 5 seconds in TNFR1/2-/- mice on day 14 after CCI. Morphological analysis of the sciatic nerve revealed similar degrees of nerve injury on the side of CCI in all groups as judged by the number of remaining intact myelinated axons in the endoneurium. However, acutely degenerating fibers were still prominent in wild-type mice on day 15 after surgery, while TNFR1-/- mice had only a few remaining degenerated axons. Instead, we observed many postphagocytotic macrophages in the endoneurium (Fig. 3), indicative of faster myelin degradation in the knock-out animals.

DISCUSSION

The proinflammatory cytokine TNF is an important mediator of inflammatory and neuropathic pain (Cunha 1992; Sommer et al. 1998). The extent of thermal hyperalgesia and mechanical allodynia after CCI of the sciatic nerve can be reduced if TNF or TNFR1 are blocked by neutralizing antibodies, whereas antibodies to TNFR2 have no effect (Sommer et al. 1998). Our study primarily revealed a reduction of the hindpaw withdrawal latency to heat in naive TNFR1-/- but elevation in naive TNFR2-/- mice. Heat hyperalgesia did not develop in TNFR1-/- mice after CCI. Paw skin temperatures were lower in TNFR1-/- mice preoperatively than in the other groups of mice. Withdrawal thresholds to innocuous mechanical stimuli were not significantly different between the groups of mice, with a trend to lower thresholds in TNFR1-/- mice. The development of mechanical allodynia was delayed in TNFR1-/- mice after CCI. We observed a trend to reduced hindpaw elevation time after stimulation with acetone in TNFR1-/- mice before CCI, but no difference between the groups after CCI.

Our data from unoperated animals suggest that TNF, acting via both receptor subtypes, has a physiological role in the regulation of cutaneous

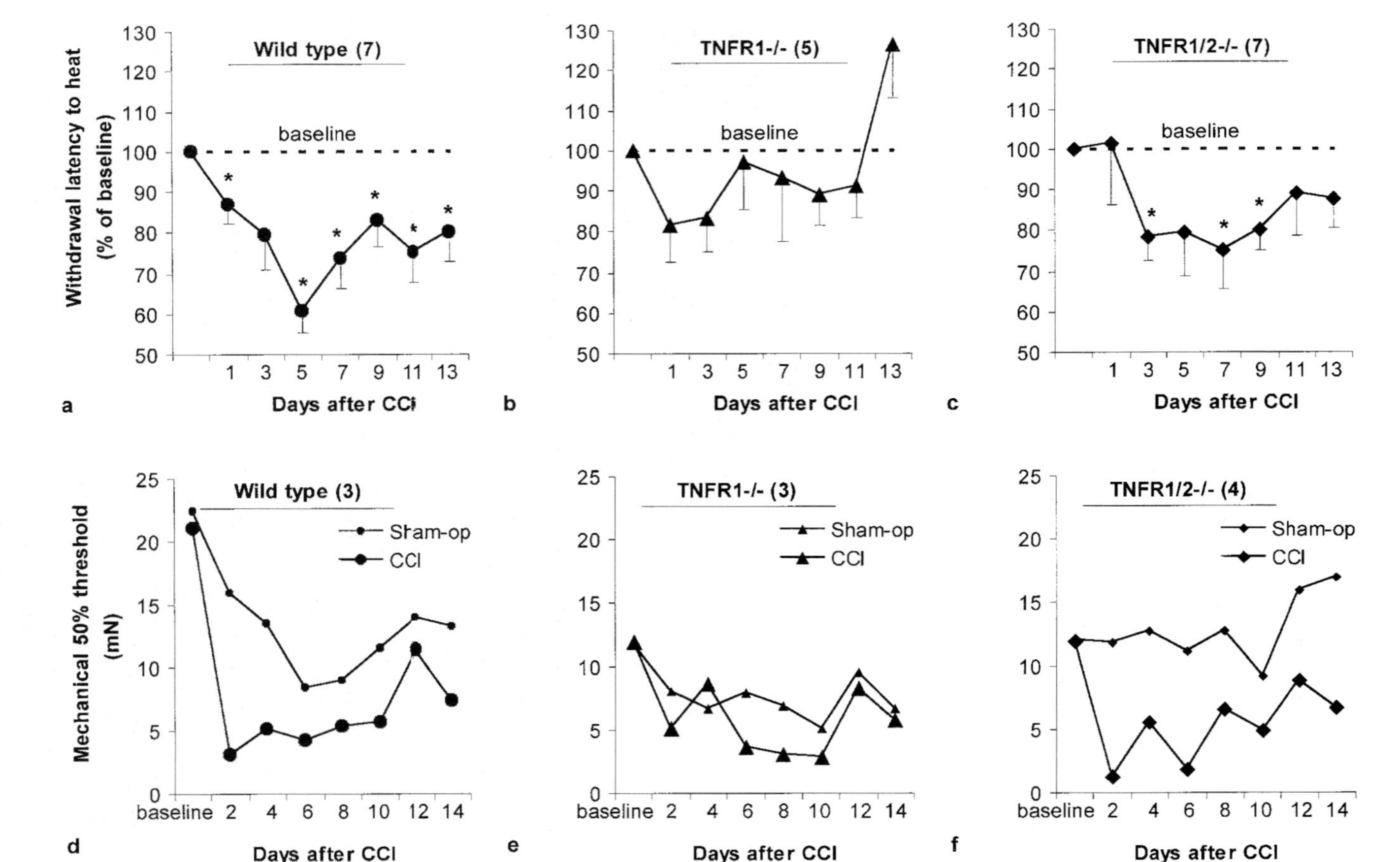
Withdrawal latency to heat (% of baseline)
Wild type (7)
TNFR1-/- (5)
TNFR1/2-/- (7)
baseline
Days after CCI
a
b
c
Mechanical 50% threshold (mN)
Wild type (3)
TNFR1-/- (3)
TNFR1/2-/- (4)
Sham-op
CCI
d
e
f

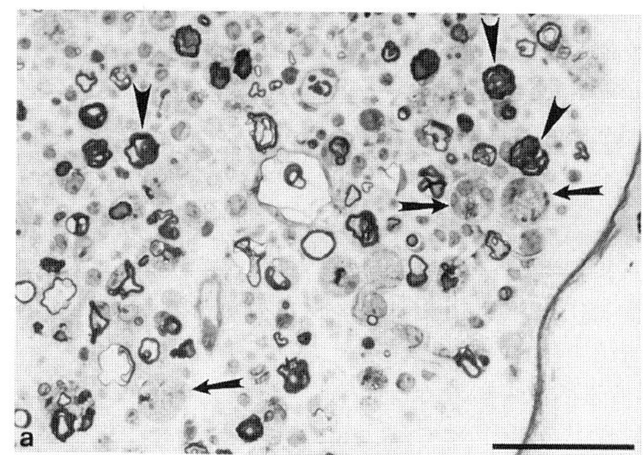

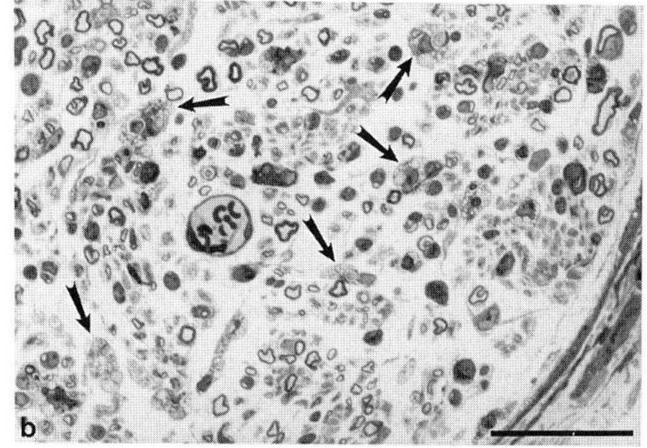

Fig. 3. Semithin sections of sciatic nerve, stained with toluidine blue, harvested on day 15 after CCI from (a) a wild-type mouse and (b) a TNFR1-/- mouse. (a) Many degenerated fibers (arrowheads) are visible in this representative wild-type mouse, with only a few postphagocytotic macrophages. (b) In the TNFR1-/- mouse, many postphagocytotic macrophages are observed (arrowheads). Myelin debris indicative of degenerating fibers is no longer visible. Bar = 50 μm.

sensitivity to heat. The effect of the two receptors seems to be antagonistic; a lack of TNFR1 reduces heat thresholds and a lack of TNFR2 elevates them. The literature suggests that the effect of TNF on skin sensitivity to heat depends on the developmental stage (Bianchi et al. 1992; Fiore et al. 1996). TNF regulates cutaneous sympathetic nerve activity (Saigusa 1989) and may have both a peripheral and a central action (Rothwell 1988). Skin temperature is positively correlated to the heat threshold, i.e., a colder paw should have a longer withdrawal latency to a given heat stimulus than does a warmer

---

← **Fig. 2.** Hindpaw withdrawal latencies to heat on the CCI side as a percentage of baseline (a–c) and mechanical 50% thresholds of the hindpaws in mN on the side of CCI compared to the sham-operated side (d–f) in wild-type and TNFR1-/- and TNFR1/2-/- mice. Values are shown at baseline (mean over 2 days of testing before CCI) and at regular intervals after CCI. (a–c) Heat hyperalgesia (asterisks: $P < 0.05$) was present in wild-type (a) and to a lesser extent in TNFR1/2-/- mice (c). In TNFR1-/- mice heat hyperalgesia was not observed (b). Data are presented as mean ± SEM. (d–f) Wild-type and TNFR1/2-/- mice had an obvious decrease of the mechanical thresholds on the side of CCI compared to baseline values and to the sham-operated side from day 1 after CCI. Mechanical thresholds were reduced only from day 6 after CCI in TNFR1-/- mice. Numbers in parentheses show number of animals tested.

paw (Luuko et al. 1994). In the TNFR1-/- mice, we observed the opposite; these animals had colder hindpaws and shorter withdrawal latencies to heat. This finding suggests either that the primary afferent heat-sensitive neurons are more sensitive in TNFR1-/- mice, or that central processing of heat stimuli is enhanced in these animals. Studies are investigating the first possibility.

The finding of a reduced heat hyperalgesia after CCI in TNFR1-/- mice must be considered with care because of the small number of animals tested (n = 5 vs. n = 7 in wild-type mice and TNFR1/2-/-). Nevertheless, this result corresponds with our previous data showing reduced thermal hyperalgesia after epineurial treatment with antagonistic antibodies to TNFR1 (Sommer et al. 1998). However, we did not measure skin temperatures in those experiments and therefore do not know whether the epineurial antibody treatment had any influence on them. Also, the lack of a TNF receptor during development may lead to compensatory changes or other developmental abnormalities that warrant caution in comparing the results to those obtained in the adult animal. TNF has some benefit in the regeneration of an injured motor nerve (Chen et al. 1996). Our preliminary morphometric data do not favor a delay in regeneration in the receptor-deficient mice. In contrast, phagocytotic activity of macrophages seemed to be more efficient in TNFR1-/- mice. This finding will require evaluation in a larger series of experiments.

In conclusion, mice deficient in TNF receptors display different cutaneous sensitivity to heat and abnormalities of skin temperature. Furthermore, they are less prone to the development of thermal hyperalgesia after nerve injury. Future investigations must determine whether central or peripheral nervous mechanisms are responsible for these abnormalities.

ACKNOWLEDGMENTS

We thank B. Dekant and L. Biko for technical assistance and A. Spahn for help with statistical analysis. This work was supported by funds from Volkswagenstiftung (C. Vogel) and Deutsche Forschungsgemeinschaft SFB 353 (T. Lindenlaub).

REFERENCES

Bennett GJ, Xie YK. A peripheral mononeuropathy in rat that produces disorders of pain sensation like those seen in man. *Pain* 1988; 33:87–107.

Bianchi M, Sacerdote P, Ricciardi-Castagnoli P, Mantegazza P, Panera AE. Central effects of tumor necrosis factor α and interleukin-1α on nociceptive thresholds and spontaneous locomotor activity. *Neurosci Lett* 1992; 148:76–80.

Chaplan SR, Bach F W, Pogrel J W, Chung JM, Yaksh TL. Quantitative assessment of tactile allodynia in the rat paw. *J Neurosci Methods* 1994; 53:55–63.

Chen LE, Seaber AV, Wong GH, Urbaniak JR. Tumor necrosis factor promotes motor functional recovery in crushed peripheral nerve. *Neurochem Int* 1996; 29:197–203.

Choi Y, Yoon YW, Na HS, Kim SH, Chung JM. Behavioral signs of ongoing pain and cold allodynia in a rat model of neuropathic pain. *Pain* 1994; 59:369–376.

Cunha FQ, Poole S, Lorenzetti BB, Ferreira SH. The pivotal role of tumor necrosis factor alpha in the development of inflammatory hyperalgesia. *Br J Pharmacol* 1992; 107:660–664.

Dixon W. The up-and-down method for small samples. *J Am Statist Assoc* 1965; 60:967–978.

Erickson SL, de Sauvage FJ, Kikly K, et al. Decreased sensitivity to tumour-necrosis factor but normal T-cell development in TNF receptor-2-deficient mice. *Nature* 1994; 372:560–563.

Fiore M, Probert L, Kollias G, et al. Neurobehavioral alterations in developing transgenic mice expressing TNF-α in the brain. *Brain Behav Immun* 1996; 10:126–138.

George A, Schmidt C, Weishaupt A, Toyka KV, Sommer C. Serial determination of tumor necrosis factor-alpha content in rat sciatic nerve after chronic constriction injury. *Exp Neurol* 1999; 160:124–132.

Hargreaves K, Dubner R, Brown F, Flores C, Joris J. A new and sensitive method for measuring thermal nociception in cutaneous hyperalgesia. *Pain* 1988; 32:77–88.

Luuko M, Konttinen Y, Kemppinen P, Pertovaara A. Influence of various experimental parameters on the incidence of thermal and mechanical hyperalgesia induced by a constriction mononeuropathy of the sciatic nerve in lightly anesthetized rats. *Exp Neurol* 1994; 128:143–154.

Rothe J, Lesslauer W, Lötscher H, et al. Mice lacking the tumour necrosis factor receptor 1 are resistant to TNF-mediated toxicity but highly susceptible to infection by Listeria monocytogenes. *Nature* 1993; 364:798–802.

Rothwell NJ. Central effects of TNF alpha on thermogenesis and fever in the rat. *Biosci Rep* 1988; 8:345–352.

Saigusa T. Participation of interleukin-1 and tumor necrosis factor in the responses of the sympathetic nervous system during lipopolysacharide-induced fever. *Pflügers Arch* 1989; 416:225–229.

Sommer C, Marziniak M. Experimental painful mononeuropathy: inhibitors of TNF-α-production induce a decrease in hyperalgesia and an increase of spinal met-enkephalin. *Soc Neurosci Abstracts* 1996; 22:511.

Sommer C, Schäfers M. Painful mononeuropathy in C57Bl/Wld mice with delayed Wallerian degeneration: differential effects of cytokine production and nerve regeneration on thermal and mechanical hypersensitivity. *Brain Res* 1998; 784:154–162.

Sommer C, Schmidt C, George A, Toyka KV. A metalloprotease-inhibitor reduces pain associated behavior in mice with experimental neuropathy. *Neurosci Lett* 1997; 237:45–48.

Sommer C, Schmidt C, George A. Hyperalgesia in experimental neuropathy is dependent on the TNF receptor 1. *Exp Neurol* 1998; 151:138–142.

Correspondence to: Claudia Sommer, Dr. med., Neurologische Klinik der Universität, Bayerische Julius-Maximilians-Universität, Josef-Schneider-Str. 11, 97080 Würzburg, Germany. Tel: 49-931-201-2621; Fax: 49-931-201-2697; email: sommer@mail.uni-wuerzburg.de.

Proceedings of the 9th World Congress on Pain, Progress in Pain Research and Management, Vol. 16, edited by M. Devor, M.C. Rowbotham, and Z. Wiesenfeld-Hallin, IASP Press, Seattle, © 2000.

25

Neurogenic Inflammation following Intradermal Injection of Capsaicin Is Partially Mediated by Dorsal Root Reflexes

Qing Lin, Jing Wu, and William D. Willis

Department of Anatomy and Neurosciences, University of Texas Medical Branch, Galveston, Texas, USA

Inflammation triggered by substances released from sensory nerve terminals is referred to as neurogenic inflammation. Components of neurogenic inflammation include arteriolar vasodilation and plasma extravasation (Szolcsányi 1996). Neurogenic inflammation is initiated by the effector function of small myelinated and unmyelinated nociceptive primary afferent terminals (Lewis 1927; Jancsó et al. 1967) that release vasoactive peptides following injury to peripheral tissue (Colpaert et al. 1983; Brain and Williams 1985; Ferrell and Russell 1986; Lewin et al. 1992). These inflammatory agents may sensitize primary afferent nociceptors (Schaible and Schmidt 1985), and secondarily may sensitize nociceptive neurons in the spinal dorsal horn (Simone et al. 1991; Dougherty and Willis 1992). Peripheral and central sensitization would exacerbate pain perception.

Neurogenic inflammation in the skin has been attributed to axon reflexes (Lewis 1927). However, our group has shown that neurogenic inflammation in the knee joint is controlled by dorsal root reflexes (DRRs) (Sluka et al. 1995; Willis 1999). DRRs are nerve impulses generated in the spinal cord due to an excessive primary afferent depolarization (PAD). These impulses travel antidromically along primary afferent fibers (Eccles et al. 1961).

Recently we examined the role of DRRs in neurogenic inflammation in the skin (Lin et al. 1999). A useful experimental method for inducing cutaneous neurogenic inflammation is the intradermal injection of capsaicin (CAP) (Szolcsányi 1996). CAP causes vasodilation if the cutaneous sensory innervation is intact (Bernstein et al. 1981; Carpenter and Lynn 1981). To evoke an acute inflammation, CAP was injected intradermally into the plantar skin of the foot in rats. The flare (a major characteristic of inflammation) was evaluated by measuring changes in cutaneous blood flow in the foot.

METHODS

Male Sprague-Dawley rats (n = 60, 250–350 g) were anesthetized with sodium pentobarbital (50 mg·kg^{-1}, intraperitoneally [i.p.]) during initial surgery. Anesthesia was maintained by continuous intravenous infusion of pentobarbital (5–8 mg·kg^{-1}·h^{-1}, intravenously [i.v.]). Once a stable surgical anesthesia was reached, animals were paralyzed with pancuronium (0.3–0.4 mg·h^{-1}, i.v.) and ventilated artificially. End-tidal CO_2 was kept between 3.5 and 4.5%. Rectal temperature was maintained near 37°C by a servo-controlled heating blanket.

Cutaneous blood flow was measured in the plantar skin of the foot with laser Doppler flowmeter probes (Moor Instruments, UK). Blood flow, detected as blood cell flux by the flowmeter, was processed by a computer analysis system (CED1401 *plus*, Cambridge Electronic Design Limited, UK) and was shown as a voltage level. A volume of 25 µL of CAP, dissolved in Tween 80 (polyoxyethylene, Fisher Scientific) (7%) and saline (93%) to a concentration of 1%, was injected intradermally into the plantar surface of the foot. The flare reaction following CAP injection was detected at distances up to 30 mm away from the CAP injection site (Fig. 1A,B). The maximal reaction was recorded about 15–20 mm away from the injection site (Probe II; see Fig. 1A).

The following manipulations were performed to determine whether elimination of presumed DRRs would reduce the flare reaction produced by CAP injection. In two groups of rats, either the femoral and sciatic nerves were sectioned ipsilaterally or dorsal roots L3–S1 were cut, respectively, before CAP injection. For control purposes, surgery was performed in another two groups. In an additional five groups of experimental animals, prior to CAP injection the spinal cord was pretreated with $GABA_A$, $GABA_B$, non-NMDA, or NMDA-receptor antagonists by intrathecal infusion of bicuculline (5 µg), phaclofen (15 µg), CNQX (6-cyano-7-nitroquinoxaline-2,3-dione, 0.1 µg), or AP7 (D(–)-2-amino-7-phosphonoheptanoic acid, 4 µg), respectively, at L4–6 levels. Drugs were dissolved in artificial cerebrospinal fluid (ACSF) in a volume of 15 µL and were given intrathecally 20 minutes prior to CAP injection. The same volume of ACSF was used in another control group of animals.

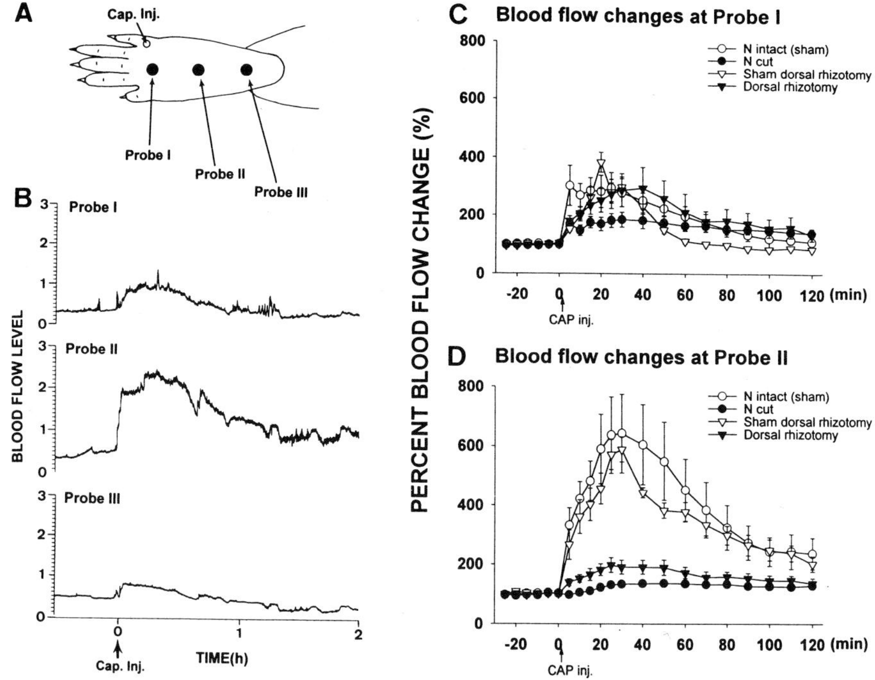

Fig. 1. (A) Schematic diagram showing measurements of blood flow in the foot skin. Laser doppler probes were placed on the plantar skin at 5, 15–20, and 30 mm from the site of an intradermal injection of capsaicin (CAP). (B) Blood flow recorded from Probes I, II, and III following CAP injection. (C,D) Blood flow changes at different times following CAP injection at 5 mm (C) and 15–20 mm (D). Data are from animals with the sciatic and femoral nerves cut (n = 6), with dorsal rhizotomy (n = 6), or with sham surgery (n = 14). Reprinted from Lin et al. (1999), with permission.

Electrophysiological observations of DRRs were performed by recording the antidromic activity from the central stumps of cut dorsal roots in other groups of rats separate from those used for blood flow measurements. After CAP injection, the spinal cord was post-treated with the same drugs to see whether they reduced the DRRs.

RESULTS

EFFECTS OF NERVE SECTIONING OR DORSAL RHIZOTOMY

Fig. 1C,D shows the changes in cutaneous blood flow recorded 5 mm (Probe I, shown in Fig. 1A) and 15–20 mm (Probe II, shown in Fig. 1A) away from the CAP injection spot, respectively. In control animals with sham surgery without cutting the sciatic and femoral nerves (n = 7), an elevated blood flow was seen at both sites following CAP injection, but the increased blood flow at the Probe II site was much larger than that at Probe I. After the sciatic and femoral nerves were sectioned (*n* = 6), the enhanced blood flow recorded from Probe II was nearly completely blocked ($P = 0.002$). However, there was no statistical difference in peak increases measured by Probe I between the nerve-sectioned and sham-operated groups ($P = 0.11$). An extensive dorsal rhizotomy gave identical results (Fig. 1D). Control experiments in six rats showed that the same volume of vehicle injected intradermally into the foot caused no significant change in blood flow.

EFFECTS OF ANTAGONISTS OF GABA AND EXCITATORY AMINO ACID RECEPTORS

Fig. 2A,B shows the changes in cutaneous blood flow at Probes I and II following intradermal CAP injection in control animals given intrathecal injections of ACSF and in animals given intrathecal injections of bicuculline, phaclofen, CNQX, or AP7. Spinal pretreatment with ACSF did not affect the blood flow response evoked by CAP injection. However, pretreatment with bicuculline, CNQX, or AP7 attenuated markedly the blood flow responses recorded from Probe II (Fig. 2B; $P = 0.0004$, 0.009, and 0.015, respectively). The responses at Probe I, near the CAP injection site, were also reduced slightly (Fig. 2A), but the changes did not reach statistical significance. Pretreatment with phaclofen, a $GABA_B$-receptor antagonist, did not significantly change blood flow responses.

DORSAL ROOT REFLEXES AFTER INTRADERMAL CAPSAICIN

DRRs recorded from the central stumps of dorsal root filaments were enhanced following intradermal injection of CAP. Spontaneous reflexes and DRRs evoked by cutaneous stimulation were reduced when the spinal cord was post-treated with bicuculline, CNQX, or AP7, but not phaclofen (Fig. 2C,D).

Fig. 2. (A,B) Blood flow changes in the foot skin at different times following CAP injection and effects of intrathecal pretreatment of the spinal cord with $GABA_A$, $GABA_B$, non-NMDA-receptor, and NMDA-receptor antagonists. The sites for blood flow measurements were as in Fig. 1C,D. (C,D) Changes in dorsal root reflexes following CAP injection and effects of post-treatment with GABA and EAA receptor antagonists. Panel C shows the spontaneous discharges, and panel D the discharges evoked by applying von Frey hairs of increasing bending force to the foot skin. The responses to CAP injection were expressed as a percentage of baseline, with baseline set at 100%. *, $P < 0.05$; **, $P < 0.01$; ***, $P < 0.001$, compared to the baseline level of the same group. +, $P < 0.05$; ++, $P < 0.01$; +++, $P < 0.001$, compared to the value at the same time point after CAP injection in the ACSF group. Reprinted from Lin et al. (1999), with permission. →

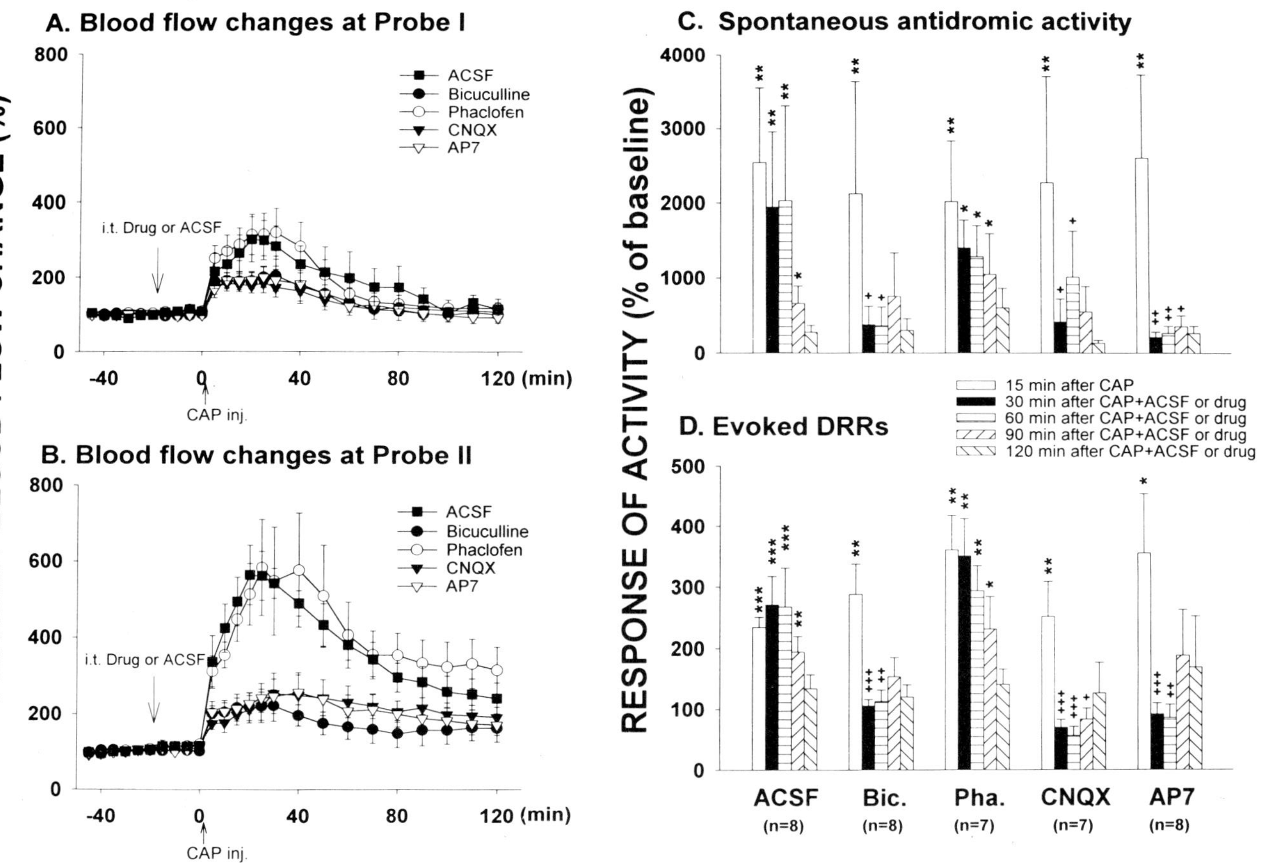
A. Blood flow changes at Probe I
B. Blood flow changes at Probe II
PERCENT BLOOD FLOW CHANGE (%)
ACSF
Bicuculline
Phaclofen
CNQX
AP7
i.t. Drug or ACSF
CAP inj.
(min)
C. Spontaneous antidromic activity
D. Evoked DRRs
RESPONSE OF ACTIVITY (% of baseline)
15 min after CAP
30 min after CAP+ACSF or drug
60 min after CAP+ACSF or drug
90 min after CAP+ACSF or drug
120 min after CAP+ACSF or drug
ACSF (n=8)
Bic. (n=8)
Pha. (n=7)
CNQX (n=7)
AP7 (n=8)

DISCUSSION

The cutaneous vasodilation that follows intradermal injection of CAP is dramatically attenuated by peripheral nerve section or by dorsal rhizotomy. Since the peripheral arborizations of the sensory receptors would have been unaffected by the lesions, our observations do not support the view that neurogenic inflammation depends substantially on peripheral axon reflexes. Vasodilation mediated by axon reflexes is presumably restricted to a localized area, the size of which coincides with the afferent receptive fields (Gee et al. 1997). The nociceptors in the rat foot have receptive fields smaller than 6 mm^2 in area (Bharali and Lisney 1992). Our new findings are that (1) the blood flow that could be measured 15–20 mm away from the CAP injection site was increased more than that recorded at a site within 5 mm of the injection site; (2) proximal sectioning of peripheral nerves or dorsal rhizotomy nearly completely abolished the CAP-evoked increase in blood flow at the distal site, but the change in blood flow near the injection site was only slightly affected; and (3) more importantly, blockade of spinal $GABA_A$, non-NMDA, or NMDA receptors reduced dramatically the CAP-evoked increase in blood flow at the distal site, although the enhanced response near the injection site was only slightly decreased. These observations are consistent with previous findings in relation to acute arthritis (Sluka and Westlund 1993; Sluka et al. 1993), except that AP7 was not effective in reducing the knee joint swelling and joint temperature increase in arthritis. We conclude that the widespread vasodilation in the skin distal to the injury (CAP injection) site involves a spinally mediated mechanism that triggers DRRs in

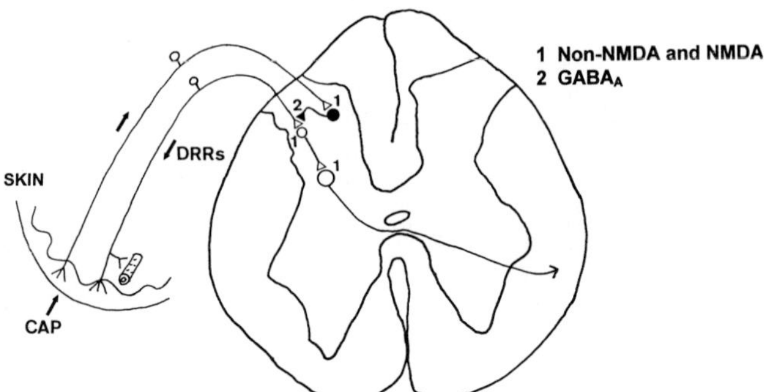

Fig. 3. Proposal for the dorsal horn circuits that produce primary afferent depolarization (PAD) and generate dorsal root reflexes (DRRs). The terminals of two primary afferent fibers are shown to innervate the skin at the CAP injection site and at a site away from the injection site. CAP injection activates dorsal horn circuits that cause DRRs, producing vasodilation in the skin away from the injection site. Reprinted from Lin et al. (1999), with permission.

large numbers of primary afferent fibers to cause the release of vasoactive substances in the skin (Willis et al. 1998; Willis 1999).

In the same model, enhanced DRRs were recorded from the cut central ends of dorsal roots at the L4–6 level or of skin nerves after intradermal injection of CAP. The enhanced DRRs were blocked pharmacologically by post-treatment of the spinal cord with antagonists of $GABA_A$ and excitatory amino acids (EAAs). CNQX and bicuculline are both known to reduce PAD (Levy et al. 1971; Evans and Long 1989), and in the arthritis experiments they blocked the DRRs that could be evoked after the onset of inflammation (Rees et al. 1995). Therefore, we suggest that generation of DRRs is an important factor in acute cutaneous neurogenic inflammation. The dorsal horn circuits that produce DRRs in cutaneous nerve fibers presumably involve $GABA_A$, non-NMDA, and NMDA receptors (Fig. 3). When irritated, the primary afferent fibers activate GABAergic interneurons by release of EAAs to initiate PAD via activation of $GABA_A$ receptors on primary afferent terminals. DRRs are generated when PAD becomes excessive; they propagate peripherally to trigger the release of inflammatory agents in the periphery and consequently cause neurogenic inflammation.

ACKNOWLEDGMENTS

This work was supported by Recruitment Grant 2517-98 (the Sealy Memorial Endowment Fund for Biomedical Research) and NIH Grant NS09743.

REFERENCES

Bernstein JE, Swift RM, Soltani K, Lorincz AL. Inhibition of axon reflex vasodilatation by topically applied capsaicin. *J Invest Derm* 1981; 76:394–395.

Bharali LAM, Lisney SJW. The relationship between unmyelinated afferent type and neurogenic plasma extravasation in normal and reinnervated rat skin. *Neuroscience* 1992; 47:703–712.

Brain SD, Williams TJ. Inflammatory oedema induced by synergism between calcitonin gene-related peptide (CGRP) and mediators of increased vascular permeability. *Br J Pharmacol* 1985; 86:855–860.

Carpenter SE, Lynn B. Vascular and sensory responses of human skin to mild injury after topical treatment with capsaicin. *Br J Pharmacol* 1981; 73:755–758.

Colpaert FC, Donnerer J, Lembeck F. Effects of capsaicin on inflammation and on substance P content of nervous tissues in rats with adjuvant arthritis. *Life Sci* 1983; 32:1827–1834.

Dougherty PM, Willis WD. Enhanced responses of spinothalamic tract neurons to excitatory amino acids accompany capsaicin-induced sensitization in the monkey. *J Neurosci* 1992; 12:883–894.

Eccles JC, Kozak W, Magni F. Dorsal root reflexes of muscle group I afferent fibres. *J Physiol* 1961; 159:128–146.

Evans RH, Long SK. Primary afferent depolarization in the rat spinal cord is mediated by pathways utilising NMDA and non-NMDA receptors. *Neurosci Lett* 1989; 100:231–236.

Ferrell WR, Russell NJ. Extravasation in the knee induced by antidromic stimulation of articular C fibre afferents of the anaesthetized cat. *J Physiol* 1986; 379:407–416.

Gee MD, Lynn B, Cotsell B. The relationship between cutaneous C fibre type and antidromic vasodilatation in the rabbit and the rat. *J Physiol* 1997; 503:31–44.

Jancsó N, Jancsó-Gábor A, Szolcsányi J. Direct evidence for neurogenic inflammation and its prevention by denervation and pretreatment with capsaicin. *Br J Pharmacol* 1967; 31:138–151.

Levy RA, Repkin AH, Anderson EG. The effects of bicuculline on primary afferent terminal excitability. *Brain Res* 1971; 32:261–265.

Lewin GR, Lisney SJW, Mendell LM. Neonatal anti-NGF treatment reduces the A delta and C fiber evoked vasodilator responses in rat skin: evidence that nociceptor afferents mediate antidromic dilatation. *Eur J Neurosci* 1992; 4:1213–1218.

Lewis T. *The Blood Vessels of the Human Skin and Their Responses*. London: Shaw & Sons, 1927.

Lin Q, Wu J, Willis WD. Dorsal root reflexes and cutaneous neurogenic inflammation following intradermal injection of capsaicin in rats. *J Neurophysiol* 1999; 82:2602–2611.

Rees H, Sluka KA, Westlund KN, Willis WD. The role of glutamate and GABA receptors in the generation of dorsal root reflexes by acute arthritis in the anaesthetised rat. *J Physiol* 1995; 484:437–445.

Schaible H, Schmidt RF. Effects of an experimental arthritis on the sensory properties of fine articular afferent units. *J Neurophysiol* 1985; 54:1109–1122.

Simone DA, Sorkin LS, Oh U, et al. Neurogenic hyperalgesia: central neural correlates in responses of spinothalamic tract neurons. *J Neurophysiol* 1991; 66:228–246.

Sluka KA, Westlund KN. Centrally administered non-NMDA but not NMDA receptor antagonists block peripheral knee joint inflammation. *Pain* 1993; 55:217–225.

Sluka KA, Willis WD, Westlund KN. Joint inflammation and hyperalgesia are reduced by spinal bicuculline. *Neuroreport* 1993; 5:109–112.

Sluka KA, Willis WD, Westlund KN. The role of dorsal root reflexes in neurogenic inflammation. *Pain Forum* 1995; 4:141–149.

Szolcsányi J. Neurogenic inflammation: reevaluation of axon reflex theory. In: Geppetti P, Holzer P (Eds). *Neurogenic Inflammation*. New York: CRC Press, 1996, pp 33–42.

Willis WD. Dorsal root potentials and dorsal root reflexes: a double-edged sword. *Exp Brain Res* 1999; 124:395–421.

Willis WD, Sluka KA, Rees H, Westlund KN. A contribution of dorsal root reflexes to peripheral inflammation. In: Rudomin P, Romo R, Mendell LM (Eds). *Presynaptic Inhibition and Neural Control*. New York: Oxford University Press, 1998, pp 407–423.

Correspondence to: William D. Willis, MD, PhD, Department of Anatomy and Neurosciences, University of Texas Medical Branch, 301 University Boulevard, Galveston, TX 77555-1069, USA. Tel: 409-772-2103; Fax: 409-772-4687; email: wdwillis@utmb.edu.

Proceedings of the 9th World Congress on Pain, Progress in Pain Research and Management, Vol. 16, edited by M. Devor, M.C. Rowbotham, and Z. Wiesenfeld-Hallin, IASP Press, Seattle, © 2000.

26

Hyperalgesia Generated by the Sympatho-Adrenal System

Wilfrid Jänig,[a] Sacha G. Khasar,[b] Jon D. Levine,[b] and Fred J.-P. Miao[b]

[a]*Physiological Institute, Christian-Albrechts University, Kiel, Germany;* [b]*Departments of Anatomy, Medicine, and Oral Surgery and Division of Neuroscience, Biomedical Sciences Program, and NIH Pain Center (UCSF), University of California, San Francisco, California, USA*

The sympathetic nervous system is involved in the regulation of a large variety of mechanisms that adapt the organism to external demands. Pain is one component of these protective reactions (Jänig and McLachlan 1992, 1999); however, the sympathetic nervous system is not normally involved in the generation or exacerbation of pain. Under certain pathological conditions seen in patients with complex regional pain syndromes (CRPS) and other neuropathic pain syndromes, however, activity in the sympathetic neurons may generate *sympathetically maintained pain* (SMP). Clinical observations, experimental investigations on humans, and experimental studies on animals show that following trauma with nerve lesions (e.g., in CRPS, type II), SMP is dependent on direct or indirect coupling between sympathetic neurons and afferent neurons and that the latter express adrenoceptors. Thus, SMP is believed to be dependent on ongoing activity in nociceptive afferent neurons that is maintained by sympathetic activity. The mechanism of SMP that occurs in CRPS, type I, which develops after trauma without obvious nerve lesion, is still a puzzle. However, convincing evidence shows that SMP depends on activity in the sympathetic neurons innervating the affected extremity (Stanton-Hicks et al. 1995; Jänig et al. 1996; Jänig and Stanton-Hicks 1996; Baron et al. 1999).

The sympatho-adrenal (SA) system also provides catecholamines that could contribute to SMP (Khasar et al. 1999). We tested the hypothesis that mechanical hyperalgesic behavior can be generated or enhanced by activation of the SA system.

SUBDIAPHRAGMATIC VAGOTOMY ENHANCES BRADYKININ-INDUCED HYPERALGESIA

Injection of bradykinin (BK) in the skin of dorsal hindpaw of rats leads to a decrease of the withdrawal threshold of the hindpaw to mechanical stimulation (BK-induced mechanical hyperalgesia). This type of experimentally induced enhanced nociception is mediated by the B2 BK receptor (Khasar et al. 1995). It does not occur when BK is injected subcutaneously (Khasar et al. 1993), or when BK is injected into sympathectomized rats and rats blocked by indomethacin. Cutaneous nociceptors are believed to be sensitized by prostaglandin released from sympathetic varicosities or from other cells (for discussion see Jänig et al. 1999; Khasar et al. 1993, 1995, 1998a).

Gebhart and Randich have shown that electrical stimulation of abdominal vagal afferents inhibits nociceptive behavior and transmission of nociceptive impulses in the lumbar dorsal horn of rats (Gebhart and Randich 1992; Randich and Gebhart 1992). If ongoing activity in abdominal vagal afferents exerts continuous inhibition of nociceptive impulse transmission in the dorsal horn, interruption of these afferents by subdiaphragmatic vagotomy should enhance or induce hyperalgesic behavior. This was indeed the case: a week after subdiaphragmatic vagotomy, but not immediately, the baseline paw-withdrawal threshold was significantly decreased and BK-induced hyperalgesia was significantly enhanced (Khasar et al. 1998a,b).

ENHANCED HYPERALGESIA AFTER VAGOTOMY IS LARGELY DEPENDENT ON THE SA SYSTEM

Further experimental investigations revealed, to our surprise, that only a small component of the vagotomy-induced hyperalgesia can be explained by removal of ongoing inhibition acting at the dorsal horn neurons. Removal of the adrenal medulla (5 weeks before the behavioral experiments) or denervation of the adrenal medulla (cutting the preganglionic axons innervating the cells) largely prevented vagotomy-induced enhancement of hyperalgesia (Khasar et al. 1998b; Jänig et al. 1999).

This observation led to an experiment showing that the vagotomy-induced decrease in baseline paw-withdrawal threshold and the enhancement of BK-induced hyperalgesia are induced by an endocrine signal released from the adrenal medulla. We studied paw-withdrawal threshold to mechanical stimulation at baseline and after intracutaneous injection of 1 ng BK, a low dose that normally does not decrease paw-withdrawal threshold over 5

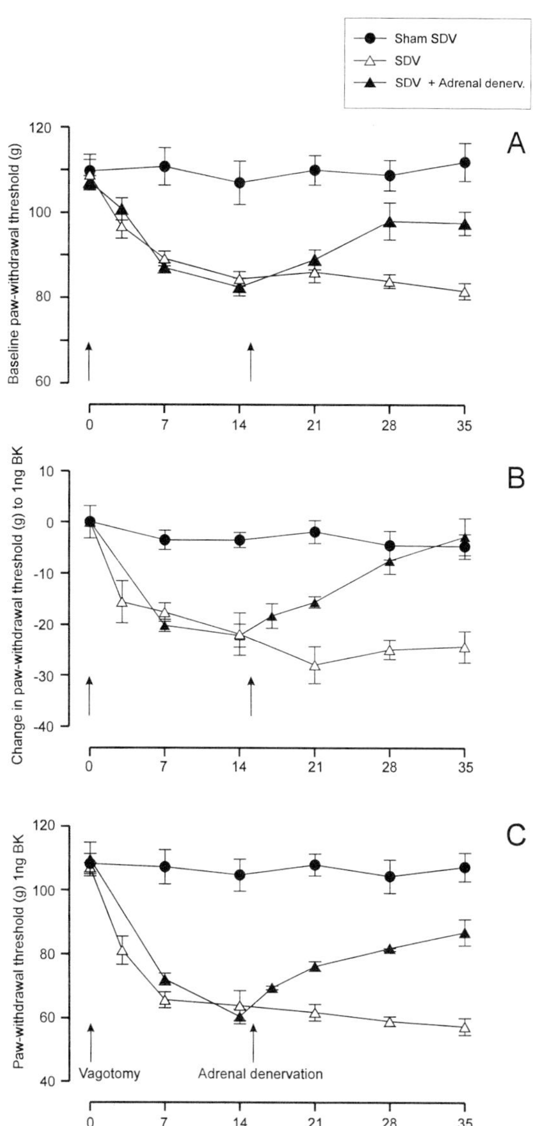

Fig. 1. (A) Baseline paw-withdrawal threshold, (B) difference between paw-withdrawal threshold and baseline and in response to 1 ng BK injected intradermally, and (C) total change of paw-withdrawal threshold in response to intradermal injection of 1 ng BK in rats before and 7–35 days after subdiaphragmatic vagotomy (SDV) (open triangles, n = 6), before and 7–35 days after sham vagotomy (closed circles, n = 8), and in rats that were first vagotomized and whose adrenal medullae were denervated 14 days after vagotomy and measurements taken up to 35 days after initial surgery (closed triangles, n = 6). Ordinate scale is threshold in grams. Data of the sham vagotomy and vagotomy groups were significantly different 7 days after vagotomy ($P < 0.01$). Data of vagotomized rats with denervated adrenal medulla and rats that were only vagotomized were significantly different on days 28 and 35 ($P < 0.01$). Data between sham-vagotomized rats and vagotomized rats in which the adrenal medullae were denervated were not significantly different on days 28 and 35 ($P > 0.05$). Modified from Khasar et al. (1998b).

weeks in three groups of rats. The first group underwent vagotomy alone and the second, vagotomy followed after 2 weeks by denervation of the adrenal medulla. Sham-operated animals served as controls (Fig. 1). Vagotomy caused a decrease in the paw-withdrawal threshold to BK that was reversed by adrenal denervation (Fig. 1). These results can be interpreted as follows: vagotomy activates the SA system, leading to release of an endocrine signal that sensitizes cutaneous nociceptors for mechanical stimuli; denervation of the adrenal medulla removes the signal and reverses the sensitization of the nociceptors.

The time course of the hypothetical sensitization of cutaneous nociceptors by the signal released by the adrenal medulla and of its reversal (after denervation of the adrenal medulla) is slow. Thus, this signal must act over many days on the nociceptors or associated cells in the skin, in order to be effective (i.e., to sensitize nociceptors); alternatively, it could be assumed that activity in the preganglionic sympathetic neurons activating adrenal medulla cells increases slowly over days. However, the latter possibility is unlikely for two reasons: first, denervation of the adrenal medulla did not

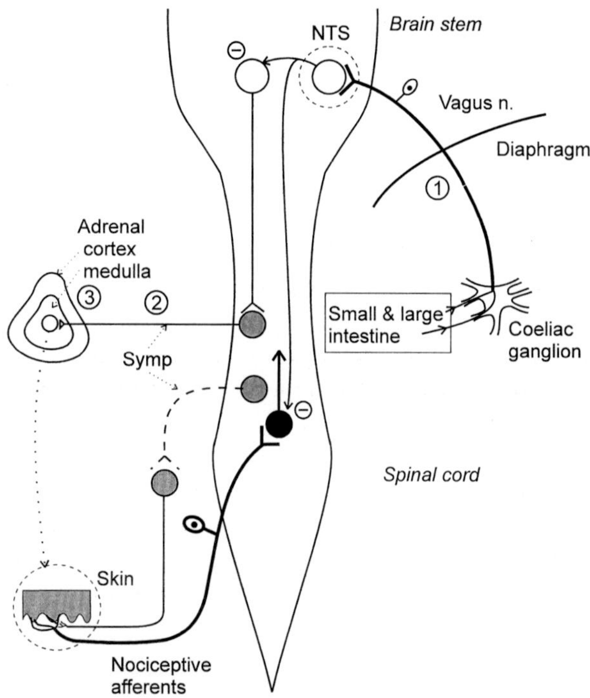

Fig. 2. Summary scheme of afferent, central, and efferent pathways that may be involved in decrease of baseline threshold and of BK-induced paw-withdrawal threshold following subdiaphragmatic vagotomy. Activity in vagal afferents that innervate small and large intestines and project to the nucleus of the solitary tract (NTS) centrally inhibit the pathway to preganglionic neurons innervating the adrenal medulla and neurons of the nociceptive system, e.g., in the dorsal horn. Interruption of these afferents leads to disinhibition of the central pathway to the preganglionic neurons innervating the adrenal medulla and of the central nociceptive system. Interruption was caused by (1) subdiaphragmatic vagotomy and (2) removal or (3) denervation of the adrenal medulla. Modified from Khasar et al. (1998b).

immediately reverse the decreased paw-withdrawal threshold (Fig. 1); second, adrenoceptor blockers (injected intracutaneously) did not reverse the decreased paw-withdrawal threshold (S.G. Khasar et al., unpublished data). This would be expected if the signal from the adrenal medulla were epinephrine and had to act over a prolonged time to induce nociceptor sensitization.

CONCLUSIONS

The experiments reported here indicate the existence of a novel mechanism by which the sympathetic nervous system might be involved in the generation of pain. These experiments have several implications (Fig. 2): (1) The sensitivity of nociceptors can be changed from remote parts of the body (e.g., the viscera) via the SA system. The sympatho-neural system (e.g., sympathetic neurons innervating the skin) is probably not involved. (2) Although the central mechanisms that increase activity in sympathetic neurons innervating the adrenal medulla after vagotomy are unknown, it is not far-fetched to assume that the brain can also use these mechanisms to change the sensitivity of nociceptors. (3) The change of sensitivity of nociceptors is slow and takes days to weeks to develop. The signal from the adrenal medulla is epinephrine and/or another substance. (4) It is unclear whether nociceptors are generally involved or only a subpopulation of nociceptors. It is furthermore unclear whether the signal from the adrenal medulla acts directly on the nociceptors or indirectly via other cells in the microenvironment of the nociceptors.

Mechanisms of pain involving the SA system may operate in such ill-defined pain syndromes as irritable bowel syndrome, functional dyspepsia, fibromyalgia, chronic fatigue syndrome, and illness behaviors (Wolfe et al. 1990; Mayer and Raybould 1993; Goebell et al. 1998). Further implications of our experiments with respect to vagal afferents are concerned are discussed elsewhere (Khasar et al. 1998a,b; Jänig et al. 1999).

ACKNOWLEDGMENT

Supported by NIH grant AR32634.

REFERENCES

Baron R, Levine JD, Fields HL. Causalgia and reflex sympathetic dystrophy: does the sympathetic nervous system contribute to the generation of pain? *Muscle Nerve* 1999; 22:678–695.

Gebhart GF, Randich A. Vagal modulation of nociception. *Am Pain Soc J* 1992; 1:26–32.

Goebell H, Holtmann G, Talley N (Eds). *Functional Dyspepsia and Irritable Bowel Syndrome: Concepts and Controversies*. Dordrecht: Kluwer Academic, 1998.

Jänig W. Pain and the sympathetic nervous system: pathophysiological mechanisms. In: Bannister R, Mathias CJ (Eds). *Autonomic Failure,* 4th ed. Oxford: Oxford University Press, 1999, pp 99–108.

Jänig W, McLachlan EM. Characteristics of function-specific pathways in the sympathetic nervous system. *Trends Neurosci* 1992; 15:475–481.

Jänig W, McLachlan EM. Neurobiology of the autonomic nervous system. In: Bannister R, Mathias CJ (Eds). *Autonomic Failure*, 4th ed. Oxford: Oxford University Press, 1999, pp 3–15.

Jänig W, Stanton-Hicks M (Eds). *Reflex Sympathetic Dystrophy: A Reappraisal,* Progress in Pain Research and Management, Vol. 6. Seattle: IASP Press, 1996.

Jänig W, Levine JD, Michaelis M. Interaction of sympathetic and primary afferent neurons following nerve injury and tissue trauma. *Prog Brain Res* 1996; 112:161–184.

Jänig W, Khasar SG, Levine JD, Miao FJ-P. The role of vagal visceral afferents in the control of nociception. In: Mayer EA, Saper CB (Eds). The biological basis for mind body interaction. *Prog Brain Res* 1999; 122:271–285.

Khasar SG, Green PG, Levine JD. Comparison of intradermal and subcutaneous hyperalgesic effects of inflammatory mediators in the rat. *Neurosci Lett* 1993; 153:215–218.

Khasar SG, Miao FJ-P, Levine JD. Inflammation modulates the contribution of receptor-subtypes to bradykinin-induced hyperalgesia in the rat. *Neuroscience* 1995; 69:685–690.

Khasar SG, Miao FJ-P, Jänig W, Levine JD. Modulation of bradykinin-induced mechanical hyperalgesia in the rat skin by activity in the abdominal vagal afferents. *Eur J Neurosci* 1998a; 10:435–444.

Khasar SG, Miao FJ-P, Jänig W, Levine JD. Vagotomy-induced enhancement of mechanical hyperalgesia in the rat is sympathoadrenal-mediated. *J Neurosci* 1998b; 18:3043–3049.

Khasar SG, McCarter G, Levine JD. Epinephrine produces a beta-adrenergic receptor-mediated mechanical hyperalgesia and in vitro sensitization of rat nociceptors. *J Neurophysiol* 1999; 81:1004–1112.

Mayer EA, Raybould HE (Eds). *Basic and Clinical Aspects of Chronic Abdominal Pain.* Pain Research and Clinical Management, Vol. 9. Amsterdam: Elsevier, 1993.

Randich A, Gebhart GF. Vagal afferent modulation of nociception. *Brain Res Rev* 1992; 17:77–99.

Stanton-Hicks M, Jänig W, Hassenbusch S, et al. Reflex sympathetic dystrophy: changing concepts and taxonomy. *Pain* 1995; 63:127–133.

Wolfe F, Smythe HA, Yunus MB, et al. The American College of Rheumatology 1990 criteria for the classification of fibromyalgia: report of the multicenter criteria committee. *Arthritis Rheum* 1990; 33:160–172.

Correspondence to: Wilfrid Jänig, Dr med, Physiologisches Institut, Christian-Albrechts-Universität zu Kiel, Olshausenstr. 40, 24098 Kiel, Germany. Tel: 431-8802036, Fax: 431-8802036, e-mail: w.janig@physiologie.uni-kiel.de.

Proceedings of the 9th World Congress on Pain,
Progress in Pain Research and Management,
Vol. 16, edited by M. Devor, M.C. Rowbotham, and
Z. Wiesenfeld-Hallin, IASP Press, Seattle, © 2000.

27

Blockade of Diabetic, Chemotherapeutic, and NGF-Induced Pain by Antisense Knockdown of PN3/SNS, a TTX-Resistant Sodium Channel

Frank Porreca,[a] Michael H. Ossipov,[a] Josephine Lai,[a] Sandra Wegert,[a] Di Bian,[a] Scott Rogers,[b] Patrick Mantyh,[b] Sanja Novakovic,[c] and John C. Hunter[c]

[a]*Departments of Pharmacology and Anesthesiology, University of Arizona Health Sciences Center, Tucson, Arizona, USA;* [b]*Department of Preventative Science, University of Minnesota, Minneapolis, Minnesota, USA;* [c]*Center for Biological Research, Roche Bioscience, Palo Alto, California, USA*

The neuropathic pain state is characterized by intense paroxysmal pain that may be triggered by normally innocuous stimuli. The abnormal pain syndromes most commonly associated with neuropathic pain are tactile allodynia, where normal touch is perceived as painful, and thermal hyperalgesia, where perception of noxious thermal stimuli is greatly exaggerated. Common causes of neuropathic pain include physical trauma to a peripheral nerve or the consequences of diabetes, AIDS, or radiotherapy (Portenoy et al. 1996).

An important aspect of abnormal neuronal activity associated with neuropathic pain is repetitive, spontaneous firing of primary afferent neurons. This increased spontaneous and persistent afferent discharge is believed to drive the development of hypersensitivity of spinal neurons and result in a condition of central sensitization (Devor and Seltzer 1999). A prominent molecular basis for the abnormal, repetitive firing of injured primary afferent neurons in many neuropathic conditions is an accumulation and increased membrane density of sodium channels at focal sites of injury. This state leads to a lower threshold for action potential generation and the generation of ectopic impulses (England et al. 1996). Accumulating converging evidence indicates that the tetrodotoxin-resistant (TTX-r) PN3 or sensory-neuron-specific (SNS) sodium channel may be an important factor in the development of signs of neuropathic pain (Sangameswaran et al. 1996; Novakovic et al. 1998). In normal adult dorsal root ganglion (DRG) neurons, the more slowly inactivating, rapidly repriming TTX-r current appears predominantly in a subpopulation of small-diameter, unmyelinated, capsaicin-sensitive neurons. The properties of this channel, together with its discrete localization to peripheral, sensory neurons, suggest that a PN3 inhibitor may alleviate chronic pain states, especially neuropathic pains, which are often resistant to clinical interventions (Elliott and Elliott 1993; Sangameswaran et al. 1996; Novakovic et al. 1998; Rush et al. 1998). We had previously demonstrated that the repeated administration of antisense oligodeoxynucleotide (ODN) to mRNA for PN3 both prevented and reversed tactile allodynia and thermal hyperalgesia in rats with L5/L6 spinal nerve ligation (SNL) (Porreca et al. 1999). This effect correlated with a loss of expression of PN3 protein in the DRG, and was not produced by mismatch ODN. The studies we describe here further explore the effect of inhibition of PN3 expression on behavioral manifestations (tactile allodynia and thermal hyperalgesia) evoked by different neuropathic conditions.

METHODS

Male Sprague-Dawley rats weighing 200–250 g were used in these studies. The Institutional Animal Care and Use Committee of the University of Arizona approved all experiments. Any animals in obvious distress or showing signs of morbidity were humanely killed.

Diabetic neuropathy. Diabetic neuropathy in rats was induced by a single i.p. injection of streptozotocin (75 mg/kg) (Courteix et al. 1993). Blood glucose levels were determined weekly with Ames Dextrostix and a reflectance colorimeter. Only rats with blood glucose levels of >14 mM at the end of 4 weeks were used in the studies. Bilateral thermal hyperalgesia and mechanical allodynia had fully developed within 4 weeks of streptozotocin injection.

Vincristine-induced neuropathy. Male rats received injections of 0.1 mg/kg of vincristine followed by 0.5 mL of saline into a tail vein. Injections were given once daily on days 1 through 5 and 8 through 12. Control rats received a similar protocol of saline injections.

NGF-induced neuropathy. Intraplantar nerve growth factor (NGF) was given daily at 100 ng in 50 μL, and thermal hyperalgesia and tactile allodynia were monitored. NGF treatment was stopped on the 10th day in the group receiving NGF alone, and recovery from the allodynic and hyperalgesic state was monitored (Amann et al. 1996).

Evaluation. To assess tactile allodynia (i.e., decreased threshold to paw withdrawal following probing with non-noxious mechanical stimuli) we measured the withdrawal of the paw ipsilateral to the site of nerve injury in response to probing with a series of eight calibrated von Frey filaments. Each filament was applied perpendicularly to the plantar surface of the ligated paw of rats kept in suspended wire-mesh cages. Withdrawal threshold was determined by sequentially increasing and decreasing the stimulus strength ("up-down" method), analyzed by a Dixon nonparametric test as described by Chaplan and colleagues (1994) and expressed as the mean withdrawal threshold.

We assessed thermal hyperalgesia by measuring paw-withdrawal latencies to a radiant heat source applied to the plantar surface of one hindpaw of rats contained within plexiglass enclosures on a clear glass plate maintained at 30°C (Hargreaves et al. 1988). A maximal cut-off of 40 seconds prevented tissue damage. Hyperalgesia was indicated by a significant ($P \leq 0.05$) decrease in paw-withdrawal latency compared to normal control animals.

Cannulation and ODN administration. We administered halothane anesthesia to all rats before implanting catheters (PE-10, 8 cm) for intrathecal (i.t.) injections. The phosphodiester antisense (5´-TCC-TCT-GTG-CTT-GGT-TCT-GGC-CT-3´) and mismatch (5´-TCC-TTC-GTG-CTG-TGT-TCG-TGC-CT-3) ODNs were screened against known sequences to ensure lack of overlap with sequences for other known proteins. All ODNs were reconstituted in nuclease-free water, and i.t. injections were given in a volume of 5 µL followed by a 9-µL flush. Rats received twice-daily injections (45 µg) of either antisense or mismatch ODNs and were evaluated daily for allodynia and hyperalgesia. We stopped injecting ODNs and monitored the reversibility of effects. Since the DRG lie within the dura mater, in a space continuous with the intrathecal space and sharing the same cerebrospinal fluid, we believe that antisense/mismatch oligonucleotides were delivered to, and acted on, primary sensory neurons in the DRG.

RESULTS

Diabetic neuropathy. A single injection of 75 mg/kg i.p. of streptozotocin produced signs of diabetic neuropathy by the fourth week, including bilateral tactile allodynia and thermal hyperalgesia. Twice-daily injections of antisense ODN to PN3 reversed tactile allodynia and thermal hyperalgesia

(Fig. 1) by approximately the fifth day. Mismatch ODN or saline did not produce any changes in paw-withdrawal thresholds or latencies in rats with diabetic neuropathy (Fig. 1). Termination of the antisense ODN injections allowed a return of tactile allodynia and thermal hyperalgesia.

Vincristine-induced neuropathy. Intravenous vincristine produced bilateral tactile allodynia and thermal hyperalgesia within 4 days of the first injection. The twice-daily spinal administration of PN3 antisense ODN caused a significant elevation in paw-withdrawal thresholds to probing with von Frey filaments and in paw-withdrawal latencies to radiant heat by the end of the sixth day of ODN treatment (Fig. 2). Discontinuation of the antisense ODN led to a restoration of signs of neuropathic pain. Mismatch ODN to PN3 produced no changes in tactile allodynia or thermal hyperalgesia in rats receiving vincristine (Fig. 2).

NGF-induced neuropathy. As expected, NGF (but not saline) elicited hyperalgesia within 2 hours after the first administration and a sustained allodynia that developed by day 3 in the injected, but not contralateral, paw. The NGF-induced allodynia and thermal hyperalgesia were both reversed by PN3 antisense, but not mismatch ODN (data not shown). Discontinuation of

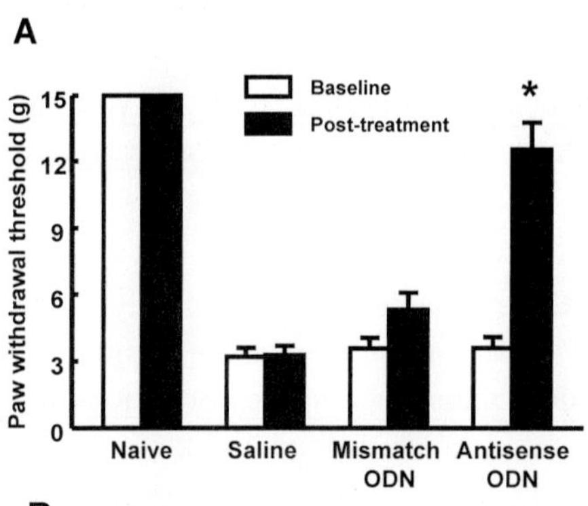

Fig. 1. Diabetic neuropathy was induced with streptozotocin. Tactile allodynia (A) and thermal hyperalgesia (B) were present. The b.i.d. i.t. injection of antisense, but not mismatch, ODN to PN3 or saline, significantly reversed the developed tactile allodynia and thermal hyperalgesia. Reversal was maximal on day 6 of ODN injections. Asterisk (*) indicates significant ($P \leq 0.05$) change from pre-ODN baseline.

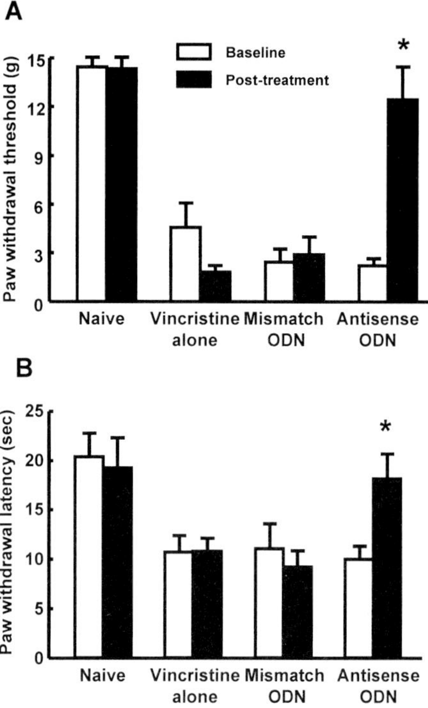

Fig. 2. Tactile allodynia (A) and thermal hyperalgesia (B) were induced by repeated daily i.v. injections of vincristine (0.1 mg/kg). The b.i.d. i.t. injection of antisense, but not mismatch, ODN to PN3 or saline, significantly reversed the developed tactile allodynia and thermal hyperalgesia. Reversal was maximal on day 3 of ODN injections. Asterisk (*) indicates significant ($P \leq 0.05$) change from pre-ODN baseline.

antisense ODN injections restored tactile allodynia and thermal hyperalgesia. Mismatch ODN did not change behavioral responses to tactile or thermal stimuli.

DISCUSSION

The i.t. administration of ODNs has proven to be a valuable tool to alter the expression of proteins in the spinal cord, the DRG, and peripheral nerve terminals (Bilsky et al. 1996; Khasar et al. 1996). The reversal of allodynia and hyperalgesia in rats with spinal nerve injury coupled with the selective "knockdown" of PN3 immunoreactivity in the lumbar DRG neurons by antisense, but not mismatch, ODN to the PN3 sodium channel supports the applicability of this technique as indicated by previous findings (Porreca et al. 1999). These initial observations provide confirmatory evidence that the antisense ODN treatment targeting PN3 expression was effective in reversing diverse types of neuropathic pain. Along with the previous observations that antisense ODN to PN3 did not affect the expression of the TTX-sensitive sodium channels PN1 or PN4 (see Porreca et al. 1999), our current study bolsters the argument that antisense ODN administration does not nonspecifically elicit changes in behaviorally determined thresholds to noxious and non-noxious sensory stimuli in normal or nerve-injured animals. It seems that "knockdown" of a functionally important protein (PN3) is required for these effects to occur.

Our study extends the importance of the activity of PN3 sodium channels to neuropathy relevant to disease states in addition to traumatic peripheral nerve injury. Hyperglycemia, tactile allodynia, and thermal hyperalgesia developed within 3 weeks of a single injection of streptozotocin, in accordance with the established literature, and allowed us to test the relevance of PN3 expression in a model of diabetic neuropathy (Courteix et al. 1983). Similarly, repeated injections of vincristine provided a model of neuropathic pain induced by cancer chemotherapy (Tanner et al. 1998) and allowed us to assess the potential relevance of PN3 expression. Both manifestations of neuropathic pain behavior measured—tactile allodynia and thermal hyperalgesia—were reversibly blocked by treatment with antisense, but not mismatch ODN to PN3. These results strongly implicate this TTX-r sodium channel in neuropathic pain behavior of organic origins, and indicate that possible changes in PN3 expression are not solely due to a physical injury to the peripheral nerve. Importantly, in both of these models, treatment with the mismatch ODN had no significant effect on the level of tactile allodynia or thermal hyperalgesia observed, again attesting to a specific action of antisense ODN to PN3, and not to a nonspecific artifact caused by repeated ODN injections.

Given that NGF regulates PN3 expression (Dib-Hajj 1998), and that neuropathic pain states are associated with NGF release (Amann et al. 1996), NGF-induced alterations in the expression of PN3 may be a common feature of neuropathic pain. Our findings support this view. We have shown that NGF produces a clear tactile allodynia and thermal hyperalgesia. The spinal administration of antisense, but not mismatch, ODN to PN3 blocked these signs of neuropathic pain. Again, as with the other models employed in this study, cessation of antisense ODN injections reversed the loss of these signs of neuropathic pain.

In summary, the PN3 sodium channel may underlie neuropathic pain states derived from significantly different and clinically relevant causes. Antisense ODN-induced reduction of PN3 protein in sensory neurons relieved established neuropathic pain resulting from physical (i.e., traumatic nerve injury) or organic (i.e., diabetic neuropathy and cancer chemotherapy) peripheral nerve injury, without altering normal non-noxious or noxious sensory functions (data not shown). Together, these data suggest that a selective inhibitor of PN3 expression or function may offer pain relief in a wide variety of neuropathic conditions or in countering the painful side effects associated with NGF-trophic activity (Blesch et al. 1998). A critical issue is the restricted expression of PN3 to sensory neurons; thus, the effects of inhibiting PN3 function would most likely be analgesic without the side effects associated with current therapies.

ACKNOWLEDGMENT

Research was supported in part by Roche Biosciences.

REFERENCES

Amann R, Sirinathsinghji DJS, Donnerer J, Liebmann I, Schuligoi R. Stimulation by nerve growth factor of neuropeptide synthesis in the adult rat in vivo: bilateral response to unilateral intraplantar injections. *Neurosci Lett* 1996; 203:171–174.

Bennett GA. Neuropathic pain. In: Wall PD, Melzack R (Eds). *Textbook of Pain*. Edinburgh: Churchill Livingstone,1994, pp 201–224.

Bilsky EJ, Wang T, Lai J, Porreca F. Selective blockade of peripheral delta opioid agonist induced antinociception by intrathecal administration of delta receptor antisense oligodeoxynucleotide. *Neurosci Lett* 1996; 220:155–158.

Blesch A, Grill RJ, Tuszynski MH. Neurotrophin gene therapy in CNS models of trauma and degeneration. *Prog Brain Res* 1998; 117:473–484.

Chaplan SR, Bach FW, Pogrel JW, Chung JM, Yaksh TL. Quantitative assessment of tactile allodynia in the rat paw. *J Neurosci Methods* 1994; 53:55–63.

Courteix C, Eschalier A, Lavarenne J. Streptozocin-induced diabetic rats: behavioral evidence for a model of chronic pain. *Pain* 1993; 53:81–88.

Devor M, Seltzer Z. Pathophysiology of damaged nerves in relation to chronic pain. In: Wall PD, Melzack R (Eds). *Textbook of Pain*, 4th ed. London: Churchill Livingstone, 1999, pp 129–164.

Dib-Hajj SD, Black JA, Cummins TR, et al. Rescue of alpha-SNS sodium channel expression in small dorsal root ganglion neurons after axotomy by nerve growth factor *in vivo*. *J Neurophysiol* 1998; 79:2668–2676.

Elliott AA, Elliott JR. Characterization of TTX-sensitive and TTX-resistant sodium currents in small cells from adult rat dorsal root ganglia. *J Physiol* 1993; 463:39–56.

England JD, Happel LT, Kline DG, et al. Sodium channel accumulation in humans with painful neuromas. *Neurology* 1996; 47:272–276.

Hargreaves K, Dubner R, Brown F, Flores C, Joris J. A new and sensitive method for measuring thermal nociception in cutaneous hyperalgesia. *Pain* 1988; 32:77–88.

Khasar SG, Gold MS, Dastmalchi S, Levine JD. Selective attenuation of mu-opioid receptor-mediated effects in rat sensory neurons by intrathecal administration of antisense oligodeoxynucleotides. *Neurosci Lett* 1996; 218:17–20.

Matzner O, Devor M. Hyperexcitability at sites of nerve injury depends on voltage-sensitive Na^+ channels. *J Neurophysiol* 1994; 72:349–359.

Novakovic SD, Tzoumaka D, Mcgivern E, et al. Distribution of the tetrodotoxin-resistant sodium channel, PN3, in rat sensory neurons in normal and neuropathic conditions. *J Neurosci* 1998; 18:2174–2187.

Porreca F, Lai J, Bian D, et al. A comparison of the potential role of the tetrodotoxin-insensitive sodium channels, PN3/SNS and NaN/SNS2, in rat models of chronic pain. *Proc Natl Acad Sci USA* 1999; 96:7640–7644.

Portenoy RK. Neuropathic pain. In: Portenoy RK, Kanner RM (Eds). *Pain Management: Theory and Practice*. Philadelphia: F.A. Davis, 1996, pp 83–125.

Rush AM, Brau ME, Elliott AA, Elliott JR. Characterization of multiple sodium current subtypes in small cells from adult rat dorsal root ganglia. *J Physiol* 1998; 551:771–789.

Sangameswaran L, Delgado SG, Fish LM, et al. Structure and function of a novel voltage-gated, tetrodotoxin-resistant sodium channel specific to sensory neurons. *J Biol Chem* 1996; 271:5953–5956.

Tanner KD, Reichling DB, Levine JD. Nociceptor hyper-responsiveness during vincristine-induced painful peripheral neuropathy in the rat. *J Neurosci* 1998; 18:6480–6491.

Wall PD, Gutnick M. Properties of afferent nerve impulses originating from a neuroma. *Nature* 1974; 248:740–743.

Correspondence to: Frank Porreca, PhD, Department of Pharmacology, University of Arizona Health Sciences Center, Tucson, AZ 85724, USA. Tel: 520-626-7421; Fax: 520-626-4182; email: frankp@u.arizona.edu.

Proceedings of the 9th World Congress on Pain,
Progress in Pain Research and Management,
Vol. 16, edited by M. Devor, M.C. Rowbotham, and
Z. Wiesenfeld-Hallin, IASP Press, Seattle, © 2000.

28

The Effect of Lamotrigine and Morphine on Neuropathic Pain in the Rat

Susanne D. Collins,[a] Nick M. Clayton,[a]
Malcolm Nobbs,[b] and Chas Bountra[a]

[a]Neuroscience Unit, and [b]Medicinal Chemistry, Glaxo Wellcome Medicines Research Centre, Stevenage, Hertfordshire, United Kingdom

Peripheral nerve injury may result in chronic neuropathic pain, which is characterized by spontaneous burning pain with accompanying hyperalgesia and allodynia (Mitchell 1872). The mechanisms underlying neuropathic pain are poorly understood, and until recently there has been little in the way of effective treatment within the clinic. The most commonly used experimental model of mononeuropathy in the rat is the Chronic Constriction Injury (CCI) technique as described by Bennett and Xie (1988). Clinical painful neuropathies have a much reduced sensitivity to the two major classes of analgesics—opioids (Arnér and Meyerson 1988) and nonsteroidal anti-inflammatory drugs (Max et al. 1988). However, drugs that act through a frequency-dependent sodium channel blockade (e.g., carbamazepine; Zakrzewska and Patsalos 1992) have recently been shown to possess analgesic properties in neuropathic pain. The sodium channel blocker 4030W92 [R(–)Diamino-5-(dichlorophenyl)-6-fluromethylpyrimidine] antagonizes tetrodotoxin-sensitive and -insensitive voltage-gated sodium channels (Trezise et al. 1998), and has previously been shown to have significant analgesic activity in this model of neuropathic pain in the rat (Collins et al. 1998). In addition, the novel anticonvulsant lamotrigine (Zakrzewska et al. 1997), another sodium channel blocker (Gardiner et al. 1998), is increasingly proving to be a drug of choice to alleviate the symptoms of various neuropathic pain states in humans.

The aim of the present study was to compare current treatments for neuropathic pain that are commonly used in the clinic, using CCI, a rat model of peripheral mononeuropathy.

METHODS

ANIMALS USED

All procedures involving the use of animals were approved by the Home Office and were carried out in accordance with the requirements of the project license. Male random hooded rats (RH) (180–200 g) were used in all experiments (supplied by the rodent breeding unit at GlaxoWellcome). Animals were housed in groups of five and fed on RMI Chow pelleted diet, with free access to water.

SURGICAL TECHNIQUE

Briefly, under isoflurane anesthesia, the left sciatic nerve was exposed at mid-thigh level and four loose ligatures of chromic gut (4.0) were tied around it. The wound was then closed and secured using suture clips. The sham-operated animals underwent the same surgical technique, except the sciatic nerve was not ligated. For each study, 40 animals were divided into groups of 10. The rats were allowed a period of 7 days to recover from the surgery before behavioral testing began. Chronic dosing commenced after a further week when the mechanical hypersensitivity had reached a stable maximum.

BEHAVIORAL TESTING

The effect of each compound on CCI -induced decrease in mechanical paw-withdrawal threshold was measured using an algesymeter (Randall and Selitto 1957). In brief, an increasing weight was applied (16 g/second) to the dorsal surface of each hindpaw until the rat attempted to remove the paw. The increasing weight was halted at this point, and the weight recorded and expressed as mechanical paw-withdrawal threshold. The maximum weight applied in this model was 250 g.

STATISTICAL ANALYSIS

Statistical analysis was carried out to compare the difference between the drug-treated and vehicle-treated group using unpaired Student's *t* test ($P < 0.05$ was considered significant).

RESULTS

The doses used in these studies were high, being determined from previous "in house" data and doses known to be efficacious in the clinical treatment of neuropathic pain.

Morphine (3 mg/kg), when administered chronically (3 times daily) by the subcutaneous route for a period of 5 days (days 12–16 postoperative), had only a small effect on the CCI-induced decrease in paw-withdrawal threshold. A small, significant reversal (12%; $P < 0.05$) was observed 5 hours after a single administration on day 12 postoperative, but was not maintained throughout the dosing period (see Fig. 1). The animals were only dosed with morphine for 5 days because no significant effect was observed during this time when compared to the vehicle-treated CCI group. In addition, side effects such as sedation and catatonia were evident in some of the animals being treated with morphine.

Chronic dosing with lamotrigine (30 mg/kg, twice daily, days 13–24 postoperative) by the oral route fully reversed (by day 16) the CCI -induced characteristic decrease in paw-withdrawal threshold to that of the sham-operated animals (91 ± 10 g vs. 92.5 ± 3 g, respectively [mean ± SEM], both n = 10; $P < 0.05$). The analgesic effects of lamotrigine appeared to be maintained following cessation of the treatment, until day 37 postoperative (see Fig. 2).

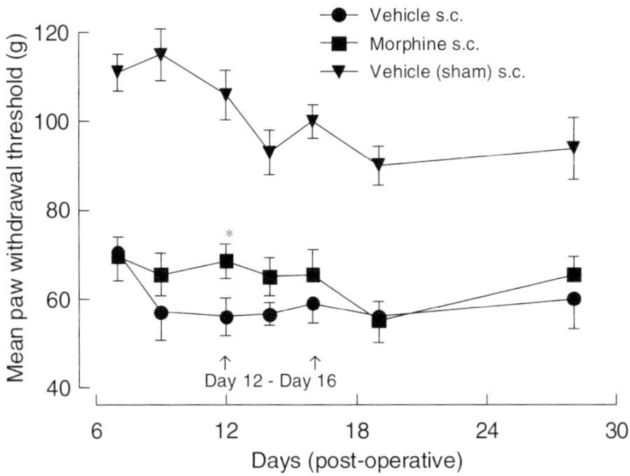

Fig. 1. Morphine (3 mg/kg t.i.d., s.c.) had a limited effect on the mechanical paw-withdrawal threshold of the paw with chronic constriction injury (CCI) ipsilateral to the sciatic nerve ligation (values depict mean ± SEM for n = 10 rats per group; $^*P < 0.05$ compared with the vehicle-treated, nerve-ligated group).

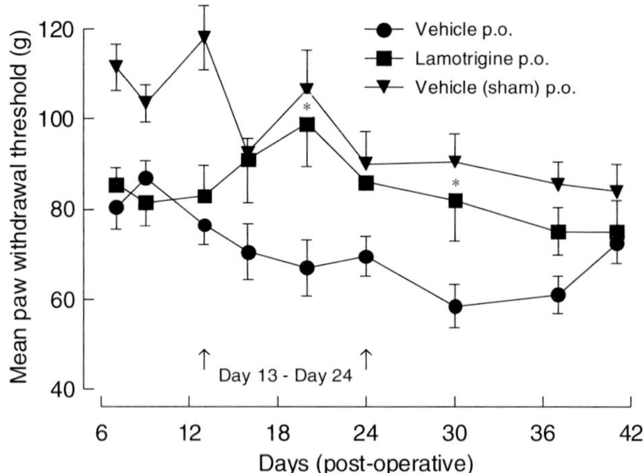

Fig. 2. Lamotrigine (30 mg/kg b.i.d., p.o.) reversed and maintained the mean mechanical paw-withdrawal threshold following ligation of the sciatic nerve. All thresholds are for the paw corresponding to the ligated side (values depict mean ± SEM for n = 10 rats per group; *$P < 0.05$ compared with the vehicle-treated, nerve-ligated group).

DISCUSSION

These studies demonstrated that the CCI model of peripheral mononeuropathy in the rat produces a significant and long-lasting hypersensitivity, similar to that observed in clinical neuropathies. The dose of lamotrigine used in these studies was based on previous data generated "in house" using the carrageenan model of acute inflammatory pain, where 30 mg/kg p.o. was required to produce a significant effect. We are unable to predict whether lower doses of lamotrigine would also be as effective in this model, although clinical data would suggest it is highly likely.

The use of morphine in the clinic for the treatment of neuropathic pain is limited due to significant side effects at efficacious doses. In the CCI model, morphine produced an initial reversal of the mechanical hypersensitivity, but this was not maintained. Chronic dosing with morphine was terminated early as significant side effects such as sedation were observed in some of the rats.

The novel anticonvulsant lamotrigine is increasingly proving to be a drug of choice in the clinic for the treatment of neuropathic pain. Although it has demonstrated some analgesic activity in several neuropathic pain states, dose escalation over several weeks is often required to achieve maximum benefit and minimum side effects (Eisenberg et al. 1998). These studies demonstrated that a high dose of lamotrigine was effective in reversing the CCI -induced decrease in paw-withdrawal threshold. Clinical treatment of neuropathic pain requires several days of chronic dosing before an analgesic effect is observed; this was also the case in the CCI model. The analgesic effects of lamotrigine were maintained following cessation of the treatment for several days. No apparent side effects were observed with lamotrigine during chronic dosing.

Several clinical studies (e.g., Zakrzewska et al. 1997) have already demonstrated that lamotrigine has clinical utility in the treatment of some neuropathic pain states. The above animal studies further support the use of lamotrigine in the treatment of neuropathic pain.

ACKNOWLEDGMENTS

This study was supported by Glaxo Wellcome Research and Development.

REFERENCES

Arnér S, Meyerson BA. Lack of analgesic effect of opioids on neuropathic and idiopathic forms of pain. *Pain* 1988; 33:11–23.

Bennett GJ, Xie YK. A peripheral mononeuropathy in rat that produces disorders of pain sensation like those seen in man. *Pain* 1988; 33:87–107.

Collins SD, Clayton NM, Nobbs M, Bountra C. The effect of 4030W92, a novel sodium channel blocker on the treatment of neuropathic pain in the rat. *Br J Pharmacol* 1998; (Suppl 16P):125.

Eisenberg E, Alon N, Ishay A, Daoud D, Yarnitsky D. Lamotrigine in the treatment of painful diabetic neuropathy. *Eur J Neurol* 1998; 5(2):167–173.

Gardiner JC, Gupta P, Butler P, Pryke JG, Roffey SJ. The sodium channel modulators, lamotrigine and 4030W92 block ectopic discharge originating in rat sciatic neuromas. *Br J Pharmacol* 1998; (Suppl 39P):125.

Max MB, Schafer SC, Culnane M, Dubner R, Gracely RH. Association of pain relief with drug side effects in postherpetic neuralgia: a single-dose study of clonidine, codeine, ibuprofen and placebo. *Clin Pharmacol Ther* 1988; 43(4):363–371.

Mitchell SW (Ed). *Injuries of Nerves and Their Consequences*. Philadelphia: JB Lippincott, 1872, pp 252–281.

Randall LO, Selitto JJ. A method for measurement of analgesic activity on inflamed tissue. *Arch Int Pharmacodyn* 1957; 61:409–419.

Trezise DJ, John VH, Nobbs M, Xie XM. Voltage- and use-dependent inhibition of Na^+ channels in rat sensory neurones by 4030W92, a new antihyperalgesic agent. *Br J Pharmacol* 1998; 124(5):953–963.

Zakrzewska JM, Patsalos PN. Drugs used in the management of trigeminal neuralgia. *Oral Surg Oral Med Oral Pathol* 1992; 74:439–450.

Zakrzewska JM, Chaudhry Z, Nurmikko TJ, Patton DW, Mullens EL. Lamotrigine (Lamictal) in refractory trigeminal neuralgia: results from a double-blind placebo controlled crossover trial. *Pain* 1997; 73:223–230.

Correspondence to: S.D. Collins, BSc, Neuroscience Unit, Glaxo Wellcome Medicines Research Centre, Gunnels Wood Road, Stevenage, Hertfordshire, SG1 2NY, United Kingdom. Tel: 44 (0)1438-768339; Fax: 44 (0)1438-764898; email: sdc41626@glaxowellcome.co.uk.

Proceedings of the 9th World Congress on Pain, Progress in Pain Research and Management, Vol. 16, edited by M. Devor, M.C. Rowbotham, and Z. Wiesenfeld-Hallin, IASP Press, Seattle, © 2000.

29

What Transgenic Mice Have Taught Us about Pain

Allan I. Basbaum

Departments of Anatomy and Physiology and W.M. Keck Foundation Center for Integrative Neuroscience, University of California, San Francisco, California, USA

Recent years have seen significant advances in our understanding of the nociceptive circuits through which injury messages are processed. Of particular interest is the growing evidence that injury induces long-term changes in the organization of dorsal horn neurons, creating a state of hyperexcitability that facilitates the processing of nociceptive messages (Dubner and Basbaum 1994). These changes are presumed to underlie the clinical conditions of allodynia, in which innocuous stimuli induce pain, and hyperalgesia, where noxious stimuli produce exacerbated pain. Because the development of new therapeutic approaches to treating these conditions requires a detailed understanding of their pharmacological basis, it is not surprising that the predominant focus has been on identifying antagonists to various molecules (neurotransmitter receptors, ion channels, second messenger molecules, etc.). More recently, however, many researchers have turned to the analysis of mice with specific gene deletions. This chapter will discuss the different approaches that have been used, including overexpression of genes and specific gene deletion.

ADVANTAGES AND DISADVANTAGES OF TRANSGENIC MICE IN THE STUDY OF PAIN

Why bother making and studying a knockout mouse when pharmacological antagonists are available? Given that generating mice with specific gene deletions is both time-consuming and expensive, the question is reasonable. There are, in fact, several reasons. First, there are no specific pharmacological antagonists; at best they are relatively selective. Moreover, what is selective today may turn out to be far from selective after further study. For example, many β-adrenergic antagonists, although very useful drugs, can "cross over" to some extent to α-adrenergic receptors. Targeting of antagonists to central sites may also be difficult if the drugs do not cross the blood–brain barrier. Furthermore, if the contribution of specific receptor subtypes is to be defined, the great multiplicity of receptors identified by molecular cloning will require the development of many new antagonists. By contrast, subtypes of different receptors or enzymes can readily be studied by deletion of single genes.

Specificity is not the only reason for using transgenics. The half-life of most antagonists limits the types of experiments that can be performed. For example, to study the effect of blocking a particular receptor on the consequences of peripheral nerve injury, it may be necessary to use continuous long-term administration. This is difficult to achieve with available technology (although slow-release systems have been developed). By knocking out a particular gene, it is possible to permanently eliminate the protein product of interest. Most importantly, the specificity of the knockout cannot be matched by pharmacological antagonism.

Of course, problems may arise when using knockout mice, including potential developmental abnormalities induced by the gene deletion and concerns about genetic background. The fact that some knockouts are lethal indicates that gene deletion may induce significant changes during development. In some cases an animal may have survived because a compensatory event substituted for the loss of the particular gene and its protein product. If that compensation persists into adulthood, it may mask the phenotype of the gene deletion, leading to an erroneous conclusion about the contribution of the particular gene product to pain processing.

New approaches make it possible to avoid the problem of compensatory responses that occur during development. This is achieved by creating inducible knockouts, a condition in which the gene can be deleted in the adult. Typically the targeted gene is arranged so that it can be deleted, usually by injecting a drug that triggers its excision (see Stark et al. 1998, for example). In some respects this approach is comparable to the use of antisense oligonucleotides, which reduce the expression of a particular gene at a given time, usually in the adult. With antisense, the effect is of limited duration. Eventually the antisense is degraded and a new message can be translated. An important concern, sometimes overlooked in the use of inducible knockouts, is that only newly synthesized protein is affected. A certain amount of time should be allowed for degradation of the already synthesized protein. With a neurotransmitter receptor molecule, which probably has a relatively long half-life, the induced knockout could take significant time to manifest.

Another legitimate concern is that the phenotype of the knockout mice may vary because of differences in the genetic background of the mouse. This problem is difficult to avoid and should be kept in mind, particularly when comparing the phenotypes of mice generated on different backgrounds. Jeffrey S. Mogil discusses a related concern in greater detail in his chapter in this volume, namely that the pain behavior of different strains of mice in response to various types of noxious stimuli differs considerably, but predictably. For certain tests, a particular strain of mice may be advantageous. Typically, knockout mice are generated on a 129 genetic background, not the ideal mouse in which to study pain behavior. For this reason, the offspring are often backcrossed to other strains, most commonly C57Bl/6. If the behavior of the mice with the gene deletion is similar on two different backgrounds, researchers can have more confidence that the particular gene was indeed the critical contributor to the phenotype.

Many knockouts have been developed for the study of pain. These include knockouts of growth factors and their receptors (see below), the two cannabinoid receptor subtypes, and all of the opioid receptors, as well as genes that encode the endogenous opioids, enkephalin, dynorphin, and β-endorphin. Recent studies have addressed the consequences of deleting genes that code for different α-adrenergic and glutamate receptor subtypes. The results of many of these studies are discussed in detail elsewhere (see reviews by Mogil et al. 1996; Mogil and Grisel 1998; Mogil et al. 2000). In this chapter, I have chosen examples that illustrate interesting advantages of transgenic technology. The examples are conditions in which the molecular approach provides information that is not available with conventional pharmacological antagonism. The two approaches are not mutually exclusive, however. If the molecular approach points to the importance of a particular molecule to nociceptive processing, the goal would be to develop a selective antagonist that could be used clinically.

TERMINOLOGY

Before discussing these examples, some definitions are in order. "Transgenic" is a generic term. We are dealing with transgenics when we are studying a mouse in which a particular gene has been deleted, or a mouse in which a novel gene has been inserted or overexpressed (i.e., so that its protein product is generated in abundance). The transgene refers to the gene that has been inserted. Commonly, however, the term "transgenic mice" refers to animals in which a gene has been inserted randomly into the genome, usually by injecting the gene, in an appropriate plasmid, into the oocyte. In some cases researchers insert the gene coupled to a known promoter, or at least a gene sequence believed to contain promoter elements. The promoter refers to the part of the gene that normally controls expression of the gene. For example, if we wanted to express gene X, but only in cells in which the μ-opioid receptor is expressed, we would create a construct that couples the μ-opioid receptor promoter to gene X. Proteins (transcription factors) that are uniquely expressed in subsets of neurons activate the promoter. This results in cell-specific expression of the gene that is controlled by that promoter. Often promoters are not available, or the promoter sequence that has been defined does not produce sufficiently strong expression. A more general, strong promoter could then be used that ensures high levels of gene transcription and thus high levels of the desired protein. Viral promoters, such as the cytomegalovirus (CMV) promoter, are commonly used in such studies. Under these conditions the protein is likely to be expressed in all cell types, including neurons and glia.

USING TRANSGENICS TO OVEREXPRESS PAIN-RELEVANT GENES

Using these different constructs it is possible to insert new genes, delete existing ones, or overexpress endogenous genes. The following discussion illustrates an excellent example in which overexpression of an endogenous gene provided new insights into the factors that contribute to injury-induced neuropathic pain. Considerable evidence has shown that injury to peripheral nerve can induce a neuropathic pain condition associated with thermal and mechanical allodynia and hyperalgesia (Bennett and Xie 1988; Dubner and Basbaum 1994; Kim et al. 1997; Malmberg and Basbaum 1998). Furthermore, there is evidence that the pain phenotype is sometimes sympathetically maintained, i.e., it is exacerbated by increased activity of sympathetic efferents (Wall and Gutnick 1974; Sato and Perl 1991; Devor et al. 1994). The mechanisms by which the sympathetic efferents mediate the injury-evoked changes are many, including sprouting at the level of the injured nerve (Fried et al. 1991), upregulation of adrenergic receptors on the primary afferent nociceptors (Birder and Perl 1999), and sprouting in the dorsal root ganglion (DRG), notably around large-diameter cell bodies (McLachlan et al. 1993). Normally, sympathetic postganglionic efferents found in the DRG arborize around blood vessels. After peripheral nerve injury, these catecholaminergic axons sprout extensively within the ganglion and eventually innervate large DRG neurons (McLachlan et al. 1993). Because Aβ-mediated allodynia is commonly observed after peripheral nerve injury (Price et al. 1989), the latter observation was of particular interest. It suggested that the sympathetic efferents contributed to the increased activity of large-diameter afferents, via their abnormal regulation of the cell bodies of the Aβ afferents.

Because of the evidence for sprouting of sympathetic efferents, many studies have focused on the possible contribution of neurotrophins, i.e., growth factors that influence the development of primary afferent and sympathetic efferents (Otten et al. 1980). Of particular interest are studies of Davis and Albers and their colleagues (Davis et al. 1994), who examined the effect of overexpressing nerve growth factor (NGF). In addition to its developmental role, NGF can direct the growth of injured peripheral nerve fibers (Ramer and Bisby 1999). Because peripheral injection of NGF can induce a hyperalgesic condition (Lewin et al. 1993), an interesting possibility was that nerve injury alters NGF expression, and that this in turn directs the sprouting in the DRG.

In an ideal world, this hypothesis could be tested by injecting an antagonist that would selectivity block the trkA receptor, which is targeted by NGF. Unfortunately, pharmacological antagonists of the trkA receptor have not yet been developed. Mice in which the gene has been deleted that encodes NGF or the trkA receptor have been developed, but this knockout is either lethal or produces such profound abnormalities that the mechanism of nerve-injury-induced sprouting cannot be studied (Smeyne et al. 1994; Silos-Santiago et al. 1995; de Castro et al. 1998).

To overcome these limitations, Davis et al. (1994) generated a mouse that overexpresses NGF. They hypothesized that the involvement of NGF could be determined by studying the consequences of having too much NGF. They reasoned that overexpression of NGF might recapitulate the conditions typically produced by nerve injury. To prevent overexpression of NGF throughout the brain and periphery (which would occur if a nonselective viral promoter, such as CMV, were used to drive expression), Davis's team used a promoter that is specific to keratinocytes (Davis et al. 1994), i.e., to cells that are only found in skin; this strategy restricted overexpression of NGF to the skin. Critical to their experiment was that the NGF that was synthesized by the keratinocytes was processed normally and that it was secreted. This resulted in constitutive expression of NGF throughout development and in the adult. Peripheral nerve endings (some of which express the trkA receptor) were thus constantly exposed to high levels of NGF. When NGF binds the trkA receptor, the NGF–trkA complex is internalized by the peripheral terminals of sensory and sympathetic nerve terminals and is retrogradely transported to the cell bodies, where it influences cell function, including expression of genes involved in the survival of the neuron.

What then was the consequence of increasing the exposure of DRG and sympathetic neurons to retrogradely transported NGF?

The phenotype of the NGF overexpressers was interesting in several respects. First, the number of neurons in the adult sensory and sympathetic ganglia was greatly increased in comparison to animals that expressed normal levels of NGF (Albers et al. 1994). Presumably this is because the apoptosis (i.e., cell death) that typically occurs during development failed to occur when high levels of NGF persisted throughout development. Second, not only did the authors find upregulation of NGF message in the keratinocytes, as expected, but this was associated with dramatically increased peripheral nerve innervation in the skin (Davis et al. 1997) and with increased numbers of specific subtypes of nociceptor (Stucky et al. 1999). Third, the animals were clearly hyperalgesic (Davis et al. 1993), in the absence of injury. The hyperalgesia effectively mimicked what is produced by exogenous administration of NGF in adult animals. Finally, and most interestingly, the anatomical features of the nerve injury phenotype appeared to be recapitulated in the NGF-overexpressing mice. Specifically, the authors found a dramatic increase of the sympathetic innervation of DRG cells, as occurs after peripheral nerve injury (Davis et al. 1994). Of course, in this case there was no peripheral nerve injury. The pattern of sprouting in the two conditions, however, was not identical. Thus, the hyperinnervation in the NGF overexpressers was not selectively targeted to the large-diameter cell bodies. On the contrary, it was focused on DRG neurons that expressed the trkA receptor, namely, the small-diameter, peptide-synthesizing nociceptors (Davis et al. 1998). Clearly, nerve-injury-induced and NGF-overexpression-induced sprouting of sympathetic efferents are not identical.

These experiments provide an important example of the power of transgenics. Davis's team not only uncovered an interesting consequence of excess production of NGF, but more importantly, perhaps, established that increased NGF production is not the sole explanation for the anatomical (sprouting) and behavioral (hyperalgesic) consequences of peripheral nerve injury. Although the phenotype of the animal did not precisely mimic what occurs following injury, the use of transgenic approaches provided important information about the regulation of neuronal sprouting in the DRG. Future studies must address the factors that direct sprouting of sympathetic efferents to cell bodies of large-diameter afferents. One possibility is that injury results in abnormal expression of NGF by the large-diameter afferents; this could "guide" the sprouting that is induced in sympathetic nerves when they are injured. In fact, several recent studies have demonstrated that injury to peripheral nerves can significantly alter the neurochemical phenotype of large-diameter afferents. For example, after peripheral nerve injury, large-diameter DRG neurons begin to express substance P, a peptide transmitter that is usually restricted to small-diameter afferents (Noguchi et al. 1995), as well as neuropeptide Y, a peptide not normally found in DRG neurons (Wakisaka et al. 1991). Given the plasticity of large-diameter afferents, it is possible that they begin to synthesize molecules that can direct sympathetic sprouting. It will be of particular interest in future studies to address the extent to which NGF overexpression alters the neurochemical phenotype of large-diameter afferents, whether or not nerve injury was induced.

USING TRANSGENIC TECHNOLOGY TO KNOCK OUT PAIN-RELEVANT GENES

As noted above, in the typical transgenic, the transgene is expressed randomly or is targeted to a subset of neurons, by choosing an appropriate promoter and making it part of the transgene. A variation on the transgenic overexpresser is the "knock-in." In this situation, the goal is to express a particular gene, but under the control of an endogenous promoter, so that cellular expression is controlled. For example, researchers may wish to label neurons in which the μ-opioid receptor is expressed by having a fluorescent protein synthesized in tandem with the μ-opioid receptor. For this gene construct to be appropriately transcribed, it is critical to have the exogenous gene precisely inserted into the genome, i.e., it must be "knocked in" to a particular locus, not randomly inserted. This is achieved through homologous recombination, whereby the construct will effectively substitute for the endogenous gene, provided there is enough sequence similarity between the exogenous gene and the endogenous gene. When homologous recombination is successful, the exogenous gene comes under the control of the promoter that drives the endogenous gene. Provided the endogenous promoter is sufficiently "strong," there can be expression of the exogenous gene, for example, the fluorescent marker. Few knock-in mice have been generated specifically for the study of pain, but the approach may prove incredibly valuable for studying circuits in the dorsal horn. For example, to characterize the axonal arborization of neurons that express the μ-opioid receptor, it is possible to knock in a marker that is targeted specifically to the axons of neurons that express that receptor. The approach involves knocking in "tau," an axonal microtubule protein localized to axons, into the opioid receptor locus. By linking the tau to an observable marker (such as green fluorescent protein), the axon can be visualized in sections from adult animals. This technique has been used to trace the axonal arborization of olfactory neurons (Mombaerts et al. 1996). In effect, this approach uses transgenic technology as a very powerful anatomical tool.

TRANSGENIC KNOCKOUT MICE

Knockouts are a variation of the knock-in. In this case, homologous recombination is used to delete a gene of interest, whereby an inactive or marker gene is knocked in for the gene that is to be deleted. The inactive gene substitutes precisely, and in every cell, for the deleted gene. As noted above, many genes have already been knocked out in mice. Only some of these genes have proved relevant to nociceptive processing. In some studies the intent was to test the involvement of a particular gene product in pain processing. In other cases, the pain-relevant phenotype was discovered during the experiment, i.e., the deletion was originally made for a different purpose. In the following section I describe studies performed in our laboratory on such knockout mice. Although these animals have been described in previous reports, I will discuss their phenotypes in detail, not only because they provide insights into the contribution of particular molecules, but also because each illustrates particular advantages that knockout technology brings to the study of pain.

The first illustration of the utility of transgenic mice is a general one that addresses the use of antibodies to study the organization of pain-relevant circuitry. Clearly, much of our understanding of the distribution of neurotransmitters and neurotransmitter receptors comes from immunohistochemical studies. Of particular interest are studies that have demonstrated colocalization of primary afferent peptides with particular neurotransmitter receptors. The reliability of the conclusions that are drawn from these studies is only as good as the antibodies that were used to define the neurochemistry of the circuits. Unfortunately, the problem described above concerning the nonselectivity of most pharmacological antagonists also occurs, to some extent, with antibodies. Although antibodies are raised with the intention of localizing specific molecules, the fact is that they recognize small peptide sequences, which may not only occur in the molecule (e.g., receptor) of interest. In other words, they may crossreact with many unknown molecules. The typical controls that are performed involve incubating the antibody with the molecule of interest. If the antibody was raised against a peptide sequence found within the particular molecule, then the absorption may be performed with excess peptide. Elimination of immunostaining in either case would typically lead to the conclusion that the antibody has recognized the molecule in the tissue. Unfortunately, that conclusion may be incorrect. If the antibody crossreacted with a molecule that contains the peptide sequence (epitope) that was recognized by the antibody, then the absorption controls would eliminate this inappropriate staining too, because the peptide blocks binding of the antibody. In other words, absorption controls only establish that the antibody recognizes the particular epitope; they do not demonstrate that a particular molecule was recognized.

Here is where tissue from transgenic mice can be incredibly valuable. If an antibody against the μ-opioid receptor is used to immunostain tissue from mice with a deletion of the gene that encodes that receptor, there should be no staining. Immunostaining tissue from an appropriate knockout mouse provides the most accurate way to gauge the specificity of antisera. Any residual staining must have resulted from crossreactivity of the antibody with other molecules. Given that so much of our information about the neurochemical circuitry of the dorsal horn depends on antisera, it will be of great value to study existing antisera in mice in which the protein product of the putative target gene has been deleted.

The next example of the usefulness of transgenic approaches to the study of pain comes from studies of mice that carry a deletion of the preprotachykinin (PPT) gene, which encodes for the tachykinin peptides, substance P (SP) and neurokinin A (NKA). Numerous studies have implicated SP in the production of pain. It is synthesized by a subset of small-diameter DRG neurons (Levine et al. 1993) and is transported to the central and peripheral terminals of primary afferent C fibers, where it is stored in dense-core vesicles. Its contribution to nociceptive processing is further indicated by the fact that noxious stimulation (or stimulation of peripheral nerves at C-fiber intensities) evokes the release of SP into peripheral tissue (Grutzner et al. 1992) and into the spinal cord cerebrospinal fluid (CSF) (Yaksh et al. 1980; Duggan et al. 1988). Furthermore, iontophoresis of SP excites nociresponsive neurons of the dorsal horn (Radhakrishnan and Henry 1993), and intrathecal injection of SP evokes behaviors that have been interpreted as pain (Cridland and Henry 1986). Finally, because there is evidence that SP is an agonist at the neurokinin-1 (NK1) receptor (Maggi 1995), it is of interest that studies using relatively selective NK1-receptor antagonists have shown some reduction of injury-induced pain behaviors (Yamamoto and Yaksh 1992; Yashpal et al. 1993).

Given that we have so much information about the contribution of SP to nociceptive processing, we might ask why anyone should bother making a mouse that can no longer synthesize the molecule. Perhaps the most important reason can be appreciated by examining the complexity of the primary afferent terminal. The predominant excitatory neurotransmitter of small-diameter primary afferents, indeed of all afferents, is glutamate. Glutamate is localized to small, clear vesicles within the same terminals that contain the dense-core vesicles that store the peptides (De Biasi and Rustioni 1988). There is little doubt that acute pain is generated, to a large extent, by the release of glutamate, which in turn binds to glutamate receptors. The latter are located on dorsal horn nociresponsive interneurons and projection neurons (Tölle et al. 1993). It is likely that the first consequence of glutamate release is the depolarization of postsynaptic neurons via an action at AMPA-type glutamate receptors. The released glutamate also binds to N-methyl D-aspartate (NMDA)-type glutamate receptors. With persistent or very intense stimulation, this receptor is activated, in part secondary to AMPA-mediated depolarization of the postsynaptic neuron. Binding to the NMDA receptor triggers many of the long-term changes that underlie the central sensitization of dorsal horn neurons and the resultant development of allodynia and hyperalgesia (Woolf and Thompson 1991; Basbaum and Woolf 1999).

Under what conditions then does SP come into play? Some studies have demonstrated that SP can enhance the action of glutamate (Randic et al. 1990; Dougherty et al. 1993), but when does this occur? Is SP released under both acute and prolonged stimulus conditions? Is there a differential contribution of SP in the setting of injury? Because it is difficult to sustain antagonist action, it is difficult to assess the contribution of peptides over long periods of time, as during persistent injury. For example, although there is pharmacological evidence that the NK1 receptor contributes to the central sensitization to noxious/injury stimuli (Ma and Woolf 1997), it is not clear that SP and the NK1 receptor also contribute to the allodynia that occurs when injury persists. Finally, and perhaps most importantly, we must not forget that the dense-core vesicle not only stores SP, but also contains NKA (the other tachykinin product of the PPT-A gene), calcitonin gene-related peptide (CGRP), and even some neurotrophins, such as brain-derived neurotrophic factor. Can we assume that SP and NKA exert identical central effects? This is unlikely, for several reasons. First, although SP predominantly targets the NK1 receptor, NKA is more promiscuous, having relatively high affinity for the three neurokinin receptors, NK1, 2, and 3. Furthermore, based on studies of Duggan and colleagues (1990), it is likely that the central actions of NKA are considerably more diffuse (in a topographic/spatial sense) than those of SP because NKA is less susceptible to the endopeptidases that rapidly degrade SP.

The construct that we used to generate the knockout mice targeted both the SP- and NKA-encoding exons (Cao et al. 1998). This ensured that neither tachykinin was produced in the knockout mice. We first tested the response of the mice to stimuli that were close to the nociceptive threshold (i.e., the intensity at which nocifensive behaviors are first induced). The knockout mice were identical to the wild-type animals in these tests. We presume that glutamate mediates behaviors generated when the noxious stimulus is near threshold. This is consistent with other studies that reported that release of SP from small-diameter primary afferents occurs at higher frequencies and intensities than that which is required to evoke the release of glutamate (Marvizon et al. 1997). In contrast to the similarity of the knockout and wild-type mice with near-threshold stimuli, we observed a significant decrease in pain behavior compared to wild-type animals when the stimulus intensity was increased. Interestingly, there appeared to be a window of stimulus intensities that did not induce "increased" pain behavior, e.g., shorter latency responses. At the highest intensities tested, we observed that the behavior once again more closely approximated that of the wild type. Presumably, other neurotransmitters or sensitization of dorsal horn neurons sustained the behaviors in the absence of the tachykinins.

We also found that neither the thermal nor the mechanical allodynia that developed after tissue or nerve injury, with inflammation induced by complete Freund's adjuvant (CFA) or with partial sciatic nerve section, respectively, was altered in the PPT-A knockout mice. The mice showed a profound allodynia despite the loss of the tachykinins, and were equivalent in this respect to wild-type mice. Based on these results, we concluded that tissue- and nerve-injury-induced allodynia are mediated by release of glutamate from the primary afferents, secondary to a central sensitization of dorsal horn neurons that was triggered by the injury. That conclusion is of course consistent with the view that glutamate is critical for stimuli that are either innocuous or slightly into the noxious range. It should be emphasized that we did not test our animals for hyperalgesia (i.e., exaggerated pain responses to noxious stimuli). Because tachykinins are released when stimuli are very intense (Yaksh et al. 1980), it is likely that the development of hyperalgesia would be reduced in the PPT-A mutant mice. This conclusion about the requirement of intense stimuli to evoke the release of SP and NKA is also consistent with our studies of the internalization of the NK1 receptor in response to natural stimuli (Mantyh et al. 1995). We found that only intense, noxious stimuli consistently induced NK1-receptor internalization in dorsal horn neurons. This was so even under conditions in which there was significant hindpaw inflammation (Abbadie et al. 1997).

How do these results compare with those obtained with antagonists of the NK1 receptor? As noted above, the antagonist studies are somewhat difficult to interpret because of variability of the antagonists (early versions had significant calcium channel blocking activity), mode of administration (systemic versus intrathecal), or because of the particular pain model that was studied. A more telling comparison, however, can be made with mice in which the gene that encodes the NK1 receptor was deleted (De Felipe et al. 1998). In fact, the phenotypes of the NK1 and PPT-A mutant mice differed considerably. Most importantly, in contrast to the PPT-A knockout animals, mice with a deletion of the NK1 receptor gene did not show deficits in acute pain behaviors in response to thermal or mechanical stimuli. Both animals, however, did show decreased responses to the selective C-fiber activator capsaicin, and both showed an almost complete absence of neurogenic inflammation.

What can account for these striking differences? Fig. 1 illustrates, in a highly schematic form, major elements at the primary afferent, peptide-containing terminal in the superficial dorsal horn. In the "normal" condition (i.e., in the absence of gene deletion), the terminal releases glutamate, which can target multiple glutamate receptors, (none of which are illustrated), as well as the peptides, SP and NKA. The latter can activate the postsynaptic neuron via multiple tachykinin receptor subtypes (Fig. 1A). To simplify the figure, I have placed the three major subtypes (NK1, 2, and 3) on a single postsynaptic neuron, but these are probably distributed among projection neurons and interneurons. In the PPT-A knockout mice, both SP and NKA are absent (Fig. 1C). Thus, no primary afferent tachykinin peptide influence is possible. The NK3 receptor will be targeted by neurokinin B (NKB), a natural ligand with high affinity for the NK3 receptor, but NKB is not found in primary afferents. Compare this arrangement with what occurs in the NK1-receptor knockout mice (Fig. 1B). Here the tachykinins will be released from the primary afferent terminal, as in the wild-type mice. Although they can no longer target the NK1 receptor, they may still act upon NK2 and NK3 receptors (Fig. 1B). Moreover, because NKA can diffuse considerable distances from its site of release (Duggan et al. 1990), its "sphere of influence" is not affected. It is not surprising, therefore, that the PPT-A and NK1 receptor mutant mice are not identical.

These studies illustrate how studies in transgenic mice can reveal features of the neurochemistry of nociceptive processing that could not be surmised exclusively from the use of antagonists. Obviously it will be important to perform studies with a combination of antagonists directed against the multiple neurokinin receptors. These will provide information that will help decipher the mechanisms that underlie the difference between deleting ligands and receptors in the mutant mice.

As noted above, one of the more surprising results in the PPT-A knockout mice was that neither tissue-injury-induced nor nerve injury-induced thermal or mechanical allodynia was altered in the mutant animals. Although compensatory responses during development may have masked this pheno-

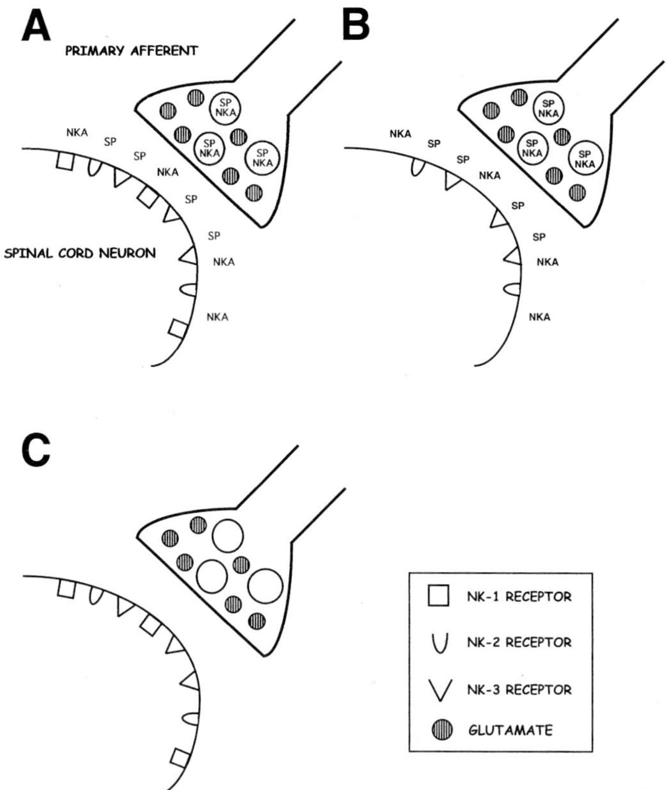

Fig. 1. Diagrams illustrating some differences between deleting a gene that encodes a neurotransmitter receptor (in this case the NK1 receptor) and deleting a gene that encodes the precursor for the neurotransmitter peptides that target the receptor. (A) The normal terminal of small-diameter primary afferents contains glutamate, in small clear vesicles, and the preprotachykinin (PPT-A) products, substance P (SP) and neurokinin A (NKA), in dense-core vesicles. Also depicted is a postsynaptic dorsal horn neuron that for simplicity's sake expresses all three neurokinin receptors on its surface. Importantly, SP and NKA can target each of the three neurokinin receptors, albeit with different affinities. (B) In a mouse with a deletion of the NK1 receptor, the tachykinins may still influence the postsynaptic neurons, via the remaining NK2 and NK3 receptors. (C) In contrast, when the PPT-A gene is deleted, there is no possible primary afferent-derived tachykinin influence upon the dorsal horn neurons.

type, we believe that changes downstream of the primary afferent may be more critical to the development of central sensitization and to its behavioral correlate, lowered nociceptive thresholds. In fact, many studies have implicated a variety of second messenger systems in the development of central sensitization. Of particular interest is the contribution of the lipid- and Ca^{2+}-dependent protein kinases C (PKC). Using very nonselective blockers or activators of PKC, which do not distinguish among the many isoforms of this enzymes, several laboratories have provided evidence that injury-induced facilitation of nociceptive processing can be reduced (Coderre 1992; Mao et al. 1992, 1993; Yashpal et al. 1995).

Given that the different isoforms of PKC are expressed throughout the brain and spinal cord as well as in peripheral tissue, including non-neuronal cells, it is difficult to discern the mechanism through which these pharmacological manipulations influence pain processing. Transgenic mice with highly specific deletions of isoforms of PKC offer a valuable tool. For several reasons, our studies focused on the contribution of the gamma isoform of PKC (Malmberg et al. 1997). First, in contrast to the other isoforms, PKCγ is not expressed until after birth; thus, the developmental consequences of gene deletion can be avoided. Furthermore, PKCγ is only expressed in neurons. Most importantly perhaps, in the spinal cord, PKCγ is found exclusively in a population of interneurons in the inner part of the substantia gelatinosa, lamina II. Finally, PKCγ is the only PKC isoform that is not found in DRG neurons. Thus, any phenotype that is identified in PKCγ mutant mice could be interpreted as arising from a distinct group of spinal cord interneurons, rather than be attributed to changes in the properties of primary afferents or of dorsal horn projection neurons.

In contrast to the phenotype of the PPT-A mutant mice, we found that acute pain processing was entirely normal in the mice with a deletion of the gene that encodes PKCγ (Malmberg et al. 1997). This was true for noxious thermal, mechanical, and chemical stimuli, whether they were applied to visceral or somatic tissue. By contrast, in a mouse model of neuropathic pain that is produced by partial sciatic nerve section, we found a remarkable difference in the magnitude of the resultant mechanical and thermal allodynia. Within 24 hours of nerve injury, wild-type mice show a profound drop in the mechanical and thermal threshold for evoking withdrawal of the hindpaw. In the PKCγ mutant mice, however, at most a mild allodynia developed. Because the allodynia is presumed to arise from nerve-injury-induced central sensitization of dorsal horn neurons such that normally innocuous stimuli can now evoke nocifensive reflexes, these results pointed to the PKCγ interneuron as critical. Clearly, these conclusions could not have been established in pharmacological studies; there are no selective inhibitors of PKCγ. Taken together, these results offer an excellent example of how transgenic technology can provide insights into pain mechanisms that would not be possible with other approaches. Obviously, the development of selective antagonists of PKCγ or of the membrane protein to which the activated form of the kinase binds will greatly facilitate analyses of PKCγ's contribution to pain mechanisms, but until that development, the knockout mice provide the best alternative.

In summary, I believe that transgenic technology has clearly had a very positive influence on pain research. There are many caveats of which we must be aware. However, it is certain that the transgenic mice (overexpressers, knock-ins, and knockouts) can provide information that is very difficult to collect by more traditional approaches. Until much more selective pharmacological antagonists are developed, studies with these mice will continue to provide important insights into pain mechanisms.

ACKNOWLEDGMENT

This work was supported by NIH grants NS14627, NS21445, DE08973, and DA08377.

REFERENCES

Abbadie C, Trafton J, Liu H, Mantyh PW, Basbaum AI. Inflammation increases the distribution of dorsal horn neurons that internalize the neurokinin-1 receptor in response to noxious and non-noxious stimulation. *J Neurosci* 1997; 17:8049–8060.

Albers KM, Wright DE, Davis BM. Overexpression of nerve growth factor in epidermis of transgenic mice causes hypertrophy of the peripheral nervous system. *J Neurosci* 1994; 14:1422–1432.

Basbaum AI, Woolf CJ. Pain. *Curr Biol* 1999; 9:R429–431.

Bennett GJ, Xie Y-K. A peripheral mononeuropathy in rat that produces disorders of pain sensation like those seen in man. *Pain* 1988; 33:87–107.

Birder LA, Perl ER. Expression of alpha$_2$-adrenergic receptors in rat primary afferent neurones after peripheral nerve injury or inflammation. *J Physiol (Lond)* 1999; 515:533–542.

Cao YQ, Mantyh PW, Carlson EJ, et al. Primary afferent tachykinins are required to experience moderate to intense pain. *Nature (Lond)* 1998; 392:390–394.

Coderre TJ. Contribution of protein kinase C to central sensitization and persistent pain following tissue injury. *Neurosci Lett* 1992; 140:181–184.

Cridland RA, Henry JL. Comparison of the effects of substance P, neurokinin A, physalaemin and eledoisin in facilitating a nociceptive reflex in the rat. *Brain Res* 1986; 381:93–99.

Davis BM, Lewin GR, Mendell LM, Jones ME, Albers KM. Altered expression of nerve growth factor in the skin of transgenic mice leads to changes in response to mechanical stimuli. *Neuroscience* 1993; 56:789–792.

Davis BM, Albers KM, Seroogy KB, Katz DM. Overexpression of nerve growth factor in transgenic mice induces novel sympathetic projections to primary sensory neurons. *J Comp Neurol* 1994; 349:464–474.

Davis BM, Fundin BT, Albers KM, et al. Overexpression of nerve growth factor in skin causes preferential increases among innervation to specific sensory targets. *J Comp Neurol* 1997; 387:489–506.

Davis BM, Goodness TP, Soria A, Albers KM. Over-expression of NGF in skin causes formation of novel sympathetic projections to trkA-positive sensory neurons. *Neuroreport* 1998; 20:1103–1107.

De Biasi S, Rustioni A. Glutamate and substance P coexist in primary afferent terminals in the superficial laminae of spinal cord. *Proc Natl Acad Sci USA* 1988; 85:7820–7824.

de Castro F, Silos-Santiago I, Lopez de Armentia M, Barbacid M, Belmonte C. Corneal innervation and sensitivity to noxious stimuli in trkA knockout mice. *Eur J Neurosci* 1998; 10:146–152.

De Felipe C, Herrero JF, O'Brien JA, et al. Altered nociception, analgesia and aggression in mice lacking the receptor for substance P. *Nature (Lond)* 1998; 392:394–397.

Devor M, Janig W, Michaelis M. Modulation of activity in dorsal root ganglion neurons by sympathetic activation in nerve-injured rats. *J Neurophysiol* 1994; 71:38–47.

Dougherty PM, Palecek J, Zorn S, Willis WD. Combined application of excitatory amino acids and substance P produces long-lasting changes in responses of primate spinothalamic tract neurons. *Brain Res Rev* 1993; 18:227–246.

Dubner R, Basbaum AI. Spinal dorsal horn plasticity following tissue or nerve injury. In: Wall PD, Melzack R (Eds). *The Textbook of Pain,* 3rd ed. London: Churchill-Livingstone, 1994, pp 225–241.

Duggan AW, Hendry IA, Morton CR, Hutchison WD, Zhao ZQ. Cutaneous stimuli releasing immunoreactive substance P in the dorsal horn of the cat. *Brain Res* 1988; 451:261–273.

Duggan AW, Hope PJ, Jarrott B, Schaible HG, Fleetwood WS. Release, spread and persistence of immunoreactive neurokinin A in the dorsal horn of the cat following noxious cutaneous stimulation. Studies with antibody microprobes. *Neuroscience* 1990; 35:195–202.

Fried K, Govrin-Lippman R, Rosenthal F, Ellisman MH, Devor M. Ultrastructure of afferent axons endings in a neuroma. *J Neurocytol* 1991; 20:682–701.

Grutzner EH, Garry MG, Hargreaves KM. Effect of injury on pulpal levels of immunoreactive substance P and immunoreactive calcitonin gene-related peptide. *J Endo* 1992; 18:553–557.

Kim KJ, Yoon YW, Chung JM. Comparison of three rodent neuropathic pain models. *Exp Brain Res* 1997; 113:200–206.

Levine JD, Fields HL, Basbaum AI. Peptides and the primary afferent nociceptor. *J Neurosci* 1993; 13:2273–2286.

Lewin GR, Ritter AM, Mendell LM. Nerve growth factor-induced hyperalgesia in the neonatal and adult rat. *J Neurosci* 1993; 13:2136–2148.

Ma QP, Woolf CJ. Tachykinin NK1 receptor antagonist RP67580 attenuates progressive hypersensitivity of flexor reflex during experimental inflammation in rats. *Eur J Pharmacol* 1997; 322:165–171.

Maggi CA. The mammalian tachykinin receptors. *Gen Pharmacol* 1995; 26:911–944.

Malmberg AB, Basbaum AI. Partial injury to the sciatic nerve in the mouse: neuropathic pain behavior and dorsal horn plasticity. *Pain* 1998; 76:215–222.

Malmberg AB, Chen C, Tonegawa S, Basbaum AI. Preserved acute pain and reduced neuropathic pain in mice lacking PKCγ. *Science* 1997; 278:279–283.

Mantyh PW, DeMaster E, Malhotra A, et al. Receptor endocytosis and dendrite reshaping in spinal neurons after somatosensory stimulation. *Science* 1995; 268:1629–1632.

Mao J, Price DD, Mayer DJ, Hayes RL. Pain-related increases in spinal cord membrane-bound protein kinase C following peripheral nerve injury. *Brain Res* 1992; 588:144–149.

Mao J, Mayer DJ, Hayes RL, Price DD. Spatial patterns of increased spinal cord membrane-bound protein kinase C and their relation to increases in ^{14}C-2-deoxyglucose metabolic activity in rats with painful peripheral mononeuropathy. *J Neurophysiol* 1993; 70:470–481.

Marvizon JCG, Martinez V, Grady EF, Bunnett NW, Mayer EA. Neurokinin 1 receptor internalization in spinal cord slices induced by dorsal root stimulation is mediated by NMDA receptors. *J Neurosci* 1997; 17:8129–8136.

McLachlan EM, Janig W, Devor M, Michaelis M. Peripheral nerve injury triggers noradrenergic sprouting within dorsal root ganglia. *Nature (Lond)* 1993; 363:543–546.

Mogil JS, Grisel JE. Transgenic studies of pain. *Pain* 1998; 77:107–128.

Mogil JS, Sternberg WF, Marek P, et al. The genetics of pain and pain inhibition. *Proc Natl Acad Sci USA* 1996; 93:3048–3055.

Mogil JS, Yu L, Basbaum AI. Pain genes: natural variation and transgenic mutants. *Ann Rev Neurosci* 2000; 23:777–811.

Mombaerts P, Wang F, Dulac C, et al. Visualizing an olfactory sensory map. *Cell* 1996; 87:675–686.

Noguchi K, Kawai Y, Fukuoka T, Senba E, Miki K. Substance P induced by peripheral nerve injury in primary afferent sensory neurons and its effect on dorsal column nucleus neurons. *J Neurosci* 1995; 15:7633–7643.

Otten U, Goedert M, Mayer N, Lembeck F. Requirement of nerve growth factor for development of substance P-containing sensory neurones. *Nature (Lond)* 1980; 287:158–159.

Price DD, Bennett GJ, Rafii A. Psychophysical observations on patients with neuropathic pain relieved by a sympathetic block. *Pain* 1989; 36:273–288.

Radhakrishnan V, Henry JL. Excitatory amino acid receptor mediation of sensory inputs to functionally identified dorsal horn neurons in cat spinal cord. *Neuroscience* 1993; 55:531–544.

Ramer MS, Bisby MA. Adrenergic innervation of rat sensory ganglia following proximal or distal painful sciatic neuropathy: distinct mechanisms revealed by anti-NGF treatment. *Eur J Neurosci* 1999; 11:837–846.

Randic M, Hecimovic H, Ryu PD. Substance P modulates glutamate-induced currents in acutely isolated rat spinal dorsal horn neurones. *Neurosci Lett* 1990; 117:74–80.

Sato J, Perl ER. Adrenergic excitation of cutaneous pain receptors induced by peripheral nerve injury. *Science* 1991; 251:1608–1610.

Silos-Santiago I, Molliver DC, Ozaki S, et al. Non-TrkA-expressing small DRG neurons are lost in TrkA deficient mice. *J Neurosci* 1995; 15:5929–5942.

Smeyne RJ, Klein R, Schnapp A, et al. Severe sensory and sympathetic neuropathies in mice carrying a disrupted Trk/NGF receptor gene. *Nature (Lond)* 1994; 368:246–249.

Stark KL, Oostings RS, Hen R. Inducible knockout strategies to probe the functions of 5-HT receptors. *Ann NY Acad Sci* 1998; 861:57–66.

Stucky CL, Koltzenburg M, Schneider M, et al. Overexpression of nerve growth factor in skin selectively affects the survival and functional properties of nociceptors. *J Neurosci* 1999; 19:8509–8516.

Tölle TR, Berthele A, Zieglgänsberger W, Seeburg PH, Wisden W. The differential expression of 16 NMDA and non-NMDA receptor subunits in the rat spinal cord and in periaqueductal gray. *J Neurosci* 1993; 13:5009–5028.

Wakisaka S, Kajander KC, Bennett GJ. Increased neuropeptide Y (NPY)-like immunoreactivity in rat sensory neurons following peripheral axotomy. *Neurosci Lett* 1991; 124:200–203.

Wall PD, Gutnick M. Properties of afferent nerve impulses originating from a neuroma. *Nature (Lond)* 1974; 248:740–743.

Woolf CJ, Thompson S. The induction and maintenance of central sensitization is dependent on N-methyl-D-aspartic acid receptor activation: implications for the treatment of post-injury pain hypersensitivity states. *Pain* 1991; 44:293–299.

Yaksh TL, Jessell TM, Gamse R, Mudge AW, Leeman SE. Intrathecal morphine inhibits substance P release from mammalian spinal cord in vivo. *Nature (Lond)* 1980; 286:155–157.

Yamamoto T, Yaksh TL. Effects of intrathecal capsaicin and an NK-1 antagonist, CP,96-345, on the thermal hyperalgesia observed following unilateral constriction of the sciatic nerve in the rat. *Pain* 1992; 51:329–334.

Yashpal K, Radhakrishnan V, Coderre TJ, Henry JL. CP-96,345, but not its stereoisomer, CP-96,344, blocks the nociceptive responses to intrathecally administered substance P and to noxious thermal and chemical stimuli in the rat. *Neuroscience* 1993; 52:1039–1047.

Yashpal K, Pitcher GM, Parent A, Quirion R, Coderre TJ. Noxious thermal and chemical stimulation induce increases in ^{3}H-phorbol 12,13-dibutyrate binding in spinal cord dorsal horn as well as persistent pain and hyperalgesia, which is reduced by inhibition of protein kinase C. *J Neurosci* 1995; 15:3263–3272.

Correspondence to: Allan I. Basbaum, PhD, Department of Anatomy, University of California, San Francisco, 513 Parnassus Avenue, Box 0452, San Francisco, CA 94143, USA. Tel: 415-476-5270; Fax: 415-476-4845; e-mail: aib@phy.ucsf.edu.

Proceedings of the 9th World Congress on Pain,
Progress in Pain Research and Management,
Vol. 16, edited by M. Devor, M.C. Rowbotham, and
Z. Wiesenfeld-Hallin, IASP Press, Seattle, © 2000.

30

Spinal Substance P Receptor Expression and Internalization in Acute, Short-Term, and Long-Term Inflammatory Pain States

Prisca Honoré and Patrick W. Mantyh

Neurosystems Center, Departments of Preventive Sciences, Psychiatry, and Neuroscience, and Cancer Center, University of Minnesota, Minneapolis, Minnesota; and Molecular Neurobiology Laboratory, VA Medical Center, Minneapolis, Minnesota, USA

Chronic inflammation is responsible for various persistent pain states, including arthritis, back pain, and temporomandibular joint disorder. Although significant progress has been made in understanding the peripheral inflammatory response, the neurochemical changes within the spinal cord that are involved in the generation and maintenance of chronic inflammatory pain are poorly understood. In response to persistent inflammatory pain, normally innocuous sensory stimuli are perceived as painful (allodynia), and mildly noxious sensory stimuli are perceived as highly painful (hyperalgesia). Both hyperalgesia and allodynia are thought to arise from a sensitization of peripheral nociceptors (peripheral sensitization) and of spinal dorsal horn neurons (central sensitization) (Treede et al. 1992).

In an effort to understand the mechanisms involved in the peripheral and central sensitization associated with acute, short-term, and long-term inflammatory pain, we explored the expression and internalization of the substance P receptor (SPR; also called the neurokinin 1 [NK1] receptor) in the spinal dorsal horn of the rat (Mantyh et al. 1995, 1997; Allen et al. 1997). Using well-characterized experimental models, we induced inflammatory pain by unilateral subcutaneous (s.c.) injection of formalin, carrageenan, or complete Freund's adjuvant (CFA) into the hindpaw. In addition, we examined the neurochemical changes in an animal model of polyarthritis induced by CFA injection into the base of the tail. Each of these inflammatory models is characterized by a different onset and time course of nociceptive inputs and responses. Finally, we evaluated the effects of non-noxious and noxious mechanical stimulation in animals injected with carrageenan and CFA. We compared the previous electrophysiological and behavioral data with the alterations in the amount and site of release of substance P (SP) from primary afferent neurons, the number and location of SPR-expressing spinal neurons that are thus activated, and the populations of neurons showing upregulation of the SPR.

ACUTE INFLAMMATORY PAIN

Formalin induces a stereotypical biphasic response, consisting of an early, brief, painful response followed by a prolonged period of tonic (persistent) pain (Dubuisson and Dennis 1977; Dickenson and Sullivan 1987a,b). Although it is generally agreed that the first phase results from a direct action of formalin on nociceptive primary afferent fibers, the factors contributing to the second phase have not been fully defined. In formalin-injected rats we observed significant SPR internalization in lamina I of the spinal dorsal horn at the end of the first phase (8 minutes), a time where there was almost no detectable peripheral edema. At 1 hour following the initial injection, SPR internalization was still observed in most lamina I SPR immunoreactive (-ir) neurons; by that time significant peripheral edema had developed.

It is of interest to compare this pattern of internalization with that produced by a single injection of capsaicin (Mantyh et al. 1995). Capsaicin induces a rapid, marked SPR internalization that is confined to lamina I neurons and is largely resolved at 1 hour post-injection. In contrast, 1 hour after formalin injection, a significant SPR internalization persists in lamina I neurons, suggesting an ongoing release of SP from primary afferent terminals. These results suggest ongoing primary afferent input from C fibers and release of SP in the spinal cord during both the first and second phases of the formalin response. These data agree with previous reports demonstrating that SPR antagonists could block both the first and second phases of the formalin response in spinal neurons (Chapman and Dickenson 1993) and that peripheral injection of local anesthetics after the end of the first phase reduces the electrophysiological, behavioral, and anatomical correlates of the second phase (Dickenson and Sullivan 1987a; Taylor et al. 1995; Puig and Sorkin 1996; Abbadie et al. 1997a). These results provide further evidence that a major component of the second phase of the formalin response is due to ongoing activity of primary afferent neurons. Together these results suggest that the neurochemical signature of acute inflammation is similar to, although with a longer time course than, the reaction produced by a brief chemical noxious stimulus, i.e., a stimulus that produces acute pain under nonpathological conditions.

SHORT-TERM INFLAMMATORY PAIN

In rats injected with carrageenan, peripheral edema, allodynia, and hyperalgesia had fully developed within 3 hours of injection. In this condition, SPR internalization was observed early (10 minutes after injection) in dendrites and in a few lamina I SPR-ir neurons. This finding indicates that SP release occurs in the early stage of carrageenan inflammation. However, there is a major difference between carrageenan-induced inflammation (short-term) and formalin-induced inflammation (acute). We found that formalin injection induced SPR internalization in lamina I neurons, even at 1 hour post-injection, whereas there was no evidence of ongoing SPR internalization at 3 hours post-carrageenan injection. This lack of ongoing SPR internalization suggests either that there was no significant release of SP (using SP-induced SPR internalization as an assay of SP release) from primary afferents, even though a significant edema had developed by this time, or that the system had desensitized, i.e., the receptor no longer responded. This absence of ongoing SPR internalization agrees with the observation that there is no spontaneous activity of dorsal horn neurons 3 hours after carrageenan injection (Stanfa et al. 1992; see however Kocher et al. 1987), although many spinal neurons express the FOS protein in laminae I–II and III–IV 3 hours after carrageenan injection (Honore et al. 1995, 1997). If spinal FOS induction is a reflection of neuronal activation (Hunt et al. 1987; Munglani and Hunt 1995; Doyle and Hunt 1999), it seems reasonable to conclude that nociceptive input from the periphery to the spinal cord must be maintained during the development of carrageenan inflammation. Whether this is due to SP that is released immediately after carrageenan injection or to other neurotransmitters such as excitatory amino acids, remains unclear.

What is apparent at 3 hours post-carrageenan injection is that normally non-noxious mechanical stimulation of the carrageenan-inflamed hindpaw, which does not induce SPR internalization in normal animals, now induces massive SPR internalization in lamina I neurons. Furthermore, noxious mechanical stimulation, which induces SPR internalization only in lamina I in normal animals, now induces SPR internalization in neurons of laminae I and III–IV.

A key question raised by these observations is whether these laminae III–IV SPR-ir neurons are activated by increased release and diffusion of SP from terminals that reside in laminae I–II, or by de novo synthesis and release of SP from primary afferent neurons that terminate in laminae III–IV. Following peripheral inflammation, an increase has been reported in SP synthesis by small DRG neurons that normally synthesize SP (Donnerer et al. 1993; Galeazza et al. 1995) and by large DRG neurons (Neumann et al. 1996). Release of SP by Aβ fibers could explain the SPR internalization observed in laminae III–IV after non-noxious stimulation in long-term inflammatory pain (Abbadie et al. 1997b). However, 3 hours after carrageenan injection, there would appear to be insufficient time for de novo synthesis and transport of SP from primary afferent cell body to the terminals in the spinal cord.

These data suggest that the SPR internalization observed in lamina I following normally innocuous stimulation and the increased SPR internalization observed in laminae I–II and III–IV following noxious stimulation are due primarily to peripheral sensitization that manifests itself as a greater release and diffusion of SP from primary afferent neurons that normally express SP. This increase in SP release from primary afferent fibers could allow SP to diffuse significantly farther, resulting in a switch from synaptic to volume neurotransmission (Agnati et al. 1995; Zoli et al. 1998). Because SP would diffuse and interact with SPRs at both synaptic and extrasynaptic sites, this increased release of SP from primary afferent fibers could also explain why there is significantly greater SPR internalization in lamina I SPR neurons after noxious stimulation under inflammatory conditions. Based on these observations, we suggest that this neurochemical signature of short-term inflammation is characterized by a lack of spontaneous SP release from primary afferents, as reflected by the lack of ongoing SPR internalization, a lack of SPR upregulation, and a switch from synaptic to volume transmission. Thus, more SPR-ir spinal neurons in a wider area are activated in response to innocuous or noxious stimuli.

LONG-TERM INFLAMMATORY PAIN

CFA-induced unilateral inflammation and adjuvant-induced polyarthritis are two of the most commonly used models of long-term inflammatory pain. These animal models elicit peak symptoms at 3 and 21 days, respectively. Similarities in the neurochemical signature of short- and long-term inflammatory pain include the lack of ongoing SPR internalization in basal unstimulated condition and an increase in the number and location of the spinal neurons that show SPR internalization in response to either normally non-noxious or noxious stimuli.

The major difference in the spinal cords of animals with short- vs. long-term inflammation is that the latter is associated with significant upregulation of the SPR on neurons in lamina I of the spinal cord. The increase in SPR mRNA observed in the spinal cord several days after peripheral inflammation has been blocked by morphine or SPR antagonists (Noguchi et al. 1988; McCarson and Krause 1994, 1995, 1996), which suggests that SP release or SPR activation is necessary for SPR upregulation. However, both in chronic inflammatory pain, which is associated with an increase in SP in primary afferents (Lembeck et al. 1981; Donaldson et al. 1992), and after nerve injury, which is associated with a decrease of SP in primary afferents (Noguchi et al. 1989; Garrison et al. 1993), SPR immunoreactivity increases in lamina I of the spinal dorsal horn (Abbadie et al. 1996). Additionally, while cAMP has been reported to be involved in the regulation of SPR expression, SPR activation leads to the production of inositol phosphates, suggesting that SP is not the major regulator of SPR expression. These findings suggest that while SP could contribute to SPR upregulation, other neurotransmitters, acting directly on SPR-ir neurons or indirectly via the release of yet unknown factors, must be involved.

If there is a significant upregulation of the SPR in lamina I neurons in long-term inflammation, does it alter the response properties of these neurons? Several electrophysiological studies have shown that the response of spinal cord neurons to peripheral stimuli increases in an inflammatory pain state (Hylden et al. 1989; Haley et al. 1990; Simone et al. 1991; Dougherty et al. 1992; Stanfa et al. 1992; Urban et al. 1993; Neugebauer et al. 1994). This increased responsiveness is hypothesized to be largely mediated by a facilitated transmission through the N-methyl D-aspartate (NMDA) receptor. SPR activation leads to the generation of diacyl glycerol and inositol triphosphate, inducing an increase in intracellular calcium and a synergistic facilitation of the activity of protein kinase C. In turn, protein kinase C induces phosphorylation of the NMDA receptors, counteracting the magnesium block and allowing the receptors to operate at a more negative potential (for review see Urban et al. 1994; Yaksh et al. 1995; Urban and Gebhart 1998; Millan 1999). These data suggest that SPR activation enhances NMDA-receptor-mediated events and that the combined activation of SPR and NMDA receptors leads to increased neuronal excitability. The SPR upregulation observed in long-term inflammatory pain states may therefore contribute to the central sensitization that accompanies such pain.

CONCLUSIONS

Previous experimental and clinical studies have suggested distinctive differences between acute and chronic pain, including the shift from a sensitization of primary afferent neurons to a sensitization of spinal cord neurons. What is unique about the present approach is the ability to visualize and quantify neurochemical changes at the single-cell and intracellular level as a pain "moves" from the acute to the long-term state. These results suggest that SPR internalization might serve as a marker of the contribution of ongoing primary afferent input to acute or persistent pain states. A similar approach to understanding the changes that other neurotransmitter/receptor systems undergo as a pain moves from acute to chronic should provide insight into the mechanisms involved in the generation and maintenance of chronic pain.

ACKNOWLEDGMENTS

This work was supported by a Merit Review from the Veterans Administration, the Spinal Cord Society, NIH grants NS23970, AG11852, DA11986, and training grant DEO7288.

REFERENCES

Abbadie C, Brown JL, Mantyh PW, Basbaum AI. Spinal cord substance P receptor immunoreactivity increases in both inflammatory and nerve injury models of persistent pain. *Neuroscience* 1996; 70:201–209.

Abbadie C, Taylor BK, Peterson MA, Basbaum AI. Differential contribution of the two phases of the formalin test to the pattern of c-fos expression in the rat spinal cord: studies with remifentanil and lidocaine. *Pain* 1997a; 69:101–110.

Abbadie C, Trafton J, Liu H, Mantyh PW, Basbaum AI. Inflammation increases the distribution of dorsal horn neurons that internalize the neurokinin-1 receptor in response to noxious and non-noxious stimulation. *J Neurosci* 1997b; 17:8049–8060.

Agnati LF, Zoli M, Stromberg I, Fuxe K. Intercellular communication in the brain: wiring versus volume transmission. *Neuroscience* 1995; 69:711–726.

Allen BJ, Rogers SD, Ghilardi JR, et al. Noxious cutaneous thermal stimuli induce a graded release of endogenous substance P in the spinal cord: imaging peptide action in vivo. *J Neurosci* 1997; 17(15):5921–5927.

Chapman V, Dickenson AH. The effect of intrathecal administration of RP67580, a potent neurokinin 1 antagonist on nociceptive transmission in the rat spinal cord. *Neurosci Lett* 1993; 157:149–152.

Dickenson AH, Sullivan AF. Peripheral origins and central modulation of subcutaneous formalin-induced activity of rat dorsal horn neurons. *Neurosci Lett* 1987a; 83:207–211.

Dickenson AH, Sullivan AF. Subcutaneous formalin-induced activity of dorsal horn neurones in the rat: differential response to an intrathecal opiate administered pre or post formalin. *Pain* 1987b; 30:349–360.

Donaldson LF, Harmar AJ, McQueen DS, Seckl JR. Increased expression of preprotachykinin, calcitonin gene-related peptide, but not vasoactive intestinal peptide messenger RNA in dorsal root ganglia during the development of adjuvant monoarthritis in the rat. *Mol Brain Res* 1992; 16:143–149.

Donnerer J, Schuligoi R, Stein C, Amann R. Upregulation, release and axonal transport of substance P and calcitonin gene-related peptide in adjuvant inflammation and regulatory function of nerve growth factor. *Reg Peptides* 1993; 46:150–154.

Dougherty PM, Sluka KA, Sorkin LS, Westlund KN, Willis WD. Enhanced responses of spinothalamic tract neurons to excitatory amino acids parallel the generation of acute arthritis in the monkey. *Brain Res* 1992; 17:1–13.

Doyle CA, Hunt SP. Substance P receptor (neurokinin-1)-expressing neurons in lamina I of the spinal cord encode for the intensity of noxious stimulation: a c-Fos study in rat. *Neuroscience* 1999; 89:17–28.

Dubuisson D, Dennis SG. The formalin test: a quantitative study of the analgesic effects of morphine, meperidine, and brain stem stimulation in rats and cats. *Pain* 1977; 4:161–174.

Galeazza MT, Garry MG, Yost HJ, et al. Plasticity in the synthesis and storage of substance P and calcitonin gene-related peptide in primary afferent neurons during peripheral inflammation. *Neuroscience* 1995; 66:443–458.

Garrison CJ, Dougherty PM, Carlton SM. Quantitative analysis of substance P and calcitonin gene-related peptide immunohistochemical staining in the dorsal horn of neuropathic MK-801-treated rats. *Brain Res* 1993; 607:205–214.

Haley JE, Sullivan AF, Dickenson AH. Evidence for spinal N-methyl-D-aspartate receptor involvement in prolonged chemical nociception in the rat. *Brain Res* 1990; 518:218–226.

Honore P, Buritova J, Besson JM. Carrageenin-evoked c-Fos expression in rat lumbar spinal cord: the effects of indomethacin. *Eur J Pharmacol* 1995; 272:249–259.

Honoré P, Buritova J, Fournié-Zaluski MC, Roques BP, Besson J-M. Antinociceptive effects of RB101, a complete inhibitor of enkephalin-catabolizing enzymes, are enhanced by a CCK_B receptor antagonist as revealed by noxiously-evoked spinal c-Fos expression in the rat. *J Pharmacol Exp Ther* 1997; 281:208–217.

Hunt SP, Pini A, Evan G. Induction of *c-fos*-like protein in spinal cord neurons following sensory stimulation. *Nature* 1987; 328:632–634.

Kocher L, Anton F, Reeh PW, Handwerker HO. The effect of carrageenin-induced inflammation on the sensitivity of unmyelinated skin nociceptors in the rat. *Pain* 1987; 29:363–373.

Lembeck F, Donnerer J, Colpaert FC. Increase of substance P in primary afferent nerves during chronic pain. *Neuropeptides* 1981; 1:175–180.

Mantyh PW, DeMaster E, Malhotra A, et al. Receptor endocytosis and dendrite reshaping in spinal neurons after somatosensory stimulation. *Science* 1995; 268:1629–1632.

Mantyh PW, Rogers SD, Honoré P, et al. Inhibition of hyperalgesia by ablation of lamina I spinal neurons expressing the substance P receptor. *Science* 1997; 278:275–279.

McCarson KE, Krause JE. NK-1 and NK-3 type tachykinin receptor mRNA expression in the rat spinal cord dorsal horn is increased during adjuvant or formalin-induced nociception. *J Neurosci* 1994; 14:712–720.

McCarson KE, Krause JE. The formalin-induced expression of tachykinin peptide and neurokinin receptor messenger RNAs in rat sensory ganglia and spinal cord is modulated by opiate preadministration. *Neuroscience* 1995; 64:729–739.

McCarson KE, Krause JE. The neurokinin-1 receptor antagonist LY306,740 blocks nociception-induced increases in dorsal horn neurokinin-1 receptor gene expression. *Mol Pharmacol* 1996; 50:1189–1199.

Millan MJ. The induction of pain: an integrative review. *Prog Neurobiol* 1999; 57(1):1–164.

Munglani R, Hunt SP. Molecular biology of pain. *Br J Anaesth* 1995; 75:186–192.

Neugebauer V, Lucke T, Grubb B, Schaible HG. The involvement of N-methyl-D-aspartate (NMDA) and non-NMDA receptors in the responsiveness of rat spinal neurons with input from the chronically inflamed ankle. *Neurosci Lett* 1994; 170:237–240.

Neumann S, Doubell TP, Leslie T, Woolf CJ. Inflammatory pain hypersensitivity mediated by phenotypic switch in myelinated primary sensory neurons. *Nature* 1996; 384:360–364.

Noguchi K, Morita Y, Kiyama H, Ono K, Tohyama M. A noxious stimulus induces the preprotachykinin-A gene expression in the rat dorsal root ganglion: a quantitative study using in situ hybridization. *Brain Res* 1988; 464:31–35.

Noguchi K, Senba E, Morita Y, Sato M, Tohyama M. Prepro-VIP and preprotachykinin mRNAs in the rat dorsal root ganglion cells following peripheral axotomy. *Mol Brain Res* 1989; 6:327–330.

Puig S, Sorkin LS. Formalin-evoked activity in identified primary afferent fibers: systemic lidocaine suppresses phase-2 activity. *Pain* 1996; 64:345–355.

Simone DA, Sorkin LS, Oh U, et al. Neurogenic hyperalgesia: central neural correlates in responses of spinothalamic tract neurons. *J Neurophysiol* 1991; 66:228–246.

Stanfa LC, Sullivan AF, Dickenson AH. Alterations in neuronal excitability and the potency of spinal mu, delta and kappa opioids after carrageenan-induced inflammation. *Pain* 1992; 50:345–354.

Taylor BK, Peterson MA, Basbaum AI. Persistent cardiovascular and behavioral nociceptive responses to subcutaneous formalin require peripheral nerve input. *J Neurosci* 1995; 15:7575–7584.

Treede RD, Meyer RA, Raja SN, Campbell JN. Peripheral and central mechanisms of cutaneous hyperalgesia. *Prog Neurobiol* 1992; 38:397–421.

Urban L, Dray A, Nagy I, Maggi CA. The effects of NK-1 and NK-2 receptor antagonists on the capsaicin evoked synaptic response in the rat spinal cord in vitro. *Reg Peptides* 1993; 46:413–414.

Urban L, Thompson SWN, Dray A. Modulation of spinal excitability: co-operation between neurokinin and excitatory amino acid neurotransmitters. *Trends Neurosci* 1994; 17:432–438.

Urban MO, Gebhart GF. The glutamate synapse: a target in the pharmacological management of hyperalgesic pain states. Glutamate synapse as a therapeutical target: molecular organization and pathology of the glutamate synapse. *Prog Brain Res* 1998; 116:407–420.

Yaksh TL, Chaplan SR, Malmberg AB. Future directions in the pharmacological management of hyperalgesic and allodynic pain states: the NMDA receptor. *NIDA Res Monogr* 1995; 147:84–103.

Zoli M, Torri C, Ferrari R, et al. The emergence of the volume transmission concept. *Brain Res Brain Res Rev* 1998; 26:136–147.

Correspondence to: Patrick W. Mantyh, PhD, Neurosystems Center, 18-208 Moos Tower, 515 Delaware Street, Minneapolis, MN 55455, USA. Tel: 612-626-0810, Fax: 612-626-2565, email: manty001@maroon.tc.umn.edu.

Proceedings of the 9th World Congress on Pain,
Progress in Pain Research and Management,
Vol. 16, edited by M. Devor, M.C. Rowbotham, and
Z. Wiesenfeld-Hallin, IASP Press, Seattle, © 2000.

31

Discrepant Results from Preclinical and Clinical Studies on the Potential of Substance P-Receptor Antagonist Compounds as Analgesics[1]

S. Boyce and R.G. Hill

Merck Sharp and Dohme Research Laboratories, Neuroscience Research Centre, Harlow, Essex, United Kingdom

Since the discovery of abundant substance P in small-diameter primary afferent fibers it has been considered a candidate neurotransmitter for pain. Support for this hypothesis comes from the excitation produced by iontophoretic application of substance P onto dorsal horn neurons (Henry 1976) and behavioral hyperalgesia induced when it is injected intrathecally (Cridland and Henry 1986). Prolonged and intense noxious stimulation causes the release of substance P in the dorsal horn of the spinal cord (Duggan et al. 1987). Substance P most avidly binds to and activates NK1 receptors, which are present on many dorsal horn neurons that respond to noxious peripheral stimulation (Mantyh and Hunt 1985). Recent immunocytochemical studies have shown that NK1 receptors become internalized following noxious peripheral stimulation and that NK1-receptor antagonists can block internalization (Mantyh et al. 1995).

In addition to its effects on spinal nociceptive processing, substance P is also released from peripheral nerve endings where it may contribute to inflammation (Shepheard et al. 1993, 1995) and immunological responses (Okayama et al. 1998). Substance P has also been implicated in the pain associated with migraine. C-fiber sensory afferents that innervate meningeal tissues contain substance P and other neuropeptides and their release may cause neurogenic inflammation that contributes to activation of nociceptive

---

[1] Mini-review based on a congress workshop.

afferents projecting to the brain stem. Such evidence contributed to the expectation that centrally acting NK1-receptor antagonists would be antinociceptive in animals, analgesic in humans, and constitute a novel class of analgesic drug. Although data from preclinical studies are supportive of analgesic potential, clinical trials have not yet shown a convincing analgesic profile for NK1-receptor antagonists. This chapter summarizes recent animal studies and clinical trials with NK1-receptor antagonists and suggests possible reasons for the apparent mismatch between preclinical and clinical studies in pain.

SPECIES DIFFERENCES IN NK1-RECEPTOR PHARMACOLOGY

One of the first problems encountered with preclinical evaluation of NK1-receptor antagonists was the marked species variation in NK1-receptor pharmacology. Compounds such as CP-96,345 (Pfizer) have high affinity for NK1 receptors expressed in human, gerbil, guinea pig, cat, and rabbit brain but low affinity for the rat/mouse receptor (Beresford et al. 1991; see Table I). This finding complicated the evaluation of high-affinity human NK1-receptor antagonists as most established antinociception assays use rats or mice. Although this problem may be overcome by administering high doses of NK1-receptor antagonists to rats or mice to achieve adequate receptor occupancy, other nonspecific pharmacological effects such as blockade of ion channels may confound the interpretation of these studies (see review by Hill and Rupniak 1999). Preclinical assessment of compounds

Table I
Species variants in NK1-receptor pharmacology

	IC_{50} for Inhibition of [^{125}I]-SP Binding (nM)				
Compound	Human	Gerbil	Guinea Pig	Rabbit	Rat
CP-96,345*	28.8	32.3	31.6	41.6	5888
MK-869	0.1	0.3	0.31	–	–
L-733,060	0.87	0.36	0.3	–	550
L-733,061	350	370	240	–	>1000
L-760,735	0.3	0.5	0.34	–	10
GR205171	0.08	0.06	0.09	–	1.4

Note: IC_{50} = median inhibitory dose. [^{125}I]-SP binding assays were performed as described by Cascieri et al. (1992). Cloned human NK1 and rat NK1 receptors were stably expressed in Chinese hamster ovary (CHO) cells. For other species, membrane homogenates were prepared from cerebral cortex.

* Data from Beresford et al. (1991).

selective for human NK1 receptors therefore necessitated development of analgesia assays in species with human-like NK1-receptor pharmacology such as guinea pigs, rabbits, or gerbils (see Table I).

In addition to high affinity at human NK1 receptors, GR205271 (Glaxo) has nanomolar affinity for the rat receptor and thus has been used as a research tool in rats (Table I). Most preclinical studies with LY303870 (Lanepitant, Eli Lilly & Co) have used rats or mice as this compound also has reasonable affinity (8.7 nM) for the rat receptor (Iyengar et al. 1997). To ensure that antinociceptive effects can be confidently attributed to NK1-receptor blockade and not to nonspecific effects, studies need to be carefully controlled where possible by use of enantiomeric pairs of compounds, one having high affinity for the NK1 receptor and the other low affinity. For example, the affinity of L-733,060 for the human NK1 receptor is 0.87 nM, compared with 350 nM for L-733,061 (Merck; Table I) (Rupniak et al. 1996). Most animal studies described in this chapter have used such enantiomeric pairs.

NK1-RECEPTOR ANTAGONISTS IN PRECLINICAL ASSAYS OF NOCICEPTION

In vivo electrophysiological studies on anaesthetized /spinalized or decerebrate/spinalized animals suggest that NK1-receptor agonists may be useful in the management of painful conditions. For example, CP-96,345 and LY303870, but not their less active enantiomers, CP-96,344 and LY396155, are potent inhibitors of the excitation of dorsal horn neurons elicited by prolonged noxious mechanical or thermal peripheral stimulation or by iontophoretic application of substance P in cats (Radhakrishnan and Henry 1991; Radhakrishnan et al. 1998), which shows that these effects are due to a specific blockade of NK1 receptors. In addition, CP-99,994 but not its less active enantiomer CP-100,263, inhibited the facilitation of a spinal flexion reflex produced by C-fiber conditioning stimulation in anaesthetized/spinalized rabbits (Boyce et al. 1993). We have also shown inhibition of wind-up of the spinal flexion reflex in decerebrate/spinalized rabbits with the clinical development compound MK-869 (L-754,030, $ID_{50} = 0.47$ mg/kg i.v.; Fig. 1A).

Despite the clear findings from electrophysiological studies, it was not until the discovery of long-acting brain-penetrant NK1-receptor antagonists such as L-733,060, or compounds with useful affinity at rat receptors like GR205171, that it was possible to demonstrate specific antinociceptive effects of NK1-receptor antagonists in studies of conscious animals following systemic administration (see review by Hill and Rupniak 1999). L-733,060 produced clear enantioselective inhibition of the late-phase nociceptive

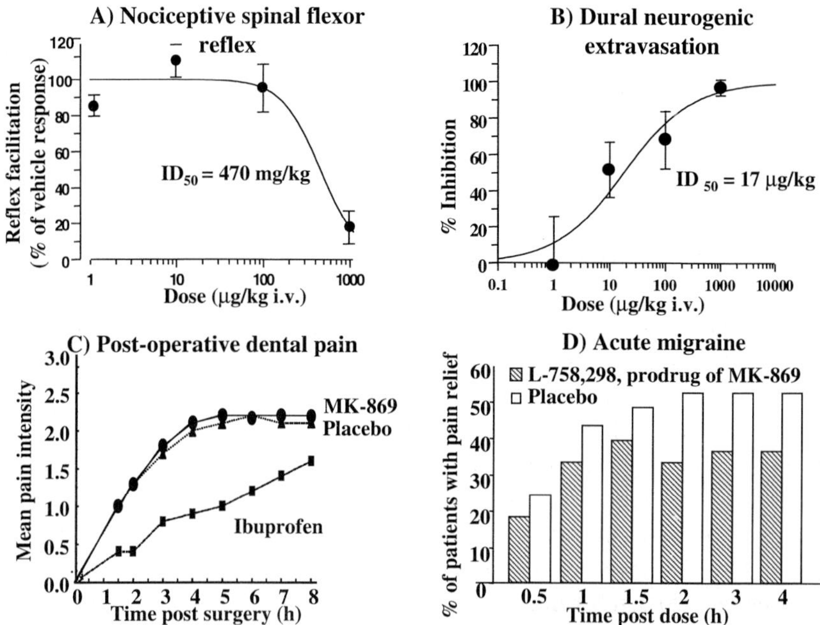

Fig. 1. (A) Inhibition of the facilitation of nociceptive spinal flexor reflex by MK-869 in decerebrate and spinalized rabbits. For methods see Boyce et al. (1999). Animals received vehicle followed by sequential rising doses of MK-869 (1–1000 μg/kg i.v.). Ten minutes after each dose a conditioning stimulus (20 shocks of 1 ms, 2 × threshold voltage for recruiting C-fiber responses, 1 Hz) was applied and the response to the next baseline stimulus was taken as the conditioned response (facilitation). The facilitation was expressed as percentage change of the vehicle response for individual animals. (B) Inhibition of dural neurogenic extravasation by MK-869 in rats. For methods see Shepheard et al. (1993). Rats received MK-869 (1–1000 μg/kg i.v.) or vehicle, and 10 minutes later dural plasma protein extravasation was evoked by electrical stimulation of the right trigeminal ganglion (5 Hz, 5 ms, 25 V for 5 minutes). Data are expressed as percentage inhibition of dural plasma protein extravasation in vehicle-treated animals. (C) Lack of effect of MK-869 in postoperative dental pain (Reinhardt et al. 1998). Patients undergoing third-molar tooth extraction were given oral MK-869 (300 mg; 2 hours prior to surgery), ibuprofen (800 mg; 30 minutes prior to surgery), or matching placebo. Efficacy was measured by time point evaluation of pain intensity for up to 8 hours postsurgery. (D) L-758,298, prodrug of MK-869, is not efficacious as an abortive migraine treatment (Norman et al. 1998). Patients with moderate to severe migraine were given intravenous infusion of L-754,298 (20, 40, or 60 mg) or placebo. Headache severity was assessed at baseline and up to 4 hours post-dose. Data are expressed as the percentage of patients reporting pain relief (only data for 60 mg dose are presented).

responses to intraplantar injection of formalin in gerbils (Rupniak et al. 1996). In the same study, the poorly brain-penetrant compound L-743,310, a potent inhibitor of peripherally mediated, NK1-receptor-agonist-induced chromodacryorrhea, failed to inhibit the late-phase response, which indicates that the antinociceptive effect of L-733,060 occurred via blockade of central NK1 receptors. Consistent with a central antinociceptive action, intrathecal injection of CP-96,345 but not its less active enantiomer CP-96,344, attenuated the late-phase response in rats (Yamamoto and Yaksh 1991). LY303870 also blocked the late phase of the formalin test in rats (Iyengar et al. 1997), although it is not clear whether this effect is mediated centrally or peripherally (Iyengar et al. 1997; Rupniak et al. 1997).

Oral administration of CP-99,994, SDZ NKT 343 (Novartis), or LY303870 also attenuates mechanical hyperalgesia induced by carrageenan in guinea pigs (Patel et al. 1996; Urban et al. 1999). The effect appears to be mediated via blockade of spinal NK1 receptors, as intrathecal but not intraplantar injection of SDZ NKT 343 reduced the hyperalgesia. We recently found that L-733,060, but not its inactive isomer L-733,061, reversed carrageenan-induced mechanical hyperalgesia in guinea pigs (Fig. 2). In addition to their effects in assays of inflammatory hyperalgesia, NK1-receptor antagonists are effective in several neuropathic pain assays. Cumberbatch et al. (1998) found that intravenous injection of GR205171, but not its inactive enantiomer L-796,325, reversed both mechanical hypersensitivity and the increase in receptive field size of dorsal horn neurons following loose ligation of the sciatic nerve in rats. Similarly, Urban et al. (1999) used partial sciatic nerve ligation in guinea pigs to show that SDZ NKT 343 and LY303870 reduced established mechanical hyperalgesia following either oral or intrathecal administration. In contrast, RPR 100,893 was only active following intrathecal administration (Urban et al. 1999), probably due to poor brain penetration

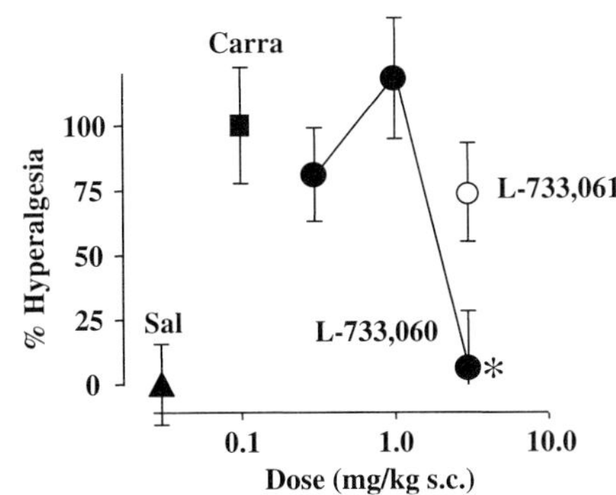

Fig. 2. Paw-withdrawal thresholds (PWT) to increasing compression of the hindpaw were measured 3 hours after intraplantar injection of carrageenan (4.5 mg into one paw) or saline (0.15 mL). L-733,060 (0.3-3 mg/kg s.c.), its less active enantiomer L-733,061 (3 mg/kg s.c.), or vehicle were administered 1 hour before the test. Hyperalgesia was defined as the difference in PWT for saline and carrageenan-injected guinea pigs. Paw pressure scores for drug-treated guinea pigs were expressed as a percentage of this response. * $P < 0.05$ compared to carrageenan/vehicle-treated guinea pigs.

when given systemically (Rupniak et al. 1997). LY303870 also reduces mechanical allodynia following spinal nerve ligation neuropathy in rats, albeit at high doses of 30 mg/kg (S. Iyengar, personal communication).

In a collaborative study we found that, in a similar manner to indomethacin, daily administration of the NK1-receptor antagonist L-760,735 (3 mg/kg s.c.) for 21 days reduced paw edema and the associated thermal and mechanical hyperalgesia in Freund's adjuvant arthritic guinea pigs (S. Boyce, S. Cruwys, and B. Kidd, unpublished observations). Consistent with these findings, Binder et al. (1999) showed that repeated administration of GR205171, but not its less active enantiomer, also reduced arthritic joint damage (joint swelling, synovitis, and bone demineralization) caused by complete Freund's adjuvant in rats. These findings suggest that NK1-receptor antagonists may possess anti-inflammatory and antinociceptive activity. The NK1-receptor antagonists RP-67,580, CP-99,994, and LY303870 are extremely potent at blocking neurogenic plasma extravasation in the dura following trigeminal ganglion stimulation in rats or guinea pigs (Shepheard et al. 1993, 1995; Phebus et al. 1997). MK-869 is also a potent inhibitor of dural neurogenic extravasation (Fig. 1B). In addition to its actions on neurogenic extravasation, CP-99,994 also reduces *c-fos* mRNA expression in the trigeminal nucleus caudalis in rats after trigeminal ganglion stimulation (Shepheard et al. 1995). Based on these findings, Shepheard et al. (1995) hypothesized that brain-penetrant NK1-receptor antagonists may have antimigraine effects peripherally through blockade of dural extravasation and centrally by inhibition of nociceptive pathways.

In summary, preclinical data support analgesic potential for NK1 antagonists. Although these agents do not display the broad spectrum of antinociceptive activity of the opiate analgesics such as morphine, (e.g., not effective in hot-plate or tail-flick tests), NK1-receptor antagonists have a profile that is comparable to that of nonsteroidal anti-inflammatory drugs (NSAIDs) such as indomethacin. NK1-receptor antagonists are also active against hyperalgesia caused by nerve injury (Table II).

CLINICAL TRIALS WITH NK1-RECEPTOR ANTAGONISTS

Despite the convincing evidence from animal studies for antinociceptive effects of NK1 antagonists, only one clinical study, with CP-99,994 in postoperative dental pain, has demonstrated analgesic activity in humans (Dionne et al. 1998). In this study, CP-99,994 was administered as an intravenous infusion over 5 hours, starting 30 minutes prior to surgery (total dose 0.75 mg/kg). CP-99,994 had comparable clinical efficacy to ibuprofen (Dionne et

Table II
Antinociceptive profile of NK1-receptor antagonists in preclinical assays

Assay	Morphine	Indomethacin	NK1 Antagonist
Tail flick/hotplate	Yes	No	No
Paw pressure	Yes	No	No
Writhing	Yes	Yes	Yes
Formalin paw	Yes	Yes	Yes
Carrageenan paw	Yes	Yes	Yes
Nerve injury	Yes	No	Yes
CFA arthritis	Yes	Yes	Yes
Reduction of facilitation of spinal nociceptive reflex	Yes	Yes	Yes
Reduces dural extravasation	Yes	Yes	Yes

al. 1998). In contrast to these findings, the long-acting orally active NK1-receptor antagonist MK-869 (300 mg p.o. given 2 hours prior to surgery), a dose established to be anti-emetic in humans (Navari et al. 1999), was ineffective in postoperative dental pain (Reinhardt et al. 1998; Fig. 1C). Similarly, CP-122,721 (200 mg p.o.; also an anti-emetic dose in humans, Gesztesi et al. 1998) had no effect in postoperative dental pain (McLean 1997). NK1-receptor antagonists have also been evaluated in patients with neuropathic pain, and MK-869 (300 mg p.o. for 2 weeks) was ineffective in patients with established postherpetic neuralgia (duration of 6 months to 6 years; Block et al. 1998). Lanepitant (LY303870; 50, 100, or 200 mg p.o. b.i.d. for 8 weeks) had no significant effect on pain intensity (daytime or night-time) when compared to placebo in patients with painful diabetic neuropathy (Goldstein and Wang 1999). Lanepitant (10, 30, 100, or 300 mg p.o. for 3 weeks) was also without effect in patients with moderate to severe osteoarthritis (Goldstein et al. 1998).

Finally, clinical trials with NK1-receptor antagonists for acute migraine and migraine prophylaxis have also been disappointing. L-758,298, an intravenous prodrug of MK-869 (20, 40, or 60 mg i.v.), failed to abort migraine pain as measured either by the time to meaningful relief or the number of patients reporting pain relief within 4 hours (Norman et al. 1998; Fig. 1D). Similarly, GR205171 (25 mg i.v.; Connor et al. 1998) and lanepitant (30, 80, or 240 mg p.o., Goldstein et al. 1997) were ineffective as abortive treatments for migraine headache. Furthermore, prophylactic administration of lanepitant (200 mg/day p.o.) for 1 month had no effect on migraine frequency and severity compared to placebo (Goldstein et al. 1999).

The lack of clinical efficacy of MK-869 or GR205171 in pain or migraine trials is not due to insufficient dose or lack of brain penetration. At the dose used in the analgesia trials, MK-869 produced antidepressant effects in patients with moderate to severe depression (Kramer et al. 1998) and prevented cisplatin-induced emesis following chemotherapy (Navari et al. 1999). Similarly, the dose of GR205171 employed in the migraine trial was based on adequate occupancy of NK1 receptors as calculated from PET studies (Connor et al. 1998). The negative findings with lanepitant may be inconclusive, however, as it has not been established that functional blockade of central NK1 receptors was achieved at the doses employed in the clinical trials. Overall, the conclusion from the clinical studies to date is that NK1-receptor antagonists are unlikely to have major utility as analgesics.

HAVE NK1-RECEPTOR ANTAGONISTS BEEN TESTED IN THE MOST APPROPRIATE CLINICAL TRIALS?

In the preclinical studies, NK1-receptor antagonists were particularly effective in assays of inflammatory pain, yet most clinical trials have addressed acute pain (dental pain or migraine). The recent findings that NK1-receptor antagonists appear to reduce arthritic joint damage and resultant hypersensitivity in animals with adjuvant arthritis suggest that these agents may be worth evaluating in rheumatoid arthritis. This concept is supported by the high expression of NK1-receptor mRNA in synovia taken from patients with rheumatoid arthritis (Sakai et al. 1998). Moreover, the signal intensities of NK1 mRNA positively correlated with serum C-reactive protein levels and radiological grade of joint destruction, which suggests that NK1-receptor gene expression may reflect the disease progression in rheumatoid arthritis. Interestingly, NK1-receptor mRNA expression was low in synovia taken from patients with osteoarthritis. Other chronic pain conditions in which NK1-receptor antagonists may be worth testing include fibromyalgia, a syndrome in which elevated levels of substance P are found in the cerebrospinal fluid (Russell et al. 1994). Recently, Littman et al. (1999) reported that the NK1-receptor antagonist CJ-11,974 (50 mg p.o. b.i.d. for 4 weeks) was able to reduce dysesthesias in patients with fibromyalgia. Although it had no significant effect on nociceptive thresholds, a subset of patients showed some improvement in pain severity, morning stiffness, and sleep disturbances. These findings warrant further investigation.

DO PRECLINICAL ANTINOCICEPTION ASSAYS RELIABLY PREDICT CLINICAL EFFICACY?

The negative results with NK1-receptor antagonists across a variety of clinical pain conditions has raised concerns as to the general relevance of animal assays and their ability to predict clinical analgesic efficacy. The most compelling preclinical evidence for antinociceptive activity of NK1-receptor antagonists comes from electrophysiological studies in which supraspinal influences have been removed by spinalization. It is possible that under these conditions the effect of substance P in the spinal cord may have greater significance than in intact animals (or humans) because of the loss of descending inhibitory controls. With regard to studies of conscious animals, many of the assays in which the NK1-receptor antagonists exhibit antinociceptive effects have been successful in predicting or confirming activity of a broad range of clinically effective analgesics. For example, the carrageenan-induced hyperalgesia and arthritis assays have been used to predict analgesic activity of NSAIDs and selective COX-2 inhibitors (Boyce et al. 1994; Chan et al. 1999). The neuropathic pain assays have demonstrated antinociceptive activity in NMDA antagonists, anticonvulsants (Boyce et al. 1999), and antidepressants (Ardid and Guilbaud 1992), and these agents have all shown some activity against neuropathic pain in humans. One possible criticism of the behavioral nociception tests is that changes in heat or mechanical thresholds are typically used as indicators of altered pain level; however, this effect may not translate to clinical efficacy for persistent pain. It thus may be important to establish new behavioral tests to measure persistent pain in animals, for example, by assessing spontaneous locomotor activity or spontaneous ultrasound vocalizations in neuropathic and arthritic animals, in an effort to more accurately predict analgesic activity in humans.

CONCLUSIONS

Although substance P, acting at NK1 receptors, appears to play an important role in pain transmission in animals, studies still need to demonstrate that blocking NK1 receptors produces clinical pain relief. Nevertheless, NK1-receptor antagonists are likely to have an important therapeutic role in the treatment of depression (Kramer et al. 1998) and cancer chemotherapy-induced emesis, particularly in the control of delayed emesis, which is poorly controlled by current anti-emetics (Navari et al. 1999).

ACKNOWLEDGMENTS

We thank our colleagues G.A. Block (migraine study) and B.J. Gertz (dental study) for the clinical data on MK-869, and S.L. Shepheard and D.J. Williamson (dural extravasation), J.M.A. Laird (spinal flexor reflex), and J.K. Webb (carrageenan) for the preclinical data.

REFERENCES

Ardid D, Guilbaud G. Antinociceptive effects of acute and 'chronic' injections of tricyclic antidepressant drugs in a new model of mononeuropathy in rats. *Pain* 1992; 49:279–287.

Beresford IJ, Birch PJ, Hagan RM, Ireland SJ. Investigation into species variants in tachykinin NK1 receptors by use of the non-peptide antagonist, CP-96,345. *Br J Pharmacol* 1991; 104:292–293.

Binder W, Scott C, Walker JS. Involvement of substance P in the anti-inflammatory effects of the peripherally selective kappa-opioid asimadoline and the NK1 antagonist GR 205171. *Eur J Neurosci* 1999; 11:2065–2072.

Block GA, Rue D, Panebianco D, SA Rienes. The substance P receptor antagonist L-754,030 (MK-0869) is ineffective in he treatment of postherpetic neuralgia. *Neurology* 1998; 4:A225.

Boyce S, Laird JMA, Tattersall FD, et al. Antinociceptive effects of NK1 receptor antagonists: comparison of behavioural and electrophysiological tests. *Abstracts: 7th World Congress on Pain*. Seattle: IASP, 1993.

Boyce S, Chan C-C, Gordon R, et al. L-745,337: a selective inhibitor of cyclo-oxygenase-2 elicits antinociception, but not gastric ulceration in rats. *Neuropharmacology* 1994; 33:1604–1611.

Boyce S, Wyatt A, Webb JK, et al. Selective NMDA NR2B antagonists induce antinociception without motor dysfunction: correlation with restricted localization of NR2B subunits in dorsal horn. *Neuropharmacology* 1999; 38:611–623.

Chan CC, Boyce S, Brideau C, et al. Rofecoxib [Vioxx, MK-0966; 4-(4′-methylsulfonylphenyl)-3-phenyl-2-(5H)-furanone]: a potent and orally active cyclooxygenase-2 inhibitor. Pharmacological and biochemical profiles. *J Pharmacol Exp Ther* 1999; 290:551–560.

Connor HE, Bertin L, Gillies, et al. Clinical evaluation of a novel, potent, CNS penetrating NK1 receptor antagonist in the acute treatment of migraine. *Cephalalgia* 1998; 18:392.

Cridland RA, Henry JL. Comparison of the effects of substance P, neurokinin A, physalaemin and eledoisin in facilitating a nociceptive reflex in the rat. *Brain Res* 1986; 381:93–99.

Cumberbatch MJ, Carlson E, Wyatt A, et al. Reversal of behavioural and electrophysiological correlates of experimental peripheral neuropathy by the NK1 receptor antagonist GR205171 in rats. *Neuropharmacology* 1998; 37:1535–1543.

Dionne RA. Clinical analgesic trials of NK1 antagonists. *Curr Opin CPNS Invest Drugs* 1999; 1:82–85.

Dionne RA, Max MB, Gordon SM, et al. The substance P receptor antagonist CP-99,994 reduces acute postoperative pain. *Clin Pharmacol Ther* 1998; 64:562–568.

Duggan AW, Morton CR, Zhao ZQ, Hendry IA. Noxious heating of the skin releases immunoreactive substance P in the substantia gelatinosa of the cat: a study with antibody microprobes. *Brain Res* 1987; 403:345–349.

Gesztesi ZS, Song D, White PF. Comparison of a new NK-1 antagonist (CP-122,721) to ondansetron in the prevention of postoperative nausea and vomiting. *Anesth Analg* 1998; 86:S32.

Goldstein DJ, Wang O. Lanepitant, an NK1 antagonist, in painful diabetic neuropathy [abstract]. *Clin Pharmacol Ther* 1999; 65.

Goldstein DJ, Wang O, Saper JR, et al. Ineffectiveness of neurokinin-1 antagonist in acute migraine: a crossover study. *Cephalalgia* 1997; 17:785–790.

Goldstein DJ, Wang O, Todd TE. Lanepitant in osteoarthritis pain. *Clin Pharmacol Ther* 1998; 63:168.

Goldstein DJ, Offen WW, Klein EG. Lanepitant, an NK1 antagonist, in migraine prophylaxis [abstract]. *Clin Pharmacol Ther* 1999; 65.

Henry JL. Effects of substance P on functionally identified units in cat spinal cord. *Brain Res* 1976; 114:439–451.

Hill RG, Rupniak NMJ. Tachykinin receptors and the potential of tachykinin antagonists as clinically effective analgesics and anti-inflammatory agents. In: Brain SD, Moore PK (Eds). *Pain and Neurogenic Inflammation.* Basel: Birkhauser, 1999, pp 313–333.

Iyengar S, Hipskind PA, Gehlert DR, et al. LY303870, a centrally active neurokinin-1 antagonist with a long duration of action. *J Pharmacol Exp Ther* 1997; 280:774–785.

Kramer MS, Cutler N, Feighner J, et al. Distinct mechanism for antidepressant activity by blockade of central substance P receptors. *Science* 1998; 281:1640–1645.

Littman B, Newton FA, Russell IJ. Substance P antagonism in fibromyalgia: a trial with CJ-11,974. *Abstracts: 9th World Congress on Pain.* Seattle: IASP Press, 1999, p 67.

Mantyh PW, Hunt SP. The autoradiographic localization of substance P receptors in the rat and bovine spinal cord and the rat and cat spinal trigeminal nucleus pars caudalis and the effects of neonatal capsaicin. *Brain Res* 1985; 332:315–324.

Mantyh PW, DeMaster E, Malhotra A, et al. Receptor endocytosis and dendrite reshaping in spinal neurons after somatosensory stimulation. *Science* 1995; 268:1629–1632.

McLean DB. Presented at American Society of Clinical Pharmacological Therapy Meeting, March, San Diego, 1997.

McLean S, Ganong AH, Seeger TF, et al. Activity and distribution of binding sites in brain of a nonpeptide substance P (NK1) receptor antagonist. *Science* 1991; 251(4992):437–439.

Navari RM, Reinhardt RR, Gralla RJ, et al. Reduction of cisplatin-induced emesis by a selective neurokinin-1-receptor antagonist. L-754,030 Antiemetic Trials Group. *N Engl J Med* 1999; 340:190–195.

Norman B, Panebianco D, Block GA. A placebo controlled, in clinic study to explore the preliminary safety and efficacy of intravenous L-758,298 (a prodrug of the NK1 receptor antagonist L-754,030) in the acute treatment of migraine. *Cephalalgia* 1998; 18:407–442.

Okayama Y, Ono Y, Nakazawa T, Church MK, Mori M. Human skin mast cells produce TNF-alpha by substance P. *Int Arch Allergy Immunol* 1998; 117(Suppl 1):48.

Patel S, Gentry CT, Campbell EA. A model for in vivo evaluation of tachykinin NK1 receptor antagonists using carrageenan-induced hyperalgesia in the guinea pig paw. *Br J Pharmacol* 1996; 117:248P.

Phebus LA, Johnson KW, Stengel PW, et al. The non-peptide NK-1 receptor antagonist LY303870 inhibits neurogenic dural inflammation in guinea pigs. *Life Sci* 1997; 60:1553–1561.

Radhakrishnan V, Henry JL. Novel substance P antagonist, CP-96,345, blocks responses of cat spinal dorsal horn neurons to noxious cutaneous stimulation and to substance P. *Neurosci Lett* 1991; 132:39–43.

Radhakrishnan V, Iyengar S, Henry JL. The nonpeptide NK-1 receptor antagonists LY303870 and LY306740 block the responses of spinal dorsal horn neurons to substance P and to peripheral noxious stimuli. *Neuroscience* 1998; 83:1251–1260.

Reinhardt RR, Laub JB, Fricke JR, Polis AB, Gertz BJ. Comparison of the neurokinin 1 antagonist, L-754,030, to placebo, acetaminophen and ibuprofen in the dental pain model. *Clin Pharmacol Ther* 1998; 63:168.

Rupniak NM, Carlson E, Boyce S, Webb JK, Hill RG. Enantioselective inhibition of the formalin paw late phase by the NK1 receptor antagonist L-733,060 in gerbils. *Pain* 1996; 67:189–195.

Rupniak NM, Tattersall FD, Williams AR, et al. In vitro and in vivo predictors of the anti-emetic activity of tachykinin NK1 receptor antagonists. *Eur J Pharmacol* 1997; 326:201–209.

Russell IJ, Orr MD, Littman B, et al. Elevated cerebrospinal fluid levels of substance P in patients with the fibromyalgia syndrome. *Arthritis Rheum* 1994; 37:1593–1601.

Sakai K, Matsuno H, Tsuji H, Tohyama M. Substance P receptor (NK1) gene expression in synovial tissue in rheumatoid arthritis and osteoarthritis. *Scand J Rheumatol* 1998; 27:135–141.

Shepheard SL, Williamson DJ, Hill RG, Hargreaves RJ, The non-peptide neurokinin1 receptor antagonist, RP 67580, blocks neurogenic plasma extravasation in the dura mater of rats. *Br J Pharmacol* 1993; 108:11–12.

Shepheard SL, Williamson DJ, Williams J, Hill RG, Hargreaves RJ. Comparison of the effects of sumatriptan and the NK1 antagonist CP-99,994 on plasma extravasation in dura mater and c-fos mRNA expression in trigeminal nucleus caudalis of rats. *Neuropharmacology* 1995; 34:255–2561.

Urban L, Gentry C, Patel S, Kox A. Selective NK1 receptor antagonists block neuropathic and inflammatory pain in the guinea pig. *Abstracts: 9th World Congress on Pain*. Seattle: IASP Press, 1999, p 40.

Yamamoto T, Yaksh TL Stereospecific effects of a nonpeptidic NK1 selective antagonist, CP-96,345: antinociception in the absence of motor dysfunction. *Life Sci* 1991; 49:1955–1963.

Correspondence to: R.G. Hill, BPharm, PhD, Merck Sharp and Dohme Research Laboratories, Neuroscience Research Centre, Terlings Park, Eastwick Road, Harlow, Essex CM20 2QR, United Kingdom. email: hillr@merck.com.

Proceedings of the 9th World Congress on Pain,
Progress in Pain Research and Management,
Vol. 16, edited by M. Devor, M.C. Rowbotham, and
Z. Wiesenfeld-Hallin, IASP Press, Seattle, © 2000.

32

Receptive Field Properties and Spike-Burst Responses to Intracellular Current Injection in Dorsal Horn Neurons

Han-Rong Weng and Patrick M. Dougherty

Departments of Neurosurgery and Neuroscience, The Johns Hopkins University School of Medicine, Baltimore, Maryland, USA

The responses of cells in the dorsal horn to peripheral stimuli are determined by monosynaptic input from primary afferent fibers as well as polysynaptic inputs from spinal interneurons and cells in more rostral forebrain sites (Wall 1989; Willis and Coggeshall 1991). These influences are notoriously changeable, and vary according to previous peripheral inputs and the level of attention, arousal, and anesthesia (Cervero et al. 1976; Bushnell et al. 1984; Collins 1987). The net effect is that input to a given cell from a given stimulus applied to a fixed site on skin might increase, decrease, appear, or disappear, depending on many conditions. One example of this plasticity that is particularly pertinent to pain mechanisms is the dorsal horn sensitization, or increased excitability of the spinal cord, that occurs after peripheral injury (see Dubner 1991, for review).

Dynamic regulation of biophysical properties of cells, such as membrane potential and membrane resistance, is the most likely mechanism by which the functional class of dorsal horn cells is rapidly regulated (Woolf and King 1987, 1989). This hypothesis is consistent with observations that sensitization-induced increases in excitability of neurons, as well as secondary hyperalgesia in humans, are produced by depolarization of spinal neurons from sustained nociceptor discharges (LaMotte et al. 1988). The key neurotransmitter receptor systems involved in the sensitization cascade, the N-methyl-D-aspartate (NMDA) glutamate receptors and the neurokinin 1 and 2 receptors (see Dougherty et al. 1994 and Dougherty and Raja 1999 for reviews), produce direct changes in membrane potential and resistance and also activate protein kinase systems that have further influences on these properties of cells (see Millan 1999 for review). Finally, regulation of the electrical properties of cells is sufficiently rapid to account for the known time courses of the onset and reversal of sensitization and hyperalgesia (LaMotte et al. 1988).

To better assess the membrane properties of dorsal horn neurons in pain transmission, we have recently adapted whole-cell patch-clamp recording techniques for in vivo analysis in intact rats (Ferster and Jagadeesh 1992; Jagadeesh et al. 1992, 1993; Nelson et al. 1994; Light and Willcockson 1996; Moore and Nelson 1998). In the present study we examined the baseline receptive field properties of dorsal horn neurons and tested for correlation of these properties to the spike-burst responses of cells to intracellular current injection.

METHODS

SURGICAL PREPARATION

Rats were anesthetized with either urethane (1.25 g/kg) or sodium pentobarbital (50.0 mg/kg) by intraperitoneal injection. Intravenous, arterial, and endotracheal catheters were inserted. Adequacy of anesthesia was determined by establishment of areflexia to all sensory stimuli (e.g., no flexor withdrawal or pupillary dilation, and no change of heart rate, expired CO_2, or blood pressure). Once under deep anesthesia, the animals were paralyzed with pancuronium (2.0 mg/kg, i.v.) and a partial lumbar laminectomy was performed to expose the L6–S1 region of the lumbar spinal cord. The rat was mounted in a stereotaxic and a spinal frame. The spinal cord was covered with warmed, oxygenated artificial cerebrospinal fluid (ACSF; 120 mM NaCl, 2.5 mM KCl, 1.25 mM NaH_2PO_4*H_2O, 26 mM $NaHCO_3$, 1.5 mM $MgSO_4$, 2.5 mM $CaCl_2$, and 10 mM dextrose).

SINGLE-NEURON, WHOLE-CELL PATCH RECORDINGS

Glass micropipettes (Drummond Scientific Company, Broomall, Pennsylvania; #9-000-2312, 0.060 inch outer diameter, 0.0445 inch inner diameter) were fashioned (Narishige Model PP-830 microelectrode puller) with a tip size of 0.75–1.0 μm (estimated by bubble pressure [Mittman et al. 1987]). Micropipettes were filled with a solution designed to approximate the internal environment of neurons (130 mM K-gluconate, 5 mM NaCl, 1 mM $CaCl_2$, 1 mM $MgCl_2$, 11 mM EGTA, 10 mM HEPES, 1 mM GTP, 0.01 mM GMP, and 2 mM Mg-ATP [adjusted to 280 milliosmoles]). Electrical resistance of filled micropipettes ranged from 6 to 8 MΩ. The electrodes were mounted in a carrier (Warner Instruments E45W-MxxPH), and 15–50 millibars positive pressure was applied. The electrode was advanced into the dorsal horn with a hydraulic microdrive (David Kopf Model 640) while 0.1 nA square negative current pulses (AMPI Master 8) were applied at 1 Hz. The electrode potential was amplified (Adams List SEC 05L/H), and unfiltered DC potential was monitored on a digital oscilloscope (Nicolet 4094) and also captured and analyzed on a personal computer (Spike 2, Version 2.6, Cambridge Electronics Devices). An AC-coupled output was further amplified (Axon Instruments CyberAmp 380), filtered (20 kHz, 300 Hz), and displayed on a separate oscilloscope (Hitachi VC-6155). As a single cell was approached, positive pressure was released and a gigaohm seal was allowed to form. Negative pressure was applied to the electrode as necessary to encourage seal formation. Once the seal was stable, a negative pressure transient was used to rupture the cell membrane and establish whole-cell recording. Spike duration, amplitude, membrane potential, and access resistance were monitored throughout all recordings to ensure the integrity of each cell.

A soft brush was used to briefly stimulate multiple areas on the skin of the hindlimb. Identified responsive areas were re-tested while the responses to 5 seconds of brush stimulation were collected while depressing a foot pedal connected to a 5-V source. Pinch of the skin with a calibrated forceps (6 N/mm^2), painful when placed on human skin, was tested in the same manner. After the initial characterization of receptive field properties, a set of 10 positive and 10 negative current pulses, 500 ms in duration, incremented in 0.1-nA steps, were delivered at 3.0-s intervals. Additional positive current steps were added as necessary to provoke spike-burst discharges of cells. Membrane potential was sampled at 50 kHz and stored for offline analysis with appropriate software (Signal Version 1.6, Cambridge Electronic Devices).

The rats were killed at the conclusion of each experiment without regaining consciousness. A fatal overdose of barbiturate was given (100 mg, i.v.), followed by exsanguination, and perfusion with 4% paraformaldehyde. This method is considered quick and painless, and is approved by the American Medical Veterinarians Association.

DATA ANALYSIS AND INTERPRETATION

Cells were classified by statistical off-line, within-cell analysis of action potential responses to cutaneous stimuli. The numbers of action potentials evoked at each cutaneous site were sorted into 100-ms bins for the duration of each stimulus. These data were compared to the numbers of spontaneous discharges sorted into an equal number of 100-ms bins using a one-way analysis of variance. Cells were defined as nociceptive specific (NS) when action potential responses to pinch (6 N/mm^2) significantly differed from background, but responses to brush did not. Low-threshold (LT) cells were those with a significant increase in firing to brush but without further increase to the compressive stimuli. Wide-dynamic-range (WDR) cells were defined as those with a significant increase in firing to mechanical stimuli and a further significant increase in firing rate with increasing stimulus intensity.

RESULTS

A total of 23 neurons were studied, including 9 LT, 7 WDR, and 7 NS neurons. The average depths of recording of the groups of neurons were as follows: LT neurons averaged 130 ± 8.8 μm (mean ± SD; range 52–224 μm), WDR cells 150 ± 35 μm (range 110–286 μm), and NS cells 88 μm ± 31 μm from the surface (range 58–92 μm) of the spinal cord.

A representative example of a whole-cell recording from an LT neuron in the intact spinal dorsal horn of an anesthetized rat is shown in Fig. 1. Four distinct types of electrical activity were observed following application of mechanical stimuli to skin. The most central zone was often an area from which action potentials were provoked, as indicated for the cell in Fig. 1 by the black shaded region. The depolarizations provoked by innocuous brushing often showed pronounced excitatory potentials: a burst of action potentials was observed on the peak, followed by a pronounced hyperpolarization. In some cells these hyperpolarizations exceeded the baseline potential and appeared both before and after the excitatory wave. A second zone, composed only of subliminal non-spike-generating excitatory potentials, was observed in nearly all cells. In some cases cells were observed that did not have an active action-potential zone, but which nevertheless showed this subliminal excitatory input. A third zone from which inhibitory potentials in exclusion of excitatory events were provoked was less frequently observed. Finally, stimuli applied to a fourth zone, not observed in this example but in other cells, yielded a prolonged hyperpolarization of cells but without obvious isolated inhibitory potentials.

After measuring receptive field properties, we explored the responses of 15 cells to intracellular current injection. Fig. 2 shows representative examples of three of the four patterns of spike-burst responses defined by Lopez-Garcia and King in vitro (1994) that we observed in vivo. Type I responses consisted of sustained discharges following current injection (cell 1, line 1), although in the case of cell 2 (line 2) this train came only after a prolonged delay. Type II responses are illustrated in line 3, where intracellular current provoked spike bursts. Type III responses are shown at the left trace of line 4, where a single action potential is provoked by current injection. Continued increases in current intensity caused the cell to discharge more spikes and to assume a type II spike-burst pattern. Since we have always observed single-spike (type III) responses to assume a burst pattern (type II) when the current is sufficiently increased, we are beginning to question the validity of categorizing single spikes as a separate response type. It may be more appropriate to consider these as a subtype of burst (type II) responses. Type IV responses are not shown, although we observed these on one occasion. In this cell a burst of action potentials with release of hyperpolarizing current steps was observed. The numbers of discharges increased as a function of the current intensity.

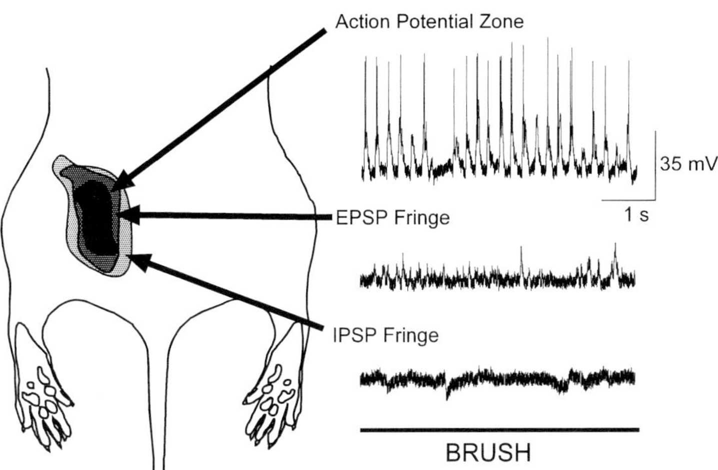

Fig. 1. Representative intracellular whole-cell patch clamp recordings from a low-threshold (LT) dorsal horn neuron in an intact anesthetized rat that illustrates the three most commonly observed types of electrical activity provoked by cutaneous stimuli. Application of innocuous brush to the center region of the receptive field, shown on the drawing of the hindlimb as the black filled region, provoked pronounced excitatory post-synaptic potentials with action potentials on the crests that were followed by pronounced hyperpolarizing events. The responses to noxious pinch were not characterized by these pronounced depolarization–hyperpolarization events. Surrounding the action potential zone, an area was identified from which subliminal excitatory inputs were provoked, indicated here by the dark gray area. Finally, a region from which inhibitory potentials were provoked could also often be identified (light gray). As indicated in the figure, the orientation of these zones in the representative cell appeared as concentric areas around the center action potential zone. However, the margins for the subliminal excitatory and the inhibitory areas were often very irregular and overlapped to a great extent. EPSP = excitatory postsynaptic potential; IPSP = inhibitory postsynaptic potential.

A clear correlation between spike-burst and functional class (LT, WDR, NS) has not emerged. The type I response was observed most frequently (in 11 of 15 cells, including cells of each functional class). Type II responses were shown by one LT and one WDR neuron, while type III (n = 1) and type IV (n = 1) responses were only observed in NS cells.

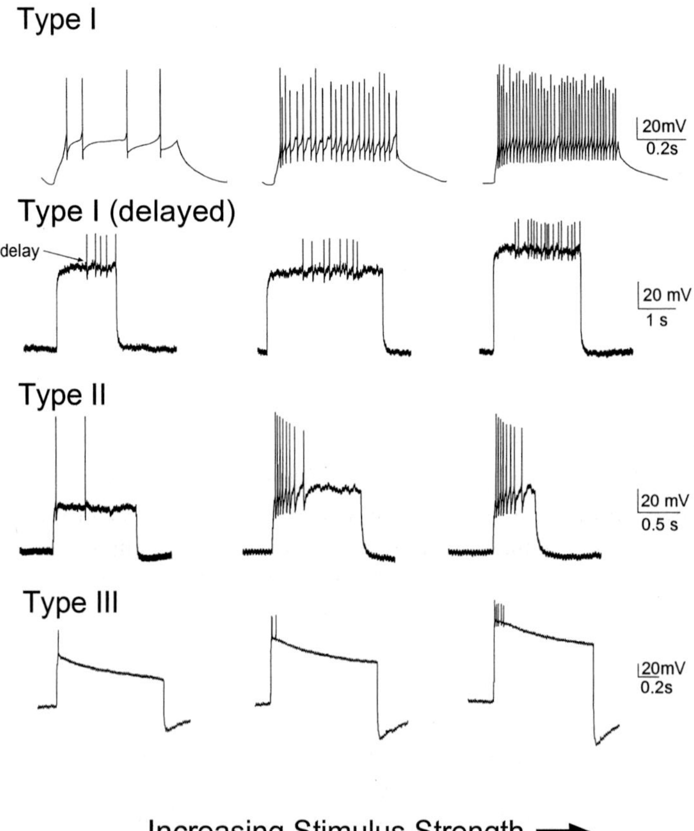

Fig. 2. Representative examples of the three most commonly observed spike-burst responses of cells provoked by depolarizing intracellular current injection. The top two lines show type I responses composed of sustained, regenerating spike trains. The second line shows an example of a type I response that occurred following a significant delay, which suggests that the recording site was distant from the spike-initiation zone. Type II responses, shown in line 3, are characterized by a self-limited burst of action potentials (also commonly referred to as spike frequency adaptation). Finally, at the left of line 4, a single-spike, type III response to current injection is shown. However, as shown to the right of this line, in our hands type III responses could be converted to either type I or II responses by sufficiently increasing current strength.

DISCUSSION

Recent technical advances in several laboratories have proven the feasibility of intracellular recording of neurons in vivo using whole-cell patch clamp (Neher and Sakman 1976). Whole-cell patch recording is an exciting technical advance over the traditional impalement of cells with sharp, high-impedance electrodes (Ferster and Jagadeesh 1992; Jagadeesh et al. 1992, 1993; Nelson et al. 1994; Light and Willcockson 1996; Moore and Nelson 1998). Whole-cell patch clamp provides a more detailed and accurate measure of biophysical properties than is possible with traditional high-impedance microelectrodes, due to the patch electrode's larger tip size and consequent reduced series resistance (Sigworth 1986). Additionally, cell stability is improved because the damage associated with impalement is markedly reduced or eliminated (Neher 1982; Neher and Marty 1982). These advantages may have contributed to our preliminary success in sampling spinal neurons of superficial lamina, traditionally among the most difficult to impale successfully. Low-resistance electrodes allow more precise current and voltage-clamp studies that would otherwise be subject to bias using high-resistance probes. The large tip size of patch-clamp electrodes offers the potential for rapid introduction of chemical probes to intracellular ion channels and enzyme systems and the passive infusion of anatomic labels (Pusch and Neher 1988; Ransom and Sontheimer 1992). Although this feature also has the potential pitfall of dialyzing neurons, we have observed in our preliminary studies that prolonged, stable recordings can be achieved when secondary cell metabolites such as ATP are included in the internal electrode solution. Finally, patch clamp allows the sampling or removal of cellular contents for later chemical, molecular, or genetic analysis (Lambolez et al. 1995).

Our initial results in adapting this approach in intact rodent dorsal horn neurons have shown that receptive field properties of cells can be explored in great detail. Dorsal horn cells of all functional classes (LT, WDR, and NS) have shown up to three types of electrical activity following application of stimuli to the skin, as illustrated in Fig. 1. It will be of interest in future studies to determine the influence of sensitizing injuries, such as intradermal capsaicin, within these specific zones on the responses of dorsal horn cells.

This study explored the responses of cells to intracellular current pulses. Our goal was to determine whether the receptive field and spike-burst responses to intracellular current injection show correlation. However, our present results indicate that in fact the majority of neurons show type I responses to intracellular current injection, regardless of functional class. Type III and IV responses were observed only in NS cells; however, this preliminary observation will require validation in further studies.

ACKNOWLEDGMENTS

This work was supported by NS-32386 and by the Blaustein Pain Research Fund.

REFERENCES

Bushnell MC, Duncan GH, Dubner R, He LF. Activity of trigeminothalamic neurons in medullary dorsal horn of awake monkeys trained in a thermal discrimination task. *J Neurophysiol* 1984; 52:170–187.

Cervero F, Iggo A, Molony V. Effects of noxious stimulation of the skin on transmission through the spinocervical tract. *J Physiol (Lond)* 1976; 263:135–136.

Collins JG. A descriptive study of spinal dorsal horn neurons in the physiologically intact, awake, drug-free cat. *Brain Res* 1987; 416:34–42.

Dougherty PM, Mittman S, Sorkin LS. Hyperalgesia and amino acids. Receptor selectivity based on stimulus intensity and a role for peptides. *APS J* 1994; 3:240–248.

Dougherty PM, Li YJ, Lenz FA, Rowland L, Mittman S. Correlation of effects of general anesthetics on somatosensory neurons in the primate thalamus and cortical power. *J Neurophysiol* 1997; 77:1375–1392.

Dougherty PM, Raja SN. The neurochemistry of somatosensation. In: Benzon H, Raja SN, Strichartz GR, Borsook D (Eds). *Essentials of Pain Medicine and Regional Anesthesia.* New York: Saunders, 1999, pp 7–9.

Dubner R. Neuronal plasticity and pain following peripheral tissue inflammation or nerve injury. In: Bond MR, Charlton JE, Woolf CJ (Eds). *Proceedings of the VIth World Congress on Pain.* Amsterdam: Elsevier, 1991, pp 263–276.

Ferster D, Jagadeesh B. EPSP-IPSP interactions in cat visual cortex studied with *in vivo* whole-cell patch recording. *J Neurosci* 1992; 12:1262–1274.

Jagadeesh B, Gray CM, Ferster D. Visually evoked oscillations of membrane potential in cells of cat visual cortex. *Science* 1992; 257:552–554.

Jagadeesh B, Wheat HS, Ferster D. Linearity of summation of synaptic potentials underlying direction selectivity in simple cells of the cat visual cortex. *Science* 1993; 262:1901–1904.

Lambolez B, Audinat E, Bochet P, Rossier J. Patch-clamp recording and RT-PCR on single cells. In: Boulton A, Baker G, Walz W (Eds). *Patch-Clamp Applications and Protocols.* Totowa, NJ: Humana Press, 1995, pp 193–231.

LaMotte RH, Simone DA, Baumann TK, Shain CN, Alreja M. Hypothesis for novel classes of chemoreceptors mediating chemogenic pain and itch. In: Dubner R, Gebhart GF, Bond MR (Eds). *Proceedings of the Vth World Congress on Pain.* Amsterdam: Elsevier, 1988, pp 529–540.

Light AR, Willcockson HH. In vivo whole-cell recordings from spinal substantia gelatinosa (lamina II) neurons of adult rats. *Soc Neurosci Abstr* 1996; 22:861.

Lopez-Garcia JA, King AE. Membrane properties of physiologically classified rat dorsal horn neurons *in vitro*: correlation with cutaneous sensory afferent input. *Eur J Neurosci* 1994; 6:998–1007.

Millan MJ. The induction of pain: an integrative review. *Prog Neurobiol* 1999; 57:1–164.

Mittman S, Flaming DG, Copenhagen DR, Belgum JH. Bubble pressure measurement of micropipette tip outer diameter. *J Neurosci Methods* 1987; 22:161–166.

Moore CI, Nelson SB. Spatio-temporal subthreshold receptive fields in the vibrissa representation of rat primary somatosensory cortex. *J Neurophysiol* 1998; 80:2882–2892.

Neher E. Unit conductance studies in biological membranes. *Tech Cell Physiol* 1982; P121:1–16.

Neher E, Sakman B. Single channel currents recorded from membrane of denervated frog muscle fibers. *Nature* 1976; 260:799–802.

Neher E, Marty A. Discrete changes of cell membrane capacitance observed under conditions of enhanced secretion in bovine adrenal chromaffin cells. *Proc Natl Acad Sci USA* 1982; 79:6712–6716.

Nelson S, Toth L, Sheth B, Sur M. Orientation selectivity of cortical neurons during intracellular blockade of inhibition. *Science* 1994; 265:774–777.

Pusch M, Neher E. Rates of diffusional exchange between small cells and a measuring patch pipette. *Pflugers Arch Physiol* 1988; 411:204–211.

Ransom BR, Sontheimer H. Cell-cell coupling demonstrated by intracellular injection of the fluorescent dye Lucifer yellow. In: Kettenmann H, Grantyn R (Eds). *Electrophysiological Methods for In Vitro Studies in Vertebrate Neurobiology*. New York: Plenum Press, 1992, pp 3–35.

Sigworth FJ. The patch-clamp is more useful than anyone had expected. *Federation Proc* 1986; 45:2673–2677.

Wall PD. The dorsal horn. In: Wall PD, Melzack R (Eds). *The Textbook of Pain*. Edinburgh: Churchill Livingstone, 1989, pp 102–111.

Willis WD, Coggeshall RE. *Sensory Mechanisms of the Spinal Cord*. New York: Plenum Press, 1991, 485 pp.

Woolf CJ, King AE. Physiology and morphology of multireceptive neurons with C-afferent fiber inputs in the deep dorsal horn of the rat lumbar spinal cord. *J Neurophysiol* 1987; 58:460–479.

Woolf CJ, King AE. Subthreshold components of the cutaneous mechanoreceptive fields of dorsal horn neurons in the rat lumbar spinal cord. *J Neurophysiol* 1989; 62:907–916.

Correspondence to: Patrick M. Dougherty, PhD, Departments of Neurosurgery and Neuroscience, The Johns Hopkins University School of Medicine, Meyer 5-109, 600 N. Wolfe Street, Baltimore, MD 21287, USA. Tel: 410-955-7078; Fax: 410-955-1032; email: pmd@research.med.jhu.edu.

Proceedings of the 9th World Congress on Pain,
Progress in Pain Research and Management,
Vol. 16, edited by M. Devor, M.C. Rowbotham, and
Z. Wiesenfeld-Hallin, IASP Press, Seattle, © 2000.

33

Differential Spinal Release of Amino Acid Neurotransmitters following Selective Activation of C or Aδ Thermonociceptors

David C. Yeomans,[a,b] Ying Lu,[a] Michael Peters,[a]
Michael Whitely,[b] and Charles E. Laurito[b]

*Departments of [a]Anatomy and Cell Biology and [b]Anesthesiology,
University of Illinois at Chicago, Chicago, Illinois, USA*

Activation of nociceptive primary afferents (nociceptors) induces the release of neurotransmitters, which then interact with postsynaptic membrane receptors. Among these neurotransmitters are numerous peptides and amino acids. It is likely, however, that not all nociceptor categories use the same constellation of transmitters. This distinction among nociceptors is widely recognized for peptide transmitters (e.g., Lawson 1995). For example, substance P appears to be released by activation of unmyelinated, but not myelinated thermonociceptors (Zachariou et al. 1997). Thus, different nociceptor types make and release different ensembles of neurotransmitters.

Perhaps less widely recognized are potentially important differences in the distribution and release of excitatory amino acid neurotransmitters (EAAs). The two principle EAAs, glutamate (GLU) and aspartate (ASP), are both found in small-diameter sensory afferents (Tracey et al. 1991). However, Westlund and associates (1989) have demonstrated immunohistochemically that ASP is preferentially located in the thinnest (unmyelinated) fibers while GLU is distributed more uniformly among fiber sizes. Although both ASP and GLU are released by electrical stimulation of the sciatic nerve at A-fiber intensity, the stronger C-fiber stimulus prompts a significantly greater relative release of ASP (Kangrga and Randic 1991). In addition, ASP release increased more than that of GLU following perfusion of dorsal root ganglia with capsaicin, which activates and sensitizes C nociceptors (Kangrga and Randic 1991). Similarly, Dougherty et al. (1992) reported that intradermal injections of capsaicin increased the responses of dorsal horn neurons to ASP much more than responses to GLU. Finally, while both GLU and ASP are released in the dorsal horn by intradermal injection of formalin, the release of ASP is sensitive to the sodium channel blocker tetrodotoxin, whereas the evoked release of GLU is not (Skilling et al. 1988). These data indicate that the distribution and release of ASP and GLU may differ among nociceptors. This chapter describes experiments intended to determine whether ASP and GLU are differentially released in the spinal cord when Aδ- or C-fiber nociceptors are separately activated.

METHODS

DORSAL HORN PERFUSION

Male Sprague-Dawley rats (350–400 g, Charles River) were anesthetized with pentobarbital (50 mg/kg). A laminectomy exposed the lumbar enlargement; the dura matter was then incised, and the dorsal roots were reflected toward the midline. Following surgery, the rats were placed in a spinal frame. A push-pull cannula mounted on a stereotaxic electrode holder was lowered approximately 700 μm into the dorsal horn (laminae I–III) at the entry zone of the fourth lumbar dorsal root on the side ipsilateral to the hindpaw to be stimulated. The cannula is made from two 27-g needles (Monoject #401) whose ends had been sharpened and bent to form a perfusion chamber (McCarson and Goldstein 1991). A peristaltic pump was used to perfuse artificial cerebrospinal fluid (aCSF) through the cannula at a rate of 30 μL/min, such that the 200-μL samples were collected over 6.66 minutes. The aCSF contained 128.5 mM NaCl, 3.0 mM KCl, 21 mM $NaHCO_3$, 0.25 mM NaH_2PO_4, 3.4 mM glucose, 1.15 mM $CaCl_2$, and 0.8mM $MgCl_2$. Before the aCSF entered the cannula it was warmed to 37°C with the pH maintained at 7.4 by bubbling it with 95% O_2 and 5% CO_2.

CHROMATOGRAPHY

Amino acids were assayed by high-performance liquid chromatography (HPLC) according to a method similar to that described by Graser et al. (1985). External standards containing 1, 5, 10, or 20 ng of authentic amino acid (Altech) were run prior to and following perfusate assay. Samples (20 μL) of perfusate or standard were reacted with 1.0 μL of *o*-phthaldialdehyde/3-mercaptoproprionic acid reagent (Sigma) for derivitization. After 1 minute, a 20.0-μL sample was injected into the HPLC, which used a reversed-phase C_{18} column (Waters, 3.9 × 150 mm). Amino acids were then quantitated by absorbance at 340 nm (Waters 2487). The samples were separated with a mobile phase gradient using the following solutions: 12.5 mM $NaPO_4$, pH 7.2, and a 50% v/v mixture of 12.5 mM $NaPO_4$ and acetonitrile. Peaks for both ASP and GLU appeared during the first 5 minutes following sample application when the mobile phase was isocratic phosphate buffer. Thereafter a steep gradient (ending in 50% acetonitrile) was initiated to flush the column prior to the next sample. This procedure allowed for detection of ASP and GLU at a sensitivity of 0.5–2.0 ng per sample. We used a PC-based data acquisition and analysis system (Millennium, Waters) to quantify EAAs based on linear relationships between peak areas and amounts of standards.

NOCICEPTIVE STIMULATION

The focused beam of light from a preheated 250-W projection bulb provided noxious radiant heat. The heat intensity was set to one of two values by adjusting the source voltage of the bulb to produce surface skin heating rates of 0.9° and 6.5°C/second, respectively (Yeomans and Proudfit 1994), which activate C or Aδ nociceptors, respectively (Yeomans and Proudfit 1996). The basal release of neurotransmitter was monitored for 40 minutes prior to stimulation. In one group of rats a hindpaw was heated at the high rate for 5 seconds and in another group of rats a hindpaw was heated at the low rate for 20 seconds. Stimuli were presented repeatedly with a 2-minute interstimulus interval for a total of 20 minutes. After the stimulus period, samples were taken for an additional 20 minutes to determine whether EAA levels would return to prestimulus baseline levels. Animals were then killed by overdose with pentobarbital (75 mg/kg, i.p.), and the lumbar spinal cord was removed and fixed with 4% paraformaldehyde for later histological confirmation of the perfusion site in the dorsal horn. All experimental methods were approved by the University of Illinois Animal Care Committee.

RESULTS

Examination of the spinal cords after each experiment indicated that perfusion sites were consistently within the superficial dorsal horn. Basal EAA levels were clearly within the limits of detection by this measurement method; basal GLU levels were 3–4 times those of ASP (Table I). Low-rate (C) stimulation evoked similar, significant ($P < 0.05$, Student's t test) increases in measurable GLU and ASP (64% and 60%, respectively; Fig. 1) in spinal cord perfusates. Interestingly, while GLU recovered to basal levels during the 20-minute post-stimulation period, ASP decreased to about 28%

Table I
Mean dorsal horn release of excitatory amino acids following selective C or Aδ thermostimulation (SEM in parentheses)

Heating Rate	Condition	Glutamic Acid (pg/20 μL)	Aspartic Acid (pg/20 μL)
Low (C)	Baseline	4057.7 (812.5)	939.7 (204.8)
Low (C)	Stimulation	6640.8 (2023.6)	1503.0 (298.7)
Low (C)	Post-stimulation	4341.6 (765.4)	673.0 (121.5)
High (Aδ)	Baseline	2706.8 (522)	968.2 (241.2)
High (Aδ)	Stimulation	4498.7 (780.3)	1030.9 (279.6)
High (Aδ)	Post-stimulation	3439.9 (789.4)	1089.4 (236.4)

less than the prestimulus period. High-rate (Aδ) thermostimulation significantly ($P < 0.05$, Student's t) increased GLU (by 66%) but not ASP levels (7%; Fig. 2) in perfusates. GLU returned to levels close to prestimulus values. These data are consistent with our hypothesis that C thermostimulation evokes GLU and ASP release, whereas Aδ activation releases GLU, but not ASP, from dorsal horn terminals.

DISCUSSION

Several steps are necessary for the transfer of information on noxious events from the periphery to cells in the spinal cord dorsal horn. The energy imparted to the system from the outside stimulus must be transduced to

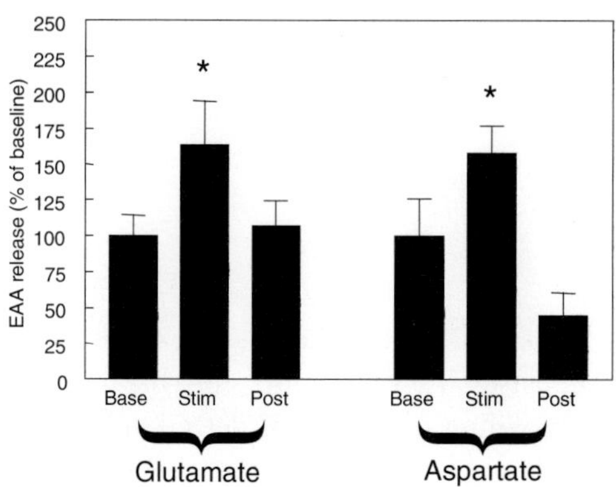

Fig. 1. GLU and ASP release in the dorsal horn of the spinal cord prior to (base), during (stim), and following (post) repetitive radiant *low*-rate heating of the hindpaw. Values are expressed as percentage increase over baseline.

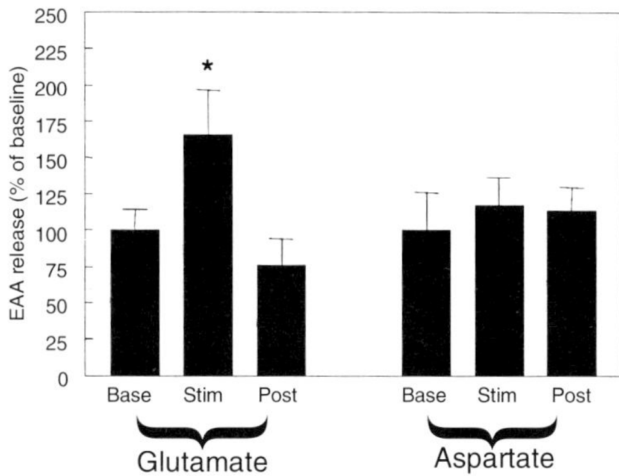

Fig. 2. GLU and ASP release in the dorsal horn of the spinal cord prior to (base), during (stim), and following (post) repetitive radiant *high*-rate heating of the hindpaw. Values are expressed as percentage increase over baseline.

action potentials, which are then conducted to the central terminals of the afferents. The information these afferents carry is then conveyed through the release of neurotransmitters to secondary cells in the spinal cord dorsal horn. For nociceptors, these neurotransmitters include several peptides, which appear to convey messages concerning strong or prolonged noxious events, and also EAAs, which rapidly convey messages concerning onset of pain and are involved in persisting pain (see Wilcox 1991; Dickenson et al. 1997). Clear distinctions emerge in the neurotransmitters used during different types of nociception. For example, somatostatin release appears to be involved in mechanical, but not thermal nociception (Morton et al. 1989). Thus, different types of noxious stimulation may activate different populations of primary afferents, which, in turn may release different neurotransmitters. A good example is the release of substance P by activation of C-fiber but not Aδ-fiber thermonociceptors (Zachariou et al. 1997). Thus, these studies demonstrate clear precedence for differential central release of neurotransmitters by different nociceptor types.

The results presented here indicate that similar distinctions may also exist for amino acid neurotransmitters. These experiments demonstrate that, while stimuli that activate C-fiber thermonociceptors induce the spinal release of GLU and ASP, selective thermal stimulation of Aδ afferents evokes the release of GLU, but not ASP. Thus, the release of ASP by thermal stimulation may be used as a marker for C, but not Aδ stimulation.

These results carry implications for some of the distinctions observed in EAA antinociceptive pharmacology. GLU and ASP, released by A- or C-fiber nociceptors, may act at different EAA receptors in the spinal cord to mediate nociception. Both GLU and ASP can bind to all three of the main classes of ionotropic EAA receptors, including NMDA (N-methyl-D-aspartate), kainate, and AMPA (DL-α-amino-3-hydroxy-5-methyl-isoxazole-proprionate) (see Wilcox 1991). Evidence suggests that activation of different nociceptors releases EAAs that act at different postsynaptic EAA receptors. For example, Dougherty et al. (1992) reported that ASP mimicked the synthetic derivative NMDA in excitatory effects on dorsal horn cells and that those effects were preferentially blocked by the NMDA antagonist AP7, but not the kainate/AMPA antagonist CNQX. GLU, however, mimicked the effects of kainate, which were blocked by CNQX, but not AP7. These authors also reported that, while both AP7 and CNQX were highly effective at blocking responses to noxious heating of the skin, CNQX, but not AP7, also blocked responses to noxious and innocuous mechanical stimuli. This result is consistent with our preliminary behavioral findings that intrathecal application of the NMDA antagonist AP5 selectively attenuates C-fiber-mediated thermonociception, whereas kainate and AMPA antagonists were equally potent analgesics for Aδ and C thermonociception (D.C. Yeomans et al., unpublished observations). These data suggest that activation of C thermonociceptors may evoke the release of ASP, which acts at least partially at NMDA receptors to excite postsynaptic neurons. In contrast, both C and Aδ thermonociceptors may release GLU, which acts at least partly at postsynaptic kainate or AMPA receptors. Thus, differential release of EAA neurotransmitters following activation Aδ- or C-fiber nociceptors could be used as an index of primary afferent presynaptic function, and pharmacologically-induced changes in EAA release can be used as an index of differential presynaptic modulation of Aδ and C nociceptors.

ACKNOWLEDGMENTS

This work was supported by PHS grant DA08256 to D.C. Yeomans.

REFERENCES

Dickenson AH, Chapman V, Green GM. The pharmacology of excitatory and inhibitory amino acid-mediated events in the transmission and modulation of pain in the spinal cord. *Gen Pharmacol* 1997; 28:633–638.

Dougherty PM, Palecek J, Paleckova V, Sorkin LL, Willis WD. The role of NMDA and Non-NMDA excitatory amino acid receptors in the excitation of primate spinothalamic tract neurons by mechanical, chemical, thermal, and electrical stimuli. *J Neurosci* 1992; 12:3025–3041.

Graser TA, Godel HG, Albers S, Földi P, Fürst P. An ultra rapid and sensitive high-performance liquid chromatographic method for determination of tissue and plasma free amino acids. *Analyt Biochem* 1985; 151:142–152.

Kangrga I, Randic M. Outflow of endogenous aspartate and glutamate from the rat spinal dorsal horn in vitro by activation of low- and high-threshold primary afferent fibers: modulation by δ-opioids. *Brain Res* 1991; 553:347–352.

Lawson SN. Neuropeptides in morphologically and functionally identified primary afferent neurons in dorsal root ganglia: substance P, CGRP and somatostatin. *Prog Brain Res* 1995; 104:161–173.

McCarson K, Goldstein BD. Release of SP into the superficial dorsal horn following nociceptive activation of the hindpaw of the rat. *Brain Res* 1991; 568:109–115.

Morton CR, Hutchison WD, Hendry IA, Duggan AW. Somatostatin: evidence for a role in thermal nociception. *Brain Res* 1989; 488:89–96.

Skilling SR, Smullin DH, Beitz AJ, Larson AA. Extracellular amino acid concentrations in the dorsal spinal cord of freely moving rats following veratridine and nociceptive stimulation. *J Neurochem* 1988; 51:127–132.

Tracey DJ, De Biasi S, Phend K, Rustioni A. Aspartate-like immunoreactivity in primary afferent neurons. *Neuroscience* 1991; 40:673–686.

Westlund NK, McNeill DL, Patterson JT, Coggeshall R. Aspartate immunoreactive axons in normal L4 dorsal roots. *Brain Res* 1989; 489:347–351.

Wilcox GL. Excitatory neurotransmitters and pain. In: Bond MR, Charlton JE, Woolf CJ (Eds). *Proceedings of the VIth World Congress on Pain*. Amsterdam: Elsevier, 1991, pp 97–117.

Yeomans DC, Proudfit HK. Characterization of the foot withdrawal response to noxious radiant heat. *Pain* 1994; 59:85–94.

Yeomans DC, Proudfit HK. Nociceptive responses to high or low rates of noxious cutaneous heating are mediated by different nociceptors in the rat: electrophysiological evidence. *Pain* 1996; 68:141–150.

Zachariou V, Goldstein B, Yeomans DC. Differential release of Substance P in rat spinal cord dorsal horn by different rates of noxious radiant heating of the hindpaw. *Brain Res* 1997; 752:143–150.

Correspondence to: David C. Yeomans, PhD, Department of Anatomy and Cell Biology (MC 512), 808 S. Wood Street, Chicago, IL 60612, USA. Tel: 312-996-7223; Fax: 312-413-0354; email: yeomans@uic.edu.

Proceedings of the 9th World Congress on Pain,
Progress in Pain Research and Management,
Vol. 16, edited by M. Devor, M.C. Rowbotham, and
Z. Wiesenfeld-Hallin, IASP Press, Seattle, © 2000.

34

Antisense Knockdown of mGluR1 Reverses Hyperalgesia and Allodynia Associated with an Established Neuropathic Injury in Rats

Marian E. Fundytus,[a,b] James L. Henry,[a]
Andy Dray,[b] and Terence J. Coderre[c]

[a]*Department of Physiology, McGill University, Montreal, Quebec, Canada;* [b]*Astra Research Centre Montreal, St Laurent, Quebec, Canada;* [c]*Pain Mechanisms Laboratory, Clinical Research Institute of Montreal, Montreal, Quebec, Canada*

Nerve injury often results in chronic neuropathy, which can cause neuropathic pain, characterized by spontaneous pain, hyperalgesia (increased responsiveness to noxious stimuli), and allodynia (painful response to normally innocuous stimuli). Neuropathic pain is very difficult to treat, often being unresponsive to opioids (MacDonald 1991; McQuay et al. 1992; Cherny et al. 1994).

A role for the excitatory amino acid glutamate in neuropathic pain has been well established. Glutamate release is enhanced in the spinal cords of neuropathic rats (Al-Ghoul et al. 1993). Moreover, antagonism of one type of glutamate receptor, the N-methyl-D-aspartate (NMDA) receptor, attenuates neuropathic pain in rats (Yamamoto and Yaksh 1992; Mao et al. 1993; Kim et al. 1997; Fisher et al. 1998), as well as humans (Sosnowski 1993; Mercadante et al. 1995; Mercadante 1996). However, use of NMDA-receptor antagonists, in doses sufficient to produce analgesia, is often associated with side effects in rats (Cahusac et al. 1984), as well as humans (Klepstad et al. 1990; Eide et al. 1995, Max et al. 1995).

In addition to acting on ionotropic NMDA receptors, glutamate also acts at metabotropic glutamate receptors (mGluRs), which are directly coupled, via guanine nucleotide regulatory (G) proteins, to intracellular second messengers. The mGluRs are divided into three groups based on sequence homology, signal transduction mechanisms, and receptor pharmacology (Hayashi et al. 1994). We have examined the role of group I mGluRs (mGluR1 and mGluR5) in neuropathic pain. Group I mGluRs are positively coupled to phosphatidylinositol hydrolysis; thus, the activation of these receptors leads to the translocation and activation of protein kinase C (PKC). We have previously shown that pretreatment with an antisense oligonucleotide targeting mGluR1 prevents the development of hyperalgesia and allodynia, attenuates heightened sensitivity to the excitatory effects of intrathecal NMDA, and restores opioid efficacy, while reducing mGluR1 protein and PKC activation in neuropathic rats (Fundytus et al. 1997, 1998; M.E. Fundytus, K. Yashpal, J.-G. Chabot, et al., unpublished manuscript). In this chapter, we describe the reversal of hyperalgesia and allodynia in neuropathic rats by antisense oligonucleotide knockdown of mGluR1, demonstrating that mGluR1 is also involved in the maintenance of neuropathic pain.

METHODS

Subjects. We used male Long Evans rats, weighing 300–350 g at the time of surgery. Rats were housed 3–4 animals per cage, on a 12:12 hour light:dark cycle, with food and water available ad libitum. All procedures were approved by the Clinical Research Institute of Montreal Animal Care Committee.

Oligonucleotides. An antisense (AS) oligonucleotide (AS: 5′-GAG CCG GAC CAT TGT GGC-3′) was designed to be complementary to base pairs 371–388 of the rat mGluR1 gene, RATGPCR. A control missense (MS) oligonucleotide was designed that had exactly the same bases as the AS sequence, with four base pairs mismatched (MS: 5′-GAG CCG AGC ACT GTG TGC-3′).

Surgery. Rats were rendered neuropathic by placing a 2-mm length of PE90 polyethylene tubing around one sciatic nerve (Mosconi and Kruger 1996). Intrathecal (i.t.) catheters, attached to Model 2001 Alzet osmotic mini-pumps (ALZA Corp., Palo Alto, California), were implanted 5 days after nerve injury. Rats were continuously infused for 7 days (from days 5 to 12 after nerve injury) with either artificial cerebrospinal fluid (ACSF), or AS or MS oligonucleotides at doses of 50 μg/day.

Sensitivity tests. Testing was performed prior to any surgery or treatment (baseline), 4 days after nerve injury, and 8, 12, and 18 days after nerve injury. Mechanical sensitivity was measured by applying thin filaments (von Frey hairs) to the plantar surface of the hindpaw and calculating the 50% response (withdrawal) threshold by the up-down method (Chaplan et al.

1994). Mechanical allodynia was assessed by calculating the percentage decrease in 50% response threshold compared to baseline.

Heat sensitivity was measured by applying a focused point of radiant heat to the plantar surface of the hindpaw (Hargreaves et al. 1988), and measuring the withdrawal latency. Heat hyperalgesia was assessed by calculating the percentage decrease in response latency compared to baseline.

Cold sensitivity was measured by placing rats in a 1 cm deep, 1°C water bath for 75 seconds and counting the number of responses (hindpaw lifts) during the test period. Cold hyperalgesia was assessed by calculating the increase in response frequency compared to baseline. Each rat was tested in all three paradigms, allowing sufficient time between tests to avoid interferences or carry-over effects (i.e., three groups of rats).

RESULTS

Fig. 1 depicts mechanical sensitivity in neuropathic rats treated with AS, MS, or ACSF. Four days after nerve injury, prior to intrathecal infusion of

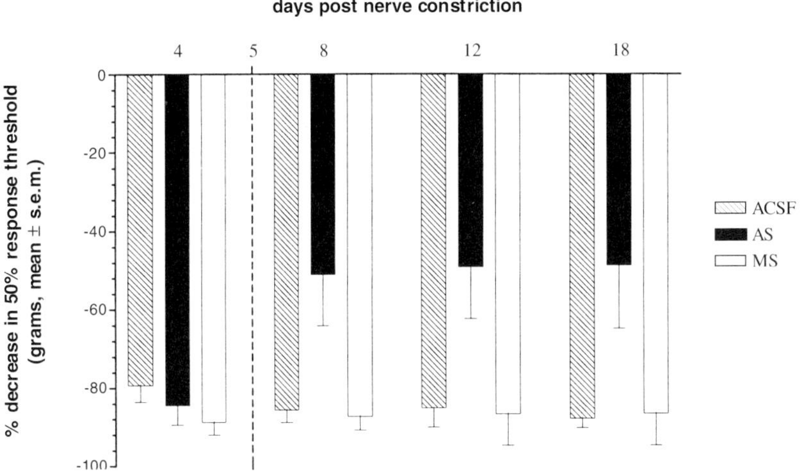

Fig. 1. Mechanical allodynia in neuropathic rats treated with i.t. antisense (AS), missense (MS), or artificial cerebrospinal fluid (ACSF), as indicated by mean percentage decrease in 50% response threshold (measured in grams) to von Frey hair stimulation of the plantar surface of the hindpaw. There was a significant day by i.t. treatment interaction ($F_{6,42} = 3.35$, $P < 0.05$). All rats displayed mechanical allodynia 4 days after nerve injury, indicated by a large decrease in 50% response threshold from baseline. Drug infusion began on day 5 after nerve injury (indicated by the dotted line), and on days 8–18 after nerve injury, post hoc tests showed that AS-treated rats displayed a significantly attenuated reduction in 50% response threshold compared to ACSF- and MS-treated rats.

oligonucleotides, all rats displayed mechanical allodynia as indicated by a large decrease in 50% response threshold from baseline. Drug infusion began on day 5 after nerve injury. On days 8–18 after nerve injury (3–13 days after initiation of oligonucleotide infusion), ACSF- and MS-treated rats were still allodynic, as indicated by a continued large decrease in 50% response threshold. In contrast, mechanical allodynia was reduced in AS-treated rats, as indicated by an attenuated reduction in 50% response threshold.

Fig. 2 shows heat sensitivity in neuropathic rats treated with AS, MS, or ACSF. Four days after nerve injury, all rats displayed heat hyperalgesia. On days 8–18 after nerve injury, ACSF- and MS-treated rats continued to display heat hyperalgesia, whereas heat hyperalgesia was reversed in AS-treated rats.

Fig. 3 illustrates the cold sensitivity in neuropathic rats treated with AS, MS, or ACSF. Four days after nerve injury all rats displayed cold hyperalgesia, as indicated by a large increase in the number of responses in the cold water bath. On days 8–18 after nerve injury, ACSF- and MS-treated animals continued to display cold hyperalgesia, whereas this was reversed in AS-treated rats, as indicated by a reduced frequency of responding.

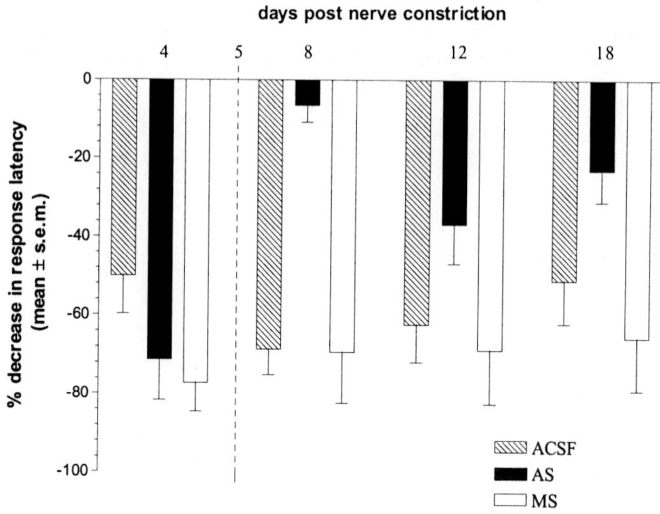

Fig. 2. Heat hyperalgesia in neuropathic rats treated with i.t. AS, MS, or ACSF as indicated by mean percentage decrease in response latency to focused radiant heat applied to the plantar surface of the hindpaw. There was a significant i.t. treatment by day interaction ($F_{6,42} = 6.22$, $P < 0.05$). All rats displayed heat hyperalgesia 4 days after nerve injury, indicated by a large decrease in response latency from baseline. Drug infusion began on day 5 (indicated by the dotted line), and on days 8–18 after nerve injury, post hoc tests showed that AS-treated rats exhibited a significantly attenuated reduction in response latency, compared to ACSF- and MS-treated rats.

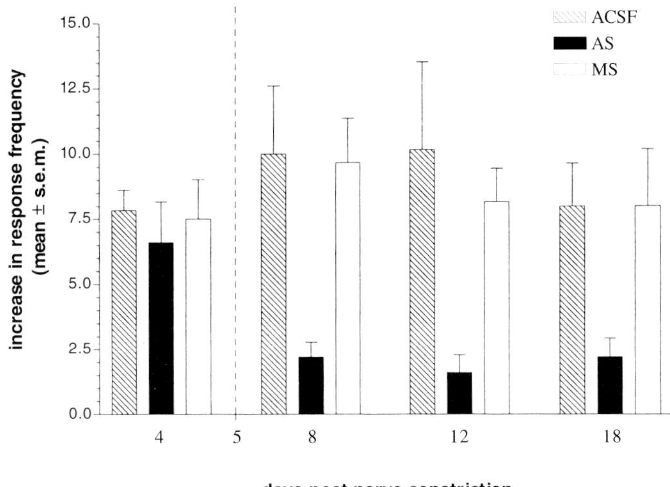

Fig. 3. Cold hyperalgesia in neuropathic rats treated with i.t. AS, MS, or ACSF, as indicated by increase in number of responses (hindpaw lifts) when rats stood in a 1 cm deep, 1°C water bath for 75 seconds. There was a significant i.t. treatment by day interaction ($F_{6,42} = 2.30$, $P = 0.05$). All rats displayed cold hyperalgesia 4 days after nerve injury, indicated by a large increase in response frequency. Drug infusion began on day 5 (indicated by the dotted line), and on days 8–18 after nerve injury, post hoc tests indicated that AS-treated rats exhibited a significantly attenuated increase in response frequency, compared to ACSF- and MS-treated rats.

DISCUSSION

In the present study we have shown that antisense oligonucleotide knockdown of mGluR1 *reverses* the mechanical allodynia and hot and cold hyperalgesia associated with nerve injury in rats. These results suggest that mGluR1 is involved in the *maintenance* of neuropathic pain. Previous results from our laboratory, showing a reduction in allodynia and hyperalgesia in nerve-injured rats with antisense oligonucleotide pretreatment, indicated that mGluR1 is involved in the *development* of neuropathic pain (Fundytus et al. 1997). Previous studies also showed that antisense oligonucleotide knockdown of mGluR1 restored opioid sensitivity in neuropathic rats (Fundytus et al. 1998; M.E. Fundytus et al., unpublished manuscript). Reduction of mGluR1 protein in the lumbar spinal cord, following intrathecal mGluR1 antisense oligonucleotide treatment, was verified by Western blot analysis (Fundytus et al. 1997, 1998). Using a [^{3}H]phorbol 12,13 dibutyrate ([^{3}H]PDBu) binding assay, a functional reduction of mGluR1 was also demonstrated by showing that enhanced PKC activity associated with neuropathic pain was attenuated by mGluR1 antisense oligonucleotide treatment (Fundytus et al. 1997,

1998). Thus, we propose that mGluR1 is a viable new target for drug development in the treatment of neuropathic pain.

ACKNOWLEDGMENTS

M.E. Fundytus was supported by an MRC/PMAC Post-doctoral Fellowship with J.L. Henry, sponsored by the ASTRA Research Centre Montreal. This research was supported by the ASTRA Research Centre Montreal and by the Medical Research Council (MRC) of Canada grants to J.L. Henry and T.J. Coderre. T.J. Coderre is an MRC scientist. The authors wish to thank Dr. Claes Wahlestedt and Dr. Francois Denis for their valuable advice on antisense oligonucleotide technology, and Dr. Robert Day for his valuable advice on Western blot analysis.

REFERENCES

Al-Ghoul WM, Li Volsi G, Weinberg RJ, Rustioni A. Glutamate immunocytochemistry in the dorsal horn after injury or stimulation of the sciatic nerve of rats. *Brain Res* 1993; 30:453–459.

Cahusac PMB, Evans RH, Hill RG, Rodriquez RE, Smith DAS. The behavioral effects of an N-methylaspartate receptor antagonist following application to the lumbar spinal cord of conscious rats. *Neuropharmacology* 1984; 23:719–724.

Chaplan SR, Bach FW, Pogrel JW, Chung JM, Yaksh TL. Quantitative assessment of tactile allodynia in the rat paw. *J Neurosci Methods* 1994; 53:55–63.

Chaplan SR, Malmberg AB, Yaksh TL. Efficacy of spinal NMDA receptor antagonism in formalin hyperalgesia and nerve injury evoked allodynia in the rat. *J Pharmacol Exp Ther* 1997; 280:829–838.

Cherny NI, Thaler HT, Friedlander-Klar H, et al. Opioid responsiveness of cancer pain syndromes caused by neuropathic or nociceptive mechanisms: a combined analysis of controlled, single-dose studies. *Neurology* 1994; 44:857–861.

Eide K, Stubhaug A, Oye I, Brevik H. Continuous subcutaneous administration of the N-methyl-D-aspartic acid (NMDA) receptor antagonist ketamine in the treatment of post-herpetic neuralgia. *Pain* 1995; 61:221–228.

Fisher K, Fundytus ME, Cahill CM, Coderre TJ. Intrathecal administration of the mGluR compound, (S)-4CPG, attenuates hyperalgesia and allodynia associated with sciatic nerve constriction injury in rats. *Pain* 1998; 77:59–66.

Fundytus ME, Fisher K, Dray A, Henry JL, Coderre TJ. Antisense oligonucleotides targeting group I mGluRs attenuate nerve constriction-induced hyperalgesia and allodynia. *Soc Neurosci Abstr* 1997; 23:1013.

Fundytus ME, Dray A, Henry JL, Coderre TJ. An antisense oligonucleotide targeting $mGluR_1$ restores opioid sensitivity in neuropathic rats. *INRC'98* (International Narcotics Research Conference Abstract), 1998, p 42.

Hargreaves K, Dubner R, Brown F, Flores C, Jores J. A new and sensitive method for measuring thermal nociception in cutaneous hyperalgesia. *Pain* 1988; 32:77–88.

Hayashi Y, Sekiyama N, Nakanishi S, et al. Analysis of agonist and antagonist activities of phenylglycine derivatives for different cloned metabotropic glutamate receptor subtypes. *J Neurosci* 1994; 14:3370–3377.

Kim YI, Na HS, Yoon YW, et al. NMDA receptors are important for both mechanical and thermal allodynia from peripheral nerve injuries in rats. *Neuroreport* 1997; 8:2149–2153.

Klepstad P, Maurset A, Moberg ER, Oye I. Evidence for a role for NMDA receptors in pain perception. *Eur J Pharmacol* 1990; 187:513–518.

MacDonald N. Opiate-resistant pain: a therapeutic dilemma. *Recent Results Cancer Res* 1991; 121:24–35.

Mao J, Price DD, Hayes RL, et al. Intrathecal treatment with dextrorphan or ketamine potently reduces pain-related behaviors in a rat model of peripheral mononeuropathy. *Brain Res* 1993: 605:164–168.

Max MB, Byas-Smith MG, Gracely RH, Bennett GJ. Intravenous infusion of the NMDA antagonist, ketamine, in chronic posttraumatic pain with allodynia: a double-blind comparison to alfentanil and placebo. *Clin Neuropharmacol* 1995; 18:360–368.

McQuay HJ, Jadad AR, Carroll D, et al. Opioid sensitivity of chronic pain: a patient-controlled analgesia method. *Anaesthesia* 1992; 47:757–767.

Mercadante S. Ketamine in cancer pain: an update. *Palliat Med* 1996; 10:225–230.

Mercadante S, Lodi F, Sapio M, Calligra M, Serretta R. Long-term ketamine subcutaneous continuous infusion in neuropathic pain. *J Pain Symptom Manage* 1995; 10:564–568.

Mosconi T, Kruger L. Fixed-diameter polyethylene cuffs applied to the rat sciatic nerve induce a painful neuropathy: ultrastructural morphometric analysis of axonal alterations. *Pain* 1996; 64:37–57.

Sosnowski M. Pain management: physiopathology, future research and endpoints. *Supportive Care Cancer* 1993; 1:79–88.

Yamamoto T, Yaksh TL. Spinal pharmacology of thermal hyperesthesia induced by constriction injury of sciatic nerve. *Pain* 1992; 49:121–128.

Correspondence to: Marian E. Fundytus, PhD, Department of Oncology, Division of Palliative Care, McGill University, 687 Pine Avenue West, Montreal, Quebec, Canada H3A 1A1. Tel: 514-842-1231 ext. 6610; Fax: 514-843-1471; email: marian.fundytus@muhc.mcgill.ca.

Proceedings of the 9th World Congress on Pain, Progress in Pain Research and Management, Vol. 16, edited by M. Devor, M.C. Rowbotham, and Z. Wiesenfeld-Hallin, IASP Press, Seattle, © 2000.

35

Spinal Cholecystokinin Systems in Two Models of Neuropathic Pain in the Rat

M. Pohl,[a] J.M. Antunes-Bras,[a] M.-A. Coudoret,[b] A.-M. Laporte,[a] J.-J. Benoliel,[a] M. Hamon,[a] A. Eschalier,[b] and F. Cesselin[a]

[a]*INSERM U-288, Faculty of Medicine, Pitié-Salpêtrière, Paris Cedex, France;* [b]*INSERM EPI 9904, Faculty of Medicine, Clermont-Ferrand Cedex, France*

A large body of evidence suggests that central cholecystokininergic neurotransmission contributes to neuropathic pain's relative resistance to the analgesic action of opioids. Indeed, expression of the gene encoding proCCK has been reported to be increased in dorsal root ganglia (DRG) after sciatic nerve section in rats (Xu et al. 1993). Both the levels of CCK-B receptor mRNA in DRG and the density of CCK-B receptors within the dorsal horn of the spinal cord are enhanced in this model of neuropathic pain (Zhang et al. 1993; Antunes-Bras et al. 1999). However, autotomy behavior, frequently observed after sciatic nerve section, can be prevented by combined treatment with morphine and a CCK-B receptor antagonist, CI-988 (Xu et al. 1993). In addition, probably via blockade of the anti-opioid properties of CCK, CI-988 relieves the allodynia-like symptoms in another model of neuropathic pain using ischemia-induced spinal cord lesions (Xu et al. 1994).

Diabetes is associated with neuropathic pain in some patients, and alterations in the analgesic potency of morphine have been reported in the relevant model of this disease in rats (Forman et al. 1986; Courteix et al. 1993). We investigated whether chronic pain associated with streptozotocin-induced diabetes in rats (Courteix et al. 1993) also involves alterations in central CCKergic neurotransmission, similar to those observed after peripheral nerve lesions.

MATERIALS AND METHODS

Animals. Male Sprague-Dawley rats (Charles River, France), weighing 180–200 g, were used. Some animals were deeply anesthetized and given two tight ligatures on the exposed right sciatic nerve; approximately 5 mm of the nerve was excised between these ligatures, and the incision was sutured. In other animals, diabetes was induced by intraperitoneal injection of streptozotocin (75 mg/kg) dissolved in distilled water. Blood glucose levels were measured 1 week later using a reflectance colorimeter; only rats with final blood glucose levels of ≥14 mM were included in the study. Axotomized and diabetic animals were allowed 14 days for recovery before the experiments were performed.

All the procedures involving animals and their care were conducted in conformity with institutional guidelines and national laws and policies.

Dissection of spinal cord and DRG. All animals were killed by decapitation. The whole spinal cord was removed at cold temperatures (0°–4°C), as described elsewhere (Cesselin et al. 1984). In axotomized rats, the cervical (C5–T1) and lumbar (L3–L5) enlargements were divided into their left and right parts by a sagittal cut, and then into their dorsal and ventral zones by a horizontal cut passing through the ependymal canal. DRG (L4–L6) were removed in the lumbar region (Pohl et al. 1990). In diabetic animals, cervical and lumbar enlargements of the spinal cord were divided only into their dorsal and ventral parts.

Tissues for RNA extractions were immediately frozen in liquid nitrogen, then stored at –80°C until use. For autoradiographic experiments, the lumbar enlargement was frozen in isopentane cooled to –40°C with dry ice.

Radioimmunoassay of CCK-like material. Dissected tissues were homogenized in 5 volumes (v/w) of 0.1 M HCl and heated for 15 minutes at 95°C. After centrifugation (38,000 *g*, 10 minutes, 4°C), the supernatant was adjusted to pH 7.0 with 1 M Tris base, and the resulting precipitate was spun down at 6000 *g* for 10 minutes at 4°C. Proteins were quantified in each pellet by the method of Lowry et al. (1951), with bovine serum albumin (BSA) as the standard. CCK-like material (CCK-LM) content in each spinal tissue extract (6000 *g* clear supernatant) was assayed in duplicates at three appropriate dilutions (Benoliel et al. 1992). Radioiodinated human gastrin (~2000 Ci/mmol, CEA, Saclay, France) was used as a tracer.

Quantitative RT-PCR analysis of PRO-CCK and CCK-B receptor mRNAs. Total RNA, extracted from dissected pieces of the spinal cord and DRG according to Chomczynski and Sacchi (1987), was quantified using as reference a scale of total RNA prepared on cesium chloride gradient (Chirgwin et al. 1979) and estimated from optical density measurement at 260 nm.

Reverse transcription polymerase chain reaction (RT-PCR) was performed on 0.5 μg of total RNA (or 2 μg for amplification of proCCK in DRG) in the presence of various amounts (0.04–3.75 fg) of an internal synthetic standard RNA prepared according to the PCR MIMIC construction kit (Clontech). The standard fragments were amplified with the same sets of proCCK- or CCK-B receptor-specific primers as for the respective cDNAs (Antunes-Bras et al. 1999). Reverse-transcribed RNAs were amplified with 30 PCR cycles (96°, 58°, and 72°C; 1 minute each) according to the Access RT-PCR system instructions (Promega). The RT-PCR products were electrophoresed in 1.2% agarose gel stained with ethidium bromide, and quantified with a gel analyzer (GDS 5000, UVP, Cambridge, United Kingdom).

CCK-B receptor autoradiography. Experiments were carried out as described by Antunes-Bras et al. (1999). Briefly, sections (20 μm) on gelatin-coated glass slides were preincubated in 50 mM Tris-HCl, pH 7.4, for 30 minutes at room temperature, and then incubated for 60 minutes under the same conditions except that the (fresh) buffer was supplemented with 5 mM $MgCl_2$, 0.5 mg/mL bacitracin, 0.05% BSA, and 0.2 nM of the tritiated CCK-B receptor agonist [^{3}H]pBC 264 (40–70 Ci/mmol, New England Nuclear). Nonspecific binding was estimated on adjacent sections processed through the same steps, except that a saturating concentration (1 μM) of CCK was added to the incubation medium. After washing, slides were dried in a stream of cold air, and then tightly apposed to ^{3}H Hyperfilm (Amersham) in the dark for 4 months at 4°C. Autoradiographic films were developed, and quantified using a BIOCOM densitometer.

Expression of results and statistical calculations. CCK-LM levels in tissues were calculated as picograms of peptide equivalents, i.e., the amount of authentic peptide producing the same displacement of the [^{125}I]probe as the endogenous immunoreactive material in the samples. Data are presented as means ± SEM. Statistical analyses were performed using ANOVA followed by Fisher's protected least significant differences (PLSD) test or Student's *t* test. $P > 0.05$ was considered to be nonsignificant.

RESULTS

Tissue levels of CCK-LM in the spinal cord. Unilateral sciatic nerve section had no effect on CCK-LM levels in either the ipsilateral or contralateral quadrants of both the dorsal and the ventral parts of the cervical and lumbar enlargements. Similarly, CCK-LM levels in the spinal cord of diabetic animals did not differ from those measured in controls (Table I).

Table I
Levels of CCK-like material (CCK-LM) in the contralateral and ipsilateral dorsal and ventral quadrants of the spinal cord in rats with unilateral sciatic nerve section, and in the dorsal and ventral parts of the spinal cord in diabetic and control animals

	CCK-LM (pg/mg protein)					
	Sciatic Nerve Section		Diabetic		Control	
	Dorsal	Ventral	Dorsal	Ventral	Dorsal	Ventral
Cervical						
Contralateral	560 ± 13	232 ± 26	590 ± 40	240 ± 20	550 ± 34	210 ± 17
Ipsilateral	615 ± 26	197 ± 15				
Lumbar						
Contralateral	580 ± 48	236 ± 25	610 ± 52	270 ± 44	570 ± 42	280 ± 44
Ipsilateral	604 ± 52	209 ± 22				

Note: Two weeks after induction of diabetes or section of the right sciatic nerve, the whole spinal cord was removed. The cervical and lumbar segments were immediately dissected and separated into their dorsal and ventral halves in diabetic or in control animals. In axotomized rats, spinal cord segments were first divided into left and right parts, which were then separated into dorsal and ventral zones. CCK-LM levels are expressed as picograms of peptide equivalents per milligram of protein. Each value is the mean ± SEM of 10–15 independent determinations.

Concentrations of pro-CCK and CCK-B receptor mRNAs in the lumbar cord and DRG. Sciatic nerve section had no effect on proCCK-mRNA concentrations in either the dorsal or ventral parts of the lumbar spinal cord. Similarly, spinal proCCK-mRNA levels were unchanged in diabetic rats as compared to controls. In DRG of both axotomized and diabetic rats, proCCK-mRNA concentrations also did not differ from the control values (data not shown).

The levels of CCK-B receptor mRNA in spinal tissues were altered neither by sciatic nerve section nor by streptozotocin-induced diabetes (Fig. 1A). Similarly, in lumbar DRG of diabetic rats, CCK-B receptor mRNA concentrations did not significantly differ from the control values. In contrast, in axotomized rats, a ~70% increase in CCK-B receptor mRNA levels was observed in DRG on the lesioned side (Fig. 1B).

Autoradiographic labeling of CCK-B receptors in the dorsal horn. The labeling of CCK-B receptors by [^{3}H]pBC 264 in superficial layers of the lumbar dorsal horn was 2.6 times greater on the lesioned side compared with the intact side in axotomized rats and with both sides in control rats. By contrast, no significant changes in the labeling of these receptors were observed after streptozotocin-induced diabetes. In both control and diabetic rats, only low levels of [^{3}H]pBC 264 specific binding were observed within the superficial layers of the lumbar dorsal horn (Fig. 2).

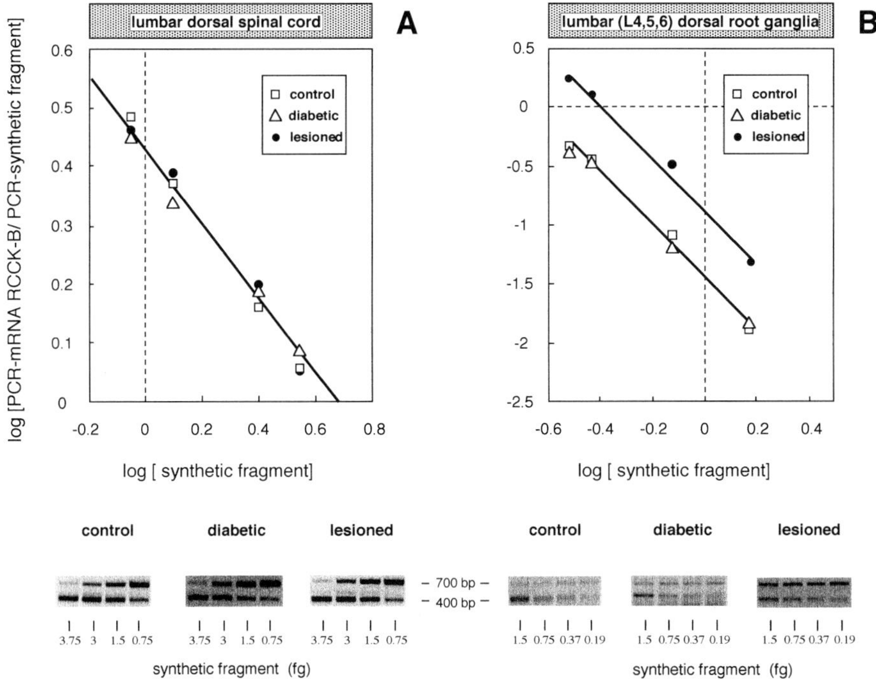

Fig. 1. Quantitative RT-PCR of CCK-B receptor mRNA (A) in the dorsal part of the lumbar spinal cord of control and diabetic rats, and the dorsal quadrant ipsilateral to the lesion in axotomized rats, and (B) in lumbar DRG in the same animals. Total RNA (500 ng) from spinal cord and DRG (ipsilateral to the lesion in axotomized rats) and four serial dilutions of the synthetic fragment (see Materials and Methods) were successively reverse transcribed and amplified for 30 cycles using specific primers. PCR products were then electrophoresed in 1.2% ethidium bromide-stained agarose gel. The logarithmic ratio of the levels (optical density measurements) of the PCR product of RCCK-B mRNA (660 base pairs) over those of the PCR product of the synthetic fragment (440 base pairs) is plotted against the logarithm of each serial dilution of the synthetic standard (measured in femtograms). At the equivalence point (0 on the ordinate), equimolar concentrations of RCCK-B mRNA and synthetic RNA were reverse transcribed and amplified.

DISCUSSION

Unilateral sciatic nerve section had no effect on spinal levels of proCCK mRNA or CCK-LM in the spinal cord of adult rats (see also McGregor et al. 1984; Antunes-Bras et al. 1999). In addition, quantitative RT-PCR measurements revealed no changes in proCCK mRNA levels in DRG of axotomized rats. This suggests that the axotomy-induced change in the expression of the proCCK gene in DRG, previously reported by Xu et al. (1993) using

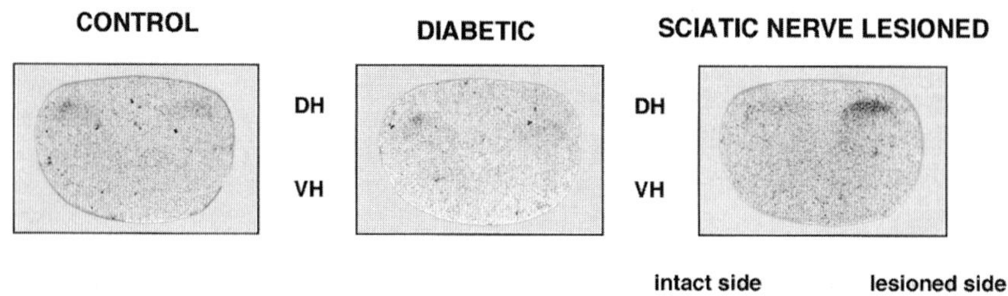

Fig. 2. Autoradiographic labeling of CCK-B receptors in the spinal cord of control, diabetic, and axotomized rats. Lumbar (L3–L5) spinal cord sections from control, diabetic, and unilaterally sciatic nerve-sectioned rats were incubated with 0.2 nM [^{3}H]pBC 264 for 60 minutes as described in Materials and Methods. Autoradiograms were obtained after exposure to ^{3}H Hyperfilm (Amersham) for 4 months. DH = dorsal horn; VH = ventral horn.

semiquantitative in situ hybridization, probably involves only a discrete increase in proCCK mRNA levels, too small to be quantified. Similarly, the concentrations of CCK-LM and proCCK mRNA in both spinal cord and DRG of diabetic rats remained indistinguishable from control values. In contrast, unilateral sciatic nerve section resulted in enhanced CCK-B receptor mRNA levels in DRG, associated with a marked increase of CCK-B receptor labeling in the ipsilateral dorsal horn, in agreement with previous data (Zhang et al. 1993; Antunes Bras et al. 1999). However, in diabetic animals none of the latter parameters were modified as compared to healthy control rats.

Thus, in spite of several similar changes in peripheral sensory nerves following axotomy and induction of diabetes (reduced availability of target-derived NGF, decreased substance P and calcitonin gene-related peptide expression in DRG, and nerve degeneration [see Brewster et al. 1994]), the spinal CCK systems are differentially affected in these two models of neuropathic pain. In sciatic nerve-sectioned rats, upregulation of CCK-B receptors (but not of CCK synthesis) probably contributes to an increased spinal CCKergic neurotransmission, whereas in diabetic animals, the unchanged CCK-related parameters indicate that spinal CCKergic neurotransmission was unaltered as compared to controls. This suggests that the reduced analgesic efficacy of morphine cannot be ascribed to enhanced spinal CCK neurotransmission in streptozotocin-induced diabetes. Further studies should explore which among the profound metabolic changes associated with the disease are relevant to the well-established relative insensitivity of diabetic rats to opiates.

ACKNOWLEDGMENT

This research was supported by grants from INSERM and Institut UPSA de la Douleur. J.M. Antunes-Bras was the recipient of a MENESR fellowship during this project.

REFERENCES

Antunes-Bras JM, Laporte AM, Benoliel JJ, et al. Effects of peripheral axotomy on cholecystokinin neurotransmission in the rat. *J Neurochem* 1999; 72:858–867.

Benoliel JJ, Bourgoin S, Mauborgne A, et al. GABA, acting at both $GABA_A$ and $GABA_B$ receptors, inhibits the release of cholecystokinin-like material from the rat spinal cord *in vitro*. *Brain Res* 1992; 590:255–262.

Brewster WJ, Fernyhough P, Diemel LT, et al. Diabetic neuropathy, nerve growth factor and other neurotrophic factors. *Trends Neurosci* 1994; 8:321–325

Cesselin F, Bourgoin S, Artaud F, Hamon M. Basic and regulatory mechanisms of *in vitro* release of met-enkephalin from the dorsal zone of the rat spinal cord. *J Neurochem* 1984; 43:763–773.

Chirgwin JJ, Przybyla AE, Mc Donald RJ, Rutter WJ. Isolation of biologically active ribonucleic acid from sources enriched in ribonuclease. *J Biochem* 1979; 18:5294–5299.

Chomczynski P, Sacchi N. Single-step method of RNA isolation by acid guanidinium thiocyanate-phenol-chloroform extraction. *Anal Biochem* 1987; 162:156–159.

Courteix C, Eschalier A, Lavarenne J. Streptozotocin-induced diabetic rats: behavioural evidence for a model of chronic pain. *Pain* 1993; 53:81–88.

Forman LJ, Lewis SEM, Vasilenko P. Streptozotocin diabetes alters immunoreactive-endorphin levels and pain perception after 8 weeks in female rats. *Diabetes* 1986; 35:1309–1313.

Lowry OH, Rosebrough NJ, Farr AL, Randall RJ. Protein measurement with the Folin phenol reagent. *J Biol Chem* 1951; 193:265–275.

McGregor GP, Gibson SJ, Sabate IM, et al. Effect of peripheral nerve section and nerve crush on spinal cord neuropeptides in the rat: increased VIP and PHI in the dorsal horn. *Neuroscience* 1984; 13:207–216.

Pohl M, Benoliel JJ, Bourgoin S, Lombard MC, et al. Regional distribution of calcitonin gene-related peptide-, substance P-, cholecystokinin-, Met^5-enkephalin-, and dynorphin A(1–8)-like materials in the spinal cord and dorsal root ganglia of adult rats: effects of dorsal rhizotomy and neonatal capsaicin. *J Neurochem* 1990; 55:1122–1130.

Xu XJ, Puke MCC, Verge VMK, Wiesenfeld-Hallin Z. Up-regulation of cholecystokinin in primary sensory neurons is associated with morphine insensitivity in experimental neuropathic pain in the rat. *Neurosci Lett* 1993; 152:129–132.

Xu XJ, Hao JX, Seiger A, et al. Chronic pain-related behaviors in spinally injured rats: evidence for functional alterations of the endogenous cholecystokinin and opioid systems. *Pain* 1994; 56:271–277.

Zhang X, Dagerlind A, Elde RP, et al. Marked increase in cholecystokinin B receptor messenger RNA levels in rat dorsal root ganglia after peripheral axotomy. *Neuroscience* 1993; 57:227–233.

Correspondence to: Michel Pohl, MD, INSERM U-288, Faculté de Médecine Pitié-Salpêtrière, 91, Boulevard de l'Hôpital, 75634 Paris Cedex 13, France. Tel.: 33-1-40-77-97-08; Fax: 33-1-40-77-97-90; email: pohl@ext.jussieu.fr.

Proceedings of the 9th World Congress on Pain,
Progress in Pain Research and Management,
Vol. 16, edited by M. Devor, M.C. Rowbotham, and
Z. Wiesenfeld-Hallin, IASP Press, Seattle, © 2000.

36

Long-Lasting Analgesia following TENS and Acupuncture: Spinal Mechanisms beyond Gate Control

Jürgen Sandkühler

Physiology and Pathophysiology Institute, University of Heidelberg, Heidelberg, Germany

Stimulation of sensory nerve fibers can alleviate acute and chronic pain. The application of thermal or tolerably painful stimuli (e.g., via acupuncture needles) has a long-standing tradition in pain therapy. Shortly after the formulation of the gate control theory (Melzack and Wall 1965), a new form of afferent stimulation was successfully introduced into clinical practice: the excitation of thick, myelinated Aβ fibers, either by transcutaneous electrical nerve stimulation (TENS), by dorsal column stimulation, or by mechanical excitation of sensory nerve endings during vibratory stimuli (Wall and Sweet 1967).

Two basically distinct forms of TENS have proven clinically useful. First, stimulation at a high frequency (e.g., at 100 Hz) and low intensity evokes paresthesia but no painful sensations. This form of stimulation recruits only Aα/β fibers and typically produces an analgesia or hypoalgesia throughout the duration of stimulation. Analgesia that lasted up to 2 hours after termination of stimulation was, however, achieved in less than 20% of patients (Johnson et al. 1991). Thus, this form of paresthetic TENS is used in a patient-controlled administration for several hours every day. In animal experiments the antinociceptive effect can be blocked by the $GABA_A$-receptor antagonist bicuculline (Duggan and Foong 1985). This form of low-intensity, high-frequency, paresthetic TENS is best explained by a spinal segmental mechanism involving an inhibitory, probably GABAergic interneuron as described in the gate control theory (see Fig. 1A; Melzack and Wall 1965).

The second form of TENS requires stimulation at an intensity that produces tolerable pain that most likely involves afferent Aδ fibers. This mildly

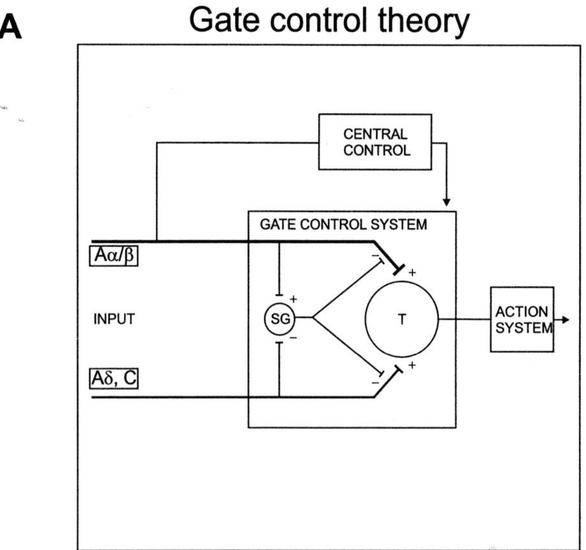

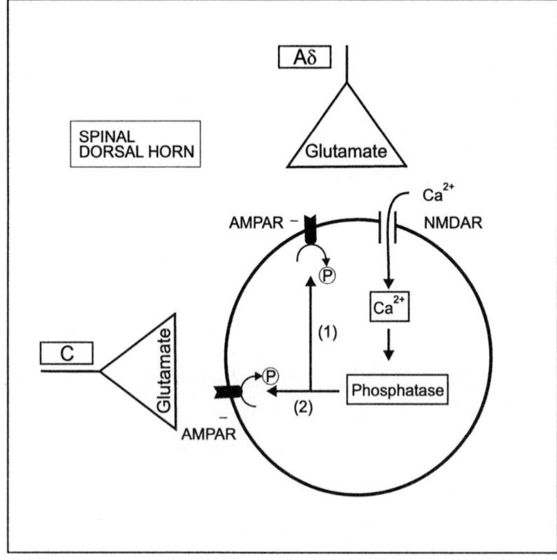

Fig. 1. Afferent-induced analgesia involves two fundamentally different mechanisms in spinal dorsal horn. (A) Conditioning stimulation of Aα/β fibers excites (+) small interneurons in substantia gelatinosa (SG) of spinal dorsal horn that exert inhibitory effects (–) on presynaptic nerve terminals of Aδ and C fibers (presynaptic inhibition). Alternatively, inhibition of spinal nociceptive projection neuron (T) may be postsynaptic (not shown) (gate control theory). (B) Conditioning stimulation of Aδ fibers induces release of glutamate from nerve terminals in superficial spinal dorsal horn that activates ionotropic glutamate receptors of the NMDA subtype (and mGluRs, not shown). This

painful TENS is tolerated if applied at relatively low frequencies (1–10 Hz) (Ishimaru et al. 1995); it is typically used for approximately 15 minutes, several times a week (Melzack 1975). This painful form of TENS (or electroacupuncture) may achieve the best analgesic effect only after repetitive stimulations over several weeks. If produced, analgesia typically outlasts the duration of conditioning stimulation by hours or days; pain reduction may be permanent in some fortunate patients (Thorsen and Lumsden 1997). This form of long-lasting analgesia, requiring mildly painful therapeutic stimulation, cannot be explained by the gate control theory.

We propose a cellular mechanism in the spinal dorsal horn that may underlie the long-lasting analgesia following painful TENS and electroacupuncture: low-frequency stimulation of Aδ fibers can induce long-term depression (LTD) of synaptic strength in fine primary afferent nerve fibers (see Fig. 1B). This form of afferent-induced spinal antinociception does not require activation of $GABA_A$ receptors but rather activation of ionotropic and metabotropic glutamate receptors.

METHODS

This section briefly reviews our methods, which are described in detail elsewhere (Sandkühler et al. 1997; Liu et al. 1998).

IN VIVO EXPERIMENTS

Adult male Sprague-Dawley rats (250–350 g) were anesthetized with urethane (1.5 g/kg, i.p.). The lumbar enlargement of the spinal cord was exposed by laminectomy. The left sciatic nerve was dissected free for bipolar electrical stimulation. Spinal field potentials were evoked by electrical stimulation of the sciatic nerve and were recorded with tungsten microelectrodes (impedance 1–3 MΩ). Single square cathodal pulses (7–20 V, 0.5 ms, at 60-second intervals) delivered to the sciatic nerve were used as test stimuli. To induce LTD of C-fiber-evoked field potentials we used conditioning stimu-

---

leads to a moderate increase in free cytosolic Ca^{2+} concentration that is sufficient to activate protein phosphatases. The dephosphorylation of synaptic proteins (e.g., of ionotropic glutamate receptors of the AMPA subtype) leads to the depression of synaptic strength for prolonged periods (e.g., by reduction of postsynaptic AMPA-receptor-gated excitatory currents [–]).This LTD may be homosynaptic in nature if dephosphorylation is restricted to the synapses of Aδ fibers that were active during conditioning stimulation (1). LTD is labeled heterosynaptic when increase of Ca^{2+} and activation of phosphatases is sufficient to also affect synapses of C fibers that were not active during conditioning stimulation (2).

lation of A fibers in sciatic nerve. For controlled superfusion of the spinal cord at the recording segment, we used a specially synthesized silicone rubber to form a small well on the cord dorsum at the recording segments (Beck et al. 1995).

IN VITRO EXPERIMENTS

The L4 to S1 segments of lumbosacral spinal cord of 17- to 28-day-old rats were excised with long (8–15 mm) dorsal roots attached. We used transverse slices (400–500 μm thick) with one bisected dorsal root attached. Oxygenated recording solution (33°C) consisted of: 124 mM NaCl, 1.9 mM KCl, 1.2 mM KH_2PO_4, 2.4 mM $CaCl_2$, 1.3 mM $MgSO_4$, 26 mM $NaHCO_3$, and 10 mM glucose, at pH 7.4, osmolarity 310–320 mosmol/kg. Intracellular recordings were made with sharp microelectrodes (170 MΩ) and a high-input impedance bridge amplifier (Axoclamp 2B, Axon Instruments). Each dorsal root half was stimulated independently through a suction electrode with isolated current stimulators. Only excitatory postsynaptic potentials (EPSPs) that were evoked by Aδ fibers were investigated further. Test pulses of 0.1 ms were given at 60-second intervals unless stated otherwise. Conditioning stimulation was applied to one dorsal root half (900 pulses of 0.1-ms duration at 0.7 mA were given at 1 Hz). Cathodal DC current (up to 0.1 nA) was passed into the cell during the course of the experiment to maintain membrane hyperpolarization typically between –75 and –85 mV (Sandkühler et al. 1997).

DRUGS

Drugs and their sources were as follows: D-2-amino-5-phosphonovaleric acid (D-AP5, 50 μM, Cambridge Research Biochemicals); bicuculline methiodide (bicuculline, 5 or 10 μM, Sigma); strychnine (2 or 4 μM, Sigma); (S)-α-methyl-4-carboxyphenylglycine ((S)-MCPG, 1 mM, Tocris); (S)-4-carboxyphenylglycine ((S)-4C-PG, 200 μM, Tocris); (RS)-α-tethylserine-O-phosphate monophenyl ester (MSOPPE, 200 μM, Tocris); (RS)-α-methylserine-O-phosphate (MSOP, 200 μM, Tocris); (1S, 3R)-1-amino-cyclopentane-1,3-dicarboxylic acid ((1S, 3R)-ACPD, 100 μM, Tocris); pertussis toxin (PTX, 1 or 2 μg/mL, Sigma).

DATA ANALYSIS

In each experiment, we averaged the amplitudes of five consecutive C-fiber-evoked field potentials, collected at 60-second intervals. We used nonparametric ANOVA (Kruskal-Wallis test) for statistical analysis and considered $P \leq 0.05$ as significant.

Two consecutive EPSPs were averaged and synaptic strength was quantified by measuring the peak amplitude and initial slope of averaged EPSPs. The mean values of four to seven averaged, consecutive test responses recorded prior to conditioning stimulation served as controls. We assessed significant changes from controls by comparing the values of four consecutive responses 23–30 minutes after conditioning stimulation. We used the nonparametric Wilcoxon rank test for statistical comparisons and considered $P \leq 0.05$ as significant. All values were expressed as mean ± SEM.

RESULTS

LONG-TERM DEPRESSION OF SYNAPTIC STRENGTH IN FINE PRIMARY AFFERENTS

Stimulation of a dorsal root in vitro or sciatic nerve in vivo at low intensities insufficient to recruit Aδ fibers consistently failed to induce LTD of synaptic strength either in Aδ (Sandkühler et al. 1997) or in C fibers (Liu et al. 1998). Only by increasing the intensity of conditioning stimulation to also recruit Aδ fibers in dorsal roots (10 V or 0.7 mA, 0.1-ms pulses given at 1 Hz for 15 minutes) could we induce a homosynaptic LTD at synapses of Aδ fibers in vitro (Fig. 2A). When conditioning stimulation of A fibers, including Aδ fibers in sciatic nerve, was delivered in bursts (10 V, 0.1-ms pulses, 100 Hz for 1 second repeated at 0.1 Hz for 15 minutes), a putatively heterosynaptic LTD of C-fiber-evoked field potentials was induced in vivo (Fig. 2B).

Conditioning stimulation of Aδ fibers not only depressed normal synaptic transmission in Aδ and in C fibers for prolonged periods (LTD), but also normalized synaptic strength after long-term potentiation (LTP) had been induced at C-fiber synapses. A robust LTP to 216 ± 22% of control (n = 5) was induced in vivo by high-frequency, high-intensity stimulation of sciatic nerve at C-fiber strength. Two sessions of 15 minutes conditioning stimulation of Aδ fibers normalized synaptic strength (to 105 ± 22% of control) (Fig. 3) (Liu et al. 1998). LTP at synapses of C-fiber afferents is considered a synaptic mechanism of central sensitization leading to hyperalgesia (Sandkühler 1996). Thus, conditioning stimulation of Aδ fibers may not only have long-lasting analgesic effects but may also *reverse* some forms of hyperalgesia.

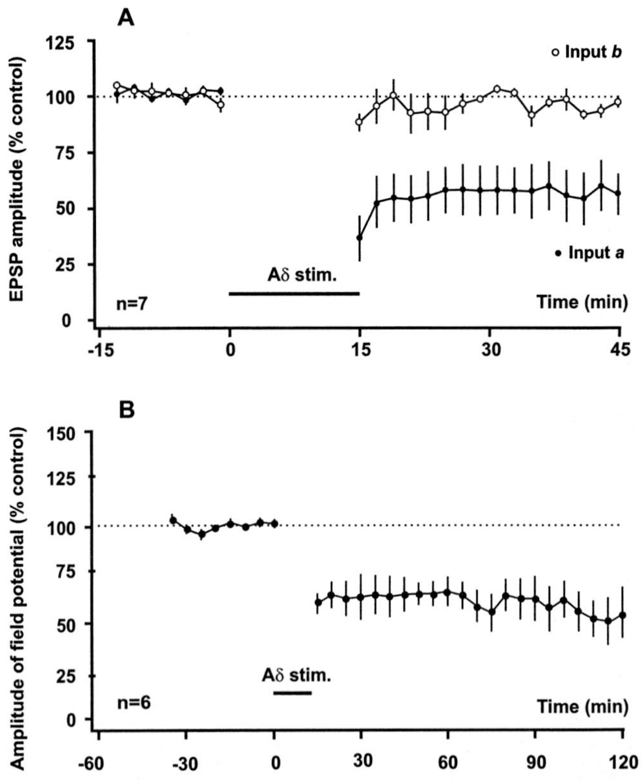

Fig. 2. Conditioning stimulation of Aδ fibers induces long-term depression (LTD) of synaptic strength in spinal dorsal horn. (A) Homosynaptic LTD at spinal synapses of afferent Aδ fibers. In a spinal cord slice preparation with one bisected dorsal root, intracellular recordings were made from neurons with monosynaptic input from both dorsal root halves (inputs *a* and *b*). EPSPs were recorded in response to inputs *a* and *b*. Conditioning low-frequency stimulation (Aδ-stim, 1 Hz, 15 minutes) was applied to one dorsal root half only (input *a*). This induced an LTD in input *a* without affecting synaptic strength in the unconditioned input *b*, i.e., LTD was homosynaptic in nature. (B) LTD at spinal synapses of afferent C fibers. In urethane-anesthetized rats, C-fiber-evoked field potentials were recorded in the superficial spinal dorsal horn in response to supramaximal electrical stimulation of sciatic nerve. Conditioning burst-like, high-frequency stimulation (Aδ-stim, 100 Hz for 1 minute repeated at 0.1 Hz for 15 minutes) of Aδ fibers in the sciatic nerve depressed synaptic strength in C fibers for prolonged periods. This LTD is probably heterosynaptic in nature. To directly prove a heterosynaptic LTD would, however, require intracellular recordings of spinal neurons with monosynaptic input from Aδ and C fibers.

TONIC DESCENDING INHIBITION MODULATES DIRECTION OF SYNAPTIC PLASTICITY IN THE SPINAL CORD

Descending systems originating at brainstem sites exert mainly inhibitory effects on nociceptive neurons in spinal dorsal horn (Fields and Basbaum

1978). The effect of conditioning Aδ-fiber stimulation critically depends upon the integrity of these descending pathways. With the spinal cord and descending pathways intact, burst-like stimulation at Aδ-fiber strength reliably induced an LTD of synaptic strength in C fibers (to 61 ± 15% of control, $n = 9$). In contrast, when the spinal cord was cut rostral to the recording site, the same conditioning stimulation now no longer produced an LTD but rather an LTP of synaptic strength in C fibers (to 187 ± 19% of control, $n = 5$). Thus, the effect of conditioning afferent stimulation depends on both the parameters of conditioning stimulation and the balance between the activity in inhibitory and in excitatory systems in spinal cord.

NEUROPHARMACOLOGY OF SPINAL LONG-TERM DEPRESSION INDUCED BY AFFERENT STIMULATION

Bath application of $GABA_A$-receptor antagonist bicuculline (5 μM) plus glycine receptor antagonist strychnine (2 μM) did not affect induction of LTD in vitro: results showed depression to 53 ± 8% of control ($n = 6$) as compared to a depression to 41 ± 10% of control ($n = 8$) in normal recording solution. Thus, neither $GABA_A$ nor glycine receptors are required for induction of LTD.

Bath application of NMDA-receptor antagonist D-AP5 (50 μM) in vitro or superfusion of spinal cord at the recording segment in vivo with D-AP5 (100 μM) abolished induction of LTD at spinal synapses of Aδ or C fibers, which suggests that these forms of spinal LTD require activation of NMDA receptors. In addition, co-activation of G-protein-coupled group I and group II mGluRs is necessary for induction of LTD at spinal synapses of Aδ fibers in vitro. Bath application of selective group I mGluR antagonist (S)-4-CPG (200 μM) or group II mGluR antagonist MSOPPE (200 μM) blocked induction of LTD (to 93 ± 12%, $n = 5$, and to 104 ± 8%, $n = 5$, respectively) by stimulation of Aδ fibers.

PHARMACOLOGICAL ACTIVATION OF LONG-TERM DEPRESSION IN THE SUPERFICIAL SPINAL DORSAL HORN

All previously described forms of LTD in the superficial spinal dorsal horn were induced by conditioning stimulation of primary afferent Aδ fibers. We have now identified a new form of spinal LTD that is induced pharmacologically by activation of mGluRs in the absence of impulses in presynaptic nerve fibers. Bath application of nonselective group I/group II mGluR agonist ACPD (100 μM) induced a robust LTD at synapses of Aδ fibers (to 72 ± 4% of control, $n = 8$) in the presence of bicuculline (5 μM) and strychnine (2 μM). This LTD was independent of NMDA-receptor

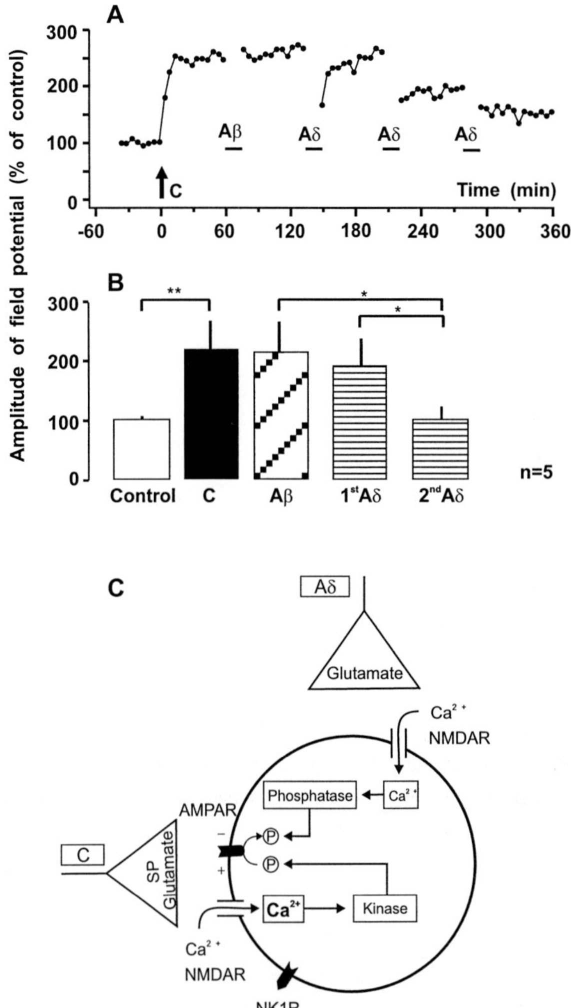

Fig. 3. Long-term potentiation (LTP) and depotentiation of synaptic strength at afferent C fibers. In urethane-anesthetized rats, C-fiber-evoked field potentials were recorded in the superficial spinal dorsal horn in response to supramaximal electrical stimulation of the sciatic nerve. Conditioning high-frequency stimulation of afferent C fibers in sciatic nerve (arrow in A) induced an LTP in this experiment to about 250% of control. Low-intensity conditioning stimulation of Aβ fibers (0.3-V, 0.1-ms pulses, 100 Hz for 1 second repeated at 0.1 Hz for 15 minutes) failed to affect synaptic strength. When stimulation intensity was raised to also recruit Aδ fibers (10 V, as above), previously potentiated synaptic strength gradually returned to normal. (B) Mean values from five experiments. (C) Putative signal transduction pathways of LTP and depotentiation in nociceptive spinal dorsal horn neurons are depicted. High-frequency conditioning stimulation of C fibers expressing substance P (SP) leads to a strong increase in $[Ca^{2+}]_i$ via activation of NMDAR and NK1R. This strong increase in $[Ca^{2+}]_i$ is sufficient to activate protein kinases that phosphorylate synaptic proteins (e.g., AMPA

activation, as bath application of D-AP5 (50 μM) failed to affect LTD (to 60 ± 11% of control, *n* = 5). G proteins sensitive to pertussis-toxin are not required for ACPD-induced LTD, as preincubation of spinal cord slice for at least 2 hours with pertussis toxin (1 or 2 μg/mL) did not affect induction of LTD (to 55 ± 8% of control, *n* = 5). Blockade of phospholipase C by U73122 but not its inactive enantiomer U73343 abolished LTD induction (101 ± 3% of control, *n* = 5), which suggests involvement of pertussis-toxin-insensitive G proteins that activate phospholipase C.

DISCUSSION

Clinically relevant afferent-induced analgesia can be achieved by excitation of various types of afferent nerve fibers (Aα/β, Aδ, or C fibers) or sensory nerve endings including low-threshold mechanoreceptors, nociceptors, and thermoreceptors. Paresthetic TENS will selectively recruit Aα/β fibers, while mildly painful TENS and some forms of electroacupuncture involve excitation of Aδ fibers. Vibratory stimuli selectively activate rapidly adapting mechanoreceptors, while needle acupuncture may in addition excite mechanosensitive and polymodal Aδ- and C-fiber nociceptors (reviewed by Kawakita and Gotoh 1996). Some forms of physical therapy will excite warm or cold receptors or low-threshold mechanoreceptors. From a practical and scientific point of view it is desirable to classify the various forms of treatment according to the afferent fiber type that induces the analgesia. However, at present afferent-induced analgesia is grouped according to the organizational level into segmental, propriospinal, and supraspinal descending forms.

SYNAPTIC LONG-TERM DEPRESSION OR GATE CONTROL IN SPINAL DORSAL HORN

We propose that electrical stimulation of Aα/β fibers induces a fundamentally different form of analgesia as compared to analgesia induced by excitation of all A fibers including Aδ fibers. The short-lasting analgesia produced by paresthetic TENS (i.e., at a low intensity and at high frequency) or by vibratory stimuli is best explained by mechanisms similar to those described in the gate control theory and that involve inhibitory, probably

---

receptors). This will potentiate synaptic strength. In contrast, conditioning stimulation of Aδ fibers leads to a moderate increase in $[Ca^{2+}]_i$ that is insufficient for activation of protein kinases, but will activate protein phosphatases that dephosphorylate synaptic proteins and thereby normalize synaptic strength (depotentiation).

GABAergic interneurons. In contrast, the same mechanisms cannot satisfactorily explain the long-lasting analgesia that requires tolerably painful therapeutic stimulation and recruitment of Aδ fibers. This form of analgesia can be better explained by an LTD of neurotransmission in primary afferent Aδ and C fibers in the superficial spinal dorsal horn.

SOURCES OF VARIABILITY OF AFFERENT-INDUCED ANALGESIA

It is a common clinical observation that the analgesia achieved by afferent stimulation can vary considerably between and within patients. None of the present models of spinal analgesia could adequately explain this observation. We have now found that induction of putatively heterosynaptic LTD is favored by intact descending inhibition in spinal cord and that during complete interruption of descending inhibitory pathways the same conditioning stimulation that previously induced an LTD may lead to the induction of LTP (Liu et al. 1998). Thus, identical conditioning stimulation may not always have the same effects at different levels of inhibition in spinal cord. If these mechanisms also apply to pain patients, we should use *painful* TENS preferentially when a postsynaptic inhibition in superficial spinal cord favors the induction of LTD. This may be achieved by the use of a *sequential* TENS.

SEQUENTIAL TENS (PARESTHETIC TENS FOLLOWED BY PAINFUL TENS)

Sequential TENS that involves two periods of stimulation with different parameters may be most efficacious if paresthetic TENS is used first (period 1), immediately followed by painful TENS (period 2). In the first period of stimulation a gate-control-like inhibition is activated in spinal cord and in the second period an LTD is induced. TENS applied in this sequence has two beneficial effects: (1) paresthetic TENS in period 1 induces an immediate inhibition by activation of GABAergic interneurons. The postsynaptic inhibition that remains during painful TENS in period 2 favors the induction of LTD. (2) Since analgesia that is induced by paresthetic TENS is still present during the second period, the patients will tolerate higher frequencies of painful TENS. Since Aδ-fiber stimulation at higher frequencies induces a heterosynaptic LTD at Aδ- and at C-fiber terminals as opposed to homosynaptic LTD that is induced by lower frequencies of stimulation, the analgesic effect would be expected to be stronger. Sequential TENS that employs similar stimulation parameters is presently in clinical use (Ghoname et al. 1999). The rational for this approach can now be explained at the synaptic level. We might predict that not only TENS but also electro-acupuncture and some forms of needle acupuncture could be more efficacious when applied immediately after a period of paresthetic TENS (Kawakita and Gotoh 1996).

ACKNOWLEDGMENTS

This work was supported by grants from the Deutsche Forschungsgemeinschaft (Sa 435/9-2 and Sa 435/10-2) and by the Pain Research Program of the Medical Faculty, University of Heidelberg.

REFERENCES

Beck H, Schröck H, Sandkühler J. Controlled superfusion of the rat spinal cord for studying non-synaptic transmission: an autoradiographic analysis. *J Neurosci Methods* 1995; 58:193–202.

Duggan AW, Foong FW. Bicuculline and spinal inhibition produced by dorsal column stimulation in the cat. *Pain* 1985; 22:249–259.

Fields HL, Basbaum AI. Brainstem control of spinal pain-transmission neurons. *Annu Rev Physiol* 1978; 40:217–248.

Ghoname ES, Craig WF, White PF, et al. The effect of stimulus frequency on the analgesic response to percutaneous electrical nerve stimulation in patients with chronic low back pain. *Anesth Analg* 1999; 88:841–846.

Ishimaru K, Kawakita K, Sakita M. Analgesic effects induced by TENS and electroacupuncture with different types of stimulating electrodes on deep tissues in human subjects. *Pain* 1995; 63:181–187.

Johnson MI, Ashton CH, Thompson JW. An in-depth study of long-term users of transcutaneous electrical nerve stimulation (TENS). Implications for clinical use of TENS. *Pain* 1991; 44:221–229.

Kawakita K, Gotoh K. Role of polymodal receptors in the acupuncture-mediated endogenous pain inhibitory systems. *Prog Brain Res* 1996; 113:507–523.

Liu X-G, Morton CR, Azkue JJ, Zimmermann M, Sandkühler J. Long-term depression of C-fibre-evoked spinal field potentials by stimulation of primary afferent Aδ-fibres in the adult rat. *Eur J Neurosci* 1998; 10:3069–3075.

Melzack R. Prolonged relief of pain by brief, intense transcutaneous somatic stimulation. *Pain* 1975; 1:357–373.

Melzack R, Wall PD. Pain mechanisms: a new theory. *Science* 1965; 150:971–979.

Sandkühler J. Neurobiology of spinal nociception: new concepts. *Prog Brain Res* 1996; 110:207–224.

Sandkühler J, Chen JG, Cheng G, Randic M. Low frequency stimulation of afferent Aδ-fibers induces long-term depression of primary afferent synapses with substantia gelatinosa neurons in the rat. *J Neurosci* 1997; 17:6483–6491.

Thorsen SW, Lumsden SG. Trigeminal neuralgia: sudden and long-term remission with transcutaneous electrical nerve stimulation. *J Manipulative Physiol Ther* 1997; 20:415–419.

Wall PD, Sweet WH. Temporary abolition of pain in man. *Science* 1967; 155:108–109.

Correspondence to: Jürgen Sandkühler, MD, PhD, Universität Heidelberg, Institut für Physiologie und Pathophysiologie, Im Neuenheimer Feld 326, D-69120 Heidelberg, Germany. Tel: 49-6221-544052; Fax: 49-6221-544047; email: sandkuhler@urz.uni-heidelberg.de.

Proceedings of the 9th World Congress on Pain,
Progress in Pain Research and Management,
Vol. 16, edited by M. Devor, M.C. Rowbotham, and
Z. Wiesenfeld-Hallin, IASP Press, Seattle, © 2000.

37

Multiple Pain Pathways[1]

Luis Villanueva[a] and Peter W. Nathan[b]

[a]INSERM, U-161, Paris, France; [b]The Radcliffe Infirmary, Oxford, United Kingdom

Anatomical, electrophysiological, and more recently, functional imaging studies have shown that pain does much more than simply activate a "pain center" and that it involves a number of structures in the brain (Porro and Cavazzuti 1996; Casey 1999). Although such data reveal a multiplicity of putative ascending "pain pathways," the contribution of each to pain processing remains obscure. This chapter considers aspects of the anatomical and functional organization of networks of the central nervous system (CNS) that convey nociceptive information.

PAIN PATHWAYS IN THE ANTEROLATERAL QUADRANT OF THE SPINAL CORD

The location of the spinothalamic and relevant spinoreticular fibers in the human spinal cord is shown in Fig. 1. When this nociceptive pathway is transected, the patient is unable to feel pain from a pathological condition on the opposite side of the body, and cannot feel pain or warmth or cold when suitable stimuli are applied (White and Sweet 1969; Nathan and Smith 1979; Lahuerta et al. 1994). Although the expected sensations do not occur, evidence indicates that other spinal pathways are conveying impulses to higher centers. For instance, repetitive stimulation with noxious, hot, or cold stimuli to the parts of the body rendered analgesic by a cordotomy can cause sweating and nausea, which suggests that impulses are activating autonomic centers by pathways other than those located in the anterolateral quadrant (ALQ) of the spinal cord.

[1] Mini-review based on a congress workshop.

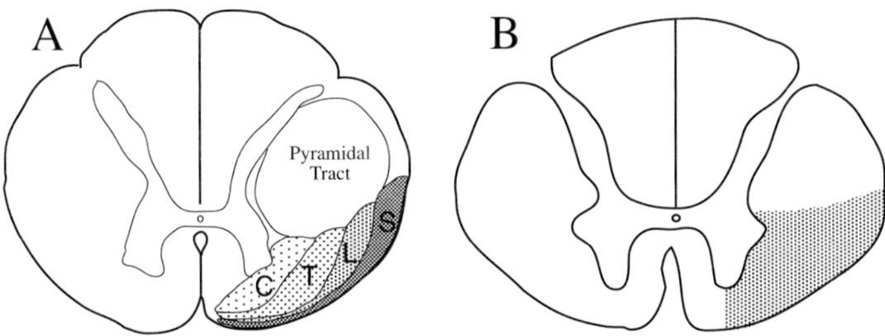

Fig. 1. Distribution of ascending axons in the spinal cord of patients based on correlations of sensory losses with the location of transections. (A) Diagram adapted from Walker (1940) showing the somatotopic distribution of axons from sacral (S), lumbar (L), thoracic (T), and cervical (C) dermatomes in the anterolateral quadrant (ALQ). A considerable overlap of fibers is observed in its ventromedial portion. (B) Diagram showing the location of ascending axons at C3 level following transections that produced long-lasting contralateral analgesia in humans.

Two questions arise. If multiple nociceptive pathways exist, how can dividing one such pathway remove the ability to feel pain? And how do pathways not ascending in the ALQ contribute to the ability to feel pain?

When the ALQ is divided, spontaneous pain can occur. Holmes (1919) termed this "pain of central origin," but it is now usually called central neuropathic or central neurogenic pain. It occurs in the part of the body that is no longer connected to ascending fibers of the ALQ, so it is apparent that pathways other than the tracts of the ALQ can be involved in the transmission of impulses that can give rise to pain. Describing this pain, Holmes writes:

> It is only necessary that stimulation of any form should be of sufficient intensity of mass, though the most severe discomfort is caused by prolonged or moving stimuli which seem to be summated until they acquire an intensity that produces much suffering.... The numerous varieties of stimuli by which pain can be produced suggest strongly that pain may not be due exclusively to impressions conveyed by the normal pain-conducting tracts.

Such pain rarely appears soon after division of the ALQ but may occur spontaneously weeks, months, or years after the occurrence of this lesion.

Holmes did not always call these sensations pain but also described them as "the most severe discomfort," and two of our patients have described them as "not pain but worse than pain." Thesc are novel sensations, and the patients find no adequate words for them. The sensations are often referred to as dysesthesiae or painful dysesthesiae. They are poorly localized and may extend over one half of the body. Following anterolateral cordotomy for painful malignant disease, patients may feel these sensations in the area of the malignant lesion. Two such patients received a spinal anesthetic that completely alleviated the sensations, which showed that they are elicited by impulses originating in the dorsal roots or the spinal cord. These dysesthesiae occur more frequently when the spinothalamic tract is sectioned in the midbrain than following transection in the spinal cord; they have not been reported following midline myelotomy.

Another kind of pain that may occur following ALQ sectioning is referred pain (Ray and Wolff 1945; Nathan 1956). One feature of this phenomenon is that the patient reports that the noxious stimulus applied in the part of the body rendered analgesic is felt elsewhere. A pinprick applied to the analgesic skin is felt as touch, and the referred pain that is felt in normally innervated parts of the body seems to come from within and spread outward to the skin, a totally new sort of sensation.

Noxious and thermal sensibility usually return within months or years of anterolateral cordotomy, even though the entire tract has been divided. This return of sensibility is probably due to conduction in the ALQ and not to the adaptation of other pathways, because these sensations have normal characteristics. White (1966) reported that a second cordotomy, performed 14 years after the first and on the same side to treat return of the original pain, again removed all pain.

Some conclusions may be drawn from these facts. The first is that to experience normal pain requires an intact pathway in the ALQ. The second is that the sensation of "not pain but worse than pain" does not occur when such pathways are intact; conduction in this system normally inhibits conduction in the other pathways used by impulses giving rise to these abnormal sensations. If cordotomy has rendered only a part of the body analgesic, then these dysesthesiae occur only in the analgesic part of the body and never in the part that is still connected to the tracts of the ALQ.

EXPERIMENTAL FINDINGS IN ANIMALS

Although there are controversies concerning the functional organization of nociceptive pathways in animals, the existence of an area within the ALQ that contains the main pathways giving rise to pain has also been demonstrated in different species (see references in Vierck et al. 1986). Misinterpretations of evidence obtained from experiments on species other than humans are always possible, as obviously the animals cannot explain what they are feeling. However, D. Denny-Brown (personal communication to P.W. Nathan, 1978) described abnormal or central pain in the monkey as follows: "I do not know of course what the monkey feels but it is unpleasant (vocalizing, expression), has a longer latency than normal (1–5 seconds), spreads (as judged by scratching a larger and larger area), and lasts a long time (scratching and protests up to 10 or more seconds). Finally, it is produced by any kind of stimulus." Such good observation as this certainly allows conclusions to be drawn about differences between normal and abnormal pain—in this case, central pain. We do not know whether normal pain is always distinguished from "not pain but worse than pain" in experiments in animals, because the physiologist simply judges the presence of pain by obvious aversive reactions of the animal. Electrophysiological, high-resolution anatomical tracing and functional imaging studies are also needed to determine the detailed anatomical and functional organization of the CNS.

Several lines of evidence indicate important differences in the anatomical and functional organization of the superficial and deep dorsal horn regions that contain the populations of spinal nociceptive neurons. These differences suggest that such areas probably play different roles in the processing of nociceptive information.

Most nociceptive primary afferent fibers terminate in the superficial dorsal horn (laminae I and IIo), some Aδ fibers terminate in lamina V, and C fibers of visceral origin terminate also in laminae V–VII and X, some terminating bilaterally. Although there is no strict segregation of these two populations, studies in several species have shown that neurons activated specifically by noxious inputs ("nociceptive-specific" [NS] cells) are found mainly in the superficial dorsal horn (laminae I–II), whereas those activated by noxious and innocuous inputs ("nociceptive-nonspecific" [NNS] cells) are located mainly in deep laminae (V–VI). Moreover, another population of neurons in the ventral horn (laminae VII–VIII) responds to noxious inputs from widespread areas of the body (see references in Willis and Coggeshall 1991).

THE SUPERFICIAL DORSAL HORN

NS neurons are located mainly in lamina I, but this area also contains NNS cells and neurons that respond specifically to cold. NS cells have small cutaneous receptive fields and are activated by Aδ and C fibers from different origins, which is consistent with the viscerosomatic convergence shown by many of these neurons. The restricted cutaneous receptive fields and the somatotopic organization indicate that NS neurons are suitable for signaling spatial and temporal features of nociceptive information. These neurons encode the intensity of both thermal and mechanical stimuli, but within a narrower range of responses than is found for NNS neurons of the deep dorsal horn. Lamina I cells probably contribute to systems that relay pain and thermal sensations to the brain as they respond to both kinds of stimuli.

Transections of the ALQ that abolish pain arising from pathological conditions are associated with loss of thermal sensations at approximately the same levels at which analgesia occurs. In this regard, Craig (1996) has shown that labeled ascending spinothalamic axons following injections in lamina I in monkeys cross at or just rostral to the segment of origin and ascend contralaterally in the middle of the lateral funiculus. In fact, some variability occurs between species and spinal cord levels in the location of ascending axons from lamina I. In the rat, these axons have a large dorsoventral dispersion within the lateral funiculus, some being located quite dorsally. It would be interesting to compare the location of NS axons with those of thermoreceptive cells; both early and recent studies have suggested that thermoreceptive ALQ axons are located more dorsally than nociceptive axons originating from various dermatomes. Thus, it seems that thermal and pain sensations are closely linked, both anatomically and functionally, perhaps because both sensations are useful for homeostasis.

As illustrated in Fig. 2, lamina I neurons terminate in several areas of the CNS that are important for processing signals relevant for homeostasis. For example, they establish propriospinal connections with the sympathetic thoracolumbar system, which provides the basis for somatosympathetic reflexes. At the medullary level, lamina I neurons establish connections with neurons in the ventrolateral medulla and in the caudal portion of the nucleus of the solitary tract, two regions involved in cardiorespiratory regulation. Among the densest projections from lamina I neurons are the lateral parabrachial (PB) area and to a lesser extent the ventrolateral periaqueductal gray matter (PAG). Bernard et al. (1996) have shown that a large proportion of PB neurons are driven by Aδ and C fibers and respond to thermal and mechanical stimuli within noxious ranges. A smaller proportion of these neurons also respond to cooling. The receptive fields of spinoparabrachial neurons are generally small, whereas those for PB neurons are larger, probably indicating the heterotopic convergence of lamina I inputs onto this region. The nociceptive (lateral) PB area projects densely to the central nucleus of the amygdala and the bed nucleus of the stria terminalis, areas that are probably involved in anxiety and reactions to fear; it also projects to the hypothalamic ventromedial nucleus, which participates in defensive/aggressive behavior and the regulation of energy metabolism. In addition, the PB nociceptive area receives a major visceral/autonomic input from the nucleus of the solitary tract, which indicates that PB neurons would also participate in autonomic aspects of pain.

The lateral and ventrolateral columns of the PAG that receive lamina I projections contain different groups of neurons that, when activated, produce antinociceptive and well-defined cardiovascular and defensive reactions such

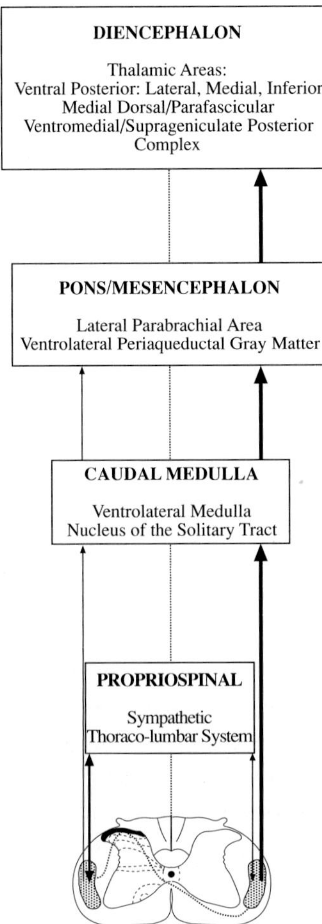

Fig. 2. Main supraspinal projections from lamina I neurons. Lamina I neurons send signals from noxious and thermal inputs to spinal, bulbar, and telencephalic regions implicated in autonomic, emotional, and somatosensory processing. Rather than only subserving pain processing, these circuits could contribute to sustain basic emotional and motivational states (Craig 1996). Arrow sizes indicate the relative density of lamina I projections.

as decreases in blood pressure, hyporeactive immobility, avoidance behavior, and vocalization, as well as a more general emotional state of fear and anxiety (Depaulis and Bandler 1991). Thus, the lamina I/PAG pathway could participate in feedback mechanisms involved in autonomic, aversive, and antinociceptive responses to strong nociceptive stimulation.

THE DEEP DORSAL HORN

Most NNS neurons are concentrated in lamina V, although NNS cells have also been found in laminae I, IV, and VI. Studies in both anesthetized and awake animals have shown that NNS neurons have a greater ability to encode noxious stimuli with a wide range of response levels than do NS neurons (see references in Le Bars et al. 1986; Willis and Coggeshall 1991).

NNS neurons receive Aβ, Aδ, and C-fiber inputs, and respond to a large range of mechanical stimuli, from innocuous to strong nociceptive stimuli. They also respond to a variety of other stimuli (innocuous or noxious thermal and chemical stimuli), and show viscerosomatic convergence. The excitatory peripheral fields of NNS neurons are usually larger than those of NS cells, although they are still compatible with a moderate degree of stimulus location. Neurons presenting larger receptive fields and activated by noxious inputs also have been found in the ventral horn, notably in lamina VII and around the central canal (lamina X) at thoracic, lumbar, and sacral levels. Many of these cells also receive viscerosomatic convergence (see references in Cervero and Morrison 1986).

The precise sites of termination of laminae V–VII nociceptive neurons are still largely unknown because most of the available data come from retrograde tracing. However, preliminary anterograde tracing studies have shown that a high proportion of these neurons project within the ALQ. Several lines of evidence indicate that the largest number of inputs to the brain comes from the upper cervical cord and a smaller number from caudal spinal regions. It is possible that at least part of the caudal ascending nociceptive information may relay at upper cervical levels, given that these areas contain both the majority of spinothalamic, spinoreticular, and spinomesencephalic afferents and neurons with heterosegmental, widespread receptive fields (see references in Willis and Coggeshall 1991). This observation suggests a common functional organization of several ascending somatosensory pathways that could explain the widespread relief of pain, including pain from caudal segments of the body, in patients following commissural myelotomy of the upper cervical spinal cord (Hitchcock 1970, 1974; Cook et al. 1984).

As illustrated in Fig. 3, laminae V–VII neurons project to several brainstem reticular areas that are among their densest targets. The medullary reticular formation may play a key role as a relay for nociceptive signals because most ALQ ascending axons, in both animals and humans, terminate within this area (see references in Bowsher 1976). Moreover, below the upper cervical segments, deep dorsal horn cells constitute the great majority of spinal afferents to the reticular formation (Willis and Coggeshall 1991). As most nociceptive reticular units recorded in older studies showed irregular responses and changes in excitability and presented some degree of heterosensory convergence, it was concluded that the reticular formation did not play a specific role in the processing of pain. This proposal has been challenged by data from rat studies showing that neurons within the medullary subnucleus reticularis dorsalis (SRD) respond selectively to the activation of peripheral Aδ fibers or of Aδ and C fibers from the whole body surface,

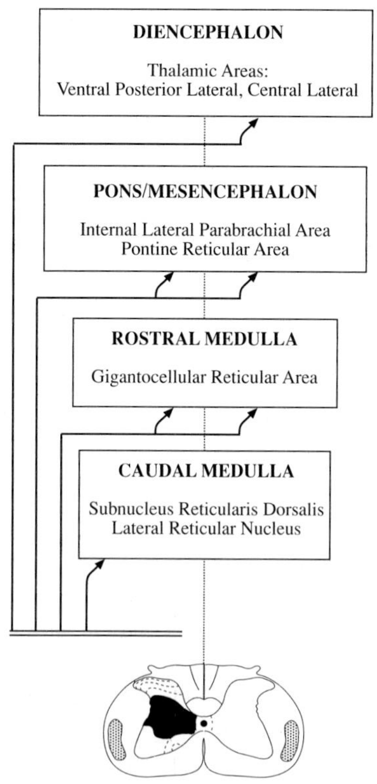

Fig. 3. Main supraspinal projections from deep dorsal horn neurons. Deep dorsal horn neurons are able to convey a variety of signals originating either from the external environment (through the skin) or from the internal organs. They send inputs to several regions implicated in somatosensory, motor, arousal, and attentional processing of nociceptive inputs. Like lamina I cells, deep dorsal horn neurons are implicated not only in pain processing but also in creating a basic somesthetic activity necessary for homeostatic regulation (Le Bars et al. 1986).

encode the intensity of natural noxious stimuli, and are activated via spinal pathways ascending in the ALQ. Neurons with similar properties also have been recorded in the monkey SRD (Villanueva et al. 1996).

OTHER PUTATIVE PAIN PATHWAYS IN THE WHITE MATTER OF THE CORD

THE DORSOLATERAL FUNICULUS

Some authors have reported that in various species, many ascending axons from lamina I neurons are located in the dorsolateral white matter. In fact, it has been claimed that some of the axons from lamina I neurons in rats ascend in the most dorsal part of the lateral funiculus (McMahon and Wall 1988), an area that does not have to be transected to produce relief of pain in humans (Nathan 1990). Yet, electrophysiological and behavioral data in animals show that dorsolateral lesions increase nociceptive reactions, probably by disrupting tonically active descending antinociceptive pathways (Vierck et al. 1986). Moreover, an anterograde tracing study in monkeys showed a different distribution of the thalamic projections of dorsal as opposed to ventral spinothalamic axons within the ALQ. Dorsal spinothalamic axons lie at the level of the denticulate ligament and terminate preferentially in ventrocaudal thalamic areas often referred to as the suprageniculate/posterior complex. On the other hand, spinothalamic axons ventral to the denticulate ligament terminate predominantly in the main portion of the ventral posterolateral thalamus (Ralston and Ralston 1992). The question of whether a "dorsolateral" ascending nociceptive pathway exists may be merely a semantic problem given that both anterograde and retrograde tracing studies in monkeys have shown that lamina I spinothalamic axons are located more laterally than those arising from deep dorsal horn neurons. Lamina I spinothalamic axons are in an area ventral to the region occupied by the lateral corticospinal tract and are still within the ALQ (Ralston and Ralston 1992; Apkarian 1995; Craig 1996).

THE DORSAL COLUMNS AND VISCERAL PAIN

Recent studies in rats have shown a visceral nociceptive pathway that activates gracile neurons (Berkley and Hubscher 1995; Willis et al. 1999). As illustrated in Fig. 4A, the ascending axons that activate these neurons following either stimulation of reproductive pelvic viscera or colorectal distension are confined to the fasciculus gracilis. Moreover, clinical findings showing a relief of pelvic cancer pain following restricted transections have prompted the proposal that an important visceral nociceptive pathway in humans is confined to the medial aspect of the dorsal columns (Willis et al. 1999). In addition, the suppression of ventroposterolateral (VPL) thalamic responses to colorectal distension following dorsal column lesions in rats led Willis to state that this pathway is more important than the ALQ for transmitting visceral nociceptive signals to VPL, whereas the ALQ may be more important for transmitting cutaneous nociceptive information. Willis concluded that the visceral inputs traveling in the dorsal columns could either cooperate with direct spinal pathways to produce the perceptions of touch and pain or serve as an alternative nociceptive pathway to the spinothalamic tract. However, if there are two nociceptive pathways conducting impulses that cause visceral pain, then the removal of one should either have no effect or some effect in reducing the pain. This effect should be present immediately after one of the pathways has been cut. Return of the ability to feel normal pain months or even years after anterolateral cordotomies does not imply that alternative nociceptive pathways are conducting impulses giving rise to pain. It means that we are facing the usual problem of the anatomical and physiological changes that occur following division of any pathway in the nervous system.

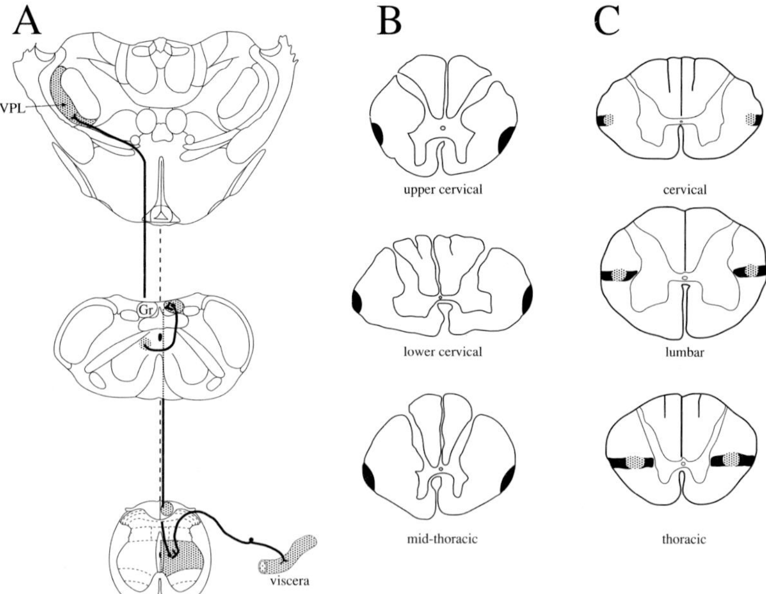

Fig. 4. (A) The putative visceral nociceptive pathway in the dorsal columns. It has been proposed that noxious inputs from viscera are relayed in laminae VII and X neurons whose ascending axons are confined near the midline of the dorsal columns. These axons terminate in the medullary nucleus gracilis (Gr), which conveys these inputs to the thalamic ventral posterolateral (VPL) nucleus (Willis et al. 1999). (B) The location of centripetal fibers subserving micturition and sensations of temperature and pain from the lower end of the ureter and from the bladder and urethra in humans (Nathan and Smith 1951). (C) The location of centripetal fibers subserving defecation (dotted areas) and sensations of pain from the rectum and anus (black areas) on the lateral surface of the cord. The efferent fibers for voluntary control probably lie in the dotted region, and those for autonomic control in the more central black area (Nathan and Smith 1953). The sensation giving rise to the desire to micturate or defecate is unilateral—much to the surprise of one of our patients who had cordotomy (a professor of neurosurgery).

Only ignorance of the clinical literature would lead to the conclusion that the dorsal columns have nothing to do with pain. The pain of distorted posture that can occur as a phantom sensation following amputation is relieved by cutting the dorsal columns (Rabiner and Browder 1948; Cook and Browder 1965). In fact, the dorsal columns not only convey ascending inputs to the brain but also contain direct descending spinal projections originating from the dorsal column nuclei (DCN) and terminating in dorsal horn laminae I and V (Villanueva et al. 1995). In addition, the ventral DCN region where most spinally projecting cells are located is an important target for corticobulbar projections. Thus, the spinal output could be modulated not only directly by the spinally projecting DCN neurons, but indirectly through cortical DCN influences (Canedo 1997). The information traveling in the DCN could be under the influence of inputs from several levels including the cerebral cortex, which suggests that DCN neurons integrate information from several ascending and descending systems. It may well be that transections confined to the dorsal columns not only disrupt an ascending pathway but also interfere with descending modulatory mechanisms. An improved knowledge of these influences might help us understand the complex modifications of sensory perception that follow lesions of the dorsal columns in humans, including changes in tactile sensations, tactile and postural hallucinations, and increases in sensations of pain, tickle, warmth, and cold. Thus, the clinical effects of lesions of the dorsal columns are much more complicated than those of lesions of the ALQ. Perhaps this accounts for the neglect of a series of papers published by German neurologists (see references in Nathan et al. 1986).

The history of cordotomy is the history of the removal of visceral pain by transecting the spinothalamic tract. The first cordotomies were usually designed to remove visceral pain, and the success of this operation has been amply confirmed throughout the 20th century. Cordotomy has been performed far more frequently for pain arising in the viscera than for somatic pain. Although in some cases the pain was caused by spread of a carcinoma to the posterior thoracic or abdominal wall and the pleura or peritoneum, in most cases the operation stopped pain from the kidneys, ureter, bladder, urethra, testes, ovaries, uterus, vagina, stomach, duodenum, pancreas, and small and large intestines, as well as the pain from malignant tissue invading bone, sacral and brachial plexus, and all afferent peripheral nerves.

Fig. 4B–C illustrates spinal cord sections from patients who had anterolateral cordotomy to relieve visceral pain associated with cancer (Nathan and Smith 1951, 1953). These examples demonstrate that information about sensation is far from simple. Examinations and tests were done before and after cordotomy, which was either unilateral or bilateral. The bladder was examined by cystoscopy, and attempts were made to induce pain by indenting and stretching the ureteric orifices, the neck of the bladder, the trigone, and the bladder walls. Sensations of pain, touch, warm, and cold in the urethra were noted. The patients were also asked to observe what they felt when they passed urine voluntarily or involuntarily. Solutions at various temperatures were introduced into the bladder. As illustrated in Fig. 4B, the afferent pathways subserving the sensations of pain from the lower end of the ureter, bladder, and urethra, and the sensation of temperature from the urethra lie on the surface of the cord approximately opposite the posterior angle of the anterior horn. However, the patients in whom the ALQ were divided bilaterally may retain the sensation that micturition is impending, that it is progressing, and that is has ceased. These sensations are doubtless due to impulses arising in the urethral mucosa, the external sphincter, and the large group of perineal muscles that act synergically with the sphincter. Such impulses probably travel via the dorsal columns. The sensation underlying the desire to micturate depends on ALQ fibers; their position is shown in Fig. 4B. Tests of rectal and anal sensation produced similar results. Following bilateral cordotomy incisions involving the areas shown in Fig. 4C, the pressure in a rectal balloon could be raised maximally without prompting a desire to defecate and without producing pain. Most patients regained some degree of anal sensation; although sensations of warmth, cold, and pain remained lost to them, those of touch and stretch recovered or were never lost. Similar to sensory input giving rise to the need to micturate, the pathway necessary for supplying information that the rectum needs emptying lies in the sacral region of the ALQ, as shown in Fig. 4C.

SPINAL PROJECTIONS TO THE DIENCEPHALON: ITS RELEVANCE TO NOCICEPTIVE PROCESSING

Although lateral, medial, and posterior thalamic areas receive lamina I projections and precisely encode different intensities of noxious stimuli, recordings in anesthetized and awake monkeys have revealed important differences between these areas. Many neurons in the medial dorsal/parafascicular (Pf) and ventromedial thalamus are modality specific, showing either nociceptive or thermal responses. The receptive fields of ventromedial cells in monkeys are restricted, whereas those from Pf cells are often large. The borders of these receptive fields and the magnitudes of their evoked responses change with the monkey's behavioral state (Bushnell 1995). These features may indicate that the Pf cells are better suited to behavioral reactions, thus strongly implicating these regions in the affective-emotional aspects of pain. This suggestion is supported by their cortical connectivity and by functional imaging studies. Ventromedial cells project to the mid/anterior insular cortex, an area that is activated by both innocuous and noxious thermal stimuli in humans and that has been implicated in the affective components of pain based on its projections to various limbic structures such as the amygdala and perirhinal cortex. Pf cells project to area 24 of the cingulate cortex, the activity of which appears to be more selectively modulated by noxious stimuli. In fact, this is a functionally heterogeneous area constituted by adjacent zones that have been implicated in attentional, motor, and autonomic reactions, which might allow it to elicit various behavioral reactions (Devinsky et al. 1995).

By contrast, in ventroposterior thalamic areas, most neurons are of wide dynamic range, have receptive fields that are not modified by the behavioral state, and are smaller than those of spinal or medullary dorsal horn projecting neurons (Bushnell 1995). These findings suggest that ventral posterior areas may subserve spatial discrimination. These regions project to the primary somatosensory cortex, and functional imaging studies have shown that noxious and innocuous stimuli similarly activate the contralateral S1 cortex, indicating a coexistence of pain and tactile representation in this area. Furthermore, single-unit recordings from a ventrocaudal region of the thalamus in humans showed neurons that could be activated by noxious stimuli, and stimulation of this region induced thermal or painful sensations (Lenz and Dougherty 1997).

Taken together, these data show that the fine encoding properties or the fact that thalamic neurons receive direct lamina I inputs alone cannot account for the sensory-discriminative aspects of pain, because encoding is shared by all (thalamic and also lower CNS) regions implicated in pain processing. Moreover, the ventral posterior thalamic areas, which are the best candidates for discrimination, can discharge with higher instantaneous frequency to innocuous than to noxious stimulation in awake monkeys. Thus, it is likely that modulatory mechanisms or the concomitant activity of multiple neuronal populations could determine the final pain perception.

Although the ventral posterior and central lateral thalamus are among the direct diencephalic targets from deep dorsal horn neurons, numerous findings indicate that the main nociceptive inputs to the thalamus from these neurons are relayed within the medullary reticular formation. A thalamic nociceptive region that receives dense brainstem reticular nociceptive afferents is the lateral Pf, which projects notably to the dorsolateral striatum and motor cortices. These connections could mediate some arousal or motor reactions following noxious stimulation. Recent studies have shown that the ventromedial thalamic area (VM*l*) in the rat conveys and encodes cutaneous nociceptive inputs from the SRD to layer I of the whole dorsolateral neocortex (Monconduit et al. 1999). As VM*l* neurons are activated from the entire body surface, they might be part of a network that allows nociceptive signals to modify cortical activity in a wide area.

In conclusion, the concomitant activity of widespread cortical regions elicited by nociceptive spinoreticulothalamic networks may be essential for modifying behavioral levels of arousal and attention, and for the planning of programmed movements. This observation confirms several findings suggesting that alterations in the firing of large ensembles of thalamocortical cells are associated with changes in different states of consciousness (Steriade et al. 1997). This would explain, for instance, functional imaging findings that showed that a single calibrated noxious stimulus not only activates several cortical areas, but also elicits an increasing number of active thalamic and cortical regions as the stimulus increases in intensity (Derbyshire et al. 1997).

CONCLUDING REMARKS

One problem of sensory transmission is the large number of pathways from the dorsal roots to the brain. We do not understand how these pathways and the information they are conveying are related. There are multiple pathways for the defense reaction, but are there multiple pathways for feeling pain? These pathways are not exactly "pain tracts." And yet, when both ALQs of the cord are transected, analgesia and thermanesthesia occur below the level of transection.

Although "pain tracts" and "pain system" are common concepts presented in textbooks, they are known to be wrong; they are retained because they are simple. The idea of a specialized chain of neurons from the periphery to the cortex, or of separated unidirectional pathways that convey the information that inevitably produces the sensory experience of pain, is obsolete. Perhaps the simplest reason is that the brain has many ways and strategies for modifying incoming information, and that sensation is not merely a facsimile in consciousness of every stimulus to the CNS. Selection is the main characteristic of sensation, and thus by means of facilitation and inhibition the brain increases or decreases the efficacy of certain inputs to the nervous system.

The sensory pathways that convey nociceptive impulses collect information simultaneously from many sources. This basic somesthetic activity is not only relevant for pain but could have a role in a continual transmission of information relevant to the integrity of the body. This information is constantly selected and modulated in the context of an appropriate response.

To study the basic reflexes of movement, Sherrington cut anterior and posterior roots to leave only a few nerves intact. He referred to this and to other less simplified portions of the nervous system on which he worked as "the preparation." When one day he was taken to the ward by the neurosurgeon G. Jefferson and was shown some interesting features related to his work, he exclaimed: "How marvellous to have a preparation that can speak." To understand and perhaps solve some of the problems of pain, investigation of the preparation that can speak—usually referred to as a human being—is essential.

ACKNOWLEDGMENTS

L. Villanueva was supported by CNRS, INSERM, and l'Institut UPSA de la douleur.

REFERENCES

Apkarian AV. Thalamic anatomy and physiology of pain perception. In: Besson JM, Guilbaud G, Ollat H (Eds). *Forebrain Areas Involved in Pain Processing*. Paris: John Libbey Eurotext, 1995, pp 93–118.

Berkley K, Hubscher CH. Are there separate central nervous system pathways for touch and pain? *Nat Med* 1995; 1:766–773.

Bernard JF, Bester H, Besson JM. Involvement of the spino-parabrachio-amygdaloid and hypothalamic pathways in the autonomic and affective emotional aspects of pain. In: Holstege G, Bandler R, Saper CB (Eds). *The Emotional Motor System*, Progress in Brain Research, Vol. 107. Amsterdam: Elsevier, 1996, pp 243–255.

Bowsher D. Role of the reticular formation in responses to noxious stimulation. *Pain* 1976; 2:361–378.

Bushnell MC. Thalamic processing of sensory-discriminative and affective-motivational dimensions of pain. In: Besson JM, Guilbaud G, Ollat H (Eds). *Forebrain Areas Involved in Pain Processing*. Paris: John Libbey Eurotext, 1995, pp 63–77.

Canedo A. Primary motor cortex influences on the descending and ascending systems. *Prog Neurobiol* 1997; 51:287–335.

Casey KL. Forebrain mechanisms of nociception and pain: analysis through imaging. *Proc Natl Acad Sci USA* 1999; 96:7668–7674.

Cervero F, Morrison JFB (Eds). *Visceral Sensation*, Progress in Brain Research, Vol. 67. New York: Elsevier, 1986.

Cook AW, Browder EJ. Functions of posterior columns in man. *Arch Neurol* 1965; 12:72–79.

Cook AW, Nathan PW, Smith MC. Sensory consequences of commissural myelotomy. A challenge to traditional anatomical concepts. *Brain* 1984; 107:547–568.

Craig AD. An ascending general homeostatic afferent pathway originating in lamina I. In: Holstege G, Bandler R, Saper CB (Eds). *The Emotional Motor System*, Progress in Brain Research, Vol. 107. Amsterdam: Elsevier, 1996, pp 225–242.

Depaulis A, Bandler R (Eds). *The Midbrain Periaqueductal Gray Matter. Functional, Anatomical, and Neurochemical Organization*, NATO ASI Series A: Life Sciences, Vol. 213. New York: Plenum, 1991.

Derbyshire SWG, Jones AKP, Gyulai F, et al. Pain processing during three levels of noxious stimulation produces differential patterns of central activity. *Pain* 1997; 73:431–445.

Devinsky O, Morrell MJ, Vogt BA. Contributions of anterior cingulate cortex to behaviour. *Brain* 1995; 118:279–306.

Hitchcock E. Stereotactic cervical myelotomy. *J Neurol Neurosurg Psychiatry* 1970; 33:224–230.

Hitchcock E. Stereotactic myelotomy. *Proc Roy Soc Med* 1974; 67:771–772.

Holmes G. Pain of central origin. In: *Contributions to Medical and Biological Research*, Vol. 1. New York: Paul B. Hoeber, 1919, pp 235–246.

Lahuerta J, Bowsher D, Lipton S, Buxton PH. Percutaneous cervical cordotomy: a review of 181 operations on 146 patients with a study on the location of "pain fibers" in the C-2 spinal cord segment of 29 cases. *J Neurosurg* 1994; 80:975–985.

Le Bars D, Dickenson AH, Besson JM, Villanueva L. Aspects of sensory processing through convergent neurons. In: Yaksh TL (Ed). *Spinal Afferent Processing*. New York: Plenum, 1986, pp 467–504.

Lenz FA, Dougherty PM. Pain processing in the human thalamus. In: Steriade M, Jones EG, McCormick DA (Eds). *Thalamus: Experimental and Clinical Aspects.* New York: Elsevier, 1997, pp 617–651.

McMahon SB, Wall PD. The significance of plastic changes in lamina I systems. In: Cervero F, Bennett GJ, Headley PM (Eds). *Processing of Sensory Information in the Superficial Dorsal Horn of the Spinal Cord*, NATO ASI Series A: Life Sciences. New York: Plenum, 1988, pp 249–271.

Monconduit L, Bourgeais L, Bernard JF, Le Bars D, Villanueva L. Ventromedial thalamic neurons convey nociceptive signals from the whole body surface to the dorsolateral neocortex. *J Neurosci* 1999; 19:9063–9072.

Nathan PW. Reference of sensation at the spinal level. *J Neurol Neurosurg Psychiatry* 1956; 19:88–100.

Nathan PW. Comments on 'a dorsolateral spinothalamic tract in macaque monkey' by Apkarian and Hodge. *Pain* 1990; 40:239–240.

Nathan PW, Smith MC. The centripetal pathway from the bladder and urethra within the spinal cord. *J Neurol Neurosurg Psychiatry* 1951; 14:262–280.

Nathan PW, Smith MC. Spinal pathways subserving defaecation and sensation from the lower bowel. *J Neurol Neurosurg Psychiatry* 1953; 16:245–256.

Nathan PW, Smith MC. Clinico-anatomical correlation in anterolateral cordotomy. In: Bonica JJ, Liebeskind JC, Albe-Fessard DG (Eds). *Advances in Pain Research and Therapy.* New York: Raven, 1979, pp 921–926.

Nathan PW, Smith MC, Cook AW. Sensory effects in man of lesions of the posterior columns and of some other afferent pathways. *Brain* 1986; 109:1003–1041.

Porro CA, Cavazzutti M. Functional imaging studies of the pain system in man and animals. In: Carli G, Zimmermann M (Eds). *Towards the Neurobiology of Chronic Pain.* Progress in Brain Research, Vol. 110. New York: Elsevier, 1996, pp 47–62.

Rabiner AM, Browder J. Concerning the conduction of touch and deep sensibilities through the spinal cord. *Trans Am Neurol Assoc* 1948; 73:137–142.

Ralston HJ, Ralston DD. The primate dorsal spinothalamic tract: evidence for a specific termination in the posterior nuclei (Po/SG) of the thalamus. *Pain* 1992; 48:107–118.

Ray BS, Wolff HG. Studies on pain. 'Spread of pain'; evidence on site of spread within the neuraxis of effects of painful stimulation. *Arch Neurol Psychiatry* 1945; 53:257–261.

Steriade M, Jones EG, McCormick DA (Eds). *Organisation and Function*, Thalamus, Vol. 1. New York: Elsevier, 1997.

Vierck CJ, Greenspan JD, Ritz LA, Yeomans DC. The spinal pathways contributing to the ascending conduction and the descending modulation of pain sensations and reactions. In: Yaksh TL (Ed). *Spinal Afferent Processing.* New York: Plenum, 1986, pp 275–329.

Villanueva L, Bernard JF, Le Bars D. Distribution of spinal cord projections from the medullary subnucleus reticularis dorsalis and the adjacent cuneate nucleus: a phaseolus vulgaris leucoagglutinin (PHA-L) study in the rat. *J Comp Neurol* 1995; 352:11–32.

Villanueva L, Bouhassira D, Le Bars D. The medullary subnucleus reticularis dorsalis (SRD) as a key link in both the transmission and modulation of pain signals. *Pain* 1996; 67:231–240.

Walker AE. The spinothalamic tract in man. *Arch Neurol Psychiatry* 1940; 43:284–298.

White JC. Cordotomy. Assessment of its effectiveness and suggestions for its improvement. *Clin Neurosurg* 1966; 15:1–19.

White JC, Sweet WH. *Pain and the Neurosurgeon: a Forty-Year Experience.* Springfield, IL: Charles C. Thomas, 1969.

Willis WD, Coggeshall RE. *Sensory Mechanisms of the Spinal Cord*, 2nd ed. New York: Plenum Press, 1991.

Willis WD, Al-Chaer ED, Quast MJ, Westlund KN. A visceral pain pathway in the dorsal column of the spinal cord. *Proc Natl Acad Sci USA* 1999; 96:7675–7679.

Correspondence to: Luis Villanueva, DDS, PhD, INSERM, U-161, 2 rue d'Alésia, 75014 Paris, France. Fax: 33-145-881-304; email: luisvil@broca.inserm.fr.

Proceedings of the 9th World Congress on Pain, Progress in Pain Research and Management, Vol. 16, edited by M. Devor, M.C. Rowbotham, and Z. Wiesenfeld-Hallin, IASP Press, Seattle, © 2000.

38

Multiplicity and Plasticity of Descending Modulation of Nociception: Implications for Persistent Pain[1]

Ke Ren,[a] Min Zhuo,[b] and William D. Willis[c]

[a]*Department of Oral and Craniofacial Biological Sciences, University of Maryland Dental School, Baltimore, Maryland;* [b]*Department of Anesthesiology, Washington University School of Medicine, St. Louis, Missouri; and* [c]*Department of Anatomy and Neuroscience, Marine Biomedical Institute, The University of Texas Medical Branch, Galveston, Texas, USA*

Brainstem descending pathways constitute a major mechanism for modulating nociceptive transmission at the spinal level. As proposed by Melzack and Wall (1965), central signals arising from the brain can influence afferent input at the "earliest synaptic levels of the somesthetic system." Descending pain modulation can account, in part, for the variant relationship between noxious stimuli and the sensations they produce. Earlier studies documented that: (1) the critical sites for morphine-produced antinociception are midbrain periaqueductal gray (PAG) and the adjacent hypothalamic periventricular area (Tsou and Jang 1964); (2) stimulation of the PAG can produce analgesia in rats (Reynolds 1969) and that PAG stimulation activates a normal function of the brain (Mayer et al. 1971; Mayer and Liebeskind 1974); and (3) there exist endogenous opioid peptides (Hughes et al. 1975). The framework for an endogenous descending pain-inhibitory system has now been well established (Fig. 1) (Fields and Basbaum 1978; Basbaum and Fields 1984; Gebhart 1986; Fields et al. 1991; Willis and Westlund 1997).

Recent studies have resulted in two conceptual advances in understanding the function of the endogenous pain-modulating circuitry. First, the control of pain is not necessarily only inhibitory. Incoming nociceptive input is

[1] Mini-review based on a congress workshop.

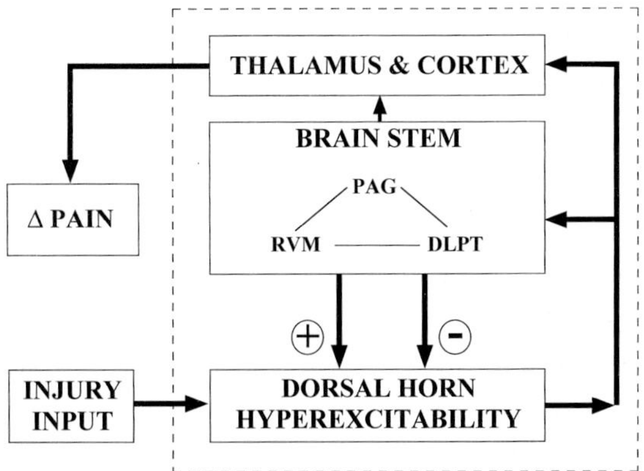

Fig. 1. Diagram illustrating the brainstem descending nociceptive modulatory system. The midbrain periaqueductal gray (PAG), the rostral ventromedial medulla (RVM), and the dorsolateral pontomesencephalic tegmentum (DLPT) are major components of the descending pathways. The PAG has connections with RVM and DLPT, and both RVM and DLPT project to the spinal dorsal horn. An enhanced primary afferent input after injury may lead to dorsal horn hyperexcitability and produce dynamic changes in excitability of descending pathways. The net effect of descending modulation depends on a balance between inhibitory (–) and facilitatory (+) input to the spinal cord. An increase in descending facilitatory modulation may lead to the development of persistent pain.

also subject to facilitatory descending modulation that may lead to the development of pathological conditions such as allodynia and hyperalgesia. Second, the endogenous pain-modulating circuitry is not fixed. This view is derived from studies using animal models of persistent pain. Dramatic plastic change occurs in the potency of descending modulation following peripheral tissue injury. This chapter will briefly discuss these new findings in the context of multiplicity and plasticity of endogenous pain-modulating pathways.

BIDIRECTIONAL DESCENDING MODULATION

In addition to demonstrating well-known inhibitory control, several early studies indicated that supraspinal structures can also exert facilitatory influences on nociceptive transmission at the spinal level. Excitation and inhibition of dorsal horn neurons can be produced by stimulation of the dorsolateral funiculus (DLF) of the spinal cord (Dubuisson and Wall 1979; McMahon and Wall 1988), nucleus raphe magnus (NRM) (Dubuisson and Wall 1980), and nucleus gigantocellularis (NGC) (Haber et al. 1980). Even microinjection of morphine into the NRM facilitates C-fiber responses of some dorsal horn nociceptive neurons (Le Bars et al. 1980). Although in most cases, it is not clear whether facilitation occurs on inhibitory interneurons whose excitation may result in subsequent inhibition, Haber et al. (1980) demonstrated the NGC-stimulation-produced excitation of primate spinothalamic tract neurons, indicating descending facilitation of nociceptive transmission.

Further evidence for facilitation and inhibition of nociceptive transmission came from neuronal recordings from the rostral ventromedial medulla (RVM). The RVM includes the NRM and adjacent lateral reticular formation, a nuclear complex that plays a key role in mediating descending control of nociceptive transmission (Basbaum and Fields 1984). Comparison of RVM neuronal activity with the occurrence of nociceptive reflexes in lightly anesthetized rats allowed identification of three classes of neurons (Fields et al. 1983a). One type of cell typically shows a burst of activity just prior to the onset of the tail flick from a noxious heat stimulus, thus named an "on-cell." Another type of cell exhibits a pause in activity less than a second before the tail flick and is called an "off-cell." The activity of the third class of cell, "neutral cell," exhibits no clear relationship to nociceptive reflexes. The firing profiles of on- and off-cells suggest that they are involved in facilitation and inhibition of nociceptive processes. In fact, both RVM on- and off-cells project to the spinal cord, particularly laminae I, II, and V of the dorsal horn (Fields et al. 1995), and are modulated by PAG stimulation and opioids (Fields et al. 1983b; Vanegas et al. 1984; Fields et al. 1991). Interestingly, μ- and κ-opioid receptor agonists may produce opposing actions on RVM pain-modulating neurons. Activation of the κ receptor hyperpolarizes RVM neurons that are disinhibited through the inhibition of a second-class of neuron (on-cells) by μ-opioid receptors (Pan et al. 1997). This κ effect reverses the analgesic effect of μ opioids. The finding of on- and off-cells in the RVM provides a cellular mechanism for descending facilitatory and inhibitory modulation of spinal pain transmission. The descending facilitation parallels inhibition and is an active process. The enhanced nociceptive responsiveness in morphine-dependent rats after treatment with opioid-receptor antagonists is accompanied by an increased RVM on-cell firing (Bederson et al. 1990).

The biphasic descending modulation of nociception has been systematically analyzed. It appears that some sites in the rostral medulla play an essential role in this balanced descending modulation. Depending on the intensities used, stimulation of the NGC, RVM region facilitates and inhibits nociceptive reflexes and responses of dorsal horn nociceptive neurons (Zhuo and Gebhart 1992, 1997). Depending on location, relatively lower and higher intensities of stimulation facilitate and inhibit nociception, respectively. RVM neurons may exert bidirectional control of nociception through descending serotonergic pathways (Zhuo and Gebhart 1991) and via the A7 catecholamine cell group. Enkephalin-containing neurons in the RVM project to the A7 cell group, and microinjection of morphine in the A7 cell group facilitates and inhibits spinal nociception mediated by α_1 and α_2 adrenoceptors (Holden et al. 1999). It is interesting that both facilitatory and inhibitory pathways can be triggered by activation of visceral afferents. Under certain circumstances, vagal afferent stimulation also facilitates the nociceptive tail-flick reflex and dorsal horn nociceptive neuronal activity (Ren et al. 1988, 1989). The neural relays involved in vagal afferent-produced facilitation and inhibition also include sites within the RVM (Ren et al. 1990). Thus, spinal nociceptive processing is subject to bidirectional control from supraspinal sites, and the intensity of perceived pain is fine-tuned by descending pathways.

Although specific, distinct individual modulatory neural circuits may be responsible for multiple phases of descending modulation, it is rather surprising that the most studied facilitatory sites in the rostral medulla generally overlap with the sites that also produce descending inhibition. It is not clear how and why a manipulation at the same site, such as electrical stimulation given at lesser or greater intensities, or receptor agents administered at lower or high doses, should produce opposing effects on nociceptive transmission. Pain-modulating neurons of different modalities intermingle within the RVM and the membrane properties of on- and off-cells are similar (Zagon et al. 1997). It appears that the net effect of excitation of brainstem nuclei is related to differential activation of subsets of neurons with different connections and different combinations of neurotransmitter receptors.

DESCENDING INPUT AND PERSISTENT PAIN

The influence of endogenous descending pain control systems on spinal cord activity following peripheral tissue injury is a topic of increasing interest. Persistent tissue or nerve injury results in an increased peripheral barrage of nerve impulses into the spinal cord that leads to hyperexcitability of dorsal horn nociceptive neurons or central sensitization (see Dubner 1991; Woolf and Thompson 1991; Dubner and Ruda 1992). These changes also lead to increased neuronal activity at supraspinal sites and presumably contribute to alterations in pain sensation and related responses.

Studies using animal models of persistent pain provide evidence that the net effect of descending modulation after tissue injury is inhibitory. Multiple descending pathways travel in the DLF of the spinal cord. Removal of descending pathways in the DLF potentiates inflammatory hyperalgesia (Ren and Dubner 1996). Complete spinalization with lidocaine leads to a further increase in dorsal horn hyperexcitability in hind paw-inflamed rats, as indicated by dorsal horn nociceptive neurons with increased background activity, enlarged receptive fields, and increased responses to noxious stimuli (Ren and Dubner 1996). FOS protein expression, a marker of neuronal activation (Hunt et al. 1987), is further increased in spinally transected and inflamed rats (Ren and Ruda 1996). MacArthur et al. (1999) showed that the levels of prodynorphin mRNA and dynorphin peptide are further increased in hind paw-inflamed rats after spinal transection. Descending modulation triggered by diffuse noxious inhibitory controls from the inflamed joint is also enhanced within the acute phase of inflammation (Danziger et al. 1999). These findings demonstrate that descending pathways are activated by tissue injury to dampen or counteract the cascade of events that ultimately contribute to the development of inflammatory hyperalgesia.

The specific sites of origin of some of these effects have been identified. Of primary interest are sites in the brain stem including the pontine locus ceruleus/subceruleus (LC/SC) and medullary structures such as NRM and the NGC. These sites coincide with well-established brainstem sites for descending modulation (Fields and Basbaum 1978; Jones and Gebhart 1986). Lesioning of LC/SC or NRM potentiated inflammatory hyperalgesia (Tsuruoka and Willis 1996a,b; Wei et al. 1999a). Microinjection of lidocaine into the NRM in adjuvant-inflamed rats increased activity in over 75% of the spinal dorsal horn neurons (Ren and Dubner 1996). Following lesions of the NRM by a selective neurotoxin, 5,7-DHT, which destroys serotonin-containing axons descending to the spinal dorsal horn, FOS protein significantly increased in all laminae of the dorsal horn on the ipsilateral and contralateral sides in animals in which the neurotoxin was injected into the NRM. Bilateral LC/SC lesions by microinjections of a noradrenergic neurotoxin, DSP-4, also increased inflammation-induced spinal FOS expression. Interestingly, the pattern of elevation of FOS expression in inflamed rats induced by the NRM and LC/SC lesions was similar to that produced by DLF and ventrolateral funiculus (VLF) lesions, respectively (Wei et al. 1998, 1999a).

Further studies suggest that descending serotonergic and noradrenergic pathways differentially suppress the responses of spinal neurons, including spinoparabrachial neurons, in the deep and superficial dorsal horn (Wei et al. 1999a,b). The NRM 5,7-DHT lesion as compared to a vehicle lesion resulted in a significant two-fold increase in the percentage of double-labeled (FOS-expressing projection neurons with FOS protein immunolabel and Fluoro-Gold retrograde label) neurons in lamina V after inflammation. There were no significant differences in the percentage of double-labeled projection neurons in laminae I–II and lamina X. In contrast to the NRM serotonergic lesions, DSP-4 significantly increased the percentage of double-labeled neurons in the superficial laminae. The findings indicate that the descending 5-HT and noradrenergic effects are lamina selective. These results demonstrate that multiple specific brainstem sites are involved in descending modulation of inflammatory hyperalgesia. Both NRM and LC/SC descending pathways are major sources of enhanced net inhibitory modulation in inflamed animals.

Importantly, descending input also exerts a facilitatory effect following persistent tissue injury. In contrast to potentiation of hyperalgesia and FOS expression after NRM and LC/SC lesions, chemical lesions of NGC and NGC pars alpha in the rostral medulla led to opposite effects (Wei et al. 1999a). The NGC lesions were made with ibotenic acid that produces excitotoxic destruction of the neurons. Two to three days after ibotenic acid injection, complete Freund's adjuvant was injected into one hindpaw and behavioral hyperalgesia was examined. Lesioned animals showed an increase in the paw-withdrawal latency following a noxious thermal stimulus as compared to vehicle controls, which indicates a reduction in the hyperalgesia and a marked reduction in FOS protein expression bilaterally in all laminae of the spinal cord after NGC lesions (Fig. 2). Furthermore, if the NGC lesion was extended to involve the NRM, the behavioral hyperalgesia and inflammation-induced FOS expression were similar to that in vehicle-injected rats (Fig. 2). These results suggest that the net descending effects from NGC were facilitatory and that NGC facilitates the central sensitization seen at the spinal level. In addition, lesions of the rostral medial medulla or RVM that included NGC inhibited secondary hyperalgesia produced by the application of mustard oil (Urban et al. 1996; Urban and Gebhart 1999), further

---

Fig. 2. Effects of the rostral ventromedial medulla nuclei lesions on inflammation-induced hyperalgesia and spinal FOS protein expression. (A) The hyperalgesia was significantly attenuated in nucleus gigantocellularis (NGC) ibotenic acid (IBO)-lesioned rats 2–24 hours after the injection of the inflammatory agent, complete Freund's adjuvant (CFA), as compared to vehicle-injected controls ($^{+}$ $P < 0.05$, $^{+++}$ $P < 0.001$). In NGC/NRM (nucleus raphe magnus) IBO-lesioned rats, the hyperalgesia was not significantly different from the vehicle-injected rats but significantly greater than that in NGC IBO-lesioned rats at 24 hours (** $P < 0.01$) post-CFA. (B) The number of FOS-positive (FOS-LI) neurons in different regions of the spinal cord from the vehicle-injected, the NGC-lesioned, and the NGC/NRM-lesioned animals. Compared to the vehicle control, the NGC lesions produced a reduction of FOS labeling in the spinal cord 24 hours following inflammation. This effect was reversed by the NGC/NRM lesions. Symbols denote significant differences: *, NGC lesions vs. vehicle; #, the NGC/NRM lesions vs. vehicle; +, the NGC lesions vs. NGC/NRM lesions. Single symbol: $P < 0.05$; double symbols: $P < 0.01$; triple symbols: $P < 0.001$. Adapted from Wei et al. (1999a), with permission. ⟶

supported the hypothesis that this region is involved in the facilitation of hyperalgesia. The facilitatory effect may also originate from other sites (e.g., the medullary dorsal reticular nucleus, Almeida et al. 1999) and the supraspinal facilitatory control may be modality selective (Bian et al. 1998; Kauppila et al. 1998). Spinalization blocked secondary mechanical allodynia and mechanical hyperexcitability of spinal nociceptive neurons produced by mustard oil, but resulted in facilitation of the thermal tail-flick reflex (Mansikka and Pertovaara 1997; Pertovaara 1998). However, hindpaw formalin-induced facilitation of the tail-flick reflex was prevented by spinal transection or RVM lesion (Wiertelak et al. 1994, 1997). When compared to

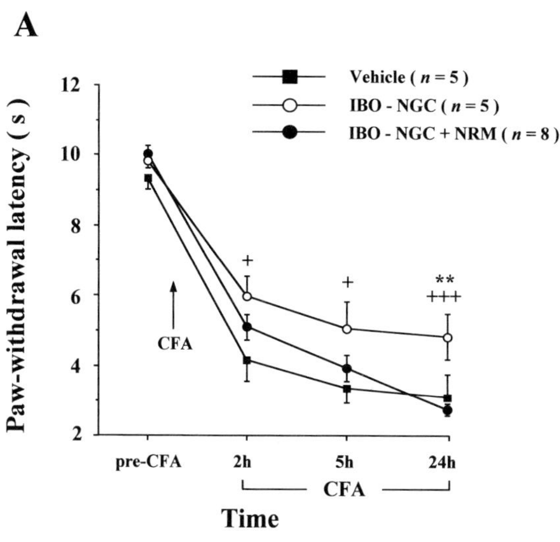

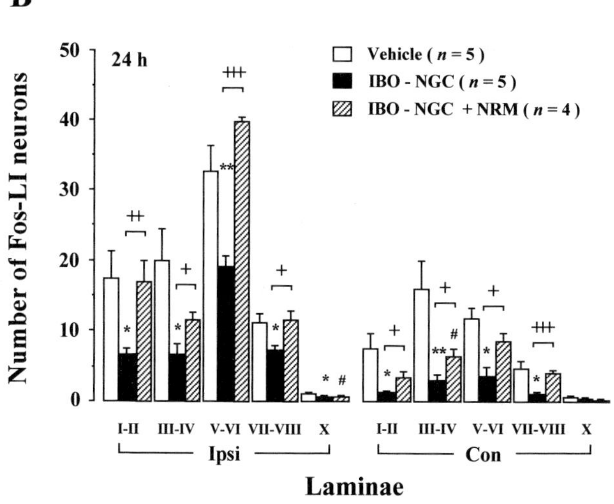

primary hyperalgesia, the secondary hyperalgesia appears to rely more on a supraspinal loop (Urban and Gebhart 1999).

It appears, then, that supraspinal mechanisms contribute to the dorsal horn hyperexcitability and development of hyperalgesia following tissue injury. Both facilitatory and inhibitory circuitry may be activated by ascending input after injury (Herrero and Cervero 1996; Gozariu et al. 1998) and the final outcome of an injury will much depend on the balance between the descending facilitatory and inhibitory input. It is possible that severe persistent pain may be enhanced when the facilitatory network overrides the inhibition.

DYNAMIC CHANGES IN DESCENDING MODULATION DURING DEVELOPMENT OF HYPERALGESIA

Inflammatory models of hyperalgesia have been used extensively in recent years. Rats with inflammatory hyperalgesia exhibit an increased sensitivity to opioid analgesics (Neil et al. 1986; Hylden et al. 1991; Kayser et al. 1991). Typically, the dose-response curve for opioids from the inflamed hyperalgesic paw has a leftward shift compared to the noninflamed paw (Hylden et al. 1991; Ren et al. 1992b). This phenomenon has attracted attention for over a decade. Kayser et al. (1991) suggested that this increased opioid sensitivity in inflamed animals was related to a peripheral mechanism as it is significantly attenuated after local injections of very low doses (0.5–1 μg) of naloxone. Recent observations indicate that the increased opioid sensitivity after inflammation may also reflect changes in central pain-modulating pathways. Hurley and Hammond (1998) have demonstrated enhancement of the descending inhibitory effects of μ and δ_2 opioid receptor agonists microinjected into the RVM during the development and maintenance of persistent inflammatory hyperalgesia.

As described above, compared to naive animals receiving the same treatment, interruption of descending pathways leads to a further increase in spinal hyperexcitability and behavioral hyperalgesia after a unilateral hindpaw inflammation. In cats with knee joint inflammation, tonic descending inhibition is apparently greater in neurons with input from the inflamed knee as revealed by reversible spinalization with a cold block (Cervero et al. 1991; Schaible et al. 1991). In hindpaw-inflamed rats, local anesthesia of the NRM results in a further increase in dorsal horn nociceptive neuronal activity (Ren and Dubner 1996). In noninflamed animals, however, lidocaine injection in the NRM or medullary raphe lesions do not result in an increase in background activity and noxious heat-evoked responses of dorsal horn neurons (Hall et al. 1981; Gebhart et al. 1983; Ren et al. 1990), which suggests that those spinal nociceptive neurons were not under tonic inhibition from the NRM, or that other descending pathways become more active to compensate for the loss of NRM-mediated inhibition. Thus, there is an important difference in the operation of descending pathways between inflamed and noninflamed naive animals. The descending circuitry appears to be actively involved in modulating inflammation-induced dorsal horn hyperexcitability. The implication of these results is that the descending pathways become more active in response to inflammation, and the whole descending system may be maximally activated by the persistent peripheral afferent barrage.

Studies of dorsal horn neuronal activity indicate that the enhancement of descending inhibition during the development of inflammation is progressive (Schaible et al. 1991). In spinally transected rats, the induction of FOS protein expression in the spinal cord is significantly increased following 3 days of persistent inflammation, compared to intact and inflamed control rats. However, this increase in FOS protein expression is not detectable at 2 hours after the introduction of inflammation (Ren and Ruda 1996). The potency of descending modulation can be directly compared between nociceptive responses of the inflamed and noninflamed paws and tail in lightly anesthetized rat preparations (Terayama et al. 1999). Stimulating the NRM in noninflamed naive rats revealed a significantly lower threshold current for complete inhibition of the nociceptive tail-flick reflex than that for inhibition of the nocifensive paw-withdrawal response. The stimulus-response (S-R) function for tail-flick inhibition was located to the left of that for the paw-withdrawal inhibition, which indicates that the NRM-produced inhibition is more potent against the tail-flick reflex in normal animals. Following a unilateral hindpaw inflammation, the S-R curve for the inflamed paw was initially shifted to the right of the noninflamed paw at 3 hours and then gradually shifted to the left to reach the location of the S-R curve for the tail-flick inhibition (Terayama et al. 1999). At 24 hours after inflammation, the S-R curve for the inflamed paw remained to the left of the noninflamed paw, and the relationship of the S-R curves between inflamed and noninflamed paws was similar to that of the opioid dose-response curves in inflamed rats (Hylden et al. 1991). These results suggest biphasic temporally related changes in NRM stimulation-produced inhibition during the development of inflammation. The descending inhibition decreases in the early period and gradually increases as inflammation persists. In the chronic stage of inflammation (1–4 weeks after induction), descending modulation appears to return to the normal level (Tsuruoka and Willis 1996b; Danziger et al. 1999).

These findings provide evidence for dynamic, time-dependent changes in the excitability of brainstem pain-modulating pathways following persistent tissue injury. The excitability of descending pathways is enhanced during the course of inflammation and hyperalgesia. This activity-induced plasticity in pain-modulating circuitry complements the activity-dependent neuronal plasticity in ascending pain transmission pathways (Dubner and Ruda 1992).

CONCLUDING REMARKS

The demonstration of the sites of origin of descending inhibition and facilitation provides a more complete picture of the body's endogenous pain-modulating system. While the pain-inhibitory circuitry is relatively well understood, we still know little about the organization and functional significance of the facilitatory network. From a physiological point of view, the facilitation of nociception helps the body to maintain normal pain sensitivity that is essential for survival. The simultaneous descending excitatory and inhibitory inputs contribute to a balance between perception and suppression of noxious events. It is important to appreciate that the pain-modulating system changes dramatically after injury. Brainstem descending inhibitory and facilitatory pathways concurrently activate and the interaction between these pathways will dictate, or affect, the development of spinal hyperexcitability and hyperalgesia. Thus, descending pathways control both the intensity of perceived pain under normal conditions and persistent pain following injury. The dynamic plasticity of descending pathways may sometimes render the system vulnerable and lead to pathological consequences. The imbalance between these modulatory pathways may be one mechanism contributing to variability in acute and chronic pain conditions. For patients suffering from deep pains such as temporomandibular disorders, fibromyalgia, and low back pain, the diffuse nature and amplification of persistent pain, in part, may be the result of a net increase in endogenous facilitation.

ACKNOWLEDGMENTS

We thank Drs. R. Dubner and H.L. Fields for their comments on this manuscript. The authors' work has been supported by NIH grants (DE11964, DA10275, to K. Ren; DA10833, NS38680 to M. Zhuo; and NS09743 to W.D. Willis).

REFERENCES

Almeida A, Storkson R, Lima D, Hole K, Tjolsen A. The medullary dorsal reticular nucleus facilitates pain behaviour induced by formalin in the rat. *Eur J Neurosci* 1999; 11:110–122.

Basbaum AI, Fields HL. Endogenous pain control systems: brainstem spinal pathways and endorphin circuitry. *Annu Rev Neurosci* 1984; 7:309–338.

Bederson JB, Fields HL, Barbaro NM. Hyperalgesia following naloxone-precipitated withdrawal from morphine is associated with increased on-cell activity in the rostral ventromedial medulla. *Somatosens Motor Res* 1990; 7:185–203.

Bian D, Ossipov MH, Zhong C, Malan TP Jr , Porreca F. Tactile allodynia, but not thermal hyperalgesia, of the hindlimbs is blocked by spinal transection in rats with nerve injury. *Neurosci Lett* 1998; 241:79–82.

Cervero F, Schaible H-G, Schmidt RF. Tonic descending inhibition of spinal cord neurones driven by joint afferents in normal cats and in cats with an inflamed knee joint. *Exp Brain Res* 1991; 83:675–678.

Danziger N, Weil-Fugazza J, Le Bars D, Bouhassira D. Alteration of descending modulation of nociception during the course of monoarthritis in the rat. *J Neurosci* 1999; 19:2394–2400.

Dubner R. Neuronal plasticity and pain following peripheral tissue inflammation or nerve injury. In: Bond MR, Charlton JE, Woolf CJ (Eds). *Proceedings of the 6th World Congress on Pain*. Amsterdam: Elsevier Science, 1991, pp 263–276.

Dubner R, Ruda MA. Activity-dependent neuronal plasticity following tissue injury and inflammation. *Trends Neurosci* 1992; 15:96–103.

Dubuisson D, Wall PD. Medullary raphe influences on units in laminae 1 and 2 of cat spinal cord. *J Physiol (Lond)* 1979; 300:33P.

Dubuisson D, Wall PD. Descending influences on receptive fields and activity of single units recorded in laminae 1, 2 and 3 of cat spinal cord. *Brain Res* 1980; 199:283–298.

Fields HL, Basbaum AI. Brainstem control of spinal pain-transmission neurons. *Annu Rev Physiol* 1978; 40:217–248.

Fields HL, Bry J, Hentall I, Zorman G. The activity of neurons in the rostral medulla of the rat during withdrawal from noxious heat. *J Neurosci* 1983a; 3:2545–2552.

Fields HL, Vanegas H, Hentall ID, Zorman G. Evidence that disinhibition of brain stem neurones contributes to morphine analgesia. *Nature* 1983b; 306:684–686.

Fields HL, Heinricher MM, Mason P. Neurotransmitters in nociceptive modulatory circuits. *Annu Rev Neurosci* 1991; 14:219–245.

Fields HL, Malick A, Burstein R. Dorsal horn projection targets of ON and OFF cells in the rostral ventromedial medulla. *J Neurophysiol* 1995; 74:1742–1759.

Gebhart GF. Modulatory effects of descending systems on spinal dorsal horn neurons. In: Yaksh TL (Ed). *Spinal Afferent Processing*. New York: Plenum, 1986, pp 391–416.

Gebhart GF, Sandkuhler J, Thalhammer JG, Zimmermann M. Inhibition of spinal nociceptive information by stimulation in midbrain of the cat is blocked by lidocaine microinjected in nucleus raphe magnus and medullary reticular formation. *J Neurophysiol* 1983; 50:1446–1459.

Gozariu M, Bouhassira D, Willer JC, Le Bars D. The influence of temporal summation on a C-fibre reflex in the rat: effects of lesions in the rostral ventromedial medulla (RVM). *Brain Res* 1998; 792:168–172.

Haber LH, Martin RF, Chung JM, Willis WD. Inhibition and excitation of primate spinothalamic tract neurons by stimulation in region of nucleus reticularis gigantocellularis. *J Neurophysiol* 1980; 43:1578–1593.

Hall JG, Duggan AW, Johnson SM, Morton CR. Medullary raphe lesions do not reduce descending inhibition of dorsal horn neurones of the cat. *Neurosci Lett* 1981; 7:25–29.

Herrero JF, Cervero F. Supraspinal influences on the facilitation of rat nociceptive reflexes induced by carrageenan monoarthritis. *Neurosci Lett* 1996; 209:21–24.

Holden JE, Schwartz EJ, Proudfit HK. Microinjection of morphine in the A7 catecholamine cell group produces opposing effects on nociception that are mediated by alpha1- and alpha2-adrenoceptors. *Neuroscience* 1999; 91:979–990.

Hughes J, Smith TW, Kosterlitz HW, et al. Identification of two related pentapeptides from the brain with potent opiate agonist activity. *Nature* 1975; 258:577–580.

Hunt SP, Pini A, Evan G. Induction of c-Fos-like protein in spinal cord neurons following sensory stimulation. *Nature* 1987; 328:632–634.

Hurley RW, Hammond DL. Enhancement of the antinociceptive effects of supraspinally administered μ and δ_2 opioid receptor agonists under conditions of persistent inflammatory nociception. *Soc Neurosci Abstr* 1998; 24:891.

Hylden JLK, Thomas DA, Iadarola MJ, Dubner R. Spinal opioid analgesic effects are enhanced in a model of unilateral inflammation/hyperalgesia: possible involvement of noradrenergic mechanisms. *Eur J Pharmacol* 1991; 194:135–143.

Jones SL, Gebhart GF. Quantitative characterization of coeruleospinal inhibition of nociceptive transmission in the rat. *J Neurophysiol* 1986; 56:1397–1410.

Kauppila T, Kontinen VK, Pertovaara A. Influence of spinalization on spinal withdrawal reflex responses varies depending on the submodality of the test stimulus and the experimental pathophysiological condition in the rat. *Brain Res* 1998; 797:234–242.

Kayser V, Chen YL, Guilbaud G. Behavioural evidence for a peripheral component in the enhanced antinociceptive effect of a low dose of systemic morphine in carrageenin-induced hyperalgesic rats. *Brain Res* 1991; 560:237–244.

Le Bars D, Dickenson AH, Besson JM. Microinjection of morphine within nucleus raphe magnus and dorsal horn neurone activities related to nociception in the rat. *Brain Res* 1980; 189:467–481.

MacArthur L, Ren K, Pfaffenroth E, Franklin E, Ruda MA. Descending modulation of opioid-containing nociceptive neurons in rats with peripheral inflammation and hyperalgesia. *Neuroscience* 1999; 88:499–506.

Mansikka H, Pertovaara A. Supraspinal influence on hindlimb withdrawal thresholds and mustard oil-induced secondary allodynia in rats. *Brain Res Bull* 1997; 42:359–365.

Mayer DJ, Liebeskind JC. Pain reduction by focal electrical stimulation of the brain: an anatomical and behavioral analysis. *Brain Res* 1974; 68:73–93.

Mayer DJ, Wolfle TL, Akil H, Carder B, Liebeskind JC. Analgesia from electrical stimulation in the brainstem of the rat. *Science* 1971; 174:1351–1354.

McMahon SB, Wall PD. Descending excitation and inhibition of spinal cord lamina I projection neurons. *J Neurophysiol* 1988; 59:1204–1219.

Melzack R, Wall PD. Pain mechanisms: a new theory. *Science* 1965; 10:971–979.

Neil A, Kayser V, Gacel G, Besson J-M, Guilbaud G. Opioid receptor types and antinociceptive activity in chronic inflammation: both kappa and mu opiate agonistic effects are enhanced in arthritic rats. *Eur J Pharmacol* 1986; 130:203–208.

Pan ZZ, Tershner SA, Fields HL. Cellular mechanism for anti-analgesic action of agonists of the k-opioid receptor. *Nature* 1997; 389:382–385.

Pertovaara A. A neuronal correlate of secondary hyperalgesia in the rat spinal dorsal horn is submodality selective and facilitated by supraspinal influence. *Exp Neurol* 1998; 149:193–202.

Ren K, Dubner R. Enhanced descending modulation of nociception in rats with persistent hindpaw inflammation. *J Neurophysiol* 1996; 76:3025–3037.

Ren K, Ruda MA. Descending modulation of Fos expression after persistent peripheral inflammation. *Neuroreport* 1996; 7:2186–2190.

Ren K, Randich A, Gebhart GF. Vagal afferent modulation of a nociceptive reflex in rats: involvement of spinal opioid and monoamine receptors. *Brain Res* 1988; 446:285–294.

Ren K, Randich A, Gebhart GF. Vagal afferent modulation of spinal nociceptive transmission in the rat. *J Neurophysiol* 1989; 62:401–405.

Ren K, Randich A, Gebhart GF. Electrical stimulation of cervical vagal afferents. I Central relays for modulation of spinal nociceptive transmission. *J Neurophysiol* 1990; 64:1098–1114.

Ren K, Hylden JLK, Williams GM, Ruda MA, Dubner R. The effects of a non-competitive NMDA receptor antagonist, MK-801, on behavioral hyperalgesia and dorsal horn neuronal activity in rats with unilateral inflammation. *Pain* 1992a; 50:331–344.

Ren K, Williams GM, Hylden JLK, Ruda MA, Dubner R. The intrathecal administration of excitatory amino acid receptor antagonists selectively attenuated carrageenan-induced behavioral hyperalgesia in rats. *Eur J Pharmacol* 1992b; 219:235–243.

Reynolds DV. Surgery in the rat during electrical analgesia induced by focal brain stimulation. *Science* 1969; 164:444–445.

Schaible HG, Neugebauer V, Cervero F, Schmidt RF. Changes in tonic descending inhibition of spinal neurons with articular input during the development of acute arthritis in the cat. *J Neurophysiol* 1991; 66:1021–1032.

Taylor BK, Basbaum AI. Neurochemical characterization of extracellular serotonin in the rostral ventromedial medulla and its modulation by noxious stimuli. *J Neurochem* 1995; 65:578–589.

Terayama R, Ren K, Dubner R. Dynamic changes in descending modulation during the development of inflammatory hyperalgesia: role of rostral ventromedial medulla (RVM). *Soc Neurosci Abstr* 1999; 25:1676.

Tsou K, Jang CS. Studies on the site of analgesic action of morphine by intracerebral microinjections. *Sci Sinica* 1964; 13:1099–1109.

Tsuruoka M, Willis WD. Bilateral lesions in the area of the nucleus locus coeruleus affect the development of hyperalgesia during carrageenan-induced inflammation. *Brain Res* 1996a; 726:233–236.

Tsuruoka M, Willis WD. Descending modulation from the region of the locus coeruleus or nociceptive sensitivity in a rat model of inflammatory hyperalgesia. *Brain Res* 1996b; 743:86–92.

Urban MO, Gebhart GF. Supraspinal contributions to hyperalgesia. *Proc Natl Acad Sci USA* 1999; 96:7687–7692.

Urban MO, Jiang MC, Gebhart GF. Participation of central descending nociceptive facilitatory systems in secondary hyperalgesia produced by mustard oil. *Brain Res* 1996; 37:83–91.

Vanegas H, Barbaro NM, Fields HL. Midbrain stimulation inhibits tail-flick only at currents sufficient to excite rostral medullary neurons. *Brain Res* 1984; 321:127–133.

Wei F, Ren K, Dubner R. Inflammation-induced Fos protein expression in the rat spinal cord is enhanced following dorsolateral or ventrolateral funiculus lesions. *Brain Res* 1998; 782:136–141.

Wei F, Dubner R, Ren K. Nucleus reticularis gigantocellularis and nucleus raphe magnus in the brain stem exert opposite effects on behavioral hyperalgesia and spinal Fos protein expression after peripheral inflammation. *Pain* 1999a; 80:127–141.

Wei F, Dubner R, Ren K. Laminar-selective noradrenergic and serotoninergic modulation includes spinoparabrachial cells after inflammation. *Neuroreport* 1999b; 10:1757–1761.

Wiertelak EP, Furness LE, Horan R, et al. Subcutaneous formalin produces centrifugal hyperalgesia at a non-injected site via the NMDA-nitric oxide cascade. *Brain Res* 1994; 649:19–26.

Wiertelak EP, Roemer B, Maier SF, Watkins LR. Comparison of the effects of nucleus tractus solitarius and ventral medial medulla lesions on illness-induced and subcutaneous formalin-induced hyperalgesias. *Brain Res* 1997; 748:143–150.

Willis WD, Westlund KN. Neuroanatomy of the pain system and of the pathways that modulate pain. *J Clin Neurophysiol* 1997; 14:2–31.

Woolf CJ, Thompson SW. The induction and maintenance of central sensitization is dependent on N-methyl-D-aspartic acid receptor activation; implications for the treatment of post-injury pain hypersensitivity states. *Pain* 1991; 44(3):293–299.

Zagon A, Meng X, Fields HL. Intrinsic membrane characteristics distinguish two subsets of nociceptive modulatory neurons in rat RVM. *J Neurophysiol* 1997; 78:2848–2858.

Zhuo M, Gebhart GF. Spinal serotonin receptors mediate descending facilitation of a nociceptive reflex from the nuclei reticularis gigantocellularis and gigantocellularis pars alpha in the rat. *Brain Res* 1991; 550:35–48.

Zhuo M, Gebhart GF. Characterization of descending facilitation and inhibition of spinal nociceptive transmission from the nuclei reticularis gigantocellularis and gigantocellularis pars alpha in the rat. *J Neurophysiol* 1992; 67:1599–1614.

Zhuo M, Gebhart GF. Biphasic modulation of spinal nociceptive transmission from the medullary raphe nuclei in the rat. *J Neurophysiol* 1997; 78:746–758.

Correspondence to: Ke Ren, PhD, 666 W. Baltimore Street, Room 5A26, University of Maryland Dental School, Baltimore, MD 21201, USA. Tel: 410-706-3250; Fax: 410-706-4172; email: kren@umaryland.edu.

Proceedings of the 9th World Congress on Pain, Progress in Pain Research and Management, Vol. 16, edited by M. Devor, M.C. Rowbotham, and Z. Wiesenfeld-Hallin, IASP Press, Seattle, © 2000.

39

Quantitative Sensory Testing in Patients with Painful or Painless Syringomyelia

Didier Bouhassira,[a,b] Nadine Attal,[a] Louis Brasseur,[a] and Fabrice Parker[c]

[a]*Pain Evaluation and Treatment Unit, Ambroise Paré Hospital, Boulogne, France;* [b]*INSERM, U-161, Paris, France;* [c]*Neurosurgery Department, Kremlin-Bicêtre Hospital, le Kremlin-Bicêtre, France*

The pathophysiology of central pain remains an enigma. Since the thorough description of central pain at the beginning of the 20th century, the main pathophysiological hypotheses have revolved around two concepts: "irritation" and "disinhibition" (Head and Holmes 1911; Garcin 1937; Riddoch 1938; White and Sweet 1969; Pagni 1989). Recent studies based on quantitative sensory testing in patients with spinal or brain injuries (Beric et al. 1988, Boivie et al. 1989; Leijon et al. 1989; Vestergaard et al. 1995; Bowsher 1996) have suggested that a lesion anywhere in the spinothalamocortical pathway is a necessary condition for the development of central pain. These patients almost always have increased thermal thresholds within the painful area, while symptoms suggestive of a lesion of the dorsal column/medial lemniscus system are milder and less frequently observed. It has thus been proposed that central pain might result from a central misinterpretation of sensory information due to the (hypothetical) inhibitory effects of the spinothalamic system on the dorsal column epicritic system. However, it is difficult to appreciate the exact pathophysiological role of a lesion of the spinothalamocortical tract, since most of the relevant studies were performed in selected patients with pain symptoms (see, however, Andersen et al. 1995). In a recent study in patients with spinal cord injury, Eide et al. (1996) reported that sensory deficits were not different between painful and nonpainful areas of denervated skin; they concluded that a lesion of the spinothalamic tract is probably not a sufficient condition for the development of central pain syndromes. In addition, these authors observed that spontaneous pains were generally associated with evoked pains (i.e., allodynia and/or hyperalgesia); this finding suggests that other mechanisms were involved, such as hyperexcitability (i.e., central sensitization) of central nociceptive neurons. This hyperexcitability might be mediated by NMDA-receptor activation, since pain symptoms were reduced after ketamine administration (Eide et al. 1995).

Pain symptoms of various kinds (headache, musculoskeletal pain, and visceral pain) have been observed in up to 90% of patients with syringomyelia, but the most disabling are neuropathic pains, which affect up to 40% of these patients (Milhorat et al. 1996). Like other central pain syndromes, due to either spinal or brain injuries, these neuropathic pains are among the most difficult to treat (Yezierski 1996). A lesion of the spinothalamic tract fibers is always a feature of this neurological syndrome. To reinvestigate the role of spinothalamic lesions in central pain, we used quantitative sensory tests to compare the distribution of sensory deficits and pain symptoms in consecutive patients with painful or painless syringomyelia.

METHODS

PATIENTS

Twenty-one consecutive patients (7 women, 14 men; mean age 39 ± 13.2 years; median duration of symptoms 6 years), who presented with clinical and radiological evidence of syringomyelia, were recruited for the study from an initial group of 23 patients. Etiology of the disease included type I Chiari malformation (n = 15 patients), sometimes associated with scoliosis (n = 2), trauma (n = 4), dorsolumbar scoliosis (n = 1), and arachnoiditis (n = 1). Most patients (n = 19) presented with cervical or cervicodorsal syrinx, while two patients presented with dorsolumbar syringomyelia. Two patients were excluded from the analysis because magnetic resonance imaging (MRI) showed pure Chiari malformation with virtual syrinx, and they had no clinical symptoms of syringomyelia. None of the patients had been regularly taking analgesics before evaluation, and none were on medication at the time of evaluation.

EXTENSION OF SENSORY DEFICITS

Extension of thermal stimuli was initially determined by means of two thermo-rollers (Somedic) set at constant temperatures of 40°C (heat) and 25°C (cold). The determination was completed by measuring detection thresholds to warm and cold stimuli, using a thermotest (see below) to confirm the highest and lowest area of the syrinx. Since most sensory deficits had asymmetrical distribution, we defined a metameric score, corresponding to the sum of affected right and left dermatomes (for example, a T5–T6 left and T5 right thermal deficit was assigned a score of 3). However, since the area of dermatomes is different for upper and lower limbs, and in order to avoid bias, this score was not determined for patients with dorsolumbar syrinx and lower limb deficits. Examination of sensory abnormalities also included evaluation of fine tactile deficits (graphesthesia, detection of movement direction), touch (using a cotton swab), pinprick (using a pinwheel), and proprioceptive deficits (detection of joint position, stereognosis). The extension of sensory deficits to pinprick, gross tactile stimulation, and thermal stimuli was determined for each patient.

PSYCHOPHYSICAL MEASURES

Psychophysical tests were performed in a quiet room at a constant temperature (22°C). Measurements were performed in the area of maximal thermal deficit and in a normal area for all patients. In patients with pain symptoms, measurements were performed in both the area of maximal spontaneous pain and an adjacent lesioned but nonpainful area. Detection and pain thresholds to mechanical stimuli were assessed with calibrated von Frey hairs (0.057–140 g), as described previously (Attal et al. 1998, 1999). The force required to bend the filaments was then converted into logarithmic units. After pain thresholds had been determined, suprathreshold stimuli were applied in a pseudorandom order using selected von Frey filaments. After each stimulus, the patients were asked to quantify the pain intensity on a visual analogue scale (VAS). Thermal sensations (warm and cold detection and pain thresholds) were assessed with a thermotest (Somedic AB, Stockholm, Sweden), using the Marstock method (Fruhstorfer et al. 1976). Thermal stimuli (5°–48°C) were applied according to a method described previously (Hansson and Linbdlom 1992; Attal et al. 1998, 1999). Vibration thresholds were determined using a vibrameter (Somedic), according to the method of limits.

EVALUATION OF SPONTANEOUS PAIN AND TACTILE ALLODYNIA

Patients with pain symptoms were asked to report their neuropathic pain intensity at the time of evaluation as well as mean and maximal pain over the previous 24 hours. Pain intensity was assessed using a 10-cm VAS graduated from 0 (no pain) to 10 (worst possible pain). Other types of pain, i.e., nociceptive pains, were recognized but not analyzed in depth. Tactile (dynamic) allodynia was considered to be present if a clear sensation of pain was evoked by stroking the skin three times with a brush. The intensity of allodynia within the area of maximal pain was marked on a VAS (as the mean of two consecutive VAS scores).

STATISTICAL ANALYSES

Data provided by the entire group are expressed as means ± 1 SD. Wilcoxon's signed rank test was used for comparison of paired data. Relationships between two variables were tested by the Kendall rank correlation (τ). Analysis of variance (ANOVA), with the Fisher's post hoc least significant difference test, was used for intergroup comparisons. In all instances, $P < 0.05$ was regarded as significant.

RESULTS

All the patients presented with thermal (warm and cold) and mechanical (pinprick) deficits; in some patients deficits were confined to cervicodorsal ($n = 15$), cervical ($n = 4$), and dorsolumbar dermatomes ($n = 2$). The thermal deficit was bilateral in 16 patients and unilateral (in accordance with the paramedian right or left extension of the syrinx shown by MRI) in 5 patients. Most patients ($n = 13$) also showed other deficits concerning tactile sensibility as assessed with von Frey hairs ($n = 10$), vibration perception ($n = 6$), graphesthesia ($n = 5$), detection of movement direction ($n = 3$) and joint position ($n = 3$), and stereognosis ($n = 3$).

COMPARISON OF PATIENTS WITH AND WITHOUT PAIN

Ten patients presented with painful and 11 with painless syringomyelia. There was no significant difference between patients with and without pain as regards age, mean duration of syrinx, or etiology of the syrinx. Analysis of sensory deficits showed no significant differences between both groups of patients regarding thermal deficits (warm and cold detection thresholds, heat and cold pain thresholds), and mechanical and vibration deficits in the area of maximal deficits. Moreover, the extension of thermal and mechanical deficits was not significantly different between the two groups of patients. Finally, the proportion of patients with impairment of graphesthesia and of detection of movement direction and joint position was similar between the two groups.

RELATIONSHIP BETWEEN PAINS AND SENSORY DEFICITS

Ten patients presented with spontaneous pain at the time of evaluation (mean VAS score = 4.7 ± 1.3; mean maximal pain over 24 hours = 7.4 ± 2.2). Pain was most commonly described as a continuous burning pain (n = 8), often associated with paroxysmal lancinating pain (n = 7). In 8 out of 10 patients, the area of maximal pain was confined within the area of maximal thermal deficit. However, in two patients with unilateral deficit, the area of maximal pain was localized on the "normal side," where no thermal or mechanical deficits were evident. No significant difference was detected regarding the thermal and mechanical deficits between the area of maximal pain and an adjacent nonpainful area (Fig. 1). No correlation was observed between the intensity of spontaneous pain and the magnitude of thermal and mechanical deficits in the area of maximal pain. In addition, impairments of graphesthesia and of detection of movement direction were similar in the two areas.

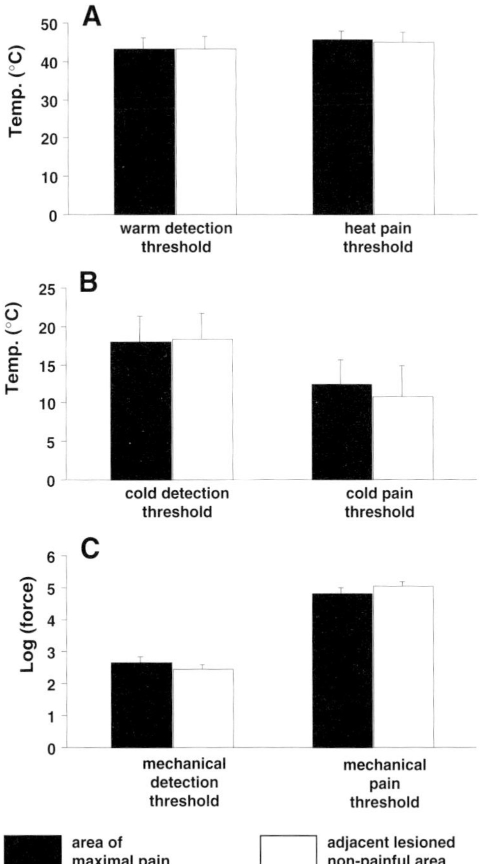

Fig. 1. (A,B) Thermal and (C) mechanical detection and pain thresholds observed in the area of maximal spontaneous pain and an adjacent lesioned but nonpainful area in patients with painful syringomyelia. Mechanical thresholds are graphed as logarithmic transformations of the force required to bend calibrated von Frey hairs (see *Methods*). Means and SD are shown.

Patients in pain were very heterogeneous as regards their thermal and mechanical pain thresholds and their responses to suprathreshold stimuli applied within the area of maximal pain (Fig. 2). They could be classified within two distinct categories. One group of patients (n = 5) had "pure" spontaneous ongoing pain that was located within an area of profound thermal deficits, as indicated by the measurements of both the detection and pain thresholds and by the stimulus-response curves evoked by thermal and mechanical stimuli. In such patients, the stimulus-response curves within the area of maximal pain were not significantly different from those observed within an adjacent nonpainful lesioned area. All these patients also presented some symptoms suggestive of dorsal column lesion (i.e., impairments of graphesthesia, and of detection of movement direction, vibration thresholds, or joint position). In sharp contrast, a second group of patients (n = 5) showed dramatically different patterns of stimulus-response curves to thermal and mechanical stimuli, suggestive of hyperalgesia. As a group,

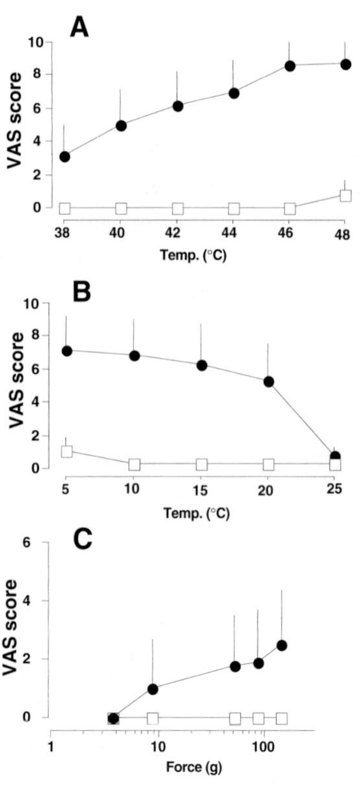

Fig. 2. Stimulus-response curves for (A) heat, (B) cold, and (C) mechanical stimuli observed in the area of maximal spontaneous pain in patients with "pure" spontaneous pain and patients with spontaneous pain associated with evoked pains. Means and SD are shown.

these patients had less severe sensory deficits. Thermal deficits in the painful area were lower in this group as compared to patients with "pure" spontaneous pain (warm thresholds were 35.5° ± 0.3°C versus 46.6° ± 5.9°C; cold thresholds were 29° ± 0.3°C versus 13.2° ± 7.1°C, respectively). Some of these patients showed reduced pain thresholds, suggestive of allodynia, when tested by different stimuli: dynamic mechanical stimuli (n = 3 patients), static mechanical stimuli (n = 3), cold (n = 3), and heat (n = 2). Two patients had a second area of evoked pain (cold or mechanical allodynia/hyperalgesia) that did not coexist spatially with that of spontaneous pain, but was located in junctional areas between normal and lesioned areas. Finally, only one of these patients presented with some form of "dorsal column deficit" within the painful area (i.e., impairment of tactile thresholds and graphesthesia in the area of maximal pain).

DISCUSSION

Authors of previous investigations in patients with central pain due to stroke or spinal cord injury have concluded, based on the use of quantitative sensory tests, that these patients have thermal deficits but a relative preservation of fine tactile and vibratory sensations (Beric et al. 1988; Boivie et al. 1989; Leijon et al. 1989; Vestergaard et al. 1995; Bowsher 1996). Lesions of the spinothalamic system, regardless of level, were thought to constitute a necessary condition for the development of neuropathic pains in these patients. These data provided some support for the "imbalance theory," suggesting that the mechanisms of central pain result from an imbalance in sensory information conveyed by the residual dorsal column system and an impaired spinothalamic system.

In the present study, in agreement with recent previous studies (e.g., Bowsher 1996), we observed that central pain symptoms were most commonly confined within the area of maximal thermal deficit. To further evaluate the correlation between pain and sensory deficits, we used two different approaches. First, for each patient we compared the magnitude of thermal and mechanical deficits between an area of maximal spontaneous pain and an adjacent lesioned but nonpainful area. In accordance with previous results (Eide et al. 1996), we did not find a significant difference in the magnitude of thermal or mechanical deficits between these two body areas. Second, we compared the magnitude and extension of thermal and mechanical deficits between patients with syringomyelia with and without pain, matched by age, duration, and etiology of the syrinx. We failed to observe an overall significant difference in the extent or magnitude of thermal or mechanical deficits between these two groups of patients. Thus, the present data primarily suggest that a lesion of the spinothalamic tract is a necessary, but probably not a sufficient, condition to account for central pain in these patients.

However, patients with painful syringomyelia appeared to be quite heterogeneous in their responses to thermal and mechanical stimuli in their area of spontaneous pain. In some patients, spontaneous pain was observed in an area of profound thermal sensory deficit and hypoalgesia, as indicated by the stimulus-response curves in the 5°–48°C range. In these patients, similar deficits and hypoalgesia were observed in an adjacent nonpainful area. In contrast, in a second group of patients, spontaneous ongoing pains were associated with increased responses to suprathreshold thermal (notably cold) or mechanical stimuli in their area of maximal pain. Some of these patients also had allodynia to tactile or thermal stimuli in their painful area (i.e., reduction of pain threshold). These two subgroups of patients were also different in other respects. Thermal deficits were more pronounced in patients with "pure" spontaneous pain and were always associated with other deficits, suggesting an extension of the lesion toward the dorsal horn of the spinal cord and/or the dorsal column.

It is thus likely that the pathophysiological mechanisms of central pain are different in these two subgroups of patients. It might be proposed that the "pure" spontaneous pains observed in our first subgroup of patients, whose deficits suggested of a dorsal extension of the syrinx, involved a disturbance of segmental modulatory systems and/or descending inhibitory controls traveling within the dorsal and dorsolateral quadrant of the spinal cord. Interestingly, Milhorat et al. (1996) observed lesions involving the dorsolateral quadrant of the spinal cord in 84% of the patients presenting with syringomyelia associated with "central dysesthetic pain." In contrast, in our second subgroup of patients, spontaneous and evoked pains might involve other mechanisms such as a hyperexcitability of nociceptive neurons at the spinal and/or supraspinal levels. Indeed, these patients' symptoms were similar to those described in other studies (e.g., Eide et al. 1996) and were reminiscent of the behavioral changes observed in animal models of ischemic or excitotoxic spinal cord injury, thus showing evidence of hyperexcitability of nociceptive dorsal horn neurons (Yezierski 1996). However, in contrast to what has been described in animals, such sensitization did not seem to be generalized in our patients, since none of them presented with hyperalgesia to any type of stimulus. In addition, on rare occasions, allodynia and hyperalgesia were not associated with spontaneous pain and were located not within the area of maximal deficit, but at the junction between the normal and lesioned area, which suggests that still other mechanisms might be involved.

In conclusion, the present results suggest that patients with painful syringomyelia fall at least into two broad categories, presumably with different pathophysiological mechanisms. Such heterogeneity has also been emphasized in some patients with neuropathic pain due to peripheral nerve lesions (Fields et al. 1998), and is highly probable in other groups of neuropathic pain patients. Our results may be relevant from a therapeutic point of view, as they suggest that treatment plans should be specific to the different subtypes of painful syringomyelia.

ACKNOWLEDGMENT

This work was supported by l'Institut UPSA de la Douleur.

REFERENCES

Andersen G, Vestergaard K, Ingerman-Nielsen M, Jensen TS. Incidence of central post-stroke pain. *Pain* 1995; 61:187–193.

Attal N, Brasseur B, Parker F, Chauvin M, Bouhassira D. Effects of the anticonvulsant gabapentin on neuropathic peripheral and central pain: a pilot study. *Eur Neurol* 1998; 40:191–200.

Attal N, Brasseur L, Chauvin M, Bouhassira D. Effects of single and repeated applications of eutectic mixture of local anesthetics (EMLA®) cream on spontaneous and evoked pains in patients with postherpetic neuralgia. *Pain* 1999; 81:203–210.

Beric A, Dimitrijewic MR, Lindblom U. Central dysesthesia syndrome in spinal cord injury patients. *Pain* 1988; 34:109–116.

Boivie J, Leijon G, Johansson I. Central post-stroke pain—a study of the mechanisms through analyses of the sensory abnormalities. *Pain* 1989; 37:173–185.

Bowsher D. Central pain: clinical and physiological characteristics. *J Neurol Neurosurg Psychiatry* 1996; 61:62–69.

Eide PK, Stubhaug A, Stenehjem AE. Central dysesthesia pain after traumatic spinal cord injury is dependent on N-methyl-D-aspartate receptor activation. *Neurosurgery* 1995; 37:1080–1087.

Eide PK, Jorum E, Stenehjem AE. Somatosensory findings in patients with spinal cord injury and central dysesthesia pain. *J Neurol Neurosurg Psychiatry* 1996; 60:411–415.

Fields HL, Rowbotham M, Baron R. Postherpetic neuralgia: irritable nociceptors and deafferentation. *Neurobiol Dis* 1998; Oct 5(4):209–227.

Fruhstorfer H, Lindblom U, Schmidt WG. Method for quantitative estimation of thermal thresholds in patients. *J Neurol Neurosurg Psychiatry* 1976; 39:1071–1075.

Garcin R. La douleur dans les affections organiques du système nerveux central [Pain in organic diseases of the central nervous system]. *Rev Neurol* 1937; 68:105–153.

Hansson P, Lindblom U. Hyperalgesia assessed with quantitative sensory testing in patients with neurogenic pain. In: Willis WD (Eds). *Hyperalgesia and Allodynia.* New York: Raven Press, 1992, pp 335–343.

Head H, Holmes G. Sensory disturbances from cerebral lesions. *Brain* 1911; 34:102–254.

Leijon G, Boivie J, Johansson I. Central post-stroke pain—neurological symptoms and pain characteristics. *Pain* 1989; 36:13–25.

Milhorat TH, Kotzen RM, MU HTM, Capocelli AL, Milhorat RH. Dysesthetic pain in patients with syringomyelia. *Neurosurgery* 1996, 38:940–947.

Pagni CA. Central pain due to spinal cord and brain stem damage. In: Wall PD, Melzack R (Eds). *Textbook of Pain*. Edinburgh: Churchill Livingstone, 1989, pp 636–655.

Riddoch G. The clinical features of central pain. *Lancet* 1938; 234:1093–1098, 1150–1156, 1205–1209.

Vestergaard K, Nielsen J, Andersen G, et al. Sensory abnormalities in consecutive, unselected patients with central post-stroke pain. *Pain* 1995; 61:177–186.

White JC, Sweet WH. *Pain and the Neurosurgeon: A Forty-Year Experience*. Springfield, IL: Charles C. Thomas, 1969, p 93.

Yezierski RP. Pain following spinal cord injury: the clinical problem and experimental studies. *Pain* 1996; 68:185–194.

Correspondence to: Didier Bouhassira, MD, PhD, INSERM, U-161, 2, rue d'Alésia, 75014 Paris, France. Tel: 33-1-40789350; Fax: 33-1-45881304; email: bouhassira@broca.inserm.fr.

Proceedings of the 9th World Congress on Pain,
Progress in Pain Research and Management,
Vol. 16, edited by M. Devor, M.C. Rowbotham, and
Z. Wiesenfeld-Hallin, IASP Press, Seattle, © 2000.

40

The Ventromedial Thalamus: A Link for Noxious Cutaneous Inputs from the Whole Body Surface

Lénaïc Monconduit, Laurence Bourgeais, Jean-François Bernard, Daniel Le Bars, and Luis Villanueva

INSERM U-161, Paris, France

The spino-reticulo-thalamic system plays a significant role in pain processing because in addition to the direct transfer of nociceptive information to the diencephalon by spinal pathways, pain information relays also occur within the medullary reticular formation (Mehler et al. 1960, Bowsher 1976). In contrast to other rostral brainstem nociceptive reticular neurons, neurons in the rat's medullary subnucleus reticularis dorsalis (SRD) respond selectively to the activation of peripheral Aδ and C fibers from any part of the body and encode the intensity of noxious cutaneous and visceral stimuli (Villanueva et al. 1996). Anatomical studies have shown that the SRD projects densely to the lateral half of the ventromedial thalamus (VM*l*; Villanueva et al. 1998). VM*l* projections are distributed as a compact band in layer I of the rostral-most part of the whole dorsolateral frontal cortex. This projection most notably includes the premotor and motor cortices, and to a lesser extent the somatosensory cortex (Herkenham 1986; Arbuthnott et al. 1990; Desbois and Villanueva 1998).

Our study investigated the somatosensory properties of VM neurons. We systematically recorded all the neurons in the VM and surrounding regions that responded to calibrated cutaneous stimuli. In an additional series of experiments, we investigated whether nociceptive responses in the VM*l* were relayed at the medullary level. Finally, we tested whether VM*l* neurons could be driven antidromically from the cortex.

METHODS

All the animal experiments were approved by our local animal care committee, and adhered to the guidelines of the IASP. Unitary extracellular recordings were made in 147 rats anesthetized with halothane (0.5–0.7%) in a mixture of 2/3 nitrous oxide to 1/3 oxygen, paralyzed with gallamine triethiodide, and artificially ventilated. Electrodes were inserted between 1–2 mm lateral to midline and 2.8–3.8 mm posterior to the bregma (Paxinos and Watson 1997). Neurons were characterized according to their responses to innocuous and noxious cutaneous electrical, thermal, and mechanical stimuli. In some experiments, poststimulus histograms of VM*l* responses elicited by repetitive suprathreshold percutaneous electrical stimulation of the limbs were built from 30 trials before, during, and 30–40 minutes following a microinjection of the NMDA antagonist MK-801 (20 mM; 0.2 μL) within the medullary SRD. Some neurons were identified by antidromic activation following stimulation of layer I of the dorsolateral frontal cortex by a pair of aligned electrodes, inserted 4–5 mm rostral to the bregma and 2–3 mm lateral to the midline.

RESULTS

A total of 135 units responding to cutaneous stimulation were recorded in an area 3.1–3.8 mm caudal to the bregma and 1.4–2 mm lateral to the midline. This region corresponds to the VM*l* thalamic nucleus. All these neurons were excited from the skin but did not respond to any innocuous stimuli, noxious cold, or to proprioceptive stimuli (joint movements). By contrast, all the VM*l* neurons responded to noxious natural stimuli (thermal or mechanical) when applied to cutaneous tissues anywhere on the body.

All the VM*l* cells were excited by percutaneous electrical stimuli no matter which part of the body was stimulated. As shown in single sweep recordings from an individual cell in Fig. 1A, the application of suprathreshold percutaneous electrical stimuli to the limbs elicited two peaks of activation at different, but fixed, latencies for all VM*l* neurons studied. The mean differences in latency from the base and tip of the tail for the earlier and late peaks were 8.7 ± 0.6 ms and 129 ± 14.7 ms, respectively, which correspond to a peripheral conduction velocity of 12.9 ± 0.9 m/s and 1.0 ± 0.2 m/s. As shown in Fig. 1B, the VM*l* neurons had clear monotonic stimulus-response relationships following thermal or mechanical stimulation. A direct relationship can be seen between the intensity of mechanical stimuli in the 4–32 N/cm^2 range and the number of action potentials evoked. When

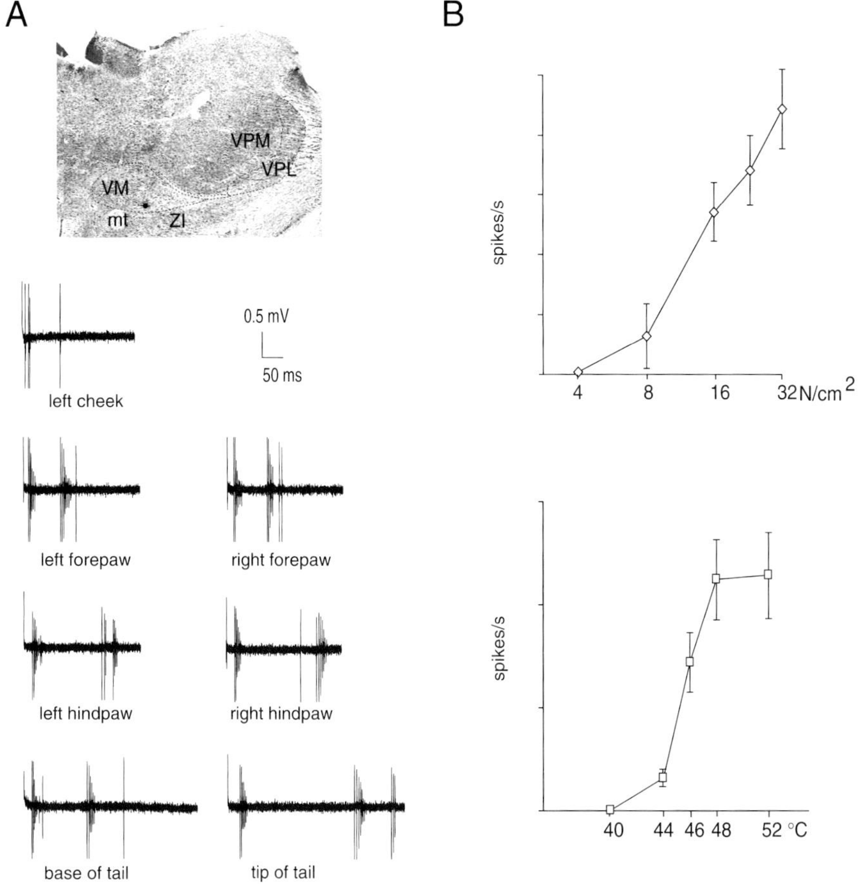

Fig. 1. (A) Single-sweep recordings showing Aδ- and C-fiber-evoked responses of a lateral ventromedial thalamus (VM) neuron (black dot) following supramaximal percutaneous electrical stimulation (2-ms square-wave pulses) of different parts of the body. VPL = ventroposterolateral thalamic nucleus; VPM = ventroposteromedial thalamic nucleus; mt = mamillothalamic track; ZI = zona incerta. (B) Cumulative results showing the magnitudes of the responses of VM*l* neurons to graded mechanical (n = 7) or thermal (n = 16) stimulation of the ipsilateral hindpaw. Adapted from Monconduit et al. (1999).

graded thermal stimuli were applied, the VM*l* discharges increased monotonically within the range of 44°–48°C; beyond this, a plateau was observed. Since these neurons are confined to a region receiving afferents from the contralateral SRD (Villanueva et al. 1998), we examined whether inactivation of this medullary structure could modify the responses of VM*l* neurons. Aδ- and C-fiber responses were strongly depressed following microinjec-

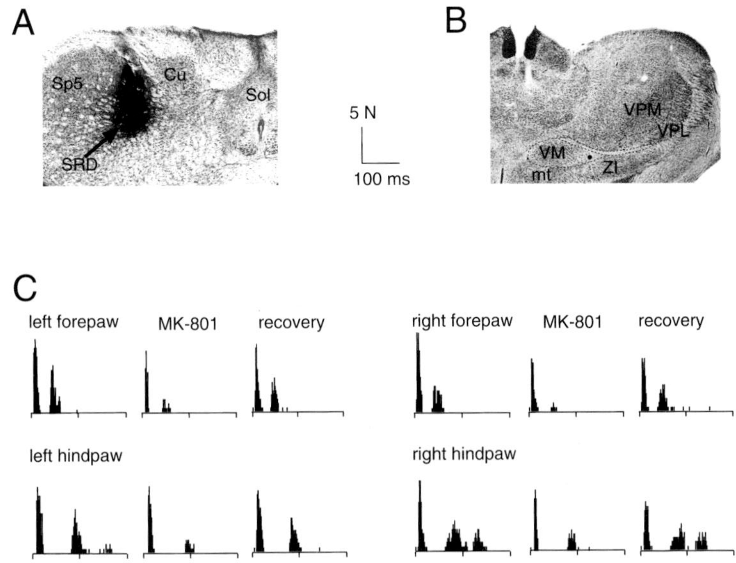

Fig. 2. Example of the effects of a microinjection of MK-801 (20 mM; 0.2 μL) into the left subnucleus reticularis dorsalis (SRD) (A), on the responses of a neuron recorded in the right VM*l* (B) to supramaximal percutaneous electrical stimulation of the four limbs (C). (A) Sp5 = trigeminal nucleus caudalis; Cu = cuneate nucleus; Sol = nucleus of the solitary tract; (B) abbreviations as in Fig. 1A. Adapted from Monconduit et al. (1999).

tions of the NMDA antagonist, MK-801, into the SRD (Fig. 2). The maximum effect was obtained with a volume of 0.2 μL. Injections of MK-801 into adjacent structures did not modify VM*l* responses.

As shown in the individual example in Fig. 3A, the application of repetitive electrical stimuli to layer I of the frontal cortex produced an antidromic response with a constant latency in the VM*l*. In all 16 nociceptive units in the VM*l* that we studied in this way, the antidromic spikes followed high-frequency stimulation (200–400 Hz; Fig. 3B) and showed collision within the $2t + r$ period (Fig. 3C).

DISCUSSION

This study reveals a population of neurons within the VM*l* thalamic nucleus that selectively conveys and encodes cutaneous nociceptive information from the whole body toward layer I of the anterior cortex. The calculation of the differences in the latencies of responses elicited from the tip and base of the tail revealed that VM*l* neurons were exclusively driven by

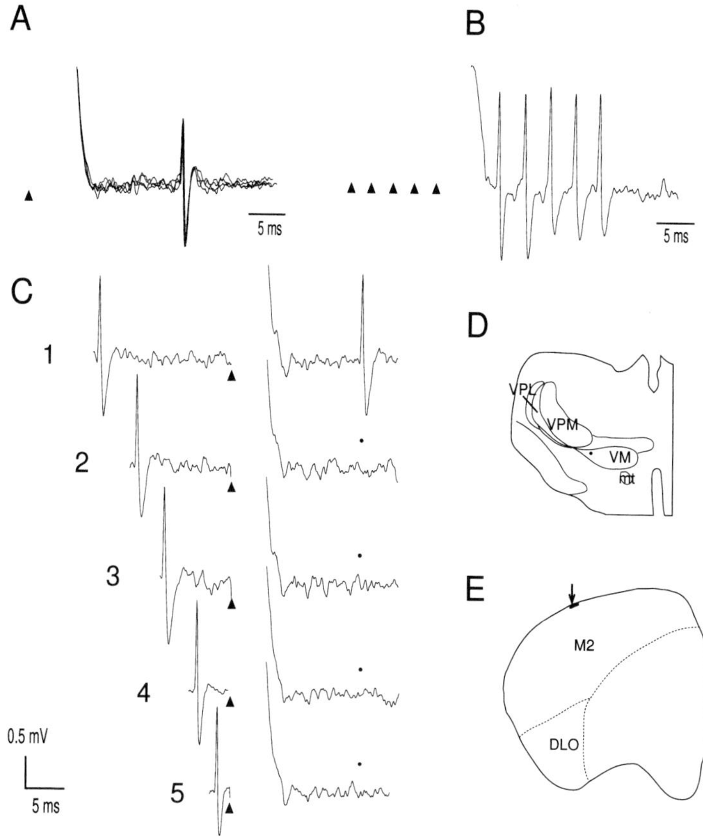

Fig. 3. Antidromic activation of a VM*l* neuron from the cortex. (A) Antidromic spikes. Note the overlapping of four antidromic spikes, indicating the stability of the latency of this response. (B) High-frequency stimulation (5 pulses, 333 Hz; timings indicated by triangles). (C) Collision test. The antidromic spike collided systematically with an orthodromic spike (spontaneous or evoked by peripheral stimulation) at an interval of less than $2t + r$, where t = the antidromic latency and r = refractory period. Filled circles show the expected timing of the antidromic spike if collision had not occurred. Triangles indicate the timing of the stimuli. (D) Location of the recording site in the VM*l* at bregma –3.6. (E) Location of the antidromic stimulation site in layer I of the dorsolateral anterior cortex, at bregma 4.2. DLO = dorsolateral orbital cortex. Adapted from Monconduit et al. (1999).

activities in Aδ and C fibers. In addition, our data suggest that Aδ- and C-fiber cutaneous polymodal nociceptors have a prominent role in activating VM*l* neurons in that they share several common features: (1) a monotonic increase in their responses to graded electrical and natural stimuli; (2) a linear relationship between the evoked firing rate and the intensities of both thermal and mechanical stimuli within noxious ranges, and (3) in some cases, the development of residual activity or after-discharges following strong noxious stimulation.

Several reasons lead us to believe that nociceptive activity in the VM*l* arises primarily from monosynaptic inputs from the contralateral medullary SRD. Indeed, a strong reduction in VM*l* responses was obtained only when MK-801 injections were confined to the dorsal half of the contralateral SRD; injections into adjacent areas were without effect. Interestingly, this medullary region, the SRD, is a principal target for afferents from the deep dorsal horn (Almeida et al. 1995; Raboisson et al. 1996), contains most of the SRD neurons with heterosegmental nociceptive convergence (Villanueva et al. 1988), and projects densely to the contralateral VM*l* (Villanueva et al. 1998).

CONCLUSIONS

Our findings suggest that VM*l* neurons relay widespread nociceptive inputs from the medullary reticular formation to the whole of layer I of the dorsolateral neocortex. In all mammals including humans, the pyramidal cell—the main output neuron in the neocortex—invariably has its apical dendrites oriented to the pial surface and contacts layer I (Cajal 1972; Marín-Padilla 1998). Our findings could provide an anatomical and functional basis for any signal of cutaneous pain to alter cortical activity in a universal way, namely by contacting the distal ends of apical dendrites of pyramidal cells in layer I.

Thus, the VM*l* may constitute an important thalamic branch of what was originally termed the "ascending reticular activating system" (Morison and Dempsey 1942; Moruzzi 1949; Jasper 1961). This hypothesis is also consistent with the fact that stimulation of VM neurons in the cat causes depolarization of cortical layer I cells and elicits recruiting responses in the anterior cortex (Glenn et al. 1982). This reticulo-thalamo-cortical network may allow any signal of pain to gain access to widespread areas of the neocortex and thus help prime the cortex for attentional reactions or the coordination of motor responses.

ACKNOWLEDGMENTS

The authors are grateful to Ms. J. Martin, Ms. F. Roudier, and Mr. R. Rambur for technical support. This work was supported by l'INSERM and l'Institut UPSA de la Douleur.

REFERENCES

Almeida A, Tavares I, Lima D. Projection sites of superficial or deep dorsal horn in the dorsal reticular nucleus. *Neuroreport* 1995; 6:1245–1248.

Arbuthnott GW, MacLeod NK, Maxwell DJ, Wright AK. Distribution and synaptic contacts of the cortical terminals arising from neurons in the rat ventromedial thalamic nucleus. *Neuroscience* 1990; 38:47–60.

Bowsher D. Role of the reticular formation in responses to noxious stimulation. *Pain* 1976; 2:361–378.

Cajal SR. *Histologie du Système Nerveux de l'Homme et des Vertébrés* [Histology of the Nervous System of Man and the Vertebrates], Vols. I, II. Madrid: Instituto Ramón Cajal. [Reprinted from the original 1911 edition.] Paris: Maloine, 1972.

Desbois C, Villanueva L. Cortical projections from the ventromedial thalamic nucleus in rats: a study of the reticulo-thalamo-cortical nociceptive system. *Forum Eur Neurosci Abstr* 1998; 22:155.

Glenn LL, Hada J, Roy JP, Deschênes M, Steriade M. Anterograde tracer and field potential analysis of the neocortical layer I projection from nucleus ventralis medialis of the thalamus in cat. *Neuroscience* 1982; 7:1861–1877.

Herkenham M. New perspectives on the organization and evolution of nonspecific thalamocortical projections. In: Jones EG, Peters A (Eds). *Cerebral Cortex, Sensory-Motor Areas and Aspects of Cortical Connectivity*, Vol. 5. New York: Plenum, 1986, pp 403–445.

Jasper HH. Thalamic reticular system. In: Sheer DE (Ed). *Electrical Stimulation of the Brain.* Austin: University of Texas, 1961, pp 277–287.

Marín-Padilla M. Cajal-Retzius cells and the development of the neocortex. *Trends Neurosci* 1998; 21:64–71.

Mehler WR, Feferman ME, Nauta WJH. Ascending axon degeneration following antero-lateral cordotomy, an experimental study in the monkey. *Brain* 1960; 83:718–751.

Monconduit L, Bourgeais L, Bernard JF, Le Bars D, Villanueva L. Ventromedial thalamic neurons convey nociceptive signals from the whole body surface to the dorsolateral neocortex. *J Neurosci* 1999; 19:9063–9072.

Morison RS, Dempsey EW. A study of thalamo-cortical relations. *Am J Physiol* 1942; 135:281–292.

Moruzzi G, Magoun HW. Brain stem reticular formation and activation of the EEG. *Electroencephalogr Clin Neurophysiol* 1949; 1:445–473.

Paxinos G, Watson C (Ed). *The Rat Brain in Stereotaxic Coordinates*, 3rd ed. New York: Academic, 1997.

Raboisson P, Dallel R, Bernard JF, Le Bars D, Villanueva L. Organization of efferent projections from the spinal cervical enlargement to the medullary subnucleus reticularis dorsalis and the adjacent cuneate nucleus: a PHA-L study in the rat. *J Comp Neurol* 1996; 367:503–517.

Villanueva L, Bouhassira D, Bing Z, Le Bars D. Convergence of heterotopic nociceptive information onto subnucleus reticularis dorsalis neurons in the rat medulla. *J Neurophysiol* 1988; 60:980–1009.

Villanueva L, Bouhassira D, Le Bars D. The medullary subnucleus reticularis dorsalis (SRD) as a key link in both the transmission and modulation of pain signals. *Pain* 1996; 67:231–240.

Villanueva L, Desbois C, Le Bars D, Bernard JF. Organization of diencephalic projections from the medullary subnucleus reticularis dorsalis and the adjacent cuneate nucleus: a retrograde and anterograde tracer study in the rat. *J Comp Neurol* 1998; 390:133–160.

Correspondence to: Luis Villanueva, DDS, PhD, INSERM U-161, 2 rue d'Alésia, 75014 Paris, France. Tel: 33-1-4078-9387; Fax: 33-1-4588-1304; email: luisvil@broca.inserm.fr.

Proceedings of the 9th World Congress on Pain,
Progress in Pain Research and Management,
Vol. 16, edited by M. Devor, M.C. Rowbotham, and
Z. Wiesenfeld-Hallin, IASP Press, Seattle, © 2000.

41

Thalamic Stimulation-Evoked Pain and Temperature Sites in Pain and Non-Pain Patients

Jonathan O. Dostrovsky,[a,c] Marosh Manduch,[a] Karen D. Davis,[b,c] Ron R. Tasker,[b] and Andres M. Lozano[b,c]

Departments of [a]Physiology and [b]Surgery, University of Toronto, and [c]Toronto Western Research Institute, Toronto, Ontario, Canada

The ventrocaudal nucleus of the thalamus (Vc) is the major relay site for innocuous cutaneous mechanoreceptor signals on their way from the periphery to cortex. The thalamic regions involved in processing nociceptive and thermoreceptive information are still not firmly established, but the Vc may be an important relay site for these modalities (Willis 1985, 1997). In addition, several other thalamic regions, in particular the region posterior and inferior to the Vc that contains the ventroposterior inferior nucleus (VPI) and posterior ventromedial nucleus (VMpo), have also been implicated (Apkarian and Shi 1994; Craig et al. 1994; Craig and Dostrovsky 1999; Davis et al. 1999). Our study sought to gain further insights into the regions involved in the thalamic processing of pain and temperature and whether changes occur in chronic pain patients. Toward this goal we analyzed thalamic microstimulation-evoked pain and temperature sites in pain and non-pain patients undergoing functional stereotactic surgery.

METHODS

We obtained data from 537 electrode trajectories passing through the thalamus in 49 movement disorder (motor group) and 37 chronic pain patients undergoing stereotactic thalamotomy or chronic-stimulation electrode implantation for treatment of tremor or chronic pain. The chronic pain patient group was divided into nonstroke pain (NSP, n = 26) and poststroke pain (PSP, $n = 11$) patients according to their diagnoses. All patients consented to the procedures, which were approved by the Human Experimentation Committee of the University of Toronto.

The methods employed have been described previously (Lenz et al. 1988; Davis et al. 1996) and are mentioned only briefly here. The coordinates of the initial microelectrode track were determined from a stereotactic atlas of the human thalamus in conjunction with the locations of the anterior and posterior commissures (AC, PC) obtained from computer tomography (CT) or magnetic resonance imaging (MRI) scans. The initial target site was usually located within the Vc, 14 or 15 mm lateral to the midline. Subsequent electrode trajectories were chosen according to the physiological findings for each patient and the specific objectives of the surgical procedure.

We used tungsten microelectrodes for neuronal recording and stimulation. We determined the receptive fields of the neurons from responses to various voluntary and passive movements, tapping or lightly brushing the skin, or applying deep pressure. Electrical stimuli (1-second trains of 0.2-ms, 300-Hz pulses) were delivered through the recording microelectrode at 0.5–1-mm intervals along the electrode trajectory. After each stimulus, the patient was asked to describe the quality of any perceived sensations and comment as to whether it was painful or not. We noted the threshold and location of the evoked sensation on the patient's body. The location of the Vc nucleus was inferred from the portion of the electrode trajectory where cells responded to cutaneous mechanical stimulation and where microstimulation at low currents (typically 5–20 μA) elicited paresthesia in the region of the neuronal receptive fields. The pain and temperature sensations evoked at sites located inferior or posterior to the Vc were deemed to lie in the posteroinferior region.

The sites where stimulation evoked pain or thermal sensations were localized with respect to the Vc and reconstructed on computer-generated sagittal maps. We measured the anterior-posterior and superior-inferior coordinates of each pain and thermal site with respect to PC and the AC–PC line, respectively. To normalize the coordinates for interpatient differences in brain size, we multiplied them by a normalization factor (patient's AC–PC length/standard AC–PC length of 23 mm). We then plotted the pain and temperature sites on a sagittal plane, where a line drawn parallel to the AC–PC line and traversing through the site of the most ventral tactile response represented the ventral Vc border. A line perpendicular to the AC–PC line and passing through the site of the most posterior tactile response in the Vc depicted the posterior Vc. If no tactile-responsive neurons were present on that electrode trajectory, the sites were plotted in relation to Vc borders determined from the nearest adjacent sagittal plane containing a trajectory passing through the Vc. The pain/temperature sites were also plotted in a coronal plane in which the stereotactic medial-lateral coordinates of each trajectory were adjusted according to the functional somatotopy of the Vc. Statistical analysis of incidence used the χ-square test.

RESULTS

Pain or temperature (warm or cold) sensations were evoked at 6.6% of the 5842 sites stimulated. Some of these sites were located in the Vc (7.8%), but most (84%) were in the posteroinferior region. Analysis of the data according to patient group and region revealed a marked increase in incidence of sites in the Vc where stimulation evoked pain in the PSP group compared with the other two groups ($P < 0.0001$) (Fig. 1a). In contrast, the incidence of stimulation-evoked innocuous thermal sensations in the Vc did not differ significantly ($P > 0.05$) among the three patient groups.

In the posteroinferior region a large increase in the incidence of stimulation-evoked pain sites also occurred in PSP patients compared with the other two groups ($P < 0.001$) (Fig. 1b). However, in contrast to the Vc, the posteroinferior region had a significantly lower incidence of temperature sensations in PSP than in NSP patients ($P < 0.001$) or movement disorder patients ($P < 0.001$).

The locations of sites where pain, warm, and cold sensations were evoked in all three groups were reconstructed in the sagittal and coronal planes. Fig. 2 provides an example of the distribution of these sites in the sagittal plane in the motor group. The vertical and horizontal axes represent the posterior and inferior borders of the Vc, respectively. The locations of sites where stimulation evoked painful or thermal sensations were collapsed across all lateralities onto a single sagittal plane. In general, the distribution of sites for each modality was comparable, although cold sites were almost exclusively located posterior to the Vc. Most sites were concentrated in the region 1–3 mm inferior and posterior to the inferior and posterior border of the Vc.

Analysis of sites in the mediolateral axis revealed that most of the pain sites located within the Vc extended about 2 mm medial or lateral to the face/hand border. In contrast, most of the warm sites were located in the medial-inferior quadrant ($P < 0.0001$). We observed the same trend for the cold sites, although it failed to reach statistical significance ($P = 0.06$, Fisher exact probabilities test).

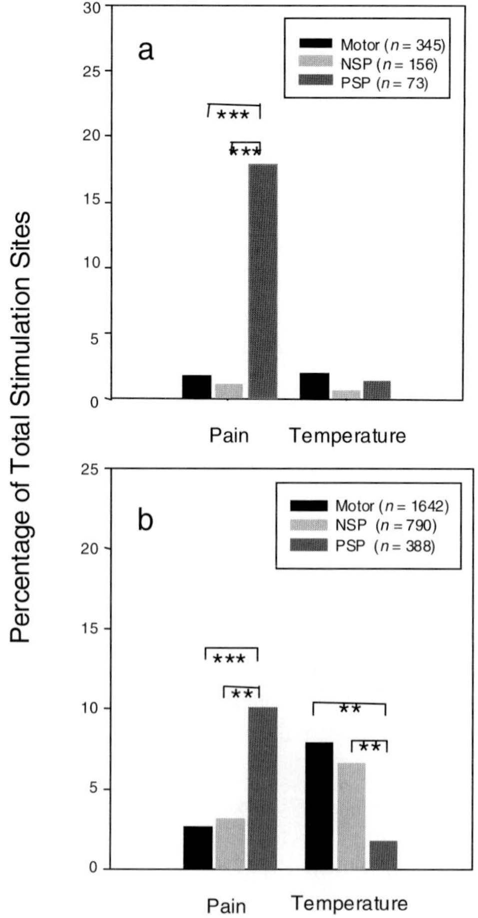

Fig. 1. Bar graphs showing the incidence of sites in (a) the ventrocaudal nucleus (Vc) and (b) the posteroinferior region where stimulation evoked sensations of pain or innocuous temperature in each of the three patient groups. Motor = movement disorder group; NSP = nonstroke pain group; PSP = poststroke pain group.

DISCUSSION

The two major findings of this study were that (1) most thalamic sites where microstimulation can evoke sensations of pain or temperature were located posterior and/or inferior to the Vc, and (2) poststroke pain patients had a marked increase in incidence of pain sites, especially in the Vc, and a decrease in temperature sites.

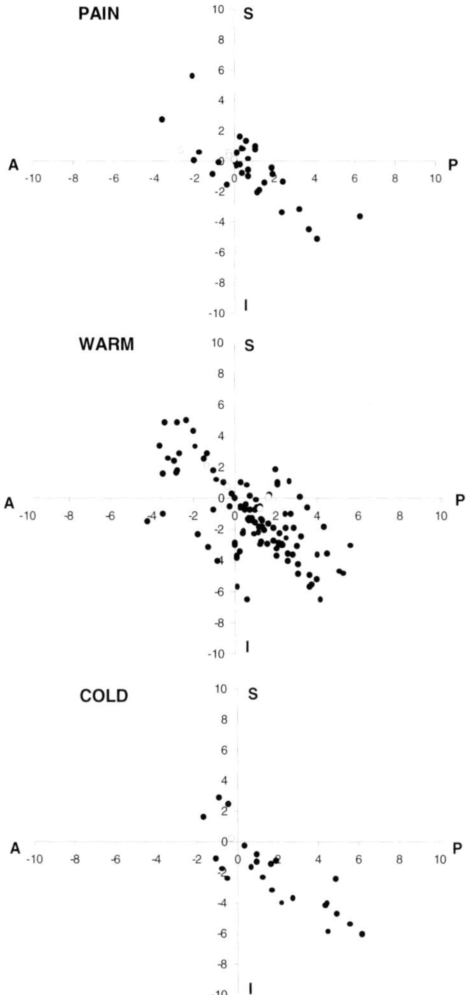

Fig. 2. Scatter plots in the sagittal plane showing the locations of the stimulation sites evoking pain, warm, or cold sensations in the motor group of patients. Open circles represent sites within the Vc. The x-axis is parallel to the AC–PC line; $x = 0$ represents the posterior border of Vc and $y = 0$ represents the ventral border of Vc. A = anterior; I = inferior; P = posterior; S = superior. Scale is in millimeters.

Several previous studies have reported that stimulation in the thalamus can evoke pain sensations. The first such report, by Hassler (1970), concluded with little supporting evidence that pain was evoked by stimulation in the parvocellular portion of the Vc (Vcpc), which lies directly inferior to the Vc. Short reports by Halliday and Logue (1972) and Dostrovsky et al.

(1992) subsequently supported this proposal. More recently, Lenz and colleagues (1993) published a detailed study showing that pain and temperature sensations could be evoked by stimulation in the posteroinferior region and to a lesser extent in the Vc. Our present study extends these findings by performing a more extensive analysis and attempting to improve on the localization by correcting the stimulation site locations, based on physiological findings, both in the inferior-superior as well as anterior-posterior axes.

Both our study and previous studies have shown that the major thalamic region from where pain and temperature sensations can be evoked is the posteroinferior region. However, in the absence of histological confirmation of stimulation sites and given the problem of activation of axons of passage, it is difficult to conclude with certainty which nuclei are involved in mediating these sensations. Some are probably due to activation of neurons in the VMpo nucleus. The VMpo in the monkey contains a high concentration of nociceptive and thermospecific neurons and is a major target of spinothalamic tract neurons originating in lamina I of the spinal and medullary dorsal horns (Craig et al. 1994). Our recent demonstration of cooling-specific neurons in this region and of the elicitation of cold sensations after microstimulation at such sites provides strong support for an involvement of VMpo in mediating the sensation of cold (Davis et al. 1999). Nevertheless, many of our stimulation sites were clearly lateral to the location of VMpo and thus must have activated neurons in the VPI or axons of spinothalamic tract neurons terminating in the VPI and/or Vc, or possibly also axons of VMpo neurons ascending to the cortex.

The marked increase in incidence of stimulation-evoked pain in the Vc of PSP patients compared with the other two groups confirms the findings of Davis et al. (1996) and extends them by also showing an increase in the posteroinferior region. Of interest was the finding of a marked reduction in temperature sites. This reduction might be due to damage to the temperature pathway, as it is well documented that PSP patients frequently have deficits in temperature perception. Alternatively, as suggested by Lenz et al. (1998) based on their somewhat similar findings, perhaps the activity of innocuous thermoreceptive neurons gives rise to painful sensations in these patients. The findings of increased incidence of pain sites in the Vc suggests that in PSP patients, perhaps due to loss of inhibition and/or sensitization, normally subthreshold activation of nociceptive neurons or excitation of innocuous tactile neurons can give rise to painful sensations. Our findings thus suggest that alterations in the thalamocortical processing of these signals may be involved in mediating central pain.

ACKNOWLEDGMENTS

The authors thank Helen Belina for help with the figures. Supported by NIH NS36824.

REFERENCES

Apkarian AV, Shi T. Squirrel monkey lateral thalamus. I. Somatic nociresponsive neurons and their relation to spinothalamic terminals. *J Neurosci* 1994; 14:6779–6795.

Craig AD, Bushnell MC, Zhang E-T, Blomqvist AA. Thalamic nucleus specific for pain and temperature sensation. *Nature* 1994; 372:770–773.

Craig AD, Dostrovsky JO. Medulla to Thalamus. In: Wall PD, Melzack R (Eds). *Textbook of Pain.* Edinburgh: Churchill-Livingstone, 1999, pp 183–214.

Davis KD, Kiss ZHT, Tasker RR, Dostrovsky JO. Thalamic stimulation-evoked sensations in chronic pain patients and in nonpain (movement disorder) patients. *J Neurophysiol* 1996; 75:1026–1037.

Davis KD, Lozano RM, Manduch M, et al. Thalamic relay site for cold perception in humans. *J Neurophysiol* 1999; 81:1970–1973.

Dostrovsky JO, Wells FEB, Tasker RR. Pain sensations evoked by stimulation in human thalamus. In: Inoki R, Shigenaga Y, Tohyama M (Eds). *Processing and Inhibition of Nociceptive Information,* International Congress Series 989. Amsterdam: Excerpta Medica, Elsevier Science, 1992, pp 115–120.

Halliday AM, Logue V. Painful sensations evoked by electrical stimulation in the thalamus. In: Somjen GG (Ed). *Neurophysiology Studied in Man.* Amsterdam: Excerpta Medica, 1972, pp 221–230.

Hassler R. Dichotomy of facial pain conduction in the diencephalon. In: Hassler R, Walker AE (Eds). *Trigeminal Neuralgia.* Philadelphia: Saunders, 1970, pp 123–138.

Lenz FA, Dostrovsky JO, Kwan HC, et al. Methods for microstimulation and recording of single neurons and evoked potentials in the human central nervous system. *J Neurosurg* 1988; 68:630–634.

Lenz FA, Seike M, Richardson RT, et al. Thermal and pain sensations evoked by microstimulation in the area of human ventrocaudal nucleus. *J Neurophysiol* 1993; 70:200–212.

Lenz FA, Gracely RH, Baker FH, Richardson RT, Dougherty PM. Reorganization of sensory modalities evoked by microstimulation in region of the thalamic principal sensory nucleus in patients with pain due to nervous system injury. *J Comp Neurol* 1998; 399:125–138.

Willis WD Jr. The Pain System. The neural basis of nociceptive transmission in the mammalian nervous system. In: Gildenberg PL (Ed). *Pain and Headache.* Basel: S. Karger, 1985, pp 1–346.

Willis WD. Nociceptive functions of thalamic neurons. In: Steriade M, Jones EG, McCormick DA (Eds). *Thalamus, Vol. II, Experimental and Clinical Aspects.* Amsterdam: Elsevier, 1997, pp 373–424.

Correspondence to: Jonathan O. Dostrovsky, PhD, Dept. of Physiology, Medical Sciences Building, Room 3305, 1 King's College Circle, University of Toronto, Toronto, Ontario, Canada M5S 1A8. Tel: 416-978-5289; Fax: 416-978-4940; email: j.dostrovsky@utoronto.ca.

Proceedings of the 9th World Congress on Pain,
Progress in Pain Research and Management,
Vol. 16, edited by M. Devor, M.C. Rowbotham, and
Z. Wiesenfeld-Hallin, IASP Press, Seattle, © 2000.

42

Plasticity of the Inhibitory Circuitry of the Primate Ventrobasal Thalamus following Lesions of Somatosensory Pathways

Diane D. Ralston,[a] Patrick M. Dougherty,[b]
Fred A. Lenz,[b] Han-Rong Weng,[b] Charles J. Vierck,[c]
and Henry J. Ralston[a]

[a]Department of Anatomy, University of California, San Francisco, California, USA; [b]Department of Neurosurgery, Johns Hopkins University School of Medicine, Baltimore, Maryland, USA; [c]Department of Neuroscience, University of Florida, Gainesville, Florida, USA

Spinal cord injury is a frequent cause of chronic pain that is characterized by dysesthesias and a decrease in pain and temperature sensations mediated by pathways in the anterolateral quadrant. The patient may describe a painful limb as being numb, despite allodynia and hyperalgesia in the same extremity (Boivie et al. 1989). In thalamic recordings from humans with chronic pain following peripheral or central neural injury, Lenz and his colleagues have found an enlarged region in the ventrobasal complex (VB) from which microstimulation can elicit a report of burning pain (Lenz et al. 1998b) and heightened burst activity of thalamic neurons following innocuous stimulation of the painful body part. These investigators have postulated that such findings in humans may result from reduced GABA-mediated inhibition of thalamic neurons (Lenz et al. 1998a). These and other studies have led to the hypothesis that central pain following damage to one or more of the somatosensory systems of the central nervous system (CNS) is due to reduced GABAergic inhibition at thalamic and cortical levels (Canavero and Bonicalzi 1998). We have focused our attention on the GABA immunoreactive (GABA-ir) interactions as we have previously shown that this inhibitory circuitry decreases following medial lemniscal lesions (Ralston et al. 1996).

About 50% of neurons of monkey somatosensory thalamus (VB) respond to peripheral noxious stimuli, and most are located in the caudal, ventral region of VB to which project noxious-specific neurons of lamina I of the dorsal horn. It is precisely this area in which noxious-responding thalamic neurons in humans are found (Lenz et al. 1998b). We examined the VB in three animals with chronic (>1 year) lesions of one dorsal spinal quadrant and the contralateral anterolateral quadrant at midthoracic levels. These lesions resulted in the deafferentation of the hindlimb representation within one VB. The macaques subsequently were examined for their ability to detect electrical stimulation of either lateral calf. We performed terminal physiological and anatomical experiments to examine the functional properties of the VB neurons and the circuitry of the thalamus that serves these functions.

METHODS

Three adult macaque monkeys (*M. arctoides*) had lesions of one dorsal and dorsolateral column and the contralateral spinothalamic tract at spinal segments T9–T11 in separate surgical procedures spaced months apart and conducted under general anesthesia. The animals were tested for the next 47–50 weeks following the second surgical procedure. The animals were trained to detect and crudely localize electrical stimulation of each leg. The detection task provided food reinforcement if the animal pulled one of two levers within 2 seconds after onset of electrical stimulation. The stimulus consisted of a maximum of four 10-ms constant current pulses at 2 Hz. Stimulus intensity varied between sessions and ranged from 0.1 to 15 mA. The correct lever was located on the side stimulated.

Following behavioral analyses the animals entered the acute anatomical and neurophysiological studies. Two days before terminal physiological recording, the animals were anesthetized and 5% wheat germ lectin conjugated to horseradish peroxidase (WGA-HRP) was injected bilaterally into nucleus gracilis. For physiological recordings, the monkeys were anesthetized with sodium pentobarbital (35.0 mg/kg, i.v.) and then maintained by constant infusion (5 $mg \cdot kg^{-1} \cdot h^{-1}$). We used stereotaxic methods to record from neurons in the VB. We defined the receptive field of each neuron and plotted the area on a standard surface map of the monkey. A series of graded mechanical stimuli ranging from innocuous to noxious were applied to the upper and lower extremities of the deafferented and normal sides, and the responses were recorded and analyzed. The bottom of the last tract was marked by a direct-current lesion. The monkey was euthanized by pentobarbital overdose and perfused intracardially with heparinized phosphate-buffered saline (PBS) followed by mixed aldehydes (2% paraformaldehyde, 2% glutaraldehyde). The brain and spinal cord were removed and post-fixed in mixed aldehydes overnight and then transferred to cold PBS. Spinal cord, brainstem, and thalamic specimens were subsequently serially sectioned in the coronal plane on a vibratome at 50 μm and processed for light and electron microscopic histochemistry.

For the anatomical studies, we tested sections of VB for the presence of HRP reaction product. VB regions showing HRP labeling following injections of the tracer into nucleus gracilis were embedded and thin-sectioned for study by electron microscopy (EM). We stained thin sections with an immunogold-labeled antibody to GABA and counted the numbers of GABA-immunoreactive (GABA-ir) profiles in the deafferented and normal VB of each animal.

For the physiological studies, we constructed accumulated frequency histograms (100-ms bins) and counted numbers of action potentials (spikes) in evoked responses and across 30 seconds of spontaneous activity. Neurons were classified based on response to mechanical stimuli and by location of cutaneous receptive field. Four classes of neurons were defined based on responses to mechanical stimuli. Low-threshold (LT) neurons were defined as those responding strongly to brush but with only weak responses (10% or less of brush response) to the compressive stimuli (Dougherty et al. 1997). Multireceptive (MR) neurons were defined as those responding to both innocuous and noxious stimuli, but not increasing discharge with graded stimulation intensity. Wide-dynamic-range (WDR) neurons were defined as those responding to innocuous and noxious stimuli and also showing a significant increase of responses with increasing stimulation intensity. Nociceptive-specific (NS) neurons, those defined as responding only to noxious stimuli, were not encountered in this sample. Neurons were further grouped based on location of cutaneous receptive field. Thalamic neurons with receptive fields on the forelimb or forepaw were considered as a baseline group outside the area affected by the lesion, while those with receptive fields on the hindlimb or hindpaw were considered as within the area of thalamus affected by the lesion.

Comparisons between groups of cells were initiated by calculating the total number of spikes (less background) evoked by each stimulus. These responses were combined for various groups and differences determined by analysis of variance with post hoc adjusted comparisons (Neuman-Keuls procedure). We use the Fisher exact probabilities test to compare receptive field sizes among groups.

RESULTS

Behavioral studies. Preoperatively, each animal could detect single pulses of electrocutaneous stimulation on either lateral calf at intensities of less than 1 mA. Postoperatively, detection thresholds were unchanged for stimulation contralateral to the dorsal quadrant lesion but were elevated for each animal for stimulation ipsilateral to the dorsal quadrant lesion (and contralateral to the anterolateral spinal lesion). However, stimulus intensities that activate nociceptors were reliably detected for stimulation of either leg. At stimulus intensities ranging from 7 to 15 mA, the average percentage of correct detections was 95.9% for stimulation of the leg with input to intact lemniscal and spinothalamic pathways and 81.4% for stimulation of the leg with input to interrupted lemniscal and spinothalamic pathways. All animals correctly localized the side of postoperative stimulation by responding to a lever located on the side of stimulation. Therefore, spinal pathways outside the distribution of the classical lemniscal and spinothalamic pathways can support detection and crude localization of cutaneous stimulation, despite profound deafferentation of the contralateral ventrobasal thalamus (see below). Alternatively, given the possibility that a few lemniscal or spinothalamic axons were spared by the lesions in each animal, the results show that sparse lemniscal or spinothalamic input to the cerebrum can support detection of cutaneous stimulation.

Anatomical studies. Thalamic tissue was examined by electron microscopy with post-embedding techniques for GABA-ir. The two major classes of GABA-ir synaptic profiles (Fig. 1) are axon terminals (F) derived primarily from neurons of the thalamic reticular nucleus and presynaptic dendrites (PSDs) of the local circuit interneurons within the thalamus. We observed a decrease in the numbers of GABA-ir thalamic reticular axonal terminals and local circuit presynaptic dendritic profiles on the deafferented side when compared with the animals' normal side. Counts of synaptic types, in nearly 110,000 μm^2 of tissue, in the normal and deafferented VB of each of the three monkeys revealed a reduction in both elements of the GABA-ir circuitry, F-axon terminals and the PSDs, on the deafferented side compared to the normal side. More than 550 GABA-ir profiles were counted in the normal VB and 470 in the deafferented VB.

When the counts of the three animals were pooled, the difference between the two sides was statistically significant ($P < 0.05$) (Fig. 2).

Physiological studies. We examined 121 neurons, 63 from the normal VB and 58 from the VB of the deafferented side. The cells of the intact VB were almost equally divided between those with receptive fields on the forelimb (31) and those with receptive fields on the hindlimb (32); combined,

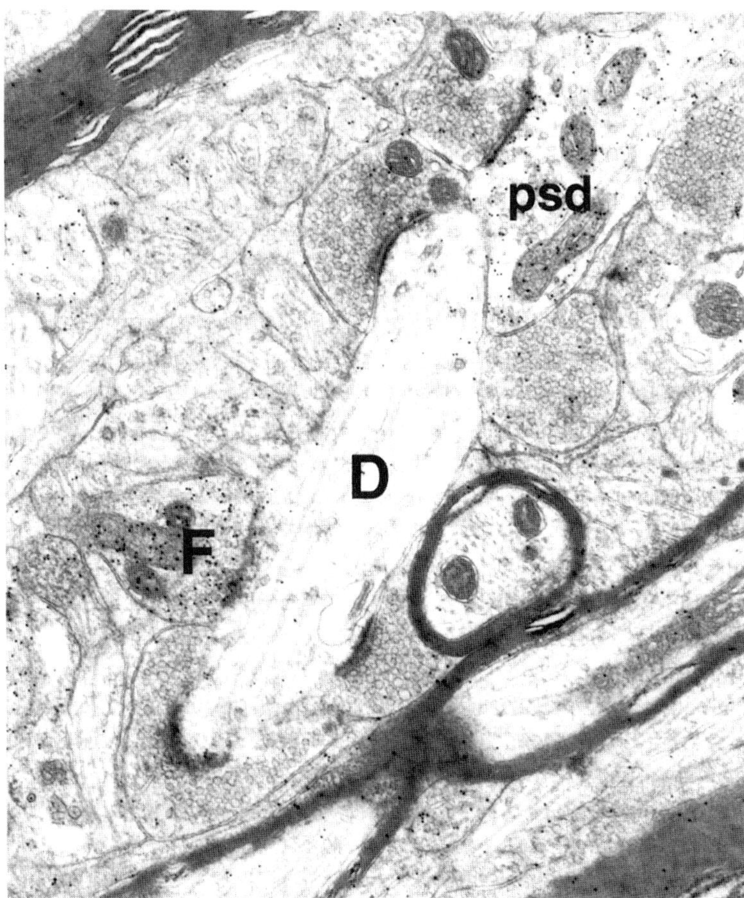

Fig. 1. Electron micrograph of the major types of GABA-ir synaptic profiles in the ventrobasal complex (VB). The presence of GABA antibody is revealed by the multiple 10-nm gold particles overlying the GABA-ir structures. A GABA-ir axon (F) contacts a thalamocortical relay cell dendrite (D). A GABA-ir profile (PSD) that is typical of presynaptic dendrites of local circuit interneurons is also present. Both the F and PSD GABA-ir synapses are reduced in number following spinal cord lesions (× 22,000).

these included 21 LT neurons and 42 MR cells. Of the neurons from the deafferented VB, 32 had receptive fields located on the forelimb (above the lesion); these included 28 cells with an LT profile and 4 cells with an MR profile. The remaining cells were sampled from VB regions lateral to the forelimb representation, and had no receptive fields. These cells were presumably deafferented neurons that formerly had hindlimb receptive fields.

Comparison of the cells from the deafferented VB with those from intact animals showed two types of changes: (1) changes in responsiveness to

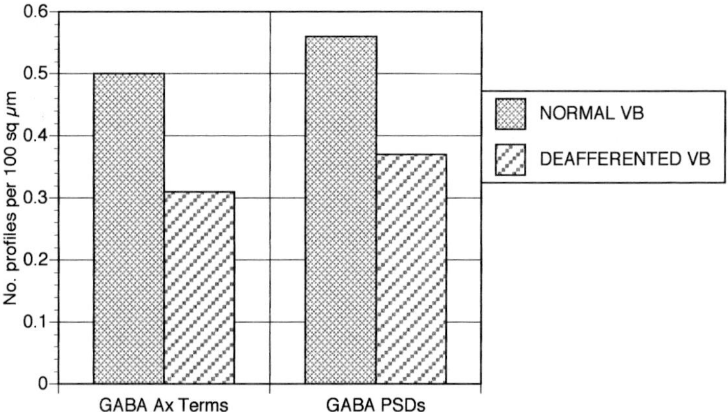

Fig. 2. Counts of the numbers (per 100 μm^2) of GABA-ir axon terminals (F profiles) and presynaptic dendrites (PSD) in normal and deafferented VB. The counts are pooled from the three animals studied. Both the F and PSD types of synaptic profiles are significantly reduced in number (unpaired t test: $P < 0.05$).

cutaneous stimuli, and (2) changes in evoked and spontaneous spike train properties. The evoked responses were increased for MR cells with forelimb receptive fields compared to intact animals, while as noted above, cells in the presumed hindlimb representation showed no responses to cutaneous stimuli. Thus, cells in both compartments of VB on the lesioned side showed changes in responses to cutaneous stimuli, but these changes were specific to each compartment. Similarly, cells in both the forelimb and hindlimb representation showed changes in spike train properties, but the characteristics of these changes were distinct for each compartment. Cells in the forelimb zone showed increased spontaneous bursts and also bursts in response to cutaneous stimulation without a change in primary event (inter-burst) spike rates. In contrast, cells in the presumed hindlimb zone showed an elevated burst rate, but a very reduced primary event rate. A representative example of the change in spontaneous activity from the deafferented zone in shown in Fig. 3.

DISCUSSION

Following spinal cord lesions that interrupt the spinothalamic and dorsal column pathways, monkeys had elevated detection thresholds for cutaneous stimulation, although the animals could reliably detect moderate and high intensities of stimulation and could identify the side stimulated. Elec-

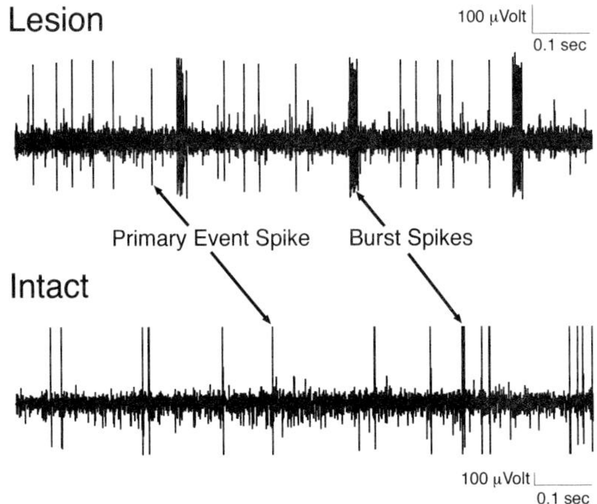

Fig. 3. Representative analogue recordings of VB neurons from macaques with combined lesions of the contralateral dorsal column pathway (fasciculus gracilis) and the ipsilateral anterolateral quadrant (upper trace) and from intact animals (lower trace). The arrows indicate spikes within bursts and some that are outside bursts (primary event rate).

tron microscopy demonstrated that GABA-ir axon terminals and interneuronal dendrites are common elements of the synaptic population of the macaque somatosensory thalamus and are significantly reduced (>40%) in the hindlimb region of VB that has been deafferented by lesions of the spinothalamic and medial lemniscal systems. Neurons in the deafferented region of VB exhibit increased spontaneous and stimulus-evoked firing, which may be related to the significant loss of GABAergic inhibition that we have found in the same animals.

Detection of cutaneous stimulus intensities that activate nociceptors after denervation of VB by combined spinal lemniscal and spinothalamic lesions indicates preservation of pain sensitivity following spinal cord lesions that involve the spinothalamic tract, albeit with elevated thresholds. The pattern of burst firing of VPL neurons found in these monkeys with spinal cord lesions is similar to that found in patients with pain following spinal cord injury (Lenz et al. 1989, 1994). Thus, the spinal lesions preserve nociceptive sensitivity and result in abnormal discharge among neurons in the major thalamic termination of the spinothalamic pathway. Plastic changes in the inhibitory, GABA-mediated synaptic circuitry of the VPL following spinal cord injury may contribute to the initiation and maintenance of abnormal function of neurons of the somatosensory thalamus. We suggest that the significant loss of GABA-mediated inhibition is an important factor in the creation and maintenance of central deafferentation pain syndromes.

ACKNOWLEDGMENTS

Supported by NIH grants NS-21445 and NS-23347 (to D.D. Ralston and H.J. Ralston), NS-32386 (to P.M. Dougherty and F.A. Lenz); and NS-07261 (to C.J. Vierck). We thank L. Rowland, A. Milroy, and S. Canchola for their expert technical assistance.

REFERENCES

Boivie J, Leijon G, Johansson I. Central post-stroke pain; a study of the mechanisms through analyses of the sensory abnormalities. *Pain* 1989; 37:173–185.

Canavero S, Bonicalzi V. The neurochemistry of central pain: evidence from clinical studies, hypothesis and therapeutic implications. *Pain* 1998; 74:109–114.

Dougherty PM, Li YJ, Lenz F A. Rowland L, Mittman S. Evidence that excitatory amino acids mediate afferent input to the primate somatosensory thalamus. *Brain Res* 1997; 278:267–273.

Lenz FA, Garonzik IM, Zirh TA, Dougherty PM. Neuronal activity in the region of the thalamic principal sensory nucleus (ventralis caudalis) in patients with pain following amputations. *Neuroscience* 1998a; 86:1065–1081.

Lenz FA, Gracely RH, Baker FH, Richardson RT, Dougherty PM. Reorganization of sensory modalities evoked by microstimulation in region of the thalamic principal sensory nucleus in patients with pain due to nervous system injury. *J Comp Neurol* 1998b; 399:125–138.

Lenz FA, Kwan HC, Dostrovsky JO, Tasker RR. Characteristics of the bursting pattern of action potentials that occurs in the thalamus of patients with central pain. *Brain Res* 1989; 496:357–360.

Lenz FA, Kwan HC, Martin R, Tasker R, et al. Characteristics of somatotopic organization and spontaneous neuronal activity in the region of the thalamic principal sensory nucleus in patients with spinal cord transection. *J Neurophysiol* 1994; 72:1570–1587.

Ralston HJ, Ohara PT, Meng XW, Wells J, Ralston DD. Transneuronal changes of the inhibitory circuitry in the macaque somatosensory thalamus following lesions of the dorsal column nuclei. *J Comp Neurol* 1996; 371:325–335.

Correspondence to: Diane Daly Ralston, PhD, Departments of Anatomy and of Neurological Surgery, University of California, San Francisco, CA 94143-0452, USA. Tel: 415-476-4400; Fax: 415-476-4845; email: ddr@phy.ucsf.edu.

Proceedings of the 9th World Congress on Pain,
Progress in Pain Research and Management,
Vol. 16, edited by M. Devor, M.C. Rowbotham, and
Z. Wiesenfeld-Hallin, IASP Press, Seattle, © 2000.

43

Migraine—A Genetic Neurovascular Channelopathy?

M.D. Ferrari, E.E. Kors, and G.M. Terwindt

Department of Neurology, Leiden University Medical Center, Leiden, The Netherlands

GENE-MAPPING APPROACHES TO MULTIFACTORIAL DISORDERS

The search for genetic risk factors for multifactorial diseases is complicated by a number of clinical, genetic, and statistical issues. Major clinical issues are how to determine whether or not a person is affected and how to distinguish likely gene carriers from possible phenocopies. While early onset and severe clinical course are traditionally regarded as indicators for a genetic background, it is unclear how this applies to episodic disorders. Do the number of attacks or their severity indicate genetic risk factors, or do they merely reflect the frequency and intensity of exposure to environmental triggers?

Once the operational criteria for disease definition have been agreed upon, the genetic strategy will depend on the available patient and family material and on the presence of likely candidate genes. When family material is abundant and candidate genes are scarce, random genome screening for linkage will be the method of choice. There is, however, considerable debate about the preferred method of analysis (parametric or nonparametric) and the statistical thresholds that provide optimal distinction between truly positive linkage signals and background noise (Thomson 1994; Lander and Kruglyak 1995; Greenberg et al. 1996; Kruglyak 1997). Linkage findings may lead to identification of *positional* candidate genes, as opposed to the *functional* candidates that originate from insights into the biochemical pathways underlying the disease. The involvement of such functional candidates may be evaluated via functional assays or by means of linkage tests in large families with several affected individuals.

A third, less commonly practiced method of identifying candidate genes for multifactorial disorders is to localize genes that cause rare Mendelian variants of that disorder. Such loci can then be evaluated as possible susceptibility loci, assuming that mutations that convey susceptibility to a complex disease are allelic to more serious gene defects leading to Mendelian segregation. We might call such candidate genes *phenotypic* candidates. Such rare variants usually have a clear inheritance pattern, and candidate loci can be identified by using regular LOD score analyses (a decimal logarithm of the odds ratio between the likelihoods of linkage and free recombination between a disease locus and a genetic marker). This approach has proven successful in the search for genes implicated in migraine.

The advantage of analysis of functional and phenotypic candidates over a genome search for positional candidates is that the former approach will involve fewer statistical tests, and that consequently a less stringent statistical correction for multiple testing is required. With respect to functional candidates, one might object that their number is a priori not strictly defined and that different investigators may favor different functional candidates. In contrast, for phenotypic candidates, the number of alternatives is usually very limited. Interpretation of a mildly significant linkage finding for a phenotypic candidate largely depends on the plausibility of a common genetic background for the common and rare variants of a disease, and on independent confirmation.

MIGRAINE, A MULTIFACTORIAL DISORDER

Migraine is an episodic neurological disorder, affecting up to 12% of males and 24% of females in the general population (Russell et al. 1995). Two main types are distinguished: migraine without aura, typically characterized by attacks of severe unilateral pulsating headache, nausea, vomiting, and photo- and phonophobia; and migraine with aura, in which the headache attacks are preceded by transient focal neurological, usually visual, aura symptoms. Visual symptoms include scintillating scotoma, blurred vision, flickering, and dark spots. Both types of migraine attacks may coexist in the same patient, but usually one type prevails. Attacks of migraine without aura occur in 67% of patients and attacks of migraine with aura in 33% (Russell and Olesen 1995). Migraine frequently runs in families, but family and segregation studies have produced conflicting results with respect to the mode of inheritance (Mochi et al. 1993; Russell and Olesen 1993; Haan et al. 1997; Stewart et al. 1997). From a large proband-oriented clinical study (Russell and Olesen 1995) it was concluded that migraine with aura is largely or exclusively determined by genetic factors, whereas migraine without aura seems to be caused by a combination of both genetic and environmental factors.

FAMILIAL HEMIPLEGIC MIGRAINE

CLINICAL FEATURES AND LINKAGE DATA

Familial hemiplegic migraine (FHM) is a rare autosomal dominantly inherited subtype of migraine with aura (Headache Classification Committee of the International Headache Society 1988). Patients with FHM have attacks of migraine with aura that are associated with hemiparesis or hemiplegia (one-sided weakness of the body). The symptoms of the headache and aura phase are otherwise similar to those of "nonhemiplegic" migraine with aura, but may last much longer. Some FHM families are also affected by progressive permanent ataxia (disturbance of co-ordination of movements). Patients with FHM may also have attacks of "nonhemiplegic" migraine, and they may have relatives who are subject to "nonhemiplegic" migraine alone. These observations strongly suggest that FHM is part of the migraine spectrum, and that genes involved in FHM are candidate genes for "nonhemiplegic" migraine with and without aura.

In approximately 50% of the reported families, FHM has been assigned to chromosome 19p13 (Joutel et al. 1994; Ophoff et al. 1994). Recently, two groups also found linkage to chromosome 1 (Ducros et al. 1997; Gardner et al. 1997). An American group showed, in one large family, an LOD score of 3.04 at $\Theta = 0.09$ with marker D1S249 on chromosome 1q31 (Gardner et al. 1997), whereas a French group showed linkage to chromosome 1q21–q23 in three FHM families (Ducros et al. 1997). Further analysis is needed to ascertain whether chromosome 1q harbors one or two FHM genes. Some FHM families are unlinked to chromosome 19 or chromosome 1; thus at least a third gene must be involved (Ducros et al. 1997).

Few clinical differences have been found between FHM families linked to chromosome 19 and those not linked to this chromosome. An exception is cerebellar ataxia, which occurs in approximately 50% of the chromosome 19-linked but in none of the unlinked families (Joutel et al. 1993, 1994; Haan et al. 1994; Ophoff et al. 1994; Elliott et al. 1996; Terwindt et al. 1996; Tournier-Lasserve 1996). Presumably, FHM and cerebellar degeneration reflect the same gene defect in chromosome 19-linked FHM families (Elliott et al. 1996; Haan et al. 1997). In addition, patients from these families are more likely to have attacks triggered by minor head trauma or attacks associated with coma in comparison to patients from families not linked to this chromosome (Terwindt et al. 1996).

MOLECULAR BIOLOGY OF CALCIUM CHANNELS

Six functional subclasses of calcium channels have been defined by electrophysiological and pharmacological criteria. The subclasses fall into two major categories: low-voltage-activated (T type) and high-voltage-activated channels (L, N, P, Q, R types) (Catterall and Striessnig 1992; Catterall 1995; Perez-Reyes and Schneider 1995; Varadi et al. 1995). Calcium channels are multiple-subunit complexes composed of a major transmembrane α_1 unit and smaller auxiliary polypeptides that include a β subunit and the disulfide-linked $\alpha_2\delta$ subunit. In skeletal muscle, a γ subunit may also form part of the channel complex. The α_1 subunit, which is the most important component, acts as a voltage sensor and forms the ion-conducting pore modified by the other subunits (Dunlap et al. 1995). Six genes (A, B, C, D, E, and S) have been identified that encode α_1 subunits (see Table I) (Catterall 1995; Perez-Reyes and Schneider 1995; Stea et al. 1995 Varadi et al. 1995). The α_1 subunit topology is very similar to the structure seen in voltage-dependent Na^+ and K^+ channels (Catterall 1995). The α_1 subunit consists of four internal homologous repeats (I–IV), each containing six putative α-helical membrane-spanning segments (S1–S6) and one pore-forming (P) segment between S5 and S6 that spans only the outer part of the transmembrane region (Guy and Durell 1996). The S4 segment contains a positively charged amino acid in every third or fourth position and is the voltage sensor for the voltage-gated ion channels (Varadi et al. 1995).

The β subunits are cytoplasmic proteins capable of modulating current amplitude, activation and inactivation kinetics, and voltage dependence when coexpressed with α_1 subunits (Schafer and Kenyon 1995). The β subunits are encoded by four different genes, all expressed in the brain (Table I).

The $\alpha_2\delta$ subunit is encoded by a single gene (Table I) and consists of glycosylated α_2 and δ proteins linked together by disulfide bonds with δ as the transmembrane protein anchor and α_2 extracellular.

Additional molecular diversity arises from alternative splicing of the α, β, and $\alpha_2\delta$ transcripts (Perez-Reyes and Schneider 1995; Schafer and Kenyon 1995). The characteristics of the different calcium channel types are primarily correlated with the different α_1 isoforms (Lory et al. 1997). The α_{1A} subunit encodes P- and Q-type calcium channels, which were originally identified in cerebellar Purkinje cells (Llinas et al. 1989) and granule cells (Zhang et al. 1993). P- and Q-type calcium channels differ in inactivation kinetics, possibly due to α_{1A} subunit splice variants (Snutch et al. 1991), post-translational modification, or the influence of an auxiliary subunit (Wheeler et al. 1995).

Table I
Calcium channel subunits

Subunit	Gene	Channel Type	Pharmacology (Blockers)	Location	Distribution	Human Disorders	Mouse Models
α_{1A}	*CACNA1A*	P/Q	ω-Agatoxin IVA; ω-Conotoxin MVIIC	19p13	Neuronal, endocrine	FHM, EA-2, SCA6	Tottering (*tg*) leaner (tg^{la})
α_{1B}	*CACNA1B*	N	ω-Conotoxin GVIA; ω-Conotoxin MVIIA	9q34	Neuronal		
α_{1C}	*CACNA1C*	L	Dihydropyridines	12p14.3	Cardiac and smooth muscle, neuronal		
α_{1D}	*CACNA1D*	L	Dihydropyridines	3p14.3	Neuronal, endocrine		
α_{1E}	*CACNA1E*	R/T	?	1q25–q31	Neuronal		
α_{1S}	*CACNA1S*	L	Dihydropyridines	1q31–q32	Skeletal muscle	HypoKK, MHS2	
β_1	*CACNB1*			17q11.2–q22	Skeletal muscle, neuronal		
β_2	*CACNB2*			10p12	Heart, aorta, neuronal		
β_3	*CACNB3*			12q13	Neuronal, aorta, trachea, lung, heart, skeletal muscle		
β_4	*CACNB4*			2q22–q23	Neuronal		Lethargic (*lh*)
$\alpha_2\delta$	*CACNA2*			7q21–q22	Skeletal muscle, heart, vascular and intestinal smooth muscle, neuronal		
γ	*CACNG*			17q24	Skeletal muscle		

Source: Reuter (1996); Tsien and Wheeler (1998).
Note: FHM = familial hemiplegic migraine; EA-2 = episodic ataxia, type 2; SCA6 = spinocerebellar ataxia, type 6; HypoKK = hypokalemic periodic paralysis; MHS2 = malignant hyperthermia susceptibility, type 2.

MUTATIONS IN THE P/Q-TYPE CALCIUM CHANNEL α_{1A} SUBUNIT GENE IN FHM

A cDNA that is highly homologous to a voltage-gated P/Q-type calcium channel α_{1A} subunit gene found in the brain of rabbits and rats was identified in humans using exon trapping (Mori et al. 1991; Starr et al. 1991; Ophoff et al. 1996). The human gene was designated *CACNL1A4,* (Diriong et al. 1995), but according to a newly proposed nomenclature the gene is called *CACNA1A* (Lory et al. 1997). The gene is transcribed specifically in the cerebellum, cerebral cortex, thalamus, and hypothalamus.

Four different missense mutations have been identified in five unrelated FHM families (see Fig. 1) (Ophoff et al. 1996). A transition from G to A was identified resulting in an arginine to glutamine substitution (R192Q) within the fourth segment of the first membrane-spanning domain (IS4). The highly conserved S4 segment is thought to be part of the voltage sensor. The second mutation occurred within the pore-forming (P) hairpin loop of the second domain, replacing a threonine residue for methionine (T666M). These conserved P segments, located between each S5 and S6 segment, are involved in the ion selectivity of ion channels and present binding sites for toxins (Guy and Durell 1996). Two other mutations were located in the sixth transmembrane-spanning segment of repeats II and IV. The IIS6 mutation was a T-to-C transition at codon 714 that resulted in a valine-to-alanine substitution (V714A). The IVS6 mutation was an A-to-C transversion at codon 1811 that resulted in a substitution of isoleucine for leucine (I1811L) and was found in two independent FHM families. The S6 mutations do not

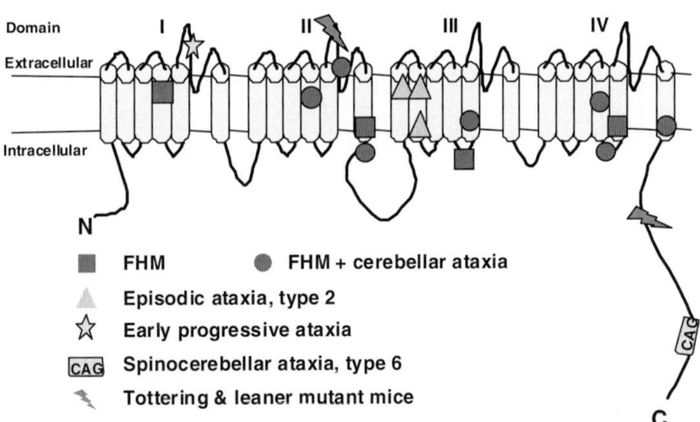

Fig. 1. Membrane topology of the α_{1A} subunit of the P/Q-type Ca^{2+} channel. The location is indicated for mutations that cause familial hemiplegic migraine (FHM), episodic ataxia, type 2 (EA-2), tottering mouse (*tg*), leaner mouse (tg^{la}), and spinocerebellar ataxia, type 6 (SCA6).

actually change the neutral-polar nature of the amino acid residues, but the original residues are conserved in all calcium channel α_1 subunit genes described (Stea et al. 1995). Residues in the S6 transmembrane segments may influence the inactivation of the calcium channel (Hering et al. 1996). The missense mutations in FHM suggest a molecular mechanism similar to what is found in other human channelopathies. Both alleles are likely to be expressed, with the allele that harbors the missense mutation resulting in gain-of-function variants of the P/Q-type calcium channels. Such mutations have been described in the α subunit of the skeletal muscle sodium channel and cause hyperkalemic periodic paralysis, paramyotonia congenita, or the sodium channel myotonias (Table II) (Hudson et al. 1995; Cannon 1996).

Table II
Heritable neurological disorders of ion channels

Disorder	Ion Channel Gene	Chromosomal Location
Hyperkalemic periodic paralysis	*SCNA4* (skeletal muscle sodium channel)	17q23–25
Paramyotonia congenita	*SCNA4*	17q23–25
Pure myotonias (fluctuans, permanens, acetazolamide-responsive)	*SCNA4*	17q23–25
Hypokalemic periodic paralysis	*CACNA1S* (skeletal muscle calcium channel)	1q31–32
Malignant hyperthermia susceptibility, type 2	*CACNA1S*	1q31–32
Familial hemiplegic migraine	*CACNA1A* (neuronal calcium channel)	19p13
Episodic ataxia, type 2	*CACNA1A*	19p13
Spinocerebellar ataxia, type 6	*CACNA1A*	19p13
Episodic ataxia, type 1	*KCNA1* (neuronal potassium channel)	12p14
Malignant hyperthermia susceptibility, type 1	*RYR1* (ryanodine calcium channel)	19q13.1
Autosomal dominant nocturnal frontal lobe epilepsy	*CHRNA4* (neuronal nicotinic acetylcholine receptor)	20q13.2–q13.3
Hyperekplexia	*GLRA1* (neuronal glycine receptor)	5q32
Thomsen's myotonia congenita	*CLCN1* (skeletal-muscle chloride channel)	7q35
Becker's myotonia congenita	*CLCN1*	7q35
Myotonia levior	*CLCN1*	7q35

Source: Stea et al. (1995); Ackerman and Clapham (1997); Ptacek (1997).
Note: All disorders have autosomal dominant inheritance except for Becker's myotonia congenita, which has autosomal recessive inheritance.

The four single mutations reported in FHM patients were introduced into the conserved rabbit α subunit. After functional expression in *Xenopus laevis* oocytes, changes in channel function were tested. Mutants T666M, V714A, and I1819L altered channel inactivation, but R192Q did not. The kinetic properties and the voltage dependence of α_{1A} Ca^{2+} channel activation were affected, resulting in a change in channel recovery and thereby altering the extent to which mutant channels accumulate in an inactivated state during rapid depolarizations. These findings agree with the hypothesis that mutations in the subunit underlie the neuronal instability that renders patients susceptible to migraine attacks triggered by neuronal stimuli such as stress or sensory afferentiation (Kraus et al. 1998).

Interestingly, the second FHM locus on chromosome 1q is located near a brain-specific R/T calcium channel α_{1E} subunit gene (*CACNA1E*). Mutation analysis has yet to disclose whether this gene is involved in chromosome 1-linked FHM families.

INVOLVEMENT OF THE P/Q-TYPE CALCIUM CHANNEL GENE ON CHROMOSOME 19 IN "NONHEMIPLEGIC" MIGRAINE

Previously, a sibling pair analysis in German families indicated that the FHM locus on chromosome 19p13 is involved in "nonhemiplegic" migraine with and without aura (May et al. 1995). However, the results were inconclusive as to the magnitude of the involvement and the relative importance of migraine with aura and migraine without aura. A second analysis of affected sibling pairs was performed in an independent additional sample of 36 extended Dutch families suffering from migraine with and without aura (Terwindt et al. 1997). Significant increased sharing of the marker alleles was confirmed in siblings who suffered from migraine with aura (maximum multipoint LOD score [MLS] = 1.29, corresponding to $P = 0.013$). No such increased sharing was found for migraine without aura. A combined analysis for both migraine types, including sibling pairs in which one individual had migraine with aura and the other migraine without aura, resulted in an even more significant increased sharing (MLS = 1.69 corresponding with $P = 0.005$). The relative risk ratio for a sibling (λ_s) to suffer from migraine with aura, defined as the increase in risk of the trait attributable to the 19p13 locus, was $\lambda_s = 2.4$. When combining migraine with and without aura, λ_s was 1.25. When we combined the results obtained in this study with those obtained by May et al. (1995), the maximum multipoint LOD score was raised to 2.27 ($P = 0.001$). These two studies provide independent evidence of the involvement of the region on chromosome 19p13 containing the P/Q-type calcium channel α_{1A} subunit gene in the etiology of migraine. The genetic contribution seems stronger for migraine with aura, however. Mutation analysis in patients with migraine has yet to reveal whether the known FHM mutations contribute to the etiology of migraine and whether other specific variants of this gene are involved in migraine with and without aura.

ROLE OF CALCIUM CHANNELS IN THE PATHOPHYSIOLOGY OF MIGRAINE

Physiologically, calcium acts as an intracellular second messenger by initiating or regulating numerous biochemical and electrical events in the cell. Calcium ions are implicated in the regulation of several enzymes and in controlling the activity of several other ion channels (Waard de et al. 1996). They also modulate many neuronal events such as neurotransmitter release (Gaur et al. 1994; Dunlap et al. 1995; Volsen et al. 1995; Uchitel et al. 1997; Wu and Saggau 1997), synaptogenesis, and neurite outgrowth (Waard de et al. 1996). P/Q-type calcium channels seem to be more effective at modulating neurotransmitter release than are other channel types (Mintz et al. 1995).

Most current models of migraine suggest that serotonin (5-hydroxytryptamine; 5-HT) has a central role in migraine pathophysiology (Ferrari and Saxena 1993). Effective specific acute antimigraine drugs all share the ability to stimulate neuronal and vascular 5-HT1 receptors, thereby inhibiting release of vasoactive neuropeptides, among other effects (Moskowitz 1992; Ferrari and Saxena 1995). Remarkably, P-type neuronal Ca^{2+} channels mediate release of neurotransmitters, including 5-HT (Codignola et al. 1993; Frittoli et al. 1994). Conversely, serotonin acts at 5-HT2c receptors to increase intracellular calcium activity in epithelial cells of the choroid plexus, both by liberating Ca^{2+} from intracellular stores and by activating a Ca^{2+} influx pathway (Watson et al. 1995). In rat motoneurons, serotonin inhibits N- and P-type calcium currents (Bayliss et al. 1995).

In the pathophysiology of migraine, cortical spreading depression may initiate migraine attacks (Lauritzen 1994). Calcium and other ion channels are important in the mechanism of cortical spreading depression (Lauritzen 1994; Shimazawa et al. 1995). Therefore, impaired function of cerebral calcium channels may facilitate the initiation of attacks.

There is also evidence of involvement of Mg^{2+} in the pathophysiology of migraine. Magnetic resonance spectroscopy studies suggest that intracellular brain magnesium is reduced in migraine patients and that the regional distribution of brain magnesium is altered in patients with FHM (Welch et al. 1992; Ramadan et al. 1996). Preliminary clinical trial data suggest that long-term administration of magnesium may reduce migraine attack frequency (Peikert et al. 1996). Interestingly, Mg^{2+} is known to interfere with Ca^{2+} channels (Altura 1985; Zhang et al. 1992).

Hormones seem to be important in migraine because there is a preponderance of females among migraine patients, and menstruation and pregnancy can affect the frequency of migraine attacks. An influence of hormones on ion channels has been considered in hypokalemic and hyperkalemic periodic paralysis (Lehmann-Horn et al. 1993; Lehmann-Horn and Rudel 1996). Joëls and Karst (1995) investigated the effects of estradiol and progesterone on voltage-gated calcium and potassium conductances in rat CA1 hippocampal neurons and concluded that long-term modulation with these hormone levels alters the calcium but not the potassium currents.

EPISODIC ATAXIA, TYPE 2

CLINICAL FEATURES AND LINKAGE DATA

Episodic ataxia (EA) is characterized by recurrent attacks of generalized ataxia and other signs of cerebellar dysfunction (Gancher and Nutt 1986). At least two autosomal dominantly inherited types of EA have been distinguished. Episodic ataxia type 1 (EA-1) is characterized by brief episodes of ataxia and dysarthria (disturbed articulation) lasting seconds to minutes, and is associated with interictal myokymia (twitching of small muscles) (Gancher and Nutt 1986). EA-1 is caused by missense mutations in a potassium channel gene (*KCNA1*) on chromosome 12p14 (Browne et al. 1994). Episodic ataxia type 2 (EA-2) is also called acetazolamide-responsive paroxysmal cerebellar ataxia (APCA), paroxysmal vestibulocerebellar ataxia (PVCA), or hereditary paroxysmal cerebellar ataxia (HPCA) (Kramer et al. 1995; Teh et al. 1995; Vahedi et al. 1995; von Brederlow et al. 1995). EA-2 is characterized by attacks of generalized ataxia, usually associated with interictal nystagmus (an eye movement disturbance). Treatment with acetazolamide is very effective in preventing attacks. Attacks typically last a few hours and can be precipitated by emotional stress, exercise, or alcoholic drinks. Clinical onset generally occurs in childhood or early adulthood (Gancher and Nutt 1986).

EA-2 was linked to the same interval on chromosome 19p as FHM (Kramer et al. 1995; Teh et al. 1995; Vahedi et al. 1995; von Brederlow et al. 1995). Notwithstanding the clinical differences between EA-2 and FHM, some similarities exist. Both are episodic disorders, and patients with EA-2 may show migraine-like features (Moon and Koller 1991; Hawkes 1992; Kramer et al. 1994; Vahedi et al. 1995; von Brederlow et al. 1995). In four families with EA-2, about half of the patients also met the International Headache Society criteria for migraine (Baloh et al. 1997). Both disorders may include progressive ataxia and dysarthria, and cerebellar atrophy may be revealed by magnetic resonance imaging (MRI) (Vighetto et al. 1988; Joutel et al. 1993; Haan et al. 1994).

MUTATIONS IN THE P/Q-TYPE CALCIUM CHANNEL α_{1A} SUBUNIT GENE IN EA-2

Because of the clinical and genetic similarities between FHM and EA-2, families with EA-2 were included in the mutation analysis of the *CACNA1A* gene. Two different truncating mutations have been identified in EA-2 families (see Fig. 1) (Ophoff et al. 1996). One mutation is a nucleotide deletion (deletion C_{4073}), causing a frame shift and a premature stop. The other mutation affects the first invariant G nucleotide of the intron consensus sequence, leading to aberrant splicing. A third mutation was seen in a patient with nonfamilial episodic vertigo and ataxia responsive to acetazolamide. A spontaneous C to T substitution resulted in an early stop codon (Yue et al. 1998). All mutations result in truncated α_{1A} subunits, which are unlikely to form functional calcium channels and may either degrade, resulting in haploinsufficiency, or negatively influence channel assembly in the membrane.

SPINOCEREBELLAR ATAXIA-6 AND THE P/Q-TYPE CALCIUM CHANNEL α_{1A} SUBUNIT GENE

The autosomal dominant spinocerebellar ataxias (SCAs) are a clinically and genetically heterogeneous group of disorders with many possible accompanying features such as ophthalmoplegia, pyramidal and extrapyramidal signs, neuropathy, dysarthria, amyotrophy, and pigmentary retinopathy (Harding 1993). Genes are located on chromosomes 6p22–p23 (SCA1) (Yakura et al. 1974; Banfi et al. 1993), 12q23–24.1 (SCA2) (Gispert et al. 1993), 14q32.1 (SCA3, also called Machado-Joseph disease) (Takiyama et al. 1993; Stevanin et al. 1994), 16q24-ter (SCA4) (Flanigan et al. 1996), 1 (SCA5) (Ranum et al. 1994), and 3p12–p21.1 (SCA7) (Benomar et al. 1995; Gouw et al. 1995; Holmberg et al. 1995). For SCA1, 2, 3, and 7, the disease-causing mutations have been identified as expanded and unstable CAG trinucleotide repeats (Orr et al. 1993; Imbert et al. 1996; Kawaguchi et al. 1996; Pulst et al. 1996; Sanpei et al. 1996; David et al. 1997). For SCA4 and 5, the disease-causing genes have yet to be identified.

Recently, six different cDNA isoforms of the *CACN1A1* gene have been reported, of which three contained a five-nucleotide insertion prior to the previously described stop codon; the insertion results in a shift of the open reading frame, and an additional stretch of the amino acid glutamine is added to the protein. (Ophoff et al. 1996; Zhuchenko et al. 1997). Small triplet expansions of the intragenic CAG repeat ranging from 21 to 30 repeat units were observed in patients with autosomal dominant cerebellar ataxia (SCA6) (Matsuyama et al. 1997; Riess et al. 1997; Zhuchenko et al. 1997), whereas normal chromosomes displayed 4–20 repeats (Ophoff et al. 1996; Ishikawa et al. 1997; Matsuyama et al. 1997; Riess et al. 1997; Zhuchenko et al. 1997). The CAG repeat length is inversely correlated with age at onset (Ishikawa et al. 1997; Matsuyama et al. 1997; Riess et al. 1997). Anticipation of the disease was observed clinically (Matsuyama et al. 1997), but no detectable intergenerational allele size change was seen in contrast to other disease-causing repeats (e.g., in other SCAs and Huntington disease). The SCA6 mutation was estimated to occur in 10% of SCA patients in Germany (Riess et al. 1997), whereas in Japan SCA6 comprised 30% of the examined ataxia patients and one homozygous case was found, suggesting a founder effect (Matsuyama et al. 1997).

Interestingly, both chromosome 19-linked FHM families and EA-2 families may develop progressive cerebellar ataxia and atrophy (Vighetto et al. 1988; Joutel et al. 1993, 1994; Haan et al. 1994; Ophoff et al. 1994; Elliott et al. 1996; Terwindt et al. 1996; Tournier-Lasserve 1996). We failed to find expansions of the intragenic CAG repeat in FHM patients with chronic cerebellar ataxia and the I1811L mutation. We therefore can conclude that the I1811L mutation causes FHM and chronic progressive cerebellar ataxia, independently of the number of CAG repeats (Terwindt et al. 1998). Recently, a family with severe progressive cerebellar ataxia was shown to have a missense mutation within the pore-forming (P) hairpin loop of the first domain, replacing a glycine by an arginine residue (Yue et al. 1997). The number of the CAG repeat was normal. In another family with a clinical diagnosis of EA-2, each affected member showed an expanded repeat of 23. No additional mutations in the gene were found (Jodice et al. 1997). This result again demonstrates the similarity of the disorders, and we might conclude that EA-2, SCA6, and FHM are part of the same spectrum.

P/Q-TYPE CALCIUM CHANNEL α_{1A} SUBUNIT GENE IN MICE WITH EPILEPSY AND ATAXIA

Simultaneously with the identification of mutations in FHM and EA-2, mutations in the *Cacna1a* gene were found in the tottering (*tg*) and leaner mouse (tg^{la}) phenotypes (Fig. 1) (Fletcher et al. 1996; Hess 1996; Doyle et al. 1997). These recessive tottering mice have been studied extensively as models for human epilepsy (Kostopoulos 1992). The mutation in the tottering mouse is a missense mutation close to the pore-forming P loop of the second transmembrane domain, very similar to one of the FHM missense mutations, and most likely affects the pore function of the P/Q-type calcium channel. The more severe leaner mouse is associated with a splice site mutation that produces an aberrant intracellular terminus and resembles the mutations found in two EA-2 families. Mutations at the mouse tottering locus result in intermittent convulsions similar to human absence epilepsy, motor seizures, and mild ataxia. The leaner (tg^{la}) mouse suffers from absence seizures, but not motor seizures. The tg^{la} mutants are more ataxic and often do not survive past weaning. The profound chronic ataxia is associated with pervasive loss of Purkinje cells and granule cells throughout the anterior cerebellum, and with reduced cerebellar size. A third mouse strain, the rolling Nagoya (tg^{rol}), presents an intermediate phenotype; the ataxia is more severe than in the *tg* mouse, motor seizures do not occur, and the mice have a normal lifespan (Fletcher et al. 1996). No mutation for the tg^{rol} mouse has yet been identified.

Tottering mutant mice have a significantly increased threshold for cortical spreading depression (C.F. Fletcher, unpublished data), a phenomenon thought to be involved in the pathophysiology of migraine. In the tottering mouse, a proliferation of noradrenaline axons arising from the locus ceruleus is considered to be one of the neuronal mechanisms that generate absence seizures (Kostopoulos 1992). Interestingly, positron emission tomography (PET) studies in acute migraine attacks suggest that the locus ceruleus and the dorsal raphe nucleus are the "migraine center" in man (Weiller et al. 1995). The tottering mice thus may serve as a model not only for epilepsy and ataxia, but also for migraine. Interestingly, a mutation in the calcium channel β_4 subunit gene has recently been associated with ataxia and seizures in the lethargic mouse (*lh*) (Burgess et al. 1997). Homozygotes of the *lh* mouse are characterized by ataxia, lethargic behavior, motor seizures, and seizures resembling absence seizures of human petit mal epilepsy (Burgess et al. 1997).

CADASIL: CLINICAL BUT NOT GENETIC OVERLAP WITH MIGRAINE

In cerebral autosomal dominant arteriopathy with subcortical infarcts and leukoencephalopathy (CADASIL), symptoms include recurrent subcortical ischemic strokes, progressive vascular dementia, and mood disorders with severe depression (Chabriat et al. 1995). Remarkably, migraine with aura occurs in many patients in CADASIL pedigrees (Jung et al. 1995; Chabriat et al. 1995; Verin et al. 1995). One CADASIL family that has been described suffered additionally from typical FHM attacks (Hutchinson et al. 1995), and members of another family linked to the CADASIL locus suffered from migraine and exhibited CADASIL-like white matter lesions on MRI (Chabriat et al. 1995). All these observations contributed to the clinical spectrum of migraine, FHM, and CADASIL. The CADASIL locus was mapped to chromosome 19 (Tournier-Lasserve et al. 1993), and CADASIL and FHM were initially considered to be allelic (Joutel et al. 1993). However, further linkage studies narrowed the CADASIL gene region and argued against allelism of CADASIL and FHM (Dichgans et al. 1996; Ducros et al. 1996). Recently, a Notch3 gene was identified in the CADASIL critical region (Joutel et al. 1996). Fifty-one unrelated CADASIL patients were screened for mutations in the Notch3 gene. Twenty-three distinct mutations were identified in 39 unrelated patients; seven mutations were recurrent without signs of a founder effect. All 23 mutations were located within the extracellular domain of the gene, which contains 34 epidermal growth factor repeats (EGF). Twenty-one are missense mutations, predicted to create or delete a cysteine residue, and the last two are splice site mutations (Joutel et al. 1997). Notch encodes for a glycosylated transmembrane receptor, which is involved in intercellular signaling essential for proper embryonic development in *Drosophila* (de Celis et al. 1994; Artavanis-Tsakonas et al. 1995). The Notch gene has closely related homologies in the nematode *Caenorhabditis elegans*, *Xenopus*, mice, and humans, which suggests that the gene's function has been widely conserved throughout evolution (de Celis et al. 1994). Another Notch-family receptor in *C. elegans*, called the sel-12 gene (Levitan and Greenwald 1995), is highly homologous to the mammalian presenilin genes, PS-1 and PS-2, which are involved in Alzheimer's disease (Cruts et al. 1996). Thus, the Notch-receptor genes are important in age-related dementia syndromes. The finding of separate genes for CADASIL and FHM show that these diseases are genetically unrelated. The question remains, however, why migraine with aura occurs so frequently in CADASIL. Unfortunately, no further genetic data are available on the families with CADASIL and (hemiplegic) migraine; however, the elucidation of the molecular mechanism underlying CADASIL may ultimately answer this question.

CONCLUSIONS AND SUMMARY

Clinical and genetic heterogeneity and the influence of environmental factors have hampered the identification of the genetic factors involved in episodic diseases such as migraine. The identification of the P/Q-type calcium channel in migraine, epilepsy, and ataxia is a leap forward in understanding these neurological channelopathies. The findings in migraine illustrate that rare, but monogenic variants of a disorder, may be successfully used to identify candidate genes for the more common, but genetically more complex, forms. Furthermore, the identification of calcium channels involved in the pathophysiology of these disorders opens new avenues for the development of prophylactic treatments.

So far, different sets of mutations in the P/Q-type calcium channel gene *CACNA1A* seem to be associated with specific clinical phenotypes, although these phenotypes may show some clinical overlap. The mechanism by which these mutations produce both episodic and chronic disorders is not yet understood. Presumably, these mutations permit proper cell function until extra- or intracellular conditions exacerbate the molecular pathology, leading to episodic failure of the channel function. In the long term, mutations may impair inactivation of the calcium channel and chronically disturb calcium homeostasis. The inability to restore the resting intracellular calcium levels may then induce a slow but progressive apoptotic neuronal cell death and eventually lead to a chronic progressive phenotype.

REFERENCES

Ackerman MJ, Clapham DE. Ion channels—basic science and clinical disease. *N Engl J Med* 1997; 336:1575–1586.

Altura BM. Calcium antagonist properties of magnesium: implications for antimigraine actions. *Magnesium* 1985; 4:169–175.

Artavanis-Tsakonas S, Matsuno K, Fortini ME. Notch signaling. *Science* 1995; 268:225–232.

Baloh RW, Yue Q, Furman JM, Nelson SF. Familial episodic ataxia: clinical heterogeneity in four families linked to chromosome 19p. *Ann Neurol* 1997; 41:8–16.

Banfi S, Chung MY, Kwiatkowski TJ, et al. Mapping and cloning of the critical region for the spinocerebellar ataxia type 1 gene in a yeast artificial chromosome contig spanning 1.2 Mb. *Genomics* 1993; 18:627–635.

Bayliss DA, Umemiya M, Berger AJ. Inhibition of N- and P-type calcium currents and the after-hyperpolarization in rat motoneurones by serotonin. *J Physiol* 1995; 485:635–647.

Benomar A, Krols L, Stevanin G, et al. The gene for autosomal dominant cerebellar ataxia with pigmentary macular dystrophy maps to chromosome 3p12–p21.1. *Nat Genet* 1995; 10:84–88.

Browne DL, Gancher ST, Nutt JG, et al. Episodic ataxia/myokymia syndrome is associated with point mutations in the human potassium channel gene, KCNA1. *Nat Genet* 1994; 8:136–140.

Burgess DL, Jones JM, Meister MH, Noebels JL. Mutation of the Ca^{2+} channel β subunit gene Cchb4 is associated with ataxia and seizures in the lethargic (lh) mouse. *Cell* 1997; 88:385–392.

Cannon SC. Ion-channel defects and aberrant excitability in myotonia and periodic paralysis. *Trends Neurosci* 1996; 19:3–10.

Catterall WA, Striessnig J. Receptor sites for Ca^{2+} channel antagonists. *Trends Pharmacol Sci* 1992; 13:256–262.

Catterall WA. Structure and function of voltage-gated ion channels. *Annu Rev Biochem* 1995; 64:493–531.

Chabriat H, Tournier-Lasserve E, Vahedi K, et al. Autosomal dominant migraine with MRI white-matter abnormalities mapping to the CADASIL locus. *Neurology* 1995; 45:1086–1091.

Chabriat H, Vahedi K, Iba-Zizen MT, et al. Clinical spectrum of CADASIL: a study of 7 families. *Lancet* 1995; 346:934–939.

Codignola A, Tarroni P, Clementi F, et al. Calcium channel subtypes controlling serotonin release from human small cell lung carcinoma cell lines. *J Biol Chem* 1993; 268:26240–26247.

Cruts M, Hendriks L, van Broeckhoven C. The presenilin genes: a new gene family involved in Alzheimer disease pathology. *Hum Mol Genet* 1996; 5:1449–1455.

David G, Abbas N, Stevanin G, et al. Cloning of the SCA7 gene reveals a highly unstable CAG repeat expansion. *Nat Genet* 1997; 17:65–70.

de Celis JF, Garcia-Bellido A. Modifications of the Notch function by Abruptex mutations in *Drosophila melanogaster*. *Genetics* 1994; 136:183–194.

Dichgans M, Mayer M, Muller-Myhsok B, Straube A, Gasser T. Identification of a key recombinant narrows the CADASIL gene region to 8 cM and argues against allelism of CADASIL and Familial Hemiplegic Migraine. *Genomics* 1996; 32:151–154.

Diriong S, Lory P, Williams ME, et al. Chromosomal localization of the human genes for α_{1A}, α_{1B}, and α_{1E} voltage-dependent Ca^{2+} channel subunits. *Genomics* 1995; 30:605–609.

Doyle J, Ren XJ, Lennon G, Stubbs L. Mutations in the CACNL1A4 calcium channel gene are associated with seizures, cerebellar degeneration, and ataxia in tottering and leaner mutant mice. *Mamm Genome* 1997; 8:113–120.

Ducros A, Joutel A, Vahedi K, et al. Familial hemiplegic migraine: mapping of the second gene and evidence for a third locus. *Cephalalgia* 1997; 17:232.

Ducros A, Nagy T, Alamowitch S, et al. Cerebral autosomal dominant arteriopathy with subcortical infarcts and leukoencephalopathy, genetic homogeneity, and mapping of the locus within a 2-cM interval. *Am J Hum Genet* 1996; 58:171–181.

Dunlap K, Luebke JI, Turner TJ. Exocytotic Ca^{2+} channels in mammalian central neurons. *Trends Neurosci* 1995; 18:89–98.

Elliott MA, Peroutka SJ, Welch S, May EF. Familial hemiplegic migraine, nystagmus, and cerebellar atrophy. *Ann Neurol* 1996; 39:100–106.

Ferrari MD, Saxena PR. On serotonin and migraine: a clinical and pharmacological review. *Cephalalgia* 1993; 13:151–165.

Ferrari MD, Saxena PR. 5-HT1 receptors in migraine pathophysiology and treatment. *Eur J Neurol* 1995; 2:5–21.

Flanigan TP, Gardner K, Alderson K, et al. Autosomal dominant spinocerebellar ataxia with sensory axonal neuropathy (SCA4): clinical description and genetic localization to chromosome 16q22.1. *Am J Hum Genet* 1996; 59:392–399.

Fletcher CF, Lutz CM, O'Sullivan TN, et al. Absence epilepsy in tottering mutant mice is associated with calcium channel defects. *Cell* 1996; 87:607–617.

Frittoli E, Gobbi M, Mennini T. Involvement of P-type Ca^{2+} channels in the K^+- and d-Fenfluramine-induced (3H)5-HT release from rat hippocampal synaptosomes. *Neuropharmacology* 1994; 33:833–835.

Gancher ST, Nutt JG. Autosomal dominant episodic ataxia: a heterogeneous syndrome. *Mov Disord* 1986; 1:239–253.

Gardner K, Ptacek LJ, Hoffman EP. A new locus for hemiplegic migraine is on chromosome 1q31. *Neurology* 1997; 49, in press.

Gaur S, Newcomb R, Rivnay B, et al. Calcium channel antagonist peptides define several components of transmitter release in the hippocampus. *Neuropharmacology* 1994; 33:1211–1219.

Gispert S, Twells R, Orozco G, et al. Chromosomal assignment of the second (Cuban) locus for autosomal dominant cerebellar ataxia (SCA2) to chromosome 12q23-24.1. *Nat Genet* 1993; 4:295–299.

Gouw LG, Kaplan CD, Haines JH, et al. Retinal degeneration characterizes a spinocerebellar ataxia mapping to chromosome 3p. *Nat Genet* 1995; 10:89–93.

Greenberg DA, Hodge SE, Vieland VJ, Spence MA. Affecteds-only linkage methods are not a panacea. *Am J Hum Genet* 1996; 58:892–895.

Guy HR, Durell SR. Three-dimensional models of ion channel proteins. In: Narahashi T (Ed). *Ion Channels*, 4th ed. New York: Plenum Press, 1996.

Haan J, Terwindt GM, Bos PL, et al. For the Dutch Migraine Genetics Research Group: familial hemiplegic migraine in The Netherlands. *Clin Neurol Neurosurg* 1994; 96:244–249.

Haan J, Terwindt GM, Ferrari MD. Genetics of migraine. In: Mathew NT (Ed). *Neurological Clinics. Advances in Headache*. Philadelphia: W.B. Saunders Co., 1997, pp 43–60.

Harding AE. Clinical features and classification of inherited ataxias. In: Harding EA, Deufel T (Eds). *Advances in Neurology*. New York: Raven Press, 1993, pp 1–14.

Hawkes CH. Familial paroxysmal ataxia: report of a family. *J Neurol Neurosurg Psychiatry* 1992; 55:212–213.

Headache Classification Committee of the International Headache Society. Classification and diagnostic criteria for headache disorders, cranial neuralgias and facial pain. *Cephalalgia* 1988; 8(S7):1–97.

Hering S, Aczel S, Grabner M, et al. Transfer of high sensitivity for benzothiazepines from L-type to class A (BI) calcium channels. *J Biol Chem* 1996; 271:24471–24475.

Hess EJ. Migraines in mice? *Cell* 1996; 87:1149–1151.

Holmberg M, Johansson J, Forsgren L, et al. Localization of autosomal dominant cerebellar ataxia associated with retinal degeneration and anticipation to chromosome 3p12-p21.1. *Hum Mol Genet* 1995; 4:1441–1445.

Hudson AJ, Ebers GC, Bulman DE. The skeletal muscle sodium and chloride channel diseases. *Brain* 1995; 118:547–563.

Hutchinson M, O'Riordan J, Javed M, et al. Familial hemiplegic migraine and autosomal dominant arteriopathy with leukoencephalopathy (CADASIL). *Ann Neurol* 1995; 38:817–824.

Imbert G, Saudou F, Yvert G, et al. Cloning of the gene for spinocerebellar ataxia 2 reveals a locus with high sensitivity to expanded CAG/glutamine repeats. *Nat Genet* 1996; 14:285–291.

Ishikawa K, Tanaka H, Saito M, et al. Japanese families with autosomal dominant pure cerebellar ataxia map to chromosome 19p13.1-p13.2 and are strongly associated with mild CAG expansions in the spinocerebellar ataxia type 6 gene in chromosome 19p13.1. *Am J Hum Genet* 1997; 61:336–346.

Jodice C, Mantuano E, Veneziano L, et al. Episodic ataxia type 2 (EA2) and spinocerebellar ataxia type 6 (SCA6) due to CAG repeat expansion in the CACNA1A gene on chromosome 19p. *Hum Mol Genet* 1997; 6:1973–1978.

Joëls M, Karst H. Effects of estradiol and progesterone on voltage-gated calcium and potassium conductances in rat CA1 hippocampal neurons. *J Neurosci* 1995; 15:4289–4297.

Joutel A, Bousser MG, Biousse V, et al. A gene for familial hemiplegic migraine maps to chromosome 19. *Nat Genet* 1993; 5:40–45.

Joutel A, Ducros A, Vahedi K, et al. Genetic heterogeneity of familial hemiplegic migraine. *Am J Hum Genet* 1994; 55:1166–1172.

Joutel A, Corpechot C, Ducros A, et al. Notch3 mutations in CADASIL, a hereditary adult-onset condition causing stroke and dementia. *Nature* 1996; 383:707–710.

Joutel A, Corpechot C, Vayssière et al. Characterization of Notch3 mutations in CADASIL patients. *Neurology* 1997; 48:1729–1730.

Jung HH, Bassetti C, Tournier-Lasserve E, et al. Cerebral autosomal dominant arteriopathy with subcortical infarcts and leukoencephalopathy: a clinicopathological and genetic study of a Swiss family. *J Neurol Neurosurg Psychiatry* 1995; 59:138–143.

Kawaguchi Y, Okamoto T, Taniwaki M, et al. CAG expansions in a novel gene for Machado-Joseph disease at chromosome 14q32.1. *Nat Genet* 1996; 14:221–227.

Kostopoulos GK. The tottering mouse: a critical review of its usefulness in the study of the neuronal mechanisms underlying epilepsy. *J Neural Transm* 1992; 35:21–36.

Kramer PL, Smith E, Carrero-Valenzuela R, et al. A gene for nystagmus-associated ataxia maps to chromosome 19p. *Am J Hum Genet* 1994; 55:A191.

Kramer PL, Yue Q, Gancher ST, et al. A locus for the nystagmus-associated form of episodic ataxia maps to an 11-cM region on chromosome 19p. *Am J Hum Genet* 1995; 57:182–185.

Kraus RL, Sinegger MJ, Glossmann H, Hering S, Striessnig J. Familial hemiplegic migraine mutations change a_{1A} Ca^{2+} channel kinetics. *J Biol Chem* 1998; 273:5586–5590.

Kruglyak L. Nonparametric linkage tests are model free. *Am J Hum Genet* 1997; 61:254–255.

Lander E, Kruglyak L. Genetic dissection of complex traits: guidelines for interpreting and reporting linkage results. *Nat Genet* 1995; 11:241–247.

Lauritzen M. Pathophysiology of the migraine aura. The spreading depression theory. *Brain* 1994; 117:199–210.

Lehmann-Horn F, Rüdel R, Ricker K. Non-dystrophic myotonias and periodic paralyses. Workshop report. *Neuromuscul Disord* 1993; 3:161–168.

Lehmann-Horn F, Rudel R. Molecular pathophysiology of voltage-gated ion channels. *Rev Physiol Biochem Pharmacol* 1996; 128:195–268.

Levitan D, Greenwald I. Facilitation of lin-12-mediated signalling by sel-12, a *Caenorhabditis elegans* S182 Alzheimer's disease gene. *Nature* 1995; 377:351–354.

Llinas RR, Sugimori M, Cherksey B. Voltage-dependent calcium conductances in mammalian neurons: the P channel. *Ann NY Acad Sci* 1989; 560:103–111.

Lory P, Ophoff RA, Nahmias J. Towards a unified nomenclature describing voltage-gated calcium channel genes. *Hum Genet* 1997; 100:149–150.

Matsuyama Z, Kawakami H, Maruyama H, et al. Molecular features of the CAG repeats of spinocerebellar ataxia 6 (SCA6). *Hum Mol Genet* 1997; 6:1283–1287.

May A, Ophoff RA, Terwindt GM, et al. Familial hemiplegic migraine locus on 19p13 is involved in the common forms of migraine with and without aura. *Hum Genet* 1995; 96:604–608.

Mintz IM, Sabatini BL, Regehr WG. Calcium control of transmitter release at a cerebellar synapse. *Neuron* 1995; 15:675–688.

Mochi M, Sangiorgi S, Cortelli P, et al. Testing models for genetic determination in migraine. *Cephalalgia* 1993; 13:389–394.

Moon SL, Koller WC. Hereditary periodic ataxias. In: Jong de JMBV (Ed). *Handbook of Clinical Neurology. Hereditary Neuropathies and Spinocerebellar Ataxias*. Amsterdam: Elsevier Science, 1991, pp 433–443.

Mori Y, Friedrich T, Kim MS, et al. Primary structure and functional expression from complementary DNA of a brain calcium channel. *Nature* 1991; 350:398–402.

Moskowitz MA. Neurogenic versus vascular mechanism of sumatriptan and ergot alkaloids in migraine. *Trends Pharmacol Sci* 1992; 13:307–311.

Ophoff RA, van Eijk R, Sandkuijl LA, et al. Genetic heterogeneity of familial hemiplegic migraine. *Genomics* 1994; 22:21–26.

Ophoff RA, Terwindt GM, Vergouwe MN, et al. Familial hemiplegic migraine and episodic ataxia type-2 are caused by mutations in the Ca^{2+} channel gene CACNL1A4. *Cell* 1996; 87:543–552.

Orr HT, Chung MY, Banfi S, et al. Expansion of an unstable trinucleotide CAG repeat in spinocerebellar ataxia type 1. *Nat Genet* 1993; 4: 221–226.

Peikert A, Wilimzig C, Köhne-Volland R. Prophylaxis of migraine with oral magnesium: results from a prospective, multi-center, placebo-controlled and double-blind randomized study. *Cephalalgia* 1996; 16:257–263.

Perez-Reyes E, Schneider T. Molecular biology of calcium channels. *Kidney Int* 1995; 48:1111–1124.

Ptacek LJ. Channelopathies: ion channel disorders of muscle as a paradigm for paroxysmal disorders of the nervous system. *Neuromuscul Disord* 1997; 7:250–255.

Pulst SM, Nechiporuk A, Nechiporuk T, et al. Moderate expansion of a normally biallelic trinucleotide repeat in spinocerebellar ataxia type 2. *Nat Genet* 1996; 14:269–276.

Ramadan NM, Barker P, Boska MD, et al. Selective occipital cortex magnesium Mg^{2+} deficiency reduction in familial hemiplegic migraine may reflect an ion channel disorder. *Neurology* 1996; A168.

Ranum LPW, Schut LJ, Lundgren JK, Orr HT, Livingston DM. Spinocerebellar ataxia type 5 in a family descended from the grandparents of President Lincoln maps to chromosome 11. *Nat Genet* 1994; 8:280–284.

Reuter H. Diversity and function of presynaptic calcium channels in the brain. *Curr Opin Neurobiol* 1996; 6:331–337.

Riess O, Schöls L, Böttger H, et al. SCA6 is caused by moderate CAG expansion in the α_{1A}-voltage-dependent calcium channel gene. *Hum Mol Genet* 1997; 6:1289–1293.

Russell MB, Olesen J. The genetics of migraine without aura and migraine with aura. *Cephalalgia* 1993; 13:245–248.

Russell MB, Olesen J. Increased familial risk and evidence of genetic factor in migraine. *BMJ* 1995; 311:541–544.

Russell MB, Rasmussen BK, Thorvaldsen P, Olesen J. Prevalence and sex-ratio of the subtypes of migraine. *Int J Epidemiol* 1995; 24:612–618.

Sanpei K, Takano H, Igarashi S, et al. Identification of the spinocerebellar ataxia type 2 gene using a direct identification of repeat expansion and cloning technique, DIRECT. *Nat Genet* 1996; 14:277–284.

Schafer WR, Kenyon CJ. A calcium-channel homologue required for adaptation to dopamine and serotonin in *Caenorhabditis elegans*. *Nature* 1995; 375:73–78.

Shimazawa M, Hara H, Watano T, Sukamoto T. Effects of Ca^{2+} channel blockers on cortical hypoperfusion and expression of c-Fos-like immunoreactivity after cortical spreading depression in rats. *Br J Pharmacol* 1995; 115:1359–1368.

Snutch TP, Tomlinson WJ, Leonard JP, Gilbert MM. Distinct calcium channels are generated by alternative splicing and are differentially expressed in the mammalian CNS. *Neuron* 1991; 7:45–57.

Starr TV, Prystay W, Snutch TP. Primary structure of a calcium channel that is highly expressed in the rat cerebellum. *Proc Natl Acad Sci USA* 1991; 88:5621–5625.

Stea A, Soong TW, Snutch TP. Voltage-gated calcium channels. In: North RA (Ed). *Handbook of Receptors and Channels. Ligand- and Voltage-Gated Ion Channels*. CRC Press, 1995, pp 113–153.

Stevanin G, Le Guern E, Ravise N, et al. A third locus for autosomal dominant cerebellar ataxia type I maps to chromosome 14q24.3-qter: evidence for the existence of a fourth locus. *Am J Hum Genet* 1994; 54:11–20.

Stewart WF, Staffa J, Lipton RB, Ottman R. Familial risk of migraine: a population-based study. *Ann Neurol* 1997; 41:166–172.

Takiyama Y, Nishizawa M, Tanaka H, et al. The gene for Machado-Joseph disease maps to human chromosome 14q. *Nat Genet* 1993; 4:300–304.

Teh BT, Silburn P, Lindblad K, et al. Familial periodic cerebellar ataxia without myokymia maps to a 19-cM region on 19p13. *Am J Hum Genet* 1995; 56:1443–1449.

Terwindt GM, Ophoff RA, Haan J, Frants RR, Ferrari MD. For the DMGRG: Familial hemiplegic migraine: a clinical comparison of families linked and unlinked to chromosome 19. *Cephalalgia* 1996; 16:153–155.

Terwindt GM, Ophoff RA, Sandkuijl LA, et al. for the DMGRG: Involvement of the familial hemiplegic migraine gene on 19p13 in migraine with and without aura. *Cephalalgia* 1997; 17:232.

Terwindt GM, Ophoff RA, Haan J, et al. Variable clinical expression of mutations in the P/Q-type calcium channel gene in familial hemiplegic migraine. *Neurology* 1998; 50:1105-1110.

Thomson G. Identifying complex disease genes: progress and paradigms. *Nat Genet* 1994; 8:108–110.

Tournier-Lasserve E, Joutel A, Melki J, et al. Cerebral autosomal dominant arteriopathy with subcortical infarcts and leukoencephalopathy maps to chromosome 19q12. *Nat Genet* 1993; 3:256–259.

Tournier-Lasserve E. Genetics of familial hemiplegic migraine. In: Sandler M, Ferrari M, Harnett S (Eds). *Migraine, Pharmacology and Genetics*. London: Chapman & Hall, 1996, pp 282–290.

Tsien RW, Wheeler DB. Voltage-gated calcium channels. In: Carafoli E, Klee CB (Eds). *Intracellular Calcium.* 1998.

Uchitel OD, Protti DA, Sanchez V, et al. P-type voltage-dependent calcium channel mediates presynaptic calcium influx and transmitter release in mammalian synapses. *Proc Natl Acad Sci USA* 1997; 89:3330–3333.

Vahedi K, Joutel A, Bogaert van P, et al. A gene for hereditary paroxysmal cerebellar ataxia maps to chromosome 19p. *Ann Neurol* 1995; 37:289–293.

Varadi G, Mori Y, Mikala G, Schwartz A. Molecular determinants of Ca^{2+} channel function and drug action. *Trends Pharmacol Sci* 1995; 16:43–49.

Verin M, Rolland Y, Landgraf F, et al. New phenotype of the cerebral autosomal dominant arteriopathy mapped to chromosome 19: migraine as the prominent clinical feature. *J Neurol Neurosurg Psychiatry* 1995; 59:579–585.

Vighetto A, Froment JC, Trillet M, Aimard G. Magnetic resonance imaging in familial paroxysmal ataxia. *Arch Neurol* 1988; 45:547–549.

Volsen SG, Day NC, McCormack AL, et al. The expression of neuronal voltage-dependent calcium channels in human cerebellum. *Mol Brain Res* 1995; 34:271–282.

von Brederlow B, Hahn AF, Koopman WJ, Ebers GC, Bulman DE. Mapping the gene for acetazolamide responsive hereditary paroxysmal cerebellar ataxia to chromosome 19p. *Hum Mol Genet* 1995; 4:279–284.

Waard de M, Gurnett CA, Campbell KP. Structural and functional diversity of voltage-activated calcium channels. In: Narahashi T (Ed). *Ionchannels.* New York: Plenum Press, 1996, pp 41–87.

Watson JA, Elliott AC, Brown PD. Serotonin elevates intracellular Ca^{2+} in rat choroid plexus epithelial cells by acting on 5-HT2C receptors. *Cell Calcium* 1995; 17:120–128.

Weiller C, May A, Limmroth V, et al. Brain stem activation in spontaneous human migraine attacks. *Nat Med* 1995; 1:658–660.

Welch KMA, Barkley GL, Ramadan NM, D'Andrea G. NMR spectroscopic and magnetoencephalographic studies in migraine with aura: support for the spreading depression hypothesis. *Path Biol* 1992; 40:349–353.

Wheeler DB, Randall A, Sather WA, Tsien RW. Neuronal calcium channels encoded by the α_{1A} subunit and their contribution to excitatory synaptic transmission in the CNS. In: Yu ACH, Eng LF, McMahan UJ, Schulman H, Shooter EM, Stadlin A (Eds). *Progress in Brain Research,* 105th ed. Amsterdam: Elsevier Science, 1995, pp 65–78.

Wu L-G, Saggau P. Presynaptic inhibition of elicited neurotransmitter release. *TINS* 1997; 20:204–212.

Yakura H, Wakisaka A, Fujimoto S, Itakura K. Hereditary ataxia and HLA genotypes. *N Engl J Med* 1974; 291:154–155.

Yue Q, Jen JC, Nelson SF, Baloh RW. Progressive ataxia due to a missense mutation in a calcium-channel gene. *Am J Hum Genet* 1997; 61:1078–1087.

Yue Q, Jen JC, Thwe MM, Nelson SF, Baloh RW. De novo mutation in CACNA1A caused acetazolamide-responsive episodic ataxia. *Am J Med Genet* 1998; 77:298–301.

Zhang A, Cheng PTO, Altura BM. Magnesium regulates intracellular free ionized calcium concentration and cell geometry in vascular smooth muscle cell. *Biophys Acta* 1992; 1134:25–29.

Zhang J-F, Randall AD, Ellinor PT, et al. Distinctive pharmacology and kinetics of cloned neuronal Ca^{2+} channels and their possible counterparts in mammalian CNS neurons. *Neuropharmacology* 1993; 32:1075–1088.

Zhuchenko O, Bailey J, Bonnen P, et al. Autosomal dominant cerebellar ataxia (SCA6) associated with small polyglutamine expansions in the α_{1A}-voltage-dependent calcium channel. *Nat Genet* 1997; 15:62–69.

Correspondence to: M.D. Ferrari, MD, PhD, Department of Neurology, Leiden University Medical Center, P.O. Box 9600, 2300 RC Leiden, The Netherlands. Fax: 31-71-524-8253; email: mferrari@neurology.azl.nl.

Proceedings of the 9th World Congress on Pain,
Progress in Pain Research and Management,
Vol. 16, edited by M. Devor, M.C. Rowbotham, and
Z. Wiesenfeld-Hallin, IASP Press, Seattle, © 2000.

44

Genetic Correlations among Common Nociceptive Assays in the Mouse: How Many Types of Pain?

Jeffrey S. Mogil

Department of Psychology and Neuroscience Program, University of Illinois at Urbana-Champaign, Champaign, Illinois, USA

A TAXONOMY OF PAIN

It is now well appreciated that pain is not a unitary phenomenon. Forty years ago, Beecher (1959) asserted that "experimental" and "pathological" pain could be differentiated based on their responsiveness to opioid analgesia. He pointed out the remarkably similar response of various pain types within the "pathological" class (e.g., traumatic pain and chronic cancer pain) to morphine or to placebo. More recent, and still controversial, reports have proposed that opioid analgesics are effective against nociceptive pain, but much less so against chronic neuropathic pain (e.g., Arnér and Meyerson 1988).

The concept of multiple pain types is reflected in the wide array of behavioral assays developed to assess nociception in laboratory animals (see, e.g., Vierck and Cooper 1984; Hammond 1989). The mechanisms underlying nociception and antinociception in some of these assays have been distinguished on the basis of anatomical, biochemical, electrophysiological, and pharmacological evidence (see Mogil et al. 1996 for review). In addition to the distinction between nociceptive and neuropathic pain noted above (see also Woolf 1995; Malmberg et al. 1997a,b), fundamental differences are proposed to exist in the processing and modulation of: (1) "first pain" versus "second pain" (Cooper et al. 1986; Taddese et al. 1995), (2) acute versus tonic nociception (Dennis and Melzack 1979; Ryan et al. 1985), (3) thermal versus nonthermal nociception (Dennis et al. 1980; Tyers 1980; Giordano and Dyche 1989; Lima et al. 1993), (4) mechanical versus chemical nociception (DeLeo et al. 1991; Lanteri-Minet et al. 1993), (5) spinally versus supraspinally mediated nociception (Konig et al. 1996; Zimmer et al. 1998), (6) low- versus high-intensity nociception (Suh et al. 1989; Yeomans et al. 1996; Cao et al. 1998), (7) deep versus superficial somatic nociception (Keay and Bandler 1993), and (8) cutaneous versus visceral nociception (McMahon 1997).

In addition, various hypersensitivity states may be dissociable. Distinctions have been made between thermal and mechanical hypersensitivity (Treede et al. 1992; Lee et al. 1994; Meller 1994), between allodynia and hyperalgesia (Lee et al. 1994), and even between types of hypersensitivity as measured on the Bennett and Xie (1988) versus the Seltzer et al. (1990) model of neuropathic pain (Yamamoto and Nozaki-Taguchi 1997).

However, there are many reasons to believe that different types of pain share underlying physiological substrates. For example, somatic nociceptive information of various stimulus modalities converges on the same "multireceptive" pain transmission neurons in the dorsal horn of the spinal cord, as do nociceptive afferents that innervate the skin and viscera (see Willis 1985). The major analgesic drug classes, opiates and nonsteroidal anti-inflammatory drugs (NSAIDs), are effective in a wide variety of different pain conditions, if not all.

Information on how many types of pain exist is crucial for several reasons. If there are many different types, then any new basic research finding that purports to have generalized relevance must be confirmed using multiple nociceptive assays. However, true mechanistic distinctions between pain types might facilitate the development of more targeted treatments. A mechanistic taxonomy of pain—or at least a classification of existing experimental pain assays in humans and animals—would thus be tremendously useful. A recent discussion group concluded that a mechanism-based taxonomy would be advantageous compared to existing labels based on anatomy ("skin" versus "viscera"), duration ("acute" versus "chronic"), or pathology ("cancer" versus "noncancer"). Such a taxonomy would distinguish between transient pain and pain caused by injury to tissues or to the nervous system (Woolf et al. 1998). My collaborators and I have attempted to determine the physiological basis of various pain types at the level of genetic (DNA sequence) variation.

GENETIC CORRELATIONS

Individual differences in pain sensitivity have a substantial genetic component (see Mogil 1999 for a recent review). Genetic variation within a species is adequately modeled by inbred laboratory mouse strains, which although all derived from a limited hybrid stock of (largely) *Mus musculus domesticus* in the early 1900s (see Silver 1995), display highly variable responses on a wide variety of traits (see, e.g., Ingram and Corfman 1980; Crawley et al. 1997). Since all members of an inbred strain are isogenic (i.e., clones), identical at all genetic loci, within-strain differences are by definition environmental in origin. In contrast, differences between strains may reflect the effects of alternate alleles of trait-relevant genes. If those genes are pleiotropic, affecting more than one trait (as virtually all genes do), the possession of a certain allele of that gene will affect each trait accordingly. Thus, panels of inbred strains can be used to establish genetic correlations among traits, subject to certain caveats (Carey 1988; Crabbe et al. 1990). If a particular inbred strain is found to be sensitive on one nociceptive assay, it should also be sensitive to other assays mediated by the same (or overlapping sets of) genes. That is, the possession of "increaser" alleles of genes mediating the first assay will also increase sensitivity in all other assays that show a positive genetic correlation (Fig. 1). Negative genetic correlations between two assays would also indicate their mediation by common genes; in this case the same allele would increase sensitivity on the first assay and decrease sensitivity on the second.

Genetic correlation between traits, in turn, implies that those traits (at least to some degree) share underlying physiological substrates (Crabbe et al. 1990). If different nociceptive assays display similar processing, they can be thought of as representing the same basic type of pain. I can think of no more fundamental approach to construct a pain taxonomy.

EXISTING DATA ON THE GENETIC CORRELATION OF NOCICEPTION

Prior to 1999, data on the genetic correlation of nociceptive sensitivity were largely based on pairwise comparisons between selectively bred lines and highly divergent inbred strains. For example, Panocka and colleagues (1986) selected outbred Swiss mice for high and low swim-stress-induced antinociception (swim SIA) on the hot-plate test. Although no selection pressure was placed on basal hot-plate sensitivity, this trait was found to co-select with swim SIA such that after five generations of breeding, hot-plate latencies in HA (high analgesia) mice were double those of LA (low analgesia) mice. Testing of sixth-generation HA and LA mice on the tail-flick test revealed similar line differences (Panocka et al. 1986), suggesting that similar genes contributed to the alterations in swim SIA, hot-plate, and tail-flick sensitivity.

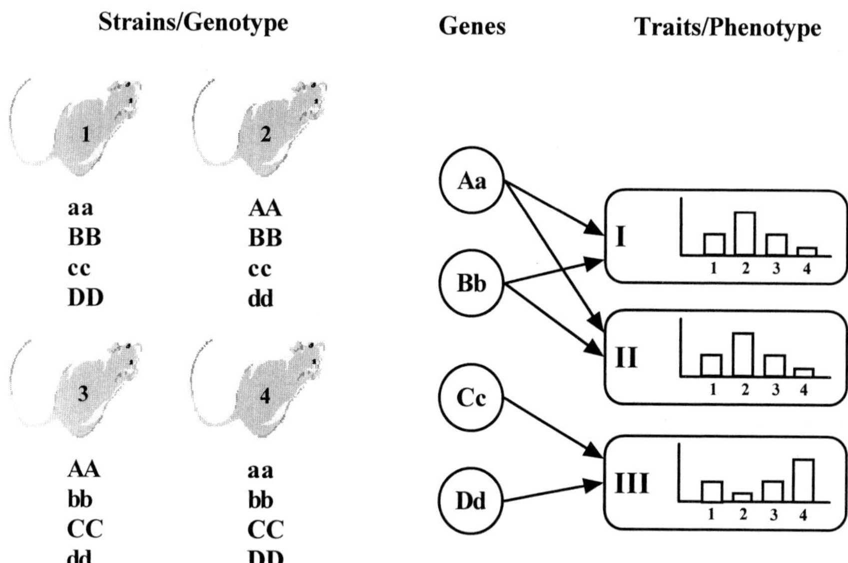

Fig. 1. Inferring genetic correlation of traits from inbred strain distributions. Assume the existence of four pain trait-relevant genes, A, B, C, and D. Each gene can exist in two allelic forms: A/a, B/b, C/c, and D/d. Four inbred mouse strains (1, 2, 3, and 4) possess each gene in one of two homozygous states (e.g., AA or aa); each strain's complete genotype is listed. If we assume that in each case, the capital letter allele is an "increaser" allele, resulting in higher trait values, three phenotypes are possible in these inbred strains for traits mediated by two genes: high (homozygous increaser alleles at both genes), medium (increaser alleles at one gene; decreaser alleles at the other), and low (decreaser alleles at both genes). To test for the genetic correlation of traits I, II, and III, therefore, we simply need to assess the phenotype of each strain on each trait. The identical phenotypic strain distributions of traits I and II indicate their common mediation by the same genes (A and B). The distinct strain distribution observed for trait III reflects its mediation by different genes (C and D).

In another example, Devor and Raber (1990) selected outbred Sabra rats for high and low propensity to autotomize after nerve transection, unfortunately also named HA (high autotomy) and LA (low autotomy). After selection became asymptotic, Devor and Raber (1990) and later Shir and colleagues (1991) tested *unoperated* HA and LA rats for mechanical and thermal sensitivity, and both found significant differences in the former (HA more sensitive than LA) and trends toward significance in the latter (data from separate experiments attained significance when pooled). This apparent correlation between basal nociceptive sensitivity and propensity to autotomize can also be seen by comparing the Lewis strain of rats (low autotomy, low thermal sensitivity) to the Sabra strain (high autotomy, high thermal sensitivity) (Y. Shir et al., unpublished observations; cf. Shir et al. 1991).

In 1996 we published a study (Mogil et al. 1996) involving four pairwise comparisons of mouse lines/strains known to display high and low morphine antinociception: (1) HA/LA (high analgesia versus low analgesia) mice (Panocka et al. 1986); (2) HAR/LAR mice, selected for high versus low antinociceptive response to the opiate levorphanol (Belknap et al. 1983); (3) DBA/2J versus C57BL/6J inbred strains, which are sensitive and resistant to opioid antinociception, respectively (see Belknap and O'Toole 1991); and (4) the μ-receptor-deficient recombinant inbred CXBK strain (Baran et al. 1975) compared to its C57BL/6J progenitor. In addition to divergent morphine antinociception, all four comparisons featured significant differences in baseline nociceptive sensitivity on the hot-plate and the hot water tail-immersion/withdrawal tests. However, no strain differed significantly from any other on the 0.6% acetic acid abdominal constriction ("writhing") assay, and the only strain differences noted on the 5% formalin test were between HAR (resistant) and LAR (sensitive) mice (Mogil et al. 1996).

Finally, in another study focusing on morphine antinociception, Elmer and colleagues (1997) tested eight different strains (inbred AKR/J, BALB/cByJ, C3H/HeJ, C57BL/6J, CBA/J, DBA/2J, and the recombinant inbred CXBH/ByJ and CXBK/ByJ strains) for sensitivity on the hot-plate test at five different temperatures (51°, 53°, 55°, 57°, and 59°C), and on the writhing test at three different concentrations of acetic acid (0.1%, 0.3%, and 0.6%). The authors noted considerable strain variability in each assay, but saw no interactions between genotype and nociceptive intensity. That is, strains differed in the location, but not the slope, of their stimulus-effect curves. This finding argues against a meaningful genetic dissociation of nociception of different intensities, at least within the range considered. Supporting our previous observations (Mogil et al. 1996), Elmer et al. (1997) also convincingly demonstrated the lack of genetic correlation (Pearson's r = 0.19, n.s.) between levels of sensitivity on the hot-plate and writhing assays.

TYPES OF NOCICEPTION

Although existing data suggested genetic correlations between certain nociceptive assays (e.g., hot-plate and tail-flick/tail-withdrawal tests) but not others (e.g., hot-plate and writhing tests), no one had ever addressed the issue systematically. Therefore, in collaboration with the laboratories of Jin Mo Chung, Marshall Devor, and Gregory Elmer, we set about testing a common set of 11 pseudorandomly chosen inbred strains (129, A, AKR, BALB/c, C3H/He, C57BL/6, C58, CBA, DBA/2, RIIIS, and SM; all "J" substrains purchased from The Jackson Laboratory, Bar Harbor, Maine) on 12 measures of nociception (acetic acid and magnesium sulfate writhing tests, autotomy, carrageenan-induced thermal hypersensitivity, peripheral nerve injury-induced thermal and mechanical hypersensitivity, early- and late-phase formalin test, hot-plate test, Hargreaves' test of thermal paw withdrawal, tail-withdrawal test, and von Frey filament test) (Mogil et al. 1999b). These assays, chosen to feature a wide range of nociceptive parameters, included nociceptive, inflammatory, and neuropathic tests, cutaneous and subcutaneous/visceral tests, and short- and long-lasting tests. Samples of 6–23 mice per strain were tested in one of our laboratories, and strain means on all 12 dependent measures were cross-correlated. Because of the large number of correlations involved, multivariate analyses (e.g., multidimensional scaling, principal components analysis) were used to represent the correlations in a two-dimensional space so that "clusters" of highly cross-correlated assays could be identified.

This effort yielded a surprisingly simple result. Using a number of different analyses, we observed that the 12 measures formed three clusters (Mogil et al. 1999c) (see Fig. 2). Cluster 1 contained the autotomy, hot-plate, Hargreaves', and tail-withdrawal tests (r = 0.21–0.85; mean: 0.48). Cluster 2 contained both phases of the formalin test and both types of writhing test (r = 0.29–0.79; mean: 0.56). Cluster 3, which was very broad compared to the others, contained the von Frey test and all three hypersensitivity measures (r = 0.00–0.60; mean: 0.33). The defining feature or dimension of each cluster represented a fundamental pain type. Thus, Cluster 1 contained all three assays employing a *thermal* noxious stimulus. The moderate-to-high correlation of autotomy with the rest of the "thermal" cluster was, of course, unexpected. Cluster 2 contained all four assays featuring spontaneously emitted responses to noxious *chemical* stimuli. This "chemical" cluster included tests of widely varying duration (<5 to >90 minutes), such that inflammation was present in some but not others. The location of the noxious chemical stimulus also did not appear to be critical, since tests featuring intraplantar injection correlated highly with those using intraperitoneal injection. Cluster 3 contained the only test of mechanical sensitivity as well as all three measures of hypersensitivity to evoked stimuli. Referring to a "mechanical + hypersensitivity" cluster, however, obscures the fact that thermal and mechanical hypersensitivity from peripheral nerve injury were in fact entirely uncorrelated (r = 0.00). This is a somewhat startling observation, since we might have expected genetic factors to similarly affect different sequelae of the *same* nerve injury. Also of considerable note were the strong negative genetic correlations between the von Frey test and members of the chemical and (especially) thermal clusters. That is, strains exhibiting

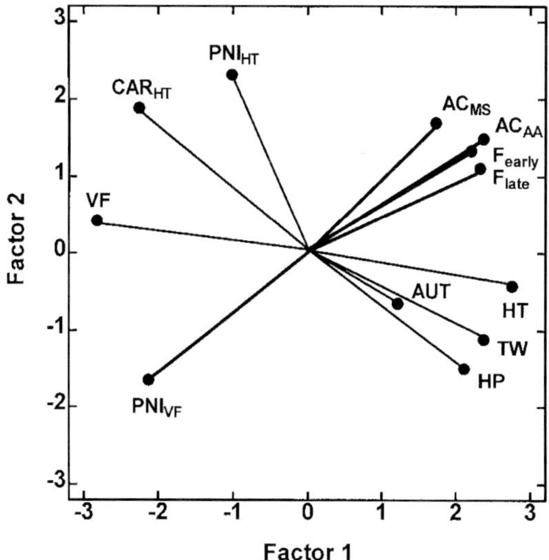

Fig. 2. Principal components analysis plot of the first two unrotated principal components for the genetic correlations between 12 dependent measures of nociception (AC_{AA} = acetic acid abdominal constriction test; AC_{MS} = magnesium sulfate abdominal constriction test; AUT = autotomy; CAR_{HT} = thermal hypersensitivity following carrageenan injection; F_{early} = formalin test, early phase; F_{late} = formalin test, late phase; HT = Hargreaves' test; HP = hot-plate test; PNI_{HT} = thermal hypersensitivity following peripheral nerve injury; PNI_{VF} = mechanical hypersensitivity following peripheral nerve injury; TW = tail-withdrawal test; VF = von Frey filament test). The angle between rays projecting to each point is representative of their cross-correlation; squared ray lengths indicate how much variance in a variable is being reconstructed by the loadings. Acute angles indicate positive correlation, 90° angles indicate no correlation, and obtuse angles indicate negative correlation. Adapted from Mogil et al. (1999c) with permission from Elsevier Science, Inc.

high sensitivity to von Frey filaments were resistant to thermal assays, and vice versa.

These findings confirm fairly common sentiment in the pain research community that the modality of the noxious stimulus (i.e., thermal, chemical, or mechanical) may largely determine the physiological mechanisms activated. At the same time, this study failed to provide evidence for other proposed distinctions. There was no indication that specific genes mediating either inflammatory or neuropathic pain exist, and no support for distinct genetic mediation of supraspinally mediated pain, long-lasting pain, or intense pain. However, our findings do not refute the possibility of such distinctions. For example, Malmberg and colleagues (1997a) observed alterations in thermal hypersensitivity following prostaglandin E_2 injection in transgenic "knockout" mice lacking the *Prkar1b* gene, encoding the type I regulatory subunit of cyclic adenosine monophosphate (cAMP)-dependent protein kinase (PKA RIβ). These mutants displayed, by contrast, entirely normal thermal hypersensitivity following nerve damage (Seltzer et al. (1990) model). Based on these findings, Malmberg et al. (1997a) concluded that this gene was involved in the mediation of inflammatory but not neuropathic nociception. This conclusion is not necessarily incompatible with our demonstration of a moderate-to-high genetic correlation between inflammatory (2% carrageenan) and neuropathic (Kim and Chung 1992 model) thermal hypersensitivity (r = 0.60). It is possible that PKA RIβ is selectively involved in inflammatory nociception, but that all the mouse strains we tested possess identical alleles of its gene.

If a gene is not polymorphic between strains, it will be effectively "invisible" to genetic correlation analysis (and also to gene-mapping efforts). This example reminds us that the demonstration of genetic correlation between nociceptive assays simply implies that some proportion of those genes *responsible for individual differences* are common to the correlated assays, not necessarily all genes. This example also illustrates the complementary roles to be played by "bottom-up" approaches to pain genetics (e.g., transgenesis, antisense studies) versus "top-down" approaches (e.g., gene mapping). The former can identify what genes are associated with a trait; the latter pinpoints which of *those* genes are associated with variability in the trait.

RELIABILITY OF GENETIC CORRELATIONS OF NOCICEPTION

The Mogil et al. (1999b,c) study was subject to a number of limitations. For practical reasons, trade-offs were made among the following competing parameters: (a) number of mice tested per strain, (b) number of strains tested, and (c) number of assays tested. Increasing sample size within a strain would increase the accuracy of the strain means obtained. Increasing the number of strains tested would improve statistical power to assess significance of strain mean correlations, although such power is inherently limited by the commercial availability of only about 30 major inbred strains (not including substrains). Finally, testing additional nociceptive assays would allow more members per cluster, increasing our confidence in each cluster's defining features, and might in addition allow the discovery of distinct clusters not apparent in the initial study. In some cases the correlations obtained may have been confounded by environmental variance and genetic × environmental interactions, given that four of the assays were performed in laboratories other than the author's. Crabbe and colleagues (1999) recently demonstrated the not insubstantial role of unidentified environmental factors in determining the behavioral responses of inbred and transgenic mice.

Data we have collected subsequent to the publication of Mogil et al. (1999b,c) are relevant to these issues. First, we have continued to collect strain survey data (using all, or large subsets, of the 11 strains considered previously, plus the C57BL/10J strain) on several neurochemically distinct antinociceptive modalities. To facilitate comparison, we measured nociception in each case on the 49°C tail-withdrawal assay. Each of these studies was performed by a different investigator (all students in the author's laboratory), at slightly different times of day, in varying seasons, and in some cases using different equipment (e.g., restrainer, heater/circulator, water bath dimensions). Unlike Crabbe and colleagues (1999), we made no heroic attempts to eliminate environmental variance. Nonetheless, correlations between the baseline nociceptive sensitivity of the 12 inbred strains on this thermal assay were consistently high. In all, we have collected 49°C tail-withdrawal data seven times in addition to Mogil et al. (1999b); of 28 possible cross-correlations, 21 exceeded $r = 0.40$ (mean: 0.63) (Flores et al. 1999; Mogil et al. 1999a; unpublished observations). In addition, we have collected strain survey data for two distinct, but putatively related thermal assays. In one case, all 12 strains were tested for sensitivity on the tail-withdrawal test using 47.5°C water. At this temperature, latencies were approximately double those at 49°C. Despite the change in noxious stimulus intensity, the correlation between the two assays was $r = 0.65$ (Mogil and Adhikari 1999). In another experiment on electroacupuncture sensitivity, baseline strain latencies in nine common strains on the radiant heat tail-flick test correlated with those on the 49°C tail-withdrawal test at $r = 0.80$ (unpublished observations).

We have also attempted to replicate findings on assays other than tail withdrawal. These replications are important because they were performed in my laboratory as opposed to other laboratories as part of the Mogil et al. (1999b) study. A strain survey of acetic acid writhing (conducted as part of a study evaluating strain differences in NSAID antinociception), using a more noxious concentration of 0.9% acetic acid, displayed a correlation with 0.6% writhing of $r = 0.91$ (unpublished observations). A strain survey of von Frey filament sensitivity, using a different set of calibrated filaments, nonetheless showed a correlation with previous strain means of $r = 0.74$ (unpublished observations). In sum, these data render confidence in the findings of our original study, and in the use of inbred mouse strains for the study of pain genetics. It is unclear why our attempts at replication were more successful than those of Crabbe and colleagues (1999); perhaps our success derives from the higher heritability of nociceptive sensitivity than many of the behavioral phenotypes studied in their experiment.

GENETIC CORRELATION OF HOT AND COLD NOCICEPTION

The clustering of hot-plate, tail-withdrawal, and Hargreaves' tests (along with autotomy) into a "thermal" cluster left open the question of whether the property of the noxious stimulus underlying the genetic correlation was heat specifically, or simply any extreme of temperature. That is, would strains sensitive to noxious heat also be sensitive to noxious cold, and vice versa? To test this question, we used the –15°C cold-water tail-withdrawal test (Pizziketti et al. 1985). This assay is advantageous because it can be performed virtually identically to the hot water version, the only differences being the use of an immersion cooler versus a heater, and of ethanol versus water. A priori, there were several reasons to believe that hot and cold water nociception would be similar, and other reasons to believe they would dissociate. For example, exposure to very cold stimuli (<0°C) is often described as "burning," although more detailed psychophysical evaluation can dissociate the two perceptions (Morin and Bushnell 1998). Although specifically cold-sensitive afferents may exist in the mouse (Koltzenburg et al. 1997), a recent study reported that noxious cold of sufficient intensity can excite *all* heat-sensitive afferents (Simone and Kajander 1996). Temperature specificity appears to be all but lost in spinal cord neurons (e.g., Kenshalo et al. 1982), but Tiseo and colleagues (1990) observed a noxious-cold-specific release of substance P in the spinal cord, in contrast to a noxious-heat-specific release of somatostatin. This same group has demonstrated a differential sensitivity of the hot-water and cold-water tail-withdrawal tests to inhibition by different opioid receptor agonists (Tiseo et al. 1988; Adams et al. 1993). Finally, functional imaging studies of heat and cold pain in humans have revealed both similarities and differences (e.g., Casey et al. 1996).

Despite the considerable evidence on both sides of this issue, the results of our study (Mogil and Adhikari 1999) were unambiguous. Correlations between mean strain withdrawal responses to –15°, 49°, and 47.5°C water (exhibiting equal grand mean latencies to –15°C) were in the range of r = 0.49–0.77. Although distinct cold nociception genes may exist, our data strongly suggest genetic and thus physiological commonality between heat and cold pain.

IS VISCERAL NOCICEPTION GENETICALLY DISTINCT?

Another question left unresolved by Mogil et al. (1999b,c) concerns visceral nociception. There is reason to believe that the processing of visceral nociception is distinct from that of somatic nociception, despite the known convergence of input to the spinal cord (Hancock et al. 1975). Many stimuli that are clearly noxious when applied to the skin (e.g., heat, cutting) are usually not perceived as painful when applied to the viscera (see Ness and Gebhart 1990; McMahon et al. 1995). In contrast to somatic pain, visceral pain is dull and poorly localized, but can be referred to somatic structures. Visceral nerves contain many fewer large myelinated fibers in comparison to cutaneous nerves, and practically no Aβ fibers (see McMahon 1997). Differential patterns of expression of the immediate early gene, *c-fos*, have been associated with somatic and visceral stimuli in the spinal cord and brainstem (Menetrey et al. 1989; Lanteri-Minet et al. 1993). Finally, a pathway in the posterior funiculus may selectively signal visceral pain (Hirshberg et al. 1996).

Although Mogil et al. (1999b,c) included the acetic acid and magnesium sulfate writhing tests, neither is a "pure" visceral assay. In both cases, the intraperitoneally injected irritants contact not only visceral tissues but also the muscle wall of the abdomen, which is of somatic origin. Our attempts to obtain reliable data in the mouse using the colorectal distention test (Anderson et al. 1987), a commonly used visceral assay in the rat, have been largely unsuccessful. However, we (and others; Olivar and Laird 1999) have succeeded in adapting for use in mice another visceral pain test developed in the rat, cyclophosphamide cystitis (Lanteri-Minet et al. 1995). Cyclophosphamide is an anticancer agent with a well-known toxic side effect on the bladder. Its metabolite, acrolein, accumulates in the bladder, and on prolonged contact with the bladder wall it generates painful cystitis. No strain of mouse we have tested so far displayed the characteristic rounded-back posture, or any other abnormal behaviors, described in rats (Lanteri-Minet et al. 1995). However, we have demonstrated a dose-dependent reduction in voluntary locomotion (with no concomitant ataxia) in cyclophosphamide-treated mice, and also dose-dependent hypersensitivity (i.e., referred pain) in the tail base region (K. Bon, C.A. Lichtensteiger, and J.S. Mogil, unpublished data).

We quantified the extent of hypolocomotion, as a surrogate for intensity of visceral nociception, in all 12 inbred strains. The dependent measure considered was percentage decrease in locomotor counts (using an automated system, with each mouse individually housed in its home cage) relative to saline-treated mice of the same strain, a variable that not unexpectedly showed large strain differences as well. The percentage of hypolocomotion did not correlate particularly well with basal locomotor activity (r = 0.33), and thus we believe that these data were not confounded by strain variability in exploratory behavior.

We found no striking correlations between cyclophosphamide hypolocomotion and any other nociceptive assay, including acetic acid writhing (r = 0.08) and magnesium sulfate writhing (r = –0.23). We tentatively conclude that genes specific to visceral nociception may exist, although this finding needs to be replicated and alternative interpretations need to be examined.

IMPLICATIONS

The finding of a restricted number of fundamental pain "types," defined largely by the modality of the noxious stimulus, has several implications. With respect to the further study of pain genetics, these data suggest that three separate gene-mapping studies need to be performed. The only nociceptive modality ever subjected to quantitative trait locus (QTL) mapping is thermal nociception (hot-plate test) (Mogil et al. 1997). In this study we demonstrated the male-specific role of the *Oprd1* gene (and its protein product, the δ_2-opioid receptor) in baseline hot-plate latencies. Efforts are presently underway in my laboratory to replicate and extend this finding using other members of the thermal cluster, the Hargreaves' and tail-withdrawal tests. Also nearing completion are QTL-mapping studies of chemical nociception using the formalin test, and of mechanical sensitivity using the von Frey filament test. Although it should be noted that QTL-mapping studies are limited to detecting genes that are polymorphic between the progenitor strains used, these experiments should provide a fairly comprehensive description of genomic regions containing genes underlying variability in nociceptive sensitivity. As predicted by the lack of correlation between thermal and chemical nociceptive assays, QTLs thus far uncovered for the formalin test are in every case distinct from those for the thermal assays (unpublished observations).

The implications of these data for humans are more tenuous. Several investigations have used various assays to uncover the correlation between experimental pain thresholds and tolerance levels in humans (e.g., Chapman and Jones 1944; Clark and Bindra 1956; Wolff and Jarvik 1964; Davidson and McDougall 1969; Harris and Rollman 1983). The findings of these studies are quite discrepant, and no consensus has ever been reached. There has certainly never been any demonstration in humans, for instance, of a negative correlation between thermal and mechanical sensitivity; indeed, Clark and Bindra (1956) observed significantly *positive* correlations between sensitivity to radiant heat and mechanical pressure. All relevant human studies were evaluating overall phenotypic correlations, including both genetic and environmental variation, whereas our studies in the mouse considered only genetic correlations. Thus, the different conclusions may reflect a species difference or the influence of shared environmental variance in the human studies. The correlations among nociceptive assays in laboratory mice (and the apparent pain taxonomy derived from them) may or may not be directly applicable to human beings. However, since the mouse is quickly becoming the preferred subject for preclinical pain research, a more complete understanding of nociceptive mechanisms in mice will undoubtedly facilitate progress in the treatment of pain in humans.

ACKNOWLEDGMENTS

The author is supported by PHS grants DA11394 and DE12735. We thank Drs. John Belknap, Bill Roberts, and Marshall Devor for helpful discussions on this topic.

REFERENCES

Adams JU, Tallarida RJ, Geller EB, Adler MW. Isobolographic superadditivity between *delta* and *mu* opioid agonists in the rat depends on the ratio of compounds, the *mu* agonist and the analgesic assay used. *J Pharmacol Exp Ther* 1993; 266:1261–1267.

Anderson R, Ness TJ, Gebhart GF. A distension control device useful for quantitative studies of hollow organ sensation. *Physiol Behav* 1987; 41:635–638.

Arnér S, Meyerson BA. Lack of analgesic effect of opioids on neuropathic and idiopathic forms of pain. *Pain* 1988; 33:11–23.

Baran A, Shuster L, Eleftheriou BE, Bailey DW. Opiate receptors in mice: genetic differences. *Life Sci* 1975; 17:633–640.

Beecher HK. Generalization from pain of various types and diverse origins. *Science* 1959; 130:267–270.

Belknap JK, O'Toole LA. Studies of genetic differences in response to opioid drugs. In: Harris RA, Crabbe JC (Eds). *The Genetic Basis of Alcohol and Drug Actions.* New York: Plenum Press, 1991, pp 225–252.

Belknap JK, Haltli NR, Goebel DM, Lamé M. Selective breeding for high and low levels of opiate-induced analgesia in mice. *Behav Genet* 1983; 13:383–396.

Bennett GJ, Xie Y-K. A peripheral mononeuropathy in rat that produces disorders of pain sensation like those seen in man. *Pain* 1988; 33:87–107.

Cao YQ, Mantyh PW, Carlson EJ, et al. Primary afferent tachykinins are required to experience moderate to intense pain. *Nature* 1998; 392:390–394.

Carey G. Inference about genetic correlations. *Behav Genet* 1988; 18:329–338.

Casey KL, Minoshima S, Morrow TJ, Koeppe RA. Comparison of human cerebral activation pattern during cutaneous warmth, heat pain, and deep cold pain. *J Neurophysiol* 1996; 76:571–581.

Chapman WP, Jones CM. Variations in cutaneous and visceral pain sensitivity in normal subjects. *J Clin Invest* 1944; 23:81–91.

Clark JW, Bindra D. Individual differences in pain thresholds. *Can J Psychol* 1956; 10:69–76.

Cooper BY, Vierck CJ, Yeomans DC. Selective reduction of second pain sensations by systemic morphine in humans. *Pain* 1986; 24:93–116.

Crabbe JC, Phillips TJ, Kosobud A, Belknap JK. Estimation of genetic correlation: interpretation of experiments using selectively bred and inbred animals. *Alcohol: Clin Exp Res* 1990; 14:141–151.

Crabbe JC, Wahlsten D, Dudek BC. Genetics of mouse behavior: interactions with laboratory environment. *Science* 1999; 284:1670–1672.

Crawley JN, Belknap JK, Collins A, et al. Behavioral phenotypes of inbred mouse strains: implications and recommendations for molecular studies. *Psychopharmacology* 1997; 132:107–124.

Davidson PO, McDougall CEA. The generality of pain tolerance. *J Psychosom Res* 1969; 13:83–89.

DeLeo JA, Coombs DW, McCarthy LE. Differential c-fos-like protein expression in mechanically versus chemically induced visceral nociception. *Mol Brain Res* 1991; 11:167–170.

Dennis SG, Melzack R. Comparison of phasic and tonic pain in animals. In: Bonica JJ (Ed). *Advances in Pain Research and Therapy,* Vol. 3. New York: Raven Press, 1979, pp 747–760.

Dennis SG, Melzack R, Gutman S, Boucher F. Pain modulation by adrenergic agents and morphine as measured by three pain tests. *Life Sci* 1980; 26:1247–1259.

Devor M, Raber P. Heritability of symptoms in an experimental model of neuropathic pain. *Pain* 1990; 42:51–67.

Elmer GI, Pieper JO, Negus SS, Woods JH. Genetic variance in innate nociception and its relationship to the potency of morphine-induced analgesia in thermal and chemical tests. *Pain* 1997; 75:129–140.

Flores CM, Wilson SG, Mogil JS. Pharmacogenetic variability in neuronal nicotinic receptor-mediated antinociception. *Pharmacogenetics* 1999; 9:619–625.

Giordano J, Dyche J. Differential analgesic actions of serotonin 5-HT_3 receptor antagonists in the mouse. *Neuropharmacology* 1989; 28:423–427.

Hammond DL. Inference of pain and its modulation from simple behaviors. In: Chapman CR, Loeser JD (Eds). *Advances in Pain Research and Therapy: Issues in Pain Management.* New York: Raven Press, 1989, pp 69–91.

Hancock MB, Foreman RD, Willis WD. Convergence of visceral and cutaneous input onto spinothalamic tract cells in the thoracic spinal cord of the cat. *Exp Neurol* 1975; 47:240–248.

Harris G, Rollman GB. The validity of experimental pain measures. *Pain* 1983; 17:369–376.

Hirshberg RM, Al-Chaer ED, Lawand NB, et al. Is there a pathway in the posterior funiculus that signals visceral pain? *Pain* 1996; 67:291–305.

Ingram DK, Corfman TP. An overview of neurobiological comparisons in mouse strains. *Neurosci Biobehav Rev* 1980; 4:421–435.

Keay KA, Bandler R. Deep and superficial noxious stimulation increases Fos-like immunoreactivity in different regions of the midbrain periaqueductal grey of the rat. *Neurosci Lett* 1993; 154:23–26.

Kenshalo DR, Jr, Leonard RB, Chung JM, Willis WD. Facilitation of the responses of primate spinothalamic cells to cold and to tactile stimuli by noxious heating of the skin. *Pain* 1982; 12:141–152.

Kim SH, Chung JM. An experimental model for peripheral neuropathy produced by segmental spinal nerve ligation in the rat. *Pain* 1992; 50:355–363.

Koltzenburg M, Stucky CL, Lewin GR. Receptive properties of mouse sensory neurons innervating hairy skin. *J Neurophysiol* 1997; 78:1841–1850.

Konig M, Zimmer AM, Steiner H, et al. Pain responses, anxiety and aggression in mice deficient in pre-proenkephalin. *Nature* 1996; 383:535–538.

Lanteri-Minet M, Isnardon P, de Pommery J, Menetrey D. Spinal and hindbrain structures involved in visceroception and visceronociception as revealed by the expression of Fos, Jun and Krox-24 proteins. *Neuroscience* 1993; 55:737–753.

Lanteri-Minet M, Bon K, de Pommery J, et al. Cyclophosphamide cystitis as a model of visceral pain in rats: model elaboration and spinal structures involved as revealed by the expression of c-Fos and Krox-24 proteins. *Exp Brain Res* 1995; 105:220–232.

Lee SH, Kayser V, Desmeules J, Guilbaud G. Differential action of morphine and various opioid agonists on thermal allodynia and hyperalgesia in mononeuropathic rats. *Pain* 1994; 57:233–240.

Lima D, Avelino A, Coimbra A. Differential activation of c-*fos* in spinal neurones by distinct classes of noxious stimuli. *Neuroreport* 1993; 4:747–750.

Malmberg AB, Brandon EP, Idzerda RL, et al. Diminished inflammation and nociceptive pain with preservation of neuropathic pain in mice with a targeted mutation of the Type I regulatory subunit of cAMP-dependent protein kinase. *J Neurosci* 1997a; 17:7462–7470.

Malmberg AB, Chen C, Tonegawa S, Basbaum AI. Preserved acute pain and reduced neuropathic pain in mice lacking PKCγ. *Science* 1997b; 278:279–283.

McMahon SB. Are there fundamental differences in the peripheral mechanisms of visceral and somatic pain? *Behav Brain Sci* 1997; 20:381–391.

McMahon SB, Dmitrieva N, Koltzenburg M. Visceral pain. *Br J Anaesth* 1995; 75:132–144.

Meller ST. Thermal and mechanical hyperalgesia: a distinct role for different excitatory amino acid receptors and signal transduction pathways? *APS J* 1994; 3:215–231.

Menetrey D, Gannon A, Levine JD, Basbaum AI. Expression of c-*fos* protein in interneurons and projection neurons of the rat spinal cord in response to noxious somatic, articular, and visceral stimulation. *J Comp Neurol* 1989; 258:177–195.

Mogil JS. The genetic mediation of individual differences in sensitivity to pain and its inhibition. *Proc Natl Acad Sci USA* 1999; 96:7744–7751.

Mogil JS, Adhikari SM. Hot and cold nociception are genetically correlated. *J Neurosci* 1999; 19:RC25(1–5).

Mogil JS, Kest B, Sadowski B, Belknap JK. Differential genetic mediation of sensitivity to morphine in genetic models of opiate antinociception: influence of nociceptive assay. *J Pharmacol Exp Ther* 1996; 276:532–544.

Mogil JS, Richards SP, O'Toole LA, et al. Genetic sensitivity to hot-plate nociception in DBA/2J and C57BL/6J inbred mouse strains: possible sex-specific mediation by δ_2-opioid receptors. *Pain* 1997; 70:267–277.

Mogil JS, Nessim LA, Wilson SG. Strain-dependent effects of supraspinal orphanin FQ/nociceptin on thermal nociceptive sensitivity in mice. *Neurosci Lett* 1999a; 261:147–150.

Mogil JS, Wilson SG, Bon K, et al. Heritability of nociception. I. Responses of eleven inbred mouse strains on twelve measures of nociception. *Pain* 1999b; 80:67–82.

Mogil JS, Wilson SG, Bon K, et al. Heritability of nociception. II. "Types" of nociception revealed by genetic correlation analysis. *Pain* 1999c; 80:83–93.

Morin C, Bushnell MC. Temporal and qualitative properties of cold pain and heat pain: a psychophysical study. *Pain* 1998; 74:67–73.

Ness TJ, Gebhart GF. Visceral pain: a review of experimental studies. *Pain* 1990; 41:167–234.

Olivar T, Laird JMA. Cyclophosphamide cystitis in mice: behavioural characterisation and correlation with bladder inflammation. *Eur J Pain* 1999; 3:141–149.

Panocka I, Marek P, Sadowski B. Inheritance of stress-induced analgesia in mice. Selective breeding study. *Brain Res* 1986; 397:152–155.

Pizziketti RJ, Pressman NS, Geller EB, et al. Rat cold water tail-flick: a novel analgesic test that distinguishes opioid agonists from mixed agonist-antagonists. *Eur J Pharmacol* 1985; 119:23–29.

Ryan SM, Watkins LR, Mayer DJ, Maier SF. Spinal pain suppression mechanisms may differ for phasic and tonic pain. *Brain Res* 1985; 334:172–175.

Seltzer Z, Dubner R, Shir Y. A novel behavioral model of causalgiform pain produced by partial sciatic nerve injury in rats. *Pain* 1990; 43:205–218.

Shir Y, Raber P, Devor M, Seltzer Z. Mechano- and thermo-sensitivity in rats genetically prone to developing neuropathic pain. *Neuroreport* 1991; 2:313–316.

Silver LE. *Mouse Genetics: Concepts and Applications*. New York: Oxford University Press, 1995.

Simone DA, Kajander KC. Excitation of rat cutaneous nociceptors by noxious cold. *Neurosci Lett* 1996; 213:53–56.

Suh HH, Fujimoto JM, Tseng LF. Differential mechanisms mediating β-endorphin- and morphine-induced analgesia in mice. *Eur J Pharmacol* 1989; 168:61–70.

Taddese A, Nah S-Y, McCleskey EW. Selective opioid inhibition of small nociceptive neurons. *Science* 1995; 270:1366–1369.

Tiseo PJ, Geller EB, Adler MW. Antinociceptive action of intracerebroventricularly administered dynorphin and other opioid peptides in the rat. *J Pharmacol Exp Ther* 1988; 246:449–453.

Tiseo PJ, Adler MW, Liu-Chen L-Y. Differential release of substance P and somatostatin in the rat spinal cord in response to noxious cold and heat; effect of dynorphin $A_{(1-17)}$. *J Pharmacol Exp Ther* 1990; 252:539–545.

Treede R-D, Meyer RA, Raja SN, Campbell JN. Peripheral and central mechanisms of cutaneous hyperalgesia. *Prog Neurobiol* 1992; 38:397–421.

Tyers MB. A classification of opiate receptors that mediate antinociception in animals. *Br J Pharmacol* 1980; 69:503–512.

Vierck CJ, Jr., Cooper BY. Guidelines for assessing pain reactions and pain modulation in laboratory animal subjects. In: Kruger L, Liebeskind JC (Eds). *Advances in Pain Research and Therapy,* Vol. 6. New York: Raven Press, 1984, pp 305–322.

Willis WD. *The Pain System.* Karger: Basel, 1985.

Wolff BB, Jarvik ME. Relationship between superficial and deep somatic thresholds of pain with a note on handedness. *Am J Psychol* 1964; 77:589–599.

Woolf CJ. Somatic pain—pathogenesis and prevention. *Br J Anaesth* 1995; 75:169–176.

Woolf CJ, Bennett GJ, Doherty M, et al. Towards a mechanism-based classification of pain? *Pain* 1998; 77:227–229.

Yamamoto T, Nozaki-Taguchi N. Effects of intrathecally administered nociceptin, an opioid receptor-like$_1$ receptor agonist, and *N*-methyl-D-aspartate receptor antagonists on the thermal hyperalgesia induced by partial sciatic nerve injury in the rat. *Anesthesiology* 1997; 87:1145–1152.

Yeomans DC, Pirec V, Proudfit HK. Nociceptive responses to high and low rates of noxious cutaneous heating are mediated by different nociceptors in the rat: behavioral evidence. *Pain* 1996; 68:133–140.

Zimmer A, Zimmer AM, Baffi J, et al. Hypoalgesia in mice with a targeted deletion of the tachykinin 1 gene. *Proc Natl Acad Sci USA* 1998; 95:2630–2635.

Correspondence to: Jeffrey S. Mogil, PhD, Department of Psychology, University of Illinois at Urbana-Champaign, 603 E. Daniel Street, Champaign, IL 61820, USA. Tel: 217-333-6546; Fax: 217-244-5876; email: jmogil@s.psych.uiuc.edu.

Proceedings of the 9th World Congress on Pain,
Progress in Pain Research and Management,
Vol. 16, edited by M. Devor, M.C. Rowbotham, and
Z. Wiesenfeld-Hallin, IASP Press, Seattle, © 2000.

45

Angiotensin-Converting Enzyme Gene Polymorphism in Patients with Neuropathic Pain

Tomomasa Kimura, Toru Komatsu, Renko Hosoda, Kimitoshi Nishiwaki, and Yasuhiro Shimada

Department of Anesthesiology, Nagoya University School of Medicine, Nagoya, Japan

The mechanism of neuropathic pain might be partly associated with sympathetic nervous system activities through the renin-angiotensin system. An insertion/deletion (I/D) gene polymorphism of the angiotensin-converting enzyme (ACE) gene present in intron 16 is a major determinant of plasma ACE activity, and previous research has shown that the DD genotype of the ACE gene has been associated with cardiovascular disease (Cambien et al. 1992). The aim of this study was to explore, in patients with neuropathic pain, whether ACE gene polymorphism is associated with genetic predisposition to neuropathic pain.

MATERIALS AND METHODS

After obtaining approval by the local review board and written informed consent, we genotyped 26 patients with complex regional pain syndrome (CRPS) for the I/D polymorphism. CRPS was diagnosed in all patients according to the standardized criteria published by the International Association for the Study of Pain (IASP; Merskey and Bogduk 1994). Patients who were taking ACE inhibitor were excluded from the study. CRPS is a new term for conditions formerly known as either reflex sympathetic dystrophy (RSD or CRPS type I) or causalgia (CRPS type II). This syndrome is often extremely painful and disabling, and is characterized by peripheral vasoconstriction and cyanotic skin, in addition to spontaneous pain and hyperalgesia. Despite many theories, the mechanism of CRPS is still unknown.

DNA was extracted from peripheral white blood cells. The 287-base pairs (bp) I/D polymorphism in intron 16 of the ACE gene was examined by polymerase chain reaction (PCR) amplification, resulting in three genotypes (DD and II homozygotes, and ID heterozygotes) (Rigat et al. 1990). PCR amplification of the I/D region of the ACE gene was performed with oligonucleotide primers (Rigat et al. 1992). The primer sequences were 5´CTGGAGACCACTCCCATCCTTTCT3´ (sense) and 5´GATATAACCATCACATTCGTCAGAT3´ (antisense). PCR was performed in a final volume of 100µL, which contained 10 µL of extracted DNA solution, 100 pmol of each primer, 200 µM each of the four deoxynucleoside triphosphates (dATP, dCIP, dGTP, dTTP), 1.5 mM $MgCl_2$, 50 mM KCl, 10 mM Tris-HCl, and 2.5 units of Taq polymerase (Boehringer Mannheim). DNA was amplified for 30 cycles, each consisting of denaturation at 93°C for 1.5 minutes, annealing at 58°C for 2 minutes, and extension at 72°C for 2 minutes. The PCR products were electrophoresed in 2% agarose gels, and DNA was visualized directly with ethidium bromide staining under UV light. The ACE gene polymorphism was characterized by three genotypes: two insertion alleles (genotype II), two deletion alleles (genotype DD), and heterozygous alleles (genotype ID). Serum ACE activity was measured by the colorimetric method (Kasahara and Ashihara 1981), and plasma renin activity and angiotensin I and II were determined by radioimmunoassay.

Differences among the three genotype groups were compared by ANOVA. The genotypic distributions were analyzed by Fisher's exact probabilities test. $P < 0.05$ was considered statistically significant.

RESULTS

The demographic characteristics and variables of the renin-angiotensin system of the neuropathic pain patients are summarized in Table I. No significant difference in arterial blood pressure, heart rate, plasma renin activity, or angiotensin I and II were detected among the ACE genotypes. Serum ACE activity was significantly higher in subjects with the ACE DD genotype than in subjects with the ID and II genotypes (Fig. 1). The distribution of the DD, ID, and II genotypes in the study group was 27%, 38% and 35%, respectively; there was an overall frequency of 46% for the *D* allele and 54% for the *I* allele. When grouped according to CRPS type, the distribution of CRPS type I was higher in those homozygous for the ACE gene deletion (86%) than in those homozygous for the ACE gene insertion (22%) ($P = 0.04$).

Table I
Demographic details and distribution of ACE gene alleles in patients with neuropathic pain with predisposition to CRPS types I and II

	ACE Genotype		
Variable	DD	ID	II
No. patients	7	10	9
Sex (M/F)	3/4	6/4	6/3
Age (y)	48 ± 16	45 ± 16	61 ± 11
SBP (mm Hg)	117 ± 14	119 ± 20	143 ± 33
DBP (mm Hg)	69 ± 11	74 ± 134	82 ± 9
Heart rate (beats/min)	80 ± 9	77 ± 17	82 ± 9
ACE (IU/L)	19.3 ± 5.1	13.8 ± 3.9*	13.5 ± 2.7*
PRA ($ng{\cdot}mL^{-1}{\cdot}h^{-1}$)	1.8 ± 2.0	3.0 ± 3.2	1.7 ± 0.7
ANG-I (pg/mL)	603 ± 226	746 ± 399	520 ± 127
ANG-II (pg/mL)	26 ± 30	35 ± 24	25 ± 12
Hypertension	2	0	2
CRPS, type I	6	6	2
CRPS, type II	1	4	7

Note: Values are mean ± SD or number. ACE: angiotensin-converting enzyme; ANG = angiotensin; CRPS: complex regional pain syndrome; DBP = diastolic blood pressure; PRA = plasma renin activity; SBP = systolic blood pressure.

* $P < 0.05$ vs. DD.

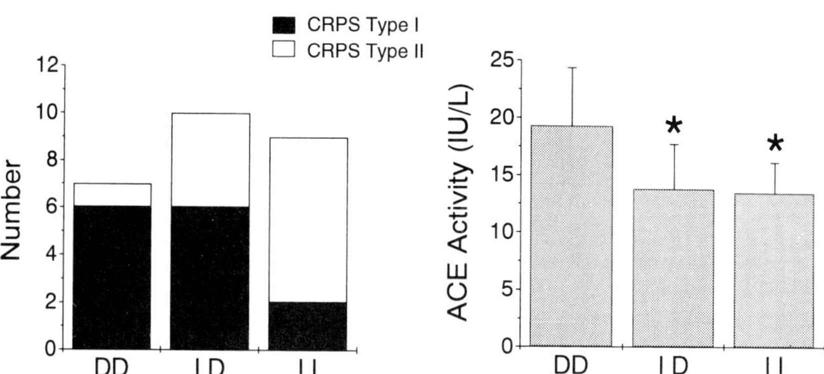

Fig. 1. Left: distribution of polymorphism of the angiotensin-converting enzyme gene. Right: comparison of serum ACE activity among the ACE genotypes. CRPS = complex regional pain syndrome; ACE = angiotensin-converting enzyme. Error bars denote SD. Asterisks denote $P < 0.05$ in comparison to the DD genotype.

DISCUSSION

Complex mechanisms and numerous pathways underlie the pathophysiology of pain perception. The cardiovascular control network shares determinants with the antinociceptive system, including various central and peripheral neurotransmitters, as well as anatomic nuclei and projections (Aicher and Randich 1990). Cardiovascular and pain-regulatory systems do not exist in isolation, but instead interact to maintain homeostasis. In addition, both in animal and human studies, hypertension has been associated with a reduced perception of painful stimuli (Guasti et al. 1998).

Activity in the renin-angiotensin system may influence the levels of peptides involved in pain processing (Fig. 2). The existence of local renin-angiotensin system components and the characteristic distribution of angiotensin II (ANG-II) receptors in the brain suggest that brain endogenous ANG-II has several roles in the central nervous system, including the central nociceptive mechanism (Takai et al. 1996).

ACE plays an important role in the production of ANG-II, which is a key component of the renin-angiotensin system; the renin-angiotensin system in general is thought to be involved in the modulation of vascular tone and in the proliferation of smooth muscle cells. The frequency of the ACE DD genotype in the study population (27%) is higher than that previously described in normal populations of Japanese people (less than 20%) (Rotimi

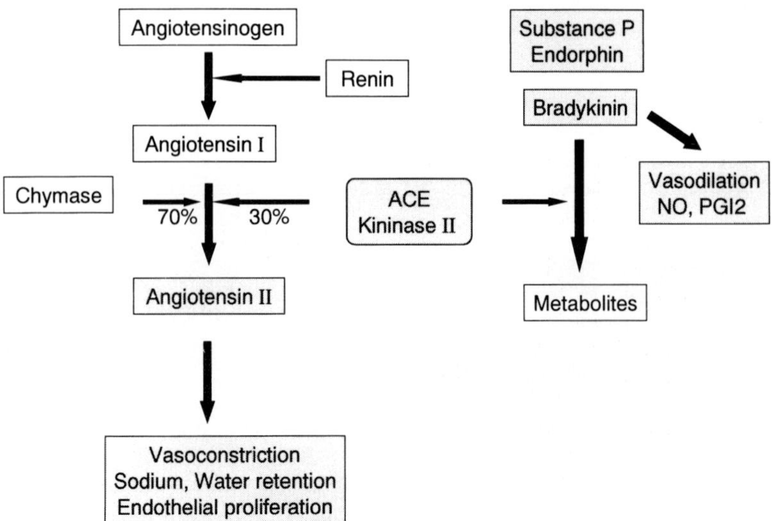

Fig. 2. Sequence of the reactions of the renin-angiotensin system with special reference to nociception. ACE = angiotensin-converting enzyme, NO = nitric oxide, PGI2 = prostaglandin I_2. Gray areas are considered to be associated with nociception.

et al. 1996; Samani et al. 1996). Further multi-center studies will be required to verify the ACE genotypic distribution in CRPS patients, since we used a small number of patients in the current study.

It is possible that the DD genotype favors the development of neuropathic pain as well as cardiovascular disease, perhaps because of higher ACE concentrations. Elevated ACE activity in these subjects may result in increased ANG-II levels in the peripheral effector site, and this putative mechanism could underlie the association between the ACE deletion polymorphism and the increased genetic risk for susceptibility to neuropathic pain. Thus, our data indicate that CRPS type I, which frequently occurs even when definitive evidence of nerve injury is lacking, might be influenced more by the renin-angiotensin system than is CRPS type II.

CONCLUSIONS

The distribution of the DD, ID, and II genotypes in the current study group was 27%, 38%, and 35%, respectively. ACE/DD genotype is a significant risk factor for CRPS type I in Japanese, perhaps through the presence of high serum ACE concentrations. We favor the hypothesis of interplay between renin-angiotensin mechanisms and intrinsic analgesic modulation in pain sensitivity in patients with neuropathic pain. Typing for ACE I/D gene polymorphism might thus be a useful predictor of neuropathic pain susceptibility.

REFERENCES

Aicher SA, Randich A. Antinociception and cardiovascular responses produced by electrical stimulation in the nucleus tractus solitarius, nucleus reticularis ventralis, and the caudal medulla. *Pain* 1990; 42:103–119.

Cambien F, Poirier O, Lecerf L, et al. Deletion polymorphism in the gene for angiotensin-converting enzyme is a potent risk factor for myocardial infarction. *Nature* 1992; 359:641–644.

Guasti L, Grimoldi P, Diolisi A, et al. Treatment with enalapril modifies the pain perception pattern in hypertensive patients. *Hypertension* 1998; 31:1146–1150.

Kasahara Y, Ashihara Y. Colorimetry of angiotensin-I converting enzyme activity in serum. *Clin Chem* 1981; 27:1922–1925.

Merskey H, Bogduk N. *Classification of Chronic Pain: Descriptions of Chronic Pain Syndromes and Definitions of Pain Terms*, 2nd ed. Seattle: IASP Press, 1994.

Rigat B, Hubert C, Alhenc-Gelas F, et al. An insertion/deletion polymorphism in the angiotensin I-converting enzyme gene accounting for half the variance of serum enzyme levels. *J Clin Invest* 1990; 86:1343–1346.

Rigat B, Hubert C, Corvol P, Soubrier F. PCR detection of the insertion/deletion polymorphism of the human angiotensin converting enzyme gene (DCP1) (dipeptidyl carboxypeptidase 1). *Nucleic Acids Res* 1992; 20:1433.

Rotimi C, Puras A, Cooper R, et al. Polymorphisms of renin-angiotensin genes among Nigerians, Jamaicans, and African Americans. *Hypertension* 1996; 27(part 2):558–563.

Samani NJ, Thompson JR, O'Toole L, et al. A meta-analysis of the association of the deletion allele of the angiotensin-converting enzyme gene with myocardial infarction. *Circulation* 1996; 94:708–712.

Takai S, Song K, Tanaka T, Okunishi H, Miyazaki M. Antinociceptive effects of angiotensin-converting enzyme inhibitors and an angiotensin II receptor antagonist in mice. *Life Sci* 1996; 59:PL331–PL336.

Correspondence to: Tomomasa Kimura, MD, Department of Anesthesiology, Nagoya University School of Medicine, Tsuruma-cho 65, Showa-ku, Nagoya 466-8550, Japan. Tel: 81-52-744-2340; Fax: 81-52-744-2342; email: tomo@med.nagoya-u.ac.jp.

Proceedings of the 9th World Congress on Pain, Progress in Pain Research and Management, Vol. 16, edited by M. Devor, M.C. Rowbotham, and Z. Wiesenfeld-Hallin, IASP Press, Seattle, © 2000.

46

Pre- but Not Postoperative Consumption of Soy Suppresses Pain Behavior following Partial Sciatic Ligation in Rats

Yoram Shir,[a] James N. Campbell,[b] Srinivasa N. Raja,[c] and Ze'ev Seltzer[d]

[a]Department of Anesthesiology and Pain Relief Unit, Hadassah University Hospital, Jerusalem, Israel; [b]Department of Neurosurgery and [c]Department of Anesthesiology, Johns Hopkins Medical Institutions, Baltimore, Maryland, USA; [d]Department of Physiology, Faculties of Medicine and Dental Medicine, Hebrew University, Jerusalem, Israel

Unilateral partial sciatic ligation (PSL) produces in rodents a model that resembles neuropathic pain in humans (Seltzer et al. 1990; Seltzer and Shir 1991). In our laboratory over the first 5 years after introduction of this model, rats with PSL injury developed signs of spontaneous pain and robust mechanical and heat hyperalgesia and allodynia. Subsequently, however, we encountered unexplained difficulties in replicating the robust expression of the original PSL model. Investigation revealed that diet critically affects sensory disorders of rats following PSL injury. Consuming diets containing soy significantly reduced the development of neuropathic sensory disorders, whereas consumption of soy-free diets produced levels of sensory disorders similar in magnitude to the original ones (Shir et al. 1997, 1998). Our current study investigated whether both phases of soy feeding (i.e., pre- vs. postinjury) are essential for suppressing the sensory disorders produced by the PSL injury.

METHODS

This study was conducted according to the regulations of the Hebrew and Johns Hopkins universities and of the national animal care and use committee for humane experimentation on animals, and in accordance with the guidelines of the International Association for the Study of Pain (Zimmermann 1983).

Eight groups of male Wistar rats (n = 10 rats/group), weighing 200–250 g at the time of surgery, were used in this study. Under ether anesthesia the right sciatic nerve was exposed high in the thigh, the dorsal one-third to one-half of the nerve thickness was tightly ligated with an 8-0 silk suture, and the wound was closed (for detailed description see Seltzer at al. 1990).

Behavioral tests. A researcher blinded to the type of diet the rats consumed determined the responses of intact and PSL-injured rats to tactile and thermal stimuli. Testing was done 1 day prior to PSL surgery and repeated on days 3, 8, and 14 thereafter. Intact rats were tested on days 13, 16, 22, and 28 of the experiment. *Tactile sensibility:* Withdrawal threshold to repetitive touch was measured with a set of nine calibrated von Frey hairs, ranging from 0.3 to 27 g. After 5 minutes of acclimation in the testing chamber the test hair was indented rapidly (twice per second) 5 times on the midplantar skin of the hindpaw until it bowed. If subthreshold, the stimulus intensity was increased by using the next hair in the series. At threshold rats responded by elevating the paw. *Noxious heat sensibility:* We used the Hargreaves device to progressively heat the midplantar area of the rat's hindpaw until the rat withdrew its paw from the stimulus. The time that lapsed between paw lifting until placing the paw back on the floor was recorded with a stop watch ("response duration"). Each paw was tested three times, alternating between the paws, with an interval of 5 minutes between tests to avoid sensitization. The response duration of each paw was calculated as the average of the three tests.

Diets. Two types of diets were compared: a diet based on soy protein (RMH-1000; PMI Feeds, St. Louis, MO; "RMH"), and a diet based on casein as its sole protein source (Bio-Serv Co., Frenchtown, NJ; "CAS"). RMH is a commercially available balanced diet, comprising 14% protein, 66% carbohydrates, 6% fat, 4.5% fiber, 8% ash, vitamins, and trace elements. Approximately 85% of the protein in RMH is derived from crude soy products. CAS is an artificial balanced diet, comprising 20% casein protein, 65% carbohydrates, 5% fat, 5% fiber, and 3.5% ash, with vitamins and trace elements (Whitten and Naftolin 1992). In unpublished preliminary experiments on nerve-injured rats fed on soy-containing diets, similar weak levels of sensory disorders were recorded for soy concentrations of 10% and 20%. We thus assumed that within the range of 10–20% soy concentration, diets based on soy are interchangeable in their ability to prevent the expression of sensory disorders in this model. Consequently, we used the RMH diet (containing 12% soy protein) in our study.

Feeding groups. We compared six different feeding regimes (Fig. 1a) in eight groups of rats. Six groups received a PSL injury and two groups remained intact to serve as controls (experiments C14/C14 and R14/R14 were

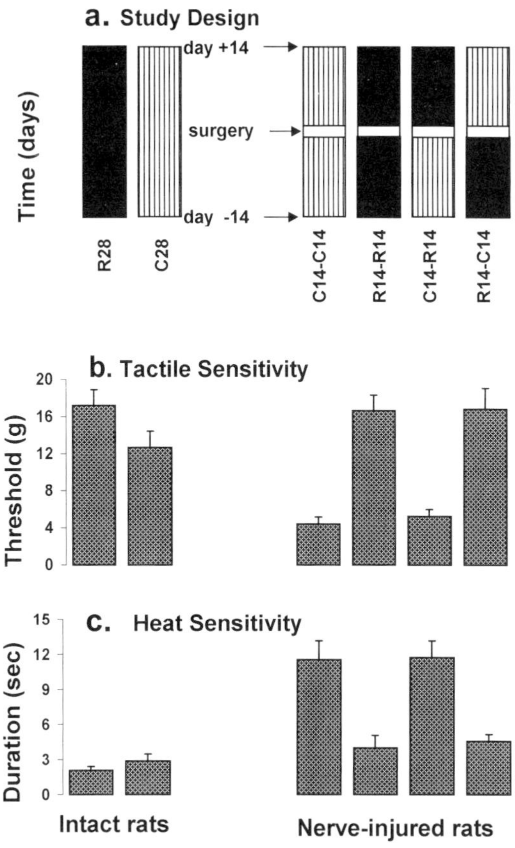

Fig. 1. Effect of diet on innocuous tactile and noxious heat sensitivities in rats. We compared soy-containing RMH diet (R; black columns) and CAS, a diet devoid of soy (C; hatched columns). (a) Study design. Onset and duration of consumption of the two diets in relation to the partial sciatic ligation (PSL) injury. R28: intact rats consuming RMH for 28 days; C28: intact rats consuming CAS for 28 days; C14/C14: PSL-injured rats consuming CAS for 14 days pre- and 14 days postoperatively; R14/R14: PSL-injured rats consuming RMH for 14 days pre- and 14 days postoperatively; C14/R14: PSL-injured rats consuming CAS for 14 days pre- and RMH for 14 days postoperatively; R14/C14: PSL-injured rats consuming RMH for 14 days pre- and CAS for 14 days postoperatively. (b) Withdrawal threshold to light touch. (c) Duration of paw lift in response to a noxious heat pulse. Columns designate the group grand average (± SEM) of the responses of intact rats on experimental days 13, 16, 22, and 28 and of operated rats on days 3, 8, and 14 after nerve injury. Compared to intact rats, low withdrawal threshold to touch and high response duration to heat in nerve-injured rats denote tactile allodynia and heat hyperalgesia, respectively.

each run using a second group of rats to reaffirm the results of the first run). From the time they were weaned until the beginning of experiments all rats were fed on the RMH diet. *Intact rats:* R28 were unoperated rats fed on RMH for 28 days (black column; Fig. 1a, left); C28 were unoperated rats fed on CAS for 28 days (hatched column; Fig. 1a, left). *Nerve-injured rats* (Fig. 1a, right): C14/C14 were fed on CAS for 14 days prior to nerve injury and for 14 days thereafter ("surgery" designates the PSL day and is considered as day 0); R14/R14 were fed on RMH for 14 days prior to nerve injury and for 14 days thereafter; C14/R14 were rats fed on CAS for 14 days prior to nerve injury and on RMH for 14 days thereafter; R14/C14 were rats fed on RMH for 14 days prior to nerve injury and on CAS for 14 days thereafter.

Data analysis. *Intact rats:* Sensitivity of each rat to tactile and noxious heat stimuli was calculated as the average threshold of both hindpaws. To simplify comparison among groups, a grand group average was calculated over all testing days. *Nerve-injured rats:* In previous research we found no correlation between preoperative tactile and heat sensitivity and postoperative mechanical allodynia and heat hyperalgesia (in preparation). Therefore, in the present study we did not use a difference score of pre- vs. post-PSL data. In addition, some rats in the PSL model develop bilateral sensory disorders (Seltzer et al. 1990). Thus, we did not use a difference score of the operated vs. the unoperated sides. Rather, to compare among groups, we represented each group by a single grand average of all postoperative testing days. Groups were compared with the Mann-Whitney U-test, corrected for ties, and adjusted for multiple comparisons when appropriate.

RESULTS

Fig. 1b,c shows that tactile withdrawal threshold and response duration to noxious heat of intact and PSL-injured rats present a similar pattern, i.e., the responses to the two sensory tests are tightly correlated. This result reaffirms previous reports (e.g., Seltzer et al. 1990). Therefore, the results of the two tests are presented together.

- Does feeding with RMH vs. CAS affect tactile and noxious heat sensibility of intact rats? (R28 vs. C28; Fig. 1b,c). The tactile withdrawal threshold and response duration of intact R28 and C28 rats were not significantly different (for touch: 17.2 ± 1.6 vs. 12.6 ± 1.7 g, respectively, $P = 0.16$; for noxious heat: 2.1 ± 0.3 vs. 2.8 ± 0.6 seconds, respectively, $P = 0.6$). Thus, diet has no significant effect on baseline tactile and noxious heat sensitivity in intact rats.

- Does RMH consumption before and after PSL injury affect sensory disorders in this model? (C14/C14 vs. R14/R14). A significant difference was noted between these feeding groups in the withdrawal threshold to touch (4.4 ± 0.7 vs. 16.6 ± 1.6 g, respectively; $P = 0.0001$) and response duration to noxious heat (11.5 ± 1.6 vs. 4.0 ± 1.0 seconds, respectively; $P = 0.0006$). Thus, the consumption of RMH, but not CAS, before and after surgery prevented the development of tactile allodynia and heat hyperalgesia.
- Does RMH suppress development of the sensory disorders when consumed postoperatively? (R14/R14 vs. C14/R14). A significant difference was noted between these feeding groups in the withdrawal threshold to touch (16.6 ± 1.6 vs. 5.2 ± 0.7 g, respectively; $P = 0.0002$) and response duration to noxious heat (4.0 ± 1.0 vs. 11.7 ± 1.4 seconds, respectively; $P = 0.0005$). Thus, pain behavior was not suppressed when RMH was consumed postoperatively only.
- Does RMH suppress development of the sensory disorders when consumed preoperatively? (R14/R14 vs. R14/C14). No significant difference was noted between these feeding groups in the withdrawal threshold to touch (16.6 ± 1.6 vs. 16.8 ± 2.3 g, respectively; $P = 0.46$) and response duration to noxious heat (4.0 ± 1.0 vs. 4.6 ± 0.6 seconds, respectively; $P = 0.32$). Thus, preoperative RMH consumption is essential for suppressing pain behavior in the PSL model.

Similar robust levels of tactile allodynia and thermal hyperalgesia developed in the groups subjected to PSL injury while fed a soy-free diet (CAS) preoperatively.

DISCUSSION

Previously we have shown that consumption of soy-based diets for at least 14 days prior to, and following a PSL injury, significantly suppressed pain-related behavior in rats. The main result of the present study is that this effect occurs only when rats consumed the soy-based diet prior to nerve injury, but not after. We are not aware of any other preemptive measure that so robustly prevents postoperative pain behavior in a model of neuropathy.

The nature of the active ingredients in soy protein that mediate pain suppression is unknown. One candidate is phytoestrogens, compounds that are abundant in soy products and possess potent estrogenic activity. Among other functions, phytoestrogens inhibit protein kinase C, implicated as an intracellular mediator of the development of abnormal pain behavior in the PSL model (Malmberg and Basbaum 1998). In addition, steroid estrogens have analgesic properties (Wardlaw et al. 1982) and block certain cytokines

(Malmberg et al. 1997) involved in neuropathic pain (Cao et al. 1998). However, results of another study do not support a role of soy phytoestrogens in suppression of pain in the PSL model (Campbell et al. 1999).

Preliminary results indicate that the pain-suppressing ingredient in soy has a short half-life, because a preoperative washout period of even a single day was sufficient to terminate the protective effect of soy (data not shown). This finding may suggest that the triggering effect of the endogenous target that mediates pain suppression is transient and limited to the very first postoperative hours. One such target could be injury discharge, a barrage of impulses emitted from damaged sensory fibers during the initial acute injury (Wall et al. 1974). However, while this signal is an important trigger of pain-related behavior in some models of neuropathy (Seltzer et al. 1991; Dougherty et al. 1992), the role of injury discharge in the PSL model is insignificant (Dougherty et al. 1992).

Nerve injury induces the production of peripherally (DiRosa et al. 1971) and centrally (Malmberg and Yaksh 1995) acting breakdown products of injured tissues, neurotrophins (Herzberg et al. 1997), free radicals, (Khalil et al. 1999) and cytokines (Sommer et al. 1998). The effect of diet on cytokine activity following tissue injury is well documented (Grimble 1992), but we are not aware of studies correlating it to soy consumption.

Our results raise the possibility that neuropathic pain in humans may be prevented by preemptive consumption of a diet rich in soy.

REFERENCES

Campbell JN, Raja SN, Shir Y. Suppression of pain behavior in mononeuropathic rats by dietary soy may not depend on phytoestrogen or protein concentrations. *Abstracts: 9th World Congress on Pain.* Seattle: IASP Press, 1999, p 146.

Cao YQ, Mantyh PW, Carlson EJ, et al. Primary afferent tachykinins are required to experience moderate to intense pain. *Nature* 1998; 392; 390–394.

DiRosa M, Giroud JP, Willoughby DA. Studies of the mediators of the acute inflammatory response induced in rats in different sites by carrageenan and turpentine. *J Pathol* 1971; 104:15–29.

Dougherty PM, Garrison CJ, Carlton SM. Differential influence of local anesthetic upon two models of experimentally induced peripheral mononeuropathy in the rat. *Brain Res* 1992; 570:109–115.

Grimble RF. Dietary manipulation of the inflammatory response. *Proc Nutr Soc* 1992; 51:285–294.

Herzberg U, Eliav E, Dorsey JM, Gracely RH, Kopin IJ. NGF involvement in pain induced by chronic constriction injury of the rat sciatic nerve. *Neuroreport* 1997; 8:1613–1618.

Khalil Z, Liu T, Helme RD. Free radicals contribute to the reduction in peripheral vascular responses and the maintenance of thermal hyperalgesia in rats with chronic constriction injury. *Pain* 1999; 79:31–37.

Malmberg AB, Basbaum AI. Partial sciatic nerve injury in the mouse as a model of neuropathic pain: behavioral and neuroanatomical correlates. *Pain* 1998; 76:215–222.

Malmberg AB, Chen C, Tonegawa S, Basbaum AI. Preserved acute pain and reduced neuropathic pain in mice lacking PKCgamma. *Science* 1997; 278:279–283.

Malmberg AB, Yaksh TL. Cyclooxygenase inhibition and the spinal release of prostaglandin E2 and amino acids evoked by paw formalin injection: a microdialysis study in unanesthetized rats. *J Neurosci* 1995; 15:2768-2776.

Seltzer Z, Shir Y. Sympathetically-maintained causalgiform disorders in a model of neuropathic pain: a review. *J Basic Clin Physiol Pharmacol* 1991; 2:18-56.

Seltzer Z, Dubner R, Shir Y. A novel behavioral model of neuropathic pain disorders produced in rats by partial sciatic nerve injury. *Pain* 1990; 43:205–218.

Seltzer Z, Beilin BZ, Ginzburg R, Paran Y, Shimko T. The role of injury discharge in the induction of neuropathic pain behavior in rats. *Pain* 1991; 46:327–336.

Shir Y, Ratner A, Raja SN, Campbell JN, Seltzer Z. The effect of diet on neuropathic pain expression in rats. In: Ayrapetyan SA, Apkarian AV (Eds). *Pain Mechanisms and Management*. New York: Ios Press, 1997, pp 139–158.

Shir Y, Ratner A, Raja SN, Campbell JN, Seltzer Z. Neuropathic pain following partial nerve injury in rats is suppressed by dietary soy. *Neurosci Lett* 1998; 240:73–76.

Sommer C, Schmidt C, George A. Hyperalgesia in experimental neuropathy is dependent on the TNF receptor 1. *Exp Neurol* 1998; 151:138–142.

Wall PD, Waxman S, Basbaum AI. Ongoing activity in peripheral nerve: injury discharge. *Exp Neurol* 1974; 45:576–589.

Wardlaw SL, Thoron L, Frantz AG. Effects of sex steroids on brain beta-endorphin. *Brian Res* 1982; 245:327–331.

Whitten PL, Naftolin F. Effects of phytoestrogen diet on estrogen-dependent reproductive processes in immature female rats. *Steroids* 1992; 57:56–61.

Zimmermann M. Ethical guidelines for investigations of experimental pain in conscious animals. *Pain* 1983; 16:109–110.

Correspondence to: Yoram Shir, MD, Department of Anesthesiology and Pain Relief Unit, Hadassah University Hospital, Jerusalem 91120, Israel. Tel: 02-677-6911; email: yshir@hadassah.org.il.

Proceedings of the 9th World Congress on Pain,
Progress in Pain Research and Management,
Vol. 16, edited by M. Devor, M.C. Rowbotham, and
Z. Wiesenfeld-Hallin, IASP Press, Seattle, © 2000.

47

Non-Invasive Brain Imaging during Experimental and Clinical Pain

M.C. Bushnell,[a,b,c] G.H. Duncan,[d] B. Ha,[c]
J.-I. Chen,[d] and H. Olausson[a]

Departments of [a]Anesthesia, [b]Dentistry, and [c]Physiology, McGill University, Montreal; and [d]Faculty of Dental Medicine, University of Montreal, Montreal, Quebec, Canada

The advent of modern non-invasive functional brain imaging in sentient humans has allowed neuroscientists to study the neural substrate for complex human behaviors, thoughts, and emotions. With these techniques we can begin to understand the neural circuitry underlying love, sadness, or the joy we feel when listening to Mozart. Pain is another complex sensory and emotional experience that we have all known in our individual and unique ways. Pain is an experience that is normally related to potential or real tissue damage, but it is highly influenced by our experiences, memories, and expectations. As characterized by Melzack (1975), pain can be described in terms of the sensations we feel—it can be burning, stinging, aching, or cutting. However, it can also be described in terms of the emotions it evokes—agonizing, fearful, or depressing (Melzack 1975). We also use pain words metaphorically to describe other negative emotional experiences that have nothing to do with tissue damage—heartache, a painful memory, or hurt feelings. Anatomical, physiological, neurochemical, and behavioral experiments in animals have taught us much about how the nervous system processes nociceptive information. However, only by examining neural activity in awake humans who can describe their pain can we begin to truly understand how the brain processes this complex experience.

BRAIN IMAGING TO IDENTIFY A COMMON NEURAL SUBSTRATE OF PAIN

Human brain activity can be imaged using several techniques, including positron emission tomography (PET), functional magnetic resonance imaging (fMRI), electroencephalographic (EEG) dipole source analysis, magnetoencephalographic analysis (MEG), and single photon emission computed tomography (SPECT). Each of these techniques has advantages and disadvantages in terms of spatial and temporal resolution, sensitivity, and cost. However, all provide measures that we can use as indirect indices of neuronal activity. Further, despite the many differences among these techniques, results derived from each are generally congruous, which helps to validate each individual method.

Pain was first imaged in the human brain in the 1970s by Lassen and colleagues (1978) using the radioisotope Xenon^{133}. This technique provided little spatial resolution, but suggested an increased blood flow to the frontal lobes during pain. The first three modern human brain imaging studies of pain were published in the early 1990s by Talbot et al. (1991) and Jones et al. (1991), using PET, and by Apkarian et al. (1991), using SPECT. Although their results differed somewhat, together these studies indicated that multiple cortical and subcortical regions are activated during the presentation of simple noxious cutaneous heat stimuli to normal subjects. Since these first studies, several others have confirmed that multiple brain regions are activated by painful cutaneous heat. As shown in Fig. 1, cortical regions most commonly identified to be activated by painful heat include the primary somatosensory cortex (S1) and secondary somatosensory cortex (S2), both probably involved in pain-related sensations, and the anterior cingulate (ACC) and insular (IC) cortices, both components of the limbic system and thus likely to play a role in the affective component of pain (Jones et al. 1991; Talbot et al. 1991; Coghill et al. 1994; Derbyshire et al. 1994; Casey et al. 1996; Craig et al. 1996; Rainville et al. 1997; Xu et al. 1997; Derbyshire and Jones 1998; Paulson et al. 1998). Subcortical activations have also been observed, most notably in the thalamus, basal ganglia, and cerebellum (Jones et al. 1991; Talbot et al. 1991; Coghill et al. 1994; Derbyshire et al. 1994; Casey et al. 1996; Craig et al. 1996).

This literature documents many differences, as well as similarities, in brain regions that are reportedly activated by pain. Some of these differences can be explained by variations in technical procedures or statistical analyses. In data analysis, different approaches are used to compare stimulation conditions; for example, some analyses use simple subtractions between conditions, whereas others use regression comparisons across multiple conditions. Methods for calculating variance and assumptions about the nature of the data also differ among laboratories. Further, although all analyses rely on a statistical determination of significance, methods of accounting for multiple comparisons vary, and thus the criteria for identifying an activation as significant are not uniform across laboratories. Finally, the power of any statistical test is influenced by the number of subjects studied, another factor that varies greatly among studies. It must be remembered that, as with any statistical test, a negative result does not mean a lack of neuronal activity in the specific region; it only means that no activation was detected using a stringent statistical requirement that biases results toward many more false negative than false positive findings.

Not all disparities among findings can be attributed to technical factors. Many differences most likely reflect the fact that we do not all have the same experience when we are presented with a painful stimulus. The pain experience will clearly vary in different experiments, depending upon the environment, experimenter, instructions, stimulus, and procedural design. However, not surprisingly, even within a single experiment in which all of the factors are standardized, there are considerable individual differences in what subjects experience, as reflected in distinctive patterns of brain activity. Fig. 2 shows heat-evoked activation in two subjects who participated in the same experiment. Both received the same instructions and were presented with the same painful heat stimulus. Both subjects showed activation in the ACC (circled areas), but one subject showed much more activation in other areas, including supplemental motor regions and widespread parietal and occipital areas, than did the other subject. Even the activation in ACC differed between the two subjects; one showed bilateral activation, whereas the other showed only significant contralateral ACC activation.

Cortical activation patterns related to many types of painful stimuli have now been studied. These stimuli include cutaneous noxious cold (Casey et al. 1996; Craig et al. 1996), electrical muscle stimulation (Svensson et al. 1997), capsaicin-evoked pain and allodynia (Iadarola et al. 1998), colonic distension (Silverman et al. 1997), esophageal distension (Aziz et al. 1997; Binkofski et al. 1998), ischemia (Crawford et al. 1993), and cutaneous injection of ethanol (Hsieh et al. 1995), as well as an illusion of pain evoked by combinations of innocuous temperatures (Craig et al. 1996). As observed in data from studies of cutaneous heat stimulation, cortical and subcortical sites likewise vary greatly in their responses to the different types of painful stimulation. These differences could be attributed to technical and statistical differences, as discussed above, or to varying pain intensities, different cognitive states, or variations specifically related to the modality of pain. Without comparing the different modalities in the same subjects and acquiring detailed evaluations of independent aspects of each individual's cognitive state, the source of the variability in results cannot be determined. However, throughout these studies many similarities accrue. The ACC shows a particularly robust activation across different stimulus modalities; almost all studies that have examined the region show a significant activation. However, the exact locus and laterality of activation vary among studies. Using the thermal grill illusion, in which the hand is placed on an alternating pattern of warm and cool metal bars to produce a feeling of burning pain, Craig et al. (1996) showed that the illusion of pain activated the ACC, whereas the individual warm and cool temperatures did not. The S1 cortex shows a less reliable pain-related activation, even though single nociceptive neurons have been identified in this region in monkeys (Kenshalo and Isensee 1983; Kenshalo et al. 1988). Only about 50% of studies imaging pain in humans show significant activation in S1 (see Bushnell et al. 1999); this variation may be due to the many factors described above.

If so many discordances can occur among subjects, studies, and types of noxious stimulation, what useful information can we learn from human brain imaging studies in terms of how pain is processed? It is important to remember that although there are great qualitative and quantitative variations among pain states, there is a common feature to all of these; that is, we describe the experience as pain. The word *pain* has evolved in all languages because it is a construct that describes experiences that have something in common. The construct of "pain" is similar to the construct of "red"; a red ball, red blood, and a red sunset are very different entities that evoke different sensory and emotional experiences, yet they are all "red." Painful distension of the esophagus, heating the skin on the foot, and injecting capsaicin into the arm are also very different experiences, but they are all "pain." By evaluating cerebral circuits, particularly those in the cerebral cortex, that are common to all of these painful conditions, we can begin to understand which neural networks are involved in the underlying experience of pain. It appears that S1, S2, ACC, and IC may all be part of a common neural substrate that could constitute the essential elements for the experience of pain. Consistent with this idea are anatomical and physiological data in humans and nonhuman primates indicating that all four of these regions receive nociceptive input via the thalamus (Gingold et al. 1991; Craig et al. 1995; Dostrovsky and Craig 1996; Apkarian and Shi 1998; Lenz et al. 1998a,b; Hutchison et al. 1999).

BRAIN IMAGING TO EXAMINE CNS ABNORMALITIES THAT CONTRIBUTE TO ALTERED PAIN PROCESSING

Some individuals have described brain imaging as the modern phrenology—a science of mapping spots in the brain that are involved in various sensory, behavioral, or cognitive processes. Despite this analogy, brain mapping serves an important function in revealing the neural networks underlying cognitive processes, as discussed above. Moreover, imaging can also examine *changes* in functions of neural regions associated with pathological states. One example of this in terms of pain processing is the observed reorganization of the S1 cortex associated with phantom limb pain. A series of studies (Flor et al. 1995, 1998; Birbaumer et al. 1997; Montoya et al. 1998) using MEG and fMRI have shown that following an upper limb amputation, the focus of activation evoked by facial stimulation in the S1 cortex shifts toward the area normally dedicated to representing the upper extremity. This reorganization is absent in amputees who do not experience phantom limb pain. Further, in cases where phantom limb pain can be temporarily blocked by local or regional anesthesia, there is a rapid change in the cortical representation of the facial area, reestablishing its expected location (Birbaumer et al. 1997).

Another pain-associated change in neural functioning is a thalamic hypoperfusion in neuropathic pain patients (Di Piero et al. 1991; Iadarola et al. 1995). This is demonstrated by a mismatch of thalamic activity between the left and right thalami during a condition of rest in patients experiencing neuropathic pain, with the thalamus contralateral to the painful area showing less activity than the ipsilateral thalamus. As concluded by Iadarola et al. (1995), this observation suggests that functional changes in thalamic nociceptive processing may provide an important contribution to the symptoms of chronic neuropathic pain.

BRAIN IMAGING TO EXAMINE MECHANISMS UNDERLYING ANALGESIC TREATMENTS

In addition to its role in revealing which neural networks subserve the pain experience, human functional brain imaging can also be used to help elucidate the mechanisms underlying a range of analgesic treatments. For example, in our laboratory, we have used functional brain imaging to examine possible mechanisms subserving the therapeutic effects of thalamic stimulation for the treatment of chronic neuropathic pain (Duncan et al. 1998). Despite its use for more than two decades, little is known about the mechanisms underlying thalamic-stimulation-produced analgesia. The original theoretical basis for this treatment was that it would produce analgesia by activating tactile thalamocortical pathways that were inactivated by nerve or neuronal damage (Mazars et al. 1960, 1974). Thus, the localization and parameters of stimulation are usually adjusted to produce a nonpainful activation within the somatosensory thalamus, so that tingling paresthesiae are referred to the painful body part. Over the years, the outcomes of this procedure have been quite equivocal, with some patients receiving excellent long-term relief and others finding the procedure totally ineffective (see Duncan et al. 1991, for review). To examine possible neural pathways evoked by thalamic stimulation that could underlie the relief some patients experience, we measured regional changes in cerebral blood flow (rCBF) in five patients who had received successful long-term pain relief with this therapy. We found that, consistent with Mazars' original idea of activating tactile thalamocortical pathways, there was some activation in S1 cortex during the stimulation. However, there was a much more robust activation in the anterior insular cortex, a region known to be activated in humans by thermal stimulation,

---

⟶

Fig. 1. Functional and anatomical MRI of a single subject exposed to a noxious heat stimulus (3 × 3 cm thermode on left leg; 46°C). Ten 9-second noxious heat stimuli and 10 9-second neutral warm stimuli (36°C) were presented sequentially with 9-second interstimulus intervals. The circled color-coded areas represent regions that show a significantly greater activation during the noxious heat than during the warm stimuli (Spearman's rank order correlation). In this subject and others, there was significant pain-related activation in (A) primary somatosensory cortex (S1), (B) secondary somatosensory cortex (S2), anterior insular cortex (IC), and cingulate cortex (ACC). Panels A and C show coronal slices (right side of brain depicted on right), and panel B shows a sagittal slice.

Fig. 2. Functional and anatomical MRI of two subjects exposed to a noxious heat stimulus on the leg (3 × 3 cm thermode, 46°C). Coronal and sagittal slices are depicted. Analysis was performed as described in Fig. 1. Both subjects showed activation in ACC (circled), but Subject A showed bilateral activation, whereas Subject B showed contralateral activation. Subject A had a more widely dispersed activation pattern, as indicated by the multiple significant activations.

Fig. 3. Pain-related activity when attention was directed to the painful stimulus (A) or to an auditory stimulus (B). Images illustrate, for each attentional state, PET data recorded during the presentation of a painfully hot stimulus (46.5°–48.5°C), compared (by subtraction) with those recorded during the presentation of a warm stimulus (32°–38°C). PET data, averaged across nine subjects, are illustrated against an MRI from one subject. Coronal slices through S1 are centered at the activation peaks. Red circles surround the region of S1. Whereas activation of S1 was significant when subjects attended to the painful stimulus (A), it did not reach significance when subjects attended to the auditory stimulus (B). A direct comparison of pain in the two attentional conditions revealed a significant difference in pain-related S1 activity during the two attentional states. Adapted from Bushnell et al. (1999).

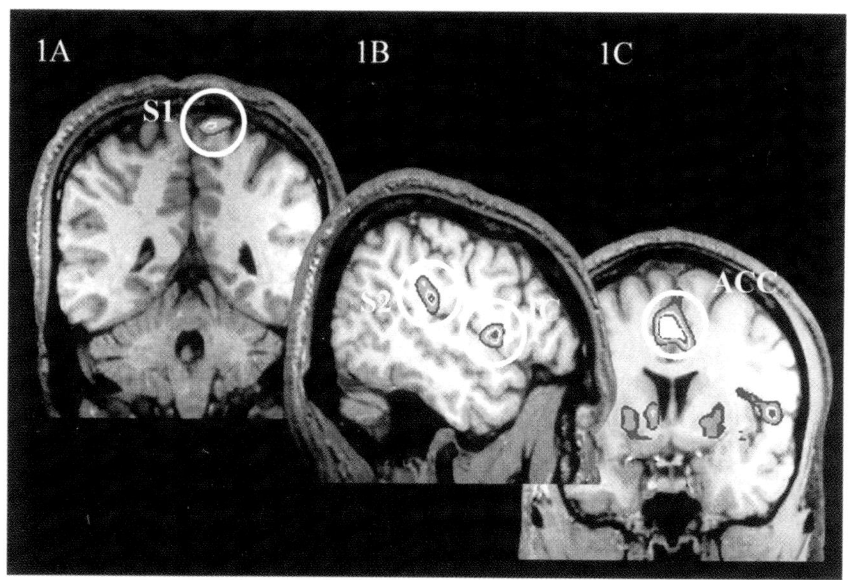
1A
1B
1C
S1
S2
ACC

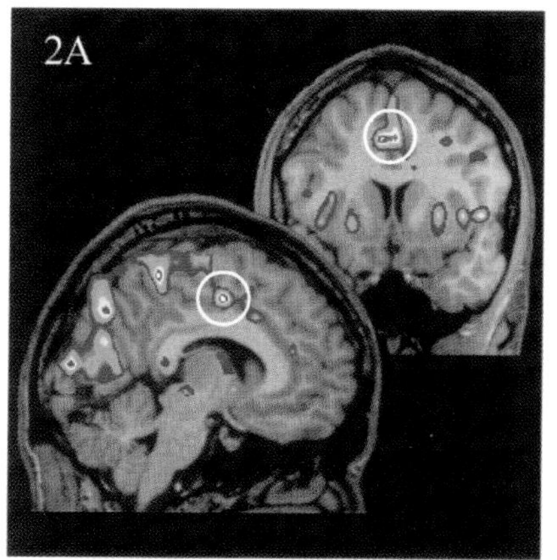
2A

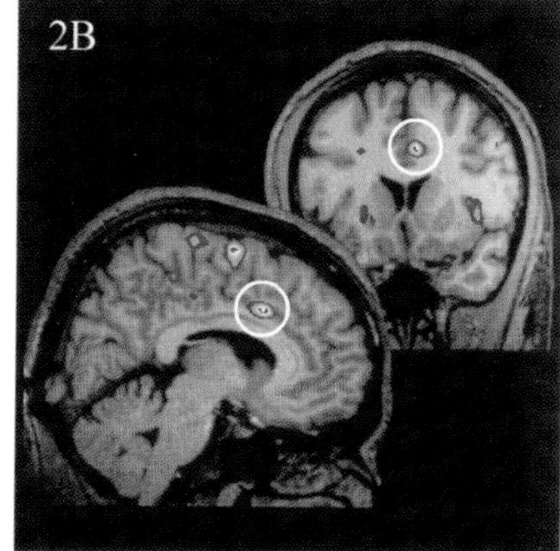
2B

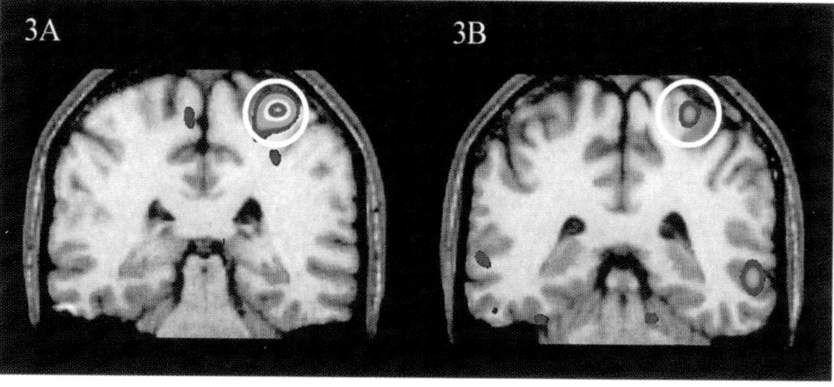
3A
3B

whether painful or innocuous (Casey et al. 1996; Craig et al. 1996). The activation of the anterior insular cortex during therapeutic thalamic stimulation suggests that activation of temperature pathways may be an important component of analgesia in these patients. This hypothesis is supported by patients' reports of stimulation-related thermal sensations (in addition to the tingling tactile paresthesiae) and by physiological and clinical data showing that pain perception is modulated by cutaneous temperature (Bini et al. 1984; Schoenfeld et al. 1985; Wahren et al. 1989; Osgood et al. 1990; Yarnitsky and Ochoa 1990; Strigo et al., in press).

Human brain imaging has also been used to reveal possible mechanisms of attentional modulation of pain (Bushnell et al. 1999; Peyron et al. 1999). When painful stimuli are presented simultaneously with either auditory or visual stimuli, and subjects are required to perform tasks that direct their attention to one or the other modality, the subjects report that the painful stimulus is less intense and less unpleasant when their attention is directed to another stimulus modality (Miron et al. 1989; Carrier et al. 1998; Bushnell et al. 1999). Fig. 3 shows that when a subject's attention is directed away from a painful stimulus, there is a significant reduction in pain-evoked S1 activity, which indicates that psychological state can alter neural activity in primary sensory processing regions of the cerebral cortex. Similar changes in pain-evoked S1 activity are observed during hypnotic suggestions that alter perceived pain intensity (Hofbauer et al. 1998; Bushnell et al. 1999), whereas hypnotic suggestions that alter the perceived unpleasantness of a painful stimulus, without changing the perceived intensity, result in a preferential modulation of pain-evoked activity in ACC (Rainville et al. 1997).

CONCLUSIONS

Results of functional brain imaging studies in humans experiencing pain indicate that a complex network of cortical and subcortical structures subserves the pain experience. The totality of the sensory and emotional experience associated with pain varies widely among individuals, as well as within the same individual at different times and in different contexts. These dissimilarities are reflected in the varying patterns of neural activation observed in different experimental studies. However, despite the distinctions among studies, many commonalities emerge, including the activation of sensory regions such as S1 and S2 and limbic areas such as ACC and IC. The degree of activation of these regions is dependent on cognitive factors, such as attentional state, that alter our perception of pain. Thus, when a patient experiences pain, whatever its origin, at least some components of this cortical network are likely to be activated.

REFERENCES

Apkarian AV, Shi T. Thalamocortical connections of the cingulate and insula in relation to nociceptive inputs to the cortex. In: Ayrapetyan SN, Apkarian AV (Eds). *Pain Mechanisms and Management*. Washington, DC: IOS Press, 1998, pp 212–220.

Apkarian AV, Shi T, Stevens RT, Kniffki K-D, Hodge CJ. Properties of nociceptive neurons in the lateral thalamus of the squirrel monkey. *Soc Neurosci Abstr* 1991; 17:838–838.

Aziz Q, Andersson JLR, Valind S, et al. Identification of human brain loci processing esophageal sensation using positron emission tomography. *Gastroenterology* 1997; 113:50–59.

Bini G, Cruccu G, Hagbarth K-E, Schady W, Torebjörk E. Analgesic effect of vibration and cooling on pain induced by intraneural electrical stimulation. *Pain* 1984; 18:239–248.

Binkofski F, Schnitzler A, Enck P, et al. Somatic and limbic cortex activation in esophageal distention: a functional magnetic resonance imaging study. *Ann Neurol* 1998; 44:811–815.

Birbaumer N, Lutzenberger W, Montoya P, et al. Effects of regional anesthesia on phantom limb pain are mirrored in changes in cortical reorganization. *J Neurosci* 1997; 17:5503–5508.

Bushnell MC, Duncan GH, Hofbauer, et al. Pain perception: is there a role for primary somatosensory cortex? *Proc Natl Acad Sci USA* 1999; 96:7705–7709.

Carrier B, Rainville P, Paus T, Duncan GH, Bushnell MC. Attentional modulation of pain-related activity in human cerebral cortex. *Soc Neurosci Abstracts* 1998; 24:1135.

Casey KL, Minoshima S, Morrow TJ, Koeppe RA. Comparison of human cerebral activation patterns during cutaneous warmth, heat pain, and deep cold pain. *J Neurophysiol* 1996; 76:571–581.

Coghill RC, Talbot JD, Evans AC, et al. Distributed processing of pain and vibration by the human brain. *J Neurosci* 1994; 14:4095–4108.

Craig AD, Krout K, Zhang E-T. Cortical projection of VMpo, a specific pain and temperature relay in primate thalamus. *Soc Neurosci Abstracts* 1995; 21:1165.

Craig AD, Reiman EM, Evans AC, Bushnell MC. Functional imaging of an illusion of pain. *Nature* 1996; 384:258–260.

Crawford HJ, Gur RC, Skolnick B, Gur RE, Benson DM. Effects of hypnosis on regional cerebral blood flow during ischemic pain with and without suggested hypnotic analgesia. *Int J Psychophysiol* 1993; 15:181–195.

Derbyshire SW, Jones AK. Cerebral responses to a continual tonic pain stimulus measured using positron emission tomography. *Pain* 1998; 76:127–135.

Derbyshire SWG, Jones AKP, Devani P, et al. Cerebral responses to pain in patients with atypical facial pain measured by positron emission tomography. *J Neurol Neurosurg Psychiatry* 1994; 57:1166–1172.

Di Piero V, Jones AKP, Iannotti F, et al. Chronic pain: a PET study of the central effects of percutaneous high cervical cordotomy. *Pain* 1991; 46:9–12.

Dostrovsky JO, Craig AD. Nociceptive neurons in primate insular cortex. *Soc Neurosci Abstracts* 1996; 22:11.

Duncan GH, Bushnell MC, Marchand S. Deep brain stimulation: a review of basic research and clinical studies. *Pain* 1991; 45:49–59.

Duncan GH, Kupers RC, Marchand S, et al. Stimulation of human thalamus for pain relief: possible modulatory circuits revealed by positron emission tomography. *J Neurophysiol* 1998; 80:3326–3330.

Flor H, Elbert T, Knecht S, et al. Phantom-limb pain as a perceptual correlate of cortical reorganization following arm amputation. *Nature* 1995; 375:482–484.

Flor H, Elbert T, Muhlnickel W, et al. Cortical reorganization and phantom phenomena in congenital and traumatic upper-extremity amputees. *Exp Brain Res* 1998; 119:205–212.

Gingold SI, Greenspan JD, Apkarian AV. Anatomic evidence of nociceptive inputs to primary somatosensory cortex: relationship between spinothalamic terminals and thalamocortical cells in squirrel monkeys. *J Comp Neurol* 1991; 308:467–490.

Hofbauer RK, Rainville P, Duncan GH, Bushnell MC. Cognitive modulation of pain sensation alters activity in human cerebral cortex. *Soc Neurosci Abstracts* 1998; 24:1135.

Hsieh J-C, Stahle-Backdahl M, Hagermark O, et al. Traumatic nociceptive pain activates the hypothalamus and the periaqueductal gray: a positron emission tomography study. *Pain* 1995; 64:303–314.

Hutchison WD, Davis KD, Lozano AM, Tasker RR, Dostrovsky JO. Pain-related neurons in the human cingulate cortex. *Nat Neurosci* 1999; 2:403–405.

Iadarola MJ, Max MB, Berman KF, et al. Unilateral decrease in thalamic activity observed with positron emission tomography in patients with chronic neuropathic pain. *Pain* 1995; 63:55–64.

Iadarola MJ, Berman KF, Zeffiro TA, et al. Neural activation during acute capsaicin-evoked pain and allodynia assessed with PET. *Brain* 1998; 121:931–947.

Jones AKP, Brown WD, Friston KJ, Qi LY, Frackowiak RSJ. Cortical and subcortical localization of response to pain in man using positron emission tomography. *Proc R Soc Lond B Biol Sci* 1991; 244:39–44.

Kenshalo DR Jr, Isensee O. Responses of primate SI cortical neurons to noxious stimuli. *J Neurophysiol* 1983; 50:1479–1496.

Kenshalo DR, Jr, Chudler EH, Anton F, Dubner R. SI nociceptive neurons participate in the encoding process by which monkeys perceive the intensity of noxious thermal stimulation. *Brain Res* 1988; 454:378–382.

Lassen NA, Ingvar DH, Skinhoj E. Brain function and blood flow: changes in the amount of blood flowing in areas of the human cerebral cortex, reflecting changes in the activity of those areas, are graphically revealed with the aid of a radioactive isotope. *Sci Am* 1978; 139:62–71.

Lenz FA, Rios M, Chau D, et al. Painful stimuli evoke potentials recorded from the parasylvian cortex in humans. *J Neurophysiol* 1998a; 80:2077–2088.

Lenz FA, Rios M, Zirh A, et al. Painful stimuli evoke potentials recorded over the human anterior cingulate gyrus. *J Neurophysiol* 1998b; 79:2231–2234.

Mazars G, Roge R, Mazars Y. Resultats de la stimulation du faisceau spino-thalamique et leur incidence sur la physiopathologie de la douleur [Effects of spino-thalamic tract stimulation on the pathophysiology of pain]. *Rev Neurol (Paris)* 1960; 103:136–138.

Mazars G, Merienne L, Cioloca C. Traitement de certains types de douleurs par des stimulateurs thalamiques implantables [Treatment of certain types of pain by implantable thalamic stimulators]. *Neuro-Chirurgie* 1974; 2:117–124.

Melzack, R. The McGill Pain Questionnaire: Major properties and scoring methods. *Pain* 1975; 1:277–299.

Miron D, Duncan GH, Bushnell MC. Effects of attention on the intensity and unpleasantness of thermal pain. *Pain* 1989; 39:345–352.

Montoya P, Ritter K, Huse E, et al. The cortical somatotopic map and phantom phenomena in subjects with congenital limb atrophy and traumatic amputees with phantom limb pain. *Eur J Neurosci* 1998; 10:1095–1102.

Osgood PF, Carr DB, Kazianis A, et al. Antinociception in the rat induced by a cold environment. *Brain Res* 1990; 507:11–16.

Paulson PE, Monoshima S, Morrow TJ, Casey KL. Gender differences in pain perception and patterns of cerebral activation during noxious heat stimulation in humans. *Pain* 1998; 76:223–229.

Peyron R, Larrea L, Grégoire MC, et al. Haemodynamic brain responses to acute pain in humans: sensory and attentional networks. *Brain* 1999; 122:1765–1780.

Rainville P, Duncan GH, Price DD, Carrier B, Bushnell MC. Pain affect encoded in human anterior cingulate but not somatosensory cortex. *Science* 1997; 277:968–971.

Schoenfeld AD, Lox CD, Chen CH, Lutherer LO. Pain threshold changes induced by acute exposure to altered ambient temperatures. *Peptides* 1985; 6:19–22.

Silverman DHS, Munakata JA, Ennes H, et al. Regional cerebral activity in normal and pathological perception of visceral pain. *Gastroenterology* 1997; 112:64–72.

Strigo I, Carli F, Bushnell MC. The effect of ambient temperature on human pain perception. *Anesthesiology;* in press.

Svensson P, Minoshima S, Beydoun A, Morrow TJ, Casey KL. Cerebral processing of acute skin and muscle pain in humans. *J Neurophysiol* 1997; 78:450–460.

Talbot JD, Marrett S, Evans AC, et al. Multiple representations of pain in human cerebral cortex. *Science* 1991; 251:1355–1358.

Wahren LK, Torebjörk E, Jorum E. Central suppression of cold-induced C fibre pain by myelinated fiber input. *Pain* 1989; 38:313–319.

Xu X, Fukuyama H, Yazawa S, et al. Functional localization of pain perception in the human brain studied by PET. *Neuroreport* 1997; 8:555–559.

Yarnitsky D, Ochoa JL. Release of cold-induced burning pain by block of cold-specific afferent input. *Brain* 1990; 113:893–902.

Correspondence to: M.C. Bushnell, PhD, Department of Anesthesia, McGill University, 687 Pine Avenue, Room F9.16, Montreal, Quebec, Canada H3A 1A1. Tel: 514-398-3493; Fax: 514-398-8241; email: bushnell@med.mcgill.ca.

Proceedings of the 9th World Congress on Pain, Progress in Pain Research and Management, Vol. 16, edited by M. Devor, M.C. Rowbotham, and Z. Wiesenfeld-Hallin, IASP Press, Seattle, © 2000.

48

fMRI of Cortical and Thalamic Activations Correlated to the Magnitude of Pain

Karen D. Davis, Chun L. Kwan, Adrian P. Crawley, and David J. Mikulis

Toronto Western Research Institute and Departments of Surgery and Medical Imaging, University of Toronto, Toronto, Ontario, Canada

Painful stimuli evoke a multitude of sensations and reactions in the sensory-discriminative, motivational-affective, and reflexive dimensions. The development of non-invasive functional magnetic resonance imaging (fMRI) allows for the study of forebrain areas during pain in awake humans (Davis et al. 1997, 1998a,b; Oshiro et al. 1998; Porro et al. 1998). Our previous fMRI studies identified activations in the thalamus, anterior cingulate cortex (ACC), anterior insula, and secondary somatosensory cortex (S2) related to the presence of long- and short-duration painful stimuli (Davis et al. 1997, 1998a,b). However, the relevance of pain-evoked activations to the multi-dimensional nature of the overall pain experience is as yet undefined. As a first step toward dissecting this issue, this fMRI study investigated whether pain-evoked activations in these areas are due to the mere presence of a painful stimulus per se or relate to the magnitude of pain experienced. We also investigated whether pain-evoked activations are related to the intensity or affect dimension of the evoked pain experience.

METHODS

Subjects. Ten healthy male (n = 6) and female (n = 4) subjects aged 21–39 years entered the study. All subjects were right-handed. Prior to imaging, test stimuli were used in each subject to ensure that the evoked pain was tolerable.

Imaging and stimulation. Functional images were obtained with a spiral sequence on a 1.5T GE echospeed MRI with the following parameters: 4 interleaves, field of view = 22 × 22 cm, voxel size = 1.7 × 1.7 × 4 mm, TE = 40 ms, TR = 480 ms for 6 axial slices (1.92 s/volume) to image the thalamus, insula, and S2 (n = 7); and 4 sagittal slices to image the ACC (n = 7) bilaterally at TR = 320 ms (1.28 s/volume). Noxious heat stimuli were applied to the right thenar eminence with an MRI-compatible Peltier-type stimulator (TSA 2001, Medoc Ltd. Advanced Medical Systems) (Davis et al. 1998a) from a base of 40°C to 48°C randomly at three ramp rates (0.3°C/s, 1°C/s, and 4°C/s). Subjects used an MRI-compatible online rating system (Davis et al. 1998b) to continuously rate their pain intensity on a scale from 0 (no pain) to 100 (maximum tolerable pain) throughout the imaging session. A vertical visual analogue scale (VAS) was back-projected from the MRI-console room onto a screen visible to the subject via the mirror mounted on the headcoil. The subject used a highly sensitive trackball device to move an arrow within the VAS to continuously register the intensity of pain throughout the experiment. We used a PC computer to sample the position of the arrow at ~2 Hz and store the data for offline analysis. For each subject we used correlation analyses to determine activations related to a hemodynamic response modeled as a gamma variate function (Cohen 1997) convolved with (1) the stimulus presentation ("boxcar" function), and (2) continuous on-line ratings of pain intensity from 0 to 100 ("ratings" function). Functional images were realigned by automated image registration (AIR) (Woods et al. 1998) and submitted to a pixel by pixel statistical analysis ("Stimulate," J.P. Strupp). Significant activations required a minimum cluster size of 2 pixels and minimum r value > 2 standard deviations above the mean r value of all brain pixels. The thalamus, anterior insula, S2, and ACC were specifically inspected for activation based on pain-related activation of these regions in previous imaging studies (Talbot et al. 1991; Coghill et al. 1994; Casey et al. 1996; Craig et al. 1996; Davis et al. 1997, 1998a,b; Svensson et al. 1997; Rainville et al. 1997; Derbyshire et al. 1997, 1998; Iadarola et al. 1998; Oshiro et al. 1998; Porro et al. 1998; Tölle et al. 1999).

Psychophysics. In separate sessions, outside the MRI environment, subjects submitted to identical heat-pain trials and rated the pain intensity in one trial and the pain affect/unpleasantness in another trial. For these non-MRI sessions, the subjects continuously rated their pain by moving a lever from 0–100 (computerized VAS, Medoc Ltd.). The position of the lever was sampled at 5 Hz and stored for offline analysis.

RESULTS AND DISCUSSION

In this study we wished to investigate the relationship between the magnitude of an evoked pain experience and the resultant thalamic and cortical activation. Total pain or pain magnitude can be viewed as a product of pain duration and intensity. One method by which different levels of heat pain can be evoked is to vary the rate of temperature change. Therefore, to evoke pain that varied in intensity and duration we delivered 48°C heat stimuli at different ascending ramp rates. Fig. 1 shows an individual example and the group mean pain ratings in response to stimuli at 0.3°, 1.0°, and 4.0°C/s. A consistent finding was that the slower heat ramps evoked pain of greater intensity (peak pain) and duration than did the faster heat ramps. This finding is particularly evident in the overall total pain (i.e., area under the curve, AUC) and peak pain, which was inversely related to the ramp rate (Fig. 1b,c). The pain intensity and affect scores were highly correlated based on the total pain (AUC) (r = 0.48) and peak pain (r = 0.68). Several groups have previously reported a strong correlation between heat-evoked pain intensity and affect (Price et al. 1987, 1989; Rainville et al. 1992; Davis et al. 1994). These findings have a direct impact on the conclusions that can reasonably be drawn from imaging studies in search of intensity-coding pain pathways. Few imaging studies have specifically addressed the separation of pain intensity from affect. Rainville et al. (1997) successfully used hypnosis to separate the intensity and affect pain components evoked by heat stimuli. Tölle et al. (1999) obtained different ratings of heat-evoked pain affect and intensity for correlational analyses of PET data by applying long, tonic heat stimuli in four repetitive scans. However, other studies that employed multiple levels of noxious stimuli have either not considered the covariance of pain-evoked affect (Porro et al. 1998) or have referred to the activations as related simply to pain perception (Apkarian et al. 1999). It is clear that affect covaries with intensity in our experimental conditions, so we have elected to use the term "pain magnitude" rather than intensity in reference to activations correlated to the subject's pain intensity ratings. In this way, we regard these activations as related to the overall magnitude of pain, which encompasses the duration, intensity, and affect of pain.

The imaging studies revealed pain magnitude-related activations in the thalamus, anterior insula, S2, and ACC of all subjects. The hemodyamic response of these activations was apparent 6–8 seconds after the stimulus or pain onset and persisted 4–8 seconds after the stimulus and pain subsided. Table I shows the incidence (across the subject pool) of activations in each

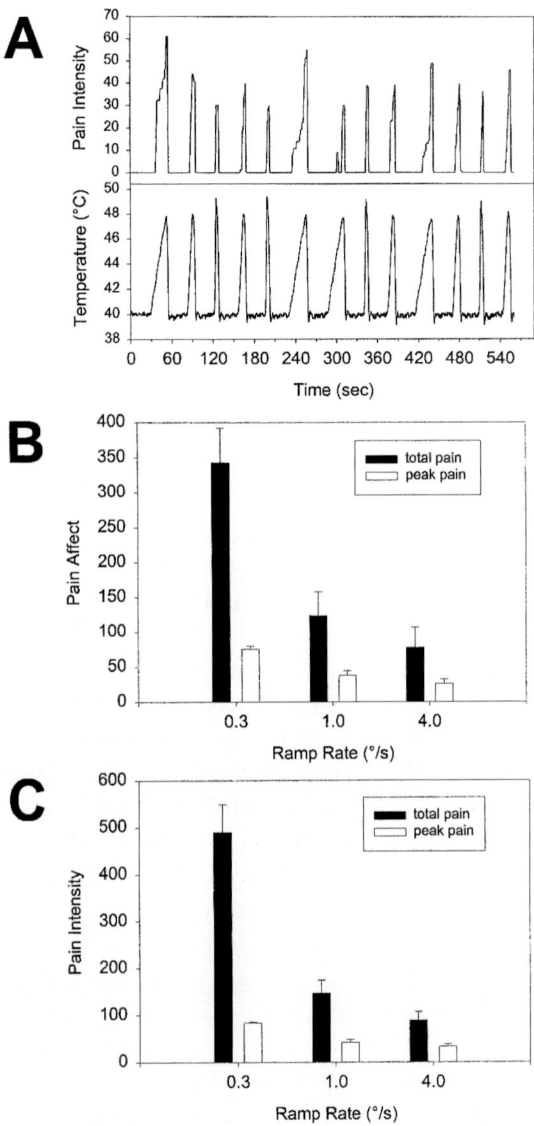

Fig. 1. (A) Continuous ratings of heat-evoked pain intensity in a representative subject evaluated outside the MRI. The ratings of pain affect (unpleasantness) in this subject were similar to the intensity ratings (not shown) (B,C). To facilitate group analyses, each subject's maximum rating was used to normalize his or her data. A high correlation was found between the summed total (area under the curve, AUC) and peak intensity and affect ratings. There was a significant difference in pain evoked by the different heat ramp rates ($P < 0.01$).

Table I
Incidence of pain-evoked activations in study (n = 7 subjects)

	Ratings Only	Boxcar Only	Ratings + Boxcar
Thalamus	7 (100%)	5 (71%)	5 (71%)
Posterior/lateral	2	3	3
Medial/anterior	6	4	3
Anterior insula	4 (57%)	7 (100%)	5 (71%)
S2 cortex	4 (57%)	5 (71%)	5 (71%)
Anterior cingulate cortex	3 (43%)	7 (100%)	5 (71%)
pACC	2	5	5
aACC	2	2	3

Note: In each selected brain region, the table shows the number (and incidence) of subjects in which pain-related activations were detected by one or both of the correlation analyses. "Ratings only" refers to the number of subjects in which activations were identified that correlated to the pain ratings but not to the boxcar function. Similarly, the "boxcar only" column gives the number (and incidence) of subjects in which activations correlated to that function (i.e., stimulus presentation) but not to the pain ratings. The "ratings + boxcar" column contains the number of subjects in which activations were identified in both analyses. Data within a row sum to >100% because each subject typically had multiple activations within a brain region. S2 = secondary somatosensory cortex; pACC and aACC = posterior and anterior part of the anterior cingulate cortex, respectively.

brain region inspected based on the "ratings" and "boxcar" correlation analyses. The data reveal that most subjects had multiple activations within each brain region, some of which correlated with the ratings while others correlated to the boxcar and still others correlated to both waveforms. An example of the thalamic, insula, and S2 correlation maps in one subject is shown in Fig. 2 (ACC sagittal maps not shown). In this subject some activations correlated specifically to the ratings, some to the boxcar, and others correlated to both the boxcar and ratings functions. For instance, several activations were identified within the anterior insula, some of which correlated only to the boxcar function while others correlated to both the boxcar and ratings function. In this subject, several thalamic activations correlated only to the ratings and one correlated only to the boxcar function.

Fig. 3 presents a schematic interpretation of possible meanings of these correlations. Activations correlated only to the stimulus boxcar likely indicate relevance to the presence of the stimulus alone. In this scenario, the MR signal intensity is elevated during pain of any magnitude (Fig. 3a). However, regions that correlated specifically to the ratings, or to both the rating and stimulus boxcar, indicate some degree of magnitude coding of the resultant pain perception (Fig. 3b,c). Activations correlated only to the ratings and not to the stimulus boxcar function indicate a magnitude coding that likely also includes a sharp stimulus-response relationship and some temporal or threshold effects.

Correlation to Boxcar

R L

Correlation to Pain Ratings

+4 +8 +12 +16 +20

○ boxcar only ○ pain only ○ boxcar + pain

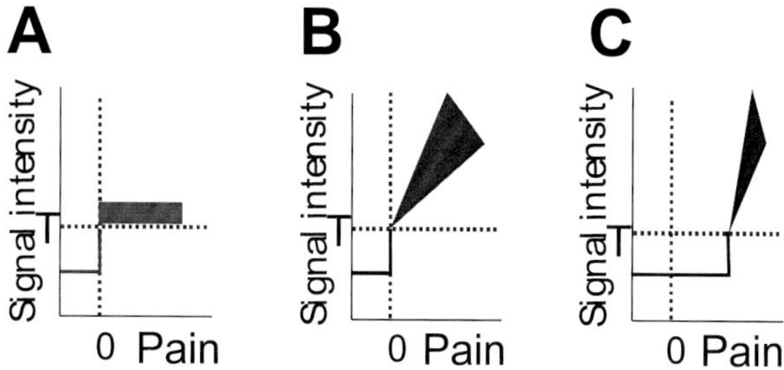

Fig. 3. An interpretation of the outcome of correlating MRI signals to the presentation of the noxious stimuli (boxcar analysis), and to the time and magnitude of the subjects' pain ratings (ratings analysis). Each region of activation correlated to either the boxcar or the ratings waveform or both. The interpretation of presence or absence of these correlations is shown to highlight a proposed dependence of pain magnitude on the signal intensity change within areas of activations during noxious stimulation. In all three scenarios depicted, the signal intensity within a region of interest is considered significantly increased from baseline above a statistical detection level T (threshold) during the evoked pain. (A) Activations that correlate to the presentation of the noxious stimulus (boxcar waveform). These regions likely have minimal or no dependence on pain magnitude. Therefore, the signal intensity would be > T at a static level at all pain intensities. (B) Regions of signal intensity change that correlated to both the stimulus boxcar and the pain ratings suggest modest dependence of signal to the evoked pain (i.e., some pain magnitude coding). (C) Regions of signal intensity changes that correlate to the pain ratings but not the boxcar could result from temporal or pain threshold effects (i.e., pain magnitude coding).

CONCLUSIONS

Pain-evoked fMRI activations correlated to ratings of pain intensity can not be attributed specifically to pain intensity due to the similarity between heat-evoked pain intensity and affect. Rather, these activations likely relate to total pain magnitude integrated over time. The data indicate that subregions within the thalamus, anterior insula, S2, and anterior cingulate may encode pain magnitude, and other subregions may be activated merely by the presence of the stimulus. The interaction and integration of these subregions likely contribute to the overall complex pain experience evoked by noxious heat stimuli.

← **Fig. 2.** Example of pain-related thalamic, S2, and insula activations in a single subject correlated only to the presence of the stimulus ("boxcar," encircled in green), only to the pain ratings (encircled in red), and to both the stimulus and ratings (encircled in blue).

ACKNOWLEDGMENTS

The authors thank Michelle Shapiro for her expert technical assistance in data acquisition and analysis. This study was supported by the Medical Research Council of Canada and the Whitehall Foundation.

REFERENCES

Apkarian AV, Darbar A, Krauss BR, Gelnar PA, Szeverenyi NM. Differentiating cortical areas related to pain perception from stimulus identification: temporal analysis of fMRI activity. *J Neurophysiol* 1999; 81:2956–2963.

Casey KL, Minoshima S, Morrow TJ, Koeppe RA. Comparison of human cerebral activation patterns during cutaneous warmth, heat pain and deep cold pain. *J Neurophysiol* 1996; 76:571–581.

Coghill RC, Talbot JD, Evans AC, et al. Distributed processing of pain and vibration by the human brain. *J Neurosci* 1994; 14:4095–4108.

Cohen MS. Parametric analysis of fMRI data using linear systems methods. *Neuroimage* 1997; 6:93–103.

Craig AD, Reiman EM, Evans A, Bushnell MC. Functional imaging of an illusion of pain. *Nature* 1996; 384:258–260.

Davis KD, Hutchison WD, Lozano AM, Dostrovsky JO. Altered pain and temperature perception following cingulotomy and capsulotomy in a patient with schizoaffective disorder. *Pain* 1994; 59:189–199.

Davis KD, Taylor SJ, Crawley AP, Wood ML, Mikulis DJ. Functional MRI of pain- and attention-related activations in the human cingulate cortex. *J Neurophysiol* 1997; 77:3370–3380.

Davis KD, Kwan CL, Crawley AP, Mikulis DJ. Functional MRI study of thalamic and cortical activations evoked by cutaneous heat, cold and tactile stimuli. *J Neurophysiol* 1998a; 80:1533–1546.

Davis KD, Kwan CL, Crawley AP, Mikulis DJ. Event-related fMRI of pain: entering a new era in imaging pain. *Neuroreport* 1998b; 9:3019–3023.

Derbyshire SWG, Jones AKP, Gyulai F, et al. Pain processing during three levels of noxious stimulation produces differential patterns of central activity. *Pain* 1997; 73:431–445.

Derbyshire SWG, Vogt BA, Jones AKP. Pain and Stroop interference tasks activate separate processing modules in anterior cingulate cortex. *Exp Brain Res* 1998; 118:52–60.

Iadarola MJ, Berman KF, Zeffiro TA, et al. Neural activation during acute capsaicin-evoked pain and allodynia assessed with PET. *Brain* 1998; 121:931–947.

Oshiro Y, Fuijita N, Tanaka H, et al. Functional mapping of pain-related activation with echo-planar MRI: Significance of the SII-insular region. *Neuroreport* 1998; 9:2285–2289.

Porro CA, Cettolo V, Francescato MP, Baraldi P. Temporal and intensity coding of pain in human cortex. *J Neurophysiol* 1998; 80:3312–3320.

Price DD, Harkins SW, Baker C. Sensory-affective relationships among different types of clinical and experimental pain. *Pain* 1987; 28:297–307.

Price DD, McHaffie JG, Larson MA. Spatial summation of heat-induced pain: influence of similes area and spatial separation of stimuli on perceived pain sensation intensity and unpleasantness. *J Neurophysiol* 1989; 1270–1279.

Rainville P, Feine JS, Bushnell MC, Duncan GH. A psychophysical comparison of sensory and affective responses to four modalities of experimental pain. *Somatosens Mot Res* 1992; 9:265–277.

Rainville P, Duncan GH, Price DD, Carrier B, Bushnell MC. Pain affect encoded in human anterior cingulate but not somatosensory cortex. *Science* 1997; 277:968–971.

Svensson P, Minoshima S, Beydoun A, Morrow TJ, Casey KL. Cerebral processing of acute skin and muscle pain in humans. *J Neurophysiol* 1997; 78:450–460.

Talbot JD, Marrett S, Evans AC, et al. Multiple representation of pain in human cerebral cortex. *Science* 1991; 251:1355–1358.

Tölle TR, Kaufmann T, Siessmeier T, et al. Region-specific encoding of sensory and affective components of pain in the human brain: a positron emission tomography correlation analysis. *Ann Neurol* 1999; 45:40–47.

Woods RP, Grafton ST, Watson JD, Sicotte NL, Mazziotta JC. Automated image registration: II. Intersubject validation of linear and nonlinear models. *J Comput Assist Tomogr* 1998; 22:153–165.

Correspondence to: Karen D. Davis, PhD, Toronto Western Hospital, Division of Neurosurgery, MP14-322, 399 Bathurst Street, Toronto, Ontario, Canada M5T 2S8. Tel: 416-603-5662; Fax: 416-603-5745; email: kdavis@playfair.utoronto.ca.

Proceedings of the 9th World Congress on Pain,
Progress in Pain Research and Management,
Vol. 16, edited by M. Devor, M.C. Rowbotham, and
Z. Wiesenfeld-Hallin, IASP Press, Seattle, © 2000.

49

The Cingulate Cortex in Acute and Chronic Pain: $H_2^{15}O$, ^{18}FDG, and ^{11}C-Diprenorphine PET Studies

Thomas R. Tölle,[a] Hans Jürgen Wester,[b] Markus Schwaiger,[b] Bastian Conrad,[a] Peter Bartenstein,[b] and Frode Willoch[b]

Departments of [a]Neurology and [b]Nuclear Medicine, Technical University, Munich, Germany

Brain imaging with positron emission tomography (PET) and functional magnetic resonance imaging (fMRI) has identified some of the principal cerebral structures activated by painful stimuli (Apkarian 1995; Casey and Minoshima 1997). Both experimental and clinical pain induce increased regional cerebral blood flow (rCBF) in the primary and secondary somatosensory cortex, prefrontal and parietal cortex, cingulate cortex, thalamus, insula, and midbrain. Interestingly, many of the neuronal structures that are centrally involved in the processing of noxious information have high levels of opioid receptors (Vogt et al. 1995).

Gross and subtle differences in central activation patterns in response to different types of pain favor the idea that specific assemblies of coherently activated brain structures are needed to portray all of the different aspects of an individual's pain (Davis et al. 1997; Rainville et al. 1997, Tölle et al. 1999). To discover whether different cortical and subcortical areas process different components of the multidimensional experience of pain, we performed two imaging studies. The first was an activation study using $H_2^{15}O$ PET and regression analysis relating noxious heat-evoked rCBF increases to ratings of pain intensity and pain unpleasantness in normal subjects. The second study involved patients with central post-stroke pain (CPSP). Their symptoms were extremely intense and unpleasant, manifesting as diffuse, mostly unilateral pain, often burning, with allodynia, hyperpathia, hypoesthesia, and hypoalgesia. We measured alterations in opioid receptor binding and glucose metabolism with the nonselective opioid receptor ligand ^{11}C-diprenorphine and ^{18}F-fluorodeoxyglucose (FDG), respectively. This chapter focuses mostly on the cingulate cortex.

MATERIALS AND METHODS

$H_2{}^{15}O$ PET activation study. Healthy male subjects (23–75 years of age, $n = 13$) received a contact heat stimulus to the right forearm. A series of heat pulses were applied (sawtooth shape with a duration of 2 seconds at base; frequency 0.5 Hz, amplitude 1.3°C). For heat pain the pulse maxima were 1°C above the individual subject's pain threshold, and for nonpainful heat, pulses were a maximum of 1°C below pain threshold. $H_2{}^{15}O$ tracer (7 mCi) was injected automatically i.v. as a semi-bolus over 30 seconds; at onset of brain activity, tracer counts were collected over 50 seconds using a ECAT Siemens 951 R/31 PET scanner operated in three-dimensional mode. Each of the two stimuli was repeated four times for 5 minutes, with treatments randomly distributed within two blocks. PET acquisitions were performed at the end of each stimulation period. After each stimulation period, the perceived intensity and unpleasantness of the pain were rated on separate visual analogue scales (VAS).

Images were coregistered, resliced, and transformed into the stereotactic space of Talairach and Tournoux, and tracer counts were normalized to the global mean (Neurostat, University of Michigan). Differences between control and activation images were analyzed with a voxel-by-voxel t statistic. Pearson's correlation analysis (with Fisher transformation) was applied to assess the relation between subjective pain intensity or unpleasantness of the pain stimulus and the degree of activation of the cerebral structures activated by the stimulus. The analysis presented here was restricted to voxels of the cingulate gyrus in which rCBF response in the across-subject analysis achieved a z-score above 1.64 when comparing the pain condition to nonpainful heat. Significance threshold was set at $P < 0.05$, corrected for multiple nonindependent comparisons (3D Hammersmith; 16 µL voxel volume and 18 mm full width at half maximum equalled a z-score of 2.2).

Opioid receptors and cerebral metabolism in CPSP patients. We studied four patients (age range 54–63 years) who had long-lasting CPSP. Two patients had a hypodense pontine lesion (one left-sided and one right-sided, as shown by magnetic resonance examination) affecting the medial lemniscus and the spinothalamic tract including trigeminal fibers rostral to the decussation. The other two patients had a right-sided hypodense lesion affecting the pulvinar region of the thalamus. The patients had left-sided ($n = 3$) or right-sided ($n = 1$) hemi-body spontaneous pain and allodynia. Spontaneous pain intensity and mechanical allodynia were rated by all patients as above 50 on the 100-mm VAS. The pain had been present for 5–12 years.

All patients underwent a dynamic ^{11}C-diprenorphine study with 90 minutes' acquisition time (25 frames from 30 seconds to 10 minutes). In addition, cerebral metabolism was investigated in two patients (right pontine lesion and right thalamic lesion) using FDG PET with acquisition times between 30 and 60 minutes post-injection (three 10-minute frames). Opioid receptor binding was quantified by means of the ratio method on a voxel-by-voxel basis according to the formula: ([voxel value] – [occipital reference value])/(occipital reference value). The FDG study was analyzed in a semi-quantitative manner summing the tracer counts over the acquisition time and normalizing the voxel counts as described below. For statistical comparisons the ^{11}C-diprenorphine and FDG data were compared to age-matched healthy control databases ($n = 12$ for ^{11}C-diprenorphin, $n = 18$ for FDG) using Neurostat. Three-dimensional stereotactic surface projections (3D-SSP) were generated. These reduce the sensitivity to atrophy or diffuse loss of the neuronal substrate (Minoshima et al. 1998). The data sets were normalized to the hemisphere with the higher average PET signal value to avoid a possible influence of functional deactivation of the cortical activity by the lesion. Each individual data set was compared voxel by voxel to the respective control groups. Predefined regions of interest over the anterior cingulate cortex (ACC) and posterior cingulate cortex (PCC) were applied on the resulting z-score maps. Scores presented are average scores in the ACC and PCC. A difference of $P < 0.05$, equivalent to a z-score of 1.8, was regarded as significant.

RESULTS

$H_2{}^{15}O$ PET activation study. The 13 normal subjects rated the "pain" stimulus as painful (VAS = 57 ± 5 mm, mean ± SEM) and unpleasant (VAS = 46 ± 5 mm), and the "heat" stimulus as neither painful nor unpleasant (VAS = 2 ± 2 mm and 0 ± 1 mm, respectively). These differences in VAS ratings between heat and pain stimulation were significant (2 × 4 MANOVA, $P < 0.001$). Pearson's linear correlation revealed significant positive correlations between rCBF increase and pain intensity and pain unpleasantness ratings (Fig. 1A,B). The correlation was significant for pain intensity in the ipsilateral posterior cingulate gyrus ($z = 2.7$; Talairach coordinates: $x = 8$, $y = -46$, $z = 34$; brain areas [BA] 23 and 31; Fig. 1A,B) but not the other

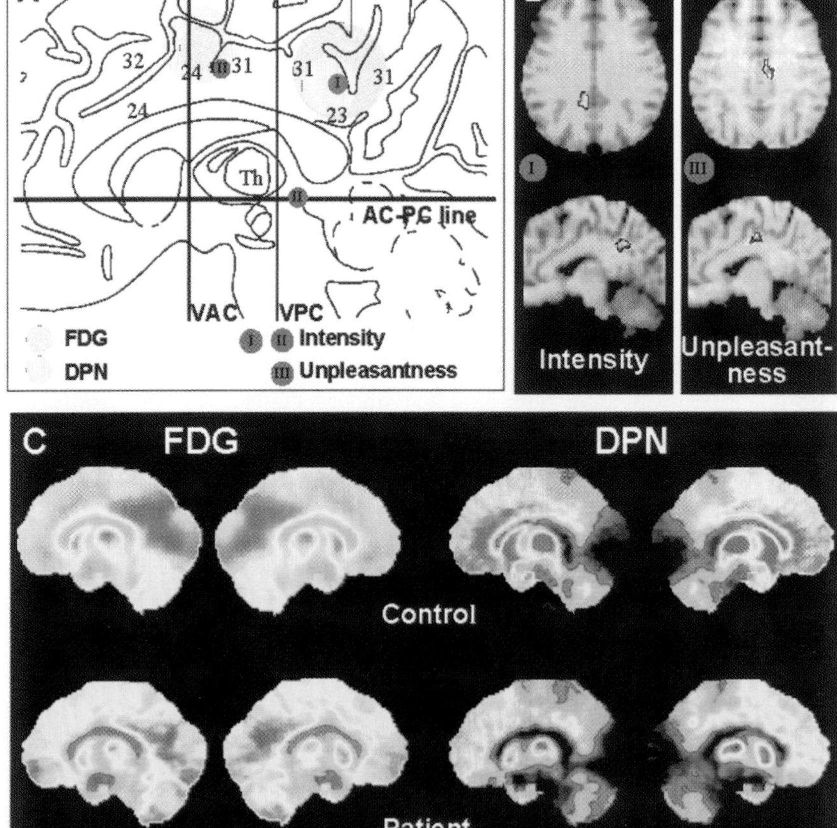

Fig 1. The composite map (A) demonstrates noxious heat-related rCBF increases correlated to pain intensity (I,II) and unpleasantness (III) from the $H_2{}^{15}O$ activation study. In addition, regions of relative hypometabolism (transparent blue) and reduced opioid receptor binding (transparent yellow) are shown in patients with central post-stroke pain (CPSP). AC-PC line = anterior-posterior commissure; Th = thalamus; VAC = vertical anterior commissure; VPC = vertical posterior commissure. (B) Focus of significant correlations from the $H_2{}^{15}O$ activation study projected onto corresponding horizontal and sagittal sections of a T1-weighted MR image. (C) Surface projections of glucose metabolism (FDG) and opioid binding (DPN) of a CPSP patient (pontine lesion) in comparison to controls.

cingulate areas studied. Positive correlations were also observed in the periventricular gray (PVG) of the midbrain (Fig. 1A) and in the ipsilateral frontal inferior cortex (BA 47, not shown). The only brain structure in which there was a significant correlation with pain unpleasantness was the contralateral posterior part of the anterior cingulate gyrus (z = 2.2; Talairach coordinates: $x = -6$, $y = -8$, $z = 30$; BA 31; Fig. 1A,B).

Opioid receptors and cerebral metabolism in CPSP patients. A pronounced relative bilateral (contralateral > ipsilateral) reduction in opioid receptor binding was seen with ^{11}C-diprenorphine in the ACC of all CPSP patients studied (Table I, Fig. 1A,C). A concurrent decrease in glucose metabolism was observed with FDG (Table I, Fig. 1A,C). However, the impaired FDG uptake and reduced ^{11}C-diprenorphine binding had different patterns. Reduction in ^{11}C-diprenorphine binding was more pronounced in anterior parts of the cingulate gyrus, whereas hypometabolism was observed mostly in the PCC, an area with lower opioid receptor density in the control subjects (Fig. 1C).

DISCUSSION

Pain-specific increases in rCBF across subjects confirmed the central involvement of the cingulate cortex in pain processing. The regression analyses support the hypothesis that spatially distinct regions within the cingulate cortex specifically process sensory and affective components of the pain experience. Pain intensity was positively correlated with the rCBF increase in the PCC. The PCC has reciprocal connections to many cerebral regions and constitutes part of a neuronal network that is involved in the monitoring and integration of sensory stimuli (Vogt et al. 1992). In contrast to the ACC, the PCC is supposed to have little relation to affect and motivation (Vogt et al. 1992). The affective aspects of pain have been allocated to different structures within the ACC. While the data of our correlation analysis favor the posterior sector of the ACC as the site for the perception of an increase in pain unpleasantness, a recent report by Rainville et al. (1997) suggests that rostral parts of the cingulate cortex play a key role in processing the pain affect because hypnosis-induced changes in the unpleasantness perception of a noxious stimulus correlate with increases of rCBF in this rostral

Table I
Average z-scores in regions of interest in the cingulate cortex from the central post-stroke pain patients in comparison to the control database. Values shown are for cerebral metabolism (FDG) and opioid receptor binding (DNP).

Region of Interest	FDG	DPN
Contralateral anterior cingulate	–1.8*	–3.7*
Ipsilateral anterior cingulate	–1.1	–1.2
Contralateral posterior cingulate	–2.5*	–1.2
Ipsilateral posterior cingulate	–2.1*	–0.3

* $P < 0.05$.

structure. However, hypnosis alone also activates the rostral ACC in that particular area, and the changes in rCBF with hypnosis-induced changes in unpleasantness perception may have been affected by attention regulation during hypnosis.

The high level of opioid binding in the ACC and the intermediate level of binding in the PCC (Vogt et al. 1995), together with observations of reduced binding in patients with inflammatory pain (Jones et al. 1994), trigeminal neuralgic pain (Jones et al. 1999), and as the present study shows, CPSP, are compatible with the assumption of a central involvement of the cingulate cortex in pain processing. Patients with CPSP had a significant decrease in diprenorphine binding only in the ACC, while statistical significance was not reached in the PCC. Jones et al. (1994) also described an exaggerated decrease of opioid binding in the ACC compared to the PCC. The most likely explanations for the decreases in receptor binding in pain-related structures are competition with the exogenous ligand due to tonic enhancement of intrasynaptic endogenous opioid peptide levels and loss of receptor binding sites caused by increased neurotransmission in the endorphinergic system. Another consequence of the increased levels of endogenous peptides may be receptor desensitization and opioid tolerance, which could also explain the poor response of CPSP patients to treatment with opioid analgesics. In patients with lateral-medullary infarct, who often describe an extremely unpleasant intense pain sensation, the mid-section of the ACC was completely unresponsive to both noxious electrical and allodynia-provoking stimulation applied on the normal and the hyperesthetic side of the body (Peyron et al. 1998). Other brain structures that received input via the spinothalamic tract such as the insula and the parietal cortex showed increased rCBF in response to an afferent barrage, so spinothalamic deafferentation is not likely to explain the absence of cingulate activation (Peyron et al. 1998).

The activation studies with acute pain showed a region-specific encoding of sensory and affective components of pain in the PCC and ACC. Monitoring glucose metabolism, which reflects total regional synaptic activity in the CNS, showed a homogenous decrease of FDG metabolism in the ACC and PCC in patients with CPSP. Interestingly, only the ACC, which encodes the affective components of pain, showed a decrease in opioid receptor binding. It remains to be shown whether differences in sensory and affective features of pain perception in various clinical pain syndromes are characterized by region-specific changes in opioid receptor binding.

ACKNOWLEDGMENT

Supported by SFB 391/C9 of the Deutsche Forschungsgemeinschaft and Norwegian Research Council (123170/320).

REFERENCES

Apkarian V. Functional imaging of pain: new insights regarding the role of the cerebral cortex in human pain perception. *Semin Neurosci* 1995; 7/4:279–293.

Casey KL, Minoshima S. Can pain be imaged? In: Jensen TS, Turner JA, Wiesenfeld-Hallin Z (Eds). *Proceedings of the 8th World Congress on Pain,* Progress in Pain Research and Management, Vol. 8. Seattle: IASP Press, 1997, pp 855–866.

Davis KD, Taylor SJ, Crawley AP, et al. Functional MRI of pain- and attention-related activations in the human cingulate cortex. *J Neurophysiol* 1997; 77:3370–3380.

Jones AKP, Cunningham VJ, Ha-Kawa S, et al. Changes in central opioid receptor binding in relation to inflammation and pain in patients with rheumatoid arthritis. *Br J Rheumatol* 1994; 33:909–916.

Jones AKP, Kitchen ND, Watabe H, et al. Measurement of changes in opioid receptor binding in vivo during trigeminal neuralgic pain using (^{11}C)Diprenorphine and positron emission tomography. *J Cereb Blood Flow Metab* 1999, 19,7:803-808.

Minoshima A, Ficaro EP, Frey KA, Koeppe RA, Kuhl DE. Data extraction from brain PET images using three-dimensional stereotactic surface projections. In: Carson RE, Daube-Witherspoon ME, Herscovitsch P (Eds). *Quantitative Functional Brain Imaging with Positron Emission Tomography*. San Diego: Academic Press, 1998, pp 133–137.

Peyron R, García-Larrea L, Grégoire MC, et al. Allodynia after lateral-medullary (Wallenberg) infarct. *Brain* 1998; 121:345–356.

Rainville P, Duncan GH, Price DD, et al. Pain affect encoded in human anterior cingulate but not somatosensory cortex. *Science* 1997; 277:968–971.

Tölle TR, Kaufmann T, Siessmeier T, et al. Region-specific encoding of sensory and affective components of pain in the human brain: a positron emission tomography correlation analysis. *Ann Neurol* 1999; 45:40–47.

Vogt BA, Finch DM, Olson CR. Functional heterogeneity in cingulate cortex: the anterior executive and the posterior evaluative regions. *Cereb Cortex* 1992; 2(6):435–443.

Vogt BA, Watanabe H, Grootoonk S, Jones AKP. Topography of diprenorphine binding in human cingulate gyrus and adjacent cortex derived from coregistered PET and MR images. *Human Brain Mapping* 1995; 3:1–12.

Correspondence to: Thomas R. Tölle, MD, PhD, Neurologische Klinik und Poliklinik, Technische Universität München, Möhlstrasse 28, 81675 Munich, Germany. Tel: 49-89-4140-4699; Fax: 49-89-4140-4867; e-mail: Thomas.Toelle@riker.neuro.med.tu-muenchen.de.

Proceedings of the 9th World Congress on Pain,
Progress in Pain Research and Management,
Vol. 16, edited by M. Devor, M.C. Rowbotham, and
Z. Wiesenfeld-Hallin, IASP Press, Seattle, © 2000.

50

Is the Cerebellum Involved in Pain?

Carl Y. Saab,[a] Ashraf A. Makki,[a] Michael J. Quast,[a] Jingna Wei,[a] Elie D. Al-Chaer,[b] and William D. Willis[a]

Departments of [a]Anatomy and Neurosciences, and [b]Internal Medicine, University of Texas Medical Branch, Galveston, Texas, USA

New evidence hinting at the involvement of the cerebellum in pain is emerging (Dey and Ray 1982; Ekerot et al. 1991; Casey et al. 1994, 1996; Svensson et al. 1997; Iadarola et al. 1998). This new aspect of cerebellar function merits further investigation and possible revision of the classical conception that the cerebellum has strictly motor functions (Holmes 1939; Eccles et al. 1967; Palay and Chan-Palay 1982). The story of the basal ganglia preaches against the labeling of centers in the brain as being exclusively "motor" or "sensory" (Saadé et al. 1996, 1999; Houk 1997). To those two classifications now need to be added the labels of "cognitive," "affective," "memory," "arousal," and so on. It is not an overestimation to declare that pain involves all these labels, and that the cerebellum processes a battery of sensory information as well (Shambes et al. 1978; Gao et al. 1996; Perciavalle et al. 1998). Thus, such an artificial dichotomy may prove to be misleading.

In our studies, which deal with animal subjects, the term nociception is preferentially used (Willis 1997). Here we need to distinguish between the second-order state of conscious perception of pain and the first-order state of physiological events (also described as nociception). The latter correlate with, but do not necessarily lead to, the former. To investigate the involvement of the cerebellum in the processing of nociceptive information, we relied on fMRI and electrophysiology experiments using rats as an animal model and capsaicin as a noxious stimulus. Investigating the first-order state of nociception allowed for elimination of stress-induced epiphenomena caused by the anticipation of the noxious stimulus, as happens in humans. In addition, the capsaicin-induced noxious stimulus paradigm in rats produced fairly consistent fMRI results.

METHODS

IMAGING PROCEDURE

Three male Sprague-Dawley rats (200–350 g) were anesthetized with 1.2–1.5% isoflurane in a mixture of oxygen and nitrous oxide (30:70). A cannula was placed in the tail vein for the delivery of 2 mg Fe/kg of a superparamagnetic iron oxide tracer (SPIO; Combidex Advanced Magnetics, Inc.). Combidex has a long vascular residence time ($t_{1/2}$ = 5 hours), thereby enhancing the signal intensity decrease in proportion to increased cerebral blood volume (van Bruggen et al. 1998). To obtain coronal multislice spin echo images (TR = 3S, TE = 65 ms, FOV = 6 × 6 cm, slice thickness = 1.6 mm) before, and at several time points after, SPIO injection, we used a 4.7 T magnet (Varian, INOVA) with a 5-cm diameter surface coil tuned to 200 MHz. The stimulation protocol consisted of placing an intradermal needle in the calf region and injecting capsaicin (50 μL of 3% i.d.) following 50 minutes of baseline measurements. Capsaicin, the active ingredient in hot peppers, elicits a sensation of burning pain, presumably by activating vanilloid receptors (VR1) found on small-diameter afferents (Tominaga et al. 1998). The effects of intradermal capsaicin injection have been well documented (Dougherty and Willis 1992) and this technique is considered a model for acute pain, hyperalgesia, and allodynia. The immediate severe pain wears off gradually to become mild within the first 5 minutes (as tested and confirmed by the first author).

Spin echo images were repeated for 120 minutes after the injection. We used "STIMULATE" software (University of Minnesota) to produce a pixel-by-pixel correlation with an idealized "half boxcar" input function (Peeters et al. 1999). The correlation coefficient (CC) image represented the "goodness of fit" between the pixel data and the input function, with CC ranging from 0 (no correlation) and 1 (perfect correlation). We then obtained a "threshold image" by including only pixels with CC ≥ 0.5. We used a *t* test and calculated significance level between signal intensity and input function to identify areas where signal intensity changed significantly ($P < 0.05$) following capsaicin injection. Gray-scale images were acquired as anatomical images on which we overlaid the color activity maps (Fig. 1, where white ovals represent the color overlays from the vermis).

SURGICAL PREPARATION FOR ELECTROPHYSIOLOGY

The same rats used for fMRI were anesthetized the following day with sodium pentobarbital (50 mg/kg i.p., followed by an infusion of 5 $mg{\cdot}kg^{-1}{\cdot}h^{-1}$, i.p.); we also anesthetized another adult naïve rat. Capsaicin effects are supposed to be reversible (see previous section), except for a region of anesthesia that may develop at the primary site of the first injection, but that is unlikely to extend beyond it. When the desired state of anesthesia was reached (as measured by the suppression of reflexes to tail pinch), a mid-sagittal incision in the head and the neck region was made for tracheotomy and artificial respiration. The head was fixed in a stereotaxic apparatus (Kopf instrument). Skin and muscles were retracted, and a craniotomy was made medially at the caudal edge of the occipital bone under the microscope. The dura was then gently excised over the caudal vermis.

RECORDING AND STIMULATION PROCEDURES

Tungsten microelectrodes with tips of about 0.5 μm diameter and 12 MΩ impedance were used for extracellular recording. We used a Spike 2 program to isolate the cerebellar units from the pyramis region of the vermis as identified by vascular patterns (Shambes et al. 1978) and we displayed them both visually and audibly using conventional techniques (Al-Chaer et al. 1998). Electrode penetrations were attempted at varied angles between transverse blood vessels that delineate the folia, so the electrodes would remain perpendicular to the cerebellar cortical surface and restricted to the layers of a specific folium. The depth of the penetrations did not exceed 1.5 mm. The receptive fields (RFs) were determined by recording the responses of cerebellar units to passive movements of the tail or flexion of the hindlimbs (MV). Cutaneous stimuli consisted of gentle brushing of the RF with a camel hair brush (BR), applying pressure or pinching to a fold of the skin using an arterial clip with a weak grip (PR), or an arterial clip with a strong grip (PI), respectively. PI is considered noxious, in contrast to BR and PR. After recording baseline activity for 1–2 minutes, we applied each stimulus for 10 seconds, followed by 10 seconds of no stimulation. Following another baseline measurement, we injected capsaicin (100 μL of 3% i.d.) within the RF. At the end of the electrophysiology experiments, recording sites were verified histologically in two of the rats by producing small electrolytic lesions.

RESULTS

Serial fMRIs collected from three rats revealed regional increases in blood volume throughout different brain areas (Fig. 1). While these regions included many cerebral cortical and subcortical structures (not shown here), the high-resolution images acquired from the cerebellar hemispheres, the

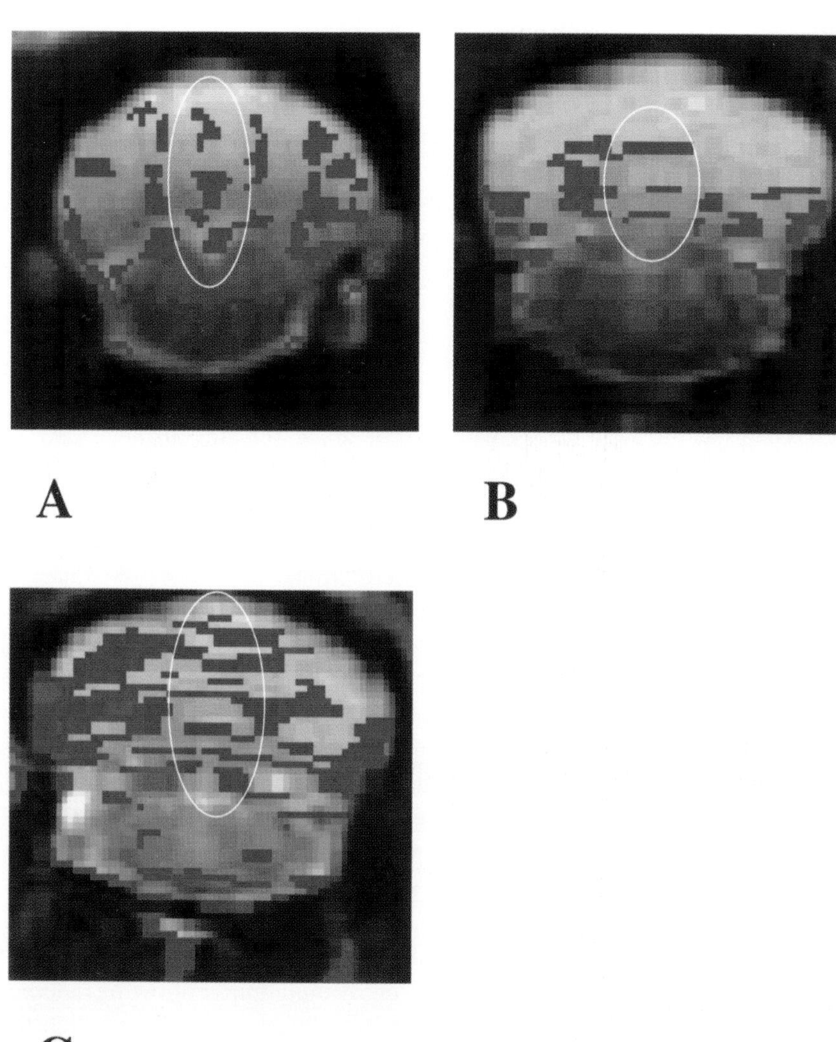

Fig. 1. Cross-sectional fMRI images obtained from the cerebellum of three rats. Ellipses indicate the location of the cerebellar vermis. Vermal areas of increased blood volume with correlation coefficient (CC) of 0.6–0.8 are shown in blue. The color map progresses to purple, which designates areas of higher correlation (CC ≥ 0.8) between blood volume increase and capsaicin injection.

paravermis and the vermis, showed a significant correlation between the event of intradermal capsaicin injection and the increase in blood volume.

In the electrophysiological experiments, we isolated 10 multiunit cell clusters that were responsive to the somatosensory stimuli applied. All clus-

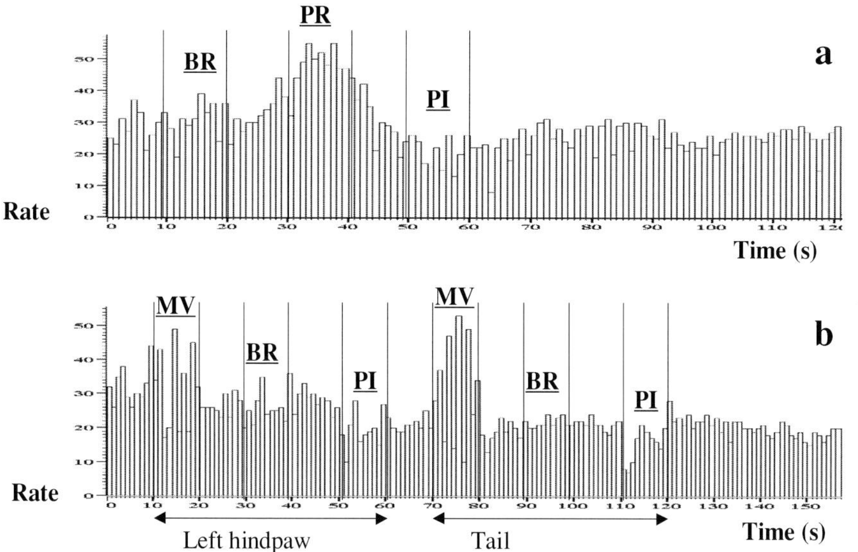

Fig. 2. Peristimulus time histograms obtained by extracellular recording from the caudal vermis of one rat at roughly the same bregma level illustrated in Fig. 1 (pyramis). The receptive fields (RFs) were localized to (a) the ankle or (b) the ankle and the tail. "Rate" indicates the sum of multiunit spikes/second plotted against time (seconds) (bin width = 1 second). Natural stimuli consisted of gentle brushing (BR), pressing (PR), pinching (PI) of the corresponding RF, or passive movement (MV) of the hindlimbs or the tail. In panel a, PR resulted in activation while PI resulted in inhibition.

ters included units responsive to the movement of the ankle joint as well as noxious stimulation of ankle skin. The recording sites corresponded mostly to the Purkinje cell layer of the pyramis folium at bregma –14 mm (Paxinos and Watson 1986). An example of the multiunit RF properties is shown in Fig. 2a; innocuous PR applied for 10 seconds increased the rate of spiking events compared to baseline, in contrast to the noxious PI, which resulted in an inhibition. Interestingly, although the responses to PR, PI, and MV were evident in most of the cases and were restricted in time to the stimulation periods, gentle BR did not seem to have any effect on the rate of spiking events. In one rat, the same multiunit group responded identically to natural stimulation of both the hindlimb and the tail, which suggested convergence of input from two RFs (Fig. 2 b).

Following intradermal capsaicin injection into the skin overlying the ankle joint, seven isolated units exhibited an immediate increase in their rate of spiking (Fig. 3a,b,c), while only three were inhibited (Fig. 3d). These positive and negative responses were grouped separately (Fig. 3e) as average percentage changes in rate relative to a normalized baseline value.

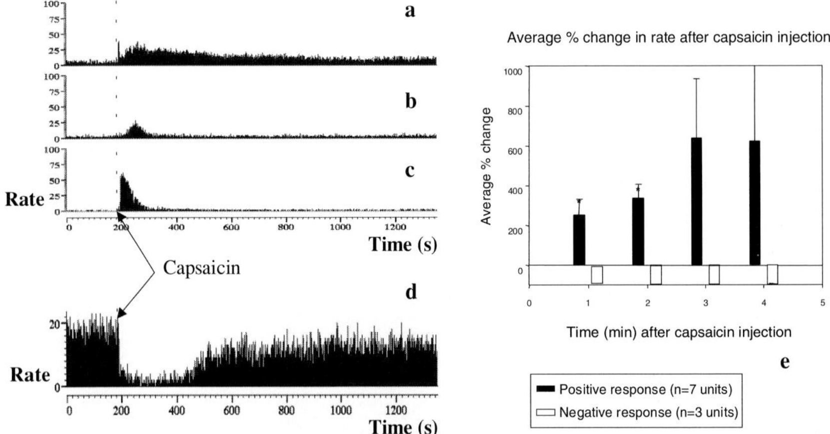

Fig. 3. Peristimulus time histograms after intradermal injection of capsaicin (denoted by arrows) into the ankle. Sample responses of single units isolated from multiunit clusters are shown separately in panels a, b, c, and d. The immediate increase in the rate of spiking (spikes/second, plotted against time in seconds) was either (a) tonic or (b,c) phasic. An inhibitory effect on an isolated single unit is shown in panel d. The average percentage increase (black bars) and decrease (white bars) in the rate of multiunit spiking events are plotted in panel e, following capsaicin injection (t = 0 minutes) and normalized to the baseline value (0%).

DISCUSSION

Previous imaging studies have described cerebellar activation during the pain experience in humans (Casey et al. 1994, 1996; Svensson et al. 1997; Iadarola et al. 1998, Coghill et al. 1999). In our study, fMRI images obtained from rats revealed nociceptive responses in the cerebellum. If we assume that the increase in blood volume is directly coupled to cellular activity, the fMRI data support the electrophysiological data, especially because we used both techniques to study the same individual rats. However, we must recognize the general limitations of the imaging techniques (Mathiesen et al. 1998). Furthermore, because of the distinction made earlier between "pain" and "nociception," we cannot declare unequivocally that the cerebellum contributes to the conscious perception of pain, although we do not dismiss this as a possibility (Schmahmann 1991, 1997a,b; Wu and Chen 1991; Fiez 1996; Wiser et al. 1998). Based on these results and recent cerebellar lesion experiments followed by behavioral assessment (C.Y. Saab et al., unpublished observations), we believe that the nociceptive input to the cerebellum may be necessary for normal pain-related behavior (Siegel and Wepsic 1974; Spiegel 1982). The evaluation of how this input translates different forms of "noxious energies" (mechanical, thermal, and chemical, either in isolation or combined) is far from complete. Because the cerebellum is endowed with a highly regular circuitry (Goldowitz and Hamre 1998; Voogd and Glickstein 1998), it is important in future studies to define accurately the position of the cells recorded relative to the electrode(s), and, when possible, to analyze their cross-correlated spiking events (McDevitt et al. 1987). This approach promises better understanding of cerebellar nociceptive processing and pain pathways.

In general, the brain areas that are involved in nociception are not exclusively "sensory"; they include the medulla, pons, midbrain, hypothalamus, basal ganglia, amygdala, and cingulate gyrus. Hence, to study the involvement of the cerebellum in such a spatially distributed system is justified, and in fact revives a century-old concept comparing cerebellar functions to those of the sensory-motor cerebrum (Russell 1894).

ACKNOWLEDGMENT

This work was supported by NIH grant NS 09743.

REFERENCES

Al-Chaer ED, Feng Y, Willis WD. A role for the dorsal column in nociceptive visceral input into the thalamus of primates. *J Neurophysiol* 1998; 79:3143–3150.

Casey KL, Minoshima S, Berger KL, et al. Positron emission tomography analysis of cerebral structures activated specifically by repetitive noxious heat stimuli. *J Neurophysiol* 1994; 71(2):802–807.

Casey KL, Minoshima S, Morrow TJ, Koeppe RA. Comparison of human cerebral activation patterns during cutaneous warmth, heat pain, and deep cold pain. *J Neurophysiol* 1996; 76(1):571–581.

Coghill RC, Sang CN, Maisoc JM, Iadarola MJ. Pain intensity within the human brain: a bilateral, distributed mechanism. *J Neurophysiol* 1999; 82:1934–1943.

Dey PK, Ray AK. Anterior cerebellum as site for morphine analgesia and post-stimulation analgesia. *Indian J Physiol Pharmacol* 1982; 26(1):3–12.

Dougherty PM, Willis WD. Enhanced responses of spinothalamic tract neurons to excitatory amino acids accompany capsaicin-induced sensitization in the monkey. *J Neurosci* 1992; 12(3):883–894.

Eccles JC, Ito M, Szentágothai J. *The Cerebellum as a Neuronal Machine*. New York: Springer-Verlag, 1967.

Ekerot CF, Garwicz M, Schouenborg J. The postsynaptic dorsal column pathway mediates cutaneous nociceptive information to cerebellar climbing fibers in the cat. *J Physiol (Lond)* 1991; 441:275–284.

Fiez JA. Cerebellar contributions to cognition. *Neuron* 1996; 16:13–15.

Gao J, Parsons LM, Bower JM, et al. Cerebellum implicated in sensory acquisition and discrimination rather than motor control. *Science* 1996; 272:545–547.

Goldowitz D, Hamre K. The cells and molecules that make a cerebellum. *Trends Neurosci* 1998; 21:375–382.

Holmes G. The cerebellum of man. *Brain* 1939; 62(1):1–30.

Houk JC. On the role of the cerebellum and basal ganglia in cognitive signal processing. *Prog Brain Res* 1997; 114:543–552.

Iadarola MJ, Berman KF, Zeffiro TA, et al. Neuronal activation during acute capsaicin-evoked pain and allodynia assessed with PET. *Brain* 1998; 121:931–947.

Mathiesen C, Caesar K, Akgören N, Lauritzen M. Modification of activity-dependent increases of cerebral blood flow by excitatory synaptic activity and spikes in rat cerebellar cortex. *J Physiol (Lond)* 1998; 512.2:555–566.

McDevitt CJ, Ebner TJ, Bloedel JR. Changes in the responses of cerebellar nuclear neurons associated with the climbing fiber response of Purkinje cells. *Brain Res* 1987; 425:14–24.

Palay SL, Chan-Palay V (Eds). *The Cerebellum: New Vistas*. New York: Springer-Verlag, 1982.

Paxinos G, Watson C. *The Rat Brain in Stereotaxic Coordinates*. San Diego: Academic Press, 1986.

Peeters RR, Verhoye M, Vos BP, et al. A patchy horizontal organization of the somatosensory activation of the rat cerebellum demonstrated by functional MRI. *Eur J Neurosci* 1999; 11:2720–2730.

Perciavalle V, Bosco G, Poppele RE. Spatial organization of proprioception in the cat spinocerebellum. Purkinje cell responses to passive foot rotation. *Eur J Neurosci* 1998; 10:1975–1985.

Russell R. Experimental researches into the functions of the cerebellum. *BMJ* 1894; 185:819–861.

Saadé NE, Shbeir SA, Atweh SF, Jabbur SJ. Effects of cerebral cortical and striatal lesions on autotomy following peripheral neurectomy in rats. *Physiol Behav* 1996; 60:559–566.

Saadé NE, Kafrouni AI, Saab CY, Atweh SF, Jabbur SJ. Chronic thalamotomy increases pain-related behavior in rats. *Pain* 1999; 83:401–409.

Schmahmann JD. An emerging concept: the cerebellar contribution to higher function. *Arch Neurol* 1991; 48:1178–1187.

Schmahmann JD. Rediscovery of an early concept. *Int Rev Neurobiol* 1997a; 41:3–27.

Schmahmann JD. The cerebrocerebellar system. *Int Rev Neurobiol* 1997b; 41:31–60.

Shambes GM, Gibson JM, Welker W. Fractured somatotopy in granule cell tactile areas of rat cerebellar hemispheres revealed by micromapping. *Brain Behav Evol* 1978; 15:94–140.

Siegel P, Wepsic JG. Alteration of nociception by stimulation of cerebellar structures in the monkey. *Physiol Behav* 1974; 13:189–194.

Spiegel EA. Relief of pain and spasticity by posterior column stimulation: a proposed mechanism. *Arch Neurol* 1982; 39:184–185.

Svensson P, Minoshima S, Beydoun A, Morrow TJ, Casey KL. Cerebral processing of acute skin and muscle pain in humans. *J Neurophysiol* 1997; 78:450–460.

Tominaga M, Caterina MJ, Malmberg AB, et al. The cloned capsaicin receptor integrates multiple pain-producing stimuli. *Neuron* 1998; 21:531–543.

Van Bruggen N, Bush E, Palmer TJ, Williams SP, de Crespigny AJ. High-resolution functional magnetic resonance imaging of the rat brain: mapping changes in cerebral blood volume using iron oxide contrast media. *J Cereb Blood Flow Met* 1998; 18:1178–1183.

Voogd J, Glickstein M. The anatomy of the cerebellum. *Trends Neurosci* 1998; 21:370–3755.

Willis WD. Pain terminology as it applies to animal experiments. *Pain Forum* 1997; 6(2):88–91.

Wiser AK, Andreasen NC, O'Leary DS, Watkins GL, Hichwa RD. Dysfunctional cortico-cerebellar circuits cause 'cognitive dysmetria' in schizophrenia. *Neuroreport* 1998; 9:1895–1899.

Wu J, Chen PX. Is the cerebellum related with pain? *Prog Physiol Sci (Sheng Li Ko Hsueh Chin Chan)* 1991; 22(3):283–284.

Correspondence to: W.D. Willis, MD, PhD, Department of Anatomy and Neurosciences, University of Texas Medical Branch, 301 University Boulevard, Galveston, TX 77555-1069, USA. Tel: 409-772-2103; Fax: 409-772-4687; email: wdwillis@utmb.edu.

Proceedings of the 9th World Congress on Pain,
Progress in Pain Research and Management,
Vol. 16, edited by M. Devor, M.C. Rowbotham, and
Z. Wiesenfeld-Hallin, IASP Press, Seattle, © 2000.

51

Visceral Hyperalgesia

Maria Adele Giamberardino

Pathophysiology of Pain Laboratory, Department of Medicine and Science of Aging, "G. D'Annunzio" University of Chieti, Italy

The clinical impact of pain arising from internal organs is far greater than that of pain of somatic origin (Bonica 1990), partly because of the high incidence of algogenic conditions affecting the viscera, but also because such conditions are often recurrent or chronic and are more likely to be life-threatening than are conditions that give rise to somatic pain (Procacci et al. 1986; Bonica 1990). Coronary heart disease, functional and organic pathologies of the gastrointestinal (GI) tract, and recurrent or chronic inflammatory processes in the pelvic domain in women are just a few examples (see Giamberardino 1999).

Despite its prominence in the clinical setting, visceral pain has traditionally been investigated to a much lesser extent than pain arising in more superficial structures, particularly the skin. One obvious reason is that access to the visceral domain is more complicated (Gebhart 1995a; Arendt-Nielsen 1997). Additional reasons lie in the particular nature of pain from internal organs, which has rendered its identification difficult and frequently has led to various misdiagnoses. Visceral pain usually has a temporal evolution, and its clinical features differ in the various phases. What is known as "true visceral pain," typical of the early stage of a visceral algogenic pathology, can be very misleading as a symptom. It is, in fact, an indistinct and poorly defined sensation, always perceived in the same site—usually the midline of the thorax or abdomen, whatever the affected organ—and is accompanied by marked autonomic signs and emotional reactions. Subsequently the symptom is referred to parietal somatic structures of the body (skin, subcutis, muscle), usually in the same metameric field as the affected organ, where it may or may not be accompanied by secondary hyperalgesia of superficial or deep body wall tissues, and thus constitutes *referred pain without hyperalgesia* or *referred pain with hyperalgesia*. At this stage, pain of visceral origin becomes sharper, better localized, and no longer accompanied by marked autonomic signs, and it may thus be difficult to differentiate from pain primarily arising in somatic structures (Lewis 1942; Lundei and Galletti 1953; Hansen and Schliack 1962; Wolff 1963; Procacci 1986; Bonica 1990).

While neglected and underestimated in the past, visceral pain has been the subject of renewed interest in research studies in recent years, as its clinical expression has been progressively better recognized and the clear need for mechanism-based therapeutic strategies has emerged (Giamberardino 1999). A great deal of the investigative effort has concentrated on phenomena of hyperalgesia, as it has become increasingly evident in patients that a painful visceral pathology frequently triggers hypersensitivity to painful stimuli at different levels, which complicates the clinical expression of visceral pain to various extents (Gebhart 1995; Koltzenburg and McMahon 1995; Vecchiet and Giamberardino 1998).

In the context of algogenic conditions affecting internal organs, the term "visceral hyperalgesia" in its strict sense should refer only to the situation in which a specific viscus becomes hyperalgesic, i.e., hypersensitive toward painful stimuli. As stated above, however, phenomena of hyperalgesia related to a visceral painful pathology are multiple and often intermingled. As a consequence, the expression "visceral hyperalgesia" has now acquired the wider meaning of *a combination of processes due to which not only the afflicted viscera but also the somatic area of referral may become hyperalgesic* (Koltzenburg and McMahon 1995; McMahon 1997; Giamberardino 1999).

Phenomena of hyperalgesia from viscera can be grouped into three main categories (Table I). The first includes hyperalgesia of an internal organ caused by inflammation or excess (repetitive and prolonged) stimulation of the same organ (strictly called visceral hyperalgesia). This is a form of primary hyperalgesia as it involves the site of injury. The second category comprises hyperalgesia of somatic tissues in the areas of referred pain from viscera. This is a form of secondary hyperalgesia as it occurs in a site other than that of the primary injury. The third category, known as viscero-visceral hyperalgesia, includes hyperalgesia of one visceral organ that manifests clinically due to an algogenic condition of another viscus whose segmental afferent innervation partially overlaps. This chapter will focus on the three categories of visceral hyperalgesia, and will present clinical examples and discuss related pathophysiological mechanisms in light of the results of the most recent experimental studies.

Table I
Categories of hyperalgesia in visceral pain

1) Hyperalgesia of a viscus from inflammation and/or excess stimulation of the same viscus (*visceral hyperalgesia*)
2) Hyperalgesia of somatic tissues in the areas of referred pain from viscera (*referred hyperalgesia from viscera*)
3) Hyperalgesia of a viscus rendered clinically manifest by an algogenic condition of another viscus (*viscero-visceral hyperalgesia*)

VISCERAL HYPERALGESIA

Visceral hyperalgesia (caused by inflammation or excess stimulation of the visceral structure) cannot be understood without recalling the modalities of nociceptive stimulation in internal organs. Viscera have long been considered insensitive to pain as they do not normally react to stimuli that are algogenic for somatic structures, such as cutting, pinching, or burning. In addition, there is often no relationship between the extent of the internal injury and the perceived visceral pain sensation (Gebhart 1995b). Adequate stimuli for viscera are of a different nature (see Bonica 1990; Cervero 1994). According to the classic definition established by Ayala (1937), Lunedei and Galletti (1953), and Procacci et al. (1978), they are subdivided into: (1) abnormal distension and contraction of the muscle walls of hollow organs, such as the ureter or the gut (the mechanism of colic); (2) rapid stretching of the capsule of solid viscera (such as the liver or the spleen); (3) abrupt anoxemia of smooth muscles; (4) formation and accumulation of pain-producing substances; (5) direct action of chemical stimuli (as in gastric acid reflux); (6) traction or compression of ligaments and vessels; (7) necrosis of some structures (such as myocardium or pancreas); and (8) inflammatory states. Inflammatory stimuli, in particular, can directly trigger pain, or, more often, render the structure hypersensitive, such that pain can now be evoked in the viscus by a stimulus that was initially nonpainful or by a lower intensity of stimulus. Algogenic substances such as kinins, 5-hydroxytryptamine, histamine, prostaglandins, and potassium released locally in the inflamed area of visceral tissues are probable mediators of the painful signals from inflamed viscera (Bonica 1990).

CLINICAL EXPRESSIONS

Inflammation. The sensitizing action of inflammation in viscera has long been known. In 1947, Wolf and Wolff demonstrated experimentally, in a subject with a large gastric stoma, that when the mucosa was healthy, pain could not be evoked by a variety of stimuli that would have been algogenic for somatic structures. However, if the mucosa was inflamed, the same stimuli became intensely painful. In 1948, Kinsella observed that squeezing the inflamed appendix provoked pain. In 1962, Teodori and Galletti investigated the sensitivity of pleura by means of electrical, thermal, and mechanical stimuli, during an intervention for section of pleural adhesions, both in normal conditions and when the serosa was inflamed. In the latter case pain was more intense, sharp, and localized than when the stimuli were applied to normal pleura.

In the clinical setting, hypersensitivity due to inflammation indeed appears to be one of the most common and best known forms of visceral hyperalgesia. Typical examples are represented by *pain upon ingestion of food or liquids at the level of the esophagus or stomach* when the mucosa is inflamed or by *pain upon bladder distension* from inflammatory processes of the lower urinary tract, such as those accompanying common infections like cystitis (Gebhart 1995a; see Vecchiet and Giamberardino 1998; Giamberardino 1999) (Table II).

Excess stimulation. Repetitive or prolonged application of a non-algogenic stimulus may also induce visceral hyperalgesia, as has been shown experimentally in humans by delivering various mechanical or electrical stimuli to various portions of the GI tract (Ness et al. 1990, 1998; Frobert et al. 1995; Arendt-Nielsen et al. 1997; Drewes et al. 1997; see also Arendt-Nielsen 1997). In particular, a classic experiment performed in 1990 by Ness and colleagues in healthy volunteers clearly demonstrated the induction of visceral hypersensitivity from repeated mechanical distension of the

Table II
Clinical examples of hyperalgesia in visceral pain

1) Visceral Hyperalgesia
- Esophageal-gastric pain at ingestion of food or liquids
- Vesical pain at bladder filling (mucosal inflammatory processes)
- Abdominal/pelvic pain in concomitance with intestinal transit (irritable bowel syndrome)

2) Referred Hyperalgesia from Viscera
- Pain upon compression of body wall tissues in:
  - thorax/left upper limb (angina, myocardial infarction)
  - lumbar region, flank, groin (renal/ureteral colic)
  - upper abdomen, right (biliary colic)
  - lower abdomen/pelvic and sacral regions (primary dysmenorrhea)

3) Viscero-visceral Hyperalgesia
- Accentuation of anginal pain in patients with coronary heart disease plus biliary calculosis (heart, gallbladder)
- Accentuation of colic pain in patients with urinary calculosis plus primary dysmenorrhea (urinary tract, female reproductive organs)

sigmoid colon. The first distension of a 25-cm tract of the organ for 30 seconds at a pressure of 60 mm Hg was not painful, but induced non-algogenic sensations in the lower abdomen, perineum, and upper part of the lumbar region. With repeated distensions, the referral areas increased progressively and the sensation became frankly painful at the 10th distension. In a later study, the same authors obtained similar results in another visceral domain, the urinary bladder (Ness et al. 1998). Repeated filling of the organ in female volunteers progressively increased the physiological and perceptual responses to pain and the extent of the somatic areas in which pain was perceived. Electrical stimulation of the GI tract also induced phenomena indicative of hypersensitivity in viscera in a study by Arendt-Nielsen et al. (1997). Continuous stimulation of the gut provoked a progressive enlargement of the referred pain area as the duration of the stimulation was increased from 30 to 120 seconds.

Irritable bowel syndrome (IBS). A very common clinical condition estimated to account for 12% of all patient visits to primary care physicians (Drossman et al. 1997) and for more than 50% of all gastroenterological consultations (see Bonica 1990), IBS is regarded as a paradigmatic clinical example of visceral hyperalgesia (Mayer and Gebhart 1993). IBS is characterized by chronic intermittent abdominal discomfort, often ameliorated by defecation, plus frequent constipation or diarrhea, in the absence of any detectable structural, inflammatory, or infectious etiology (Silverman 1999). According to several researchers, pain threshold is lowered in IBS, at least in some portions of the GI tract (references in Vecchiet and Giamberardino 1998). This would explain why patients complain of abdominal/pelvic pain in response to what are assumed to be normal, innocuous stimuli, such as intestinal transit (Thompson 1991) (Table II), and why they experience sensations reminiscent of their typical pain during sigmoid distension in the course of endoscopic examination (see Giamberardino and Vecchiet 1994; Giamberardino 1999). More than 20 years ago, Ritchie (1973) documented that IBS patients reported pain from colonic distension at lower volumes of distension than did normal patients, a finding confirmed in subsequent research by Prior et al. (1990) and Whitehead et al. (1990). Other investigators reported that IBS patients exhibit exaggerated responses to distension of various portions of the GI tract and also that the areas to which sensations are referred are significantly larger than in normal patients (see Aspirotz 1999; Giamberardino 1999). Recent years have seen more and more sophisticated techniques of mechanical distension of the GI tract, and several experimental studies using rectosigmoid balloon distension have provided evidence for both hypervigilance and inducible visceral hyperalgesia in IBS patients (Trimble et al. 1995; Munakata et al. 1997; Naliboff et al. 1997).

Trimble et al. (1995) found that IBS patients exhibited lower rectal sensory thresholds than did controls. In addition, patients had significantly lower sensory thresholds for both perception and discomfort upon balloon distension of the esophagus. Subjects with functional dyspepsia also showed enhanced esophageal sensitivity and lower sensory thresholds for rectal distension. The authors concluded that functional gastrointestinal diseases are characterized by a heightened visceral sensation that is generalized rather than site-specific.

Subsequent studies in which computerized devices made possible more standardized and controlled techniques of gut distension have challenged this assumption by showing that the altered sensitivity at gut level in IBS patients is not generalized and does not necessarily characterize all patients. Naliboff et al. (1997) concluded that IBS patients as a whole do have a greater propensity to label visceral sensations negatively and to show lower tolerance of rectal balloon distension. Only a subgroup of them, however, also have baseline rectal hypersensitivity, when this is assessed by unbiased measures of discomfort thresholds and stimulus intensity judgments.

Recent studies show that IBS patients also demonstrate altered cerebral processing of noxious events from internal organs. Silverman et al. (1997) examined changes in regional blood flow associated with perception of intestinal pain in IBS patients in comparison with controls. While in healthy individuals the perception of acute rectal pain was associated with activation of the anterior cingulate cortex (ACC), IBS patients showed an aberrant brain activation pattern, with no ACC response but instead, activation of the left prefrontal cortex both during noxious rectal distension and during anticipation of rectal pain. The ACC is a site of dense opiate binding (Jones et al. 1991a; Jones and Derbyshire 1994), and blood flow in this region increases significantly in response to analgesic doses of morphine (Jones et al. 1991b). Thus Silverman (1999) hypothesized that the failure of activation of ACC in patients with IBS expecting or receiving a painful visceral stimulus represents failure of a central pathway for descending pain inhibition.

UNDERLYING MECHANISMS

Hyperalgesia from inflammation or excess stimulation is among the most extensively investigated phenomena of hypersensitivity from a visceral domain. Proposed mechanisms are similar to those of primary cutaneous hyperalgesia (which occurs at the site of an injury) (Woolf 1983, 1984), and involve both peripheral and central sensitization (Mayer and Gebhart 1994; Cervero 1995b; see also Coutinho et al. 1998) (Table III).

Peripheral sensitization involves a lowering of the threshold of activation of nociceptors (Belmonte and Cervero 1996). This concept, applied to visceral structures, has long been a matter of debate in the scientific community (Cervero and Jänig 1992; Cervero 1994, 1996).

For quite some time there have been two different schools of thought, one in favor of the "intensity theory" and the other supporting the "specificity theory" in viscera. According to some researchers, painful stimuli in internal organs are encoded in the discharge of receptors with no background activity that respond only to high-intensity stimulation (specific nociceptors or "high-threshold receptors"); these receptors are similar to those described in the skin, muscle, and joints. Other researchers have claimed that noxious events in viscera are encoded in the intensity of discharge of the same population of receptors that also respond to innocuous events (see Giamberardino and Vecchiet 1996). Experimental evidence suggests a specific role for both mechanisms in viscera. Receptors with the characteristics of specific nociceptors, mostly high-threshold receptors sensitive to mechanical stimuli, have been identified in many visceral domains—the ureter (Sann and Cervero 1988; Cervero and Sann 1989), biliary system (Cervero 1982), small intestine (Longhurst and Dittman 1987), uterus (Berkley et al. 1988, 1993), veins (Michaelis et al. 1994), and lungs and airways (Paintal 1986; Widdicombe 1986). Intensity receptors that encode for innocuous and noxious stimuli have been documented in the testes (Kumazawa and Mizumura 1984; Kumazawa 1986). Organs such as the heart (Uchida and Murao 1975; Baker et al. 1980; Coleridge and Coleridge 1980; Malliani and Lombardi 1982), esophagus (Sengupta et al. 1989, 1990), colon (Jänig and Koltzenburg 1991; Sengupta and Gebhart 1994a), and urinary bladder (Coggeshall and Ito 1977; Häbler et al. 1993; Sengupta and Gebhart 1994b) would harbor both kinds of receptors (see also Cervero 1996). The controversy between intensity and specificity theories applied to the visceral domain has somewhat subsided in recent years, as it has become increasingly evident that both mechanisms of receptor activation play a role in visceral nociception, with a possible relative predominance of one or the other, depending on the viscus involved (Cervero and Jänig 1992).

Table III
Mechanisms of hyperalgesia in visceral pain

1) Visceral Hyperalgesia Peripheral (visceral organ) and central sensitization
2) Referred Hyperalgesia from Viscera Central sensitization (viscero-somatic convergence) Viscero-somatic reflex arcs
3) Viscero-visceral Hyperalgesia Central sensitization? (viscero-visceral convergence)

A third category of receptors likely to play an important role in visceral nociception is represented by the "silent" (or "sleeping") nociceptors. These receptors are either unresponsive or have a very high threshold for activation. However, they can be "awakened," i.e., sensitized, by prolonged noxious stimulation that is sufficient to cause inflammation or frank damage in tissues. Receptors with these characteristics were originally identified in joints (Schmidt et al. 1994) as units that could only be activated after the induction of experimental arthritis. They were subsequently also identified in viscera, i.e., the urinary bladder (Häbler et al. 1990), and recently also have been recorded in the heart (Pan and Averill 1998). In the urinary bladder it was demonstrated, in fact, that under conditions of experimental inflammation induced by chemical irritants, many unmyelinated and initially unresponsive afferents were sensitized, generating ongoing activity and in some cases showing a novel mechanosensitivity (i.e., recruitment of mechanically insensitive afferents). Some investigators have stressed the importance of silent nociceptors in visceral algogenic processes, while others believe that their role has been overestimated (see Cervero 1996).

On the whole, knowledge about the nature and characteristics of sensory receptors in viscera suggests that peripheral sensitization due to inflammation or repetitive-prolonged stimulation involves both a lowering in threshold of high-threshold receptors and the bringing into play of previously unresponsive units (silent nociceptors) (Cervero 1995b). The increased input to the CNS would then trigger neuroplastic changes that would amplify the effects of every further signal coming from the affected viscus. This process is known as *central sensitization* and involves phenomena of increased spontaneous activity of central neurons, enlarged receptive field areas, and an increase in response evoked by large- and small-caliber primary afferent fibers (Li et al. 1999).

The results of several experimental studies using animal models of visceral hyperalgesia point to a pivotal role played by N-methyl-D-aspartate (NMDA) receptors in mediating the state of central hyperexcitability (Cervero 1995a,b). NMDA-receptor agonists enhance visceral nociceptive responses (Kolhekar and Gebhart 1994, 1996), and antagonists prevent or inhibit these responses, induced in rats by visceral inflammation produced by intracolonic instillation of zymosan (Coutinho et al. 1996) or by application of turpentine in the urinary bladder (McMahon and Abel 1987; Rice and McMahon 1994). In the colonic model, visceral hyperalgesia is reflected in the facilitation of behavioral responses to colorectal distension in awake rats. In the bladder model, visceral hyperalgesia is expressed by vesical hyper-reflexia consequent to inflammation of the organ. Turpentine inflammation mimics acute cystitis in humans, but also mirrors some of the features of interstitial cystitis, a chronically painful condition, prevalent in women, that is characterized by frequency, urgency, nocturia, and pain in the suprapubic region without any documentable infection of the urine (see Jaggar et al. 1998a). In the animal model, inflammation causes an intense afferent barrage to the spinal cord, which in turn triggers a maintained increase in excitability of dorsal horn neurons (see references in Jaggar et al. 1998a). Hyper-reflexia associated with bladder inflammation in this model was prevented in a dose-dependent fashion by intrathecal application of AP-5, an NMDA-receptor antagonist (Rice and McMahon 1994).

These findings have obvious important implications for future treatment of various forms of visceral hyperalgesia. Other mediators are of potential importance in the generation of the state of central hyperexcitability at the origin of visceral hyperalgesia. Rice (1995) showed that a neuronal selective nitric oxide synthase (NOS) inhibitor, L-Ng-nitro arginine p-nitroanilide (L-Napna), prevented the development of hyper-reflexia subsequent to bladder inflammation from turpentine in the rat, while it had no effect on vesical reflexes under normal conditions. These results indicate that spinal NOS does not play a role in the generation of normal bladder reflexes, but does modulate them during vesical inflammation. Jaggar et al. (1998a) recently explored the role of the two bradykinin receptors (B1 and B2) in generating signs of visceral hyperalgesia in this same model (viscero-visceral hyper-reflexia [VVH] and plasma extravasation). The authors showed that a B2-receptor antagonist was able to prevent and reverse the VVH caused by inflammation. In contrast, a B1-receptor antagonist did not prevent the VVH, but only attenuated it at a relatively late stage, i.e., when administered 5 hours post-inflammation. Neither prevention nor reversal of the VVH from turpentine inflammation was associated with prevention of plasma extravasation into the bladder tissue. These results led the authors to conclude that VVH and tissue inflammation responses are mediated by different mechanisms. In addition, turpentine-induced VVH appears to be attenuated by the cannabinoid anandamide and by the putative CB2-receptor agonist palmitoyl-ethanolamide (Jaggar et al. 1998b). This result confirms the analgesic potential of endogenous ligands at cannabinoid receptor sites.

Several experimental studies have explored the *role of supraspinal centers* in the generation of visceral hyperalgesia. Based on previous research suggesting that the dorsal column (DC) plays an important role in the processing of visceral pain, Al-Chaer et al. (1997) explored electrophysiologically the activity of cells in the nucleus gracilis (NG) in rats subjected to graded colon distension before and after colon inflammation caused by injection of mustard oil (MO). The authors found that colon inflammation with MO lowered the threshold and increased the responses of viscerosensitive

NG cells to colorectal distension. The heightened responses to visceral stimuli of the NG neurons were abolished by a lesion of the dorsal column at the T10 level. Similar observations were made in a separate study of viscerosensitive thalamic nucleus ventroposterolateralis (VPL) neurons (Al-Chaer et al. 1996). According to the authors, the combined results of these two studies "provide a plausible mechanism to explain the central processing and the channels for primary hyperalgesia within the gastrointestinal tract" (Al-Chaer et al. 1997).

Supraspinal descending influences also are possible contributors to visceral hyperalgesia. Coutinho et al. (1998), for instance, have shown the existence of descending modulatory influences on visceral hyperalgesia induced by intracolonic instillation of zymosan in the rat. Two mutually opposing, simultaneous modulatory influences descend from the brainstem rostral ventromedial medulla (RVM): a facilitatory component mediated by activation of NMDA receptors in the RVM and production of nitric oxide, and an inhibitory component mediated by activation of non-NMDA receptors in the RVM. The selective block of one component unmasked the other, which suggests a simultaneous activation of both of them due to inflammation of the colon.

REFERRED HYPERALGESIA FROM VISCERA

As mentioned above, in the areas of referred pain from viscera, hypersensitivity of body wall tissues (skin, subcutis, and muscle) often arises, especially following prolonged or repeated internal algogenic processes. This hypersensitivity is mainly localized in the muscles, where it is often associated with a state of sustained contraction, but is sometimes extended to the overlying subcutis and skin (Procacci et al. 1986; Giamberardino 1999).

Although referred hyperalgesia from viscera is widely known clinically, it has been investigated in controlled conditions by relatively few research groups. Italy has a long tradition in this field (from Lunedei and Galletti to Vecchiet, Procacci, and Giamberardino). Research has focused on characterizing this phenomenon in patients in standardized trials and, more recently, on investigating its pathophysiological mechanisms in experimental studies.

CLINICAL EXPRESSIONS

There are numerous clinical examples of referred hyperalgesia occurring in the course of a visceral algogenic process. A typical example can often be observed during myocardial infarction (Giamberardino and Vecchiet 1996; Foreman 1999). In the early phases, true visceral pain is perceived in the lowest sternal or epigastric areas and sometimes also in the interscapular region; the symptom has only vague localization and an oppressive or constrictive quality, generally accompanied by pallor, profuse sweating, nausea, and vomiting, with associated strong alarm reactions (a feeling of impending death). After a period varying from 10 minutes to several hours, however, the pain reaches the structures of the body wall. Such referred pain becomes sharper in quality, tends to be located in the thoracic region, either anteriorly or posteriorly, and very often extends to the upper limbs (mostly on the left side). Hyperalgesia, mostly at the muscle level, accompanies the symptoms, so that additional stimuli exerted on the area of referral increase the pain. Hyperalgesia mainly involves the pectoralis major and muscles of the interscapular region and forearm. The trapezius and deltoid muscles are less frequently involved. In a minor percentage of cases, pain is also referred to the skin, within dermatomes C8–T1 on the ulnar side of the arm and forearm, and hyperalgesia is found at the same level (Procacci et al. 1986).

Similarly, patients affected with other painful pathologies of internal organs will develop tenderness in the referred pain area. For instance, patients with urinary colics typically display hypersensitivity in muscles of the lumbar region (oblique muscles, quadratus lumborum), and sometimes also in those of the ipsilateral flank and groin area. Patients with biliary calculosis present exquisite tenderness of body wall tissues in the upper right abdominal quadrant (rectus abdominis, upper part), while women suffering from recurrent/chronic pain from their reproductive organs display hypersensitivity in the muscles of the lower abdomen (rectus abdominis, lower part) and pelvic area (Bonica 1990) (Table II).

Several clinical procedures can identify hyperalgesia in the three body wall tissues: the dermographic and Head's procedures for the skin, pinch palpation for the subcutis, and manual compression for the muscle (see Giamberardino and Vecchiet 1996). The Italian literature describes several maneuvers that were specifically designed to detect referred deep hyperalgesia from various organs. "Giordano's maneuver," for instance, reveals deep muscle hypersensitivity in patients with algogenic pathologies of the urinary tract; a clean blow is dealt to the lumbar region (L1) with the ulnar edge of the hand, which provokes a vigorous painful reaction by the patient in the case of hyperalgesia (see Vecchiet et al. 1989). Similarly, Murphy's sign reveals referred muscle hyperalgesia in painful pathologies of the gallbladder; firm digital pressure is applied at the level of the cystic point (at the level of junction of the 10th rib with the outer margin of the rectus abdominis muscle) while the patient is asked to inhale deeply (this puts the rectus abdominis muscle under contraction) (Bonica 1990). If the muscle is hyperalgesic, the breath is briskly interrupted by the intense pain perceived by the patient. Hyperalgesia from painful conditions from the female reproductive organs is typically found by palpating Galletti's point, an abdominal site 4 cm lateral to the navel, on the left side. Firm digital compression at this level typically evokes intense pain, especially in women affected with recurrent/chronic forms of pain from their reproductive area (see Giamberardino et al. 1997b).

Quantification of somatic hyperalgesia. While these clinical techniques are useful for rapidly detecting hyperalgesia in routine medical practice, they do not allow precise assessment of its degree. One way of measuring hypersensitivity in somatic wall tissues is evaluation of pain threshold (the least experience of pain that can be recognized; Merskey and Bogduk 1994) using various instrumental procedures: (a) thermal stimuli (thermal algometer for skin); (b) mechanical stimuli (von Frey hairs for skin, pinch algometer for subcutis, myometer for muscle); (c) chemical stimuli (injections of algogenic substances of progressively increasing concentrations for both subcutis and muscle); and (d) electrical stimuli (for skin, subcutis, and muscle) (Arendt-Nielsen 1997; Vecchiet et al. 1998). Our group has long employed the electrical stimulation technique, since it offers the advantage that thresholds can be measured differentially in the three layers (with surface electrodes for the skin and needle electrodes isolated along their whole length except at the tip for subcutis and muscle). By gradually increasing the intensity of the current, different and typical sensations can be elicited in the three tissues: pricking pain for the skin, linearly radiating prickling pain for the subcutis, and cramplike pain for the muscle. The threshold of these sensations is measured in the tissues by the method of limits (Vecchiet et al. 1989).

By combining this technique with clinical procedures to detect hypersensitivity (often incorporating measurement of pain threshold to mechanical stimulation), our group has performed numerous clinical studies in patients affected with various pathologies of internal organs, particularly of the urinary tract, biliary tract, and female reproductive organs. Our main aim has been to establish a relationship between the appearance, degree, and duration of the referred hyperalgesic phenomena and the algogenic potential of the primary visceral pathology.

Urinary calculosis. Studies performed in patients with urinary calculosis illustrate this category of hyperalgesia (Giamberardino and Vecchiet 1995). Patients affected with calculosis of the upper urinary tract of one side who had previously experienced two or three colic episodes were examined in the pain-free interval. The typical lumbar area of pain referral (metamere L1) was examined bilaterally for hyperalgesia (Vecchiet et al. 1989). Pain threshold to electrical stimulation decreased significantly ipsilaterally to the affected ureter as compared to the contralateral side and to values recorded at the same level in control subjects. This hypersensitivity proved to be very slight in the skin and moderate in the subcutis, but very marked in the muscle, indicating a prominent involvement of deep tissues of the body wall. Subsequent studies found that patients who had suffered from a high number of colics had a greater decrease in pain threshold, mostly at the muscle level, than did patients who had experienced only a few episodes (Vecchiet et al. 1990). Further research was conducted in patients who had previously suffered from colics due to calculosis of one upper urinary tract but had eliminated the stone spontaneously through the urine 3–10 years prior to examination (Vecchiet et al. 1992). Results revealed that hyperalgesia was still present in at least one of the somatic tissues of the body wall (predominantly the muscle) in 90% of the patients, 25% of whom had hyperalgesia of all three types of tissue. Some patients, especially those still presenting marked hyperalgesia in the muscle, reported that they periodically suffered from colic-type pain in spite of having no current instrumental evidence of a new calculosis or of any other organic alteration at the level of the urinary tract. In those patients still displaying muscle hyperalgesia, either with or without spontaneous pain, muscle electrical stimulation for threshold measurement frequently evoked a kind of pain that was described in terms of a "renal colic," similar to the pain experienced before the stone had been eliminated (and different from the typical sensation evoked by the procedure, i.e., a fairly well-localized, cramp-like pain).

Similar results were found in urinary colic patients who had undergone extracorporeal shock-wave lithotripsy (ESWL) (Giamberardino et al. 1994). ESWL is a technique increasingly used for elimination of urinary stones. For research purposes, it is useful in representing an experimental model of stone elimination in humans. Examination of patients before and after partial or total elimination of stone fragments allows researchers to monitor the evolution in time of the referred hyperalgesic component in relation to the primary visceral focus. Patients selected for ESWL were evaluated at lumbar level before treatment; all patients showed hyperalgesia of body wall tissues (particularly the muscle) ipsilaterally to the affected ureter. On examination after partial elimination of stone fragments 1 month subsequent to treatment, these patients showed a rise in pain threshold in the three tissues. At complete stone elimination, 8 months after treatment, thresholds were further increased but still remained significantly lower than normal, mostly at the muscle level.

Overall, the studies on patients with urinary calculosis show that referred somatic hyperalgesia (a) is mostly confined at the muscle level, within the metameric field of the viscus in question; (b) is already detectable in the very first phases of the painful experience; (c) is accentuated by the repetition of the painful episodes; and (d) outlasts not only the spontaneous pain but also the presence of the primary pathology in the visceral domain.

In an attempt to correlate the development of referred hyperalgesia to the presence and extent of spontaneous pain, we performed further studies in patients with urinary calculosis who had never suffered from colic (calculosis was occasionally discovered through ultrasounds or X-rays performed for different clinical reasons). No muscle hyperalgesia was detectable in the expected area of pain referral in these patients. This result suggests that it is the perceived visceral pain, and not the visceral pathology, that determines the occurrence of referred hyperalgesia and its degree and duration (see Giamberardino et al. 1999). The extent of the perceived pain also seems to play a major role in this process, as suggested by the comparison between spontaneous and ESWL-promoted stone elimination. Residual referred muscle hyperalgesia was much greater in patients who had expelled the stone spontaneously than in those who had eliminated the stone after ESWL fragmentation. A specific difference between these two populations of patients depends on the fact that spontaneous stone expulsion usually elicits excruciating pain, whereas elimination of fragments after ESWL is only mildly painful and sometimes even painless (Giamberardino et al. 1994). The different afferent visceral barrage in the two cases is possibly the fundamental factor in conditioning the outcome of the referred phenomena.

Biliary calculosis. Results similar to those obtained in urinary calculosis were found in patients with biliary calculosis, another extremely common painful visceral pathology that frequently causes colic pain (Bonica 1990). In patients with biliary calculosis who had suffered from colics in the past, thresholds were measured at the level of the cystic point, the typical site of pain referral from the gallbladder, and in the contralateral symmetrical site (Vecchiet et al. 1996; Vecchiet and Giamberardino 1998; Giamberardino 1999; Giamberardino et al. 1999). These thresholds, always evaluated in the pain-free interval, were significantly lower in the cystic point than contralaterally, mostly in deep tissues and in particular the muscle. The threshold decrease was significantly more pronounced in patients who had suffered from a high number of colics compared to those who had experienced only a few episodes. Thus, the extent of muscle hyperalgesia appeared to be a function of the pain experienced; as in patients with urinary calculosis, the hyperalgesia was a long-lasting phenomenon, persisting beyond the duration of the spontaneous pain. The dependence of hyperalgesia upon perception of spontaneous visceral pain was confirmed in these patients. In fact, thresholds measured in subjects affected with biliary stones who had never suffered from colic were within normal range. In contrast, thresholds in patients with painful dysfunction of the gallbladder but with no organic visceral pathology were significantly lower than normal. These findings once again confirm the assumption that it is the pain originating from the viscus and not the organic pathology that determines the occurrence, extent, and persistence of hyperalgesia.

Primary dysmenorrhea. A careful analysis of the referred component of a visceral algogenic pathology was also performed in women affected with primary dysmenorrhea (painful menstruation), a condition estimated to occur in approximately 50% of all menstruating women (Ylikorkala and Dawood 1978). In a study comparing dysmenorrheic and nondysmenorrheic women, pain thresholds to electrical stimulation were measured in the referred pain area (two symmetrical sites in the abdomen, 4 cm lateral to the navel) and also in two control sites on limbs (at the deltoid and quadriceps level) in the skin, subcutis, and muscle. Measurement was performed in four different phases of the menstrual cycle, i.e., in a 28-day cycle: menstrual, days 2–6; periovulatory, days 12–16; luteal, days 17–22; premenstrual, days 25–28 (Giamberardino et al. 1997b). The most interesting results concerned the muscle. Thresholds varied throughout the cycle, with lowest values always in the perimenstrual phase and highest always in the luteal phase, whatever the body site. In dysmenorrheic women the monthly trend was more accentuated, and the threshold decrease in the perimenstrual phase more pronounced. Thresholds in the abdomen in dysmenorrheic women were significantly lower than in nondysmenorrheic women, not only close to the painful period (perimenstrual phase) but also in the other phases (periovulatory, luteal). Muscle pain thresholds were significantly lower in the abdomen than in the limbs, particularly in dysmenorrheic women. There was also a direct linear correlation between the pain threshold decrease in the perimenstrual period and the intensity of the menstrual pain, both in nondysmenorrheic and dysmenorrheic women (normal women usually experience some degree of pain during menses, although of mild intensity). Further studies were conducted in different groups of women who had suffered from dysmenorrhea for a progressively higher number of years, which corresponds to a progressively higher number of painful episodes, given the recurrent nature of this painful condition (see Giamberardino et al. 1999). The results showed that the extent of pain threshold decrease at the muscle level in the perimenstrual phase was greater in those who had suffered from dysmenorrhea for many years than in those who had experienced it for only a few years. Studies of dysmenorrhea have thus confirmed the finding in other visceral pathologies that referred hyperalgesia from viscera is mostly a muscle phenomenon, that its extent is a function of the pain previously experienced by the patient, and that its duration is prolonged, i.e., outlasts the phase of spontaneous pain.

Trophic changes. In the areas of pain referral from viscera, typical *trophic* changes can be found in addition to the sensory changes in body wall tissues, consisting of thickening of subcutis and reduced thickness of muscle (Vecchiet and Giamberardino 1998; Giamberardino 1999). These changes can be detected by simple clinical tests, such as pincer palpation, but can be more easily detected and quantified by using instrumental procedures such as ultrasound evaluation of subcutis and muscle thickness (and also of muscle section area, when anatomically possible). Our group has documented trophic changes in patients with various pathologies of internal organs. Subjects suffering from urinary colics from calculosis presented a significantly increased thickness of subcutis and a significantly decreased thickness of muscle (obliquus externus) on the affected side compared to the contralateral side (Vecchiet et al. 1990; Vecchiet and Giamberardino 1998). Similarly, in patients with gallbladder calculosis, we found a significantly increased thickness of subcutis and significantly decreased thickness of muscle at the level of the cystic point compared to the contralateral symmetric side (Vecchiet et al. 1996; Giamberardino et al. 1999). As for the hyperalgesia, these trophic changes appeared to be a function of the algogenic potential of the internal disease. In fact, they were not detectable in patients with biliary calculosis who had never experienced any pain, while they were present in patients affected with painful gallbladder dysfunction (M.A. Giamberardino, unpublished observation).

UNDERLYING MECHANISMS

The most credited hypothesis about mechanisms of referred hyperalgesia from viscera attributes the phenomenon to a process of central sensitization that takes place in the CNS and is triggered by the massive afferent visceral barrage upon convergent viscerosomatic neurons (Cervero 1993) (Table III).

Viscerosomatic convergence, in fact, is the rule in visceral pain, as many electrophysiological studies in animals have demonstrated, at both the spinal and supraspinal levels (Pomeranz et al. 1968; Willis and Coggeshall 1991; see also Wall 1993; Kawakita et al. 1997; Ito 1998). As discussed above, central sensitization involves phenomena of increased activity and excitability of neurons; this process has been documented in cases of referred hyperalgesia from viscera in electrophysiological studies on animal models (see Giamberardino 1999). One such model was devised by our group (Giamberardino et al. 1990, 1995) and subsequently adopted by other laboratories (Laird et al. 1997; Roza et al. 1998). This model of experimental ureteric calculosis in rats mimics urinary colics and referred lumbar muscle hyperalgesia in humans. Rats in which an artificial stone was formed in the upper third of one ureter showed behavioral signs indicative of both direct visceral pain and referred hyperalgesia of the oblique musculature. For several days subsequent to the intervention, in fact, the animals presented multiple complex behavioral "crises" whose characteristic movements and postures were suggestive of urinary colics in patients, as shown by long-term videorecording. Along with the crises, which were mostly concentrated during the first 3–4 days, calculosis rats showed referred muscle hypersensitivity, as evidenced by a significant decrease in the vocalization threshold to electrical stimulation (considered as an equivalent of the pain threshold in humans) at the level of the obliquus externus muscle (the same muscle involved in patients with urinary stones) ipsilateral to the affected ureter. This threshold decrease appeared as soon as the first day after stone implantation and lasted over a week, although it peaked on the second to third day. The extent of the maximal threshold decrease was positively correlated with the number of painful "crises" shown by the animal. Thus, as in patients, referred muscle hyperalgesia is an early process, accentuated by repetition of the visceral pain episodes, and lasts for a long time, sometimes even beyond the presence of the stone in the urinary tract. In fact, hypersensitivity is often detectable up to the last day of evaluation, even in rats that proved to have eliminated the stone through urination (i.e., the stone was no longer detectable in the urinary tract on autopsy). Electrophysiological evidence at the spinal cord level (the lowest thoracic segments) in this animal model provides a further indication that a condition of central sensitization takes place as a consequence of the massive afferent barrage from the viscus. In fact, neurons receiving input from the hyperalgesic muscle (Giamberardino et al. 1996, 1997) and from the affected ureter (Roza et al. 1998) showed signs of both hyperactivity and hyperexcitability. The extent of this sensitization in the spinal cord was proportional to the degree of muscle hyperalgesia behaviorally evaluated in the rats prior to the electrophysiological experiment.

As mentioned in the previous sections, mechanisms underlying the central neuronal changes in visceral nociception have been explored in a number of experimental studies on animal models of hypersensitivity from internal organs (references in Giamberardino 1999). As a result of these studies, and similar to the findings for visceral hyperalgesia, NMDA receptors have been suggested to play an important role in generating the changes in central hyperexcitability that mediate referred hyperalgesia from viscera (see Cervero 1995a).

One crucial point concerning the pathophysiology of referred phenomena from viscera is the fact that hyperalgesia is a persistent phenomenon, which outlasts not only the spontaneous pain but also often the presence of the primary focus in the visceral domain. The main issue of debate regarding the process of central sensitization is whether central changes, once established, persist over time and become relatively independent of the primary peripheral, "macroscopic" focus that originally triggered them, or whether they require continued input from the periphery (Coderre et al. 1992; Wall 1993; Cervero 1995b; Devor 1997).

Several experimental studies in animals have shown that a nociceptive input from deep structures (and visceral organs *are* deep structures) is much more powerful than an input from cutaneous structures in creating central plastic changes of long duration (Wall and Woolf 1984; Woolf and Wall 1986). It is thus plausible that input from viscera could trigger changes that might outlive the peripheral event. However, it cannot be excluded that several clinically inapparent peripheral changes at the visceral level continue to act even after apparent removal of the visceral focus, and sustain the central changes. The results of recent studies on ureter motility in rats with artificial ureteral calculosis, which found abnormal hypermotility persisting long after stone elimination (Laird et al. 1997), indeed suggest that various "clinically inapparent" peripheral visceral changes are likely to outlast the presence of the primary focus and thus maintain the state of central hyperexcitability via persistence of the peripheral drive.

The contribution of further mechanisms in the genesis of referred hyperalgesia from viscera cannot be ruled out. Algogenic conditions could develop at the periphery (i.e., the referred area), with subsequent excitation of pain receptors, because of several viscerocutaneous and visceromuscular reflexes that are triggered by the afferent visceral barrage (see Procacci et al. 1986; Giamberardino and Vecchiet 1996) (Table III). Referred hyperalgesia would thus be produced by activation of a reflex arc, of which the afferent branch is represented by sensory afferent fibers from the viscera, while the efferent branch differs for superficial and deep somatic tissues. Some authors have concluded that hyperalgesia and related trophic phenomena at skin level are induced by sympathetic efferents (Penfield 1925; Davis and Pollock 1930; Procacci et al. 1986); an experimental, local anesthetic block of the sympathetic ganglia in patients led to the disappearance of or a marked decrease in referred pain, hyperalgesia, and dermographic alterations (Galletti and Procacci 1966). In contrast, hyperalgesia in muscle is caused by somatic efferents in this view. These are responsible for a sustained contraction that in turn sensitizes muscular nociceptors and becomes a new source of pain. The muscle contraction that occurs subsequent to noxious visceral stimulation was illustrated in a classic experiment by McLellan and Goodell in 1943. Upon electrical stimulation of the pelvis and ureter in patients, muscles on the abdominal wall on the stimulated side remained contracted and began to ache 30 minutes later. The aching increased over the following 6 hours, with tenderness persisting until the next day. It must be noted, however, that sustained contraction is not always documented in cases of referred hyperalgesia, even though it is a frequent finding. Therefore, while local sensitization of nociceptors via a reflex arc may contribute in some cases, it certainly is not the sole mechanism.

The reflex arc hypothesis has yet to be confirmed experimentally; apart from the clinical research reported above, few experimental studies have specifically addressed this issue. Some results in the rat model of ureteric calculosis indicate that a reflex mechanism could play a role in the generation of referred hyperalgesia from viscera. In fact, some degree of hyperactivity and hyperexcitability was found in neurons with input from the hyperalgesic muscle located in the intermediate region of the cord (at the level of the lowest thoracic segments), where the cells of origin of the sympathetic outflow are situated (Giamberardino et al. 1996). It is clear, however, that more studies are needed to test this hypothesis.

In this regard, further animal models of this condition will be of particular value. One such model, established recently by Wesselmann and Lai (1997), reproduces persistent pain from the female reproductive organs through injection of mustard oil into one uterine horn. Rats with experimental uterine inflammation showed signs both of direct visceral pain (major episodes of movements and postures of the rat resembling those of rats with experimental calculosis) and of referred hyperalgesia of the flank musculature ipsilateral to the inflamed uterine horn (Wesselmann et al. 1998). In the areas of referred muscle hyperalgesia in rats with uterine inflammation, neurogenic plasma extravasation in the skin has also been documented, in the first experimental evidence of trophic changes in sites of referred pain from viscera (Wesselmann and Lai 1997). This animal model thus seems particularly useful for investigation of mechanisms other than central sensitization as the basis of referred phenomena from internal organs.

VISCERO-VISCERAL HYPERALGESIA

Viscero-visceral hyperalgesia is undoubtedly the least investigated form of visceral hyperalgesia. Yet clear examples in patients show that the pain reactivity of one visceral domain can be enhanced by an algogenic process in another internal organ. This phenomenon usually involves viscera with at least partially overlapping innervation (see Vecchiet and Giamberardino 1998; Giamberardino 1999).

CLINICAL EXPRESSIONS

Although systematic studies have not yet been conducted, it is not unusual to observe in the clinical setting that patients with ischemic heart disease who are also affected with gallbladder calculosis complain of a higher number of anginal attacks than do patients with ischemic heart disease and a normal gallbladder. The gallbladder and heart do in fact have a partially overlapping central projection (at the T5 level). Another example is the interaction between pathologies of the urinary tract and female reproductive organs, such as dysmenorrhea and urinary calculosis.

A recent epidemiological study by our group (Giamberardino et al. 1998a,c; Giamberardino 1999), which used an ad hoc questionnaire in fertile women, both nondysmenorrheic and dysmenorrheic, found a viscero-visceral interaction between the female reproductive organs and the urinary tract (common spinal segments T10–L1) (Table II). Fertile women affected with urinary calculosis (and a tendency to repeated colic episodes) who were also dysmenorrheic manifested a higher number of colics than did nondysmenorrheic women with urinary calculosis of comparable characteristics, when examined in a retrospective study over 3 years. A prospective evaluation, over a period of 2 years, revealed that the women manifested their urinary colic preferentially in one specific phase of their monthly cycle; this tendency was more pronounced if they also suffered from dysmenorrhea. In particular, the dysmenorrheic women could typically be divided into two subgroups: in the first, the colics always occurred premenstrually, while in the second they always occurred at mid-cycle, around the time of ovulation. These data indicate that colic pain from the urinary tract was preferentially manifested in periods of the cycle when the input from the female reproductive organs was greatly enhanced by pelvic congestion (around either menstruation or ovulation).

In addition to a higher number of urinary colics, dysmenorrheic women also presented a much greater degree of referred muscle hyperalgesia at the lumbar level, that is in the area of pain referral from the urinary tract, than did nondysmenorrheic women who had experienced a comparable number of colics. Thus, referred hyperalgesia from the urinary tract was notably enhanced by the inflammatory condition of the reproductive organs.

UNDERLYING MECHANISMS

Viscero-visceral hyperalgesia is a complex form of hypersensitivity that is likely to be mediated by more than one mechanism. It takes place preferentially among visceral organs that share, at least in part, their central projection, so it is plausible that phenomena of central sensitization play an important role (Table III). Hyperactivity and hyperexcitability could involve viscero-visceral convergent neurons at the central level. Viscero-visceral convergences have, in fact, been documented in electrophysiological studies in animals, for instance between the gallbladder and heart (Foreman 1989) (which would explain the frequent interaction between pathologies of these two organs), and between the colon/rectum, urinary bladder, vagina, and uterine cervix (Berkley et al. 1993a,b; see also Ness and Gebhart 1990) (which would explain the clinical interaction between female reproductive organs and the urinary tract). The increased input from one visceral domain could trigger changes in the excitability of these neurons and thus enhance the central effect of the input from the second visceral domain.

This hypothesis, however, must be verified experimentally, and other possible mechanisms could also be implicated. It would thus be of great importance to have a reliable animal model of the viscero-visceral hyperalgesia that is observed in patients. One such model has recently been set up to reproduce the characteristics of the viscero-visceral interaction between the female reproductive organs and the urinary tract. Our group combined the model of urinary calculosis in rats with a model of experimental endometriosis established by Wood et al. (1995) and Bradshaw and Berkley (1996). Endometriosis was chosen because it is a very frequent cause of secondary dysmenorrhea in women (Bonica 1990). Preliminary data in this model have shown that rats with experimental endometriosis plus urinary stones display a significantly higher number and duration of typical ureteral crises than do rats with sham endometriosis plus urinary stones. In addition, they also show a much higher degree of referred muscle hyperalgesia than do sham endometriosis rats (Giamberardino et al. 1998a,b, 1999). This model thus represents the experimental counterpart of the clinical condition, and may be a useful tool for further investigation of the underlying mechanisms.

CONCLUSIONS

Clinical evidence and controlled studies in patients and human volunteers have clearly shown that phenomena of hyperalgesia from internal organs have multiple expressions, since they involve not only the visceral domains primarily affected by the algogenic pathologies but also the somatic domain in the site of pain referral. The different categories of hyperalgesia from viscera are likely to be sustained by diverse pathophysiological mechanisms (Table III), as suggested by the outcome of studies on animal models of the various conditions.

Some of these mechanisms, i.e., those underlying visceral hyperalgesia according to its strict definition, have been fairly thoroughly investigated. Other mechanisms that are responsible for referred hyperalgesia from viscera are still incompletely clarified, in spite of a relatively vigorous research effort in this direction, especially in recent years. The mechanisms of viscerovisceral hyperalgesia are only just beginning to be explored, as the nature and importance of this form of hypersensitivity are becoming progressively more evident in the clinical setting.

Clarification of the pathophysiology of these phenomena of hyperalgesia from viscera is undoubtedly fundamental to the development of therapeutic strategies that are not merely symptomatic, and will also help clinicians better identify the target and most appropriate timing of treatment.

However, while distinguishing different categories of hyperalgesia is useful for research purposes, it is extremely important never to forget that clinically, these categories can often intermingle. Together they give rise to the patient's global pain experience, which is ultimately what clinicians are called on in their daily practice to diagnose, to differentiate from other conditions, often in difficult circumstances, and finally to treat.

ACKNOWLEDGMENTS

The author wishes to thank Professor Leonardo Vecchiet, Director of the Semeiotica Medica at the "G. D'Annunzio" University of Chieti, for valuable suggestions and critical revision of the manuscript.

REFERENCES

Al-Chaer ED, Westlund KN, Willis WD. Potentiation of thalamic responses to colorectal distension by visceral inflammation. *Neuroreport* 1996; 7:1635–1639.

Al-Chaer ED, Westlund KN, Willis WD. In: Jensen TS, Turner JA, Wiesenfeld-Hallin Z (Eds). *Proceedings of the 8th World Congress on Pain,* Progress in Pain Research and Management, Vol. 8. Seattle: IASP Press, 1997, pp 839–853.

Arendt-Nielsen L. Induction and assessment of experimental pain from human skin, muscle and viscera. In: Jensen TS, Turner JA, Wiesenfeld-Hallin Z (Eds). *Proceedings of the 8th World Congress on Pain,* Progress in Pain Research and Management, Vol. 8. Seattle: IASP Press, 1997, pp 393–425.

Arendt-Nielsen L, Drewes AM, Hansen JB, Tage-Jensen U. Plasticity of gut pain in man: an experimental investigation using short and long duration transmucosal electrical stimulation. *Pain* 1997; 69:255–262.

Aspirotz F. Dimensions of gut dysfunction in irritable bowel syndrome: altered sensory function. *Can J Gastroenterol* 1999; 13(A):12–14.

Ayala M. Douleur sympathique et douleur viscérale [Sympathetic pain and visceral pain]. *Rev Neurol* 1937; 68:222–242.

Baker DG, Coleridge HM, Coleridge JCG, Nerdrum T. Search for a cardiac nociceptor: stimulation by bradykinin of sympathetic afferent nerve endings in the heart of the cat. *J Physiol (Lond)* 1980; 302:519–536.

Belmonte C, Cervero F (Eds). *Neurobiology of Nociceptors*. Oxford: Oxford University Press, 1996.

Berkley KJ, Robbins A, Sato Y. Afferent fibers supplying the uterus in the rat. *J Neurophysiol* 1988; 59:142–163.

Berkley KJ, Robbins A, Sato Y. Functional differences between afferent fibers in the hypogastric and pelvic nerves innervating female reproductive organs in the rat. *J Neurophysiol* 1993; 69:533–544.

Berkley KJ, Hubscher CH, Wall PD. Neuronal responses to stimulation of the cervix, uterus, colon and skin in the rat spinal cord. *J Neurophysiol* 1993a; 69:533–544.

Berkley KJ, Guilbaud G, Benoist JM, Gautron M. Responses of neurons in and near the thalamic ventrobasal complex of the rat to stimulation of uterus, cervix, vagina, colon and skin. *J Neurophysiol* 1993b; 69:557–568.

Bonica JJ (Ed). *The Management of Pain*. Philadephia: Lea & Febiger, 1990.

Bradshaw HB, Berkley KJ. Effects of estrous stage and endometriosis on escape response to vaginal distention and vaginal tone in the awake rat. *Abstracts: 8th World Congress on Pain*. Seattle: IASP Press, 1996, p 247.

Cervero F. Afferent activity evoked by natural stimulation of the biliary system in the ferret. *Pain* 1982; 13:137–151.

Cervero F. Pathophysiology of referred pain and hyperalgesia from viscera. In: Vecchiet L, Albe-Fessard D, Lindblom U, Giamberardino MA (Eds). *New Trends in Referred Pain and Hyperalgesia*, Pain Research and Clinical Management, Vol. 7. Amsterdam: Elsevier, 1993, pp 35–46.

Cervero F. Sensory innervation of the viscera: peripheral basis of visceral pain. *Physiol Rev* 1994; 74(1):95–138.

Cervero F. Mechanisms of visceral pain: past and present. In: Gebhart GF (Ed). *Visceral Pain*, Progress in Pain Research and Management, Vol. 5. Seattle: IASP Press, 1995a, pp 25–40.

Cervero F. Visceral pain: mechanisms of peripheral and central sensitization. *Ann Med* 1995b; 2:235–239.

Cervero F. Visceral nociceptors. In: Belmonte C, Cervero F (Eds). *Neurobiology of Nociceptors*. New York: Oxford University Press, 1996, pp 220–240.

Cervero F, Jänig W. Visceral nociceptors: a new world order. *Trends Neurosci* 1992; 15:374–378.

Cervero F, Sann H. Mechanically evoked responses of afferent fibers innervating the guinea-pig's ureter: an in vitro study. *J Physiol Lond* 1989; 412:245–166.

Coderre TJ, Katz J, Vaccarino AL, Melzack R. Contribution of central neuroplasticity to pathological pain: review of clinical and experimental evidence. *Pain* 1992; 52:259–285.

Coggeshall RE, Ito H. Sensory fibers in ventral roots L7 and S1 in the cat. *J Physiol (Lond)* 1977; 267:215–235.

Coleridge HM, Coleridge JCG. Cardiovascular afferents involved in regulation of peripheral vessels. *Annu Rev Physiol* 1980; 42:413–427.

Coutinho SV, Meller ST, Gebhart GF. Intracolonic zymosan produces visceral hyperalgesia in the rat that is mediated by spinal NMDA and non-NMDA receptors. *Brain Res* 1996; 736:7–15.

Coutinho SV, Urban MO, Gebhart GF. Role of glutamate receptors and nitric oxide in the rostral ventromedial medulla in visceral hyperalgesia. *Pain* 1998; 78:59–69.

Davis L, Pollock LJ. The peripheral pathway for painful sensations. *Arch Neurol Psychiatry* 1930; 24:883–898.

Devor M. Central versus peripheral substrates of persistent pain: which contributes more? *Behav Brain Sci* 1997; 20:446.

Drewes AM, Arendt-Nielsen L, Jensen JH, et al. Experimental pain in the stomach: a model based on electrical stimulation guided by gastroscopy. *Gut* 1997; 41(6):753–757.

Drossman DA, Whitehead WE, Camilleri M. Irritable bowel syndrome: a technical review for practice guideline development. *Gastroenterology* 1997; 112:2120–2137.

Foreman RD. Organization of the spinothalamic tract as a relay for cardiopulmonary sympathetic afferent fiber activity. *Prog Sens Physiol* 1989; 9:1–51.

Foreman RD. Mechanisms of cardiac pain. *Annu Rev Physiol* 1999; 61:143–147

Frobert O, Arendt-Nielsen L, Bak P, Funk J, Bakker JP. Oesophageal sensation assessed by electrical stimuli and brain evoked potentials: a new model for visceral nociception. *Gut* 1995; 37:603–609.

Galletti R, Procacci P. The role of the sympathetic system in the control of somatic pain and of some associated phenomena. *Acta Neuroveg* 28; 1966:495–500.

Gebhart GF (Ed). *Visceral Pain.* Progress in Pain Research and Management, Vol. 5. Seattle: IASP Press, 1995a.

Gebhart GF. Visceral nociception: consequences, modulation and the future. *Eur J Anaesthesiol* 1995b; 12(10):24–27.

Giamberardino MA. Recent and forgotten aspects of visceral pain. *Eur J Pain* 1999; 3:77–92.

Giamberardino MA, Vecchiet L. Visceral pain, referred hyperalgesia and outcome: new concepts. *Eur J Anaesthesiol* 1995; 12(10):61–66.

Giamberardino MA, Vecchiet L. Pathophysiology of visceral pain. *Curr Rev Pain* 1996; 1:23–33.

Giamberardino MA, Vecchiet L, Albe-Fessard D. Comparison of the effects of ureteral calculosis and occlusion on muscular sensitivity in rats. *Pain* 1990; 43:227–234.

Giamberardino MA, Vecchiet L. Experimental studies on pelvic pain. *Pain Rev* 1994; 1:102–115.

Giamberardino MA, de Bigontina P, Martegiani C, Vecchiet L. Effects of extracorporeal shock-wave lithotripsy on referred hyperalgesia from renal/ureteral calculosis. *Pain* 1994; 56:77–83.

Giamberardino MA, Valente R, de Bigontina P, Vecchiet L. Artificial ureteral calculosis in rats: behavioural characterization of visceral pain episodes and their relationship with referred lumbar muscle hyperalgesia. *Pain* 1995; 61:459–469.

Giamberardino MA, Dalal A, Valente R, Vecchiet L. Changes in activity of spinal cells with muscular input in rats with referred muscular hyperalgesia from ureteral calculosis. *Neurosci Lett* 1996; 203:89–92.

Giamberardino MA, Valente R, Affaitati G, Vecchiet L. Central neuronal changes in recurrent visceral pain. *Int J Clin Pharmacol Res* 1997a; 17(2/3):63–66.

Giamberardino MA, Berkley KJ, Iezzi S, de Bigontina P, Vecchiet L. Pain threshold variations in somatic wall tissues as a function of menstrual cycle, segmental site and tissue depth in non-dysmenorrheic women, dysmenorrheic women and men. *Pain* 1997b; 71:187–197.

Giamberardino MA, Affaitati G, Lerza R, Vecchiet L, Berkley KJ. The impact of painful pelvic conditions on pain of urological origin: human and animal studies. *Abstracts: 4th Italian Congress of "Neuroscience and Pain" Group*. Siena, 1998a, pp 23–24.

Giamberardino MA, Affaitati G, Vecchiet L, Berkley KJ. Effects of endometriosis on pain behaviours induced by ureteral calculosis in female rats. *J Musculoskeletal Pain* 1998b; 6(2):172.

Giamberardino MA, de Laurentis S, Affaitati G, et al. The impact of menstrual cycle upon pain perception from urinary calculosis. *Dolor* 1998c; 13:32.

Giamberardino MA, Berkley KJ, Affaitati G, Lerza R, Vecchiet L. The influence of endometriosis on pain behaviors induced by ureteral calculosis in female rats. *Abstracts: 9th World Congress on Pain,* Seattle: IASP Press, 1999, p 392.

Giamberardino MA, Affaitati G, Iezzi S, Vecchiet L. Referred muscle pain and hyperalgesia from viscera. *J Musculoskeletal Pain* 1999; 7(1/2):61–69.

Häbler H-J, Jänig W, Koltzenburg M. Activation of unmyelinated afferent fibers by mechanical stimuli and inflammation of the urinary bladder in the cat. *J Physiol (Lond)* 1990; 425:545–562.

Häbler H-J, Jänig W, Koltzenburg M. Myelinated primary afferents of the sacral spinal cord responding to slow filling and distension of the urinary bladder. *J Physiol (Lond)* 1993; 463:449–460.

Hansen K, Schliack H. *Segmentale Innervation: Ihre Bedeutung für Klinik und Praxis*. Stuttgart: Thieme, 1962, pp 166–325.

Ito SI. Possible representation of somatic pain in the rat insular visceral sensory cortex: a field potential study. *Neurosci Lett* 1998; 24:171–174.

Jaggar SI, Habib S, Rice ASC. The modulatory effects of Bradykinin B1 and B2 receptor antagonists upon viscero-visceral hyper-reflexia in a rat model of visceral hyperalgesia. *Pain* 1998a; 75:169–176.

Jaggar SI, Hasnie FS, Sellaturay S, Rice ASC. The anti-hyperalgesic actions of the cannabinoid anandamide and the putative CB2 receptor agonist palmitoylethanolamide in visceral and somatic inflammatory pain. *Pain* 1998b; 76:189–199.

Jänig W, Koltzenburg M. Receptive properties of sacral primary afferent neurons supplying the colon. *J Neurophysiol* 1991; 65:1067–1077.

Jones AKP, Derbyshire SWG. Positron emission tomography as a tool for understanding the cerebral processing of pain. In: Boivie J, Hansson P, Lindblom U (Eds). *Touch, Temperature, and Pain in Health and Disease: Mechanisms and Assessments,* Progress in Pain Research and Management, Vol. 3. Seattle: IASP Press, 1994, pp 491–520.

Jones AKP, Friston KJ, Qi LY. Sites of action of morphine in the brain. *Lancet* 1991a; 338:825.

Jones AKP, Qi LY, Fujirawa T. In vivo distribution of opioid receptors in man in relation to the cortical projections of the medial and lateral pain systems measured with positron emission tomography. *Neurosci Lett* 1991b; 126:25–28.

Kawakita K, Sumiya E, Murase K, Okada K. Response characteristics of nucleus submedius neurons to colo-rectal distension in the rat. *Neurosci Res* 1997; 28:59–66.

Kinsella VJ. *The Mechanism of Abdominal Pain*. Sydney: Australasian Medical Publishing Company, 1948.

Kolhekar R, Gebhart GF. NMDA and quisqualate modulation of visceral nociception in the rat. *Brain Res* 1994; 561:215–226.

Kolhekar R, Gebhart GF. Modulation of spinal nociceptive transmission by NMDA receptor activation in the rat. *J Neurophysiol* 1996; 75:2344–2351.

Koltzenburg M, McMahon SB. Mechanically insensitive primary afferents innervating the urinary bladder. In: Gebhart GF (Ed). *Visceral Pain,* Progress in Pain Research and Management, Vol. 5. Seattle: IASP Press, 1995, pp 163–192.

Kumazawa T. Sensory innervation of reproductive organs. In: Cervero F, Morrison JFB (Eds). *Visceral Sensation,* Progress in Brain Research, Vol. 67. Amsterdam: Elsevier, 1986.

Kumazawa T, Mizumura K. Functional properties of the polymodal receptors in the deep tissues. In: Hamann W, Iggo A (Eds). *Sensory Receptor Mechanisms*. Singapore: World Scientific Publishing Company, 1984, pp 1193–1202.

Laird JMA, Roza C, Cervero F. Effects of artificial calculosis on rat ureter motility: peripheral contribution to the pain of ureteric colic. *Am J Physiol* 1997; 272:R1409–R1416.

Lewis T. *Pain*. New York: Macmillan, 1942, pp 118–172.

Li J, Simone DA, Larson AA. Windup leads to characteristics of central sensitization. *Pain* 1999; 79:75–82.

Longhurst JC, Dittman LE. Hypoxia, bradykinin and prostaglandins stimulate ischemically sensitive visceral afferents. *Am J Physiol Heart Circ Physiol* 1987; 253:H556–H567.

Lunedei A, Galletti R. Il meccanismo di insorgenza del dolore dei visceri nei suoi recenti sviluppi [Mechanisms of pain from viscera: recent advances]. *Rass Neurol Veg* 1953;10:3–22.

Malliani A, Lombardi F. Consideration of the fundamental mechanisms eliciting cardiac pain. *Am Heart J* 1982; 103:575–578.

Mayer EA, Gebhart G. Functional bowel disorders and the visceral hyperalgesia hypothesis. In: Mayer EA, Raybould HE (Eds). *Basic and Clinical Aspects of Chronic Abdominal Pain,* Pain Research and Clinical Management, Vol. 9. Amsterdam: Elsevier, 1993, pp 3–28.

Mayer EA. Gebhart GF. Basic and clinical aspects of visceral hyperalgesia. *Gastroenterology* 1994; 107:271–293.

McLellan AM, Goodell H. Pain from the bladder, ureter and kidney pelvis. *Proc Assoc Res Nerv Ment Dis* 1943; 23:252–262.

McMahon SB. Are there fundamental differences in the peripheral mechanisms of visceral and somatic pain? *Behav Brain Sci* 1997; 20:381–391.

McMahon SB, Abel C. A model for the study of visceral pain states: chronic inflammation of the chronic decerebrate rat urinary bladder by irritant chemicals. *Pain* 1987; 28:109–127.

Merskey H, Bogduk N. *Classification of Chronic Pain: Descriptions of Chronic Pain Syndromes and Definitions of Pain Terms,* 2nd ed. Seattle: IASP Press, 1994.

Michaelis M, Göder M, Häbler H-J, Jänig W. Properties of afferent nerve fibers supplying the saphenous vein in the cat. *J Physiol (Lond)* 1994; 474:233–243.

Munakata J, Naliboff B, Harraf F, et al. Repetitive sigmoid stimulation induces rectal hyperalgesia in patients with irritable bowel syndrome. *Gastroenterology* 1997; 112:55–63.

Naliboff BD, Munakata J, Fullerton S, et al. Evidence for two distinct perceptual alterations in irritable bowel syndrome. *Gut* 1997; 51:505–512.

Ness TJ, Gebhart GF. Visceral pain: a review of experimental studies. *Pain* 1990; 41:167–234.

Ness TJ, Metcalf AM, Gebhart GF. A psychophysiological study in humans using phasic colonic distension as a noxious visceral stimulus. *Pain* 1990; 43:377–386.

Ness TJ, Richter HE, Varner RE, Fillingim RB. A psychophysical study of discomfort produced by repeated filling of the urinary bladder. *Pain* 1998; 76:61–69.

Paintal AS. The visceral sensations: some basic mechanisms. In: Cervero F, Morrison JFB (Eds). *Visceral Sensation,* Progress in Brain Research, Vol. 67. Amsterdam: Elsevier, 1986, pp 3–19.

Pan H-L, Averill D. Functional properties of silent cardiac sympathetic afferents in cats. *FASEB J* 1998; 12(5):399.

Penfield W. Neurological mechanism of angina pectoris and its relation to surgical therapy. *Am J Med Sci* 1925; 170:864–873.

Pomeranz B, Wall PD, Weber WV. Cord cells responding to fine myelinated afferents from visceral muscle and skin. *J Physiol (Lond)* 1968; 199:511–532.

Prior A, Maxton DG, Whorwell PJ. Anorectal manometry in irritable bowel syndrome: differences between diarrhea and constipation predominant subjects. *Gut* 1990; 31(4):458–462.

Procacci P, Maresca M, Zoppi M. Visceral and deep somatic pain. *Acupunct Electrother Res* 1978; 3:135–160.

Procacci P, Zoppi M, Maresca M. Clinical approach to visceral sensation. In: Cervero F, Morrison JFB (Eds). *Visceral Sensation,* Progress in Brain Research, Vol. 67. Amsterdam: Elsevier, 1986, pp 21–28.

Rice AS. Topical spinal administration of a nitric oxide synthase inhibitor prevents the hyper-reflexia associated with a rat model of persistent visceral pain. *Neurosci Lett* 1995; 187:111–114.

Rice ASC, McMahon SB. Pre-emptive intrathecal administration of an NMDA receptor antagonist (AP-5) prevents hyper-reflexia in a model of persistent visceral pain. *Pain* 1994; 57:335–340.

Ritchie J. Pain from distension of the pelvic colon by inflating a balloon in the irritable bowel syndrome. *Gut* 1973; 14:125–132.

Roza C, Laird JMA, Cervero F. Spinal mechanisms underlying persistent pain and referred hyperalgesia in rats with an experimental ureteric stone. *J Neurophysiol* 1998; 79:1603–1612.

Sann H, Cervero F. Afferent innervation of the guinea-pig's ureter. *Agents Actions* 1988; 25:243–245.

Schmidt RF, Schaible H-G, Messlinger K, et al. Silent and active nociceptive structure, functions, and clinical implications. In: Gebhart GF, Hammond DL, Jensen TS (Eds). *Proceedings of the 7th World Congress on Pain,* Progress in Pain Research and Management, Vol. 2. Seattle: IASP Press, 1994, pp 213–250.

Sengupta JN, Gebhart GF. Characterization of mechanosensitive pelvic nerve afferent fibers innervating the colon of the rat. *J Neurophysiol* 1994a; 71:2046–2060.

Sengupta JN, Gebhart GF. Mechanosensitive properties of pelvic nerve afferent fibers innervating the urinary bladder of the rat. *J Neurophysiol* 1994b; 72:2420–2430.

Sengupta JN, Kauvar D, Goyal RK. Characteristics of vagal esophageal tension-sensitive afferent fibers in the opossum. *J Neurophysiol* 1989; 61:1001–1010.

Sengupta JN, Saha JK, Goyal RK. Stimulus-response function studies of esophageal mechanosensitive nociceptors in sympathetic efferents of opossum. *J Neurophysiol* 1990; 64:796–812.

Silverman DHS. Cerebral activity in the perception of visceral pain. *Curr Rev Pain* 1999; 3(4):290–299.

Silverman DH, Munakata JA, Ennes H, et al. Regional cerebral activity in normal and pathological perception of visceral pain. *Gastroenterology* 1997; 112:64–72.

Teodori U, Galletti R. *Il Dolore nelle Affezioni degli Organi Interni del Torace* [Pain in Pathologies of Internal Organs of the Thorax]. Rome: Pozzi, 1962.

Thompson WG. Irritable bowel syndrome. In: Philips SF, Pemberton JH, Shorter RG (Eds). *The Large Intestine: Physiology, Pathophysiology and Disease.* New York: Raven, 1991, pp 593–610.

Trimble KC, Farouk R, Pryde A, Douglas S, Heading RC. Heightened visceral sensation in functional gastrointestinal disease is not site-specific. Evidence for a generalized disorder of gut sensitivity. *Dig Dis Sci* 1995; 40:1607–1613.

Uchida Y, Murao S. Acid-induced excitation of afferent cardiac sympathetic nerve fibers. *Am J Physiol* 1975; 228:27–33.

Vecchiet L, Giamberardino MA, de Bigontina P. Referred pain from viscera: when the symptom persists despite the extinction of the visceral focus. In: Sicuteri F, Terenius L, Vecchiet L, Maggi CA (Eds). *Pain Versus Man,* Advances in Pain Research and Therapy, Vol. 20. New York: Raven Press, 1992, pp 101–110.

Vecchiet L, Giamberardino MA. Clinical and pathophysiological aspects of visceral hyperalgesia. In: De Vera JA, Parris W, Erdine S (Eds). *Management of Pain. A World Perspective. III.* Bologna: Monduzzi, 1998, pp 214–230.

Vecchiet L, Giamberardino MA, Dragani L, Albe-Fessard D. Pain from renal/ureteral calculosis: evaluation of sensory thresholds in the lumbar area. *Pain* 1989; 36:289–295.

Vecchiet L, Giamberardino MA, Dragani L, Galletti R, Albe-Fessard D. Referred muscular hyperalgesia from viscera: clinical approach. In: Lipton S, Tunks E, Zoppi M (Ed). *The Pain Clinic.* Advances in Pain Research and Therapy, Vol. 13. New York: Raven Press, 1990, pp 175–182.

Vecchiet L, Iezzi S, Giamberardino MA. Relationship between occurrence of biliary colics and sensory/trophic changes in abdominal parietal tissues in patients with gallbladder calculosis. *Abstracts: 8th World Congress on Pain.* Seattle: IASP Press, 1996, pp 255–256.

Vecchiet L, Pizzigallo E, Iezzi S, et al. Differentiation of sensitivity in different tissues and its clinical significance. *J Musculoskeletal Pain* 1998; 6:33–45.

Wall PD. Neurophysiological mechanisms of referred pain and hyperalgesia. In: Vecchiet L, Albe-Fessard D, Lindblom U, Giamberardino MA (Eds). *New Trends in Referred Pain and Hyperalgesia,* Pain Research and Clinical Management, Vol. 7. Amsterdam: Elsevier, 1993, p 312.

Wall PD, Woolf CJ. Muscle but not cutaneous C-afferent input produces prolonged increases in the excitability of the flexion reflex in the rat. *J Physiol (Lond)* 1984; 356:443–458.

Wesselmann W, Lai J. Mechanisms of referred visceral pain: uterine inflammation in the adult virgin rat results in neurogenic plasma extravasation in the skin. *Pain* 1997; 73:309–317.

Wesselmann U, Czakanski PP, Affaitati G, Giamberardino MA. Uterine inflammation as a noxious visceral stimulus: behavioral characterization in the rat. *Neurosci Lett* 1998; 246:73–76.

Whitehead WE, Holtkotter B, Enck P, et al. Tolerance for rectosigmoid distension in irritable bowel syndrome. *Gastroenterology* 1990; 98:1187–1192.

Widdicombe JG. Sensory innervation of the lungs and airways. In: Cervero F, Morrison JFB (Eds). *Visceral Sensation,* Progress in Brain Research, Vol. 67. Amsterdam: Elsevier, 1986, pp 49–64.

Willis WD, Coggeshall RE. *Sensory Mechanisms of the Spinal Cord.* New York: Plenum Press, 1991.

Wolf S, Wolff HG. *Human Gastric Function. An Experimental Study of a Man and His Stomach.* New York: Oxford University Press, 1947.

Wolff HG. *Headache and Other Head Pain.* New York: Oxford University Press, 1963, pp 28–46.

Wood E, Pauley S, Bradshaw H, et al. Vaginal allodynia and hyperalgesia in rats with endometriosis and after pre-senescent ovariectomy. *Soc Neurosci Abstr* 1995; 21:388.

Woolf CJ. Evidence for a central component of post-injury pain hypersensitivity. *Nature* 1983; 306:686–688.

Woolf CJ. Long term alterations in the excitability of the flexion reflex produced by peripheral tissue injury in the chronic decerebrate rat. *Pain* 1984; 18:325–343.

Woolf CJ, Wall PD. Relative effectiveness of C primary afferent fibers of different origins in evoking a prolonged facilitation of the flexion reflex in the rat. *J Neurosci* 1986; 6:1433–1442.

Ylikorkala O, Dawood MY. New concepts in dysmenorrhea. *Am J Obstet Gynecol* 1978; 130:833–847.

Correspondence to: Maria Adele Giamberardino, MD, Via Carlo de Tocco n. 3, 66100 Chieti, Italy. Tel/Fax (laboratory): 39-0871-565286; email: mag@unich.it.

Proceedings of the 9th World Congress on Pain,
Progress in Pain Research and Management,
Vol. 16, edited by M. Devor, M.C. Rowbotham, and
Z. Wiesenfeld-Hallin, IASP Press, Seattle, © 2000.

52

Urogenital Pain Syndromes in Men and Women[1]

Ursula Wesselmann

Blaustein Pain Treatment Center, Departments of Neurology and Biomedical Engineering, The Johns Hopkins University School of Medicine, Baltimore, Maryland, USA

Chronic nonmalignant pain syndromes (of more than 6 months' duration) of the urogenital area in men and women are focal pain syndromes that are well described, but poorly understood. The urogenital area is often considered taboo in our society, and many patients are embarrassed to suffer from a chronic pain syndrome in this particular area of the body. Except in cases in which a specific secondary cause can be identified, the etiology of chronic urogenital pain often remains unknown. Rarely are these pain syndromes the manifestation of a psychiatric disease in the absence of an organic basis. Currently available treatment options are empirical only. Although complete cures are uncommon, some pain relief can be provided to almost all patients using currently available treatment strategies. The purpose of this chapter is to highlight the clinical presentation of common pain syndromes of urogenital origin (vulvodynia, orchialgia, urethral syndrome, prostatodynia, and perineal pain) and to discuss pain management options.

UROGENITAL NEUROBIOLOGY

The urogenital floor is a highly specialized area of the body that is responsible for a host of basic biological functions including defecation, micturition, copulation, and reproduction. Precise nervous system control, together with endocrine and other local control mechanisms, is required for the coordination of these different functions. Compared to other areas of the

[1] Mini-review based on a congress workshop.

body, there has been little research on the neuroanatomy, neurophysiology, and neuropharmacology of the perineum. The complexity of the perineum, which carries out many different specialized functions, may largely account for the slow progress in our understanding of the neurobiology of this area. In addition, this area of the body is often considered taboo, which might be another reason why research on this topic has been neglected.

A detailed review of the neurobiology of the pelvic floor is provided elsewhere (Burnett and Wesselmann 1999; Wesselmann and Burnett 1999). Briefly, the innervation of the urogenital floor is served by both components of the autonomic nervous system, the sympathetic and parasympathetic divisions, as well as the somatic nervous system (De Groat 1994; Hoyle et al. 1994); see Figs. 1 and 2. Sensations from the urogenital floor are mainly conveyed via the sacral afferent parasympathetic system (spinal cord levels S2 to S4), with a far lesser afferent supply from afferents traveling with the thoracolumbar sympathetics (spinal cord levels T10–L2) (Jänig and Koltzenburg 1993). When evaluating patients with urogenital pain syndromes, it is important to know that in contrast to other areas of the urogenital floor, sensations of the testis and epididymis may predominantly involve thoracolumbar afferents (Jänig and Koltzenburg 1993, see Fig. 1). The inferior hypogastric plexus is the major neuronal coordinating center that supplies the urogenital floor. The inferior hypogastric plexus receives both sympathetic (the superior hypogastric plexus and its caudal extension, the hypogastric plexus, and the sympathetic chain ganglia) and parasympathetic input (pelvic splanchnic nerve) (De Groat 1994).

Somatic efferent and afferent innervation to the perineum originates from sacral spinal cord levels S2 to S4 (Figs. 1 and 2). Sacral nerve roots emerge from the spinal cord to form the sacral plexus, giving rise to the pudendal nerve (Elbadawi 1996). The pudendal nerve also receives postganglionic axons from the caudal sympathetic chain ganglia (De Groat 1994). It runs medial to the internal pudendal vessels along the lateral wall of the ischiorectal fossa, dorsal to the sacrospinous ligament. The first branch to split off becomes the dorsal nerve of the penis (or clitoris), and the remaining pudendal nerve fibers distribute a medial branch to the anal canal, dorsal branches to the urethral sphincter, and dorsolateral branches to the anterior perineal musculature. The posterior perineal musculature is supplied by nerves originating predominantly from sacral level S4. Branches of the S4–S5 nerve roots form the coccygeal plexus, distributing fibers to the perineal, perianal, and scrotal (labial) skin (Matzel et al. 1990). The central projections of afferents traveling in the pelvic splanchnic nerve and in the pudendal nerve overlap within the spinal cord (Figs. 1 and 2), allowing integration of somatic and parasympathetic motor activity. Thus, stimulation of afferents in one area of the urogenital floor can influence the efferent output to another region (Jänig et al. 1991). This might explain why patients with chronic urogenital pain syndromes often complain about changes in bowel or urinary bladder motility or in sexual function and why clinical examination sometimes reveals increased pelvic floor muscle tone.

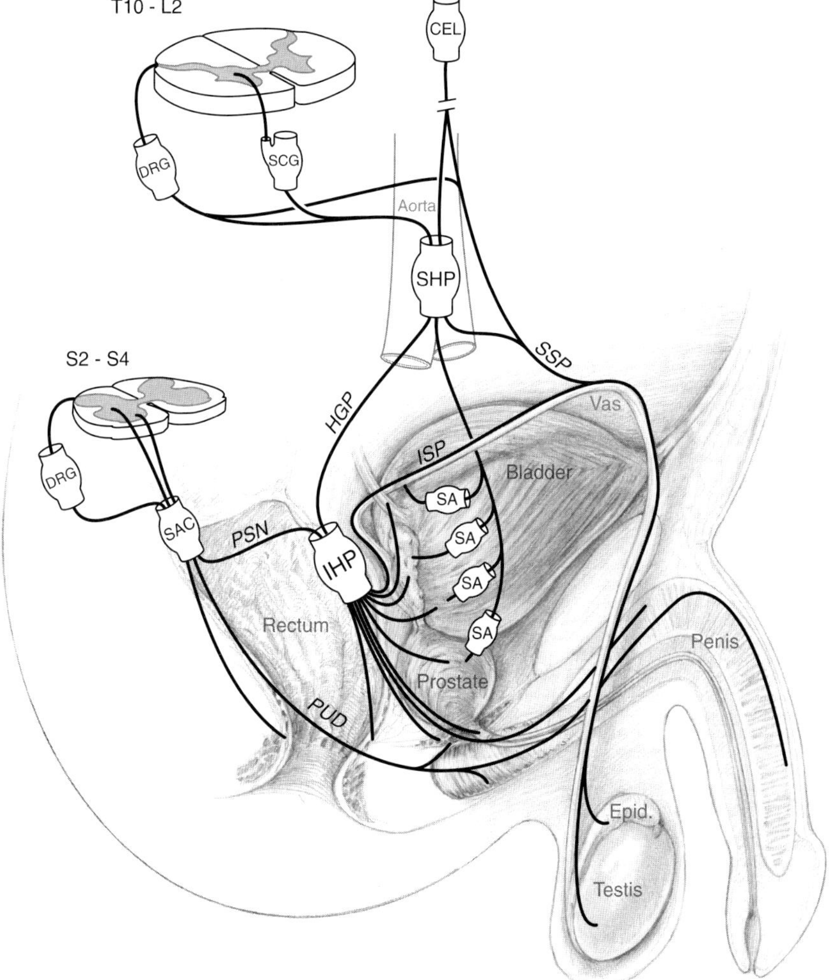

Fig. 1. Schematic drawing showing the innervation of the urogenital area in males. Although this diagram attempts to show the innervation in humans, much of the anatomical information is derived from animal data. CEL = celiac plexus, DRG = dorsal root ganglion, HGP = hypogastric plexus, IHP = inferior hypogastric plexus, ISP = inferior spermatic plexus, PSN = pelvic splanchnic nerve, PUD = pudendal nerve, Epid. = epididymis, SA = short adrenergic projections, SAC = sacral plexus, SCG = sympathetic chain ganglion, SHP = superior hypogastric plexus, SSP = superior spermatic plexus. Reprinted from Wesselmann et al. (1997), with permission.

Neuropeptide release appears to account for perineal sensations (Jänig and Koltzenburg 1993). Numerous peptides have been associated with afferent pathways of the urogenital floor, although a preponderance of evidence supports the roles of substance P and calcitonin gene-related peptide (CGRP) as primary chemicals released from these sensory neurons (De Groat 1987).

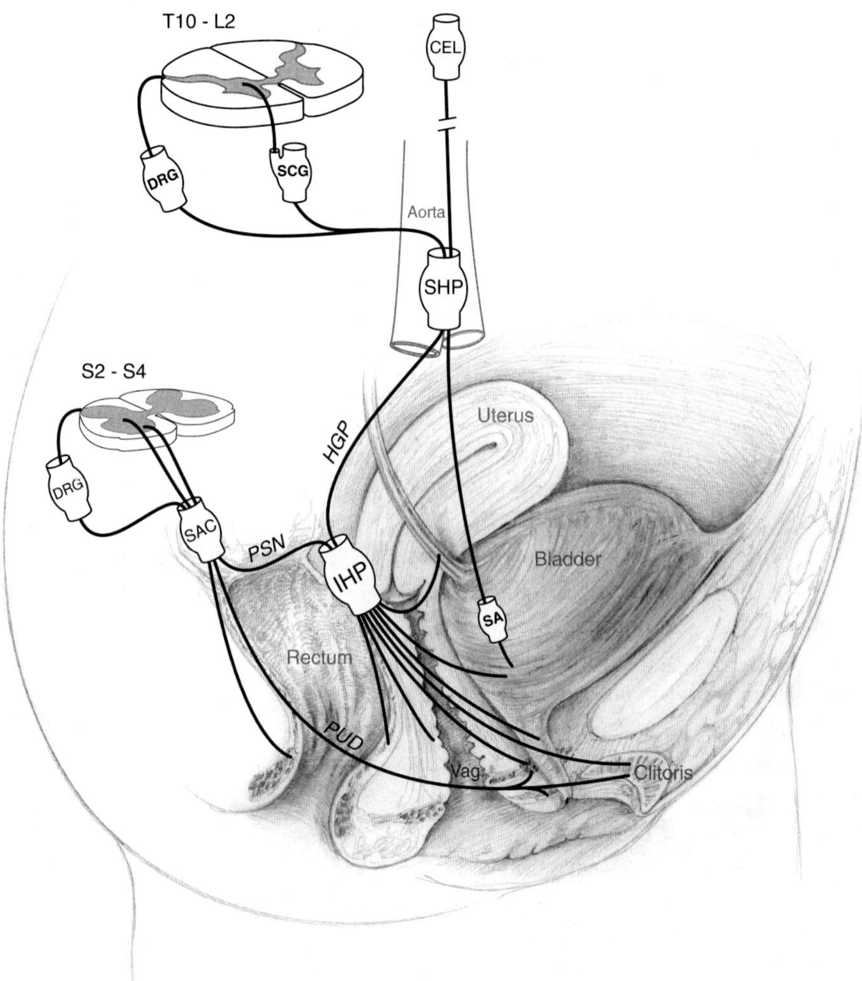

Fig. 2. Schematic drawing showing the innervation of the urogenital area in females. Although this diagram attempts to show the innervation in humans, much of the anatomical information is derived from animal data. CEL = celiac plexus, DRG = dorsal root ganglion, HGP = hypogastric plexus, IHP = inferior hypogastric plexus, PSN = pelvic splanchnic nerve, PUD = pudendal nerve, SA = short adrenergic projections, SAC = sacral plexus, SCG = sympathetic chain ganglion, SHP = superior hypogastric plexus, Vag. = vagina. Reprinted from Wesselmann et al. (1997), with permission.

CLINICAL PRESENTATION AND PAIN MANAGEMENT APPROACHES

VULVODYNIA

Hyperesthesia of the vulva was well described in American and European gynecological textbooks in the 19th century (Thomas 1880; Pozzi 1897). However, despite these early reports, the medical literature did not mention vulvar pain again until the early 1980s, when interest in this chronic pain syndrome revived. It is not clear why the syndrome had disappeared from the medical literature for almost 100 years. It is possible that the medical community denied and neglected it, or perhaps chronic vulvar pain was quite rare for a period of time. Further epidemiological studies are necessary to clarify this issue.

Vulvodynia is defined as chronic vulvar discomfort and includes several subgroups: vulvar dermatosis, cyclic vulvovaginitis, vulvar vestibulitis, vulvar papillomatosis, and dysesthetic vulvodynia (McKay 1984). The incidence and prevalence of vulvodynia are unknown. A recent survey of sexual dysfunction, analyzing data from the National Health and Social Life Survey, reported that 16% of women between the ages of 18 and 59 years living in households throughout the United States experience pain during sex (Laumann et al. 1999). However, the location and etiology of pain were not analyzed in this study. When these data were analyzed by age group, the highest number of women reporting pain during sex was in the 18–29-year-old group. It has been estimated that at least 200,000 women in the United States suffer from significant vulvar discomfort that greatly reduces their quality of life (Jones and Lehr 1994). The age distribution ranges from the 20s to late 60s (Lynch 1986; Paavonen 1995). In a general gynecological practice setting, about 15% of all patients fulfill the definition of vulvar vestibulitis, a major subgroup of vulvodynia (Goetsch 1991).

Chronic vulvodynia is often characterized by acute onset. Some patients recall frequent episodes of a vaginal infection, local treatments of the vulvar or vaginal area (application of steroid or antimicrobial cream, cryo- or laser surgery), or changes in the pattern of sexual activity, prior to the onset of vulvodynia. It will be important to elucidate why some women develop chronic vulvar pain after these events and others do not. Further, since uncomplicated vaginal infections and changes in the pattern of sexual activity are typical events during the reproductive years of any woman, epidemiological studies will have to show whether there is any link between these events and vulvodynia. Many women cannot recall any initiating event.

The pelvic examination is usually normal in women with vulvodynia, except for hyperalgesia in the vulvar area, in which case pain can easily be elicited or exacerbated by a simple "swab test," where touching the vulvar area with a moist cotton swab results in sharp, burning pain (Goetsch 1991). This "hyperalgesia" is similar to sensory findings in patients with painful neuropathies of the extremities. Recent histological studies of vaginal biopsy specimen reported vestibular neural hyperplasia in women with vulvar vestibulitis, which might provide a morphological explanation for the pain in this syndrome (Bohm-Starke et al. 1998; Westrom and Willen 1998).

Chronic infections of the vulvar area should be treated before a diagnosis of vulvodynia is made. Genital infections constitute a frequent cause of chronic vulvar pain, and a thorough evaluation is essential to rule out infections of the vulva and vagina (Mroczkowski 1998). Another frequent cause of chronic vulvar pain is vulvar dermatoses, which can often be cured with corticosteroids (Fischer et al. 1995). Unlike other vulvar pain syndromes, vulvar dermatoses are characterized by typical signs on physical examination—redness, blisters, and erosions. To confirm the diagnosis of vulvodynia, secondary causes such as gynecological infections or dermatitis must be excluded. An effective treatment plan requires a multidisciplinary approach involving the collaboration of gynecologists, dermatologists, neurologists, pain specialists, psychologists, and psychiatrists. A symptomatic pain management approach is indicated in women with vulvar vestibulitis and dysesthetic vulvodynia. Vulvar vestibulitis is characterized by entry dyspareunia. Pain is localized at the vaginal introitus, and the patient can usually point to an exact area where pain is evoked by mechanical stimuli. Gynecological examination may reveal vestibular erythema, but an infectious etiology has never been confirmed, despite numerous studies (see review in Wesselmann and Czakanski 1999). Dysesthetic vulvodynia is a subtype of vulvodynia that involves diffuse, constant hyperalgesia in the vulvar area, often extending throughout the perineum. Patients with dysesthetic vulvodynia can easily be differentiated from patients with vulvar vestibulitis because they show less focal tenderness at the vulvar vestibule on examination, and complain less about dyspareunia. Some women have features of vulvar vestibulitis as well as constant vulvar pain. The term vestibulodynia was recently coined for this symptom complex (Bornstein et al. 1997).

Many patients presenting with vulvodynia can be helped with oral medications recommended for neuropathic pain management including antidepressants, anticonvulsants, membrane-stabilizing agents, and opioids (Pavoonen 1995; Wesselmann et al. 1997). In patients with vulvar vestibulitis, where a very localized, small area is painful, topical treatment regimens such as creams with local anesthetics, aspirin, steroids, or estrogen might reduce the pain. Glazer et al. (1995) reported pain relief in over 80% of patients with vulvar vestibulitis using electromyographic biofeedback of the pelvic floor musculature. Surgical procedures have been advocated to remove the hyperalgesic skin area in patients with vulvar vestibulitis (see review in Wesselmann et al. 1997). The most commonly used procedure is perineoplasty. Risks include general anesthesia, a prolonged healing period, intraoperative bleeding, and disfigurement of the vulvar area (Goetsch 1996). A simplified surgical revision, as an alternative to this extensive surgical intervention, has been advocated by Goetsch (1996), where the painful area is excised under local anesthesia.

ORCHIALGIA

Orchialgia (chronic testicular pain) can be one of the most vexing pain problems for men and their treating physicians. Similar to women with vulvodynia, men with chronic testicular pain are usually embarrassed to talk about it. The exact incidence and prevalence of orchialgia is unknown. The majority of patients are in their mid- to late 30s (Davis et al. 1990; Costabile et al. 1991). A precipitating event that triggered the onset of the chronic pain can be recalled by only a minority of men suffering from orchialgia (Costabile et al. 1991; Wesselmann and Burnett 1996). The pain can be unilateral or bilateral and may be confined to the scrotal contents or can radiate to the groin, penis, perineum, abdomen, legs, and back. Usually no erectile or ejaculatory sexual dysfunction is associated with chronic orchialgia (Davis et al. 1990; U. Wesselmann, unpublished observation).

A careful history and physical examination are very important. A thorough urological evaluation and selected imaging studies will uncover most secondary causes of chronic testicular pain, including infection, tumor, testicular torsion, varicocele, hydrocele, spermatocele, trauma (such as a bicycle accident), and previous surgical interventions (Davis et al. 1990; Costabile et al. 1991). Testicular pain can be a sign of referred pain from the ureter, pelvic organs, hip, or intervertebral discs. Entrapment neuropathies of the ilioinguinal or genitofemoral nerve due to hernias must be considered in the differential diagnosis. Vasectomy can result in chronic orchialgia, which is probably far more common than is realized and is sometimes the subject of litigation (Selikowitz and Schned 1985; McMahon et al. 1992). Whether this postvasectomy pain syndrome is due to impairment of the genital branch of the genitofemoral nerve by sperm granuloma is the subject of controversy (Silber 1981; Yeates 1985; McCormack 1988).

If the urological evaluation is inconclusive, further gastroenterological evaluations may be necessary to rule out referred pain from the organs of the abdominal cavity. A neurological evaluation is directed toward the lumbosacral roots and the ilioinguinal, genitofemoral, pelvic, and pudendal nerves. Placebo-controlled nerve blocks with local anesthetic may help to differentiate which nerves are mediating the chronic pain. A psychological evaluation should be included in a multidisciplinary comprehensive work-up to assess the patient for depression or other psychological issues.

If the underlying cause of chronic orchialgia can be identified, it must be treated. However, in many cases no etiology can be identified (Davis et al. 1990). Hydrocele, varicocele, and spermatocele are often coincidental findings, but not the cause of orchialgia. Drastic surgical procedures have been recommended for the treatment of this syndrome, including epididymectomy and orchiectomy (Davis et al. 1990; Chen and Ball 1991). Microsurgical denervation of the spermatic cord has been suggested as an alternative to orchiectomy (Levine et al. 1996; Heidenreich et al. 1997). However, before any invasive and irreversible measures are considered for pain relief, non-invasive pain management should be attempted. It is important that the physician should not be compelled by the lack of findings to institute more invasive procedures in an effort to find a nonexistent pathological condition (Costabile et al. 1991). Urologists usually prescribe a trial of antibiotics and NSAIDs with the aim of treating a possible occult inflammatory process (Davis et al. 1990). Medications used for other chronic pain syndromes such as antidepressants, anticonvulsants, membrane-stabilizing agents, and opioids result in excellent pain relief in patients with chronic testicular pain (Costabile et al. 1991; Hagen 1993; Hayden 1993; Wesselmann et al. 1997). Transcutaneous electrical nerve stimulation (TENS) and acupuncture might be helpful (Hayden 1993; Holland et al. 1994). Sympatholytic procedures, such as a lumbar sympathetic block with local anesthetic and phentolamine infusions, have resulted in marked pain relief in a subgroup of men with orchialgia (Wesselmann et al. 1997), where the chronic pain syndrome seems to be sympathetically maintained (Wesselmann and Raja 1997).

URETHRAL SYNDROME

The term urethral syndrome was first used by Gallagher (1965) to describe a syndrome characterized by urinary urgency, frequency, dysuria and, at times, by suprapubic and back pain and urinary hesitancy in the absence of objective urological findings. This chronic pain syndrome occurs most commonly in women during the reproductive years, but it has also been seen in children; it is estimated to account for as many as five million office visits a year in the United States (Peters-Gee 1998). The etiology of this syndrome remains unclear. Although several studies have proposed that symptoms are caused by urethral obstruction and are thus surgically treatable, it is important to point out that there is rarely evidence to support an anatomically obstructive etiology. Since the symptoms are indistinguishable from those caused by urinary infections, tumors, stones, interstitial cystitis, and many other entities, it is very important to rule out these conditions before diagnosing the urethral syndrome. Urethral syndrome is thus a diagnosis of exclusion. A conservative treatment approach is recommended because this is usually as effective as surgery, less expensive, and, most importantly, less subject to risk (reviewed in Messinger 1992). Treatment strategies for the urethral syndrome include urological procedures with the aim of eliminating a presumed urethral stenosis. Systemic therapy with anticholinergics, α-adrenergic blockers, and muscle relaxants has been advocated. High rates of success were found with skeletal muscle relaxants or electrostimulation combined with biofeedback techniques (Schmidt and Tanagho 1981). In contrast to other chronic nonmalignant urogenital pain syndromes, the rates of spontaneous remission for the urethral syndrome are very high, ranging from 85% to 100% (Zufall 1978; Carson et al. 1980). However, for those patients whose symptoms persist, life can be of unrelenting agony. The high rates of spontaneous remission should not prevent physicians from realizing that these patients suffer from a chronic pain syndrome and require treatment. Physicians should encourage these patients to consider a conservative treatment approach, while exercising caution toward invasive and irreversible therapeutic procedures.

PROSTATODYNIA

"Prostatitis" is a diagnosis that is often given to patients presenting with unexplained symptoms or conditions that might originate from the prostate gland (Nickel 1998). In the United States, approximately 25% of men presenting with genitourinary tract problems are diagnosed with prostatitis (Lipsky 1989; Meares 1992). Drach et al. (1978) described four categories of prostatitis: (1) acute bacterial prostatitis, (2) chronic bacterial prostatitis, (3) nonbacterial prostatitis (including nonbacterial infections, allergic and autoimmune prostatitis), and (4) prostatodynia. Prostatodynia accounts for approximately 30% of patients presenting with prostatitis and is defined as persistent complaints of urinary urgency, dysuria, poor urinary flow, and perineal discomfort or pain, without evidence of bacteria or purulence in the prostatic fluid (Drach 1978). In addition to the perineal pain, patients often report that the pain is radiating to the lower back, suprapubic area, and groin. In contrast to patients with chronic testicular pain, those with prostatodynia often complain about pain with ejaculation (Brunner et al. 1983).

Physical examination of the prostate is typically normal. A thorough urological evaluation is indicated including urinalysis, urine culture, urine cytology, and urethral cultures (de la Rosette et al. 1993). Referred pain from the pelvic organs to the urogenital floor needs to be ruled out. Prostatodynia is a diagnosis of exclusion, where it is assumed that the chronic pain syndrome is related to the prostate, but no inflammatory prostatic process can be identified. The most frequently advocated treatment is antibiotics, despite the fact that usually no infectious etiology can be found. The urodynamic abnormalities observed in some patients with prostatodynia suggest increased sympathetic tone. Oral α-adrenergic blockers can improve the voiding abnormalities as well as pain; however, their use is often limited by side effects, most frequently hypotension (Barbalias et al. 1998). Transurethral microwave hyperthermia has been successfully used to treat nonbacterial prostatitis and prostatodynia (Nickel and Sorenson 1994). There may be an increase in pelvic floor muscle tone in patients presenting with prostatodynia, and pelvic floor relaxation techniques and muscle-relaxing agents can markedly improve symptoms (Segura et al. 1979).

PERINEAL PAIN

Perineal pain can be associated with one of the more specific pain syndromes of the urogenital area described in this chapter. These cases involve pain radiating into the perineal region. However, chronic perineal pain often is an entity of its own, although poorly defined. The differential diagnosis of chronic perineal pain is extensive, and the concerted effort of gastroenterologists, proctologists, urologists, gynecologists, and neurologists might be necessary to reach a diagnosis. Pudendal nerve blocks with local anesthetic might be helpful to assess whether the pudendal nerve contributes to the chronic pain syndrome. Pudendal nerve entrapment has been reported as a cause of perineal pain. Surgical neurolysis transposition resulted in marked pain improvement in most of the patients (Robert et al. 1993; Bensignor et al. 1996); early diagnosis of nerve entrapment yielded the best results. Imaging studies of the thoraco-lumbo-sacral spine should be considered if there is any suspicion of rare cases of meningeal cysts (Van De Kleft and Van Vyve 1993) resulting in perineal pain; surgical resection of sacral meningeal cysts has been reported to result in complete resolution of perineal pain in most of these patients (Van de Kleft and Van Vyve 1993). Patients with systemic diseases associated with painful peripheral neuropathies such as diabetes mellitus or AIDS can experience perineal pain. Ford et al. (1994, 1996) discussed perineal pain in the context of movement disorders, describing such pain as a rare feature of Parkinson's disease and as a complication of neuroleptic drug exposure ("painful tardive perineal pain syndrome").

PSYCHOLOGICAL ASPECTS OF UROGENITAL PAIN

The literature examining psychological factors in chronic urogenital pain has been reviewed in detail (Wesselmann et al. 1997). As with other chronic pain syndromes in the absence of obvious organic pathology, many studies have claimed a purely psychogenic origin of urogenital pain. Many of them neglected to examine whether the psychological findings were likely to be pre-existing or reactive. It would not be surprising or necessarily indicative of psychopathology if a patient with a chronic urogenital pain syndrome were depressed. The important questions are, was this patient depressed before the chronic pain syndrome started, and did his or her mood return to normal after successful pain therapy?

A history of sexual and physical abuse has been associated with a variety of pain syndromes (Kinzl et al. 1995), and that association appears to be especially strong with chronic pain of the sexual organs (Walker and Stenchever 1993), including urogenital pain. It is important that these issues are adequately addressed in patients with urogenital pain who report a history of physical or sexual abuse. However, patients and health care providers should be aware that a causal relationship between abuse history and development of pain is controversial and has not been confirmed unequivocally. In fact, two recent large controlled studies failed to find any association between abuse or trauma and sexual pain in women (Meana et al. 1997; Laumann et al. 1999). Several methodological limitations are inherent in the study of physical and sexual trauma. Most of the studies have used retrospective, cross-sectional designs in which the evaluation of the physical complaint and the abuse history are taken concurrently. What is not known is the validity of retrospective recall of remote abuse events. Recollection of such remote events may be accurate in some individuals, but in others it may be subject to various recall biases. Furthermore, it is important to recall the relatively high prevalence rates of physical and sexual victimization in the general population, particularly at tertiary care sites, in which many studies are conducted. A completely unexplored question is, whether physical injury to the genitourinary tract, as occurs during sexual abuse, can make the victim more likely to develop chronic urogenital pain. In summary, further research is urgently needed to assess a relationship between physical and sexual abuse and chronic urogenital pain. Considering the increasing empirical support for the multidimensional causality of chronic pain in general, it is unlikely that further investigation will yield simple linear relationships between a history of abuse and urogenital pain (Binik et al. 2000).

Health care providers treating patients with chronic urogenital pain must realize that these patients are often embarrassed to talk about pain in a location that is considered taboo. They are afraid that they might be labeled as suffering from a psychosomatic or psychiatric illness, or as hypochondriacs. They are also afraid that conclusions will be drawn about their sexual life (because the genitalia are either directly affected by the chronic pain syndrome or are close to the painful area), and such fears might further isolate them. Location of pain may be a significant predictor for appraisals of pain and disclosure of pain complaints. Klonoff et al. (1993) demonstrated that subjects asked to imagine pain in their genitals appraised themselves as more ill than if they were asked to imagine chest, stomach, head, and mouth pain. Further, subjects reported that they would be least likely to disclose genital pain and would be more worried, depressed, and embarrassed by pain in the genitals than in all other areas of the body. Chronic urogenital pain affects many aspects of a patient's life, including his or her sexual life, and it is crucial that early depressive symptoms be treated appropriately. A multidisciplinary evaluation should include a psychological or psychiatric evaluation to assess for depression early on, rather than as a last resort after other treatment approaches have failed.

CONCLUSIONS AND FUTURE DIRECTIONS

Although the chronic nonmalignant urogenital pain syndromes discussed in this chapter are well described and may be quite frequent, many of the patients suffering from them do not receive adequate pain management, and some do not receive any pain treatment at all. In many cases the clinician's focus is on finding and possibly treating the underlying etiology. Pain—the prominent symptom—is often considered only as a symptom of chronic disease, but not as a treatable entity of its own (Wesselmann 1999). In the future, treatment strategies might become available that are targeted specifically against the pathophysiological mechanisms of the chronic urogenital pain syndromes. However, while these developments may be on the horizon, it is very important to consider what can be done for these patients now. It is important for both the patient and the physician to realize that chronic urogenital pain syndromes do exist and are in fact quite common. Although these pain syndromes can rarely be cured, some relief can be provided to almost all patients by using a multidisciplinary approach including pain medications (antidepressants, anticonvulsants, membrane-stabilizing agents, and opioids), local treatment regimens, nerve blocks, selected surgical procedures, physical therapy, and psychological support (Wesselmann et al. 1997). Educating patients and their health care providers about currently available pain treatment strategies will be an important step forward because many are not aware of options that already exist.

Since the etiology of most urogenital pain syndromes is not known, further research is urgently needed to develop improved and more specific pain treatment strategies. Progress in the treatment of the chronic urogenital pain syndromes must come from both basic science and clinical research studies. It will be important to advance research on the neuroanatomy, neurophysiology, and neurochemistry of the urogenital floor, which has been neglected compared to other areas of the body. Further, better insight into the pathophysiological mechanisms of chronic urogenital pain is likely to come from the development and study of specific animal models of these chronic pain syndromes. In the clinical arena, a first step should be to develop a classification of the urogenital pain syndromes and make it available to all health care providers who are likely to see patients suffering from these pain syndromes. This will result in better recognition and diagnosis of these syndromes and will allow comparison of future case studies, in which a uniform classification of the urogenital pain syndromes should be used. The urogenital pain syndromes have not yet been included in the classification of chronic pain syndromes (Merskey and Bogduk 1994). Partial classifications have been provided for some of the pain syndromes through the urological and gynecological literature, but they are not uniformly used. Most of the clinical literature on urogenital pain consists of reports on small clinical trials or case reports, but since no common definitions of the urogenital pain syndromes exist, it is often difficult to compare clinical reports. For example, some authors use the term perineal pain exchangeably with prostatodynia in men or dysesthetic vulvodynia in women. Epidemiological studies will be important to assess the prevalence of urogenital pain syndromes and to learn about environmental and genetic factors that might be involved. Further clinical studies will be necessary to assess the characteristics of pain in these patients, and controlled clinical trials will be important, both to study the effects of currently available analgesic approaches and to explore future therapies targeted against the pathophysiological mechanisms of urogenital pain.

ACKNOWLEDGMENTS

Research in the author's laboratory is supported by National Institutes of Health grants RO1 NS36553 (NINDS/Office of Research for Women's Health) and R21 DK57315 (NIDDK), the Blaustein Pain Research Fund, and a grant from the National Vulvodynia Association.

REFERENCES

Barbalias GA, Nikiforidis G, Liatsikos EN. Alpha-Blockers for the treatment of chronic prostatitis in combination with antibiotics. *J Urol* 1998; 159:883–887.

Bensignor MF, Labat JJ, Robert R, Ducrot P. Diagnostic and therapeutic pudendal nerve blocks for patients with perineal non-malignant pain. *Abstracts: 8th World Congress on Pain*. Seattle: IASP Press, 1996, p 56.

Binik YM, Meana M, Berkley K, Khalife S. The sexual pain disorders: is the pain sexual or is the sex painful. *Ann Rev Sex Res* 2000; in press.

Bohm-Starke N, Hilliges M, Falconer C, Rylander E. Increased intraepithelial innervation in women with vulvar vestibulitis syndrome. *Gynecol Obstet Invest* 1998; 46:256–260.

Bornstein J, Zarfati D, Goldshmid N, et al. Vestibulodynia—a subset of vulvar vestibulitis or a novel syndrome. *Am J Obstet Gynecol* 1997; 177:1439–1443.

Brunner H, Weidner W, Schiefer HC. Studies on the role of ureaplasma urealyticum and mycoplasma hominis in prostatitis. *J Infect Dis* 1983; 126:807–813.

Burnett AL, Wesselmann U. Neurobiology of the pelvis and perineum: principles for a practical approach. *J Pelvic Surg* 1999; 5:224–232.

Carson CC, Segura JW, Osborne DM. Evaluation and treatment of the female urethral syndrome. *J Urol* 1980; 124:609–610.

Chen TF, Ball RY. Epididymectomy for post-vasectomy pain: histological review. *Br J Urol* 1991; 68:407–413.

Costabile RA, Hahn M, McLeod DG. Chronic orchialgia in the pain prone patient: the clinical perspective. *J Urol* 1991; 146:1571–1574.

Davis BE, Noble MJ, Weigel JW, Foret J, Mebust WK. Analysis and management of chronic testicular pain. *J Urol* 1990; 143:936–939.

De Groat WC. Neuropeptides in pelvic afferent pathways. *Experientia* 1987; 43:801–812.

De Groat WC. Neurophysiology of the pelvic organs. In: Rushton DN (Ed). *Handbook of Neuro-Urology*. New York: Marcel Dekker, 1994, pp 55–93.

de la Rosette JJMCH, Hubregtse MR, Karhaus HFM, Debruyne FMJ. Results of a questionnaire among Dutch urologists and general practitioners concerning diagnostics and treatment of patients with prostatitis syndrome. *Eur Urol* 1992; 22:14–19.

Drach GW, Fair WR, Meares EM, Stamey TA. Classification of benign diseases associated with prostatic pain: prostatitis or prostatodynia? *J Urol* 1978; 120:266.

Elbadawi A. Functional anatomy of the organs of micturition. *Urol Clin North Am* 1996; 23:177–210.

Fischer G, Spurrett B, Fisher A. The chronically symptomatic vulva: aetiology and management. *Br J Obstet Gyn* 1995; 102:773–779.

Ford B, Greene P, Fahn S. Oral and genital tardive pain syndromes. *Neurology* 1994; 44:2115–2119.

Ford B, Louis ED, Greene P, et al. Oral and genital pain syndromes in Parkinson's disease. *Mov Disord* 1996; 11:421–426.

Gallagher DJA, Montgomerie JZ, North JDK. Acute infections of the urinary tract and the urethral syndrome in general practice. *BMJ* 1965; 1:622–626.

Glazer HI, Rodke G, Swencionis C, Hertz R, Young AW. Treatment of vulvar vestibulitis syndrome with electromyographic biofeedback of pelvic floor musculature. *J Reprod Med* 1995; 40:283–290.

Goetsch MF. Vulvar vestibulitis: Prevalence and historic features in a general gynecologic practice population. *Am J Obstet Gynecol* 1991; 164:1609–1616.

Goetsch MF. Simplified surgical revision of the vulvar vestibule for vulvar vestibulitis. *Am J Obstet Gynecol* 1996; 174:1701–1707.

Hagen NA. Sharp, shooting neuropathic pain in the rectum or genitals: pudendal neuralgia. *J Pain Symptom Manage* 1993; 8:496–501.

Hayden LJ. Chronic testicular pain. *Austral Fam Phys* 1993; 22:1357–1365.

Heidenreich A, Zumbe J, Martinez F, Grozinger K, Engelmann UH. Die mikrochirurgische testikuläre Denervierung als Therapieoption der chronischen Testalgie. [Microsurgical testicular denervation as therapy option in chronic testalgia]. *Urologe A* 1997; 36:177–180.

Holland JM, Feldman JL, Gilbert HC. Phantom orchalgia. *J Urol* 1994; 152:2291–2293.

Hoyle CHV, Lincoln J, Burnstock G. Neural control of pelvic organs. In: Rushton DN (Ed). *Handbook of Neuro-Urology*. New York: Marcel Dekker, 1994, pp 1–54.

Jänig W, Koltzenburg M. Pain arising from the urogenital tract. In: Maggi CA (Ed): *Nervous Control of the Urogenital System*. Chur, Switzerland: Harwood Academic, 1993, pp 525–578.

Jänig W, Schmidt M, Schnitzler A, Wesselmann U. Differentiation of sympathetic neurons projecting in the hypogastric nerve in terms of their discharge patterns in cats. *J Physiol* 1991; 437:157–179.

Jones KD, Lehr ST. Vulvodynia: diagnostic techniques and treatment modalities. *Nurse Pract* 1994; 19:34–46.

Kinzl JF, Traweger C, Biebl W. Family background and sexual abuse associated with somatization. *Psychother Psychosom* 1995; 64:82–87.

Klonoff EA, Landrine H, Brown M. Appraisal and response to pain may be a function of its bodily location. *J Psychosom Res* 1993; 37:661–670.

Laumann EO, Paik A, Rosen RC. Sexual dysfunction in the United States. Prevalence and predictors. *JAMA* 1999; 281:537–544.

Levine LA, Matkov TG, Lubenow TR. Microsurgical denervation of the spermatic cord: a surgical alternative in the treatment of chronic orchialgia. *J Urol* 1996; 155:1005–1007.

Lipsky BA. Urinary tract infections in men. *Ann Int Med* 1989; 110:138.

Lynch PJ. Vulvodynia: A syndrome of unexplained vulvar pain, psychologic disability and sexual dysfunction. *J Reprod Med* 1986; 31:773–780.

Matzel KE, Schmidt RA, Tanagho EA. Neuroanatomy of the striated muscular anal continence mechanism: implications for the use of neurostimulation. *Dis Colon Rectum* 1990; 33:666–673.

McCormack M. Physiologic consequences and complications of vasectomy. *CMAJ (Ottawa)* 1988; 138:223–225.

McKay M. Burning vulva syndrome. *J Reprod Med* 1984; 29:457.

McMahon AJ, Buckley J, Taylor A, et al. Chronic testicular pain following vasectomy. *Br J Urol* 1992; 69:188–191.

Meana M, Binik YM, Khalife SE, Cohen D. Biopsychosocial profile of women with dyspareunia. *Obstet Gynecol* 1997; 90:583–589.

Meares EMJ. Prostatitis and related disorders. In: Walsh PC, Retik AB, Stanley TA, Vaughan EDJ (Eds). *Campbell's Urology,* 6th ed. Philadelphia: WB Saunders, 1992, pp 807–822.

Merskey H, Bogduk N. *Classification of Chronic Pain*. Seattle: IASP Press, 1994.

Messinger EM. Urethral syndrome. In: Walsh PC, Retik AB, Stanley TA, Vaughan EDJ (Eds). *Campbell's Urology,* 6th ed. Philadelphia: WB Saunders, 1992, pp 997–1005.

Mroczkowski TF. Vulvodynia—a dermatovenereologist's perspective. *Int J Dermatol* 1998; 37:567–569.

Nickel JC, Sorenson R. Transurethral microwave thermotherapy of nonbacterial prostatitis and prostatodynia: initial experience. *Urology* 1994; 44:458–460.

Nickel JC. Prostatitis—myths and realities. *Urology* 1998; 51:363-366.

Paavonen J. Diagnosis and treatment of vulvodynia. *Ann Med* 1995; 27:175–181.

Peters-Gee JM. Bladder and urethral syndromes. In: Steege JF, Metzger DA, Levy BS (Eds). *Chronic Pelvic Pain*. Philadelphia: WB Saunders, 1998, pp 197–204.

Pozzi SJ. *Traite de Gynecologie Clinique et Operatoire*. Paris: Masson, 1897.

Robert R, Brunet C, Faure A, et al. La chirurgie du nerf pudental lors de certaines algies perineales: evolution et resultats. [Pudendal nerve surgery for perineal pain syndromes: technical aspects and results]. *Chirurgie* 1993; 119:535–539.

Schmidt RA, Tanagho EA. Urethral syndrome or urinary tract infection? *Urology* 1981; 18:424–427.

Segura JW, Opitz JL, Greene LF. Prostatosis, prostatitis or pelvic floor tension myalgia? *J Urol* 1979; 122:168–169.

Selikowitz SM, Schned AR. A late post-vasectomy syndrome. *J Urol* 1985; 134:494–497.
Silber SJ. Reversal of vasectomy and the treatment of male infertility: role of microsurgery, vasoepididymostomy, and pressure-induced changes of vasectomy. *Urol Clin North Am* 1981; 8:53–62.
Thomas TG (Ed). *Practical Treatise on the Diseases of Woman*. Philadelphia: Henry C. Lea's Son, 1880, pp 145–147.
Van de Kleft E, Van Vyve M. Sacral meningeal cysts and perineal pain. *Lancet* 1993; 341:500–501.
Walker EA, Stenchever MA. Sexual victimization and chronic pelvic pain. *Obstet Gynecol Clin North Am* 1993; 20:795–807.
Wesselmann U. Guest Editorial: Pain—the neglected aspect of visceral pain. *Eur J Pain* 1999; 3:189–191.
Wesselmann U, Burnett AL. Treatment of neuropathic testicular pain. *Neurology* 1996; 46(Suppl):206.
Wesselmann U, Burnett AL. Genitourinary pain. In: Wall PD, Melzack R (Eds). *Textbook of Pain,* 4th ed. New York: Churchill Livingstone, 1999, pp 689–709.
Wesselmann U, Czakanski PP. Pain of urogenital origin. *Curr Rev Pain* 1999; 3:160–171.
Wesselmann U, Raja SN. Reflex sympathetic dystrophy and causalgia. *Anesth Clin North Am* 1997; 15:407–427.
Wesselmann U, Burnett AL, Heinberg LJ. The urogenital and rectal pain syndromes. *Pain* 1997; 73:269–294.
Westrom LV, Willen R. Vestibular nerve fiber proliferation in vulvar vestibulitis syndrome. *Obstet Gynecol* 1998; 91:572–576.
Yeates WK. Pain in the scrotum. *Br J Hosp Med* 1985; 33:101–104.
Zufall R. Ineffectiveness of treatment of urethral syndrome in women. *Urology* 1978; 12:337–339.

Correspondence to: Ursula Wesselmann, MD, Johns Hopkins Hospital, Department of Neurology, 720 Rutland Avenue, Traylor Building 604, Baltimore, MD 21205, USA. Tel: 410-614-8840; Fax: 410-955-9826; email: pain@welchlink.welch.jhu.edu.

Proceedings of the 9th World Congress on Pain, Progress in Pain Research and Management, Vol. 16, edited by M. Devor, M.C. Rowbotham, and Z. Wiesenfeld-Hallin, IASP Press, Seattle, © 2000.

53

Role of the Limbic System in Sex, Gender, and Pain[1]

Anna Maria Aloisi

Institute of Human Physiology, University of Siena, Siena, Italy

Do sex differences in pain exist? This important question still has not been answered conclusively. However, together with this question we should also ask: Why are we looking for sex differences? Clinical and animal studies strongly suggest that "something" in the central nervous system (CNS) of females causes them to develop many pain syndromes more easily than do males, or, conversely, "something" in the CNS of males allows them not to develop these syndromes.

To date, studies of pain transmission have focused on thousands of molecules whose activities have been studied prevalently in males. Gonadal hormones, which are generally considered the origin of all sex differences, have rarely been tested for their ability to modulate these activities. This big gap needs to be filled because gonadal hormones, like all steroid hormones, modify gene expression and thus affect the synthesis, metabolism, and degradation of factors that could play a determinant role in nociception. Animal and human studies show only small sex differences in behavioral responses induced by painful stimuli, but these small differences could mask very large sex differences in the brain. Indeed the "behavioral output" is rarely the only consequence of the nociceptive input; instead, it is the complex output of numerous components (e.g., emotional status, age, time of day) of which the nociceptive input represents a part.

In the following pages I will focus on the interaction between gonadal hormones and CNS circuits, not only the circuits involved in the acute response to pain, but also those in which long-lasting pain-induced modifications probably occur, such as in the limbic system.

---

[1] Mini-review based on a congress workshop.

GONADAL HORMONES AND SEX DIFFERENCES

When we look at a man and a woman, many characteristics inform us about their gender: their aspect, their voice, their way of solving problems, their sensitivity toward fine or ugly things. It seems obvious that their brains must have sex-dependent anatomical or functional characteristics. However, many years of pain research have been blind to this obvious concept. While women have always been more numerous than men in pain center populations, and women have shown pain syndromes unknown in men, animal research has failed to acknowledge this evidence. Male animals were commonly used for basic science research, while females were used for *strange* reasons, such as their ability to develop experimental arthritis more easily and faster than males (Spitzer 1999).

Today, a few years after the international warning by Karen Berkley (Berkley 1992) and Marianne Ruda (Ruda 1993) about the lack of information on sex differences in pain, many data and many reviews are available on this topic. Thus, in writing this chapter, I will not reiterate the excellent recent summary articles available on both animal and human studies (Unruh 1996; Berkley 1997; Riley et al. 1998). Rather, I will concentrate on a neuronal system in which the influence of sex appears to be particularly important but toward which pain research has only rarely directed its attention. I will report data about the limbic system, with the aim not to be exhaustive about its physiology but to provide new insight into its functional aspects, which have rarely been considered a main issue in pain research.

The limbic system is a functional circuit including several small and large nuclei (Paxinos 1995). It was first described in 1937 by Papez (Papez 1995) and, although with different interpretations about its extent, has since been described as the brain circuit involved in emotion, motivation, arousal, attention, learning, and memory. Its involvement in pain has been repeatedly suggested, and often proved, but has still not been defined precisely.

The limbic system includes areas like the septum, hippocampus, prefrontal cortex, amygdala, and hypothalamus. Indeed, each of these areas deserves a specific description of its involvement in pain, which is not possible in this mini-review. My experience and knowledge lead me to focus on the septo-hippocampal-hypothalamic system. This system includes cholinergic, glutamatergic, endorphinergic, and GABAergic neurons whose activity is strongly modulated by estrogen and androgens. The component nuclei of the limbic system contain the highest concentrations of sex-steroid-receptive cells in the CNS (Paxinos 1995). Gonadal hormones influence the development of the limbic system, and in several ways determine the number and types of neurons devoted to specific tasks and neural activities

(Pilgrim et al. 1994; Yuan et al. 1995). In experimental animals, several areas of the CNS show sex differences in many parameters, including the number of synapses and the number of neurons themselves (Kawata 1995). The hippocampus, the amygdala, and the hypothalamus are all included in the list of brain areas in which a sex difference is apparent.

With regard to the physiology of gonadal hormones, detailed descriptions of their source and action can be found in articles dealing with the reproductive apparatus. Of great interest, but practically impossible to summarize, is the series of effects exerted by gonadal hormones during development, known as "organizational effects" (Pilgrim and Hutchinson 1994). Here I will deal only with the actions of gonadal hormones in adulthood, known as "activational effects" (Pilgrim and Hutchinson 1994).

The principal androgen in males is testosterone, while in females the main estrogen is estradiol (Fig. 1). These hormones are both present in males and females, and they both contribute to most of the body functions expressed in the male and female. Gonadal hormones have both short- and long-lasting effects; the former are rapid and do not appear to affect transcription, while the latter are the classical actions of the sex steroid hormones in altering the activity of neurotransmitter/modulator systems by regulating the genomic activity of neurons (Schumacher 1990).

An interesting and important point to underline is that in the brain of the male, most of the masculinizing effects exerted by testosterone are mediated by a previous aromatization to estrogen (Pfaff and Schwartz-Giblin 1988). Moreover, in describing the actions of estradiol and testosterone, we must

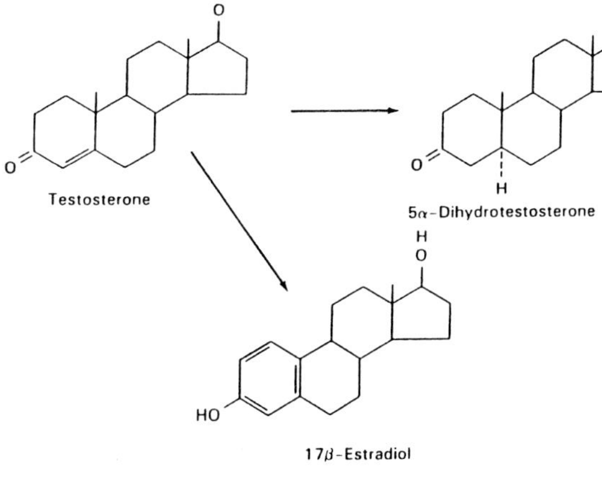

Testosterone

5α-Dihydrotestosterone

17β-Estradiol

Fig. 1. Testosterone: schematic representation of the two metabolic pathways in neurons. The enzyme 5α-reductase transforms it in 5α-dihydrotestosterone; the enzyme aromatase transforms it in 17β-estradiol.

consider that their activity is supported by the effects of numerous other steroid hormones.

In males and females, testosterone binds to an androgen receptor (AR). A single type of AR has been reported in neural tissues including the hypothalamus, cortex, amygdala, and hippocampus (Kerr et al. 1995). In rats, AR expression in peripheral tissues and the whole brain increases following gonadectomy; these increases are reversed by androgen treatment (Quarmby et al. 1990; Blok et al. 1992). Estrogens exert their action by binding to two kinds of receptor (ERα and ERβ) (Enmark and Gustafsson 1999). Loy et al. (1988) and later Maggi et al. (1989) showed that ERs are present in the hippocampus, primarily in the CA1 region but also to a lesser extent in CA3 and the dentate gyrus of male and female rats.

GONADAL HORMONES AND THE LIMBIC SYSTEM

Numerous studies have focused on ovarian steroid effects on septo-hippocampal-hypothalamic structure and function in adulthood. For androgens, little is known about the functional role of ARs in the hippocampus, although they may modulate several hippocampal-mediated behaviors, including emotionality, memory formation, and the response to novelty (Herbert 1990; Roof et al. 1992; Kerr et al. 1996a). In rats, androgens antagonized glucocorticoid action in the hippocampus by decreasing the synthesis of glucocortical receptors (GR), and thus the sensitivity of this structure to circulating glucocorticoids (Kerr et al. 1996b). These effects were related to studies demonstrating increased cell death in hippocampal pyramidal cells following chronic stress in gonadectomized animals, but not in intact or androgen-treated ones (Mizoguchi et al. 1992; McEwen 1999). Interestingly, these data are in line with findings that most of the sex differences in the number of neurons are due to the protective effect of androgens on these neurons (Kawata 1995). Indeed, the number of hypothalamic neurons and spinal cord motoneurons seems to be smaller in females because their rate of death is higher than in males. The mechanism of cell death can probably be attributed to the molecular modulation exerted by gonadal hormones on the transcription factors, such as *c-fos* and *c-myc,* known to be involved in cell death (Evan et al. 1992). Recent data from our laboratory show that gonadectomy increases choline acetyltransferase activity and *c-fos* expression in the male hippocampus (Aloisi et al. 2000) (Fig. 2).

With regard to the role played by estrogens in the hippocampus, rats clearly show a positive correlation between estrogen and dendritic spine and synapse density in the CA1 region, both after experimental manipula-

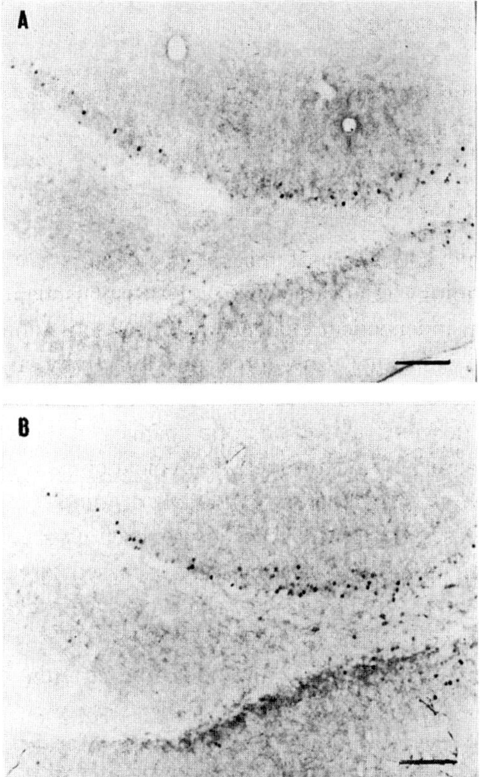

Fig. 2. *C-fos* immunoreactivity in the dentate gyrus of the hippocampus of male rats in (A) intact animals and (B) gonadectomized animals (3 weeks after surgery). The scale bar represents 100 μm.

tions and in response to natural hormonal fluctuations (Luine 1997). Indeed, in female rats the number of synapses in the hippocampus changed with the estrous cycle: the number of dendritic spines and the density of synapses in the hippocampal CA1 stratum radiatum increased during diestrus, peaked in proestrus, when estrogen and progesterone are at their highest levels, and declined by more than 30% during estrus (when estrogen and progesterone are lowest) (Woolley and McEwen 1992).

In humans, in addition to their effects throughout the body, estrogens influence cognition, mood, and subjective well-being in the perimenopausal and postmenopausal period (Gerdes et al. 1982; Luine et al. 1998). A particular role is played by the cholinergic system, which estrogens can activate at different levels: they increase nerve growth factor (NGF)-mRNA, choline acetyl transferase (ChAT)-mRNA, and trkA-mRNA expression in adult female rats (Singh et al. 1995; McMillan et al. 1996). Finally, estrogens as growth factors also induce axonal and dendritic growth of cholinergic neurons from the diagonal band of the forebrain (Gibbs 1998). In consequence, sexual dimorphism in the cholinergic septo-hippocampal pathway has been described extensively in adult rodents, based on different cholinergic markers (Aloisi 1997) and behavioral responses to cholinergic drugs (Berger-Sweeney et al. 1995).

Electrophysiological studies of the hippocampus have confirmed the activating role played by estrogens; both in vivo and in vitro, neuronal excitability increases with rising levels of estrogen. Seizure threshold is lowered during proestrus (Teresawa and Timiras 1968) and following estrogen administration to ovariectomized females (Buterbaugh and Hudson 1991). When applied to isolated rodent hippocampal neurons, 17β-estradiol potentiates the kainate-induced current (Gu et al. 1998). The action is rapid (within 3 minutes) and reversible upon removal of the steroid. The time course of estrogen potentiation is too rapid to be explained by the classical mechanism of steroid action and appears to be independent of the genomic mechanism (Moss et al. 1997).

Despite its small size, the hypothalamus strongly influences body functions and acts along different and apparently independent paths. Now well established is a sex difference in hypothalamic-pituitary-adrenal (HPA) activity, with enhanced activity in female rats. Indeed, adrenocorticotropic hormone (ACTH) and corticosterone plasma levels are higher in female than male rats under both basal and stimulated conditions (Aloisi et al. 1994). The difference appears to be due to an activational influence of female sex steroids, in addition to the inhibitory role of androgens (Handa et al. 1994; Carey et al. 1995; Patchev et al. 1998). As a consequence, fluctuations in HPA activity occur as a function of the ovarian cycle stage. The highest activity is seen at the end of the follicular phase in humans and at proestrus in rats. The ability to change the plasma levels of hormones, such as ACTH, β-endorphin, and corticosterone, gives the hypothalamus the power to modulate the way the nociceptive input can be perceived as pain. Moreover, in hypothalamic nuclei, estrogens induce important effects on substance P (SP) and nitric oxide, two molecules deeply involved in nociception. Indeed, estrogens modulate the mRNA expression and immunoreactivity of SP in the hypothalamus (Tsuruo et al. 1984; Brown et al. 1990). Estrogen receptors occur upstream from the SP promoter, which suggests the direct influence of estrogens on the gene expression of SP (Brown et al. 1990). Nitric oxide synthase activity is positively regulated by estradiol in neurons containing estrogen receptors in the medial preoptic nucleus and ventromedial nucleus of females, but not of males (Okamura et al. 1994). It would be of particular interest to ascertain whether these effects also occur in the specific nociceptive pathways.

Another important interaction occurs between gonadal hormones and immunity. Indeed, gonadal steroids seem to play a central role as predisposing factors in many forms of arthritis, with estrogens involved as immune-enhancing hormones and androgens as natural immunosuppressors (Spitzer 1999). Functional receptors for sex hormones have been described in cells involved in the immune response; after activation, the hormone receptor complex might modulate the expression of selected cytokines (Cerinic et al. 1998).

GONADAL HORMONES, THE LIMBIC SYSTEM, AND PAIN

The results of animal studies, ours and those of others, strongly indicate that painful stimuli activate hypothalamic and hippocampal neurons (Aloisi 1997). However, it appears that in their capacity to change the levels of arousal, attention, emotions (like fear and anxiety), hormones of both the HPA and hypothalamic pituitary gonadal (HPG) axes could greatly influence nociception and pain (Chapman 1996). It is common experience that when faced with a subject complaining of pain, the first thing we think of is to distract the person, i.e., to shift attention away from the body and pain and toward other things. Thus, in animals as well as in humans, different kinds of experiments have been devised to demonstrate the influence of attention on pain. In animals, the drive to eat can significantly decrease formalin-induced responses (Aloisi and Carli 1996), while in humans the request to not think about pain can change the cerebral response to pain (Peyron et al. 1999). As reported above, one of the neurotransmitters involved in processes of arousal and attention is ACh. Several methods have shown that damage to the septo-hippocampal cholinergic pathway is followed by impairment of subjects' ability to focus their attention on anything, with important consequences for learning and memory. ACh release is strongly activated by novel stimuli or stress (Perry et al. 1999). In rats a persistent painful stimulus slowly increases ACh to high levels and maintains them for a rather long period (Ceccarelli et al. 1999). These effects are strongly modulated by the estrous cycle phase, being maximal in females during proestrus/estrus (Fig. 3). Therefore, it appears that the ability of estrogens to induce higher cholinergic activity in the hippocampus can result in greater attention toward the painful stimulus and thus in a stronger perception of the stimulus itself. The sexual dimorphism shown by rats, with females having higher cholinergic activity than males, suggests a possible involvement of this pathway in the perception and persistence of pain.

In particular, we can hypothesize that life events such as strong emotions, prolonged stressful situations, or repeated mild painful episodes (i.e.,

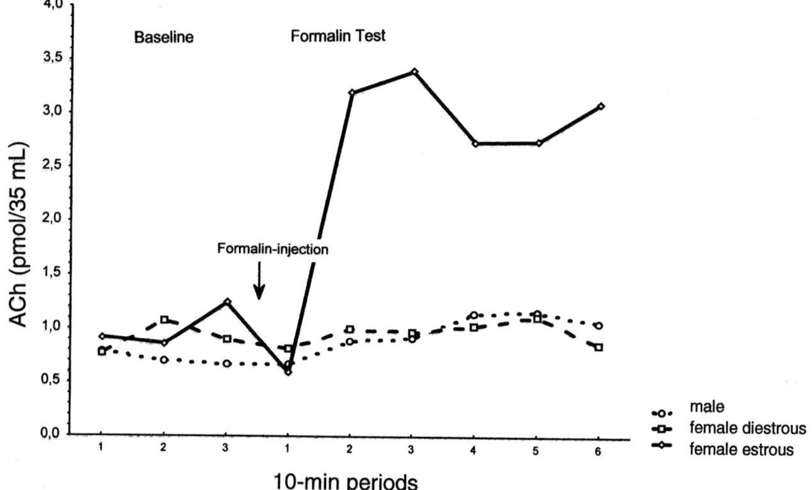

Fig. 3. Time course of ACh release during the formalin test (50 µL, 10% in the dorsal hindpaw) in male (○) and female rats. Females are divided in those belonging to estrous (◇) and diestrous (□) cycle phases.

at each menstruation) could leave greater traces in the CNS of females, especially in the limbic system. Interestingly, a recent study reported that the use of estrogens in postmenopausal hormone replacement therapy significantly increases the odds of having temporomandibular disorders, a chronic painful state that most commonly occurs in women (Meisler 1999). No animal data address the role of the hippocampus in the origin of chronic pain. However, the results of animal studies not related to pain provide some insight into these mechanisms. For instance, Tanapat et al. (1999) showed that female rats produce more dentate gyrus neurons than do males; these cells, showing characteristics of immature neurons, die if the animal is kept in deprived laboratory conditions, whereas when subjects are exposed to conditions of enhanced environmental complexity and increased learning opportunities, these neurons are preserved and are able to modulate hippocampal functions.

Other data that confirm the sex-dependent organization of the hippocampus concern glutamatergic transmission in the hippocampus, in particular the N-methyl D-aspartate (NMDA) receptor of glutamate. McEwen's laboratory has demonstrated that in the CA1 of estradiol-treated rats, pyramidal neurons increase levels of NMDA mRNA and protein (Gazzaley et al. 1996), which explains the greater sensitivity of these neurons to NMDA (Woolley et al. 1997). Warren et al. (1995) have found that induction of long-term potentiation (LTP), which depends on NMDA-receptor activation, is maximal in female rats during the afternoon of proestrus. Interestingly, in Cordoba Montoya's experiments (Cordoba Montoya and Carrer 1997), both the size of the population spike and the slope of the summed excitatory postsynaptic potential recorded in the cell body layer of CA1 of awake rats were not modified by estrogen injection in basal conditions, while these parameters were significantly greater after high-frequency stimulation of the stratum radiatum. These results show that CA1 neurons are not affected by changes in the levels of circulating estrogens, while synaptic plasticity, which is the basis of memory processes, is facilitated by estrogen treatment (Cordoba Montoya and Carrer 1997).

Opioids remain one of the most effective therapies for many forms of chronic pain. Estrogens interact with the opioid system at different levels. At supraspinal levels, one of the most important circuits able to affect nociception is the periaqueductal gray (PAG) matter and its descending pathways. PAG descending neurons are tonically inhibited by GABA neurons; β-endorphin (β-EP) inhibits GABAergic interneurons and thus frees the descending pathways. The cells of origin of all β-EP in the limbic-hypothalamic circuit are the hypothalamic arcuate nucleus cell bodies, which send widespread axonal projections to the forebrain and midbrain (Thornton et al. 1994). β-EP is a product of the hypothalamic pro-opiomelanocortin (POMC) system (Tiligada and Wilson 1990). POMC neurons contain estrogen receptors (Morrell et al. 1985) in functional relationship with opioid receptors of the μ-type. Therefore, the μ-opioid receptor (μ-OR) is an autoreceptor on POMC neurons. In the whole brain of the female rat, the number of μ-ORs fluctuates during the different phases of the estrous cycle. The predominant action of opioid peptides is to inhibit cell firing; thus the arcuate β-EP neurons are hyperpolarized by μ-OR activation via an increase of an inwardly rectifying potassium conductance (Lagrange et al. 1997). Consistent with this process, both in vivo and in vitro experiments have found that μ-OR activation decreases β-EP release from arcuate β-EP neurons, an effect counteracted by estrogen administration. In particular, Eckersell et al. (1998) showed that estrogen treatment induces the translocation of μ-OR immunoreactivity from the membrane to an internal location in steroid-sensitive cell groups of the limbic system and hypothalamus. Similarly, Limonta et al. (1987) reported a progressive decline of the number of hypothalamic μ-OR in the afternoon of proestrus, which coincides with the initiation of the luteinizing hormone (LH) surge. Thus, estrogens have two opposite effects on nociception: (1) an analgesic effect, due to the decrease of the μ-OR autoreceptor on β-EP arcuate neurons; and (2) a hyperalgesic effect, due to the LH increase, which has been described as hyperalgesic per se (Ratka et al. 1990).

Interestingly, opioid receptors in the thalamic neurons also are sensitive to circulating levels of gonadal steroids. Wardlaw et al. (1982) reported that thalamic endorphin content decreases in castrated females exposed to estrogens. Moreover, they reported that ovariectomized rats exposed to estradiol benzoate showed a rapid and reversible increase in the number of μ-OR-positive fibers, an effect prevented by naltrexone administration.

CONCLUSIONS

Gonadal hormones and acute pain are two important components of physical well-being. The gonads, through their products, are the main reproductive structures and also have important effects on cognitive functions. Acute pain should preserve the body from danger. However, clinical data show that pain can be chronic and that gonadal hormones can make it worse. Is it possible that during the reproductive period of a woman's life, the gonads work to mask pain so as to help females reproduce successfully? If so, with the huge increase in lifespan in modern times, the effects of the gonadal hormones on the septo-hippocampal/hypothalamic system may have acquired negative consequences. The "discovery" of sex differences in pain will probably be a useful tool to help us understand these phenomena, and it should be considered an asset and not, as we are used to considering it, a problem.

ACKNOWLEDGMENTS

This study was supported by Ministero Universita, Ricerca Scientifica e Tecnologica, and by the University of Siena.

REFERENCES

Aloisi AM. Sex differences in pain-induced effects on the septo-hippocampal system. *Brain Res Brain Res Rev* 1997; 25:397–406.

Aloisi AM, Carli G. Formalin pain does not modify food-hoarding behaviour in male rats. *Behav Processes* 1996; 36:125–133.

Aloisi AM, Steenbergen HL, van de Poll NE, Farabollini F. Sex-dependent effects of restraint on nociception and pituitary-adrenal hormones in the rat. *Physiol Behav* 1994; 55:789–793.

Aloisi AM, Ceccarelli I, Herdegen T. Gonadectomy and persistent pain affect hippocampal c-Fos expression in male and female rats. *Neurosci Lett* 2000; in press.

Berger-Sweeney J, Arnold A, Gabeau D, Mills J. Sex differences in learning and memory in mice: effects of sequence of testing and cholinergic blockade. *Behav Neurosci* 1995; 109:859–873.

Berkley KJ. Vive la difference! *Trends Neurosci* 1992; 15:331–332.

Berkley KJ. Sex differences in pain. *Behav Brain Sci* 1997; 20:371–380.

Blok LJ, Bartlett JMS, Bolt-De Vries J. Effect of testosterone deprivation on expression of the androgen receptor in rat prostate epididymis and testis. *Int J Androl* 1992; 15:182–198.

Brown ER, Harlan RE, Krause JE. Gonadal steroid regulation of substance P (SP) and SP-encoding messenger ribonucleic acids in the rat anterior pituitary and hypothalamus. *Endocrinology* 1990; 126:330–340.

Buterbaugh GG, Hudson GM. Estradiol replacement to female rats facilitates dorsal hippocampal but not ventral hippocampal kindled seizure acquisition. *Exp Neurol* 1991; 111:55–64.

Carey MP, Deterd CH, De Koning J, Helmerhorst F, De Kloet ER. The influence of ovarian steroids on hypothalamic-pituitary-adrenal regulation in the female rat. *J Endocrinol* 1995; 144:311–321.

Ceccarelli I, Casamenti F, Massafra C, et al. Effects of novelty and pain on behavior and hippocampal extracellular ACh levels in male and female rats. *Brain Res* 1999; 815:169–176.

Cerinic MM, Konttinen Y, Generini S, Cutolo M. Neuropeptides and steroid hormones in arthritis. *Curr Opin Rheumatol* 1998; 10:220–235.

Chapman CR. Limbic processes and the affective dimension of pain. *Prog Brain Res* 1996; 110:63–81.

Cordoba Montoya DA, Carrer HF. Estrogen facilitates induction of long term potentiation in the hippocampus of awake rats. *Brain Res* 1997; 778:430–438.

Eckersell CB, Popper P, Micevych PE. Estrogen-induced alteration of mu-opioid receptor immunoreactivity in the medial preoptic nucleus and medial amygdala. *J Neurosci* 1998; 18:3967–3976.

Enmark E, Gustafsson J. Oestrogen receptors—an overview. *J Intern Med* 1999; 246:133–138.

Evan GI, Wyllie AH, Gilbert CS, et al. Induction of apoptosis in fibroblasts by c-myc protein. *Cell* 1992; 69:119–128.

Gazzaley AH, Weiland NG, McEwen B. Differential regulation of NMDAR1 mRNA and protein by estradiol in the rat hippocampus. *J Neurosci* 1996; 16:6830–6838.

Gerdes LC, Sonnendecker EWW, Polakow ES. Psychological change effected by estrogen-progesterone and clonidine treatment in climacteric women. *Am J Obstet Gynecol* 1982; 142:98–104.

Gibbs RB. Impairment of basal forebrain cholinergic neurons associated with aging and long-term loss of ovarian function. *Exp Neurol* 1998; 151:289–302.

Gu Q, Moss RL. Novel mechanism for non-genomic action of 17 beta-oestradiol on kainate-induced currents in isolated rat CA1 hippocampal neurones. *J Physiol (Lond)* 1998; 506:745–754.

Handa RJ, Nunley KM, Lorens SA, et al. Androgen regulation of adrenocorticotropin and corticosterone secretion in the male rat following novelty and foot shock stressors. *Physiol Behav* 1994; 55:117–124.

Herbert W. Psychotropic effects of testosterone. In: Neischlag E, Behre HM (Eds). *Testosterone: Action, Deficiency, Substitution.* Springer-Verlag: New York, 1990, pp 51–71.

Kawata M. Roles of steroid hormones and their receptors in structural organization in the nervous system. *Neurosci Res* 1995; 24:1–46.

Kerr JE, Allore RJ, Beck SG, Handa RJ. Distribution and hormonal regulation of androgen receptor (AR) and AR messenger ribonucleic acid in the rat hippocampus. *Endocrinology* 1995; 136:3213–3221.

Kerr JE, Beck SG. Handa RJ. Androgens selectively modulate C-fos messenger RNA induction in the rat hippocampus following novelty. *Neuroscience* 1996a; 74:757–766.

Kerr JE, Beck SG, Handa RJ. Androgens modulate glucocorticoid receptor mRNA, but not mineralocorticoid receptor mRNA levels, in the rat hippocampus. *J Neuroendocrinol* 1996b; 8:439–447.

Lagrange AH, Ronnekleiv OK, Kelly MJ. Modulation of G protein-coupled receptors by an estrogen receptor that activates protein kinase A. *Mol Pharmacol* 1997; 51:605–612.

Limonta P, Maggi R, Dondi D, Martini L, Piva F. Gonadal steroid modulation of brain opioid systems. *J Steroid Biochem* 1987; 27:691–698.

Loy R, Gerlach JL, McEwen BS. Autoradiographic localization of estradiol-binding neurons in the rat hippocampal formation and entorhinal cortex. *Brain Res* 1988; 467:245–251.

Luine VN. Steroid hormone modulation of hippocampal dependent spatial memory. *Stress* 1997; 2:21–36.

Luine VN, Richards ST, Wu VY, Beck KD. Estradiol enhances learning and memory in a spatial memory task and effects levels of monoaminergic neurotransmitters. *Horm Behav* 1998; 34:149–162.

Maggi A, Susanna L, Bettini E, Mantero G, Zucchi I. Hippocampus: a target for estrogen action in mammalian brain. *Mol Endocrinol* 1989; 3:1165–1170.

McEwen BS. Stress and hippocampal plasticity. *Annu Rev Neurosci* 1999; 22:105–122.

McMillan PJ, Singer CA, Dorsa DM. The effects of ovariectomy and estrogen replacement on trkA and choline acetyltransferase mRNA expression in the basal forebrain of the adult female Sprague-Dawley rat. *J Neurosci* 1996; 16:1860–1865.

Meisler JG. Chronic pain conditions in women. *J Womens Health* 1999; 8:313–320.

Mizoguchi K, Kunishita T, Chui DH, Tabira T. Stress induces neuronal death in the hippocampus of castrated rats. *Neurosci Lett* 1992; 138:157–160.

Morrell JI, McGinty JF, Pfaff DW. A subset of β-endorphin- or dynorphin-containing neurons in the medial basal hypothalamus accumulates estradiol. *Neuroendocrinology* 1985; 41:417–426.

Moss RL, Gu Q, Wong M. Estrogen: nontranscriptional signaling pathway. *Recent Prog Horm Res* 1997; 52:33–68.

Okamura H, Yokosuka M, McEwen BS, Hayashi S. Colocalization of NADPH-diaphorase and estrogen receptor immunoreactivity in the rat ventromedial hypothalamic nucleus: stimulatory effect of estrogen on NADPH-diaphorase activity. *Endocrinology* 1994; 135:1705–1708.

Papez JW. A proposed mechanism of emotion. 1937. *J Neuropsychiatry Clin Neurosci* 1995; 7:103–112.

Patchev VK, Almeida OF. Gender specificity in the neural regulation of the response to stress: new leads from classical paradigms. *Mol Neurobiol* 1998; 16:63–77.

Paxinos G. *The Rat Nervous System.* San Diego: Academic Press, 1995.

Perry E, Walker M, Grace J, Perry R. Acetylcholine in mind: a neurotransmitter correlate of consciousness? *Trends Neurosci* 1999; 22:273–280.

Peyron R, Garcia-Larrea L, Gregoire MC, et al. Haemodynamic brain responses to acute pain in humans: sensory and attentional networks. *Brain* 1999; 122:1765–1780.

Pfaff DW, Schwartz-Giblin S. Cellular mechanisms of female reproductive behaviors. In: Knobil E, Neill J (Eds). *The Physiology of Reproduction.* New York: Raven Press, 1988, pp 1487–1568.

Pilgrim C, Hutchison JB. Developmental regulation of sex differences in the brain: can the role of gonadal steroids be redefined? *Neuroscience* 1994; 60:843–855.

Quarmby VE, Yarbrough WG, Lubahn DB, French FS, Wilson EM. Autologous down-regulation of androgen receptor messenger ribonucleic acid. *Mol Endocrinol* 1990; 4:22–28.

Ratka A, Simpkins JW. A modulatory role for luteinizing hormone-releasing hormone in nociceptive responses of female rats. *Endocrinology* 1990; 127:667–673.

Roof RL, Havens MD. Testosterone improves maze performance and development of a male hippocampus in females. *Brain Res* 1992; 572:310–331.

Ruda MA. Gender and pain. *Pain* 1993; 53:1–2.

Schumacher M. Rapid membrane effects of steroid hormones: an emerging concept in neuroendocrinology. *Trends Neurosci* 1990; 13:359–362.

Singh M, Meyer EM, Simpkins JW. The effect of ovariectomy and estradiol replacement on brain-derived neurotrophic factor messenger ribonucleic acid expression in cortical and hippocampal brain regions of female Sprague-Dawley rats. *Endocrinology* 1995; 136:2320–2324.

Spitzer JA. Gender differences in some host defense mechanisms. *Lupus* 1999; 8:380–383.

Tanapat P, Hastings NB, Reeves AJ, Gould E. Estrogen stimulates a transient increase in the number of new neurons in the dentate gyrus of the adult female rat. *J Neurosci* 1999; 19:5792–5801.

Teresawa S, Timiras PS. Electrical activity during the estrous cycles of the rat: cyclic changes in limbic structures. *Endocrinology* 1968; 83:207–216.

Thornton JE, Loose MD, Kelly MJ, Ronnekleiv OK. Effects of estrogen on the number of neurons expressing beta-endorphin in the medial basal hypothalamus of the female guinea pig. *J Comp Neurol* 1994; 341:68–77.

Tiligada E, Wilson JF. Ionic, neuronal and endocrine influences on the proopiomelanocortin system of the hypothalamus. *Life Sci* 1990; 46:81–90.

Tsuruo Y, Hisano S, Okamura Y, Tsukamoto N, Daikoku S. Hypothalamic substance P-containing neurons. Sex-dependent topographical differences and ultrastructural transformations associated with stages of the estrous cycle. *Brain Res* 1984; 305:331–341.

Unruh AM. Gender variations in clinical pain experience. *Pain* 1996; 65:123–167.

Riley JL 3rd, Robinson ME, Wise EA, Myers CD, Fillingim RB. Sex differences in the perception of noxious experimental stimuli: a meta-analysis. *Pain* 1998; 74:181–187.

Wardlaw SL, Thoron L, Frantz AG. Effects of sex steroids on brain beta-endorphin. *Brain Res* 1982; 245:327–331.

Warren SG, Humphreys AG, Juraska JM, Greenough WT. LTP varies across the estrous cycle: enhanced synaptic plasticity in proestrus rats. *Brain Res* 1995; 703:26–30.

Woolley CS, McEwen BS. Estradiol mediates fluctuation in hippocampal synapse density during the estrous cycle in the adult rat. *J Neurosci* 1992; 12:2549–2554.

Woolley CS, Weiland NG, McEwen BS, Schwartzkroin PA. Estradiol increases the sensitivity of hippocampal CA1 pyramidal cells to NMDA receptor-mediated synaptic input: correlation with dendritic spine density. *J Neurosci* 1997; 17:1848–1859.

Yuan H, Bowlby DA, Brown TJ, Hochberg RB, MacLusky NJ. Distribution of occupied and unoccupied estrogen receptors in the rat brain: effects of physiological gonadal steroid exposure. *Endocrinology* 1995; 136:96–105.

Correspondence to: Anna Maria Aloisi, MD, PhD, Institute of Human Physiology, University of Siena, Via Aldo Moro, 53100 Siena, Italy. email: aloisi@unisi.it.

Proceedings of the 9th World Congress on Pain,
Progress in Pain Research and Management,
Vol. 16, edited by M. Devor, M.C. Rowbotham, and
Z. Wiesenfeld-Hallin, IASP Press, Seattle, © 2000.

54

Altered CNS Processing of Nociceptive Messages from the Vagina in Rats that Have Recovered from Uterine Inflammation

Ursula Wesselmann,[a,b,c] Christin Sanders,[a] and Peter P. Czakanski[a,d]

Departments of [a]Neurology, [b]Neurological Surgery, [c]Biomedical Engineering, and [d]Gynecology and Obstetrics, The Johns Hopkins University School of Medicine, Baltimore, Maryland, USA

Chronic pelvic pain is a common, debilitating problem in women that is difficult to treat and can significantly impair quality of life. Recent epidemiological data from the United States show that 14.7% of women in their reproductive ages reported chronic pelvic pain (Mathias et al. 1996); of these, 15% reported time lost from work and 45% claimed reduced work productivity. In the United States, 10% of outpatient gynecological consultations are for chronic pelvic pain (Reiter 1990), and medical costs for outpatient visits for this pain syndrome are estimated at U.S.$881.5 million per year (Mathias et al. 1996). The personal costs to women in terms of years of suffering, disability, marital discord, loss of employment, and unsuccessful medical intervention cannot be calculated so easily.

Overall, a woman has about a 5% risk of having chronic pelvic pain in her lifetime. In patients with a previous diagnosis of pelvic inflammatory disease this risk is increased fourfold (Ryder 1996). It is not clear why about 20% of the 750,000 American women who are clinically diagnosed with pelvic inflammatory disease each year develop a chronic pelvic pain syndrome (Lipscomb and Ling 1993), despite the fact that the infection has resolved, while the majority of women recover completely. While most clinical and research efforts have focused on identifying an underlying etiology for chronic pelvic pain, recent editorials have called for a new approach in recognizing chronic pelvic pain not only as a symptom of visceral disease, but as a chronic visceral pain syndrome (Campbell and Collett 1994; Wesselmann 1999).

The neurophysiological and neuropharmacological mechanisms that mediate chronic pelvic pain are poorly understood; animal models are a necessary step to help elucidate these mechanisms. We recently developed a new model in the rat that closely resembles a state of inflammatory uterine pain (Wesselmann and Lai 1997; Wesselmann et al. 1998). Rats with uterine inflammation show abnormal behavior suggestive of visceral pain during the first 4–5 days following uterine inflammation. In the present study, we tested the hypothesis that a previous noxious uterine event (i.e., inflammation) can modify the response to noxious stimulation of the vagina, via altered processing in the central nervous system (CNS).

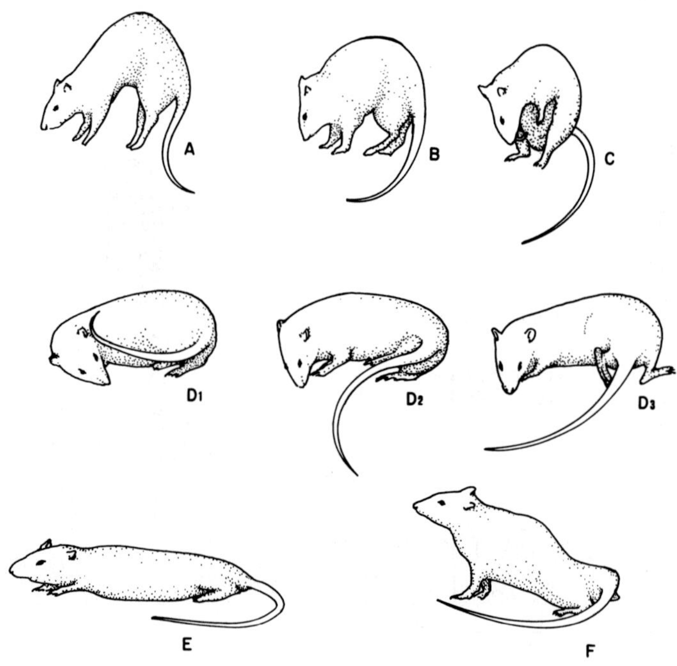

Fig. 1. Behavioral characteristics of rats with unilateral uterine inflammation. (A) hunching; (B) hump-backed position; (C) licking of the lower abdomen and/or flanks; (D) variations of the alpha-position; (E) stretching of the body; (F) squashing of the lower abdomen against the floor. (Reprinted from Wesselmann et al. 1998, with permission from Elsevier Science.)

METHODS

All experimental protocols were approved by the Animal Care and Use Committee of The Johns Hopkins University and followed the guidelines of the International Association for the Study of Pain (Zimmermann 1983). The experiments were performed on female adult virgin Sprague-Dawley rats (180–250 g). Stages of the estrous cycle were determined daily by vaginal smears until rats were killed. Experimental and control rats were matched for the stage of the estrous cycle, since the response to noxious stimulation might vary with the stage of the estrous cycle. Experimental rats (n = 5) were anesthetized on day 1 with pentobarbital (50 mg/kg intraperitoneally [i.p.]), and the uterus was chemically inflamed using mustard oil (see Wesselmann et al. 1998 for details). Briefly, a small ventral midline laparotomy was performed, and a solution of 5% mustard oil (Aldrich Chemical Co.), dissolved in mineral oil, was injected into the right uterine horn. The abdominal incision was then closed, and the rats were allowed to recover

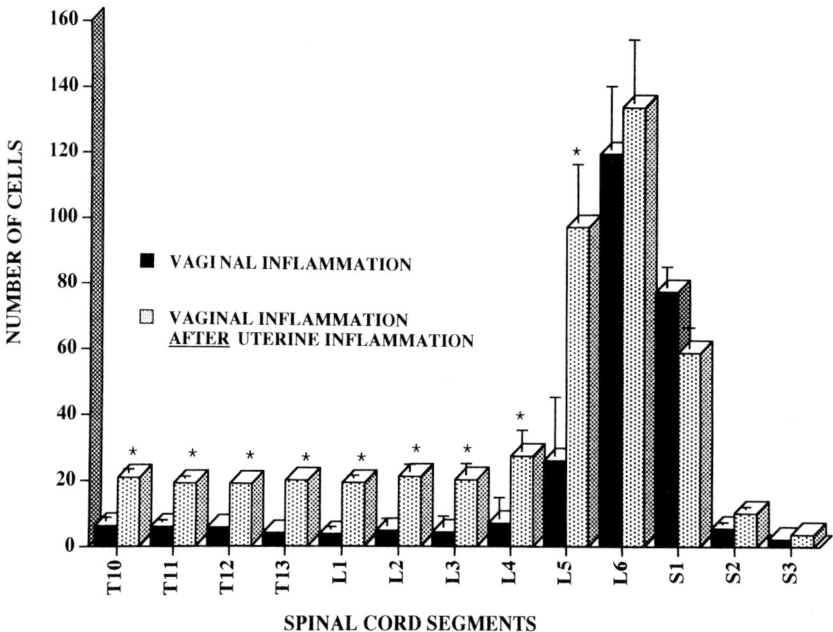

Fig. 2. Effects of previous uterine inflammation on the response to noxious vaginal stimulation, showing mean (± SEM) number of FOS-ir cells per section in spinal cord segments T10–S3 after vaginal inflammation with mustard oil (stimulus duration: 2 hours). In contrast to control rats with vaginal inflammation only, the number of FOS-ir neurons was significantly increased in response to vaginal inflammation in segments T10–L5 in rats with previous uterine inflammation. ANOVA; $^*P < 0.05$.

from anesthesia. Animal behavior was video recorded for 9 days and analyzed post hoc. Rats showed abnormal behavior indicative of visceral pain for 4–5 days post-inflammation (Wesselmann et al. 1998), and behavior then returned to normal. On day 9 post-uterine inflammation, the rats were anesthetized again (urethane; 1.1 g/kg i.p.), and the vagina was inflamed with 10% mustard oil. In control rats (n = 5) with no prior inflammation of the uterus, the vagina was likewise inflamed with mustard oil. Two hours after vaginal inflammation, all rats were killed via intracardiac perfusion with 4% formaldehyde fixative.

The uterine horns and the vagina were dissected and examined for inflammatory changes. Spinal cord segments T10–S3 were removed and post-fixed in the same fixative for 2 days, and then 50-μm transverse sections were processed for FOS protein using an antibody (rabbit anti-*c-fos*) purchased from Arnel Products and diluted at 1:40,000. The reaction product was visualized with diaminobenzidine as the chromogen. Spinal cord sections were examined using bright-field optics, and all FOS-immunoreactive (FOS-ir) cells in each section were counted. During this phase the investigators were blinded to the type of noxious stimulation under study. Cell counts in spinal cord segments T10–S3 in experimental and control rats were analyzed statistically using a factorial ANOVA (Statview 4.51; Abacus Concepts 1994). The protected least significant difference (PLSD) Fisher's test was used to determine probability values between animal groups. Significance levels were assessed at $P < 0.05$.

RESULTS

Mustard oil injection into the uterine horn and into the vagina resulted in massive inflammation in all rats. Histological examination revealed infiltration with polymorphonuclear leukocytes, edema, dilated blood vessels, and ulcerations (Wesselmann and Lai 1997).

Fig. 3. Spinal cord segments T11, T13, L2, and L4 showing the distribution of FOS-ir cells after vaginal inflammation for 2 hours in *control rats,* which received vaginal inflammation only, and *experimental rats,* which received vaginal inflammation 9 days after uterine inflammation. (A) Localization of laminae according to Molander et al. (1984). (B) Each dot represents one FOS-ir cell identified in 10 of the most heavily stained sections from each segment. Note that more FOS-ir cells were labeled in rats with vaginal inflammation after uterine inflammation than in rats with vaginal inflammation only. The majority of these neurons were located in laminae I and II. →

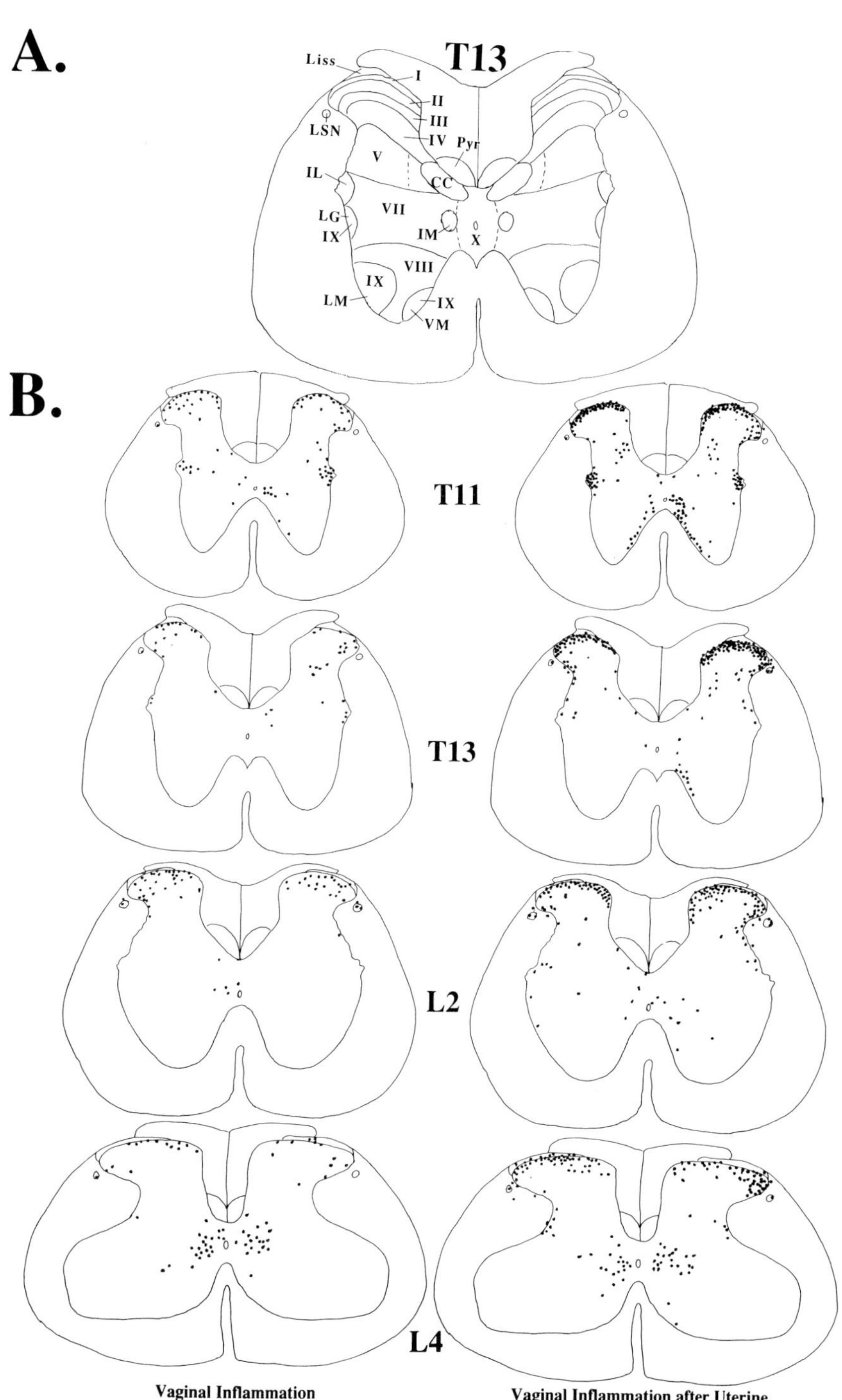
A.
T13
Liss
I
II
III
IV
Pyr
LSN
V
IL
CC
VII
LG
IX
IM
X
VIII
IX
LM
IX
VM
B.
T11
T13
L2
L4
Vaginal Inflammation
Vaginal Inflammation after Uterine Inflammation

BEHAVIORAL CHARACTERISTICS OF RATS WITH UTERINE INFLAMMATION

All experimental rats showed abnormal behavior indicative of visceral pain during the first 4–5 days following uterine inflammation. The behavioral characteristics of rats with uterine inflammation consisted of six characteristic movements (Fig. 1): hunching, hump-backed position, licking of the lower abdomen, repeated waves of contraction of the ipsilateral oblique musculature with inward turning of the ipsilateral hindlimb (alpha-position), stretching, and squashing of the lower abdomen against the floor, as described in detail elsewhere (Wesselmann et al. 1998).

QUANTITATIVE ANALYSIS OF FOS-IR CELLS IN THE SPINAL CORD

Preliminary studies have shown that there is no significant expression of *c-fos* in the spinal cord above baseline 9 days after uterine inflammation. Vaginal inflammation with mustard oil for 2 hours resulted in a marked increase of FOS-ir cells in spinal cord segments L5, L6, and S1 (pelvic nerve input) in both our experimental (vaginal inflammation on day 9 following uterine inflammation) and control (vaginal inflammation only) groups. In contrast to control rats, FOS-ir neurons were significantly increased ($P < 0.05$) in segments T10–L4 in response to vaginal inflammation in experimental rats (Fig. 2). Also, the number of FOS-ir cells in segment L5 was significantly ($P < 0.05$) higher in experimental compared to control rats (Fig. 2). The increase in FOS-ir cells in segments T10–L5 in experimental rats was mainly due to an increase in cells in laminae I and II (Fig. 3).

DISCUSSION

Our key observation was the significant increase in FOS-ir neurons in spinal cord segments T10–L5 2 hours after vaginal inflammation in rats subjected to uterine inflammation 9 days previously in comparison to control rats with vaginal inflammation only. In the rat, afferent fibers in the hypogastric and pelvic nerves convey sensory information to thoracolumbar (T13–L2) and lumbosacral (L6–S1) segments of the spinal cord (Peters et al. 1987; Nance et al. 1988; Berkley and Hubscher 1995). Fibers that innervate the uterine body and horns of adult virgin rats travel in the hypogastric nerves, and fibers that innervate the vagina travel mainly in the pelvic nerves (Berkley and Hubscher 1995). In agreement with these studies on the neural pathways of the uterus and vagina in the rat, we have previously shown that noxious uterine stimulation results in *c-fos* expression in spinal cord segments T13–L2, which receive input through the hypogastric nerve (Wesselmann et al. 1997), and in the present study we have demonstrated that noxious vaginal stimulation results in *c-fos* expression in segments L5–S1, which receive input through the pelvic nerve.

Our finding that FOS-ir neurons increased significantly in spinal cord segments T10–L5 in response to vaginal inflammation in rats 9 days post-uterine inflammation suggests that previous uterine inflammation creates a latent algogenic condition that modifies CNS processing of nociceptive information from the vagina. Thus, a noxious stimulus to one area of the reproductive tract (the uterus) influences the reactivity to subsequent stimulation of another area of the reproductive tract (the vagina), whose sensory innervation projects to adjacent spinal cord segments. Further studies on the pathophysiological mechanisms of these neuroplastic changes in the spinal cord in the rat model of pelvic pain might result in a better understanding of the pathophysiological mechanisms of chronic pelvic pain in women, and might open new perspectives for developing improved pharmacological therapies.

ACKNOWLEDGMENTS

This work was supported by National Institutes of Health grant RO1 NS36553/NINDS/Office of Research for Women's Health (U. Wesselmann), and in part by Astra Research Centre Montreal (U. Wesselmann) and the National Vulvodynia Association (U. Wesselmann).

REFERENCES

Berkley KJ, Hubscher CH. Visceral and somatic sensory tracks through the neuraxis and their relation to pain: lessons from the rat female reproductive system. In: Gebhart GF (Ed). *Visceral Pain.* Progress in Pain Research and Management, Vol. 5. Seattle: IASP Press, 1995, pp 195–216.

Campbell F, Collett BJ. Chronic pelvic pain. *Br J Anaesth* 1994; 73:571–573.

Lipscomb GH, Ling FW. Relationship of pelvic infection and chronic pelvic pain. *Obstet Gynecol Clin North Am* 1993; 20:699–708.

Mathias SD, Kuppermann M, Liberman RF, Lipschutz RC, Steege JF. Chronic pelvic pain: prevalence, health-related quality of life, and economic correlates. *Obstet Gynecol* 1996; 87:321–327.

Molander C, Xu Q, Grant G. The cytoarchitectonic organization of the spinal cord in the rat. I. The lower thoracic and lumbosacral cord. *J Comp Neurol* 1984; 230:133–141.

Nance DM, Burns J, Klein CM, Burden HW. Afferent fibers in the reproductive system and pelvic viscera of female rats: anterograde tracing and immunocytochemical studies. *Brain Res Bull* 1988; 21:701–709.

Peters LC, Kristal MB, Komisaruk BR. Sensory innervation of the external and internal genitalia of the female rat. *Brain Res* 1987; 408:199–204.

Reiter RC. A profile of women with chronic pelvic pain. *Clin Obstet Gynecol* 1990; 33:130–136.

Ryder RM. Chronic pelvic pain. *Am Fam Phys* 1996; 54:2225–2232.

Wesselmann U. Pain—the neglected aspect of visceral pain [guest editorial]. *Eur J Pain* 1999; 3:189–191.

Wesselmann U, Lai J. Mechanisms of referred visceral pain: uterine inflammation in the adult virgin rat results in neurogenic plasma extravasation in the skin. *Pain* 1997; 73:309–317.

Wesselmann U, Minson JB, Llewellyn-Smith IJ. Expression of C-FOS-like immunoreactivity in the spinal cord after noxious uterine stimulation—a model for uterine pain. *Neurology* 1997; 48(Suppl):259.

Wesselmann U, Czakanski PP, Affaitati G, Giamberardino MA. Uterine inflammation as a noxious visceral stimulus: behavioral characterization in the rat. *Neurosci Lett* 1998; 246:73–76.

Zimmermann M. Ethical guidelines for investigation of experimental pain in conscious animals. *Pain* 1983; 16:109–110.

Correspondence to: Ursula Wesselmann, MD, Johns Hopkins Hospital, Department of Neurology, 720 Rutland Avenue, Traylor Building 604, Baltimore, MD 21205, USA. Tel: 410-614-8840; Fax: 410-955-9826; email: pain@welchlink.welch.jhu.edu.

Proceedings of the 9th World Congress on Pain, Progress in Pain Research and Management, Vol. 16, edited by M. Devor, M.C. Rowbotham, and Z. Wiesenfeld-Hallin, IASP Press, Seattle, © 2000.

55

Peripheral and Central Sensitization during Migraine[1]

Rami Burstein[a,b] and Andrew Strassman[a]

[a]Department of Anesthesia and Critical Care, Beth Israel Deaconess Medical Center, and [b]Department of Neurobiology and the Program in Neuroscience, Harvard Medical School, Boston, Massachusetts, USA

Current theories on the pathophysiology of migraine propose that pain results from the activation of meningeal perivascular sensory afferents initiated by a chemical signal (Moskowitz et al. 1988). According to these theories, ions, protons, and inflammatory agents that activate and sensitize peripheral nociceptors (Handwerker and Reeh 1992; Kessler et al. 1992; Steen et al. 1992, 1995) are released in the vicinity of sensory fibers innervating the dura following an episode of cortical spreading depression (Lauritzen 1994) or neurogenic inflammation (Goadsby and Edvinsson 1993; Moskowitz and Macfarlane 1993). Although the cause of the initial release of these chemicals is unknown, a recently developed concept suggests that temporary exposure of perivascular fibers to chemical agents may alter their sensitivity to mechanical stimuli. Theoretically, it is possible that chemically mediated sensitization of dural primary afferent nociceptors can explain the hypersensitivity of migraineurs to changes in intracranial pressure (e.g., during coughing) and the throbbing nature of their pain.

A possible consequence of peripheral sensitization is the development of spontaneous activity and the anomalous bombardment of second-order neurons with impulses originating from peripheral nociceptors. Dorsal horn neurons that receive an increased number of signals from the periphery often become hyperexcitable and begin to respond to mild stimuli that do not normally activate them (Woolf 1983; Cook et al. 1986; Simone et al. 1991; Torebjörk et al. 1992; McMahon et al. 1993; Ren and Dubner 1993; Woolf and Doubell 1994; Koltzenburg et al. 1995; Woolf et al. 1995; Magerl

[1] Mini-review based on a congress workshop.

et al. 1998). Because second-order nociceptive neurons receive convergent input from cerebral blood vessels, meninges, and facial skin (Davis and Dostrovsky 1988), painful signals that arise intracranially during a migraine attack can theoretically induce changes in extracranial sensation. Such changes in extracranial sensation were described for the first time by Edward Liveing in 1873. Further documentation has been provided by a number of clinical studies on scalp tenderness during migraine (Tfelt-Hansen et al. 1981; Lous and Olesen 1982; Drummond 1987; Jensen et al. 1988, 1993; Gobel et al. 1992; Jensen 1993).

This chapter summarizes recent studies on the development of peripheral and central sensitization along the trigeminovascular pain pathway following the induction of intracranial pain in an animal model of migraine (Strassman et al. 1996; Burstein et al. 1998; Yamamura et al. 1999).

PERIPHERAL SENSITIZATION MEDIATES INTRACRANIAL (MENINGEAL) HYPERSENSITIVITY

To test the hypothesis that inflammatory agents such as histamine (HA), serotonin (5-HT), bradykinin (BK), and prostaglandins (PGE_2) can activate and sensitize trigeminal primary afferent neurons that innervate the dura, single-unit extracellular recordings were made in mechanosensitive meningeal primary afferent neurons (Strassman et al. 1996; Fig. 1A). These agents were used for the following reasons: (1) They are endogenous, and are believed to be released in the vicinity of the dural sinuses by increased plasma extravasation and mast cell degranulation induced by neurogenic inflammation (Handwerker and Reeh 1992; Hanesch et al. 1992; Moskowitz and Macfarlane 1993). (2) They can activate and sensitize somatic and visceral nociceptive primary afferent neurons (Beck et al. 1974; Mizumura et al. 1987; Neugebauer et al. 1989; Lang et al. 1990; Handwerker and Reeh 1992; Hanesch et al. 1992; Khan et al. 1992; Steen et al. 1992; Davis et al. 1993). (3) They are potent algesics in humans (Armstrong et al. 1957; Hollander et al. 1957; Guzman et al. 1962; Sicuteri 1967; Fock and Mense 1976). (4) When applied together, these agents enhance each other's effects on the nociceptors (Fock and Mense 1976; Lang et al. 1990; Kessler et al. 1992).

Meningeal nociceptors were initially identified by their responses to electrical and mechanical (Fig. 1B, 2A) stimulation of the dura overlying the ipsilateral transverse sinus. Their neuronal responses to mechanical indentation of the dura (with calibrated von Frey monofilaments); were then studied before and after the application of the inflammatory agents to the dural

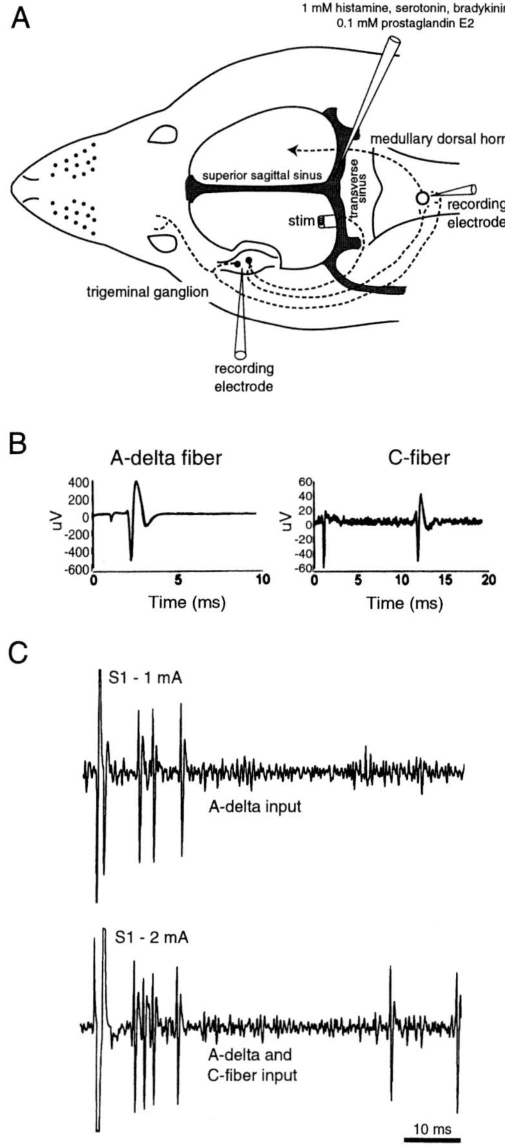

Fig. 1. Experimental setup. (A) Anatomical locations of stimulation and recording sites. (B) Responses of two trigeminal ganglion cells to single-shock stimulation of the dura overlying the ipsilateral transverse sinus. Each trace shows three superimposed sweeps. (C) Responses of two trigeminal brainstem neurons to single-shock stimulation of the dura overlying the ipsilateral transverse sinus. Adapted with permission from Strassman et al. (1996) and Burstein et al. (1998).

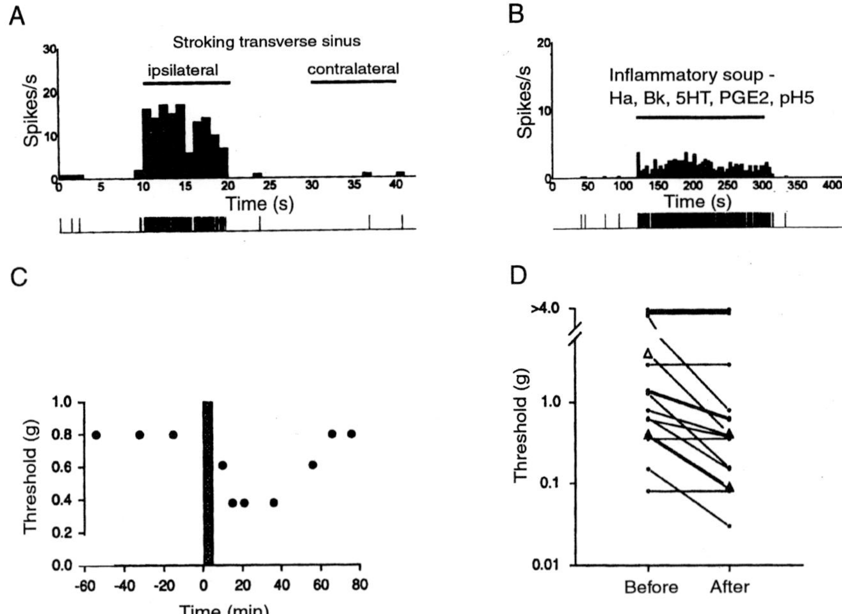

Fig. 2. The development of peripheral sensitization following chemical irritation of the dura. (A) Peristimulus time histogram showing the response of a mechanosensitive meningeal primary afferent neuron to mechanical stroking of the ipsilateral but not contralateral transverse sinus. (B) Peristimulus time histogram showing the response of a mechanosensitive meningeal primary afferent neuron to topical application of an inflammatory mediators (serotonin, bradykinin, prostaglandin E2, all 10 μM; and histamine, 100 μM, pH 5.0) to the dura overlying the ipsilateral transverse sinus. Ha = histamine; Bk = bradykinin; 5HT = serotonin. (C) Time course of the development of mechanical sensitization. In this case, the smallest force required to activate the meningeal primary afferent neuron by dural indentation with von Frey monofilaments was 0.8 g prior to the chemical stimulation (black rectangle) of the dura, and 0.4 g after chemical stimulation. (D) Individually plotted response thresholds of 17 neurons both before and after the application of inflammatory or acidic chemicals. Adapted with permission from Strassman et al. (1996).

receptive field (Fig. 2B). Prior to chemical irritation of the dura, mechanical thresholds were 0.86 ± 0.98 g (mean ± 1 SD). Following chemical irritation, 66% of the neurons became hypersensitive and started to respond to dural indentation with mechanical forces that produced minimal or no responses prior to the chemical stimulation (Fig. 2C–D). Such sensitization to mechanical stimuli was observed both in neurons that discharged in direct response to the sensitizing agent ($n = 6$) and in neurons that did not ($n = 5$).

Physiologically, these results demonstrate that the excitability of meningeal nociceptors can increase following exposure to inflammatory chemicals such as histamine, serotonin, bradykinin, and prostaglandin E_2.

The clinical implication of this *peripheral sensitization* is *intracranial hypersensitivity*. Studies have repeatedly shown that peripheral nociceptors can be silent and unresponsive under normal conditions, but active and responsive to even the mildest stimulus under pathological conditions (Cervero and Jänig 1992; Schmidt et al. 1995; Michaelis et al. 1996). In the context of migraine, sensitization of mechanosensitive meningeal nociceptors might explain how small increases in intracranial pressure during routine physical activities such as climbing stairs, bending over, and coughing (Blau and Dexter 1981; Anthony and Rasmussen 1993; Moskowitz and Macfarlane 1993) can aggravate the pain.

CENTRAL SENSITIZATION MEDIATES EXTRACRANIAL (CUTANEOUS) HYPERSENSITIVITY

To test the hypothesis that chemical activation and sensitization of trigeminal mechanosensitive meningeal primary afferent neurons can lead to activation and sensitization of second-order trigeminal brainstem neurons, we made single-unit extracellular recordings in medullary dorsal horn neurons that receive convergent input from the dura and skin (Fig. 1A,C; Burstein et al. 1998).

We recorded changes in the responsiveness of 23 (16 WDR, 5 HT, and 2 LT) trigeminal brainstem dura-sensitive neurons to mechanical stimulation of their dural receptive fields and to mechanical and thermal stimulation of their cutaneous receptive fields following local application of inflammatory mediators to the dura. Fig. 3 provides an example of the changes that occurred in an individual neuron. In this case, the threshold to mechanical stimulation of the dura was 2.35 g (3A, left) before the application of inflammatory agents to the dura, and then dropped to 0.217 g (3A, right) 20 minutes after the chemical irritation. Regarding cutaneous mechanosensitivity, the neuron responded maximally to noxious mechanical stimulation of the skin (3B, left) before the chemical stimulation of the dura. However, 25 minutes after the chemical irritation its response to brushing the cutaneous receptive field increased 4-fold, becoming as large as its response to noxious stimulation (3B, right). Regarding cutaneous thermosensitivity, prior to the chemical stimulation of the dura the threshold of this neuron to slowly heating (35–45°C) or cooling (35°–0°C) its cutaneous receptive field was 42°C (3C, left) and 21°C (3D, left) respectively. However, 30 minutes after the chemical irritation of the dura, the heat threshold dropped to 39°C (3C, right) and the cold threshold changed from 21° to 33°C (3D, right). The response magnitude to heat and cold also increased 3-fold.

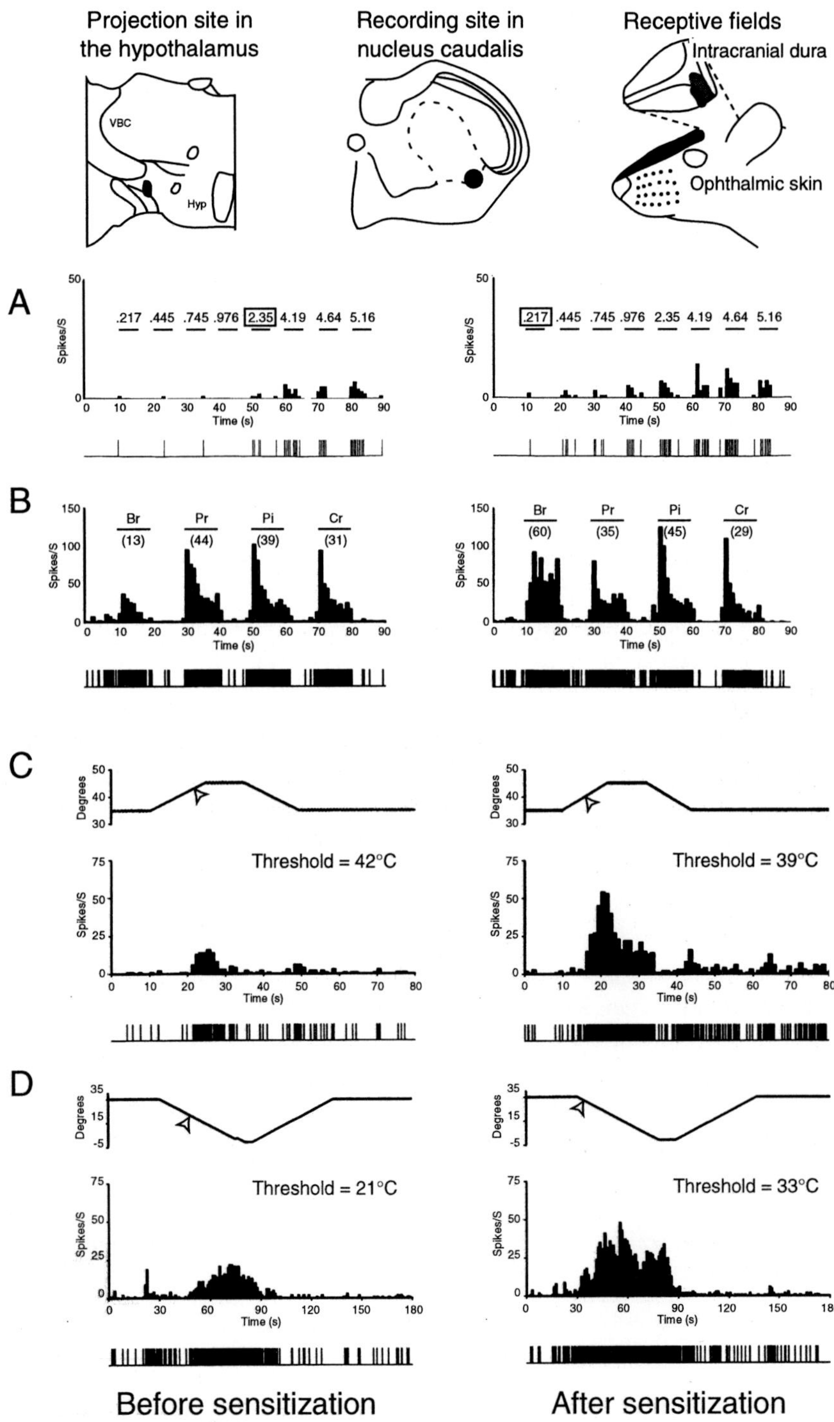

Projection site in the hypothalamus
Recording site in nucleus caudalis
Receptive fields
Intracranial dura
Ophthalmic skin
VBC
Hyp
A
.217 .445 .745 .976 2.35 4.19 4.64 5.16
Spikes/S
Time (s)
B
Br Pr Pi Cr
(13) (44) (39) (31)
(60) (35) (45) (29)
C
Degrees
Threshold = 42°C
Threshold = 39°C
D
Threshold = 21°C
Threshold = 33°C
Before sensitization
After sensitization

Following chemical stimulation of the dura, 95% of the neurons showed significant increases in sensitivity to mechanical indentation: their thresholds to dural indentation decreased from 1.57 to 0.49 g (means, $P < 0.0001$), and their response magnitudes to identical stimuli increased by 2–4-fold. Eighty percent of the neurons showed significant increases in cutaneous mechanosensitivity: their responses to brush and pressure increased 2.5-fold ($P < 0.05$) and 1.6-fold ($P < 0.05$), respectively. Seventy-five percent of the neurons showed a significant increase in cutaneous thermosensitivity: their thresholds to slow heating of the skin changed from 43.7° ± 0.7° to 40.3° ± 0.7°C (mean ± SD, $P < 0.005$), and to slow cooling from 23.7° ± 3.3° to 29.2° ± 1.8°C ($P < 0.05$). Dural receptive fields expanded within 30 minutes and cutaneous receptive fields within 2–4 hours, and ongoing activity developed in WDR and HT, but not in LT neurons.

Physiologically, these results demonstrate that brief chemical stimulation of the dura sensitizes central trigeminal neurons in addition to peripheral nociceptors. The clinical implication of *central sensitization* of neurons that receive convergent input from the dura and skin is the development of *intra- and extracranial hypersensitivity* during migraine. Sensitization of second-order nociceptive neurons in the medullary dorsal horn that receive convergent viscero-somatic input from both intra- and extracranial structures might explain how painful signals that arise from meningeal nociceptors during a migraine attack can induce changes in facial skin sensitivity: their sensitization by meningeal primary afferent nociceptors can change the way they process sensory signals arriving from the periorbital skin. Such changes in extracranial sensation during migraine have been described by Edward

---

← **Fig. 3.** The development of intracranial and extracranial hypersensitivity following chemical irritation of the dura. Comparisons of physiological responses of a dura-sensitive neuron in lamina V of the medullary dorsal horn that projects to the hypothalamus (top row). The responses of the neuron to a graded increase in the intensity of mechanical indentation of the dura (A), mechanical stimulation of the skin (B), and slowly heating (C) and cooling (D) the skin are shown before (left column) and after (right column) the irritation of the dura with the low pH buffer. Black area in the hypothalamus depicts low-threshold point for antidromic activation, black dot in the brainstem depicts recording site, black areas on the skin and dura depict sizes and locations of receptive fields prior to the chemical irritation of the dura, and gray area on the dura depicts the expanded receptive field following the chemical irritation. Numbers above lines in A indicate force of von Frey hairs (in grams), boxes in A depict the mechanical threshold, and numbers under lines in B indicate mean number of spikes per second in response to each stimulus. Arrowheads in C and D show the temperature at which a response occurred. Note the drop in the mechanical threshold of the dural receptive field, the exaggerated response to brushing the skin, and the drop in the thresholds for heating and cooling the skin. HYP = hypothalamus, Br = brush, Cr = crush, Pr = pressure, Pi = pinch, VBC = ventrobasal complex. Adapted with permission from Burstein et al. (1998).

Liveing in 1873, by clinical studies on scalp tenderness (Tfelt-Hansen et al. 1981; Lous and Olesen 1982; Drummond 1987; Jensen et al. 1988; Gobel et al. 1992; Jensen 1993; Jensen et al. 1993), and most recently by our paper on mechanical and thermal cutaneous allodynia (Burstein et al. 2000).

ENHANCED CARDIOVASCULAR RESPONSES REFLECT THE DEVELOPMENT OF CUTANEOUS ALLODYNIA

Burstein and colleagues (Yamamura et al. 1999) also sought to determine whether nonpainful stimuli such as mild dural indentation or skin brush are perceived as painful when trigeminal brainstem dura-sensitive neurons become sensitized To address this issue, they correlated sensory stimuli with cardiovascular responses (measured continuously through an intra-arterial line) and neuronal responses (measured continuously by recording from single dura-sensitive neurons) they induce. The rationale for measuring cardiovascular changes such as the pressor response was based on the notion that noxious visceral and cutaneous stimuli that cause tissue damage and pain produce pressor responses (Woodworth and Sherrington 1904). Pressor responses are a commonly used indicator of nociceptive stimulation because they can be induced by electrical stimulation of group IV muscle, cutaneous, or tooth dentin afferents (Johansson 1962; Sato and Schmidt 1973; Allen et al. 1996; Allen and Pronych 1997), noxious colorectal or

---

Fig. 4. Increased sensitivity to mechanical stimulation of the dura, and to mechanical and thermal stimulation of the facial skin following chemical stimulation of the dura. (A) Example of the changes in the minimum force required to induce blood pressure and neuronal responses before and after the chemical stimulation of the dura. Note that before chemical stimulation of the dura, neuronal and blood pressure responses were induced only by indenting the dura with a force >4 g and that 20 minutes after chemical stimulation, similar neuronal and blood pressure responses were induced by smaller (<1 g) forces as well. (B) Example of simultaneous recording of neuronal and blood pressure responses to mechanical skin stimulation showing that prior to chemical stimulation of the dura only pinch and pressure induced neuronal and blood pressure responses and that 60 minutes after the chemical stimulation similar responses were induced by brushing the skin. (C) Example of simultaneous recording of neuronal and blood pressure responses to thermal skin stimulation showing that prior to chemical stimulation of the dura neuronal and blood pressure responses were induced at 51° and 54ºC, and that afterwards they were induced by 46° and 48°C, respectively. In (A), lines above histograms indicate stimulus duration and numbers above these lines depict the force used to indent the dura. Boxes depict the mechanical threshold for eliciting the neuronal response. Numbers in parentheses indicate the magnitude of blood pressure change. In (B), lines above histograms indicate stimulus duration and numbers below these lines depict mean spikes/second. In (C), dotted lines illustrate the initiation times (vertical) and the thresholds (horizontal) of the responses. Adapted with permission from Yamamura et al. (1999). ⟶

ureter distension (Cervero 1982; Ness and Gebhart 1988; Roza and Laird 1995), and noxious chemical irritation of the cornea or nasal mucosa (Bereiter et al. 1994; Panneton and Yavari 1995).

In 24 experiments, neuronal and cardiovascular responses to mechanical and chemical stimulation of the dura (Fig. 4A), and to mechanical (Fig. 4B) and thermal (Fig. 4C) stimulation of the skin, were recorded simultaneously before, during, and after the induction of central sensitization by

A. Increased sensitivity to mechanical stimulation of the dura

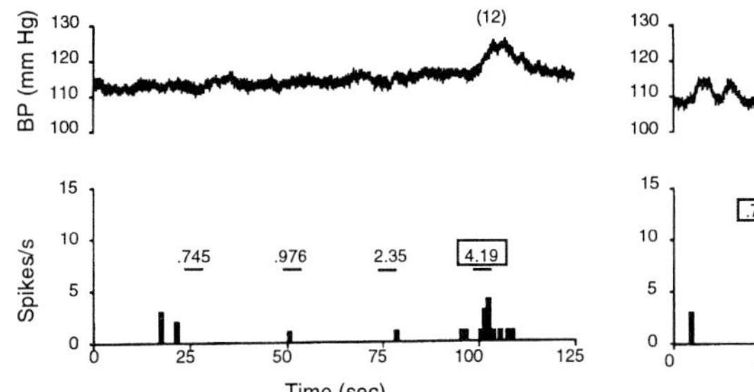

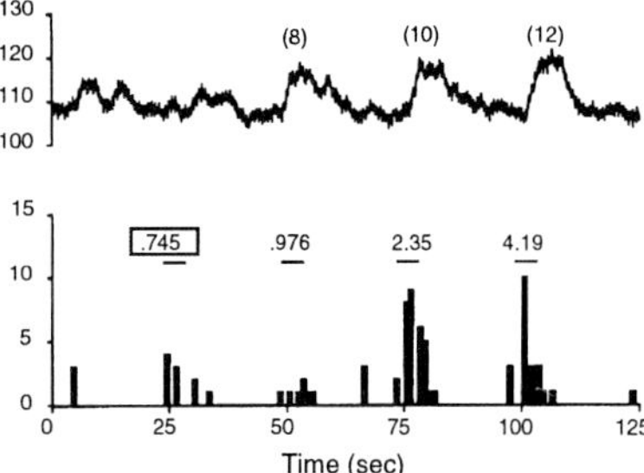

B. Increased sensitivity to mechanical stimulation of the skin

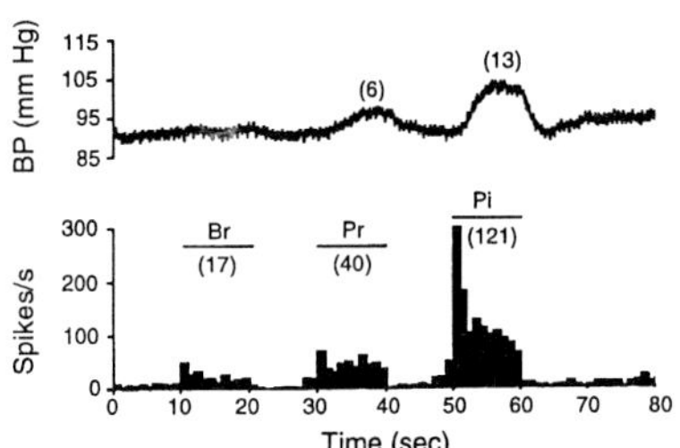

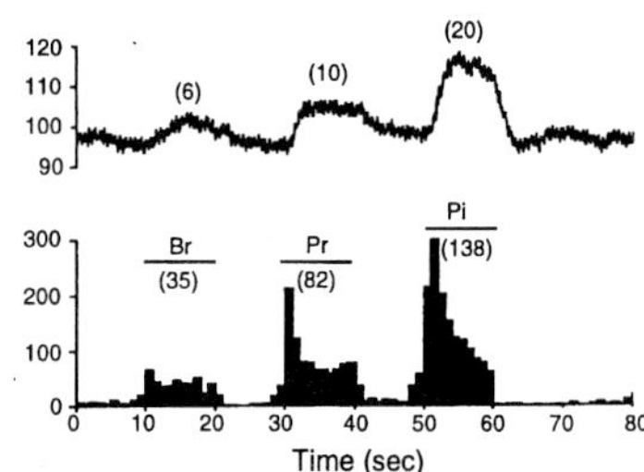

C. Increased sensitivity to thermal stimulation of the skin

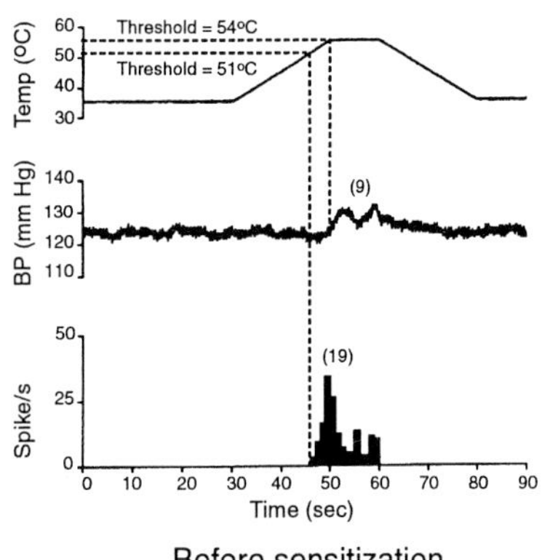

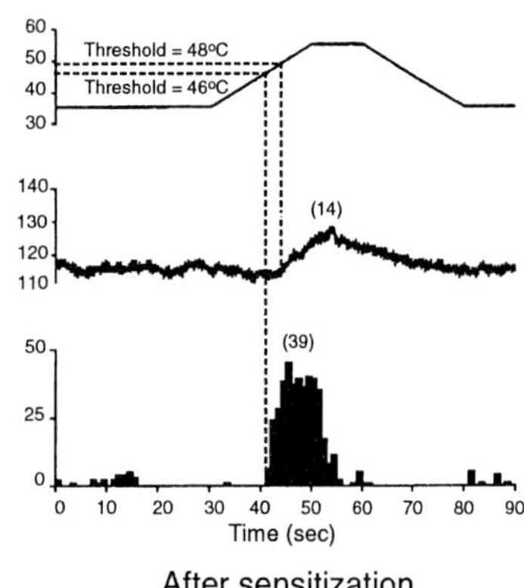

chemically stimulating the meningeal sensory fibers with the inflammatory agents described above. Prior to chemical stimulation, mechanical indentation of the dura with von Frey monofilaments induced neuronal and pressor responses when the applied forces were 2.35 g (median). The mechanical sensitivity of the dura increased significantly, however, following the chemical stimulation. About 20 minutes after the initial irritation of the dura, much smaller mechanical forces were required to induce neuronal (2.35 to 0.445 g) and pressor (2.35 to 0.976 g) responses (median ± SD, unpaired Wilcoxon signed-rank test, $P < 0.0001$). This hypersensitivity lasted nearly 7 hours. Fig. 4 illustrates a case in which thresholds for neuronal and blood pressure (BP) responses were altered by chemical stimulation. As shown in the figure, neuronal responses were short and rapidly adapting, usually outlasting the stimulus by 2–3 seconds, while pressor responses were large (8–14 mm Hg) and longer, usually outlasting the stimulus by 10–15 seconds.

Sixty minutes after chemical stimulation of the dura, a significant increase in the mechanical sensitivity of the skin manifested as increased neuronal and BP response magnitudes to brush and pressure ($P < 0.05$). Neuronal responses to brush and pressure increased 2-fold and 1.6-fold, respectively, while BP responses to brush and pressure increased 3-fold and 1.5-fold, respectively. Fig. 4B illustrates a case in which neuronal and BP responses to mechanical stimulation of the skin were altered by chemical stimulation of the dura. Neuronal responses to brush and pressure increased 2-fold, pressor responses to brush occurred only after chemical stimulation, and pressor responses to pressure and pinch increased 1.4-fold.

Prior to chemical stimulation, slow increases in skin temperature (1°C/second) induced neuronal responses at 44.8° ± 0.7°C (mean ± SE) and BP responses about 2 seconds later, at 46.5° ± 0.7°C. The magnitude of these responses was 30.0 ± 6.4 spikes/second for neuronal activation and 12.1 ± 1.4 mm Hg for BP changes. Sixty minutes following chemical stimulation of the dura, increased skin sensitivity to heat was apparent as the lowest temperature capable of initiating neuronal and BP responses dropped by 3.7° and 3.4°C (means, $P < 0.0005$), respectively. Fig. 4C illustrates a case in which neuronal and pressor response thresholds to slow heat of the cutaneous receptive field of a dura-sensitive WDR neuron in lamina V dropped by 5–6°C following chemical stimulation of the dura.

Physiologically, this study shows that when trigeminal brainstem dura-sensitive neurons become more sensitive to mechanical stimulation of the dura and to mechanical and thermal stimulation of the skin, this neuronal hypersensitivity is accompanied by parallel changes in cardiovascular responses associated with pain. The findings that in the same animal, pressor responses are induced by noxious stimuli prior to the neuronal sensitization and by both innocuous and noxious stimuli after the sensitization suggest that when neuronal hypersensitivity develops, innocuous stimuli such as skin brush and mild warming or dural indentation with small forces could be as painful as skin pinching and high heat or dural indentation with maximal forces in the absence of neuronal sensitization. In the context of migraine, we propose that changes in neuronal and cardiovascular responses to mild dural indentation, skin brushing, or low temperatures reflect the development of visceral and cutaneous allodynia and represent a shift in the perception of these stimuli from nonpainful to painful. Because innocuous stimuli such as brush are usually perceived as nonpainful when applied to control patients, but often as painful (i.e., mechanical tactile allodynia) when applied to chronic pain patients suffering from inflammatory or neuropathic pain (Bennett 1994; Dubner and Basbaum 1994), it is possible that inflammatory or neuropathic mechanisms contribute to the pathophysiology of migraine as well.

Regarding therapy, this model concurs with current practice that sensitization of meningeal nociceptors could be addressed with receptor agonists and antagonists that reduce peripheral activation of these pain fibers. The presence of central sensitization, however, calls for two additional therapeutic measures: (1) early prevention by using peripherally acting drugs (such as NSAIDs and triptans) that can block the incoming impulses from the periphery, and (2) blockade or reversal of central sensitization by drugs such as NMDA antagonists and calcium channel blockers. We do not yet have evidence that triptans can block central sensitization.

ACKNOWLEDGMENTS

Supported by NIH grants DE-10904 (National Institutes of Dental and Craniofacial Research) and NS-35611-01 (National Institutes of Neurological Disorder and Stroke).

REFERENCES

Allen GV, Pronych SP. Trigeminal autonomic pathways involved in nociception-induced reflex cardiovascular responses. *Brain Res* 1997; 754:269–278.

Allen GV, Barbrick B, Esser MJ. Trigeminal-parabrachial connections: possible pathway for nociception-induced cardiovascular reflex responses. *Brain Res* 1996; 715:125–135.

Anthony M, Rasmussen BK. Migraine without aura. In: Olesen J, Tfelt-Hansen P, Welch MA (Eds). *The Headaches*. Raven Press, 1993.

Armstrong D, Jepson JB, Keele CA, et al. Pain-producing substances in human inflammatory exudates and plasma. *J Physiol (Lond)* 1957; 135:350–370.

Beck PW, Handwerker HO, Zimmermann M. Nervous outflow from the cat's foot during noxious radiant heat stimulation. *Brain Res* 1974; 67(3):373–386.

Bennett GJ. Neuropathic pain. In: Wall PD, Melzack R (Eds). *Textbook of Pain*. Edinburgh: Churchill-Livingstone, 1994.

Bereiter DA, Hathaway CB, Benetti AP. Caudal portions of the spinal trigeminal complex are necessary for autonomic responses and display Fos-like immunoreactivity after corneal stimulation in the cat. *Brain Res.* 1994; 657:73–82.

Blau JN, Dexter SL. The site of pain origin during migraine attacks *Cephalalgia* 1981; 1(3):143–147.

Burstein R, Yamamura H, Malick A, et al. Chemical stimulation of the intracranial dura induces enhanced responses to facial stimulation in brain stem trigeminal neurons. *J Neurophysiol* 1998; 79(2):964–982.

Burstein R, Yarnitsky D, Goor-Aryeh I, et al. An association between migraine and cutaneous allodynia. *Ann Neurol* 2000; in press.

Cervero F. Afferent activity evoked by natural stimulation of the biliary system in the ferret. *Pain* 1982; 13:137–151.

Cervero F, Jänig W. Visceral nociceptors: a new world order? *Trends Neurosci* 1992; 15(10):374–378.

Cook AJ, Woolf CJ, Wall PD. Prolonged C-fibre mediated facilitation of the flexion reflex in the rat is not due to changes in afferent terminal or motoneurone excitability. *Neurosci Lett* 1986; 70(1):91–116.

Davis KD, Dostrovsky JO. Responses of feline trigeminal spinal tract nucleus neurons to stimulation of the middle meningeal artery and sagittal sinus. *J Neurophysiol* 1988; 59(2):648–666.

Davis KD, Meyer RA, Campbell JN. Chemosensitivity and sensitization of nociceptive afferents that innervate the hairy skin of monkey. *J Neurophysiol* 1993; 69(4):1071–1081.

Drummond PD. Scalp tenderness and sensitivity to pain in migraine and tension headache. *Headache* 1987; 27(1):45–50.

Dubner R, Basbaum A. I. Spinal dorsal horn plasticity following tissue or nerve injury. In: Wall PD, Melzack R (Eds). *Textbook of Pain*. Edinburgh: Churchill-Livingstone, 1994.

Fock S, Mense S. Excitatory effects of 5-hydroxytryptamine, histamine and potassium ions on muscular group IV afferent units: a comparison with bradykinin. *Brain Res* 1976; 105(3):459–469.

Goadsby PJ, Edvinsson L. The trigeminovascular system and migraine: studies characterizing cerebrovascular and neuropeptide changes seen in humans and cats. *Ann Neurol* 1993; 33(1):48–56.

Gobel H, Weigle L, Kropp P, et al. Pain sensitivity and pain reactivity of pericranial muscles in migraine and tension-type headache. *Cephalalgia* 1992; 12(3):142–151.

Guzman F, Braun C, Lim RKS. Visceral pain and the pseudoaffective response to intra-arterial injection of bradykinin and other algesic agents. *Arch Int Pharmacodyn Ther* 1962; 136:353–384.

Handwerker HO, Reeh PW. Chemosensitivity and sensitization by chemical agents. In: Willis WD (Ed). *Hyperalgesia and Allodynia*. New York: Raven Press, 1992.

Hanesch U, Heppelmann B, Messlinger K, et al. Nociception in normal and arthritic joints: structural and functional aspects. In: Willis WD (Ed). *Hyperalgesia and Allodynia*. New York: Raven Press, 1992.

Hollander W, Michaelson AL, Wilkins RW. Serotonin and antiserotonins. I. Their circulatory respiratory and renal effects in man. *Circulation* 1957; 16:246–255.

Jensen K. Extracranial blood flow, pain and tenderness in migraine. Clinical and experimental studies. *Acta Neurol Scand Suppl* 1993; 147:1–27.

Jensen K, Tuxen C, Olesen J. Pericranial muscle tenderness and pressure-pain threshold in the temporal region during common migraine. *Pain* 1988; 35(1):655–670.

Jensen R, Rasmussen BK, Pedersen B, et al. Muscle tenderness and pressure pain thresholds in headache. A population study. *Pain* 1993; 52(2):193–199.

Johansson B. Circulatory responses to stimulation of somatic afferents. *Acta Physiol Scand Suppl* 1962; 198:1–91.

Kessler W, Kirchhoff C, Reeh PW, et al. Excitation of cutaneous afferent nerve endings in vitro by a combination of inflammatory mediators and conditioning effect of substance P. *Exp Brain Res* 1992; 91(3):467–476.

Khan AA, Raja SN, Manning DC, et al. The effects of bradykinin and sequence-related analogs on the response properties of cutaneous nociceptors in monkeys. *Somatosens Mot Res* 1992; 9(2):97–106.

Koltzenburg M, Häbler HJ, Jänig W. Functional reinnervation of the vasculature of the adult cat paw pad by axons originally innervating vessels in hairy skin. *Neuroscience* 1995; 67(1):245–252.

Lang E, Novak A, Reeh PW, et al. Chemosensitivity of fine afferents from rat skin in vitro. *J Neurophysiol* 1990; 63(4):887–901.

Lauritzen M. Pathophysiology of the migraine aura. The spreading depression theory. *Brain* 1994; 117(Pt 1):199–210.

Liveing E. *On Megrim, Sick Headache*. Nijmegen: Arts & Boeve Publishers, 1873.

Lous I, Olesen J. Evaluation of pericranial tenderness and oral function in patients with common migraine, muscle contraction headache and "combination headache." *Pain* 1982; 12(4):385–393.

Magerl W, Wilk SH, Treede RD. Secondary hyperalgesia and perceptual wind-up following intradermal injection of capsaicin in humans. *Pain* 1998; 74(2–3):257–268.

McMahon SB, Lewin GR, Wall PD. Central hyperexcitability triggered by noxious inputs. *Curr Opin Neurobiol* 1993; 3(4):602–610.

Michaelis M, Häbler HJ, Jänig W. Silent afferents: a separate class of primary afferents? *Clin Exp Pharmacol Physiol* 1996; 23(2):99–105.

Mizumura K, Sato J, Kumazawa T. Effects of prostaglandins and other putative chemical intermediaries on the activity of canine testicular polymodal receptors studied in vitro. *Pflugers Arch* 1987; 408(6):565–572.

Moskowitz MA, Henrikson BM, Markowitz S, et al. Intra- and extracraniovascular nociceptive mechanisms and the pathogenesis of head pain. In: Olesen J, Edvinsson L (Eds). *Basic Mechanisms of Headache*. Elsevier, 1988.

Moskowitz MA, Macfarlane R. Neurovascular and molecular mechanisms in migraine headaches. *Cerebrovasc Brain Metab Rev* 1993; 5(3):159–177.

Ness TJ, Gebhart GF. Colorectal distension as a noxious visceral stimulus: physiologic and pharmacologic characterization of pseudoaffective reflexes in the rat. *Brain Res* 1988; 450:153–169.

Neugebauer V, Schaible HG, Schmidt RF. Sensitization of articular afferents to mechanical stimuli by bradykinin. *Pflugers Arch* 1989; 415(3):330–335.

Panneton WM, Yavari P. A medullary dorsal horn relay for the cardiorespiratory responses evoked by stimulation of the nasal mucosa in the muskrat *Ondatra zibethicus:* evidence for excitatory acid transmission. *Brain Res* 1995; 691:37–45.

Ren K, Dubner R. NMDA receptor antagonists attenuate mechanical hyperalgesia in rats with unilateral inflammation of the hindpaw. *Neurosci Lett* 1993; 163(1):22–26.

Roza C, Laird JMA. Pressor responses to distension of the ureter in anaesthetised rats: characterization of a model of acute visceral pain. *Neurosci Lett* 1995; 198:9–12.

Sato A, Schmidt RF. Somatosympathetic reflexes: afferent fibers, central pathways, discharge characteristics. *Physiol Rev* 1973; 53:916–947.

Schmidt R, Schmelz M, Forster C, et al. Novel classes of responsive and unresponsive C nociceptors in human skin. *J Neurosci* 1995; 15(1 Pt 1):333–341.

Sicuteri F. Vasoneuractive substances and their implication in vascular pain. *Res Clin Stud Headache* 1967; 1:6–45.

Simone DA, Sorkin LS, Oh U, et al. Neurogenic hyperalgesia: central neural correlates in responses of spinothalamic tract neurons. *J Neurophysiol* 1991; 66(1):228–246.

Steen KH, Reeh PW, Anton F, et al. Protons selectively induce lasting excitation and sensitization to mechanical stimulation of nociceptors in rat skin, in vitro. *J Neurosci* 1992; 12(1):86–95.

Steen KH, Steen AE, Reeh PW. A dominant role of acid pH in inflammatory excitation and sensitization of nociceptors in rat skin, in vitro. *J Neurosci* 1995; 15(5 Pt 2):3982–3989.

Strassman AM, Raymond SA, Burstein R. Sensitization of meningeal sensory neurons and the origin of headaches. *Nature* 1996; 384(6609):560–564.

Tfelt-Hansen P, Lous I, Olesen J. Prevalence and significance of muscle tenderness during common migraine attacks. *Headache* 1981; 21:49–54.

Torebjörk HE, Lundberg LE, LaMotte RH. Central changes in processing of mechanoreceptive input in capsaicin- induced secondary hyperalgesia in humans. *J Physiol (Lond)* 1992; 448:765–780.

Woodworth RS, Sherrington CS. A pseudaffective reflex and its spinal path. *J Physiol (Lond)* 1904; 31:234–243.

Woolf CJ. Evidence for a central component of post-injury pain hypersensitivity. *Nature* 1983; 306(5944):686–688.

Woolf CJ, Doubell TP. The pathophysiology of chronic pain—increased sensitivity to low threshold A beta-fibre inputs. *Curr Opin Neurobiol* 1994; 4(4):525–534.

Woolf CJ, Shortland P, Reynolds M, et al. Reorganization of central terminals of myelinated primary afferents in the rat dorsal horn following peripheral axotomy. *J Comp Neurol* 1995; 360(1):121–134.

Yamamura H, Malick A, Chamberlin NL, et al. Cardiovascular and neuronal responses to head stimulation reflect central sensitization and cutaneous allodynia in a rat model of migraine. *J Neurophysiol* 1999; 81(2):479–493.

Correspondence to: Rami Burstein, PhD, Harvard Institutes of Medicine, Room 830, 77 Avenue Louis Pasteur, Boston, MA 02115, USA. Tel: 617-667-0806, Fax: 617-975-5329, email: rburstei@bidmc.harvard.edu.

Proceedings of the 9th World Congress on Pain,
Progress in Pain Research and Management,
Vol. 16, edited by M. Devor, M.C. Rowbotham, and
Z. Wiesenfeld-Hallin, IASP Press, Seattle, © 2000.

56

A Systematic Review and League Table of Pharmacological Interventions for Acute Migraine Attack

Anna D. Oldman, Lesley A. Smith, Henry J. McQuay, and R. Andrew Moore

Pain Research, Nuffield Department of Anaesthetics, University of Oxford, The Churchill, Oxford Radcliffe Hospital, Headington, Oxford, United Kingdom

Migraine affects 17.6% of women and 6% of men, according to U.S. figures based on International Headache Society (IHS) criteria (Lipton 1993). Sixty-two percent of these individuals rely solely on over-the-counter medications when treating a migraine attack.

Various prescription and over-the-counter interventions are available for the acute treatment of migraine attacks. There is, however, little consensus on how clinically effective these interventions are, or which are the most or least effective. Decisions about what to prescribe or use to treat a migraine attack are therefore likely to be governed by other factors such as habitual prescribing patterns, limited patient knowledge, or cost. The aim of this study was to construct an evidence-based league table of the efficacy of interventions available for the acute treatment of migraine attacks.

METHODS

LITERATURE SEARCH

We searched the world literature for randomized, double-blind, placebo-controlled trials of interventions for treating acute migraine attacks. Different search strategies were used to identify eligible reports from MEDLINE (1966–September 1999), EMBASE (1980–April 1999), Biological Abstracts (1993–March 1999), the Cochrane Library (Issue 3, 1999), and the Oxford

Pain Relief Database (1950–1994) (Jadad et al. 1996a). Free text searches were undertaken with no restrictions as to language.

Inclusion criteria were: randomized allocation to treatment groups including a placebo group, double-blind design, use of IHS diagnostic criteria for migraine with or without aura (Headache Classification Committee of the IHS 1988), adult population, baseline pain of moderate or severe intensity using a 4-point standardized rating scale (0 = no pain, 1 = mild pain, 2 = moderate pain, and 3 = severe pain), dosing regimes at standard or prescribing doses, full journal publication (no abstracts or posters), extractable data for at least one efficacy measure under investigation (proportion of patients with a headache response or pain-free headache response at 2 hours).

Headache response at 2 hours was defined as the proportion of patients with headache pain reduced from moderate or severe pain to mild or no pain at 2 hours. Pain-free headache response at 2 hours was defined as the proportion of patients reporting no pain at 2 hours.

Headache response and pain-free data were extracted from all trials that met the inclusion criteria, together with study details such as dosing regimes and rescue analgesia. Trials were assigned a quality score based on a commonly used quality rating scale (Jadad et al. 1996b). For trials that followed patients for more than one attack (either parallel or crossover), data were extracted for first attack only. Trials that did not allow for this were excluded.

DATA ANALYSIS

In the primary analysis, extracted data from each report were used to calculate relative benefit and number-needed-to-treat (NNT) for headache response rate at 2 hours with 95% confidence interval (CI). Secondary analysis was NNT for pain-free headache response at 2 hours. NNTs were calculated according to Cook and Sackett (1995). A statistically significant difference from placebo was assumed when the 95% CI of the relative benefit did not include one. NNTs were not calculated when the relative benefit did not reach significance. Calculations were performed using Microsoft Excel 5.0.

RESULTS

A total of 44 trials in 39 reports were included in the meta-analyses, with a total of 57 placebo comparisons. Data were available for seven oral medications and subcutaneous and intranasal sumatriptan in a total of 14,394 patients. Of these interventions, only one was for an over-the-counter preparation. Quality scores of trials ranged from 2 to 5 (median 4).

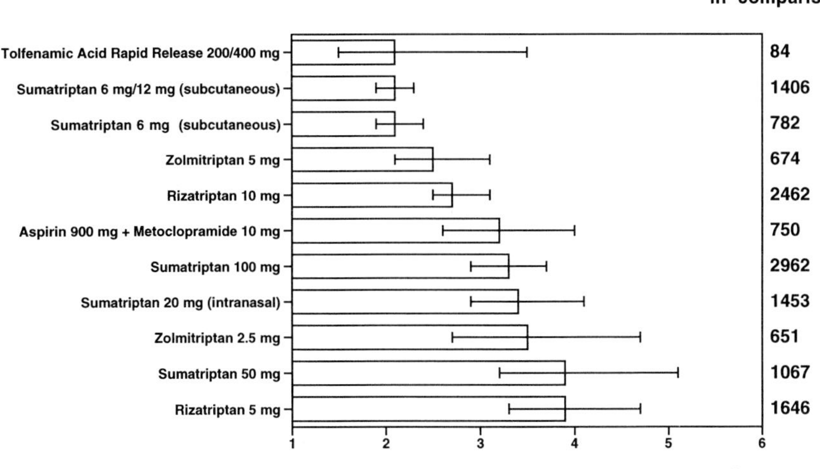

Fig. 1. League table of numbers-needed-to-treat (NNTs) for successful treatment of an acute migraine attack at 2 hours (moderate or severe pain reduced to mild or no pain). All doses oral unless otherwise stated.

HEADACHE RESPONSE AT 2 HOURS

NNTs ranged from 2.1 (1.9–2.3) to 3.9 (3.2–5.1) for headache response at 2 hours (Fig. 1; Table I). The most effective interventions were subcutaneous sumatriptan 6 mg (NNT = 2.1 [1.9–2.4]) and subcutaneous sumatriptan 6 mg with a further 6 mg given at 1 hour to patients still in pain (NNT = 2.1 [1.9–2.3]). Tolfenamic acid 200 mg (with a further 200 mg given at 1 hour to patients still in pain) had a low (good) NNT, although insufficient patients were studied for a reliable estimate (i.e., <250 patients in the comparison). Relative benefits and NNTs are listed in Table I. Cafergot (ergotamine tartrate 2 mg + caffeine 200 mg; Alliance) and naratriptan 2.5 mg were not significantly better than placebo at 2 hours on this measure.

PAIN-FREE HEADACHE RESPONSE AT 2 HOURS

NNT ranged from 2.5 (2.1–3.1) to 9.5 (6.4–1.9) for pain-free headache response at 2 hours (Table II). The subcutaneous sumatriptan interventions were the most effective interventions. Cafergot was not significantly better than placebo, and no data were available for naratriptan 2.5 mg on this measure. Insufficient patient information was available for a reliable estimate of an NNT for tolfenamic acid.

Table I

Summary of relative benefit and number-needed-to-treat (NNT; with 95% confidence intervals) for headache response at 2 hours for acute migraine interventions

Intervention	Number of Comparisons	Improved on Active	Improved on Placebo	Relative Benefit (95% CI)	NNT (95% CI)
Tolfenamic acid rapid release 200 mg/400 mg*	1	33/43	12/41	2.6 (1.6–4.3)	2.1 (1.5–3.5)
Sumatriptan 6 mg/12 mg (subcutaneous)†	3	734/923	154/483	2.5 (2.2–2.8)	2.1 (1.9–2.3)
Sumatriptan 6 mg (subcutaneous)	7	275/363	118/419	2.7 (2.3–3.2)	2.1 (1.9–2.4)
Zolmitriptan 5 mg	3	295/445	61/229	2.5 (2.0–3.1)	2.5 (2.1–3.1)
Rizatriptan 10 mg	6	1081/1582	279/880	2.1 (1.9–2.3)	2.7 (2.5–3.1)
Aspirin 900 mg + metoclopramide 10 mg	3	214/373	95/374	2.2 (1.8–2.7)	3.2 (2.6–4.0)
Sumatriptan 100 mg	12	1042/1807	312/1155	2.1 (1.9–2.3)	3.3 (2.9–3.7)
Sumatriptan 20 mg (intranasal)	6	571/907	183/546	1.9 (1.7–2.2)	3.4 (2.9–4.1)
Zolmitriptan 2.5 mg	2	279/438	74/213	1.8 (1.5–2.2)	3.5 (2.7–4.7)
Excedrin‡ (Bristol-Myers; paracetamol 500 mg + aspirin 500 mg + caffeine 130 mg)	3	358/602	204/618	1.8 (1.6–2.1)	3.8 (3.1–4.8)
Rizatriptan 5 mg	4	548/933	234/713	1.8 (1.6–2.0)	3.9 (3.3–4.7)
Sumatriptan 50 mg	5	392/711	105/356	1.8 (1.5–2.1)	3.9 (3.2–5.1)
Cafergot (ergotamine tartrate 2 mg + caffeine 200 mg)	1	58/169	19/85	1.5 (0.98–2.4)	not calculated
Naratriptan 2.5 mg	1	51/127	37/122	1.3 (0.94–1.9)	not calculated

* A further 200 mg was given at 60 minutes "if headache not improved" (28% of patients required only 200 mg).
† A further 6 mg was given at 60 minutes if patient has any pain (or, for one trial, patient has moderate or severe pain).
‡ These trials excluded migraineurs with severely debilitating attacks usually requiring bed rest, or who vomited more than 20% of the time.

Table II

Summary of relative benefit and number-needed-to-treat (NNT; with 95% confidence intervals) for pain-free headache response at 2 hours for acute migraine interventions

Intervention	Number of Comparisons	Improved on Active	Improved on Placebo	Relative Benefit (95% CI)	NNT (95% CI)
Sumatriptan 6 mg (subcutaneous)	5	119/231	35/296	4.1 (2.9–5.7)	2.5 (2.1–3.1)
Sumatriptan 6 mg/12 mg (subcutaneous)†	2	98/189	14/113	4.2 (2.5–7.2)	2.5 (2.1–3.3)
Rizatriptan 10 mg	6	630/1582	74/880	4.7 (3.7–5.9)	3.2 (2.9–3.5)
Zolmitriptan 5 mg	3	154/445	10/229	7.9 (4.2–15)	3.3 (2.8–4.0)
Tolfenamic acid rapid release 200 mg/400 mg*	1	16/43	3/41	5.1 (1.6–16)	3.4 (2.2–7.5)
Sumatriptan 20 mg (intranasal)	3	182/536	33/276	2.9 (2.0–4.0)	4.6 (3.6–6.1)
Rizatriptan 5 mg	4	284/933	65/713	3.4 (2.6–4.4)	4.7 (4.0–5.7)
Sumatriptan 100 mg	7	265/957	46/688	3.9 (2.9–5.3)	4.8 (4.1–5.7)
Zolmitriptan 2.5 mg	2	109/438	17/213	3.1 (1.9–5.1)	5.9 (4.5–8.7)
Excedrin‡ (paracetamol 500 mg + aspirin 500 mg + caffeine 130 mg)	3	128/602	43/618	3.1 (2.2–4.3)	7.0 (5.5–9.6)
Aspirin 900 mg + metoclopramide 10 mg	3	69/378	25/375	2.7 (1.8–4.2)	8.6 (6.2–14)
Sumatriptan 50 mg	3	68/380	16/218	2.4 (1.4–4.1)	9.5 (6.4 –19)
Cafergot (ergotamine tartrate 2 mg + caffeine 200 mg)	1	19/169	4/85	2.4 (0.84–6.8)	not calculated
Naratriptan 2.5 mg	none	–	–	–	–

* A further 200 mg was given at 60 minutes “if headache not improved” (28% of patients required only 200 mg).

† A further 6 mg was given at 60 minutes if patient has any pain (or, for one trial, if patient has moderate or severe pain).

‡ These trials excluded migraineurs with severely debilitating attacks usually requiring bed rest, or who vomited more than 20% of the time.

Based on the NNT 95% CIs not overlapping, there was a significant difference between a number of interventions. For example, subcutaneous sumatriptan doses, zolmitriptan 5 mg, and rizatriptan 10 mg were all significantly more effective than sumatriptan 50 mg and rizatriptan 5 mg.

CONCLUSIONS

Of the interventions included in the meta-analysis, all but Cafergot and naratriptan were significantly superior to placebo for headache response at 2 hours. Similarly, all but Cafergot and naratriptan were significantly superior to placebo for pain-free headache response at 2 hours. Some interventions offered superior efficacy; for example, subcutaneous sumatriptan and higher doses of zolmitriptan and rizatriptan. No trials of older migraine interventions met inclusion criteria for this review. Very limited data were available for over-the-counter migraine preparations, and no information was available for simple analgesics.

ACKNOWLEDGMENT

A. Oldman is supported by a grant from the BUPA Foundation.

REFERENCES

Cook RJ, Sackett DL. The number needed to treat: a clinically useful measure of treatment effect. *BMJ* 1995; 310:452–454.

Headache Classification Committee of the International Headache Society. Classification and diagnostic criteria for headache disorders, cranial neuralgias and facial pain. *Cephalalgia* 1988; 8(Suppl 7):19–28.

Jadad AR, Carroll D, Moore A, McQuay H. Developing a database of published reports of randomised clinical trials in pain research. *Pain* 1996a; 66:239–246.

Jadad AR, Moore RA, Carroll D, et al. Assessing the quality of reports of randomized clinical trials: is blinding necessary? *Control Clin Trials* 1996b; 17:1–12.

Lipton RB, Stewart WF. Migraine in the United States: a review of epidemiology and health care use. *Neurology* 1993; 43(Suppl 3):S6–S10.

Correspondence to: Anna D. Oldman, DPhil, Pain Research, Nuffield Department of Anaesthetics, University of Oxford, The Churchill, Oxford Radcliffe Hospital, Headington, Oxford OX3 7LJ, United Kingdom. Tel: 44-1865-225774; Fax: 44-1865-226978; email: anna.oldman@pru.ox.ac.uk.

Proceedings of the 9th World Congress on Pain,
Progress in Pain Research and Management,
Vol. 16, edited by M. Devor, M.C. Rowbotham, and
Z. Wiesenfeld-Hallin, IASP Press, Seattle, © 2000.

57

Peripheral Morphine Analgesia in Dental Surgery Patients

Michael Schäfer,[a] Rudolf Likar,[b] and Christoph Stein[a]

[a]Department of Anesthesiology and Intensive Care Medicine, Free University of Berlin, Berlin, Germany; [b]Department of Anesthesiology and Intensive Care Medicine, Klagenfurt, Austria

An increasing number of experimental studies show the efficacy of peripheral opioids in relieving somatic (Stein 1995) and visceral pain (Gebhart et al. 1999). This analgesic effect is elicited by peripheral mechanisms, because systemic administration of similar doses of opioids is not effective (Zhou et al. 1998) and the use of peripherally selective compounds prevents the penetration into the central nervous system (Sengupta et al. 1999). The peripheral opioid effect is dose-dependent and antagonized by naloxone; thus, it results from activation of peripheral opioid receptors (Stein et al. 1989). Correspondingly, opioid receptors have been identified on cutaneous nerve endings of sensory neurons (Stein et al. 1990; Coggeshall et al. 1997; Wenk and Honda 1999). These findings have been confirmed in recent clinical studies. One study revealed that analgesic effects of regional intravenous (i.v.) morphine (Bier's block) were exclusively due to peripheral mechanisms, demonstrated by high regional and undetectable systemic plasma levels of morphine and its metabolites (Koppert et al. 1999). Second, intra-articular administration of three different doses (1, 2, and 4 mg) of morphine or saline in patients undergoing arthroscopic knee surgery showed a dose-dependent increase in analgesic effects of morphine and a decrease in supplemental analgesic consumption (Likar et al. 1999). Third, analgesic effects of intra-articular morphine could be antagonized by co-administration of a small dose of naloxone (Stein et al. 1991). Thus, similar to the experimental studies, these findings from controlled clinical studies suggest that analgesic effects of opioids are specifically mediated by opioid receptors within peripheral tissue. Correspondingly, research has demonstrated opioid receptors on peripheral nerve endings of human synovial tissue (Stein et al. 1996).

MECHANISMS IN DENTAL PAIN

Experimental studies show that peripheral analgesic effects of opioids are present under inflammatory conditions (Zhou et al. 1998). While local administration of opioids into non-inflamed tissue does not elicit analgesia, their administration into inflamed tissue leads to enhanced analgesic efficacy early after the onset of inflammation and increases linearly with the duration of the inflammatory process (Zhou et al. 1998). Accordingly, most of the clinical studies have demonstrated peripheral analgesic effects of opioids following injury and inflammation (Stein et al. 1997). Furthermore, some of the negative results may be explained by the absence of such an inflammatory process (Bullingham et al. 1983, 1984).

In recent controlled clinical trials we have examined the relevance of the inflammatory process for the occurrence of peripheral opioid effects in humans (Likar et al. 1998; M. Schäfer et al., unpublished data). We used the clinical model of patients having dental surgery, because it comes close to our experimental animal model of unilateral rat hindpaw inflammation (Stein et al. 1988). Under normal conditions, myelinated A fibers (mostly Aδ fibers, but also Aβ fibers) are responsible for the sensitivity of dentin (rapid and sharp pain) in response to stimuli such as drilling and drying with air blasts (Figdor 1994). In contrast, under inflammatory conditions such as pulpitis, unmyelinated C fibers become activated and produce a dull pain that radiates to a wider area of the face and jaw (Figdor 1994). Accordingly, the hyperalgesia resulting from a rat hindpaw inflammation is predominantly mediated by capsaicin-sensitive primary afferent neurons (most likely C fibers) (Bartho et al. 1990; Schäfer et al. 1995). In peripheral tissue, opioid receptors have been mainly identified on nerve endings of unmyelinated C fibers (Coggeshall et al. 1997; Wenk and Honda 1999), but neither on myelinated nor sympathetic nerve fibers (Wenk and Honda 1999). Under inflammatory conditions, peripheral analgesic effects of opioids are enhanced (Antonijevic et al. 1995; Schäfer et al. 1995) and the number of opioid receptors is upregulated due to an accelerated axonal transport to the peripheral nerve endings (Hassan et al. 1993). Thus, it is conceivable that in inflammatory dental pain, locally applied opioids act on opioid receptors of unmyelinated C fibers to counteract the inflammatory tooth pain.

INFLAMMATORY VERSUS NORMAL CONDITIONS

In dental surgery patients we examined the analgesic efficacy of the local injection of 1 mg morphine (group A) versus saline (group B) in addition to the local anesthetic (1.7 mL articaine 4%) necessary for surgery. As a control, patients in the saline group received a subcutaneous injection of 1 mg morphine. The morphine and saline injections were submucosal, and followed a randomized, double-blind protocol. In the immediate postoperative period, we expected the local anesthetic to relieve pain in both groups. However, since previous clinical trials have shown a long-lasting analgesic effect of local morphine up to 24 hours (Stein 1995; Stein et al. 1997), a difference in pain intensity between the morphine and saline-treated patients should become apparent at a later time. In the first trial (trial #1), patients had a pre-existing severe inflammatory tooth pain before they were randomly assigned to either the local morphine or saline treatment (Likar et al. 1998). Patients in the second trial (trial #2) came to the hospital for elective dental surgery without overt signs of inflammation or pain (M. Schäfer et al., unpublished data). In both trials postoperative pain intensity was assessed by the visual analogue scale (VAS) and numerical rating scale (NRS) at 2, 4, 6, 8, 10, 12, 16, 20, and 24 hours postoperatively. In addition, patients recorded the occurrence of side effects and the supplemental consumption of diclofenac.

The results showed in both trials that the pain intensity was reduced in the morphine and saline-treated group up to 6–8 hours postoperatively ($P < 0.05$, repeated-measures analysis of variance [rmANOVA]), most likely due to the local anesthetic effect. In patients with severe inflammatory tooth pain (trial #1), pain intensity scores of the morphine-treated group decreased further up to 24 hours ($P < 0.05$, rmANOVA), whereas those of the saline group remained unchanged with mean VAS scores of about 30 mm. In contrast, pain intensity scores of patients who had elective dental surgery (trial #2) did not decrease significantly either in the morphine or saline group. Thus, only patients with inflammatory tooth pain had a significant benefit from 1 mg morphine added to the local anesthetic. This effect was peripherally mediated, because subcutaneous morphine was ineffective, and it lasted up to 24 hours. In addition, these patients required significantly less supplemental analgesics as rescue medication ($P < 0.05$, Student's t test). The results are in line with two previous studies demonstrating the analgesic efficacy of local fentanyl (Uhle et al. 1997) and morphine (Hargreaves et al. 1991) in patients with dental pain. However, they are at variance with one study that failed to show a significant pain reduction following third-molar surgery (Moore et al. 1994). While the former studies recruited patients with overt inflammatory signs (Hargreaves et al. 1991; Uhle et al. 1997), the latter examined patients for elective dental surgery (Moore et al. 1994).

In summary, 1 mg morphine added to the local anesthetic for dental surgery results in significant improvement of postoperative analgesia under inflammatory but not under normal conditions. Thus, similar to peripheral opioid effects in experimental studies, an inflammatory process appears to be crucial.

LOCAL VERSUS PERINEURAL ADMINISTRATION

We also compared the efficacy of additional morphine versus saline treatment in patients receiving a local articaine injection for dental surgery of the maxillary front teeth (trial #1, as presented above) with a perineural articaine injection for dental surgery of the rear mandibular teeth (trial #3). In both trials, patients presented with pre-existing severe inflammation and pain. As mentioned above, postoperative pain intensity was assessed by the VAS and NRS at 2, 4, 6, 8, 10, 12, 16, 20, and 24 hours postoperatively. In addition, patients recorded the occurrence of side effects and the supplemental consumption of diclofenac. Again, procedures were randomized and double-blind.

Similar to the above mentioned results, the pain intensity in both trials was reduced in the morphine and saline-treated group up to 6–8 hours postoperatively ($P < 0.05$, rmANOVA) due to the local anesthetic effect. While local morphine treatment provided better and more prolonged pain relief than did local saline (trial #1, see above), the perineural injection of morphine was not different from saline at any time postoperatively (trial #3) ($P > 0.05$, rmANOVA). After the local anesthetic effect had worn off, pain intensity scores remained unchanged in both groups of trial #3 ($P > 0.05$, rmANOVA). Thus, although an inflammatory process was present, the perineural injection of morphine, i.e., some distance away from the peripheral nerve endings, was ineffective. Previous reports about the perineural administration of opioids have produced conflicting results with regard to their analgesic efficacy (Picard et al. 1997). While most clinical trials failed to demonstrate significant analgesic effects following the perineural injection of an opioid alone or together with a local anesthetic (Picard et al. 1997), a few studies showed significant pain relief (Gobeaux et al. 1987; Mays et al. 1987; Boogaerts and Lafont 1991). Possible explanations for a lack of opioid analgesia are that opioid receptors are axonally transported to peripheral nerve endings (Hassan et al. 1993) and may not be functionally active during their axonal transit as compared to their final integration into the cell membrane at peripheral nerve terminals. In addition, the perineural barrier of peripheral nerves may hinder the access of opioids to the axonally transported receptors (Antonijevic et al. 1995). In contrast, this barrier is disrupted within inflamed tissue so that the access of opioids to their receptors on nerve terminals is facilitated (Antonijevic et al. 1995). Eventually, differences in the milieu of inflamed subcutaneous versus unaltered perineural tissue may lead to differences in the physical and chemical properties of administered opioid substances.

Thus, changes in the milieu of the inflamed periodontal tissue appear to be critical for the occurrence of peripheral opioid effects. The non-inflamed perineural environment along axons appears to preclude the access to and modulation of neurons by opioids.

SUMMARY

The underlying mechanisms in dental pain are similar to the well-characterized mechanisms in animal models of inflammatory pain. These mechanisms seem to involve predominantly unmyelinated C fibers that contain opioid receptors on their peripheral nerve terminals. Activation of these receptors by local administration of morphine produces clinically relevant analgesia. This effect is moderate when the opioid is given together with the local anesthetic, but is more pronounced when administered alone (Uhle et al. 1997). Similar to the experimental studies, an inflammatory process seems to be necessary for the occurrence of peripheral opioid analgesia. Administration of morphine into non-inflamed tissue or perineurally does not elicit significant analgesia. Given that most dental surgery is accompanied by an inflammatory reaction, supplemental morphine may help relieve postoperative dental pain.

REFERENCES

Antonijevic I, Mousa SA, Schäfer M, Stein C. Perineurial defect and peripheral opioid analgesia in inflammation. *J Neurosci* 1995; 15:165–172.

Bartho L, Stein C, Herz A. Involvement of capsaicin-sensitive neurones in hyperalgesia and enhanced opioid antinociception in inflammation. *Naunyn Schmiedebergs Arch Pharmacol* 1990; 342:666–670.

Boogaerts J, Lafont N. Mechanism of action and clinical use of opioids administered by the peripheral perineural route. *Cah Anesthesiol* 1991; 39:91–95.

Bullingham R, G OS, McQuay H, et al. Perineural injection of morphine fails to relieve postoperative pain in humans. *Anesth Analg* 1983; 62:164–167.

Bullingham RE, McQuay HJ, Moore RA. Studies on the peripheral action of opioids in postoperative pain in man. *Acta Anaesthesiol Belg* 1984; 35:(Suppl)285–290.

Coggeshall RE, Zhou S, Carlton SM. Opioid receptors on peripheral sensory axons. *Brain Res* 1997; 764:126–132.

Figdor D. Aspects of dentinal and pulpal pain. Pain of dentinal and pulpal origin—a review for the clinician. *Ann R Australas Coll Dent Surg* 1994; 12:131–142.

Gebhart GF, Sengupta JN, Su X. Opioids in visceral pain. In: Stein C (Ed). *Opioids in Pain Control.* Cambridge: Cambridge University Press, 1999, pp 325–334.

Gobeaux D, Landais A, Bexon G, Cazaban J, Levron JC. Addition of fentanyl to adrenalinized lidocaine for the brachial plexus block. *Cah Anesthesiol* 1987; 35:195–199.

Hargreaves K, Keating K, Cathers SJ, Dionne R. Analgesic effects of morphine after PDL injection in endodontic patients. *J Dent Res* 1991; 70:445.

Hassan AH, Ableitner A, Stein C, Herz A. Inflammation of the rat paw enhances axonal transport of opioid receptors in the sciatic nerve and increases their density in the inflamed tissue. *Neuroscience* 1993; 55:185–195.

Koppert W, Likar R, Geisslinger G, et al. Peripheral antihyperalgesic effect of morphine to heat, but not mechanical, stimulation in healthy volunteers after ultraviolet-B irradiation. *Anesth Analg* 1999; 88:117–122.

Likar R, Sittl R, Gragger K, et al. Peripheral morphine analgesia in dental surgery. *Pain* 1998; 76:145–150.

Likar R, Kapral S, Steinkellner H, et al. Dose-dependency of intra-articular morphine analgesia. *Br J Anaesth* 1999; 83:241–244.

Mays KS, Lipman JJ, Schnapp M. Local analgesia without anesthesia using peripheral perineural morphine injections. *Anesth Analg* 1987; 66:417–420.

Moore UJ, Seymour RA, Gilroy J, Rawlins MD. The efficacy of locally applied morphine in post-operative pain after bilateral third molar surgery. *Br J Clin Pharmacol* 1994; 37:227–230.

Picard PR, Tramer MR, McQuay HJ, Moore RA. Analgesic efficacy of peripheral opioids (all except intra-articular): a qualitative systematic review of randomised controlled trials. *Pain* 1997; 72:309–318.

Schäfer M, Imai Y, Uhl GR, Stein C. Inflammation enhances peripheral mu-opioid receptor-mediated analgesia, but not mu-opioid receptor transcription in dorsal root ganglia. *Eur J Pharmacol* 1995; 279:65–69.

Sengupta JN, Snider A, Su X, Gebhart GF. Effects of kappa opioids in the inflamed rat colon. *Pain* 1999; 79:175–185.

Stein C. The control of pain in peripheral tissue by opioids. *N Engl J Med* 1995; 332:1685–1690.

Stein C, Millan MJ, Herz A. Unilateral inflammation of the hindpaw in rats as a model of prolonged noxious stimulation: alterations in behavior and nociceptive thresholds. *Pharmacol Biochem Behav* 1988; 31:455–451.

Stein C, Millan MJ, Shippenberg TS, Peter K, Herz A. Peripheral opioid receptors mediating antinociception in inflammation. Evidence for involvement of mu, delta and kappa receptors. *J Pharmacol Exp Ther* 1989; 248:1269–1275.

Stein C, Hassan AH, Przewlocki R. Opioids from immunocytes interact with receptors on sensory nerves to inhibit nociception in inflammation. *Proc Natl Acad Sci USA* 1990; 87:5935–5939.

Stein C, Comisel K, Haimerl E, et al. Analgesic effect of intraarticular morphine after arthroscopic knee surgery. *N Engl J Med* 325 1991; 325:1123–1126.

Stein C, Pfluger M, Yassouridis A, et al. No tolerance to peripheral morphine analgesia in presence of opioid expression in inflamed synovia. *J Clin Invest* 1996; 98:793–799.

Stein C, Schäfer M, Cabot PJ, et al. Peripheral opioid analgesia. *Pain Rev* 1997; 4:171–185.

Uhle RA, Reader A, Nist R, et al. Peripheral opioid analgesia in teeth with symptomatic inflamed pulps. *Anesth Prog* 1997; 44:90–95.

Wenk HN, Honda CN. Immunohistochemical localization of delta opioid receptors in peripheral tissues. *J Comp Neurol* 1999; 408:567–579.

Zhou L, Zhang Q, Stein C, Schäfer M. Contribution of opioid receptors on primary afferent versus sympathetic neurons to peripheral opioid analgesia. *J Pharmacol Exp Ther* 1998; 286:1000–1006.

Correspondence to: Michael Schäfer, Dr med, Klinik für Anaesthesiologie/ Operative Intensivmedizin, Freie Universität Berlin, Klinikum Benjamin Franklin, Hindenburgdamm 30, 12200 Berlin, Germany. Tel: 49-30-8445-2731; Fax: 49-30-8445-4469; email: mischaefer@medizin.fu-berlin.de.

Proceedings of the 9th World Congress on Pain, Progress in Pain Research and Management, Vol. 16, edited by M. Devor, M.C. Rowbotham, and Z. Wiesenfeld-Hallin, IASP Press, Seattle, © 2000.

58

Cancer Pain Mechanisms and Animal Models of Cancer Pain[1]

Paul W. Wacnik,[a] George L. Wilcox,[a,b] Denis R. Clohisy,[c,d] Margaret L. Ramnaraine,[c,d] Laura J. Eikmeier,[e] and Alvin J. Beitz[e]

Departments of [a]Pharmacology, [b]Neuroscience, and [c]Orthopedic Surgery, Medical School; [d]Cancer Center; and [e]Department of Veterinary Pathobiology, School of Veterinary Medicine, University of Minnesota, Minneapolis, Minnesota, USA

Cancer is one of the three leading causes of death in industrialized nations. As treatments for infectious diseases and the prevention of cardiovascular disease continue to improve, and the average life expectancy increases, cancer is likely to become the most common fatal disease in these countries. This assessment is supported by recent studies showing that an estimated nine million new cancer cases occur every year (World Health Organization 1996). Although pain is only one of many symptoms experienced by cancer patients, it is a common distressing symptom and one that frequently affects physical functioning, social interaction, psychological status, and quality of life. In a survey of 1308 oncology outpatients being treated by the Eastern Cooperative Oncology group, 67% reported recent pain, with 36% describing pain severe enough to impair function (Cleeland et al. 1994). Globally, of the millions of patients who suffer from cancer, approximately 58% complain of intolerable pain; this incidence increases to 85% among terminal cancer patients (Foley 1985; Abram 1989; Portenoy 1989).

While several studies have shown that 85% of cancer pain can be controlled with opiates (Schug et al. 1990; Grond et al. 1993; Cherny 1994), the management of severe cancer pain may be problematic, and significant levels of distressing pain occur in the terminal stages of cancer, despite recent

[1] Mini-review based on a congress workshop.

advances in pain management (Cleeland et al. 1994; Ingham and Foley 1998). In addition, opiates, the mainstay of cancer pain therapy, have a wide range of adverse side effects (nausea, sedation, constipation, respiratory depression, and tolerance) that limit their use (Brasseur 1997). Recent work indicates that opiates have a significant immunosuppressant effect (Eisenstein and Hilburger 1998; Hall et al. 1998; Stefano 1998). This effect may interfere with the normal immune response to tumors and could potentially lead to secondary infections in cancer patients treated with such analgesics.

Given the above problems with narcotic analgesics and the failure of these drugs to produce pain relief in over 15% of cancer patients, it is important to develop other non-narcotic, alternative treatments for cancer pain (Foley 1985; Abram 1989; Portenoy 1989). A major impediment to the development of non-narcotic cancer pain therapies is our lack of knowledge of the basic mechanisms and chemical mediators that underlie cancer pain. Fifteen years ago it was assumed that most types of pain were produced by similar mechanisms and that different types of chronic pain resulted in similar changes in the central and peripheral nervous systems. However, evidence gathered over the past 5 years has underscored the association between different types of persistent pain and different types of neural plasticity in both the central and peripheral nervous systems (Dray 1996; Dray and Rang 1998; Novakovic et al. 1998). For instance, *inflammatory pain* is associated with an upregulation of the sensory-neuron-specific sodium channel, PN3, in small neurons and a downregulation in large neurons (Dray and Rang 1998). However, *neuropathic pain* is associated with a downregulation of PN3 in small neurons and a redistribution of the PN3 channel protein along sciatic nerve axons at the site of injury (Okuse et al. 1997; Dray and Rang 1998; Novakovic et al. 1998). Similarly, inflammatory pain is associated with increased substance P release and increased NK1 receptor expression, whereas neuropathic pain is associated with decreased substance P release and no increase in NK1 expression. These are but a few examples of differential regulation of channels, neuropeptides, and receptors that occurs in different persistent pain states. The neuroplasticity associated with tumor-associated nociception may differ from that associated with neuropathic nociception or inflammatory nociception and may represent a unique "pain" state.

MECHANISMS OF CANCER PAIN

Whereas many literature references assert the likely causes of cancer pain (e.g., vascular occlusion or tumor infiltration or compression of bone, soft tissue, or peripheral nerve), they fail to consider the basic mechanisms underlying the production of pain in cancer patients. This lack of mechanistic information can be largely attributed to the paucity of available information concerning the cellular mechanisms involved. Our lack of knowledge concerning the molecular and cellular mechanisms influencing the transducer function of primary afferent nociceptors innervating tumors and surrounding tissue is a clear example of our general ignorance in this area. For example, two of the most common causes of pain in cancer patients are *somatic* (nociceptive) pain resulting from bone metastasis and *neuropathic* pain resulting from injury to the peripheral nervous system (Payne 1989; Brant 1998). The mechanism underlying somatic pain is listed by the World Health Organization (1996) as "stimulation of nerve endings," whereas the mechanism underlying neuropathic pain is listed as "injury to the peripheral nerve." Clearly, this simplistic explanation fails to consider several important aspects of cancer pain: (1) Electrophysiological changes occurring in primary afferent neurons that innervate tumors; (2) tumor-induced changes in the expression of channels or receptors on the surface of primary afferent neurons; (3) mediators released by the tumor or accessory cells near the tumor that directly or indirectly affect the firing of primary afferent neurons; and (4) mediators released by nerve fibers that may affect the physiological state or growth of the tumor. This information is critical for our understanding of cancer pain and for the development of enhanced therapies for cancer pain.

In one of the few papers that attempts to discuss basic mechanisms of cancer pain, Payne (1989) indicates that prostaglandin synthesis is associated with osteolytic and osteoclastic bone changes that accompany metastatic bone cancer. He suggests that prostaglandin synthesis is important in the mechanisms of both tumor growth and pain in bone metastasis. He further postulates that tumor infiltration may be associated with inflammation and the release of algesic chemical substances (which remain to be defined) in skin, bone, and viscera, which in turn activate and sensitize nociceptors. More recent work indicates that cancer metastasis to bone can produce pain via tumor growth into the surrounding tissue, stretching of the periosteum, nerve entrapment, and pathological fractures (Diener 1996; Coleman 1997; Mundy 1997). With respect to basic mechanisms, a recent theory proposes that metastatic bone pain is produced through the release of prostaglandins, bradykinin, substance P, and histamine (reviewed in Diener 1996). However, several issues remain to be determined: (1) Which mediators are released at tumor sites in vivo? (2) Are these substances continually released over time? (3) Do different types of tumors release different types of algesic mediators in vivo? (4) Do these mediators activate or sensitize primary afferent nociceptive neurons surrounding or innervating the tumor?

PARACRINE INTERACTIONS BETWEEN TUMORS AND NERVES

The literature includes little information regarding the possible paracrine interactions between tumors and the peripheral nerves that innervate them. Such interactions may be critical to the development and progression of the nociceptive mechanisms that underlie persistent and chronic cancer pain. Much of our knowledge regarding the substances released by tumors is derived from in vitro studies on tumor cell lines (Wasilenko et al. 1997; Bell and Chaplin 1998; Nakano et al. 1998), from biochemical analysis of tumors removed from human patients or animals (Watanabe et al. 1997; Fujita et al. 1998), or from analysis of fluid samples obtained from human patients or animal models (Luo et al. 1998). Only a few studies have directly measured substances released from tumors in vivo in awake animals or humans (Blay et al. 1997), and none has directly analyzed the effect of mediators, stimulated or released by tumors, on primary afferent neurons. We will summarize the major mediators released from tumor cells and discuss their possible effect on primary afferent nociceptive neurons based on studies that have examined the effect of inflammatory mediators on nervous tissue.

Prostanoids. Prostanoids are the products of cyclooxygenase metabolism of arachidonic acid (Smith et al. 1998); they activate different second-messenger pathways via an interaction with G-protein-coupled receptors. The five major prostanoid receptors (i.e., DP, EP, FP, IP, and TP receptors) are discriminated according to differential rank orders of agonist potency for prostaglandin D_2 (PGD_2; DP receptor), PGE_2 (EP receptor), $PGF2\alpha$ (FP receptor), PGI_2 (IP receptor), and thromboxane (TP receptor), and by selectivity of synthetic agonists and antagonists (Ushikubi et al. 1995; Coleman 1997). Several recent studies have indicated that prostanoids are produced by tumor cells (Fujita et al. 1998; Hida et al. 1998; Nakano et al. 1998; Wolff et al. 1998), and a rich literature shows that prostanoids can induce pain behavior (reviewed by Bley et al. 1998; see also Murata et al. 1997).

Nerve growth factor (NGF). Nerve growth factor was characterized over four decades ago, and, like the other neurotrophins discovered subsequently, it is best known for its trophic role, including the prevention of programmed cell death in specific populations of neurons in the peripheral nervous system (PNS) (Levi-Montalcini et al. 1996; Frade and Barde 1998). NGF also regulates neuronal function, as illustrated by its role in synaptic plasticity and in pain and inflammation (reviewed by Frade and Barde 1998; see also Ma and Woolf 1997). For instance, recent evidence indicates that NGF, but not brain-derived neurotrophic factor (BDNF) or neurotrophin 3 (NT-3), selectively increases the expression of bradykinin binding sites on cultured dorsal root ganglion (DRG) neurons from adult mice via the neurotrophin receptor p75 (p75NTR) (Petersen et al. 1998). Thus, the interaction of NGF with p75NTR may be an important factor contributing to chronic pain conditions. Since several tumors express NGF (Bonetti et al. 1997; Emmett et al. 1997; Tsujino et al. 1997) or neurotrophin receptors (Nogueira et al. 1997; Descamps et al. 1998; Paul and Habib 1998; Pflug and Djakiew 1998), it is possible that tumors release this factor directly or are affected by this growth factor to release other mediators that play a role in tumor-induced nociception.

Cytokines. Cytokines are small, soluble proteins secreted by one cell that can alter the behavior or properties of the cell itself or of another cell. Cytokines affect their target cells by binding to specific receptors that belong to the hematopoetin receptor family, the tumor necrosis factor receptor (TNF-R) family, or the chemokine receptor family. Whereas several cytokines are released from tumor cell lines (e.g., interleukin [IL]-1β [Iglesias et al. 1998; Fonsatti et al. 1997], transforming growth factor [TGF]-β [Taipale et al. 1998], tumor necrosis factor [TNF]-α [Basolo et al. 1993; Pituch-Noworolska et al. 1998], IL-6 [Nasu et al. 1998; Palma and Manzini 1998], IL-8 [Miyamoto et al. 1998; Nasu et al. 1998], and granulocyte macrophage colony-stimulating factor [GM-CSF; Palma and Manzini 1998]), to our knowledge no published in vivo studies describe cytokine release from tumors in awake, freely moving animals. With respect to nociception, it is known that primary afferent neurons express several cytokine receptors (GP-130, GP-80; Gadient and Otten 1996) and that cytokines play a role in the generation of both neuropathic and inflammatory pain (Arruda et al. 1998; Palma and Manzini 1998; Sommer and Schafers 1998; Sommer et al. 1998; Laughlin et al. 2000). Therefore, it is plausible that most tumors synthesize and secrete cytokines or mediate the release of cytokines from other cells (see review by Elgert et al. 1998) and that these cytokines can affect the excitability of primary afferent neurons.

Endothelin-1. In addition to its well-known vasoconstrictor activity, endothelin (ET), via its receptor system (ET-A and ET-B), exerts various biological effects on different types of cells. With respect to the nervous system, application of ET-1 to the rat sciatic nerve produces behavioral signs of acute pain (Davar et al. 1998), and significant evidence suggests that ET-1 can produce nociception (Raffa et al. 1996; De-Melo et al. 1998) and potentiate various types of inflammatory pain (Piovezan et al. 1997; De-Melo et al. 1998). ET-1 also plays a role in tumor cell signal transduction and mitogenesis and induction of endothelial cell growth and angiogenesis in tumor growth (reviewed by Asham et al. 1998). In addition, ET-1 is produced by several types of tumor cells (Watanabe et al. 1997; Bell and Chaplin 1998) and thus is a likely mediator of nociception at tumor sites.

Other mediators. Several other potential algogens are released at tumor sites and thus may participate in tumor-induced nociception. These include bradykinin, adenosine triphosphate (ATP), histamine, serotonin, sympathomimetics, nitric oxide, protons, and other neuropeptides (Dray et al. 1994; Dray 1996). Kinins mediate inflammation, of which pain is a cardinal feature. To date, the clearest evidence for a primary role is the activation by kinins of peripherally located nociceptive receptors on C-fiber terminals that transmit and modulate pain perception (Dray 1997). This evidence is supported by the presence of bradykinin receptors on primary afferent neurons. In addition, data show that the B2 bradykinin receptor plays a role in acute inflammatory pain, while the B1 receptor plays a role in persistent hyperalgesia (Dray 1997; Hall 1997). Interestingly, in addition to their expression by primary afferent neurons, bradykinin receptors are expressed on a variety of tumor cells. Bradykinin receptors on tumor cells appear to play a role in tumor mitogenic behavior and in the regulation of permeability of brain tumor capillaries (Seufferlein and Rozengurt 1996; Clements and Mukhtar 1997; Matsukado et al. 1998). Data showing bradykinin receptors on primary afferent nociceptive neurons together with data showing increased levels of bradykinin in several tumor types support a possible role for bradykinin in cancer pain. ATP and purines, such as adenosine, are also released from tumor cells, and distinct ATP receptors are found on pain-sensing neurons (Cook et al. 1997). These data imply a role for ATP in cancer nociception, particularly via its action on P2X receptors. As in the case of bradykinin and ATP, evidence indicates that receptors for histamine, serotonin, noradrenaline, protons, and other neuropeptides are present on primary afferent nociceptive neurons (see review by Millan 1999). Given the evidence that these substances are secreted by tumor cells or that they are found at elevated levels in certain tumors, they must also be considered viable candidates for the production of cancer pain. Clearly more work is needed to define which mediators play the greatest role in the development and maintenance of cancer pain and to determine whether different tumors produce pain via the secretion of different algogens.

NEW DIRECTIONS IN CANCER PAIN RESEARCH

The 9th World Congress on Pain included a topical workshop entitled "Novel Pathophysiologic Mechanisms of Pain Due to Cancer." The workshop offered an initial examination of needs, mechanisms, and models concerning the signaling mechanisms of tumor-associated pain and analgesic strategies in palliative care. The workshop began with a clinical perspective from Eduardo Bruera, director of the Palliative Care Program, Grey Nuns

Community Hospital in Edmonton, Alberta, Canada (Vigano et al. 1998, 1999). Animal models of cancer pain may enable identification of the intercellular signaling that gives rise to cancer pain and optimization of analgesic therapy in palliative care. Gary Bennett, Department of Neurology, Allegheny University of Health Sciences, Philadelphia, described neuropathic pain resulting from immune (Eliav et al. 1999) or chemotherapeutic (Polomano et al. 1998) challenge of peripheral nerves encountered in the management of advanced cancer. In particular, vincristine, paclitaxel (Taxol), and the monoclonal antibody GD2 ganglioside produced signs of neuropathic pain in rodent models. Gudarz Davar of the Pain Research and Management Center, Department of Anesthesiology, Brigham and Women's Hospital and Harvard Medical School, Cambridge, Massachusetts, described the excitatory effects of ET-1, a putative mediator of tumor-nerve coupling, on electrical activity in peripheral nerve. Topical application of ET-1 to distal saphenous nerve activates axons as recorded in sciatic nerve (Davar et al. 1998; Fareed et al., in press). Lastly, two new behavioral models of tumor-associated pain were presented that have been described previously by members of our group (Wacnik et al. 1998, 1999). The remainder of this chapter presents some preliminary results from these models.

GOALS IN DEVELOPING AN ANIMAL MODEL OF CANCER PAIN

To optimize pain treatments in cancer patients, it is important to empirically distinguish physiological (somatogenic) pain from the psychogenic pain associated with progression of a fatal disease. Most cancer patients experience some pain as a symptom. Because much pain appears to be associated with metastatic bone disease, we chose to focus our efforts on this kind of tumor. Understanding the mechanisms underlying tumor-associated nociception and hyperalgesia requires the establishment of animal models. Recently, in collaboration with a bone metastasis laboratory (Clohisy et al. 1996), we developed mouse models of tumor-induced allodynia and hyperalgesia that permit multidisciplinary, hypothesis-based experimentation at the behavioral, biochemical, anatomical, and molecular levels (Wacnik et al. 1998, 1999). We induce hyperalgesia using syngenetic mice and tumor cells to create a reproducible progression of mechanical allodynia and hyperalgesia. We characterize these tumor-induced hyperresponsive behaviors with mechanical stimulation (von Frey filaments) to assess mechanical allodynia on the plantar surface of the hindpaw secondary to implantation of an osteolytic tumor in the femur, and with a novel assay in the forelimb in which we use grip strength to assess movement-related incidental hyperalgesia. These paradigms may provide clinically relevant animal models of cancer pain.

IN VIVO MICRODIALYSIS OF TUMORS

Cancer pain may be generated and partially maintained by the release of algesic mediators from the tumor itself. To test this hypothesis we have begun to measure basal and tumor levels of putative algesic substances in dialysate samples from the tumor site using in vivo microdialysis. Several studies have shown that various tumor cell lines and tumors secrete neuropeptides (Nesland et al. 1988; Aalto et al. 1998; El-Salhy et al. 1998). More importantly, several lines of evidence indicate that neuropeptides are mitogenic for various cell types, including tumor cells (Rozengurt and Sinnett-Smith 1983; Carney et al. 1987). Neuropeptide receptors are expressed at high density by neoplastic cells (Halmos et al. 1995; Madsen et al. 1998; North et al. 1998), and are upregulated on the peritumor vasculature (Reubi et al. 1996), and may thereby affect tumor growth (Scholar and Paul 1991; Seckl et al. 1997).

RATIONALE FOR TUMOR IMPLANTATION STRATEGY

Mouse lines and cell types. Male C3H/Hej mice (National Institutes of Health) aged 8–10 weeks and weighing 24–28 g are implanted with NCTC clone 2472 connective tissue (osteolytic) cells obtained from the ATCC (American Type Culture Collection). These cells, which are derived from a spontaneous connective tissue tumor in this mouse strain, grow easily after implantation, initiating osteolysis particularly when given intimate exposure to bony tissue (Clohisy et al. 1996). This technique produces a solid tumor only at the site of injection that eventually lyses the bone but does not metastasize systemically.

Tumor-induced incidental pain: movement-related hyperalgesia. Incidental pain is a specific type of breakthrough pain that is thought to predict poor response to routine pharmacotherapy (Bruera et al. 1989; Mercadante 1991; Ashby et al. 1992; Mercadante et al. 1992, 1994). We model movement-related pain by implanting these osteolytic syngeneic tumor cells in both humeri in the mice. We then evaluate the tumor-induced muscle hyperalgesia with a grip-force assay that quantifies in grams the peak force exerted by a mouse as it grips a wire screen attached to a force transducer. Inflammation-induced lowering in grip force has been attributed to hyperalgesia because it can be significantly reversed with analgesics (e.g., levorphanol) (Kehl et al., in press). Similarly, we interpret the drop in pulling force following tumor implantation as being due to hyperalgesia because it can be significantly reversed with traditional analgesics (morphine and clonidine).

Tumor-induced secondary mechanical hyperalgesia. In cancer patients, neuropathic-like pain may be initiated by a complex mixture of neuronal and non-neuronal tissue damage. This pain of complex origin is treated with various classes of pharmacotherapies in combination (Elliott and Foley 1989). Our model provides a means of measuring tumor-induced secondary mechanical allodynia or hypersensitivity in the mouse hindpaw, although we are unable to test for hypersensitivity at the primary tumor site. We interpret the hypersensitivity in the paw to represent secondary allodynia originating either peripherally or centrally.

METHODS FOR TUMOR IMPLANTATION AND BEHAVIORAL MEASUREMENTS

Mice were housed 10 to a cage in a temperature- and humidity-controlled environment, maintained on a 12-hour light/dark cycle, and given free access to mouse chow and water. The osteolytic cells were placed in 75-cm^2 flasks in NCTC 135 media, pH 7.35, 10% horse serum and were grown to confluence, fed, and passed once a week by a 1:4 split ratio. Tumor cells were prepared for implantation by first pouring off the media and rinsing with phosphate-buffered saline (PBS). Trypsin was then added for 5–10 minutes to detach cells from the flask. The enzymatic action was stopped with a sufficient volume of NCTC 135 medium. The cells were then counted with a hemocytometer, pelleted, resuspended and rinsed in PBS, pelleted a second time, then resuspended in a concentration of 2×10^5 cells in 20 μL of PBS.

Implantation. For humerus implantation, mice were anesthetized with 1–2% halothane for this percutaneous procedure. The deltoid tuberosity, located longitudinally midway on the anterior surface of the humerus, was located by identifying the midpoint between the two humerus articulations, proximally (glenoid cavity of the scapula) and distally (the radius and ulna). The area was then probed with a 0.3-cm^3 insulin syringe (29-gauge needle) until solid bone was encountered; the needle was then used to bore through the tuberosity and the cells were injected. This procedure distributes cells in both the bone and the surrounding muscle.

For intramuscular implantation near the humerus, unanesthetized mice were held firmly by the scruff of the neck, and cells were injected intramuscularly near the humerus of the forelimb bilaterally at a depth of approximately 5 mm.

Minor surgery was required for femur implantation of tumor cells. Mice were anesthetized as above, and the distal end of the femur was accessed through a 0.5-cm unilateral incision at the knee, in some cases cutting the patellar tendon. A 0.3-cm^3 insulin syringe with the needle aligned parallel to the femur was used to penetrate the bone and deposit the cells in the medullary space. The skin was closed with a single sterile wound clip, which was removed 2 days later. Full mobility resumed within 15 minutes of cessation of the anesthetic. This implantation technique was based on a skeletal metastasis model developed in the laboratory of D.R. Clohisy for studying tumor site mechanisms of bone destruction (Clohisy et al. 1996).

For implantation near the sciatic nerve, unanesthetized mice were held firmly by the iliac crest and cells were injected intramuscularly in the posterior biceps femoris muscle of the hindlimb unilaterally at a depth of approximately 5 mm.

Histological examination of paraffin-embedded, hemosin- and eosin-stained sections of the femur on day 21 after implantation of 2472 cells (data not shown) indicated that the cells produce nonencapsulated tumors. The individual cells are spindle-shaped, typical of a fibrosarcoma, and the tumor breaks down the bone and spreads relatively quickly from the bone into the surrounding tissue.

Grip force assay. We mimic movement-related pain in mice by repeatedly measuring the tumor-induced change in forelimb grip force (grams) produced when a mouse pulls against a force transducer. Two force transducers (DFIS series) are aligned in series, one to measure the peak force exerted by the forelimbs and the other to measure that exerted by the hindlimbs when the mouse is pulled by the tail over two meshes connected to the transducers (Kehl et al. 1999; Wacnik et al. 1999). Grip testing was conducted 4 and 2 days prior to the day of cell implantation to establish baselines. Testing was repeated every 2–3 days to follow changes in muscle sensitivity as the tumor progressed. Front paw mechanical allodynia was also tested as below (von Frey filament #2.44 exerting 0.34 mN force), but no allodynia was detected; this result rules out forepaw allodynia as the cause of the decreased grip force.

Secondary mechanical allodynia, von Frey assay. Mechanical allodynia was measured on the plantar surface of the hindpaw to determine the extent of secondary hypersensitivity associated with the hindlimb tumor. Baseline values for mechanical sensitivity to a #3.61 (2.6 mN) von Frey filament, which elicits a <20% response at baseline, were determined prior to tumor cell implantation (day 0) for each animal and for several days to several weeks after implantation as shown in the Results section. Animals were placed on a wire mesh platform and covered with a glass custard cup (Corning) and allowed to acclimate to their surroundings for a minimum of 30 minutes before testing. The filament was applied to the point of bending six times on the plantar surface of each hindpaw, and the number of positive (vigorous responses) to the filament were counted. Data were expressed as a percentage of positive responses. The mean and SEM were determined for each paw for each treatment group. Significance was determined by repeated-measures ANOVA followed by the Bonferroni post hoc test.

ANALGESICS

Effects of morphine and clonidine on tumor-induced reduction in grip strength. Bilateral osteolytic tumors implanted in both humeri in mice produce a robust and long-lasting attenuation of grip strength. We took advantage of the long-lasting effect and evaluated the efficacy and potency of both morphine and clonidine alone or in combination over a 2-week study period (days 7–21 post-implantation) in a single group of mice. We administered all drugs intraperitoneally (i.p.) in 100 μL saline following baseline grip testing. Based on preliminary studies, we concluded that the optimum time for post-drug grip measurement was 30 minutes after drug administration. We used the same-day baseline as a basis to determine what, if any, effect analgesics would have on tumor-induced reduction in grip strength. We used the following calculation in all humerus drug analyses:

Percentage increase in grip strength = (post-drug grip strength [grams]) – (same-day baseline grip strength [grams])/(same-day baseline grip strength [grams]) × 100.

Effects of morphine and clonidine on tumor-induced secondary mechanical allodynia. Unilateral implantation of osteolytic tumors in the femur produces an ipsilateral secondary mechanical allodynia that is evaluated on the plantar surface of the hindpaw with a von Frey filament. We used this method to evaluate the efficacy and potency of both morphine and clonidine alone or in combination in mice that remained allodynic, days 23–29 following the time-course analysis. To establish a uniform baseline for evaluating drug-induced changes in allodynic behaviors, all mice used were allodynic as defined by a 50% or greater response to the #3.61 von Frey filament. The #3.83 von Frey filament was used in fewer than 20% of these mice to bring their baseline to the 83–100% response level. We used the following calculation in all femur drug analyses:

Percentage inhibition = ([% response baseline] – [post-drug % response])/(% response baseline) × 100.

Statistical (isobolographic) analysis. Data describing antinociception are expressed as means of percentage inhibition (femur tumor mice) or percentage increase in grip strength (humerus tumor mice), with SEM. The median effective dose (ED_{50}) values and confidence limits were calculated according to the method of Tallarida and Murray (1987). Groups of four (femur tumor mice) or 10 (humerus tumor mice) or more animals were used for each dose and saline. For each experiment, we generated three dose-response curves. These included dose-response curves for agonist 1, agonist 2, and agonists 1 and 2 co-administered in an equi-effective dose ratio. The dose-response curves of the combination of agonist 1 and 2 were calculated twice: first in terms of the agonist 1 dose (closed circles) and second in terms of the agonist 2 dose (closed triangles). To test for synergistic interactions, the 95% confidence intervals of all dose-response curves were arithmetically arranged around the ED_{50} value using the equation ($\ln_{10} \times ED_{50}$) $\times$ (SE of log ED_{50}) (Tallarida 1992). Isobolographic analysis, the appropriate method for evaluating synergistic interactions (Tallarida and Murray 1987; Tallarida 1992), necessitates this manipulation. When testing an interaction between two drugs given in combination for synergy, additivity, or subadditivity, it is necessary to calculate a theoretical additive ED_{50} value for the combination based on the dose-response curves of each drug administered separately. This theoretical value is then compared by a *t* test ($P <$ 0.05) with the observed experimental ED_{50} value of the combination. These values are based on total dose of both drugs: in this case, the sum of the clonidine and morphine doses. An interaction is considered synergistic if the observed ED_{50} value is significantly ($P < 0.05$) less than the calculated theoretical additive ED_{50} value (Tallarida and Murray 1987; Tallarida 1992). Additivity is indicated when the theoretical and experimental ED_{50} values do not differ. An interaction is considered subadditive if the observed combined ED_{50} value is significantly ($P < 0.05$) greater than the calculated theoretical additive ED_{50} value. A complete description of the isobolographic method for evaluating drug combinations is detailed by Tallarida et al. (1989).

Collection of substances released by or near tumors using in vivo microdialysis. To examine putative algogens in the extracellular fluid of solid tumors, we implanted a microdialysis fiber into the center of the tumor or into a comparable site in control animals. The microdialysis procedure is similar to that described previously (Herzberg et al. 1996). Dialysis probes are constructed from a 6-cm length of dialysis fiber (diameter = 200 μm; molecular mass cutoff = 20–50 kDa; Amicon Vitafiber II) cannulated with a 0.005-inch (0.13-mm) diameter stainless steel wire and coated along their entire length except for a central region (2–3 mm in length) with 5-minute epoxy (Devcon) to seal the pores. A 23-gauge hypodermic needle is inserted through the center of the tumor and the dialysis probe is then inserted through the 23-gauge needle. Removal of the needle leaves the dialysis probe in place. The stainless steel wire is then removed and the free ends of the dialysis tubing are trimmed and joined to two lengths of PE tubing with epoxy. The PE tubes are then attached to a fluid swivel (Harvard Instruments), which is connected to a peristaltic pump (Rabbit Plus; Rainin Instrument Co.). Following the mouse's recovery, the dialysis tubing is perfused with a modified Ringer's solution at a flow rate of 3–5 μL/min. Following a 1-hour equilibration period, dialysis samples are collected for a period of 3–4 hours by using a Gilson fraction collector. Samples are concentrated and frozen until analysis.

Microdialysis is used in combination with mass spectrometry or with ELISA assays to analyze putative algesic agents recovered in dialysates from femur tumors and compared to dialysates obtained from control mice. Matrix-assisted laser desorption ionization (MALDI) is a recently developed soft ionization technique that, together with time-of-flight (TOF) mass spectrometry, permits detection and characterization of biopolymers such as peptides, proteins, oligosaccharides, and nucleotides, especially in mixtures and crude samples (Kaufmann 1995; de Jong 1998). The resolving power, precision, and accuracy of a simple linear MALDI-TOF spectrometer is two to four orders of magnitude better than that obtainable with gel electrophoresis. TOF analysis provides very high precision and sensitivity, allowing detection of 10–15 fmol of a peptide with a mass accuracy of 1 part in 10,000. The MALDI-TOF technique has been used successfully for the mass spectrometric analysis of intact proteins, domains, and conjugates (Kaufmann 1995; Chaurand et al. 1999). Samples are mixed with a matrix (such as dihydroxybenzoate) and dried on the target. A laser pulse vaporizes the matrix, releasing the entrapped peptide into the gas phase. A pulse of electrical potential sends the charged ions toward the detector, which measures the time of ion arrival and determines the mass-to-charge ratio. This method allows determination of the molecular mass of an array of proteins and peptides in the sample.

RESULTS AND DISCUSSION

Osteolytic 2472 sarcoma cells implanted in the femur and near the sciatic nerve of the hindlimb in C3H mice create a robust and reproducible model of tumor-induced allodynia. Fig. 1 depicts the time course of behavioral hypersensitivity to application of a #3.61 von Frey filament (2.6 mN) to the plantar surface of both hindpaws. Both femur and intramuscular implantation of the cells enhance responses to stimulation, but femur implantation produces more robust, progressively increasing responsiveness.

Fig. 2 depicts the reduction in forelimb grip force as humerus-implanted tumors progressed. In this graph, decreased force indicates hyperalgesia. Hindlimb grip strength did not change as the tumor progressed, which suggests a localized hyperalgesic state. In addition, mechanical

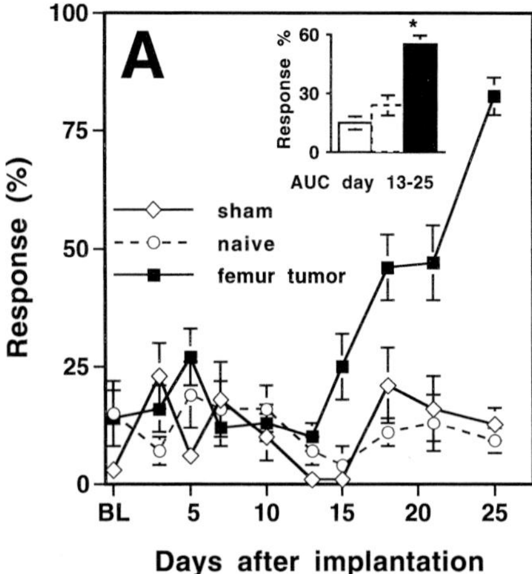

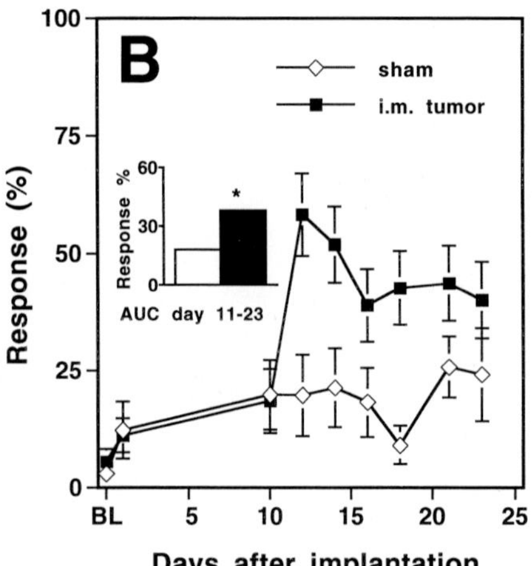

Fig. 1. Osteolytic 2472 cells implanted unilaterally in the femur (A) or i.m. near the sciatic nerve (B) of C3H/He mice produce significant mechanical allodynia (13–25 or 11–23 days, respectively, after implantation), as measured by the percentage response to a single #3.61 von Frey filament on the ipsilateral paw pad. The percentage response represents the number of positive responses divided by 6 (the total number of stimuli/paw) and multiplied by 100. The mean and SEM were calculated for each group from this percentage. The time course data were converted into a single point area under the curve (AUC) for a time period determined from preliminary experiments (data not shown) on (A) days 13–25 or (B) days 11–23 by averaging the data across the individual time points. The AUCs were then used to test for significance between groups through analysis of variance (ANOVA). The groups were further tested for differences from sham with the Bonferroni post hoc test for multiple comparisons. $P < 0.05$ (*) was considered statistically significant.

allodynia (as measured with von Frey filaments on the plantar surface of the forepaw) was not detectable (data not shown), which suggests that the decrease in grip strength is attributable to a primary effect near the tumor site. The reduction in grip force coincident with progressive tumor growth further suggests that tumor progression is responsible for the reduction in force.

Systemically administered analgesics, morphine and clonidine, attenuated tumor-induced mechanical allodynia in a dose-dependent manner (Fig. 3). The drop in grip strength was dose-dependently attenuated by either morphine or clonidine; the activity of these analgesics supports the idea that a hyperalgesic condition underlies this behavioral change (Fig. 3).

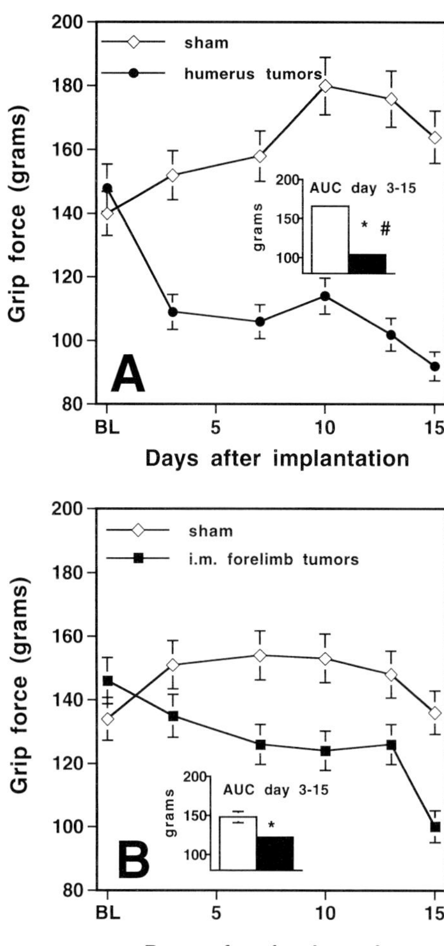

Fig. 2. Osteolytic 2472 cells implanted bilaterally (A) in the humerus or (B) i.m. near the humerus of C3H/He mice produce significant reduction in grip force (days 3–15 postimplantation) compared to their respective sham-treated controls. In addition, humerus implantation (bone involvement) was also significantly different from the i.m. implantation group. The mean and standard error of the mean (SEM) were calculated for each group from the grip response. The time course data were converted into a single point area under the curve (AUC), (A,B) for days 3–15 and by averaging the data across the individual time points. The AUCs were then used to test for significance between groups through analysis of variance (ANOVA). The tumor groups were further tested for differences from sham-treated groups with the Bonferroni post hoc test for multiple comparisons. *P* (# and *) < 0.05 was considered statistically significant.

Both systemically administered clonidine (ED_{50}: 0.14 mg/kg, 0.067–0.29) and morphine (ED_{50}: 11 mg/kg, 6.9–16) inhibited responses to mechanical stimulation (2.6 mN force) in mice with unilateral femur implantation. The clonidine:morphine equi-effective dose ratio administered was 1:110. When administered in combination, the ED_{50} values of clonidine (ED_{50}: 0.016 mg/kg, 0.011–0.03) and morphine (ED_{50}: 1.76 mg/kg, 1.26–3.0) are markedly lower than that of either agonist administered individually (Fig. 3A). This observation indicates an increase in potency for each drug administered in the presence of the other compared to each drug administered alone. Specifically, the potency of clonidine increased 8.8-fold in the presence of morphine, and likewise the potency of morphine increased 6.3-fold in the presence of clonidine. Isobolographic analysis revealed that the administra-

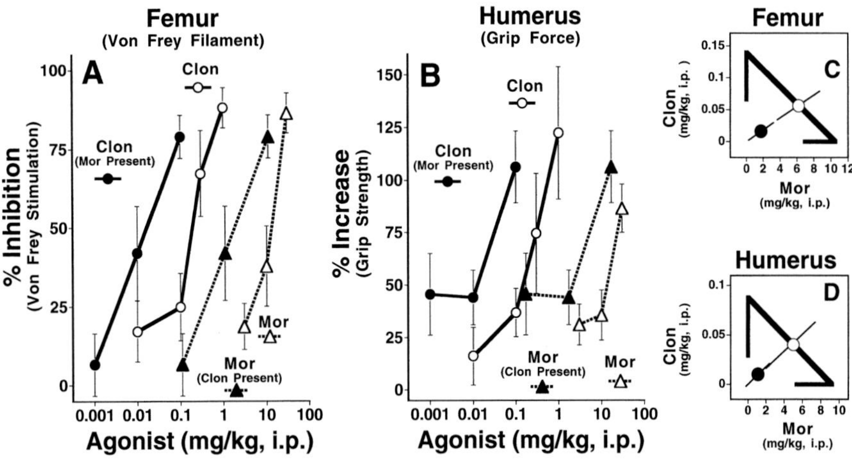

Fig. 3. Systemically administered clonidine produces antiallodynic synergy with morphine. Dose-response curves for clonidine and morphine administered i.p. separately and in combination. (A) *Femur.* Dose-response curves of the inhibition of mechanical allodynia by clonidine (open circles, ED_{50}: 0.14 mg/kg, 0.067–0.29), morphine (open triangles, ED_{50}: 11 mg/kg, 6.9–16), clonidine in the presence of morphine (closed circles, ED_{50}: 0.016 mg/kg, 0.011–0.03), and morphine in the presence of clonidine (closed triangles, ED_{50}: 1.76 mg/kg, 1.26–3.3). (B) *Humerus.* Dose-response curves for clonidine and morphine administered i.p. separately and in combination. Dose-response curves of the increased grip force effect of clonidine (open circles, ED_{50}: 0.088 mg/kg, 0.29–0.22), morphine (open triangles, ED_{50}: 9.2 mg/kg, 5.3–16), clonidine in the presence of morphine (closed circles, ED_{50}: 0.005 mg/kg, 0.0014–0.012), and morphine in the presence of clonidine (closed triangles, ED_{50}: 0.83 mg/kg, 0.25–2.8). (C,D) Isobolographic representation of the antinociceptive (% inhibition) effect of the combination of clonidine and morphine. The theoretical additive line connects the ED_{50} value of clonidine (y-axis intercept) to the ED_{50} value of morphine (x-axis intercept). The white open circle represents the theoretical additive point where the ED_{50} value of the combination would fall were the interaction merely additive. The experimentally derived ED_{50} value of the combination of clonidine and morphine is represented by the filled circle. The combination is considered synergistic when the experimental ED_{50} value differs significantly from the theoretical additive ED_{50} value (Student's t test, $P < 0.05$). (C) *Femur.* In this isobologram, the ED_{50} value of the combination of clonidine and morphine indicates that the interaction is synergistic. (D) *Humerus.* In this isobologram, the ED_{50} value of the combination of clonidine and morphine also indicates that the interaction is synergistic.

tion of clonidine-morphine combinations in mice resulted in antinociceptive dose-response curves with ED_{50} values significantly less than the calculated theoretical additive values (Fig. 3C). This result demonstrates a synergistic interaction between clonidine and morphine in attenuating the tumor-induced secondary allodynia observed in mice carrying osteolytic tumor cells in the femur.

Both systemically administered clonidine (ED_{50}: 0.088 mg/kg, 0.29–0.22) and morphine (ED_{50}: 9.2 mg/kg, 5.3–16) increased grip force strength in mice implanted bilaterally in the humerus. The clonidine:morphine equi-effective dose ratio administered was 1:127. When administered in combination, the ED_{50} values of clonidine (ED_{50}: 0.005 mg/kg, 0.0014–0.012) and morphine (ED_{50}: 0.83 mg/kg, 0.25–2.8) were markedly lower than that of either agonist administered individually (Fig. 3B). This observation indicates an increase in potency for each drug administered in the presence of the other compared to each drug administered alone. Specifically, the potency of clonidine increased 18-fold in the presence of morphine, and likewise the potency of morphine increased 11-fold in the presence of clonidine. Isobolographic analysis revealed that the administration of clonidine-morphine combinations in mice bearing osteolytic tumors resulted in antinociceptive dose-response curves with ED_{50} values significantly less than the calculated theoretical additive values (Fig. 3D). This finding demonstrates a synergistic interaction between clonidine and morphine in reversing the tumor-induced drop in grip force observed in mice bearing osteolytic tumors in the humerus.

We employed MALDI-TOF to analyze and compare the peptides present in microdialysate samples obtained from the tissue surrounding tumor-infected femur 14 days after implantation with those present in dialysates from vehicle-injected control animals. Fig. 4 presents a typical MALDI-TOF spectrum from a tumor-injected mouse compared to that from a control mouse. The lower spectrum in Fig. 4 shows that tumor dialysates have considerably more peptides present in the extracellular fluid than are present in the extracellular fluid from control animals. We can obtain structural information concerning several of these proteins by exploiting metastable post-source decay (PSD) processes; PSD allows extraction of sequence information on individual peptide fragments and proteins. Preliminary data using ELISA (Beitz and Eikmeier, unpublished data) suggest that substance P, nerve growth factor (NGF), and interleukin-10 (IL-10) are present at higher levels in tumor dialysates from mice carrying tumors in their femurs than in those obtained from control mice. These preliminary data are intriguing and suggest that several putative algogens may be elevated in or near the tumors. Further studies are being conducted to determine the presence and concentration of such algogens in this bone tumor model.

SUMMARY AND CONCLUSIONS

The relatively slow tumor growth rate or its osteolytic capabilities may account for long-lasting mechanical allodynia and movement-related hyperalgesia observed in C3H/Hej mice after implantation of osteolytic tumor cells in or near major bones. We conclude that these persistent hyper-

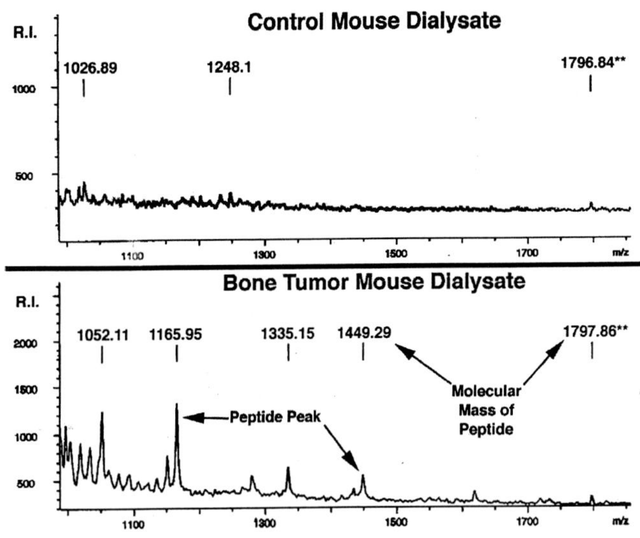

Fig. 4. MALDI-TOF mass spectrometry shows that peptides with molecular mass between 1000 and 1800 Da are present in dialysate samples obtained from tumor (bottom) and vehicle-injected control (top) mice. These spectra demonstrate that there are many more peptides present in the tumor dialysate sample (peptide peaks) than in the control sample. Some peaks are present in both the tumor and control dialysates (double asterisks). The vertical axis indicates relative intensity (RI) of the ionization signal of molecules within a sample, and the horizontal axis indicates molecular mass in daltons.

responsive states constitute animal models of chronic cancer pain. In addition, the hyperalgesia observed in these two osteolytic/C3H models are sensitive to the analgesics morphine and clonidine; the models may therefore be useful in testing other agents for therapeutic utility in control of cancer pain. The models also enable us to analyze the signaling components altered in or near tumors to test hypotheses concerning the origins of cancer pain.

ACKNOWLEDGMENTS

The laboratory of Dr. Lois Kehl, University of Minnesota School of Dentistry, contributed early access to the grip assay technique. Undergraduate research assistants Fariha Ahmed, Matthew Veldman, and Jennifer Cash contributed greatly to development of the behavioral assays used in these studies. Ms. Kristin Schreiber contributed to the final preparation of this manuscript. Dr. Carolyn Fairbanks contributed to the synergy and isobolographic analysis. Ms. Melanie Watson contributed to development of the microdialysis technique and early dialysis analysis. This research was supported in part by the Roby C. Thompson Endowment in Musculoskeletal Oncology and by seed research funds provided by the University of Minnesota Academic Health Center. P.W. Wacnik was supported by NIDR training grant NIH/5T 32-DEO 7288-02 (P. Mantyh, PI). L.J. Eikmeier was supported by NIDA training grant DA07239-09 (T.W. Molitor, PI).

REFERENCES

Aalto Y, Forsgren S, Franzen L, Henriksson R. Is radiation-induced degranulation of mast cells in salivary glands induced by substance P? *Oral Oncol* 1998; 34:332–339.

Abram SE. *Cancer Pain*. Boston: Kluwer Academic, 1989.

Arruda JL, Colburn RW, Rickman AJ, Rutkowski MD, DeLeo JA. Increase of interleukin-6 mRNA in the spinal cord following peripheral nerve injury in the rat: potential role of IL-6 in neuropathic pain. Brain Research. *Mol Brain Res* 1998; 62:228–235.

Asham EH, Loizidou M, Taylor I. Endothelin-1 and tumour development. *Eur J Surg Oncol* 1998; 24:57–60.

Ashby MA, Fleming BG, Brooksbank M, et al. Description of a mechanistic approach to pain management in advanced cancer. Preliminary report. *Pain* 1992; 51:153–161.

Basolo F, Conaldi PG, Fiore L, Calvo S, Toniolo A. Normal breast epithelial cells produce interleukins 6 and 8 together with tumor-necrosis factor: defective IL6 expression in mammary carcinoma. *Int J Cancer* 1993; 55:926–930.

Bell KM, Chaplin DJ. The effect of oxygen and carbon dioxide on tumor cell endothelin-1 production. *J Cardiovasc Pharmacol* 1998; 31:S537–S540.

Blay J, White TD, Hoskin DW. The extracellular fluid of solid carcinomas contains immunosuppressive concentrations of adenosine. *Cancer Res* 1997; 57:2602–2605.

Bley KR, Hunter JC, Eglen RM, Smith JA. The role of IP prostanoid receptors in inflammatory pain. *Trends Pharmacol Sci* 1998; 19:141–147.

Bonetti B, Panzeri L, Carner M, et al. Human neoplastic Schwann cells: changes in the expression of neurotrophins and their low-affinity receptor p75. *Neuropathol Appl Neurobiol* 1997; 23:380–386.

Brant JM. Cancer-related neuropathic pain. *Nurse Pract Forum* 1998; 9:154–162.

Brasseur L. Review of current pharmacologic treatment of pain. *Drugs* 1997; 53:10–7.

Bruera E, MacMillan K, Hanson J, MacDonald RN. The Edmonton staging system for cancer pain: preliminary report. *Pain* 1989; 37:203–209.

Carney DN, Cuttitta F, Moody TW, Minna JD. Selective stimulation of small cell lung cancer clonal growth by bombesin and gastrin-releasing peptide. *Cancer Res* 1987; 47:821–825.

Chaurand P, Luetzenkirchen F, Spengler B. Peptide and protein identification by matrix-assisted laser desorption ionization (MALDI) and MALDI-post-source decay time-of-flight mass spectrometry. *J Am Soc Mass Spectrom* 1999; 10:91–103.

Cherny NI, Portnoy RK. Practical issues in the management of cancer pain. In: Wall PD, Melzack R (Eds). *Textbook of Pain*. Edinburgh: Churchill Livingstone, 1994, pp 787–823.

Cleeland CS, Gonin R, Hatfield AK, et al. Pain and its treatment in outpatients with metastatic cancer. *N Engl J Med* 1994; 330:592–596.

Clements J, Mukhtar A. Tissue kallikrein and the bradykinin B2 receptor are expressed in endometrial and prostate cancers. *Immunopharmacology* 1997; 36:217–220.

Clohisy DR, Ogilvie CM, Carpenter RJ, Ramnaraine ML. Localized, tumor-associated osteolysis involves the recruitment and activation of osteoclasts. *J Orthop Res* 1996; 14:2–6.

Coleman RE. Skeletal complications of malignancy. *Cancer* 1997; 80:1588–1594.

Cook SP, Vulchanova L, Hargreaves KM, Elde R, McCleskey EW. Distinct ATP receptors on pain-sensing and stretch-sensing neurons. *Nature* 1997; 387:505–508.

Davar G, Hans G, Fareed MU, Sinnott C, Strichartz G. Behavioral signs of acute pain produced by application of endothelin-1 to rat sciatic nerve. *Neuroreport* 1998; 9:2279–2283.

de Jong A. Contribution of mass spectrometry to contemporary immunology. *Mass Spectrom Rev* 1998; 17:311–335.

De-Melo JD, Tonussi CR, D'Orleans-Juste P, Rae GA. Articular nociception induced by endothelin-1, carrageenan and LPS in naive and previously inflamed knee-joints in the rat: inhibition by endothelin receptor antagonists. *Pain* 1998; 77:261–269.

Descamps S, Lebourhis X, Delehedde M, Boilly B, Hondermarck H. Nerve growth factor is mitogenic for cancerous but not normal human breast epithelial cells. *J Biol Chem* 1998; 273:16659–16662.

Diener KM. Bisphosphonates for controlling pain from metastatic bone disease. *Am J Health Syst Pharm* 1996; 53:1917–1927.

Dray A. Neurogenic mechanisms and neuropeptides in chronic pain. *Prog Brain Res* 1996; 110:85–94.

Dray A. Kinins and their receptors in hyperalgesia. *Can J Physiol Pharmacol* 1997; 75:704–712.

Dray A, Rang H. The how and why of chronic pain states and the what of new analgesia therapies. *Trends Neurosci* 1998; 21:315–317.

Dray A, Urban L, Dickenson A. Pharmacology of chronic pain. *Trends Pharmacol Sci* 1994; 15:190–197.

Eisenstein TK, Hilburger ME. Opioid modulation of immune responses: effects on phagocyte and lymphoid cell populations. *J Neuroimmunol* 1998; 83:36–44.

El-Salhy M, Simonsson M, Stenling R, Grimelius L. Recovery from Marie-Bamberger's syndrome and diabetes insipidus after removal of a lung adenocarcinoma with neuroendocrine features. *J Intern Med* 1998; 243:171–175.

Elgert KD, Alleva DG, Mullins DW. Tumor-induced immune dysfunction: the macrophage connection. *J Leukocyte Biol* 1998; 64:275–290.

Eliav E, Herzburg U, Ruda MA, Bennett GJ. Neuropathic pain from an experimental neuritis of the rat sciatic nerve. *Pain* 1999; 83:169–182.

Elliott K, Foley KM. Neurologic pain syndromes in patients with cancer. *Neurol Clin* 1989; 7:333–360.

Emmett CJ, McNeeley PA, Johnson RM. Evaluation of human astrocytoma and glioblastoma cell lines for nerve growth factor release. *Neurochem Int* 1997; 30:465–474.

Fareed M, Hans G, Atanda A, Strichartz GGD, Davar G. Pharmacologic characterization of acute pain behavior produced by the application of endothelin-1 to rat sciatic nerve. *J Pain;* in press.

Foley KM. The treatment of cancer pain. *N Engl J Med* 1985; 313:84–95.

Fonsatti E, Altomonte M, Coral S, et al. Tumour-derived interleukin 1alpha (IL-1alpha) up-regulates the release of soluble intercellular adhesion molecule-1 (sICAM-1) by endothelial cells. *Br J Cancer* 1997; 76:1255–1261.

Frade JM, Barde YA. Nerve growth factor: two receptors, multiple functions. *Bioessays* 1998; 20:137–145.

Fujita T, Matsui M, Takaku K, et al. Size- and invasion-dependent increase in cyclooxygenase 2 levels in human colorectal carcinomas. *Cancer Res* 1998; 58:4823–4826.

Gadient RA, Otten U. Postnatal expression of interleukin-6 (IL-6) and IL-6 receptor (IL-6R) mRNAs in rat sympathetic and sensory ganglia. *Brain Res* 1996; 724:41–46.

Grond S, Zech D, Lynch J, et al. Validation of World Health Organization guidelines for pain relief in head and neck cancer. A prospective study. *Ann Otol Rhinol Laryngol* 1993; 102:342–348.

Hall DM, Suo JL, Weber RJ. Opioid mediated effects on the immune system: sympathetic nervous system involvement. *J Neuroimmunol* 1998; 83:29–35.

Hall JM. Bradykinin receptors. *Gen Pharmacol* 1997; 28:1–6.

Halmos G, Wittliff JL, Schally AV. Characterization of bombesin/gastrin-releasing peptide receptors in human breast cancer and their relationship to steroid receptor expression. *Cancer Res* 1995; 55:280–287.

Herzberg U, Brown DR, Mullett MA, Beitz AJ. Increased delayed type hypersensitivity in rats subjected to unilateral mononeuropathy is mediated by neurokinin-1 receptors. *J Neuroimmunol* 1996; 65:119–124.

Hida T, Yatabe Y, Achiwa H, et al. Increased expression of cyclooxygenase 2 occurs frequently in human lung cancers, specifically in adenocarcinomas. *Cancer Res* 1998; 58:3761–3764.

Iglesias M, Yen K, Gaiotti D, et al. Human papillomavirus type 16 E7 protein sensitizes cervical keratinocytes to apoptosis and release of interleukin-1 alpha. *Oncogene* 1998; 17:1195–1205.

Ingham JM, Foley KM. Pain and the barriers to its relief at the end of life: a lesson for improving end of life health care. *Hospice J* 1998; 13:89–100.

Kaufmann R. Matrix-assisted laser desorption ionization (MALDI) mass spectrometry: a novel analytical tool in molecular biology and biotechnology. *J Biotechnol* 1995; 41:155–175.

Kehl LJ, Trempe TM, Hargreaves KM. A new animal model for assessing mechanisms and management of muscle hyperalgesia. *Pain;* in press.

Laughlin TM, Bethea JR, Yezierski RP, Wilcox GL. Cytokine involvement in dynorphin-induced allodynia. *Pain* 2000; 84:159–167.

Levi-Montalcini R, Skaper SD, Dal Toso R, Petrelli L, Leon A. Nerve growth factor: from neurotrophin to neurokine. *Trends Neurosci* 1996; 19:514–520.

Luo JC, Toyoda M, Shibuya M. Differential inhibition of fluid accumulation and tumor growth in two mouse ascites tumors by an antivascular endothelial growth factor/permeability factor neutralizing antibody. *Cancer Res* 1998; 58:2594–2600.

Ma QP, Woolf CJ. The progressive tactile hyperalgesia induced by peripheral inflammation is nerve growth factor dependent. *Neuroreport* 1997; 8:807–810.

Madsen B, Georg B, Vissing H, Fahrenkrug J. Retinoic acid down-regulates the expression of the vasoactive intestinal polypeptide receptor type-1 in human breast carcinoma cell lines. *Cancer Res* 1998; 58:4845–4850.

Matsukado K, Sugita M, Black KL. Intracarotid low dose bradykinin infusion selectively increases tumor permeability through activation of bradykinin B2 receptors in malignant gliomas. *Brain Res* 1998; 792:10–15.

Mercadante S. What is the definition of breakthrough pain? *Pain* 1991; 45:107–108.

Mercadante S, Maddaloni S, Roccella S, Salvaggio L. Predictive factors in advanced cancer pain treated only by analgesics. *Pain* 1992; 50:151–155.

Mercadante S, Armata M, Salvaggio L. Pain characteristics of advanced lung cancer patients referred to a palliative care service. *Pain* 1994; 59:141–145.

Millan MJ. The induction of pain: an integrative review. *Prog Neurobiol* 1999; 57:1–164.

Miyamoto M, Shimizu Y, Okada K, et al. Effect of interleukin-8 on production of tumor-associated substances and autocrine growth of human liver and pancreatic cancer cells. *Cancer Immunol Immunother* 1998; 47:47–57.

Mundy GR. Malignancy and the skeleton. *Horm Metab Res* 1997; 29:120–127.

Murata T, Ushikubi F, Matsuoka T, et al. Altered pain perception and inflammatory response in mice lacking prostacyclin receptor. *Nature* 1997; 388:678–682.

Nakano R, Oka M, Nakamura T, et al. A leukotriene receptor antagonist, ONO-1078, modulates drug sensitivity and leukotriene C4 efflux in lung cancer cells expressing multidrug resistance protein. *Biochem Biophys Res Commun* 1998; 251:307–312.

Nasu K, Matsui N, Narahara H, Tanaka Y, Miyakawa I. Effects of interferon-gamma on cytokine production by endometrial stromal cells. *Hum Reprod* 1998; 13:2598–2601.

Nesland JM, Holm R, Johannessen JV, Gould VE. Neuroendocrine differentiation in breast lesions. *Pathol Res Pract* 1988; 183:214–221.

Nogueira E, Navarro S, Pellin A, Llombart-Bosch A. Activation of TRK genes in Ewing's sarcoma. Trk A receptor expression linked to neural differentiation. *Diagnostic Mol Pathol* 1997; 6:10–16.

North WG, Fay MJ, Longo KA, Du J. Expression of all known vasopressin receptor subtypes by small cell tumors implies a multifaceted role for this neuropeptide. *Cancer Res* 1998; 58:1866–1871.

Novakovic SD, Tzoumaka E, McGivern JG, et al. Distribution of the tetrodotoxin-resistant sodium channel PN3 in rat sensory neurons in normal and neuropathic conditions. *J Neurosci* 1998; 18:2174–2187.

Okuse K, Chaplan SR, McMahon SB, et al. Regulation of expression of the sensory neuron-specific sodium channel SNS in inflammatory and neuropathic pain. *Mol Cell Neurosci* 1997; 10:196–207.

Palma C, Manzini S. Substance P induces secretion of immunomodulatory cytokines by human astrocytoma cells. *J Neuroimmunol* 1998; 81:127–137.

Paul A, Habib F. Low-affinity nerve growth factor receptors (p75LNGFR) in human prostate tissue: stromal localisation. *Urol Res* 1998; 26:111–116.

Payne R. Cancer pain mechanisms and etiology. In: Abram SE (Ed). *Cancer Pain*. Boston: Kluwer Academic, 1989, pp 1–10.

Petersen M, Segond von Banchet G, Heppelmann B, Koltzenburg M. Nerve growth factor regulates the expression of bradykinin binding sites on adult sensory neurons via the neurotrophin receptor p75. *Neuroscience* 1998; 83:161–168.

Pflug B. Djakiew D. Expression of p75NTR in a human prostate epithelial tumor cell line reduces nerve growth factor-induced cell growth by activation of programmed cell death. *Mol Carcinog* 1998; 23:106–114.

Piovezan AP, D'Orleans-Juste P, Tonussi CR, Rae GA. Endothelins potentiate formalin-induced nociception and paw edema in mice. *Can J Physiol Pharmacol* 1997; 75:596–600.

Pituch-Noworolska A, Gawlicka M, Wotoszyn M, et al. Tumour necrosis factor alpha (TNF alpha) and leukaemic cells: secretion and response. *Clin Lab Haematol* 1998; 20:231–238.

Polomano RC, Mannes AJ, Bennett GJ. Paclitaxel-induced painful peripheral neuropathy in rats. *Soc Neurosci Abstr* 1998; 24, Part 1:381.

Portenoy RK. Cancer pain. Epidemiology and syndromes. *Cancer* 1989; 63:2298–2307.

Raffa RB, Schupsky JJ, Jacoby HI. Endothelin-induced nociception in mice: mediation by ETA and ETB receptors. *J Pharmacol Exp Ther* 1996; 276:647–651.

Reubi JC, Mazzucchelli L, Hennig I, Laissue JA. Local up-regulation of neuropeptide receptors in host blood vessels around human colorectal cancers. *Gastroenterology* 1996; 110:1719–1126.

Rozengurt E, Sinnett-Smith J. Bombesin stimulation of DNA synthesis and cell division in cultures of Swiss 3T3 cells. *Proc Natl Acad Sci USA* 1983; 80:2936–2940.

Scholar EM, Paul S. Stimulation of tumor cell growth by vasoactive intestinal peptide. *Cancer* 1991; 67:1561–1564.

Schug SA, Zech D, Dorr U. Cancer pain management according to WHO analgesic guidelines. *J Pain Symptom Manage* 1990; 5:27–32.

Seckl M J, Higgins T, Widmer F, Rozengurt E. [D-Arg1,D-Trp5,7,9,Leu11] substance P: a novel potent inhibitor of signal transduction and growth in vitro and in vivo in small cell lung cancer cells. *Cancer Res* 1997; 57:51–54.

Seufferlein T, Rozengurt E. Galanin, neurotensin, and phorbol esters rapidly stimulate activation of mitogen-activated protein kinase in small cell lung cancer cells. *Cancer Res* 1996; 56:5758–5764.

Smith JA, Amagasu SM, Eglen RM, Hunter JC, Bley KR. Characterization of prostanoid receptor-evoked responses in rat sensory neurones. *Br J Pharmacol* 1998; 124:513–523.

Sommer C, Schafers M. Painful mononeuropathy in C57BL/Wld mice with delayed Wallerian degeneration: differential effects of cytokine production and nerve regeneration on thermal and mechanical hypersensitivity. *Brain Res* 1998; 784:154–162.

Sommer C, Schmidt C, George A. Hyperalgesia in experimental neuropathy is dependent on the TNF receptor 1. *Exp Neurol* 1998; 151:138–142.

Stefano GB. Autoimmunovascular regulation: morphine and anandamide and ancondamide stimulated nitric oxide release. *J Neuroimmunol* 1998; 83:70–76.

Taipale J, Saharinen J, Keski-Oja J. Extracellular matrix-associated transforming growth factor-beta: role in cancer cell growth and invasion. *Adv Cancer Res* 1998; 75:87–134.

Tallarida RJ. Statistical analysis of drug combinations for synergism. *Pain* 1992; 49:93–97.

Tallarida R, Murray R. *Manual of Pharmacological Calculations with Computer Programs.* New York: Springer Verlag, 1987, pp 26–31.

Tallarida RJ, Porreca F, Cowan A. Statistical analysis of drug-drug and site-site interactions with isobolograms. *Life Sci* 1989; 45:947–961.

Tsujino K, Yamate J, Tsukamoto Y, et al. Establishment and characterization of cell lines derived from a transplantable rat malignant meningioma: morphological heterogeneity and production of nerve growth factor. *Acta Neuropathol* 1997; 93:461–470.

Ushikubi F, Hirata M, Narumiya S. Molecular biology of prostanoid receptors; an overview. *J Lipid Mediat Cell Signal* 1995; 12:343–359.

Vigano A, Bruera E, Suarez-Almazor ME. Age, pain intensity, and opioid dose in patients with advanced cancer. *Cancer* 1998; 83:1244–1250.

Vigano A, Dorgan M, Bruera E, Suarez-Almazor ME. The relative accuracy of the clinical estimation of the duration of life for patients with end of life cancer. *Cancer* 1999; 86:170–176.

Wacnik PW, Kehl LJ, Cash JM, et al. Incidental hyperalgesia induced by an osteolytic tumor or carrageenan in the mouse forelimb. *Soc Neurosci Abstr* 1999; (Part 1)25:686.

Wacnik PW, Kehl LJ, Trempe TM, et al. Osteolytic tumors in C3H mice promote thermal and mechanical allodynia, grip hyperalgesia and increased spinal c-fos immunoreactivity. Abstracts: *9th World Congress on Pain.* Seattle: IASP Press, 1999, p 139.

Wacnik PW, Stone LS, Laughlin TM, et al. A practical model of cancer pain: comparing different hind limb sites of melanoma cell implantation. *Soc Neurosci Abstr* 1998; 24:628.

Wasilenko WJ, Cooper J, Palad AJ, et al. Calcium signaling in prostate cancer cells: evidence for multiple receptors and enhanced sensitivity to bombesin/GRP. *Prostate* 1997; 30:167–173.

Watanabe K, Hiraki H, Hasegawa H, et al. Immunohistochemical localization of endothelin-1, endothelin-3 and endothelin receptors in human pheochromocytoma and paraganglioma. *Pathol Int* 1997; 47:540–546.

Wolff H, Saukkonen K, Anttila S, et al. Expression of cyclooxygenase-2 in human lung carcinoma. *Cancer Res* 1998; 58:4997–5001.

World Health Organization. *Cancer Pain Relief: With a Guide to Opioid Availability,* 2nd ed. World Health Organization, 1996, p 63.

Correspondence to: George L. Wilcox, PhD, Departments of Pharmacology and Neuroscience, University of Minnesota, 6-120 Jackson, 321 Church Street SE, Minneapolis, MN 55455-0217, USA. Tel: 612-625-1474; Fax: 612-625-8408; email: george@umn.edu.

Proceedings of the 9th World Congress on Pain, Progress in Pain Research and Management, Vol. 16, edited by M. Devor, M.C. Rowbotham, and Z. Wiesenfeld-Hallin, IASP Press, Seattle, © 2000.

59

Late Sequelae of Post-Mastectomy Radiotherapy

Ulf E. Kongsgaard, Bjorn Erikstein, and Stener Kvinnsland

Departments of Anesthesia and Oncology, The Norwegian Radium Hospital, Montebello, Oslo, Norway

Radiotherapy for breast cancer has long been known to reduce regional recurrence of the disease, while improvement in long-term survival has been difficult to show. However, in 1997 two studies were performed (Overgaard et al. 1997; Ragaz et al. 1997) that showed significantly prolonged overall survival in high-risk premenopausal women with breast cancer. Survival was also enhanced for postmenopausal women in the same risk group (Overgaard et al. 1999). Yet despite the clinical benefits of irradiation of breast cancer, sequelae of this treatment could compromise a patient's quality of life. We evaluated symptoms from late sequelae in breast cancer patients who had undergone two different regimes of adjuvant irradiation.

METHODS

A total of 2113 patients were treated with either 10 fractions at 4.3 gray (Gy; 1 Gy = 1 joule/kg irradiated tissue) (1496 patients) or 20 fractions at 2.5 Gy (617 patients) of radiation applied to the breast wall and/or regional lymph nodes; 450 of these patients were still alive at the end of 1996. From this group, 361 patients were examined for late side effects of radiation. Of these, 245 patients had received the 4.3 Gy and 119 the 2.5 Gy fractions. The median observation time for the latter two groups was 16 years and 10 years, respectively. Some members of the 4.3 Gy patient group were eligible for economic compensation for severe late sequelae.

The patients were examined clinically by an oncologist (for a general evaluation of sequelae), and by a physiotherapist (for evaluation of lymphedema, shoulder joint movement, and pain). Radiological evaluation of the thorax was performed by a radiologist (to assess lung fibrosis, pleural changes, and skeletal changes including rib fractures). Scores from the three different evaluations were divided into four categories: no sequelae, few sequelae, moderate sequelae, and considerable sequelae. A patient score (based on the patients' total experience), was divided into the same categories. Patients evaluated their own pain experience and the degree to which pain interfered in their life by means of the Brief Pain Inventory (BPI) (Daut et al. 1983).

RESULTS

Arm edema, fractures of the ribs, and impaired shoulder function were the three most common objective factors predicting late side effects of radiation in all patients. The incidence of significant arm edema was 4.2% in the 2.5 Gy group and 19.6% in the 4.3 Gy group, respectively; rib changes affected 1.7% and 9.5%, and impaired shoulder function 4.2% and 22.0%,

Table I
Percentage (and number) of patients with different sequelae scores in the two irradiation regimens

Score*		Irradiation Regimen					
		4.3 Gy		2.5 Gy		Total	
DocScore	No	45%	(11)	40%	(47)	16%	(58)
	Little	35%	(86)	50%	(59)	40%	(145)
	Moderate	38%	(93)	10%	(12)	29%	(105)
	Considerable	22%	(55)	0.8%	(1)	15%	(56)
PhyScore	No	1.6%	(4)	40%	(48)	14%	(52)
	Little	35%	(85)	45%	(54)	28%	(139)
	Moderate	46%	(112)	14%	(17)	35%	(129)
	Considerable	18%	(44)	0%	(0)	12%	(44)
RadScore	No	1.2%	(3)	43%	(50)	15%	(53)
	Little	54%	(132)	50%	(58)	53%	(190)
	Moderate	30%	(73)	5.1%	(6)	23%	(79)
	Considerable	14%	(35)	2.6%	(3)	11%	(38)
PatScore	No	5.3%	(13)	34%	(40)	15%	(53)
	Little	19%	(47)	43%	(51)	27%	(98)
	Moderate	43%	(105)	19%	(23)	35%	(128)
	Considerable	33%	(80)	4.2%	(5)	23%	(85)

* DocScore = score by oncologist; PhyScore = score by physiotherapist; RadScore = score by radiologist; PatScore = score by patient.

Table II
Pearson correlation (r) between the scores provided by the oncologist (DocScore), physiotherapist (PhyScore), radiologist (RadScore), and patient (PatScore)

Score	Correlation	DocScore	PhyScore	RadScore	PatScore
DocScore	Pearson correlation	–	0.808**	0.461**	0.743**
	No. patients		361	359	361
PhyScore	Pearson correlation		–	0.449**	0.690**
	No. patients			359	361
RadScore	Pearson correlation			–	0.331**
	No. patients				359

** $P \leq 0.01$ (two-tailed).

respectively. Comparison of the different scores assigned by the oncologist, the physiotherapist, the radiologist, and the patients themselves was most relevant for the purposes of our study (Table I). The group that had undergone larger fractions of irradiation had the worst outcome.

There was a strong correlation between the different score categories (Table II), independently of whether the patients had any prospect of economic compensation. Most patients had pain that interfered with their life, as evaluated by the BPI (Fig. 1). Furthermore, when the BPI score was split into pain scores (based on the four visual analogue scale [VAS] scores for pain) and reduced function scores (based on the seven VAS scores for pain

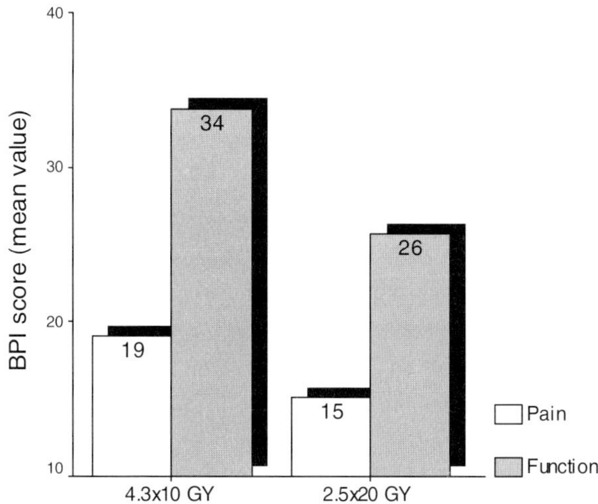

Fig. 1. Brief Pain Inventory (BPI) scores, split into pain score (based on four VAS scores for pain measurements; maximum 40 points) and reduced function score (seven VAS scores for pain interference with everyday function measurements; maximum 70 points).

interference with daily functions), there was a strong correlation with the other scores used, especially for the BPI pain score. Despite high BPI pain scores, only 134 patients (37.1%) were on pain medication. These included 53 patients (14.7%) on acetaminophen (paracetamol) and 49 patients (13.6%) on acetaminophen + codeine. Nineteen patients (5.2%) were taking aspirin or nonsteroidal anti-inflammatory drugs, four patients (1.1%) were taking antidepressants, and no patients were taking anticonvulsants. Only five patients (1.4%) were taking strong opioids.

DISCUSSION

Expectations for long-term survival have emerged in breast cancer patients treated with therapeutic radiotherapy. Therefore, late sequelae of thoracic irradiation have come under scrutiny. It is obvious that treatment may produce physical and psychological distress that could compromise a patient's quality of life.

The symptoms found in the two patient groups are typical for late sequelae of irradiation (Bentzen and Overgaard 1993). However, the incidence of arm edema, fractures of the ribs, and impaired shoulder function were well within the acceptable range for the 2.5 Gy group of patients, while as expected, patients receiving larger fractions (4.3 Gy) had more pronounced side effects.

The full range of deleterious effects has not been fully evaluated. Symptoms were most likely influenced by surgical technique (Halsted's technique), complications after surgery, rehabilitation after primary treatment, and late rehabilitation. Some side effects such as secondary nerve injury and lymphedema can be related both to surgery as well as to radiotherapy. Furthermore, such aspects as type of work and social network were not considered in this report. Although there was a correlation between all the different scoring systems used (Table II), the patient scores (both the global patient score and the BPI score) were generally higher compared to the scores performed by the oncologist, physiotherapist, and radiologist.

Several considerations should be kept in mind when using self-report measures of cancer pain and suffering: (1) Pain is multidimensional, (2) pain develops and changes over time, (3) suffering comes from many sources and involves many processes, (4) selection of assessment tool should directly reflect clinical purpose, selection of assessment tool should directly reflect definition of pain, and (5) the self-report of pain experience can be strongly affected by diverse contextual factors.

It is likely, however, that people attempted to honestly report their subjective pain experience in most cases, since the patterns of self-report scores were comparable in the two groups, despite expectations of possible economic compensation in one of the groups.

Why was consumption of traditional analgesics so low? Pain scores were relatively high, especially using the four VAS pain measurements in the Brief Pain Inventory (Fig. 1). Also, few patients used adjuvant analgesic drugs commonly used in similar pain syndromes. Several explanations could be suggested: (1) The patients have accepted suffering as part of their disease, (2) the patients have accepted suffering as part of their treatment regimen, (3) the patients have prior negative experiences with drug treatments, (4) the patients are poor responders to traditional analgesics, and (5) the patients were not referred to pain clinics or treated by pain specialists.

Although most symptoms in the two patient groups were typical for late irradiation sequelae, the pathophysiological changes comprised a group of heterogeneous disorders characterized by variable presentations and probably variable responses to treatment. This study cannot capture the full clinical dimension of the suffering from the treatment regimes used. However, based on our results, we conclude that late sequelae after adjuvant breast irradiation are associated with physical and psychological distress that compromises the quality of life and that these problems may be underestimated.

Although modern radiotherapy, with lower daily fractions and better computerized tomography planning, will reduce the deleterious effects, this report characterizes a patient group with the requirements for a thorough assessment and a possible treatment potential.

REFERENCES

Bentzen SM, Overgaard M. Early and late normal-tissue injury after postmastectomy radiotherapy. In: Hinkelbein W, Bruggmoser G, Frommhold H, Wannenmacher K (Eds). *Recent Results in Cancer Research*, Vol. 130. Berlin: Springer-Verlag, 1993, pp 59–78.

Daut RL, Cleeland CS, Flanery RC. Development of the Wisconsin Brief Pain Questionnaire to assess pain in cancer and other diseases. *Pain* 1983; 17:197–210.

Ragaz J, Jackson MJ, Le N, Plenderlith IH, et al. Adjuvant radiotherapy and chemotherapy in node-positive premenopausal women with breast cancer. *N Engl J Med* 1997; 337:956–962.

Overgaard M, Hansen PS, Overgaard J, Rose C, et al. Postoperative radiotherapy in high-risk premenopausal women with breast cancer who receive adjuvant radiotherapy. *N Engl J Med* 1997; 337:949–955.

Overgaard M, Jensen MB, Overgaard J, Rose C, et al. Postoperative radiotherapy in high-risk postmenopausal breast-cancer patients given adjuvant tamoxifen: Danish Breast Cancer Cooperative Group DBCG 82c randomised trial. *Lancet* 1999; 353:1641–1648.

Correspondence to: Ulf E. Kongsgaard, MD, PhD, Department of Anesthesia, The Norwegian Radium Hospital, Montebello, 0310 Oslo, Norway. Fax: 47-22-93-42-90; email: u.e.kongsgaard@klinmed.uio.no.

Proceedings of the 9th World Congress on Pain,
Progress in Pain Research and Management,
Vol. 16, edited by M. Devor, M.C. Rowbotham, and
Z. Wiesenfeld-Hallin, IASP Press, Seattle, © 2000.

60

Coupling of Sympathetic and Somatosensory Neurons following Nerve Injury: Mechanisms and Potential Significance for the Generation of Pain[1]

Martin Michaelis

Physiological Institute, Christian-Albrechts University, Kiel, Germany

The sympathetic nervous system has several biological functions that subserve the preservation of body homeostasis. Painful tissue-damaging events threaten the integrity of the organism and thus disturb the homeostasis. Therefore, reflex changes in sympathetic activity, which are usually evoked by noxious events, likely have a protective function (Jänig 1995). That is, under normal conditions the sympathetic nervous system *responds to pain*. However, activity in sympathetic neurons does not significantly excite somatosensory neurons. In particular, sympathetic activity *does not induce pain* (Jänig and Koltzenburg 1992).

For several syndromes that may develop following peripheral nerve trauma and are characterized by chronic pain, it has been assumed that the sympathetic nervous system is involved in the generation and maintenance of pain. The clinical phenomenology of these syndromes has been described comprehensively elsewhere (Bonica 1990; Blumberg and Jänig 1994; Baron et al. 1999). The hypothesis of a sympathetically maintained pain component in these syndromes is essentially based on observations that sympatholytic procedures lead to at least temporary pain relief (Bonica 1990; Jänig and Stanton-Hicks 1996). Pain maintained by sympathetic innervation or by circulating catecholamines has been termed *sympathetically maintained pain* (SMP) (Merskey and Bogduk 1994; Stanton-Hicks et al. 1995).

[1] Mini-review based on a congress workshop.

The realization that SMP exists inevitably led to the conclusion that a coupling between the sympathetic and sensory nervous system developed in the affected patients consequent to peripheral nerve trauma. Understanding of plastic changes occurring in the peripheral or central nervous system due to the nerve trauma, and which are the basis for the novel sympathetic-sensory coupling, is fundamental for the development of rational therapies.

Two questions immediately arise concerning (1) *where* sympathetic-sensory coupling may develop and (2) *how* activity in sympathetic neurons may affect sensory processing. This chapter reviews recent results, mostly obtained from animal studies, which yield evidence for several pathophysiological mechanisms causing sympathetic-sensory coupling under well-defined experimental conditions. These results may finally lead to a better understanding of SMP in patients.

SITES OF SYMPATHETIC-SENSORY COUPLING

In contrast to the separation of the sympathetic and the somatosensory nervous system found under normal conditions, evidence is accumulating for the development of functional sympathetic-sensory coupling consequent to a peripheral nerve injury. I use the term sympathetic-sensory coupling when evidence exists for excitatory (or inhibitory) effects on activity in sensory neurons produced by experimental stimulation of the sympathetic supply or by local or systemic application of sympathetic transmitters.

Sympathetic-sensory coupling develops following peripheral nerve injury at three different sites (Fig. 1): in a neuroma after partial or complete

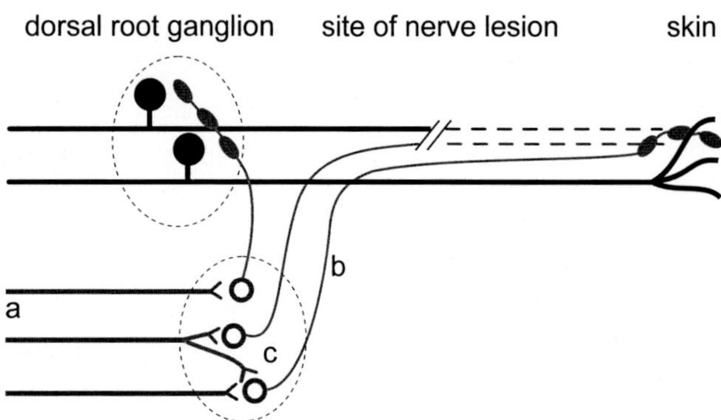

Fig. 1. Sympathetic-sensory coupling may develop in the skin following partial nerve lesion, at the site of the nerve lesion (in a nerve-end neuroma or a neuroma-in-continuity), or within a dorsal root ganglion following complete or partial nerve lesion. (a–b) pre/postganglionic sympathetic fibers; (c) paravertebral sympathetic ganglion.

nerve transection, in the skin following partial nerve lesion, and within dorsal root ganglia (DRG) containing somata of sensory neurons that have been axotomized by the nerve lesion.

THE NEUROMA

After transection of a peripheral nerve most axotomized sensory neurons start to regenerate. Some of these afferents survive, although their sprouts fail to reach target tissue but instead remained chronically trapped in a neuroma. This situation has often been experimentally mimicked by tightly ligating a nerve before cutting it. Neuroma afferents could be excited by electrical stimulation of sympathetic fibers projecting into the neuroma or by systemic or local application of catecholamines (Wall and Gutnick 1974; Devor and Jänig 1981; Scadding 1981; Blumberg and Jänig 1984; Burchiel 1984; Welk et al. 1990; Chen et al. 1996; Rubin et al. 1997). Some responding afferents had thinly myelinated or unmyelinated axons and many presumably were nociceptors (Devor and Jänig 1981; Blumberg and Jänig 1984). In patients complaining about pain originating from chronic neuromas of the nerve endings, perineuromal injections of epinephrine exacerbated the pain (Chabal et al. 1992). Nonadrenergic sympathetic transmitters (e.g., neuropeptide Y, see below) also may excite neuroma afferents, particularly in the chronic state (Jänig 1990).

THE SKIN

Receptive endings of intact cutaneous nociceptors in normal animals do not respond to catecholamines (see Jänig and Koltzenburg 1992). Sato and Perl (1991) were the first to demonstrate that under certain circumstances receptive endings of intact cutaneous nociceptors may acquire novel catecholamine sensitivity: following partial transection of a cutaneous nerve in rabbits some of the remaining intact afferents projecting through the same nerve could now be excited by electrical stimulation of the sympathetic supply or by close arterial injection of norepinephrine (NE). The coupling indeed occurred in the skin and not at the nerve lesion site, because it could be suppressed completely by infiltration of the afferent's receptive field with a local anesthetic (Sato and Perl 1991). The catecholamine sensitivity was demonstrable a few days after nerve lesion and remained for months. The excitatory effects were mediated predominantly via α_2-adrenoceptors (Sato and Perl 1991; O'Halloran and Perl 1997; Perl 1999) and were more pronounced in unmyelinated nociceptors than in thinly myelinated nociceptors (Bossut and Perl 1995).

A similar result occurred following chronic constriction injury (CCI) of the saphenous nerve in rats: a subgroup of unmyelinated fibers, which projected through the site of the constriction lesion, was excited by NE superfusion of their receptive fields (Koltzenburg et al. 1994). The report emphasized that NE-sensitive afferents exhibited low or no spontaneous activity, while spontaneous activity of higher frequency in other fibers was either unchanged or reduced by NE (Koltzenburg et al. 1994). This finding indicates that NE sensitivity is not a corollary of an increased excitability as judged by the level of spontaneous activity, but is presumably based on a specific mechanism (see below).

Axons (both of sensory and postganglionic sympathetic neurons) in major peripheral nerves do not all arise from the same spinal nerve but from two or more adjacent spinal nerves. Therefore, cutting one of these spinal nerves results in another form of partial nerve injury. When in monkeys the lumbar spinal nerve L6 was ligated, some remaining intact unmyelinated cutaneous nociceptors in the superficial peroneal nerve became sensitive to NE superfusion of their receptive field (Ali et al. 1999). In contrast to the findings in rabbits (see above), the NE effect in monkeys is predominantly mediated by α_1-adrenoceptors (Ali et al. 1999).

It is not known to date whether receptive endings of afferent fibers, which successfully regenerated after axotomy, may remain responsive to catecholamines. In some patients with SMP following nerve lesion, iontophoretic intracutaneous application of NE aggravated the pain (Torebjörk et al. 1995). However, in the clinical setting it must inevitably remain unclear whether NE excited regenerated afferents or unlesioned neighboring afferents. In one study on cats, afferent and sympathetic fibers were allowed to regenerate for more than a year after nerve transection and resuture. This study revealed that low-frequency electrical stimulation of the sympathetic supply and also systemic catecholamine injection excited some unmyelinated afferent fibers (Häbler et al. 1987). However, the study did not investigate whether the responding afferent fibers had reinnervated peripheral target tissue or whether their axon endings were chronically trapped in a neuroma-in-continuity, which had formed after nerve suture.

THE DORSAL ROOT GANGLION

Following peripheral nerve lesion, some sensory neurons start to exhibit continuous discharges that originate from the DRG (Wall and Devor 1983; Devor and Wall 1990). First indications for a sympathetic-sensory coupling within DRG came from studies showing that following transection of the sciatic nerve in rats, more than 50% of those DRG neurons exhibiting spontaneous activity responded to electrical stimulation of the sympathetic supply (McLachlan et al. 1993; Devor et al. 1994). During the first 2 months after sciatic nerve lesion, this sympathetic-sensory coupling in the DRG was predominantly excitatory; later, most sympathetically evoked responses were inhibitory (Michaelis et al. 1996). Both excitatory and inhibitory sympathetic-sensory coupling in the DRG was mainly α_2-adrenoceptor mediated (Chen et al. 1996). Intriguingly, a recent study has shown that continuing activity arises in muscle afferents but not in cutaneous afferents following transection of major branches of the sciatic nerve (Michaelis et al. 1999). Most muscle afferents with continuing activity had myelinated axons of intermediate conduction velocity, which indicates that some are likely nociceptors (Michaelis et al. 1999). In contrast to DRG neurons with spontaneous activity, excitation of afferents not exhibiting continuing activity by sympathetic stimulation was rare (Devor et al. 1994; Michaelis et al. 1996).

Evidence for an excitatory sympathetic-sensory coupling in the DRG has also been reported following CCI of the sciatic nerve (Xie et al. 1995; Petersen et al. 1996; Zhang et al. 1997) and following spinal nerve lesion (Eschenfelder et al. 1999). The coupling seems to be mainly restricted to spontaneously active DRG neurons with myelinated axons after spinal nerve and sciatic nerve lesions, whereas after CCI, excitatory responses to NE were observed in unmyelinated and in myelinated afferents (Xie et al. 1995; Zhang et al. 1997).

While we have good evidence that activation of sympathetic neurons can increase the firing frequency in many spontaneously active DRG neurons following peripheral nerve injury, the occurrence of spontaneous activity itself is probably entirely independent of the sympathetic supply. Following spinal nerve lesion in rats, no significant difference in the incidence of spontaneous activity or in firing frequency or pattern occurred in those with intact sympathetic supply compared with sympathectomized rats (Liu et al. 2000). Instead, development of spontaneous activity within DRG following peripheral nerve injury depends on an enhanced incidence of high-frequency oscillations in the membrane potential of DRG neurons (Amir et al. 1999).

MODES OF SYMPATHETIC-SENSORY COUPLING

As reviewed above, convincing experimental evidence points to α-adrenergic sympathetic-sensory coupling following nerve injury. Such coupling is not detectable under normal conditions, so injury must in some way trigger its development.

DIRECT COUPLING

An attractive hypothesis postulates that as a result of a nerve injury some afferent neurons express functional α-adrenoceptors, which then directly mediate excitatory catecholamine effects (Fig. 2; Campbell et al. 1991; Perl 1994, 1999). Support for this hypothesis comes from studies providing immunohistochemical evidence for an increased expression of α_{2A}-adrenoceptors on DRG neurons both after spinal nerve ligation (Cho et al. 1997) and after partial or complete sciatic nerve transection (Birder and Perl 1999). The increase was detected in DRG neurons of all diameters including small-diameter neurons, which were presumably nociceptors, but the increase was most prominent in medium-sized to large neurons (Birder and Perl 1999). These descriptive results raise important questions.

What is the trigger for upregulation of adrenoceptors on sensory neurons? The finding that nociceptive afferents acquired catecholamine sensitivity not only after partial nerve injury (see above) but also—albeit to a lesser degree—after sympathectomy (Bossut et al. 1996) has prompted a suggestion that a similar mechanism that induces denervation supersensitivity of autonomic effector organs following sympathetic denervation may trigger upregulation of adrenoceptors on sensory neurons (Perl 1994; 1999). This hypothesis, however, awaits direct proof.

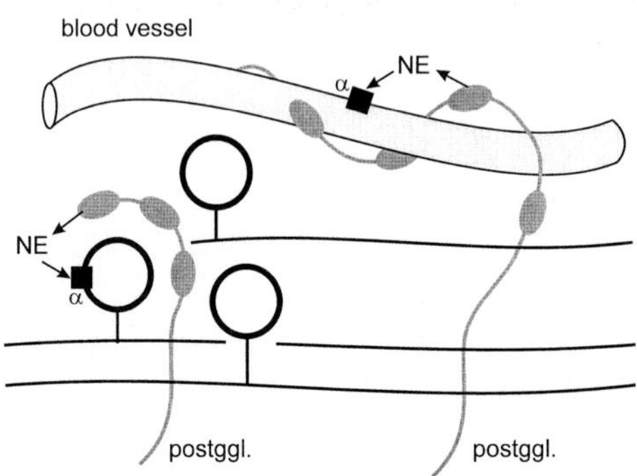

Fig. 2. Two pathophysiological mechanisms may contribute to sympathetic-sensory coupling in dorsal root ganglia following peripheral nerve lesion. *Direct coupling*: Norepinephrine (NE) released from sympathetic postganglionic (postggl.) fibers activates α-adrenoceptors, which are expressed on sensory neurons following nerve lesion. *Indirect coupling:* Some sensory neurons may become sensitive to even mild hypoxia after nerve lesion. NE activates α-adrenoceptors on vascular smooth muscle cells, thereby decreasing oxygen pressure downstream. In this way, sympathetic activity could indirectly excite sensory neurons. A similar mechanism may act in nerve-end neuromas.

How do functional adrenoceptors appear in the membrane of sensory neurons? Several possibilities exist. One is novel synthesis of adrenoceptors followed by their functional expression. Moreover, it is conceivable that adrenoceptors are already present on sensory neurons, although in a non-functional state, and that they become functional following by nerve injury. Consistent with this hypothesis, immunohistochemistry techniques have demonstrated that a subset of predominantly small, substance P-containing afferents expresses α_{2A}-adrenoceptors in intact DRG (Gold et al. 1997; Stone et al. 1998; Birder and Perl 1999). However, activation of these receptors does not induce excitatory responses, at least under normal conditions. To the contrary, adrenoreceptor activation inhibits transmitter release from central terminals of primary afferents in the spinal cord (Yaksh 1985). Perhaps nerve injury induces changes in intracellular transduction pathways so that activation of the same type of adrenoceptor mediates inhibition under normal conditions, but excitation after nerve lesion? Note also that any depolarization produced by NE will not be translated into spikes except in the presence of an axotomy-induced increase in subthreshold membrane potential oscillations (Amir et al. 1999).

Where exactly on sensory neurons are adrenoceptors expressed? The aforementioned studies provided evidence for adrenoceptor expression in DRG preparations. Therefore, these results are particularly well suited to explain sympathetic-sensory coupling in the DRG. A direct proof of adrenoceptor expression on receptive endings of uninjured cutaneous afferents, some of which acquire NE sensitivity after partial nerve lesion, is still missing.

A second line of evidence favoring the direct coupling hypothesis is based on electrophysiological experiments on dissociated DRG neurons. NE increased the excitability of lumbar DRG neurons that were obtained from rats with a prior sciatic nerve transection; NE did not change excitability of control neurons from intact rats (Abdulla and Smith 1997). This NE action is mediated by α_2-adrenoceptors and is presumably based on attenuation of a calcium-dependent potassium conductance. The strongest effects were detected in small cells and in cells from animals, that exhibited autotomy behavior. Neuropeptide Y, another sympathetic transmitter, enhances excitability of DRG neurons after nerve lesion via Y2 receptors, and likewise by attenuation of a calcium-dependent potassium conductance (Abdulla and Smith 1999). These results have been obtained on isolated DRG cells. Their relevance for stimulus encoding and signal transduction in sensory neurons in vivo has yet to be demonstrated.

INDIRECT COUPLING

A further consequence of a peripheral nerve lesion is that axotomized sensory neurons may become particularly sensitive to hypoxia. First, axon tips of many neuroma afferents respond to local ischemia (Korenman and Devor 1981; Burchiel 1984). Second, as described above, several axotomized afferents develop continuing discharges, which originate within the DRG. This ectopic activity is enhanced during periods of hypoxia; in addition, formerly silent DRG neurons begin to discharge (Burchiel 1984; Häbler et al. 1998; Eschenfelder et al. 1999; see also Häbler et al., this volume). NE and possibly other neurotransmitters released from postganglionic sympathetic neurons in the neuroma and the DRG or circulating catecholamines evoke dose-dependent vasoconstriction via activation of α-adrenoceptors on vascular smooth muscle cells (Fig. 2). It is this sympathetically induced vasoconstriction that may cause a degree of hypoxia sufficient to excite sensitive axotomized afferent neurons (Häbler et al. 1998; Eschenfelder et al. 1999). In contrast, receptive endings of spared afferents that developed catecholamine sensitivity following partial nerve injury (see above) did not respond to vigorous vasoconstriction induced by vasopressin or even to complete arterial occlusion (Sato and Perl 1991; O'Halloran and Perl 1997).

SYMPATHETIC SPROUTING IN DORSAL ROOT GANGLIA

An intriguing morphological phenomenon has been observed in DRG following peripheral nerve lesions. While in normal rat DRG only few postganglionic sympathetic fibers innervate blood vessels, they exhibit a massive sprouting response to peripheral nerve lesions and invade the DRG proper where some build up basket formations around cell bodies of DRG neurons (McLachlan et al. 1993; Chung et al. 1993; Jänig and McLachlan 1994; Chung et al. 1997; Shinder et al. 1999; for discussion of mechanisms of sympathetic sprouting in DRG see Ramer et al. 1999). These sympathetic baskets have been assumed to form the morphological basis for sympathetic-sensory coupling in DRG. However, several obstacles impede such a straightforward interpretation.

The first is that functional excitatory sympathetic-sensory coupling is evident significantly earlier than the appearance of basket formations (McLachlan et al. 1993; Devor et al. 1994; Jänig et al. 1996; Ramer and Bisby 1998). Therefore, we must conclude that the phenomenon of sympathetic baskets is unimportant for the onset of sympathetic-sensory coupling in DRG. However, sympathetic sprouting starts soon after nerve injury, so it is possible that these sprouts are important for sympathetic-sensory coupling in DRG (Ramer and Bisby 1998).

Sympathetic stimulation primarily excites neurons with myelinated axons in the DRG. Although sympathetic baskets are also usually found around large sensory neurons, it is not clear whether the responding neurons are the same ones that are surrounded by the baskets. During the first days after nerve lesion, when no baskets are present, most DRG neurons only respond when the sympathetic supply is stimulated at relatively high frequencies of 20–50 Hz (Devor et al. 1994). We could assume that once a DRG neuron is wrapped by sympathetic sprouts, a much increased concentration of transmitter now reaches the neuron so that it should already respond to low-frequency sympathetic stimulation. However, to date we have no evidence for excitatory responses in DRG neurons after low-frequency sympathetic stimulation when baskets are definitely present in the DRG (Michaelis et al. 1996). An explanation might be that only 1–2% of all DRG neurons are surrounded by baskets (McLachlan et al. 1993) and investigations to date might simply have missed those few DRG neurons surrounded by baskets.

Nevertheless, it appears worthwhile to address the question of the role of this novel anatomical arrangement in altered pain generation in patients with SMP.

CONCLUSIONS

Experimental evidence reveals the development of a variety of pathological interactions of sympathetic and sensory neurons after peripheral nerve injury. However, studies have yet to provide definite proof that any of these mechanisms underlie the maintenance of pain. Therefore, we should consider these mechanisms as proposals until careful clinical investigations have resolved their pathophysiological relevance.

Patients suffering from peripheral nerve lesions may chronically complain about spontaneous pain and different forms of hypersensitivity, e.g., to mechanical or thermal stimulation of the affected skin (see Koltzenburg 1997). Patients differ greatly with regard to the sympathetic component of the pain, i.e., each form of pain may be sympathetically maintained in one patient but sympathetically independent in others. No symptoms or diagnostic tests other than sympatholytic procedures can identify SMP. It is even more enigmatic that a particular nerve trauma may give rise to SMP in a few affected patients, but that similar trauma does not cause any form of chronic pain in most others.

This astonishing interindividual variability invites the speculation that a genetic predisposition separates patients with SMP from other persons. Evidence supporting the general idea of heritability as an important factor for the generation of chronic pain comes from a recent study on different inbred mouse strains that demonstrated remarkable differences among strains with respect to behavioral signs of continuing and evoked pain following standard nerve lesions (Mogil et al. 1999). Therefore, future investigations on patients with SMP should seriously consider the possibility that a genetic factor contributes to the underlying pathophysiology of this chronic pain condition.

ACKNOWLEDGMENTS

The author thanks Wilfrid Jänig for comments, Stefan Becker for carefully reading the manuscript, and Eike Tallone for her expert help with the illustrations. Supported by the Deutsche Forschungsgemeinschaft (Mi 457/2-1).

REFERENCES

Abdulla FA, Smith PA. Ectopic alpha 2-adrenoceptors couple to N-type $Ca2^+$ channels in axotomized rat sensory neurons. *J Neurosci* 1997; 17:1633–1641.

Abdulla FA, Smith PA. Nerve injury increases an excitatory action of neuropeptide Y and Y2 agonists on dorsal root ganglion neurons. *Neuroscience* 1999; 89:43–60.

Ali Z, Ringkamp M, Hartke TV, et al. Uninjured C-fiber nociceptors develop spontaneous activity and alpha-adrenergic sensitivity following L6 spinal nerve ligation in monkey. *J Neurophysiol* 1999; 81:455–466.

Amir R, Michaelis M, Devor M. Membrane potential oscillations in dorsal root ganglion neurons: role in normal electrogenesis and neuropathic pain. *J Neurosci* 1999; 19:8589–8596.

Baron R, Levine JD, Fields HL. Causalgia and reflex sympathetic dystrophy: does the sympathetic nervous system contribute to the generation of pain? *Muscle Nerve* 1999; 22:678–695.

Birder LA, Perl ER. Expression of alpha 2-adrenergic receptors in rat primary afferent neurones after peripheral nerve injury or inflammation. *J Physiol (Lond)* 1999; 515:533–542.

Blumberg H, Jänig W. Clinical manifestations of reflex sympathetic dystrophy and sympathetically maintained pain. In: Wall PD, Melzack R (Eds). *Textbook of Pain.* Livingstone: Churchill, 1994, pp 685–697.

Bonica JJ. Causalgia and other reflex sympathetic dystrophies. In: Bonica JJ (Eds). *The Management of Pain.* Philadelphia: Lea and Febinger, 1990, pp 220–243.

Bossut DF, Perl ER. Effects of nerve injury on sympathetic excitation of Aδ mechanical nociceptors. *J Neurophysiol* 1995; 73:1721–1723.

Bossut DF, Shea VK, Perl ER. Sympathectomy induces adrenergic excitability of cutaneous C-fiber nociceptors. *J Neurophysiol* 1996; 75:514–517.

Burchiel KJ. Spontaneous impulse generation in normal and denervated dorsal root ganglia: sensitivity to alpha-adrenergic stimulation and hypoxia. *Exp Neurol* 1984; 85:257–272.

Campbell JN, Meyer RA, Raja SN. Is nociceptor activation by alpha-1 adrenoreceptors the culprit in sympathetically maintained pain? *APS J* 1992; 1:3–11.

Chabal C, Jacobson L, Russell LC, Burchiel KJ. Pain response to perineuromal injection of normal saline, epinephrine, and lidocaine in humans. *Pain* 1992; 49:9–12.

Chen Y, Michaelis M, Jänig W, Devor M. Adrenoceptor subtype mediating sympathetic-sensory coupling in injured sensory neurons. *J Neurophysiol* 1996; 76:3721–3730.

Cho HJ, Kim DS, Lee NH, et al. Changes in the alpha 2-adrenergic receptor subtypes gene expression in rat dorsal root ganglion in an experimental model of neuropathic pain. *Neuroreport* 1997; 8:3119–3122.

Chung K, Kim HJ, Sik H, Park MJ, Chung JM. Abnormalities of sympathetic innervation in the area of an injured peripheral nerve in a rat model of neuropathic pain. *Neurosci Lett* 1993; 162:85–88.

Chung K, Yoon YW, Chung JM. Sprouting sympathetic fibers form synaptic varicosities in the dorsal root ganglion of the rat with neuropathic injury. *Brain Res* 1997; 751:275–280.

Devor M, Jänig W. Activation of myelinated afferents ending in a neuroma by stimulation of the sympathetic supply in the rat. *Neurosci Lett* 1981; 24:43–47.

Devor M, Wall PD. Cross-excitation in dorsal root ganglia of nerve-injured and intact rats. *J Neurophysiol* 1990; 64:1733–1746.

Devor M, Jänig W, Michaelis M. Modulation of activity in dorsal root ganglion (DRG) neurons by sympathetic activation in nerve-injured rats. *J Neurophysiol* 1994; 71:38–47.

Devor M, Shinder V, Govrin-Lippmann R. Sympathetic sprouting in axotomized rat DRG: ultrastructure. *Soc Neurosci Abstr* 1995; 21:894.

Eschenfelder S, Grunow B, Brinker H, et al. Neurogenic vasoconstriction in the dorsal root ganglion may play a crucial role in the sympathetic-afferent coupling after peripheral nerve injury. *Abstracts: 9th World Congress on Pain.* Seattle: IASP Press, 1999; p 298.

Gold MS, Dastmalchi S, Levine JD. Alpha 2-adrenergic receptor subtypes in rat dorsal root and superior cervical ganglion neurons. *Pain* 1997; 69:179–190.

Häbler H-J, Jänig W, Koltzenburg M. Activation of unmyelinated afferents in chronically lesioned nerves by adrenaline and excitation of sympathetic efferents in the cat. *Neurosci Lett* 1987; 82:35–40.

Häbler H-J, Liu X-G, Eschenfelder S, Jänig W. Responses of axotomized afferents to blockade of nitric oxide synthesis after spinal nerve lesion in the rat. *Neurosci Lett* 1998; 254:33–36.

Jänig W. Activation of afferent fibers ending in an old neuroma by sympathetic stimulation in the rat. *Neurosci Lett* 1990; 111:309–314.

Jänig W. Spinal cord reflex organization of sympathetic systems. *Prog Brain Res* 1996; 107:43–77.

Jänig W, Koltzenburg M. Possible ways of sympathetic afferent interaction. In: Jänig W, Schmidt RF (Eds). *Reflex Sympathetic Dystrophy. Pathophysiological Mechanisms and Clinical Implications*. Weinheim: VCH, 1992, pp 213–243.

Jänig W, McLachlan EM. The role of modifications in noradrenergic peripheral pathway after nerve lesions in the generation of pain. In: Fields HL, Liebeskind JC (Eds). *Pharmacological Approaches to the Treatment of Pain: New Concepts and Critical Issues,* Progress in Pain Research and Management, Vol. 1. Seattle: IASP Press, 1994, pp 101–128.

Jänig W, Stanton-Hicks M. *Reflex Sympathetic Dystrophy: A Reappraisal,* Progress in Pain Research and Management, Vol. 6. Seattle: IASP Press, 1996.

Jänig W, Levine JD, Michaelis M. Interactions of sympathetic and primary afferent neurons following nerve injury and tissue trauma. *Prog Brain Res* 1996; 113:161–184.

Koltzenburg M. The sympathetic nervous system and pain. In: Dickenson A, Besson J-M (Eds). *The Pharmacology of Pain,* Handbook of Experimental Pharmacology, Vol. 130. Berlin: Springer, 1997, pp 61–91.

Koltzenburg M, Kees S, Budweiser S, Ochs G, Toyka KV. The properties of unmyelinated afferents change in a chronic constriction neuropathy. In: Gebhardt GF, Hammond DL, Jensen TS (Eds). *Proceedings of the 7th World Congress on Pain,* Progress in Pain Research and Management, Vol. 2. Seattle: IASP Press, 1994, pp 511–522.

Korenman EM, Devor M. Ectopic adrenergic sensitivity in damaged peripheral nerve axons in the rat. *Exp Neurol* 1981; 72:63–81.

Liu X-G, Eschenfelder S, Blenk K-H, Jänig W, Häbler H-J. Spontaneous activity of axotomized afferent neurons after L5 spinal nerve injury in rats. *Pain* 2000; in press.

McLachlan EM, Jänig W, Devor M, Michaelis M. Peripheral nerve injury triggers noradrenergic sprouting within dorsal root ganglia. *Nature* 1993; 363:543–546.

Merskey H, Bogduk N. *Classification of Chronic Pain: Descriptions of Chronic Pain Syndromes and Definition of Terms.* Seattle: IASP Press, 1994.

Michaelis M, Devor M, Jänig W. Sympathetic modulation of activity in dorsal root ganglion neurons changes over time following peripheral nerve injury. *J Neurophysiol* 1996; 76:753–763.

Michaelis M, Liu X-G, Jänig W. Ongoing activity in axotomized DRG neurons. *J Peripher Nerv Syst* 1999; 4:148–149.

Mogil JS, Wilson SG, Bon K, et al. Heritability of nociception I: responses of 11 inbred mouse strains on 12 measures of nociception. *Pain* 1999; 80:67–82.

O'Halloran KD, Perl ER. Effects of partial nerve injury on the responses of C-fiber polymodal nociceptors to adrenergic agonists. *Brain Res* 1997; 759:233–240.

Perl ER. A reevaluation of mechanisms leading to sympathetically related pain. In: Fields HL, Liebeskind JC (Eds). *Pharmacological Approaches to the Treatment of Chronic Pain: New Concepts and Critical Issues,* Progress in Pain Research and Management, Vol. 1. Seattle: IASP Press, 1994, pp 129–150.

Perl ER. Causalgia, pathological pain, and adrenergic receptors. *Proc Natl Acad Sci USA* 1999; 96:7664–7667.

Petersen M, Zhang J, Zhang J-M, LaMotte RH. Abnormal spontaneous activity and responses to norepinephrine in dissociated dorsal root ganglion cells after chronic nerve constriction. *Pain* 1996; 67:391–397.

Ramer MS, Bisby MA. Differences in sympathetic innervation of mouse DRG following proximal or distal nerve lesions. *Exp Neurol* 1998; 152:197–207.

Ramer MS, Thompson SWN, McMahon SB. Causes and consequences of sympathetic basket formation in dorsal root ganglia. *Pain* 1999; (Suppl)6:S111–S120.

Rubin G, Kaspi T, Rappaport ZH, et al. Adrenosensitivity of injured afferent neurons does not require the presence of postganglionic sympathetic terminals. *Pain* 1997; 72:183–191.

Sato J, Perl ER. Adrenergic excitation of cutaneous pain receptors induced by peripheral nerve injury. *Science* 1991; 251:1608–1610.

Scadding JW. Development of ongoing activity, mechanosensitivity, and adrenaline sensitivity in severed peripheral nerve axons. *Exp Neurol* 1981; 73:345–364.

Shinder V, Govrin-Lippmann R, Cohen S, et al. Structural basis of sympathetic-sensory coupling in rat and human dorsal root ganglia following peripheral nerve injury. *J Neurocytol* 1999; in press.

Stanton-Hicks M, Jänig W, Hassenbusch S, et al. Reflex sympathetic dystrophy: changing concepts and taxonomy. *Pain* 1995;127–133.

Stone LS, Broberger C, Vulchanova L, et al. Differential distribution of alpha 2A and alpha 2C adrenergic receptor immunoreactivity in the rat spinal cord. *J Neurosci* 1998; 18:5928–5937.

Torebjörk E, Wahren LK, Wallin G, Hallin R, Koltzenburg M. Noradrenaline-evoked pain in neuralgia. *Pain* 1995; 63:11–20.

Wall PD, Devor M. Sensory afferent impulses originate from dorsal root ganglia as well as from the periphery in normal and nerve injured rats. *Pain* 1983; 17:321–339.

Wall PD, Gutnick M. Ongoing activity in peripheral nerves: the physiology and pharmacology of impulses originating from a neuroma. *Exp Neurol* 1974; 43:580–593.

Welk E, Leah JD, Zimmermann M. Characteristics of A- and C-fibers ending in a sensory nerve neuroma in the rat. *J Neurophysiol* 1990; 63:759–766.

Xie Y, Zhang J, Petersen M, LaMotte RH. Functional changes in dorsal root ganglion cells after chronic nerve constriction in the rat. *J Neurophysiol* 1995; 73:1811–1820.

Yaksh TL. Pharmacology of spinal adrenergic systems which modulate spinal nociceptive processing. *Pharmacol Biochem Behav* 1985; 22:845–858.

Zhang JM, Song XJ, LaMotte RH. An in vitro study of ectopic discharge generation and adrenergic sensitivity in the intact, nerve-injured rat dorsal root ganglion. *Pain* 1997; 72:51–57.

Correspondence to: Martin Michaelis, Dr med, Physiologisches Institut, Christian-Albrechts-Universität, Olshausenstr. 40, 24098 Kiel, Germany. Tel: 49-(0)431-8802029; Fax: 49-(0)431-8804580; email: m.michaelis@physiologie.uni-kiel.de.

Proceedings of the 9th World Congress on Pain,
Progress in Pain Research and Management,
Vol. 16, edited by M. Devor, M.C. Rowbotham, and
Z. Wiesenfeld-Hallin, IASP Press, Seattle, © 2000.

61

Immobility in Volunteers Transiently Produces Signs and Symptoms of Complex Regional Pain Syndrome

Stephen H. Butler,[a] Mayvor Nyman,[b] and Torsten Gordh[b]

[a]*Pain Center, University of Washington, Seattle, Washington, USA;*
[b]*Pain Center, University Hospital, Uppsala, Sweden*

This topic aroused interest at the Pain Center at the University of Washington several years ago when the 8-year-old daughter of one of the anesthesiologists fell and broke her wrist. On removal of the cast we all were impressed at the atrophy, hair growth, warmth, and stiffness. "It sure looks like RSD!" was the universal comment. Needless to say, all of these changes returned to normal in short order, and pain was never a part of the girl's symptoms. However, we began to wonder at the changes that normally occur after immobilization in casts and why they often appeared so similar to the clinical problem then called reflex sympathetic dystrophy (RSD).

The syndrome has been renamed complex regional pain syndrome, type I (CRPS-I) by the International Society for the Study of Pain (IASP; Merskey and Bogduk 1994) but many of the same ideas, especially regarding the disease model, linger on and bias therapy toward treating the sympathetic nervous system, which may or may not be involved (Bonica 1990). The obvious explanation that most of the signs and symptoms of either CRPS-I or the old RSD are merely disuse has been ignored because this theory negates the more exotic disease model so firmly entrenched in the folklore of pain therapy, especially among those who treat by procedures.

Let us summarize the IASP diagnostic criteria for CRPS-I: (1) The presence of an initiating noxious event, or a cause for immobilization. (2) Continuing pain, allodynia, or hyperalgesia in which the pain is disproportionate to any inciting event. (3) Evidence at some time of edema, changes in skin blood flow, or abnormal sudomotor activity in the region of the pain.

(4) This diagnosis is excluded by the existence of conditions that would otherwise account for the degree of pain and dysfunction.

In a previous study (Butler et al. 1996), we looked at the signs and symptoms of CRPS-I in a group of 28 patients 4–8 weeks after open reduction and internal fixation of calcaneal fractures. In the clinical examination, 24 patients had a temperature difference greater than 1°C between their feet (12 were warmer and 12 cooler in the injured foot), 23 patients had reduced range of motion, 22 had abnormal swelling, and 21 had abnormal color. Sixteen patients reported sensitivity to touch, and 10 sensitivity to cold. Of more than 800 patients with calcaneal fractures operated on by the surgeon involved, only two are known to have gone on to have a documented case of CRPS-I. One might say that all of these findings are normal postoperative signs and symptoms. All clinicians observe them, but we rarely make the association with CRPS because pain is not a primary symptom.

The study described above was presented at the 8th World Congress on Pain, where concurrently two animal studies were presented that offer insights pertinent to this subject. One study by Ushida and Willis (1996) looked at a rat contracture model with and without a fracture. Two groups of rats were immobilized for 3–4 weeks in full wrist flexion, one group without any other manipulation, the other after radius fracture. The authors demonstrated increased paw withdrawal latencies to von Frey filaments in both groups. They also showed an increase in dorsal horn wide-dynamic-range (WDR) neuron populations equally in both groups over controls. They concluded: "The increased response frequency to innocuous mechanical stimuli suggests that mechanical allodynia occurs after long term casting. In these models, sensitization or plastic changes in the characteristics of dorsal horn neurons was suggested by an increased population of WDR cells and a decreased population of LT [low-threshold] cells." The authors related this not to CRPS but to the pain on remobilization following contracture. They clearly demonstrated that dorsal horn changes occur with immobilization both with and without tissue damage, in this case a radius fracture.

The second study, by Maves and Smith (1996) looked at immobilization in rat hindpaws splinted for 1 week only. They demonstrated thermal hyperalgesia to warmth, mechanical "allodynia," and cold "allodynia." This study simplified the methods of Ushida and Willis by immobilizing a limb in a neutral position without injury. The effects seen were similar to the Ushida and Willis study in that an alteration took place in the processing of sensory data that changed non-noxious information to noxious. These models begin to approximate more closely the clinical situation in CRPS-I than do others in the literature using peripheral or nerve root lesions that have been presented as good animal representations of the syndrome. This study was an animal model of the human study we proposed years ago, to see if signs and symptoms of CRPS could be produced in human volunteers by immobilization alone.

The present study was completed in the Pain Center, University Hospital, Uppsala, Sweden after approval by the institutional ethics committee. Twenty-one volunteers were enrolled. A forearm cast (scaphoid immobilization) was placed on the nondominant arm for 4 weeks. Following removal of the cast, quantitative sensory testing (QST) was performed; subjects filled out a 10-item questionnaire on signs and symptoms of CRPS-I and completed a 5-item questionnaire on signs and symptoms of a neglect-like state (similar to that following stroke; Galer et al. 1995). A short, standardized physical examination for signs of CRPS-I was performed. The results were rather similar to those from the study of the calcaneal fracture patients, as the animal studies would suggest. On clinical examination, all 21 subjects had a temperature difference ranging from 0.5° to 2.7°C (10 were warmer and 11 cooler in the affected arm). Of these, 10 had a difference of over 1°C, and in three of these patients the difference persisted beyond 2 weeks.

Sixteen subjects had decreased range of motion of the thumb. Twelve had altered sensation to sensory testing, of whom four had summation to pinprick and another four had hyperalgesia to pinprick. Pain was only present in seven individuals—burning pain in two and aching pain in five. Eighteen subjects reported stiffness, and other symptoms of CRPS were seen in a few individuals. Fourteen subjects had signs and symptoms of a neglect-like state.

QST to determine warm and cool detection thresholds and hot and cold pain was the most accurate approach to examining sensory processing because dorsal horn neuron function could not be measured directly, as in the Ushida and Willis study. Tests were performed immediately after cast removal, using the contralateral limb as the control. The more notable findings were: (1) decreased tolerance to cold, either cold pain on the immobilized side while the control side was not painful, or pain at a higher temperature on the immobilized side (14/21); (2) increased warmth detection threshold (9/21); and (3) decreased warmth detection threshold (5/21).

These changes were maintained for as long as 5 weeks for cold pain, 3 weeks for increased warm detection threshold, and 1 week for decreased cold detection threshold. No subjects had persistent discomfort at 2 weeks, and none had persistent stiffness after 4 weeks.

Positron emission tomography (PET) studies were also conducted, but full analysis has not been completed. Differences in the patterns at rest between baseline and after casting were found that will require further study.

Many of the subjects in the study, if their presenting complaint were pain in the immobilized limb, would fit the criteria in the IASP taxonomy for CRPS-I. They all were immobilized (criterion 1). The majority (16) had hypersensitivity, at least by QST, and eight had hyperpathia or summation to pinprick (criterion 2). All had temperature differences between the limbs, although only 10 had a difference greater than 1°C. Six subjects had abnormal sweating; seven had skin, hair, or nail changes; and one had abnormal swelling (criterion 3). Finally, none had any underlying disease process that would account for ongoing pain (criterion 4).

The information presented shows clearly, both in animal and human studies, that signs and symptoms of CRPS can be seen after immobilization, with or without prior tissue damage. In the human studies, no individual went on to develop chronic pain or CRPS among the volunteers participating in the casting. In the animal studies, it is clear that dorsal horn changes occurred and that these are compatible with a change in central processing and hypersensitivity. Evidence for such changes in the human volunteers given casts without injury was provided by their history, physical examination, and QST results. These data suggest that we change our thinking about CRPS from the disease model held for so long and reconsider the signs and symptoms as the normal response to disuse. Treatment then should consist of prevention by early active rehabilitation after injury as well as aggressive active and passive physical therapy when pain, stiffness, and other complaints compatible with CRPS follow injury or immobilization.

ACKNOWLEDGMENTS

Research was funded by a county grant from the Uppsala Commun.

REFERENCES

Bonica JJ (Ed). *The Management of Pain,* 2nd ed. Philadelphia: Lea & Febiger, 1990, pp 230–241.

Butler SH, Galer BS, Benirschke S. Disuse as a cause of signs and symptoms of CRPS(I). *Abstracts: 8th World Congress on Pain.* Seattle: IASP Press, 1996, pp 401.

Galer BS, Butler SH, Jensen MP. Case reports and hypothesis: a neglect like syndrome may be responsible for the motor disturbance in reflex sympathetic dystrophy (CRPS-1). *J Pain Symptom Manage* 1995; 10:385–391.

Maves TJ, Smith B. Pain behaviors and sensory alterations following immobilization of the rat hindpaw. *Abstracts: 8th World Congress on Pain.* Seattle: IASP Press 1996, p 118.

Merskey H, Bogduk N. *Classification of Chronic Pain,* 2nd ed. Seattle: IASP Press, 1994, pp 41–43.

Ushida T, Willis WD. Effect of contracture-induced pain in rat: electrophysiological and behavioral study. *Abstracts: 8th World Congress on Pain.* Seattle: IASP Press 1996, p 6.

Correspondence to: Stephen H. Butler, MD, Multidisciplinary Pain Center, University of Washington Medical Center-Roosevelt, 4245 Roosevelt Way NE, Seattle, WA 98105, USA. Fax: 206-548-8776; email: stevpain@u.washington.edu.

Proceedings of the 9th World Congress on Pain,
Progress in Pain Research and Management, Vol. 16, edited by M. Devor, M.C. Rowbotham, and Z. Wiesenfeld-Hallin, IASP Press, Seattle, © 2000.

62

Neurogenic Vasoconstriction in the Dorsal Root Ganglion May Play a Crucial Role in Sympathetic-Afferent Coupling after Spinal Nerve Injury

Heinz-Joachim Häbler,[a] Sebastian Eschenfelder,[a] Henrike Brinker,[a] Birgit Grunow,[a] Xianguo Liu,[b] and Wilfrid Jänig[a]

[a]*Physiological Institute, Christian-Albrechts University, Kiel, Germany;* [b]*Department of Physiology, Sun Yat-sen University of Medical Sciences, Guangzhou, P.R. China*

In patients with sympathetically maintained pain, the mechanisms of sympathetic-afferent coupling are still controversial. In several animal models, electrical stimulation of sympathetic axons can activate lesioned afferents (e.g., Häbler et al. 1987; Devor et al. 1994; Xie et al. 1995) and unlesioned afferents in a partially lesioned nerve (Sato and Perl 1991). Possible sites of sympathetic-afferent coupling are the dorsal root ganglion (DRG), the lesion site, and the peripheral receptor. The underlying coupling mechanism is generally assumed to be a direct mechanism involving activation of α-adrenoceptors upregulated by afferent neurons after nerve lesion (Birder and Perl 1999). The histological substrates of sympathetic-afferent coupling are thought to be the baskets that are formed around cell bodies in the DRG by postganglionic sympathetic axons that sprout from local blood vessels after nerve lesion (McLachlan et al. 1993). However, it is known that afferents ending in a neuroma can be activated by hypoxia (Korenman and Devor 1981). Thus, an alternative possibility is that sympathetic-afferent coupling is generated indirectly and nonspecifically by neurogenic vasoconstriction in the lesioned peripheral nerve or in the DRG. After L5 spinal nerve lesion (SNL) in rats, some of the axotomized afferents develop spontaneous activity (Liu et al. 2000), which is thought to be crucial for generating and maintaining neuropathic pain behavior. Furthermore, the pain behavior in this model is believed to depend on the integrity of the sympathetic nervous system (Kim et al. 1997; but see Ringkamp et al. 1999).

The aim of the present study was to test whether, after L5 SNL, axotomized afferents respond to electrical stimulation of the lumbar sympathetic chain, and whether this response is related to neurogenic vasoconstriction in the DRG.

In anesthetized (Nembutal 60 mg/kg, i.p.) male Wistar rats the left L5 spinal nerve was ligated and cut. The final experiment was conducted 3–56 days after SNL under anesthesia (Nembutal 60 mg/kg initially i.p., and 10 mg/kg i.v. every hour), under muscular paralysis (pancuronium 1 mg/kg initially, maintenance with 0.4 mg/kg when necessary), and with artificial ventilation (with additional oxygen). Arterial blood pressure, tracheal pressure, blood gases, and blood acid-base status were monitored. Rectal temperature was kept constant at around 37°C by means of a feedback-controlled heating blanket. At the end of the experiments, the animals were killed under deep anesthesia by intravenous injection of a saturated solution of potassium chloride. All experiments were approved by the local animal care committee of the state administration and were conducted in accordance with German federal law.

After a lumbosacral laminectomy, single-fiber activity was recorded from axotomized afferent neurons in filaments split from the L5 dorsal root using conventional techniques. The lumbar sympathetic chain was cut bilaterally and stimulated electrically between ganglia of L2 and L3 at frequencies between 1 and 50 Hz (10–20 seconds' duration, supramaximal for C fibers). Vasoconstrictor drugs (N^G-nitro-L-arginine methyl ester [L-NAME], 100 μmol/kg; angiotensin II and nordrenaline, 0.5–1 μg/kg; L-8-ornithine vasopressin, 0.0025–0.5 IU) and α-adrenoceptor antagonists (α_2: yohimbine, 100–400 μg; α_1: prazosin, 50–100 μg) were injected intravenously. Blood flow was recorded from the surface of the L5 DRG using laser Doppler flowmetry (MBF3D, Moor Instruments). Vascular resistance in the DRG was calculated in arbitrary units from mean arterial blood pressure and laser Doppler flow.

Stimulation of the ipsilateral lumbar sympathetic chain at frequencies up to 50 Hz elicited graded phasic vasoconstrictions in the DRG, yet did not affect 103 of the 125 axotomized afferents (82.4%) tested (Fig. 1A). Most of the remainder were activated, but almost all at high stimulation frequencies ≥10 Hz; a few afferents were inhibited (not shown). Responsive axotomized afferents were activated by sympathetic stimulation once a critical vasoconstriction was reached in the DRG (Fig. 2). The activation of afferent fibers always followed neurogenic vasoconstriction at a latency of 10–30 seconds, depending on how fast the critical level of vascular resistance was reached.

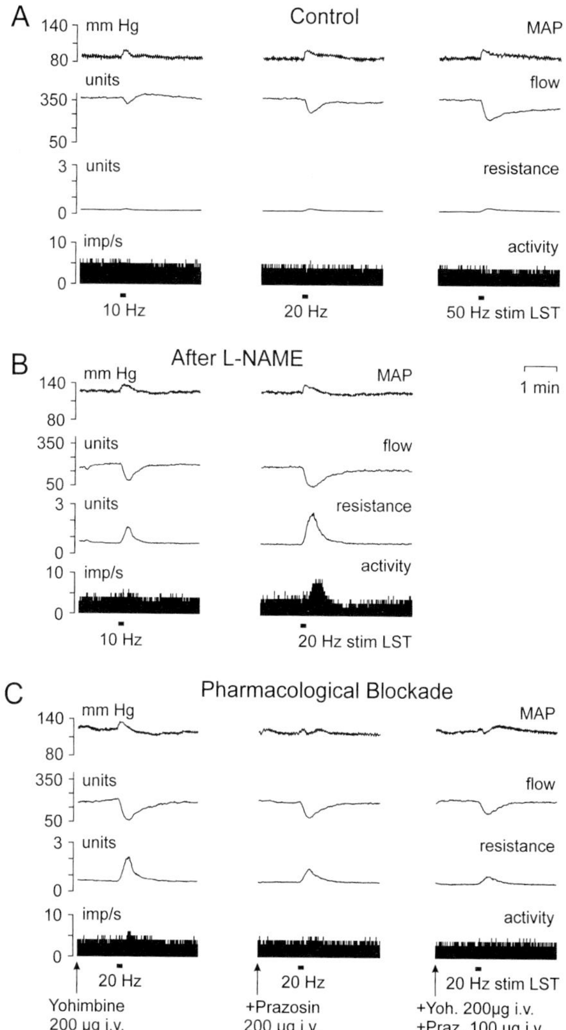

Fig. 1. (A) Lack of response of a lesioned afferent fiber to stimulation of the lumbar sympathetic trunk at frequencies up to 50 Hz (duration of impulse train = 10 s) prior to applying L-NAME. (B) Application of L-NAME induced a sustained baseline vasoconstriction in the dorsal root ganglion (DRG). Sympathetic stimulation now induced much larger phasic vasoconstrictions and activated the afferent fiber at a frequency of 10 Hz. The activation was followed by an after-depression. (C) Both yohimbine (α_2-adrenoceptor antagonist) and prazosin (α_1-adrenoceptor antagonist) reduced neuronal responses to stimulation of the sympathetic chain and neurogenic vasoconstriction in the DRG in parallel. MAP = mean arterial blood pressure; flow = blood flow in the DRG measured by laser Doppler flowmetry; resistance = calculated vascular resistance in the DRG; stim LST = stimulation of the lumbar sympathetic trunk.

The duration of afferent activation matched the time period during which phasic short-lasting vasoconstrictions exceeded this critical level. Typically, the activation was followed by an after-depression (Figs. 1B, 2).

We tested the hypothesis that a reduced baseline perfusion in the DRG may enhance the proportion of fibers that respond to a superimposed phasic vasoconstriction evoked by sympathetic stimulation. L-NAME, applied at 100 μmol/kg i.v., induced a sustained increase in vascular resistance in the DRG (Fig. 1B), but by itself did not change afferent activity (see Häbler et al. 1998). After administration of L-NAME, 25 of 36 previously unresponsive axotomized afferents were activated by sympathetic stimulation (Fig. 1B) (response incidence compared with that prior to L-NAME: $P < 0.001$, χ^2 test); the time course of the response was as described above. All afferents (n = 10) that were activated by sympathetic chain stimulation prior to L-NAME showed stronger activations and were activated at lower frequencies after L-NAME administration. Two fibers were inhibited by lumbar sympathetic trunk (LST) stimulation before and activated by it after L-NAME.

Activation of axotomized afferent neurons to sympathetic stimulation could be mimicked by i.v. injection of vasoconstrictor drugs such as angiotensin II, vasopressin, or noradrenaline. The response was thus probably caused by the vasoconstriction. Yohimbine (α_2-adrenoceptor antagonist) and prazosin (α_1-adrenoceptor antagonist) antagonized, and finally abolished, responses of axotomized afferents to sympathetic stimulation and reduced neurogenic vasoconstriction in the DRG in parallel (Fig. 1C).

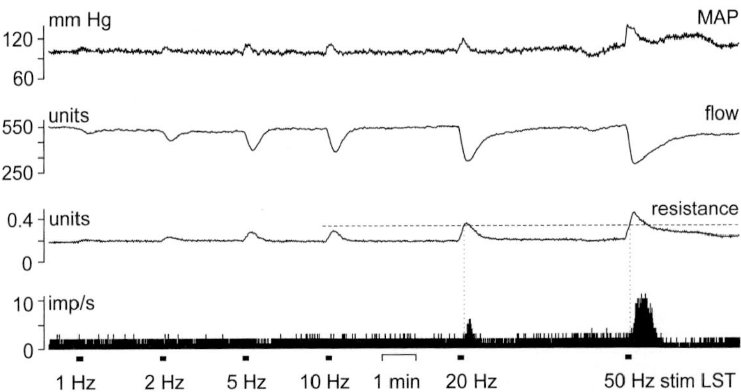

Fig. 2. Response of an axotomized afferent neuron belonging to the minority of fibers that were activated by stimulation of the lumbar sympathetic chain *without* prior application of L-NAME. Sympathetic stimulation evoked frequency-dependent phasic vasoconstrictions in the DRG. The afferent neuron responded only to the highest frequencies used (20–50 Hz). The activation occurred in parallel with vascular resistance exceeding a certain critical threshold value (broken line).

Stimulation-induced vasoconstriction in the L5 DRG was enhanced in rats with L5 SNLs as compared with unlesioned controls (Fig. 3). L-NAME not only increased baseline vascular resistance but also markedly enhanced the amplitude of stimulation-induced vasoconstrictions in the L5 DRG, indicating that stimulation of the sympathetic chain was more efficacious during pronounced vascular preconstriction in the ganglion.

In rats with L5 SNLs, ectopic activity arising in axotomized myelinated afferents is thought to be involved in the generation and maintenance of neuropathic behavior (Sheen and Chung 1992). The present results show that in this rat model of neuropathic pain, only a small percentage of axotomized afferent fibers can be activated by sympathetic stimulation. The fibers that were activated, with one exception, responded only to stimulation frequencies that are too high to occur under physiological conditions. These results are consistent with previous findings showing that in this rat model, sympathectomy changed neither the neuropathic pain behavior (Ringkamp et al. 1999) nor the rate of ectopic activity arising in axotomized afferent fibers (Liu et al. 2000). In aggregate, these results suggest that neuropathic pain behavior in this model is not dependent on the sympathetic nervous system.

Sympathetic stimulation resulted in a frequency-dependent phasic vasoconstriction in the DRG. Responses in axotomized afferent neurons were

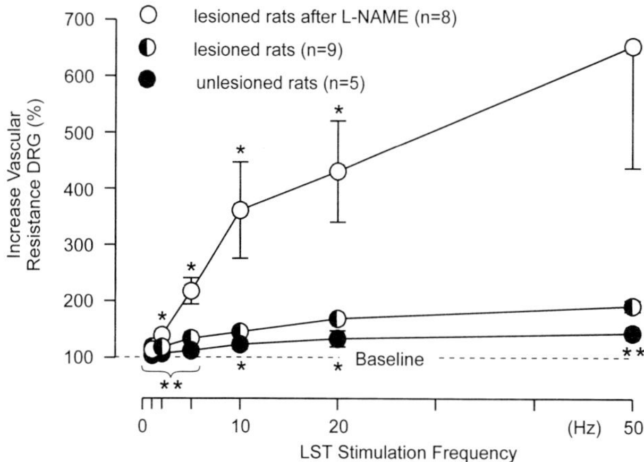

Fig. 3. Electrical stimulation of the lumbar sympathetic trunk (duration of impulse train = 10 s) induced a frequency-dependent vasoconstriction in the L5 DRG. Neurogenic vasoconstriction was significantly stronger in the L5 DRG of lesioned rats than in that of unlesioned rats (* $P < 0.05$, ** $P < 0.01$, t test). L-NAME increased baseline vasoconstriction in the DRG by 200.7 ± 35.1% (n = 8 lesioned rats). From the new baseline, stimulation-induced vasoconstrictions were markedly enhanced. Both effects probably contributed to the increased incidence of afferent neurons responding to stimulation of the lumbar sympathetic trunk after L-NAME. Data are presented as mean ± SEM.

only evoked when vascular resistance exceeded a critical level, and they reflected the time course of the evoked vasoconstriction. It was possible to convert unresponsive afferents into responders by increasing baseline vasoconstriction in the DRG of the lesioned segment. Any vasoconstrictor drug used was capable of reproducing stimulation-induced activation of axotomized afferents. Finally, α_1- and α_2-adrenoceptor antagonists antagonized both the sympathetically induced responses of lesioned afferent fibers and the vasoconstriction in the DRG in parallel. These results suggest that when sympathetic/afferent coupling occurs in the L5 SNL model, it is mainly or exclusively mediated indirectly by stimulation-induced neurogenic vasoconstriction in the DRG of the lesioned segment. Thus, the perfusion of the related DRG appears to be a crucial factor for the activation of axotomized afferents. A role for α-adrenoceptors upregulated on the afferent cell bodies after nerve lesion (Birder and Perl 1999) is not apparent from the present study. On the contrary, if this mechanism were responsible for direct sympathetic/afferent coupling, it would be difficult to explain why a 50-Hz stimulation failed to activate a given axotomized afferent before L-NAME (as in Fig. 1), but a 10-Hz stimulation was sufficient to evoke a response thereafter. As neurogenic vasoconstriction in the DRG of unlesioned rats appears to be weaker than in lesioned ones, one possibility is that sprouted sympathetic fibers forming baskets around afferent cell somata (McLachlan et al. 1993) may contribute to the enhanced vasoconstriction in the DRG of nerve-lesioned rats.

ACKNOWLEDGMENTS

We are grateful to Eike Tallone for producing the illustrations and to Sigrid Augustin for technical help in the experiments. This work was supported by the Deutsche Forschungsgemeinschaft.

REFERENCES

Birder LA, Perl ER. Expression of α_2-adrenergic receptors in rat primary afferent neurones after peripheral nerve injury or inflammation. *J Physiol* 1999; 515:533–542.

Devor M, Jänig W, Michaelis M. Modulation of activity in dorsal root ganglion (DRG) neurons by sympathetic activation in nerve-injured rats. *J Neurophysiol* 1994; 71:38–47.

Häbler H-J, Jänig W, Koltzenburg M. Activation of unmyelinated afferents in chronically lesioned nerves by adrenaline and excitation of sympathetic efferents in the cat. *Neurosci Lett* 1987; 82:35–40.

Häbler H-J, Liu X-G, Eschenfelder S, Jänig W. Responses of axotomized afferents to blockade of nitric oxide synthesis after spinal nerve lesion in the rat. *Neurosci Lett* 1998; 254:33–36.

Kim KJ, Yoon YW, Chung JM. Comparison of three rodent neuropathic pain models. *Exp Brain Res* 1997; 113:200–206.

Korenman EMD, Devor M. Ectopic adrenergic sensitivity in damaged peripheral nerve axons in the rat. *Exp Neurol* 1981; 72:63–81.

Liu X-G, Eschenfelder S, Blenk K-H, Jänig W, Häbler H-J. Spontaneous activity of axotomized afferent neurons after L5 spinal nerve injury in rats. *Pain* 2000; 84:309–318.

McLachlan EM, Jänig W, Devor M, Michaelis M. Peripheral nerve injury triggers noradrenergic sprouting within dorsal root ganglia. *Nature* 1993; 363:543–546.

Ringkamp M, Eschenfelder S, Grethel EJ, et al. Lumbar sympathectomy failed to reverse mechanical allodynia- and hyperalgesia-like behavior in rats with L5 spinal nerve injury. *Pain* 1999; 79:143–153.

Sato J, Perl ER. Adrenergic excitation of cutaneous pain receptors induced by peripheral nerve injury. *Science* 1991; 251:1608–1610.

Sheen K, Chung JM. Signs of neuropathic pain depend on signals from injured nerve fibers in a rat model. *Brain Res* 1992; 610:62–68.

Xie Y, Zhang J, Petersen M, LaMotte RH. Functional changes in dorsal root ganglion cells after chronic nerve constriction in the rat. *J Neurophysiol* 1995; 73:1811–1820.

Correspondence to: H.-J. Häbler, MD, Physiologisches Institut, Christian-Albrechts-Universität Kiel, Olshausenstrasse 40, 24098 Kiel, Germany, Tel: 431-880-2037; Fax: 431-880-2036; email: j.haebler@physiologie.uni-kiel.de.

Proceedings of the 9th World Congress on Pain,
Progress in Pain Research and Management,
Vol. 16, edited by M. Devor, M.C. Rowbotham, and
Z. Wiesenfeld-Hallin, IASP Press, Seattle, © 2000.

63

Does Regional Acute Pain in Humans Alter Regional Sympathetic Discharge?

Magnus Nordin and Mikael Elam

Department of Clinical Neurophysiology, Sahlgren University Hospital, Göteborg, Sweden

Microneurographic recordings of skin sympathetic activity (SSA) from human peripheral nerves have demonstrated that stressful events, including pain, cause generalized activation of sympathetic sudomotor and vasoconstrictor fibers (for reviews see Vallbo et al. 1979; Wallin and Elam 1997). The aim of the present study was to determine whether noxious stimulation, in addition, elicits a regional reflex, leading to stronger SSA increase in the stimulated limb than in the contralateral nonpainful limb.

Measurements of skin temperature and skin blood flow during noxious stimulation suggest the existence of regional sympathetic vasoconstrictor reflexes in humans (Magerl et al. 1990, 1994, 1996), but direct evidence from neural recordings is lacking. In the cat, electrophysiological studies have demonstrated nociceptor-driven segmental sympathetic reflexes (for reviews see Sato and Schmidt 1973; Jänig 1985). If such reflexes are present also in awake humans, they may be important in the pathogenesis of complex regional pain syndrome (CRPS) and sympathetically maintained pain.

METHODS

In 10 healthy volunteers (age 21–36 years), SSA was recorded simultaneously from the common peroneal nerve of both legs using tungsten needle electrodes (for details on microneurography and SSA, see Vallbo et al. 1979; Wallin and Elam 1997). All recordings were obtained from fascicles innervating the skin on the dorsum of the foot. SSA was identified by its characteristic discharge pattern consisting of bursts of multiunit neural impulses that occur "spontaneously" and in response to arousal stimuli and mental stress. The search for the nerve sometimes induced minor discomfort, but once left in a recording position the electrode caused no pain or other sensation. Recordings of skin perfusion (laser Doppler flowmetry) and skin resistance within the innervation zone, skin temperature on the dorsum of the foot, beat-to-beat blood pressure variations (Finapres), ECG, and respiratory chest movements were also obtained, but these data are not included in this preliminary report. The study was approved by the local human ethics committee.

Each subject was asked to lie in supine position on a couch, at an ambient temperature of 23° ± 1°C. After recording of SSA during 5 minutes of relaxation, unilateral painful stimuli were delivered, including noxious mechanical pressure on the big toe and application of mustard oil on the dorsum of the foot. Noxious pressure was exerted manually, using a wooden pencil applied onto the nailbed. The force was gradually increased during a few seconds until the subject declined further increase; the instruction was to accept pain close to tolerance level. This pressure was maintained for 30 seconds. After a period of rest a similar stimulus was given on the contralateral side. A 20 × 25 mm cotton swab soaked with 0.5 mL of mustard oil was applied for 10 minutes on one side only at the end of the experiment. The pain evoked by the stimuli was scored on a verbal rating scale from 0 to 10, where 10 represents the strongest conceivable pain.

The nerve recordings were analyzed from a mean voltage display, where the burst pattern of SSA is evident. The linear correlation between the nerve signals on the two sides was calculated for a prestimulus control period, and during stimulation (all 30 seconds of toe pressure; last 60 seconds of mustard oil; control periods of corresponding duration). The relative changes in SSA total burst area in both nerves were calculated from the same time periods. Values are reported as mean ± SD. Student's t test for paired data was used. The chosen level of significance was $P < 0.05$.

RESULTS

NOXIOUS MECHANICAL PRESSURE

The intense pain evoked by this 30-second stimulus had an acute onset. As exemplified in Fig. 1, the unilateral stimulation caused a strong increase in SSA to both legs that appeared symmetric both with respect to burst pattern and magnitude of the response. For the 10 subjects, the linear correlation between the two nerve signals was high at rest ($r = 0.80 \pm 0.08$) and did not change significantly during pain stimulation ($r = 0.79 \pm 0.09$). Although the average increase in SSA tended to be larger in the stimulated

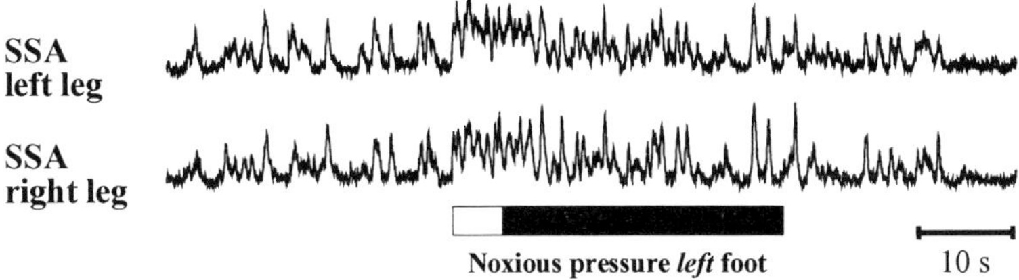

Fig. 1. Bilateral symmetric increases in peroneal nerve skin sympathetic activity (SSA) during noxious mechanical stimulation of the left big toe (pain rating 8). Open part of bar indicates initial increase in applied pressure, filled part represents the 30 seconds of constant pressure level used for analysis.

limb (+192 ± 65% vs. +162 ± 35% contralaterally), this slight asymmetry was not statistically significant ($P = 0.36$).

MUSTARD OIL

This stimulus induced a slowly increasing low to moderate pain. Even when the pain reached its peak after 10 minutes it was less intense than during noxious pressure (mean rating 3.2 vs. 6.8). As illustrated by Fig. 2, recordings showed no asymmetric change in SSA. For the 10 subjects, the linear correlation between SSA on the two sides did not change significantly between the control period ($r = 0.75 \pm 0.13$) and the 10th minute of stimulation ($r = 0.74 \pm 0.15$).

The subject whose results are shown in Fig. 2 showed no overt increase in SSA during mustard oil stimulation despite a maximal pain rating of 7. In the 10 subjects, SSA increased on the average about 30% bilaterally when

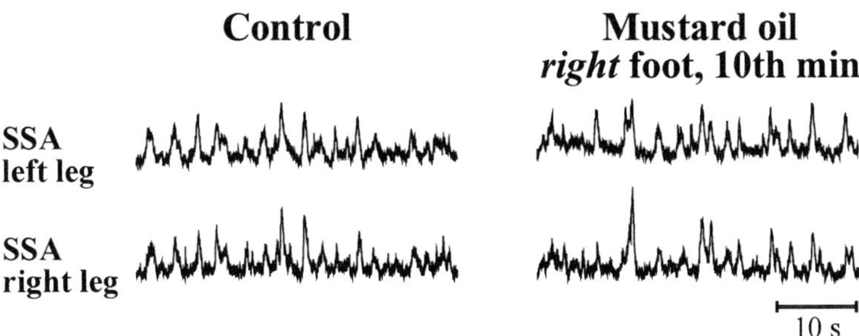

Fig. 2. In the subject shown in Fig. 1, mustard oil applied to the right foot evoked pain almost equally intense as that caused by noxious pressure (rating 7 vs. 8). Despite the similar level of pain there was no increase, nor any overt asymmetry, in skin sympathetic activity (SSA).

mustard oil was applied. However, this was apparently due to mental stress, since the rise occurred before the onset of pain (and sometimes when the subject was approached prior to any stimulation). This initial increase was followed by a gradual reduction; during the 10th minute, when the pain peaked, there was no significant change in the total amount of SSA compared to the control period, nor any significant difference between sides.

DISCUSSION

The present bilateral recordings of SSA lend no support to the existence of a regional sympathetic reflex induced by noxious mechanical or chemical stimulation. Thus, there was no significant pain-induced asymmetry in SSA burst pattern (as evidenced by linear correlation analysis) or in SSA burst size (as reflected by relative changes in burst area).

Our results seem to conflict with indirect evidence of regional sympathetic reflexes based on graded, nonhabituating cutaneous vasoconstrictor responses to noxious mechanical stimulation (Magerl et al. 1990, 1994) and small but significantly asymmetrical skin temperature changes following application of mustard oil (Magerl et al. 1994, 1996). Several reasons for this apparent discrepancy have to be considered: (1) Although bilateral SSA recordings should be a sensitive method to detect a regional reflex, our data cannot unequivocally rule out a slightly asymmetric change in *burst size*. The somewhat larger ipsilateral increase in SSA observed during noxious pressure was far from statistically significant, but warrants the inclusion of additional subjects before final publication of the study. The evidence against a regional change in SSA *burst pattern* is firmer, since the linear correlation was virtually unchanged during both types of stimulation. (2) The duration of our mechanical stimulus was 30 s. This may be too short and tends to conceal an asymmetry, since cutaneous vasoconstriction during noxious pressure (according to Magerl et al. 1994) has two phases: one initial unspecific "arousal" response and a later, somatotopically organized, tonic phase attributed to spinal processing of nociceptor input. A mechanical stimulus of 2 minutes' duration was therefore added in the course of our study and the results will be included in our final report. (3) Mustard oil was applied in a similar way, as described by Magerl et al. (1996), but the pain ratings given by our subjects were lower (3.2 on a 0–10 verbal scale compared to 65% on a visual analogue scale in Magerl's study). The lower pain rating, and other seemingly conflicting results, may be related to the fact that we chose to study the lower instead of the upper extremities. This choice was governed by the fact that SSA recordings are easier to obtain in the peroneal nerve than in the arm.

As mentioned above, SSA is derived from both vasoconstrictor and sudomotor fibers (and possibly also from vasodilator fibers; Nordin 1990; Noll et al. 1994; Sugenoya et al. 1998). It could therefore be argued that an increase in vasoconstrictor activity may be masked by a concomitant decrease in the activity of other sympathetic fibers. However, vasoconstrictor and sudomotor activity differ in burst duration (Bini et al. 1980) and degree of baroreflex modulation (cf. Wallin and Elam 1997), and a major shift between these fiber types is thus likely to be detected by linear correlation analysis.

Despite the above mentioned limitations, our results argue strongly against the existence of any pronounced regional SSA reflex induced by acute regional pain, at least where the lower limb is concerned. In particular, there were no signs of any change in SSA burst pattern. The small regional SSA reflexes that might occur seem functionally negligible compared to the strong general changes in SSA known to occur during mental stress and thermoregulation.

Autonomic phenomena in CRPS have hypothetically been attributed to a pain-induced regional increase in sympathetic neural outflow. The present study provides no evidence for such a sympathetic reflex under physiological conditions, and available studies of CRPS patients do not support the notion of regionally altered sympathetic nerve activity. Thus, Elam (1997) reported bilateral SSA recordings in three CRPS patients with marked signs of autonomic dysfunction in the affected extremity. In all patients the SSA burst pattern was similar in the two limbs, arguing against a reflex change in sympathetic outflow. In fact, the number of active sympathetic fibers seems to be *decreased* in the affected limb of such patients, according to regional plasma concentrations of catecholamines (Drummond et al. 1991). Judged from this, regional vasoconstriction in CRPS is more likely to be caused by denervation supersensitivity to noradrenaline than by a regional sympathoexcitatory reflex.

ACKNOWLEDGMENTS

The study was supported by the Swedish Medical Research Council (project 12170) and the Medical Faculty of Göteborg. We thank Tomas Karlsson and Göran Pegenius for excellent technical assistance.

REFERENCES

Bini G, Hagbarth K-E, Hynninen P, Wallin BG. Thermoregulatory and rhythm-generating mechanisms governing the sudomotor vasoconstrictor outflow in human cutaneous nerves. *J Physiol (Lond)* 1980; 306:537–552.

Drummond PD, Finch PM, Smythe GA. Reflex sympathetic dystrophy: the significance of differing plasma catecholamine concentration in affected and unaffected limbs. *Brain* 1991; 114:2025–2036.

Elam M. Is reflex sympathetic dystrophy a valid concept? *Behav Brain Sci* 1997; 20:447–448.

Jänig W. Organization of the lumbar sympathetic outflow to skeletal muscle and skin of the cat hindlimb and tail. *Rev Physiol Biochem Pharmacol* 1985; 102:119–213.

Magerl W, Geldner G, Handwerker HO. Pain and vascular reflexes in man elicited by prolonged noxious mechano-stimulation. *Pain* 1990; 43:219–225.

Magerl W, Koltzenburg M, Meyer-Jürgens D, Handwerker HO. The somatotopic organization of nociceptor-induced vascular response pattern reflects central nociceptive processing in humans. In: Gebhart GF, Hammond DL, Jensen TS (Eds). *Proceedings of the 7th World Congress on Pain,* Progress in Pain Research and Management, Vol. 2. Seattle: IASP Press, 1994, pp 843–856.

Magerl W, Koltzenburg M, Schmitz JM, Handwerker HO. *J Auton Nerv Syst* 1996; 57:63–72.

Noll G, Elam M, Kunimoto M, Karlsson T, Wallin BG. Skin sympathetic nerve activity and effector function during sleep in humans. *Acta Physiol Scand* 1994; 151:319–329.

Nordin M. Sympathetic discharges in the human supraorbital nerve and their relation to sudo- and vasomotor responses. *J Physiol (Lond)* 1990; 423:241–255.

Sato A, Schmidt RF. Somatosympathetic reflexes. Afferent fibers, central pathways, discharge characteristics. *Physiol Rev* 1973; 53:916–947.

Sugenoya J, Iwase S, Mano T, et al. Vasodilator component in sympathetic nerve activity destined for the skin of the dorsal foot of mildly heated humans. *J Physiol (Lond)* 1998; 507:603–610.

Vallbo Å, Hagbarth K-E, Torebjörk HE, Wallin BG. Somatosensory, proprioceptive and sympathetic activity in human peripheral nerves. *Physiol Rev* 1979; 59:919–957.

Wallin BG, Elam M. Cutaneous sympathetic nerve activity in humans. In: Morris JL, Gibbins IL (Eds). *Autonomic Innervation of the Skin.* Amsterdam: Harwood Academic, 1997, pp 111–132.

Correspondence to: Magnus Nordin, MD, PhD, Department of Clinical Neurophysiology, Sahlgren University Hospital, SE-413 45 Göteborg, Sweden. Tel: 46-31-3424860; Fax: 46-31-821268; email: magnus.nordin@neuro.gu.se.

Proceedings of the 9th World Congress on Pain,
Progress in Pain Research and Management,
Vol. 16, edited by M. Devor, M.C. Rowbotham, and
Z. Wiesenfeld-Hallin, IASP Press, Seattle, © 2000.

64

Pain Syndromes That May Develop as a Result of Treatment Interventions

Paolo Marchettini,[a] Fabio Formaglio,[a] Antonio Barbieri,[a] Laura Tirloni,[b] and Marco Lacerenza[a]

[a]*Pain Medicine Center, and* [b]*Department of Clinical Psychology, Scientific Institute and Hospital, San Raffaele, Milan, Italy*

DEFINITIONS

Iatrogenesis refers to a medical problem "generated or caused by medicine (or medical doctors)." The *Oxford English Dictionary* credits Bleuler for the introduction of this term in 1924 (quoted by Sharpe and Faden 1998). In reality, the tenet *"Primum non nocere"* (first do no harm) dates back to the Hippocratic era, as does the awareness that medicine can at times be dangerous for the patient.

However, what was so obvious to the Greeks, who called poison and drug by the same name (Φαρμακον = pharmacon), has been forgotten with the impressive success of modern medicine. The discovery of antibiotics and anesthesia, together with the improvement of surgical techniques, has provided such relief to mankind that physicians of the early part of this century enjoyed demigod status (Sharpe and Faden 1998). The consequent unrealistic expectations of patients and paternalistic attitudes of doctors have backfired, and today's doctor-patient relationship is undermined by litigation, causing frustration on both sides.

The time has come for patients and doctors to accept that medicine is powerful, yet potentially dangerous, and that the more powerful drugs and interventions become, the more dangerous they can be. Patients should expect side effects, and doctors must work harder to identify, control, and avoid potential risks. The 1991 Harvard Medical Press Practice Study reports that almost 70% of the iatrogenic complications that affect more than 1.3 million hospitalized patients annually are preventable (Brennan et al.

1991). Early recognition and prevention of iatrogenic problems have become even more important today, because medicine provides not only life-saving interventions, but also cosmetic services aimed at improving nonpathological conditions.

The goal of this chapter is to increase awareness that, given the arduous nature of the doctor's task and the liability of the human mind to conditioning, even gold-standard medical management and concerned physicians may contribute to the perpetuation of pain complaints. Medical interventions (diagnostic, pharmacological, anesthesiological, or surgical) may either cause or prolong chronic pain. Additionally, delayed diagnostic evaluation and medical mismanagement may perpetuate acute pain. Some harmful interventions do not imply any wrongdoing by physicians in the legal sense, since necessary drugs or surgery may inevitably cause some tissue injury. Pain syndromes can also result from psychological conditioning through patients' exposure to doctors and hospitals (Aronoff and DuPuy 1997; Kouyanou et al. 1997, 1998). This chapter will not address the legal aspects of physicians' errors of omission or commission, or with physicians' civil responsibilities (Beresford 1984).

It should be pointed out that surgery ranks with trauma as one of the most common causes of chronic pain. In a survey of patients attending pain clinics in Scotland (Crombie et al. 1998), surgery was the second most common cause of chronic pain, and contributed to it in 22% of 5130 patients. Trauma was the third most common cause of chronic pain, while degenerative diseases in general were first.

The primary cause of chronic pain induced by surgery is direct or indirect nerve injury, either acute (caused by section or ischemia) or delayed (from adhesion and entrapment) (Parks 1973). Anesthesia is also a frequent cause of painful nerve injury. Authors of a recent paper reviewing the database of closed claims in the United States found that 600 out of 4183 claims against anesthesiologists were for nerve injury (Cheney et al. 1990). Last, but not least, iatrogenesis is often the consequence of mismanagement and misdiagnosis of medical conditions. It must be emphasized that all clinicians, not only surgeons, may be responsible for causing chronic pain complaints in patients. An insightful case-controlled study on patients attending pain clinics (Kouyanou et al. 1997, 1998) documented that the patients most exposed to iatrogenic complications were those whose symptoms could not be explained by clinicians. These patients, often misdiagnosed, were more likely to receive unnecessary investigations, multiple and unsuccessful treatments, and excessive and sometimes inappropriate drug prescription. This study revealed that poor diagnostic evaluation is a major cause of iatrogenesis. Misdiagnosed patients, instead of receiving appropriate treatment, tend to be exposed to medical interventions that reinforce their beliefs and expectations, perpetuate their pain complaints through psychological conditioning, and ultimately lead to "pain behavior" (Kouyanou et al. 1997, 1998). Interestingly, even *Webster's New World Dictionary* (1980) mentions negative conditioning among the causes of iatrogenesis, defined as "a condition caused by medical treatment: said especially of imagined symptoms, ailments, or disorders induced by a physician's words or actions." It is worthwhile to underline "imagined symptoms" and "induced by a physician's words." Psychologically, an image is the construct of the unconscious. Therefore, pain experience, as with any other psychological construct, may at times be generated or induced by words.

Unnecessary medical treatments may also induce complex generalized or regional pain syndromes in predisposed subjects. Psychological factors are thus of utmost importance, even in the presence of objective nerve injury. Persons who suffer a deficit of motor or sensory function following a traumatic nerve injury often experience grief and frustration. They may be seeking understanding and compassion, and at the same time, they may turn their anger and resentment against those whom they consider responsible for their suffering. This attitude, often witnessed among accident victims, may understandably be expressed against the attending physician (or, by extension, against medical staff in general) by iatrogenic patients. Clinicians must consider the influence of psychological, emotional, social, and economic factors on the way these patients accept pain and whether it will become chronic (DeWolfe 1973). This statement should not be misunderstood to mean that we should consider all chronic neuralgias to be psychogenic. However, in the best interest of our patients, we should realize that the pain complaint may be a symbolic expression of a need for protection and care. For these patients, aggressive and invasive pain therapies must be avoided. If amplification of symptoms is suspected, we recommend a particularly conservative and reversible medical approach.

At times, injuries can offer patients "a legitimate opportunity" to adapt themselves to a "sick role." This behavior is not common, but it is probably underestimated. We have described patients suffering from an evident neurological injury (iatrogenic or not), who later developed complex sensory-motor disorders with major hysterical components (Lacerenza et al. 1996). The diagnosis of hysteria was based on strictly objective positive criteria and not simply on the absence of evidence for an organic disorder. Once again, as in the case of psychological amplification, any physician facing very atypical clinical symptom presentation should consider the possibility of coexisting physical and psychological aspects. By not taking into account the differential diagnosis between amplification, hysteria, and more rarely, malingering, physicians run the risk of overtreating their patients and thus exposing them to further harm.

IATROGENIC NERVE INJURY

Chronic iatrogenic pain may also result from direct or indirect nerve injury (Fig. 1). Compared to the number of nerve injuries provoked by surgical trauma, perioperative ischemia or compression, and delayed scar entrapment, post-injury chronic neuralgia is a rare event. Although we lack reliable clinical data, painful neuralgia following peripheral nerve injury seems to occur in about 2.5–5% of cases (Kline and Hudson 1995). The

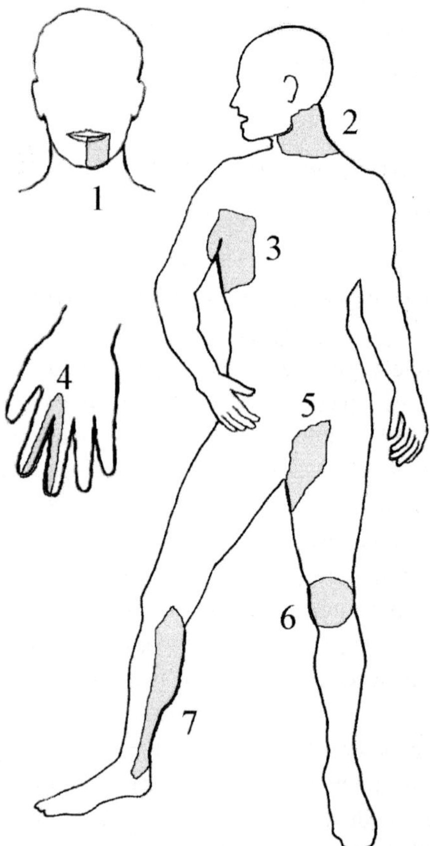

Fig. 1. The most common iatrogenic nerve injuries found in 12 years of practice at the Pain Medicine Center, Milan. (1) Alveolar nerve, (2) great auricular nerve and cutaneous branches of cervical plexus, (3) intercostobrachial nerve, (4) digital branches of the median nerve, (5) ileoinguinal nerve, (6) infrapatellar branch of the saphenous nerve, (7) saphenous nerve.

reason why few peripheral nerve injuries cause chronic pain and most do not is unknown. Perhaps the perpetuation of pain complaints requires certain biological and psychological factors at the moment of trauma, which would predispose the affected individual to the maintenance of neurological processes that ultimately are communicated as pain.

Researchers accept that the organic neurological aspects of post-injury chronic neuralgia are still unclear (Dickenson 1999). The pathophysiological mechanism that leads to chronicity may be the modification in activity of ganglion cells (Shinder and Devor 1994; Amir and Devor 1996) or central neural changes provoked by abnormal peripheral nerve afferent input (for a review, see Coderre and Katz 1997). Simultaneous recordings from ganglion and spinal cells have shown that the hyperactivity of spinal cells persists after the activity of ganglion cells has been blocked by the systemic administration of local anesthetics (Sotgiu et al. 1994). The peripheral input does play an important role, however, since it amplifies the hyperactivity in spinal neurons (Sotgiu et al. 1994). We still do not know which of these two anatomical targets has more clinical relevance; abolishing the hyperactivity of ganglion cells may be sufficient to reduce pain.

PRE-EMPTIVE AND PROPHYLACTIC ANESTHESIA

We have tentatively proposed that systemic administration of local anesthetics at the time of nerve injury could be effective against the development of chronic neuralgia (Sotgiu et al. 1995). This potential pre-emptive measure has only been demonstrated in rats with nerve ligature; pretreatment with local anesthetics completely prevented central neuronal hyperactivity and behavioral changes. Human studies are necessary to evaluate the clinical application of this prophylactic approach. The potentially protective effect of local anesthetics in surgical interventions that carry a risk for nerve injury is well worth further investigation. Of course, prophylaxis of chronic post-injury neuralgia is different from pre-emptive control of post-operative pain.

In the absence of valid pharmacological protection against the development of neuralgia, a sound preventive measure against chronic iatrogenic neuralgia would be to identify the most commonly injured nerves and the interventions most likely to cause nerve damage. For example, brachial plexus injury has drastically decreased since recognition of its incidence during general anesthesia and critical reevaluation of the most common causes of this complication. Anesthesiologists have also recommended guidelines for the careful administration of local anesthetic in peripheral nerve blocks.

The following recommendations are taken from Stöhr (1990), who reviewed the literature on the most common causes of nerve injury during local anesthesia: (a) Identify the nerve by electrical stimulation, and avoid evoking paresthesiae by searching for the nerve with a needle. (b) Do not puncture the nerve unnecessarily, and at least avoid repeated punctures. (c) Do not block nerve segments that are enclosed in rigid fascial compartments or osseous tunnels. (d) Use a blunt-tipped (45° bevel) needle for neural blockade, as recommended by Selander et al. (1977). (e) Avoid high-speed and large-volume injection in the immediate vicinity of nerve fascicles. (f) Never continue to inject local anesthetic if a patient complains of severe pain. (g) An aspiration test and an initial test dose are mandatory.

The nerves most commonly injured during medical interventions, according to Horowitz (1984), Dawson and Krarup (1989), and Sunderland (1991) are, in order of frequency: (a) brachial plexus; (b) palmar cutaneous branch of the median nerve; (c) infrapatellar cutaneous branch of the saphenous nerve; (d) ilioinguinal, iliohypogastric, genitofemoral, and femoral nerves; (e) accessory and greater auricular nerves; and (f) long thoracic nerve. In our experience, injuries to the following nerves are also frequently observed in pain clinics: (g) inferior alveolar nerve; (h) cutaneous branches of the cervical plexus; (i) intercostobrachial nerve; and (j) entire saphenous nerve of the leg.

Injuries to these nerves are rather common, and the possibility of iatrogenic neuralgia should always be considered for patients who report symptoms in the territory of innervation of the nerves following interventions in these areas.

SURGICAL AND ANESTHESIOLOGICAL INTERVENTIONS ASSOCIATED WITH NERVE INJURY

PAIN THERAPY

Nerve injuries caused by diagnostic or therapeutic interventions performed in pain clinics are not uncommon and are of great concern. Patients undergoing the following procedures to relieve or control existing pain may often end up with more pain and possibly with sensorimotor deficits.

Peripheral nerve blocks may cause permanent nerve injury either by direct traumatic needle contact or through nerve compression (Cousins and Bridenbaugh 1980; Murphy 1983; Bridenbaugh 1988). Direct traumatic injury is more likely for nerve adjacent to bone, such as the ulnar nerve at the elbow or the peroneal nerve at the knee. Indirect nerve injury may follow compression by venous punctured hematoma or by anesthetic solution injection into the unextensible epineurium.

Neurectomy may at times worsen the pain. However, in spite of contradictory opinions on the outcome of surgery for removal of stump neuromas, or neuromas in continuity, this intervention is indicated provided patients undergo accurate selection (Burchiel et al. 1993). To prevent further functional damage or worsening of the pain, surgery should be as limited as possible, avoiding intraneural dissection (Burchiel et al. 1993) or major transposition, which may cause additional ischemia.

Sympathectomy. At present, surgical sympathectomy for pain therapy is falling out of fashion, and its indication requires meticulous diagnosis. It remains acceptable for vascular pain such as Raynaud disease. Candidates for surgical sympathectomy should not only be selected by inert and active placebo controlled pharmacological sympathetic block (Verdugo et al. 1994; Verdugo and Ochoa 1995), but they should also respond positively to provocative tests. A positive diagnosis must be confirmed by recurrence of pain relieved by sympathectomy after injection of adrenergic agents. When this indication is carefully documented, the advantage of the treatment should still be weighed against the general side effects, which may include impotence (Whitelaw and Smithwick 1951), orthostatic hypotension (Hughes-Davies and Redman 1976; Löfström et al. 1980; Dondelinger and Kurdziel 1984), in rare cases paraplegia (Shallat and Klump 1971), and the puzzling condition of post-sympathectomy pain (Leriche 1949; Litwin 1962; Silverstein and Jacobson 1967; Longoni et al. 1981; Farcot et al. 1990).

Chordotomy. There is unanimous agreement that this intervention should be confined to intractable cancer. Patients affected by chronic noncancer pain who underwent chordotomy developed unpleasant dysesthesia and reappearance of the pain (post-chordotomy pain) (Lipton and McLennan 1988).

Ablative surgery for trigeminal neuralgia. Independent of the surgical technique used (balloon, injection of alcohol, or thermorhyzotomy), lesions of the fifth cranial nerve may be complicated by anesthesia dolorosa (Gybels and Sweet 1989).

Lumbar spine manipulation. A rare, but worrisome consequence of chiropractic treatment for back pain and disk herniation is cauda equina syndrome, which may cause incontinence, weakness, and sensory loss as well as chronic pain (Shapiro 1993). Exacerbation of back pain by lumbar manipulation was described by Assendelft et al. (1996).

Application or removal of epidural catheter may damage spinal roots, particularly of the lumbosacral nerve.

Surgical treatment of orofacial pain. In line with the idea that surgical intervention performed in the absence of specific indication has a poor outcome, Harris (1997) has provocatively suggested that the surgical management of idiopathic facial pain produces intractable iatrogenic pain.

ANESTHESIA

Placing patients under general anesthesia used to be frequently complicated by brachial plexus injury, while local anesthesia was a frequent cause of peripheral nerve damage (Po and Hansen 1969; Cheney et al. 1990). With more information and awareness of the problem, the incidence of these complications has decreased.

We have frequently observed lesions of the alveolar and lingual nerves in patients with chronic neuralgia as a complication of local dental anesthesia. Higher incidence of nerve injury in dental anesthesia could be due to the unextensibility of the tissues surrounding these nerves, or to dentists being less well informed of this risk compared to anesthetists.

ORTHOPEDIC AND NEUROSURGERY

Knee surgery. Incision in the area of the knee joint often causes lesion of the infrapatellar branch of the saphenous nerve, as reported by Sunderland (1991) and frequently witnessed in our clinic following arthroscopy. In our experience, this complication has increased with the widespread use of this technique.

Thoracic outlet syndrome. This is a controversial condition. As might be expected, given the lack of agreement on appropriate diagnostic criteria, the outcome of surgery is poor, with numerous complications. Of 120 patients operated for plexus entrapment pain, 47 had undergone prior surgery for the same diagnosis; of all patients, 37 had scars involving the plexus, 9 a prior major injury to the plexus, and 1 a traction injury. Prior surgery was the most common reason for intervention, followed by trauma (Kline and Hudson 1995). From a pain therapist's point of view, thoracic outlet surgery has limited usefulness even in skillful hands, as only about 50% of cases have a successful outcome.

Back surgery. Laminectomy is so often complicated by painful sequelae that it has generated an iatrogenic syndrome of its own, called "failed back surgery syndrome," which has given rise to abundant literature.

Limb amputation is also frequently followed by chronic pain (involving as many of 80% of amputees).

Carpal tunnel release. This common intervention may be complicated by partial lesion of the median and more rarely of the ulnar nerve (Goldner 1979). The median palmar branch, the recurrent thenar motor branch, and the interdigital branches are the most frequently affected (Rosenbaum and Ochoa 1993). The incidence of interdigital injury is increased with the use of endoscopic devices.

Harvesting for bone graft is one of the major causes of injury to the lateral femoral-cutaneous nerve (Weikel and Habel 1977; Moscona and Hirshowitz 1980).

Hip prosthesis often causes stretch injury of the femoral, peroneal, and sciatic nerves. The peroneal nerve also may be injured by compression in the postoperative rest period. Pain is more frequent when the cutaneous territory of the sciatic nerve is involved in the denervation.

GENERAL SURGERY AND THORACIC SURGERY

Lymph node biopsy in the neck is by far the most common cause of injury to the accessory nerve. In a series of 84 patients requiring lymph node biopsy, 42 (50%) had iatrogenic lesions to this nerve (King and Motta 1983; Swann and Heros 1985; Marini et al. 1991; Donner and Kline 1993). Iatrogenic injuries to this nerve can also result from tumor excision, carotid endarterectomy, plastic surgery (e.g., face lifts), radical neck surgery, and irradiation.

Ileoinguinal nerve lesion is an important complication, almost specific to inguinal hernioplasty. Anterior hernioplasty, requiring dissection of spermatic cord and sensory nerves, more commonly causes this injury (Sippo and Gomez 1987; Wantz 1993; Heise and Starling 1998).

Breast surgery is also reported among the common causes of chronic pain, through direct lesion or delayed entrapment of the intercostobrachial nerve (Kori et al. 1981).

Post-thoracotomy pain is reported in 9% of patients (61 out of 665 patients; Facisewzki et al. 1995). Pain may be due to intercostal nerve lesion or to traction on the brachial plexus (Berman et al. 1998). Intercostal rib resection can also cause brachial plexus injury (Horowitz 1985).

Varicose vein stripping, particularly of the saphenous vein, may frequently cause chronic pain when the saphenous nerve is injured by the surgical incisions or by the action of pulling the adjacent vein (Senegor 1991).

MANAGEMENT OF IATROGENIC NERVE INJURY

GENERAL RECOMMENDATIONS

When a nerve injury has occurred, a rational, accurate, and concerned approach may reduce the incidence of chronic pain and its psychological consequences. Early diagnosis is fundamental in reducing patient frustration and limiting the financial burden of medical management of the iatrogenic sequelae. Diagnosis of the nerve injury and also of its iatrogenic origin may be slow, sometimes because of delayed recognition, but also because symptoms may be absent for days, weeks, and sometimes months. Diagnosis may also be delayed because of immobilization by postoperative cast, bed rest, reduced activity, or excessive sedation due to anesthetic or pain medication. Also, both doctors and patients may erroneously consider neuropathic pain to be normal postoperative pain.

Once a nerve injury is suspected, clinical examination of sensory and motor function is often adequate to confirm it or rule it out. The clinical assessment should take into account that injury to motor as well as sensory nerves may cause pain. The pain may originate from tearing of the sensitive nervi nervorum, or may result from abnormal afferent activity in nociceptive muscle afferents. Pain may also be of orthopedic origin, as a consequence of ligament tearing and abnormal muscular control. In the case of iatrogenesis, it is always worthwhile to include an extensive sensory examination with identification of areas of hypoesthesia and hyperphenomena; photographs should be taken of the area of sensory disorder. We also recommend neurophysiological evaluation with quantitative sensory testing and nerve conduction studies, comparing the injured and the contralateral nerve. In case of inconsistency between clinical and neurophysiological findings, the sensory system should be explored further, for example through somatosensory evoked potentials. By analogy, the motor system should be further examined through electromyography and motor nerve conduction studies. In case of weakness of doubtful origin, comparison of electromyographic recruitment and muscle strength may allow discrimination between psychogenic and neurological weakness (Wilbourn 1995).

The purpose of a comprehensive sensorimotor examination is to provide both patient and doctor with objective identification of the neurological dysfunction. Careful evaluation allows the physician to provide a precise follow-up, which can help reassure the patient that the nerve damage is not worsening and may be improving. The evaluation also provides specific evidence in case of medicolegal assessment. A detailed clinical picture can also provide a diagnostic clue in case of late amplification of symptoms due to psychological factors or malingering. We share the recommendations of Kline (1995) for surgeons or physicians responsible for iatrogenesis: (a) Record keeping should be of the highest order. It is totally inappropriate to dictate a revision of the original note after an iatrogenic injury is discovered postoperatively. (b) Maximum care should be taken to avoid any possible alteration or loss of records, which might be interpreted against the surgeon. (c) Consultation with an expert peripheral neurologist is recommended, and the neurological examination must appear in the records.

(d) If a sharp surgical knife cut is recognizable, it is an obvious indication to proceed with immediate end-to-end reconstruction to avoid stump retraction and scar formation. Indeed, early repair may not only improve motor and sensory function, but may also alleviate pain (Kline 1985; Berman et al. 1998).

PROPOSED GUIDELINES FOR PHYSICIANS

1) Active surveillance. Ongoing records should be kept of patients' claims of nerve injuries, both painful and nonpainful. Such records will provide statistical information on the prevalence and the most common medical and surgical causes of iatrogenic nerve injuries.

2) Information. When there is even a small potential for nerve injury, physicians should always list it on the informed consent form among the possible complications (particularly for surgery or medical interventions that are not life-saving).

3) Recognition. Surgeons who perform interventions that carry the risk of nerve injury must be aware of the complex symptomatology of neuralgia, and of the possible delayed manifestation of neurological and psychogenic symptoms.

4) Diagnostic management. When nerve injury occurs, patients should undergo clinical and neurophysiological sensory testing to identify and define the location, severity, and prognosis of the lesion.

5) Psychological management. Psychological assessment and psychotherapeutic support should be provided within 6 months of the injury.

6) Medicolegal aspects. Considering that only 2.5–5% of all nerve injuries are painful, and because giving patients information may lead to negative conditioning, measures should be taken to rule out malingering and amplification of symptoms (e.g., quick evaluation of the claim, a second opinion, and sensory-motor evaluation).

The International Association for the Study of Pain should consider drafting consensus guidelines for iatrogenic pain management. Physicians are urged to avoid useless interventions that can only worsen pain, contribute to frustration and depression among patients, and foster litigation.

ACKNOWLEDGMENT

We thank Prof. José Ochoa for critical revision and fruitful discussion.

REFERENCES

Amir R, Devor M. Chemically mediated cross-excitation in rat dorsal root ganglia. *J Neurosci* 1996; 16:4733–4741.

Aronoff GM, DuPuy DN. Evaluation and management of back pain preventing disability. *J Back Muscul Rehab* 1997; 9:109–124.

Assendelft WJ, Bouter LM, Knipschild PG. Complications of spinal manipulation: a comprehensive review of the literature. *J Fam Pract* 1996; 42:475–480.

Beresford HR. Iatrogenic causalgia: legal implications. *Arch Neurol* 1984; 41:819–820.

Berman JS, Birch R, Anand P. Pain following human brachial plexus injury with spinal cord root avulsion and the effect of surgery. *Pain* 1998; 75:199–207.

Brennan TA, Leape LL, Laird NM, et al. Incidence of adverse events and negligence in hospitalized patients. Results of the Harvard Medical Practice Study I. *N Engl J Med* 1991; 324:370–376.

Bridenbaugh PO. Complications of local anesthetic neural blockade. In: Cousins MJ, Bridenbaugh PO (Eds). *Neural Blockade*, 2nd ed. Philadelphia: Lippincott, 1988.

Burchiel KJ, Johans TJ, Ochoa J. The surgical treatment of traumatic neuromas. *J Neurosurg* 1993; 78:714–719.

Cheney FW, Domino KB, Chaplan RA, Posner KL. Nerve injury associated with anesthesia: a closed claim analysis. *Anesthesiology* 1990; 4:1062–1069.

Coderre TJ, Katz J. Peripheral and central hyperexcitability: differential signs and symptoms in persistent pain. *Behav Brain Sci* 1997; 20:404–419.

Cousins MJ, Bridenbaugh PO. *Neural Blockade in Clinical Anaesthesia and Management of Pain.* Philadelphia: Lippincott, 1980.

Crombie IK, Oakley Davies HT, Macrae WA. Cut and trust: antecedent surgery among patients attending a chronic pain clinic. *Pain* 1998; 76:167–171.

Dawson DM, Krarup C. Perioperative nerve lesions. *Arch Neurol* 1989; 46:1355–1360.

DeWolfe VG. Iatrogenic and functional leg pain. *Geriatrics* 1973; 28:60–62.

Dickenson A. Pharmacological modification of electrophysiological and neurochemical aspects of hyperexcitability. In: Dickenson A, Hansson P, Jensen TS, Marchettini P (Organizers). *Pharmacological Treatment of Ongoing and Stimulus-Evoked Neuropathic Pain.* Como, Italy: IASP, August 27–29, 1999, pp 8–10.

Dondelinger R, Kurdziel JC. Percutaneous phenol neurolysis of the lumbar sympathetic chain with computed tomography control. *Ann Radiol* 1984; 27:376–379.

Donner TR, Kline DG. Extracranial accessory nerve injury. *Neurosurgery* 1993; 32:907–911.

Faciszewski T, Winter RB, Lonstein JE, Denis F, Johnson L. The surgical and medical perioperative complications of anterior spinal fusion surgery in the thoracic and lumbar spine in adults: a review of 1223 procedures. *Spine* 1995; 20:1592–1599.

Farcot JM, Grasser C, Muller JF. Post-sympathectomy pain. In: Mumenthaler M, Van Zwieten PA, Farcot JM (Eds). *Treatment of Chronic Pain.* London: Harwood Academic, 1990, pp 134–151.

Goldner JL. Causes and prevention of reflex sympathetic dystrophy. *J Hand Surg* 1979; 4:544–546.

Gybels JM, Sweet WH. Sympathectomy for pain. In: Gildenberg PL (Ed). *Neurosurgical Treatment of Persistent Pain.* Basel: Karger, 1989, pp 274–277.

Harris M. The surgical management of idiopathic facial pain produces intractable iatrogenic pain? *Br J Oral Maxillofac Surg* 1997; 35:54–58.

Heise CP, Starling JR. Mesh inguinodynia: a new clinical syndrome after inguinal herniorrhaphy? *J Am Coll Surg* 1998; 187:514–518.

Horowitz SH. Iatrogenic causalgia: classification, clinical findings, and legal ramifications. *Arch Neurol* 1984; 41:821–824.

Horowitz SH. Brachial plexus injury with causalgia resulting from transaxillary rib resection. *Arch Surg* 1985; 120:1189–1191.

Hughes-Davies DI, Redman LR. Chemical lumbar sympathectomy. *Anesthesia* 1976; 31:1068–1075.

King R, Motta G. Iatrogenic spinal accessory nerve palsy. *Ann R Coll Surg Engl* 1983; 65:35–37.

Kline DG, Hudson AR. Selected recent advances in peripheral nerve injury research. *Surg Neurol* 1985; 24:371–376.

Kline DG, Hudson AR. *Nerve Injuries*. Philadelphia: WB Saunders Company, 1995.

Kori SH, Foley KM, Posner JB. Brachial plexus lesions in patients with cancer: 100 cases. *Neurology* 1981; 31(1):45–50.

Kouyanou K, Pither CE, Wessely S. Iatrogenic factors and chronic pain. *Psychosom Med* 1997; 59:597–604.

Kouyanou K, Pither CE, Rabe-Hesketh S, Wessely S. A comparative study of iatrogenesis, medication abuse, and psychiatric morbidity in chronic pain patients with and without medically explained symptoms. *Pain* 1998; 76:417–426.

Lacerenza M, Marchettini P, Formaglio F, Castagna A, Smirne S. Chronic benign pain as ideal substrate to ignite hysteria in predisposed patients. *J Neurol* 1996; 243:352.

Leriche R. De la causalgie expérimentale. In: *La Chirurgie de la Douleur*, 3rd ed. Paris: Masson, 1949, pp 157–159.

Lipton S, McLennan JE. Percutaneous spinothalamic tractotomy: the prototype of neurosurgical pain control. In: Cousins MJ, Bridenbaugh PO (Eds). *Neural Blockade*, 2nd ed. Philadelphia: Lippincott, 1988, pp 679–690.

Litwin MS. Post-sympathectomy neuralgia. *Arch Surg* 1962; 84:591–595.

Löfström JB, Lloyd JW, Cousins MJ. Sympathetic neural blockade of upper and lower extremity. In: Cousins MJ, Bridenbaugh PO (Eds). *Neural Blockade in Clinical Anesthesia and Management of Pain*. Philadelphia: Lippincott, 1980, pp 355–382.

Longoni F, Romagnoli G, Albonico C, Montorsi M, Marstoni F. La nevralgia postsimpaticectomia lombare: nostra esperienza. *Angiologia* 1981; 33:118–122.

Marini SG, Rook JL, Green RF, Nagler W. Spinal accessory nerve palsy: an unusual complication of coronary artery bypass. *Arch Phys Med Rehab* 1991; 72:247–249.

Moscona AR, Hirshowitz B. Meralgia paresthetica: a complication of the groin flap. *Ann Plast Surg* 1980; 102:581–585.

Murphy TM. Complications of diagnostic and therapeutic nerve blocks. In: Orkin FK, Cooperman LH (Eds). *Complications in Anaesthesiology*. Philadelphia: Lippincott, 1983.

Ochoa JL, Verdugo RJ. Reflex sympathetic dystrophy: definitions and history of the ideas with a critical review of human studies. In: Low P (Ed). *The Evaluation and Management of Clinical Autonomic Disorders*. Boston: Little, Brown, 1992.

Parks BJ. Postoperative peripheral neuropathies. *Surgery* 1973; 74:348–357.

Po BT, Hansen HR. Iatrogenic brachial plexus injury: a survey of the literature and pertinent cases. *Anesth Analg* 1969; 48:915–921.

Rosenbaum RB, Ochoa JL. *Carpal Tunnel Syndrome and Other Disorders of the Median Nerve*. Boston: Butterworth-Heinemann, 1993, p 277.

Selander D, Dhuner KG, Lundborg G. Peripheral nerve injury due to injection needles used for regional anesthesia: an experimental study of the acute effects of needle point trauma. *Acta Anaesth Scand* 1977; 21:182–188.

Senegor M. Iatrogenic saphenous neuralgia: successful therapy with neuroma resection. *Neurosurgery* 1991; 28:295–298.

Shallat RF, Klump TE. Paraplegia following thoracolumbar sympathectomy: case report. *J Neurosurg* 1971; 34:569–571.

Shapiro S. Cauda equina syndrome secondary to lumbar disk herniation. *Neurosurgery* 1993; 32:743.

Sharpe VA, Faden AI. *Medical Harm, Historical, Conceptual and Ethical Dimensions of Iatrogenic Illness*. Cambridge: Cambridge University Press, 1998.

Shinder V, Devor M. Structural basis of neuron-to-neuron cross-excitation in dorsal root ganglia. *J Neurocytol* 1994; 23:515–531.

Silverstein A, Jacobson JH. Post-sympathectomy neuralgia. *Mt Sinai Hosp NY* 1967; 34:574–577.

Sippo WC, Gomez AC. Nerve entrapment syndromes from lower abdominal surgery. *J Fam Pract* 1987; 25:585–587.

Sotgiu ML, Biella G, Castagna A, Lacerenza M, Marchettini P. Different time-courses of i.v. lidocaine effect on ganglionic and spinal units in neuropathic rats. *Neuroreport* 1994; 5:873–876.

Sotgiu ML, Lacerenza M, Castagna A, Marchettini P. Pre-injury lidocaine treatment prevents thermal hyperalgesia and cutaneous thermal abnormalities in a rat model of peripheral neuropathy. *Pain* 1995, 61:3–10.

Stöhr M. Nerve Injuries after conduction block. In: Mumenthaler M, Van Zwieten PA, Farcot JM (Eds). *Treatment of Chronic Pain.* London: Harwood Academic, 1990, pp 120–126.

Sunderland T. *Nerve Injuries and Their Repair.* Edinburgh: Churchill Livingstone, 1991, pp 197–199.

Swann KW, Heros RC. Accessory nerve palsy following carotid endarterectomy: report of two cases. *J Neurosurg* 1985; 63:630–632.

Verdugo R, Ochoa JL. “Sympathetically maintained pain.” I. Phentolamine block questions the concept. *Neurology* 1994; 44:1003-1010. Comment in *Neurology* 1995; 45:1235–1237.

Verdugo R, Campero M, Ochoa JL. Phentolamine sympathetic block in painful polyneuropathies. II. Further questioning of the concept of “sympathetically maintained pain.” *Neurology* 1994; 44:1003–1010. Comment in *Neurology* 1995; 45:1235–1237.

Wantz GE. Testicular atrophy and chronic residual neuralgia as risks of inguinal hernioplasty. *Surg Clin North Am* 1993; 73:571–581.

Webster's New World Dictionary. New York: Simon & Schuster, 1980.

Weikel AM, Habel MB. Meralgia paresthetica: a complication of iliac bone procurement. *Plast Reconstr Surg* 1977; 60:572–574.

Whitelaw GP, Smithwick RH. Some secondary effects of sympathectomy with particular reference to disturbance of sexual function. *N Engl J Med* 1951; 245:121–130.

Wilbourn A. *Neurologic Clinics.* Wintraub (Ed). 1995.

Correspondence to: Paolo Marchettini, MD, Pain Medicine Center, Scientific Institute and Hospital, San Raffaele DSNP, via Prinetti 29, 20127 Milan, Italy. Fax: 39-02-2643-3394; email: marchettini.paolo@hsr.it.

Proceedings of the 9th World Congress on Pain,
Progress in Pain Research and Management,
Vol. 16, edited by M. Devor, M.C. Rowbotham, and
Z. Wiesenfeld-Hallin, IASP Press, Seattle, © 2000.

65

Mechanisms of Pain Arising from Spinal Nerve Root Compression

Cecil R. Morton,[a] Gary R. Lacey,[a] and Raymond L.G. Newcombe[b]

[a]*Division of Neuroscience, The John Curtin School of Medical Research, Australian National University, Canberra, Australia;* [b]*Canberra Regional Neurosurgical Unit, The Canberra Hospital (University of Sydney), Canberra, Australia*

Pain arising from spinal nerve root compression is a commonly observed clinical condition, but its pathogenesis is not well defined. The literature has often focused on mechanical deformation of nerve roots as the major causative factor, but considerable evidence indicates that other factors such as ischemia, edema, inflammation, and mechanical stimulation of dorsal root ganglia (DRG) can play important roles (reviewed in Rydevik et al. 1984; Garfin et al. 1995). In recent years, the use of various animal models for spinal compression syndromes has contributed significantly to our understanding of these clinical conditions (Sato et al. 1995; Yoshizawa et al. 1995; Sugawara et al. 1996; Cornefjord et al. 1997; Olmarker and Myers 1998).

The underlying neurochemical mechanisms involved in this type of pain are poorly understood. For spinal nociceptive transmission associated with peripheral activation of nociceptors, a large body of evidence supports the participation of the various neuropeptides found in DRG neurons and in the superficial dorsal horn of the spinal cord (reviewed by Levine et al. 1993). Much less information is available on a possible link between sensory neuropeptides and the pain associated with spinal compression syndromes. Experimental compression of nerve roots and DRG for 7 days increases levels of immunoreactive substance P (irSP) in DRG cell bodies and the superficial dorsal horn in rats (Badalamente et al. 1987), and in the DRG and nerve root in pigs (Cornefjord et al. 1995). In rats, irSP in the spinal dorsal horn was unaffected by brief experimental compression of the cauda equina but reduced by prolonged compression, while ir-somatostatin levels were reduced by both procedures (Kawakami and Tamaki 1992). Chronic irritation of dorsal roots in rats has been shown to increase irSP, ir-calcitonin gene-related peptide (CGRP), and ir-vasoactive intestinal polypeptide in the DRG and to slightly decrease irSP and irCGRP in the spinal cord (Kawakami et al. 1994). In patients with pain from a herniated lumbar disk, levels of irSP in the cerebrospinal fluid (CSF) increased (Sameshima 1995) or were unchanged (Lindh et al. 1997), while the activity of SP endopeptidase in CSF was lower in these patients compared with controls (Lindh et al. 1996).

We investigated the possible neurochemical mechanisms contributing to the pain associated with clinical compression syndromes, by examining the release of irCGRP within the cat spinal cord during acute mechanical compression of spinal dorsal roots.

METHODS

The experimental protocol was reviewed and approved by the Animal Experimentation Ethics Committee, Australian National University. Experiments were performed on cats (3.0–3.4 kg) anesthetized with pentobarbitone sodium (35 mg/kg i.p., maintained thereafter by 3 $mg{\cdot}kg^{-1}{\cdot}h^{-1}$ i.v. infusion). After exposure of the lumbar spinal cord and cord transection at L1, the dura mater was slit dorsally and the exposed cord surface covered with Ringer agar. Following neuromuscular paralysis (gallamine triethiodide 4 $mg{\cdot}kg^{-1}{\cdot}h^{-1}$ i.v.), the cats were artificially ventilated with air via a tracheal cannula, with end-tidal CO_2 maintained at 4%. Adequacy of anesthesia was regularly confirmed by the absence of blood pressure changes following noxious stimulation cephalic to L1.

Antibody microprobes were prepared by sequentially coating the outer surface of glass micropipettes with a siloxane polymer, protein A, and antibodies to rat CGRP (1:1500, Milab, Malmö, Sweden), as described in detail elsewhere (Duggan et al. 1988; Morton and Hutchison 1989). Following partial removal of the agar and irrigation of the cord surface with Ringer, microprobes were inserted into the lower lumbar cord through small perforations in the pia mater about midway between the lateral and median dorsal sulci at sites where innocuous mechanical hindpaw stimulation evoked maximal cord dorsum potentials. The microprobe tips were advanced to a depth of 3.0 mm. Localized, reversible pressure was applied under microscopic control to the ipsilateral dorsal roots innervating the appropriate lumbar segment by precisely controlled inflation of a balloon catheter (Microvasive, Milford, Massachusetts) positioned adjacent to the exposed roots. Microprobes were inserted into the cord for 12 minutes during inflation (compression stimulus) and deflation (control) of the balloon catheter. The tips (~15 mm) were then incubated in ^{125}I-CGRP (rat) (1700 mCi/μmol, Peninsula), diluted to 2 μCi/mL, for 36 hours and mounted next to X-ray film (Kodak NMC). Computerized microdensitometric analysis of each individual autoradiogram produced an image density scan for each microprobe, consisting of digitized optical density values plotted with respect to distance from the tip (Hendry et al. 1988). Regions of in vivo peptide release along the length of each microprobe were identifiable as relative deficits of tracer binding, producing zones of reduced optical density (peaks) on the scan. Mean scans were calculated for microprobes used under control and compression conditions, and differences in release between these groups were assessed by statistical analyses of the differences between the mean scans by calculation of t values at 16-μm intervals (Hendry et al. 1988).

Parallel in vitro assays of sensitivity were performed in each experiment by incubating (37°C, 12 minutes) the tips of prepared microprobes in known concentrations of rat CGRP (Peninsula), followed by incubation in radiolabeled CGRP for 36 hours and measurement of bound radioactivity with a gamma counter.

RESULTS

In total, 67 microprobes were analyzed: 43 probes were used to measure irCGRP release in vivo, and 24 for in vitro assays in which the binding of radiolabeled CGRP was consistently suppressed by preincubation in 10^{-7} M unlabeled rat CGRP.

The degree of inflation of the balloon catheter was monitored visually to ensure a consistent level of compression of the dorsal roots for each microprobe. Upon deflation, the extent of compression was confirmed by indentations in the dorsal roots. The mean image density scan of microprobes inserted into the spinal cord when the balloon catheter was deflated (no dorsal root compression) is shown in the upper part of Fig. 1. The mean scan features a peak centered 1.1 mm ventral to the dorsal cord surface, indicating a basal presence of irCGRP in the region of the substantia gelatinosa. The mean scan of microprobes inserted into the cord during the periods of balloon catheter inflation (dorsal root compression) is shown in the lower part of Fig. 1. The differences between these mean scans (not illustrated) were not statistically significant, indicating no increase in the basal presence of irCGRP in the substantia gelatinosa region during the acute compression stimulus of the dorsal roots.

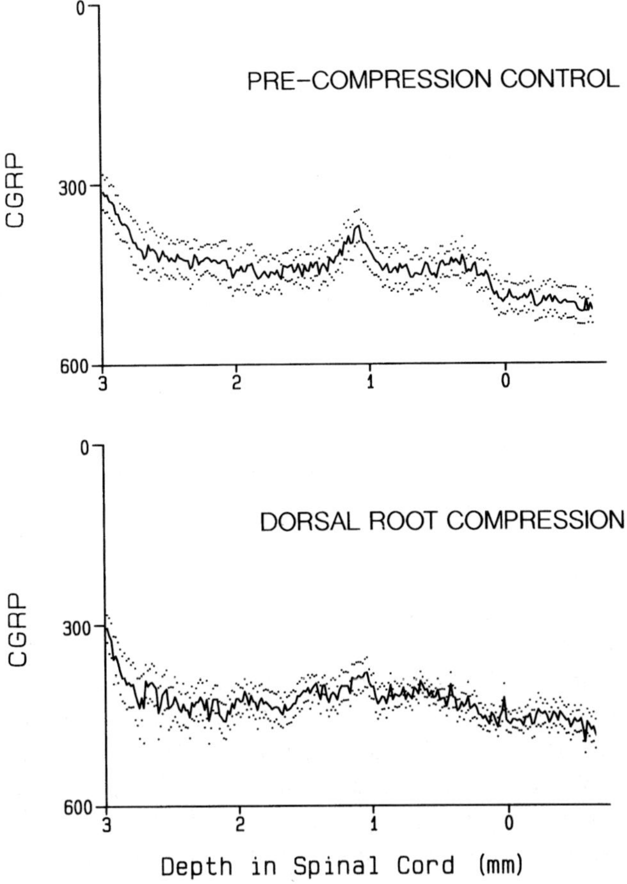

Fig. 1. Acute dorsal root compression does not affect the basal release of irCGRP in the dorsal horn. The solid lines are mean image density scans of antibody microprobe autoradiographs; the broken lines are the SEM for each mean scan. Ordinates show digitized optical density values expressed as an arbitrary gray scale (see Methods); abscissae, depth of insertion into the lower lumbar spinal cord (in millimeters), with the cord surface at 0. *Pre-compression control:* the mean scan (and SEM) of 22 microprobes detecting irCGRP release in the absence of compression of dorsal roots. *Dorsal root compression:* the mean scan (and SEM) of 21 microprobes detecting irCGRP release during acute compression of dorsal roots innervating the region from which irCGRP release was measured.

DISCUSSION

Under the present experimental conditions, release of irCGRP in the lumbar dorsal horn was not evoked by acute mechanical deformation of spinal dorsal roots. A basal presence of irCGRP was detected in the superficial dorsal horn, centered in the region of the substantia gelatinosa. The origin of this irCGRP, a consistent observation in this experimental preparation (Morton and Hutchison 1989, 1990; Morton et al. 1992), is not known, but it could derive from primary afferent fibers activated by surgical injury or by rupture of CGRP-containing neuronal structures during microprobe insertion. In this experimental model, this basal presence of irCGRP is greatly increased by activation of nociceptive afferent fibers (noxious cutaneous stimulation or high-intensity peripheral nerve stimulation), indicative of intraspinal CGRP release under conditions of acute nociception (Morton and Hutchison 1989, 1990; Morton et al. 1992). In the present experiments, however, such release was not evoked by the acute experimental compression of dorsal roots.

The present finding is consistent with the results of previous neurophysiological studies. In cats, recordings from dorsal root filaments showed lack of an injury discharge following acute root damage (Wall et al. 1974), or only transient discharges in Aα, Aβ, and Aδ fibers following mechanical stimulation of normal dorsal roots (Howe et al. 1977). Similarly, the excitatory responses evoked in wide-dynamic-range neurons of the lumbar dorsal horn of the cat by experimental dorsal root compression rapidly declined to precompression levels (Hanai et al. 1996). In contrast, acute experimental compression of DRG evoked robust, sustained firing in feline dorsal roots (Howe et al. 1977) and dorsal horn neurons (Hanai et al. 1996), and in canine dorsal roots in vitro (Sugawara et al. 1996), and the mechanical threshold for eliciting firing was much lower for the DRG than the dorsal roots. Together, the present release study and previous investigations do not favor the concept that pain occurring in acute clinical compression syndromes such as disk herniation is produced by acute mechanical stimulation of nerve roots. These data support the notion that at least the pain associated with *acute* herniated intervertebral disk might arise from either direct mechanical stimulation of the DRG by the nucleus pulposus or indirect stimulation by a traction force acting on the DRG from stretching of the nerve root (see Lindblom and Rexed 1948; Rydevik et al. 1984; Sugawara et al. 1996). In the present study, it is likely that the compression stimulus would not have been severe enough to exert such indirect force on the DRG. These microprobe experiments could be extended to examine the intraspinal release of neuropeptides during acute controlled compression of other structures such as the DRG.

Under conditions of *chronic* mechanical compression syndromes, ischemic, inflammatory, metabolic, and neurophysiological changes might participate in the pain-producing process by inducing a localized pathophysiological state at the site of injury over a period of time (reviewed in Rydevik et al. 1984 and Garfin et al. 1995). In neurophysiological experiments in animals, chronically inflamed dorsal roots display greatly increased sensitivity to controlled mechanical stimulation at the injured region, in contrast to the minimal effects observed with similar stimulation of normal roots (Howe et al. 1977). This finding suggests that root compression may play a significant role in the pathogenesis of pain in chronic compression syndromes. Long-term pathophysiological changes may also explain some of the differing results obtained in the neurochemical studies of peptides following acute and chronic compression.

In summary, the balloon catheter and the antibody microprobe are a useful combination of techniques for the experimental investigation of spinal compression syndromes in animals.

ACKNOWLEDGMENTS

This work was supported by grants from the National Health & Medical Research Council of Australia and the Australian Brain Foundation.

REFERENCES

Badalamente MA, Dee R, Ghillani R, Chien P-F, Daniels K. Mechanical stimulation of dorsal root ganglia induces increased production of substance P: a mechanism for pain following nerve root compromise? *Spine* 1987; 12:552–555.

Cornefjord M, Olmarker K, Farley DB, Weinstein JN, Rydevik B. Neuropeptide changes in compressed spinal nerve roots. *Spine* 1995; 20:670–673.

Cornefjord M, Sato K, Olmarker K, Rydevik B, Nordborg C. A model for chronic nerve root compression studies. Presentation of a porcine model for controlled, slow-onset compression with analyses of anatomic aspects, compression onset rate, and morphologic and neurophysiologic effects. *Spine* 1997; 22:946–957.

Duggan AW, Hendry IA, Green JL, Morton CR, Hutchison WD. The preparation and use of antibody microprobes. *J Neurosci Methods* 1988; 23:241–247.

Garfin SR, Rydevik B, Lind B, Massie J. Spinal nerve root compression. *Spine* 1995; 20:1810–1820.

Hanai F, Matsui N, Hongo N. Changes in responses of wide dynamic range neurones in the spinal dorsal horn after dorsal root or dorsal root ganglion compression. *Spine* 1996; 21:1408–1415.

Hendry IA, Morton CR, Duggan AW. Analysis of antibody microprobe autoradiographs by computerized image processing. *J Neurosci Methods* 1988; 23:249–256.

Howe JF, Loeser JD, Calvin WH. Mechanosensitivity of dorsal root ganglia and chronically injured axons: a physiological basis for the radicular pain of nerve root compression. *Pain* 1977; 3:25–41.

Kawakami M, Tamaki T. Morphologic and quantitative changes in neurotransmitters in the lumbar spinal cord after acute or chronic mechanical compression of the cauda equina. *Spine* 1992; 17(3S):S13–S17.

Kawakami M, Weinstein JN, Spratt KF, et al. Experimental lumbar radiculopathy. Immunohistochemical and quantitative demonstrations of pain induced by lumbar nerve root irritation of the rat. *Spine* 1994; 19:1780–1794.

Levine JD, Fields HL, Basbaum AI. Peptides and the primary afferent nociceptor. *J Neurosci* 1993; 13:2273–2286.

Lindblom K, Rexed B. Spinal nerve injury in dorso-lateral protrusions of lumbar disks. *J Neurosurg* 1948; 5:413–432.

Lindh C, Thörnwall M, Hansen A-C, et al. Neuropeptide-converting enzymes in cerebrospinal fluid. Activities increased in pain from herniated lumbar disc, but not from coxarthrosis. *Acta Orthop Scand* 1996; 67:189–192.

Lindh C, Liu Z, Lyrenas S, Ordeberg G, Nyberg F. Elevated cerebrospinal fluid substance P-like immunoreactivity in patients with painful osteoarthritis, but not in patients with rhizopatic pain from a herniated lumbar disc. *Scan J Rheumatol* 1997; 26:468–472.

Morton CR, Hutchison WD. Release of sensory neuropeptides in the spinal cord: studies with calcitonin gene-related peptide and galanin. *Neuroscience* 1989; 31:807–815.

Morton CR, Hutchison WD. Morphine does not reduce the intraspinal release of calcitonin gene-related peptide in the cat. *Neurosci Lett* 1990; 117:319–324.

Morton CR, Hutchison WD, Lacey G. Baclofen and the release of neuropeptides in the cat spinal cord. *Eur J Neurosci* 1992; 4:243–250.

Olmarker K, Myers RR. Pathogenesis of sciatic pain: role of herniated nucleus pulposus and deformation of spinal nerve root and dorsal root ganglion. *Pain* 1998; 78:99–105.

Rydevik B, Brown MD, Lundborg G. Pathoanatomy and pathophysiology of nerve root compression. *Spine* 1984; 9:7–15.

Sameshima K. Substance P-like immunoreactivity in cerebrospinal fluid in lumbar disc herniation. *Jpn Ortho Assoc J* 1995; 69:191–197.

Sato K, Konno S, Yabuki, S, et al. A model for acute, chronic, and delayed graded compression of the dog cauda equina. Neurophysiologic and histologic changes induced by acute, graded compression. *Spine* 1995; 20:2386–2391.

Sugawara O, Atsuta Y, Iwahara T, et al. The effects of mechanical compression and hypoxia on nerve root and dorsal root ganglia. *Spine* 1996; 21:2089–2094.

Wall PD, Waxman, S, Basbaum AI. Ongoing activity in peripheral nerve: injury discharge. *Exp Neurol* 1974; 45:576–589.

Yoshizawa H, Kobayashi S, Morita T. Chronic nerve root compression. Pathophysiologic mechanism of nerve root dysfunction. *Spine* 1995; 20:397–407.

Correspondence to: Cecil R. Morton, PhD, Drug Toxicology Evaluation Section, Drug Safety & Evaluation Branch, Therapeutic Goods Administration, PO Box 100, Woden ACT 2606, Australia. Tel: 61-2-62328349; Fax: 61-2-62328355; email: bob.morton@health.gov.au.

Proceedings of the 9th World Congress on Pain,
Progress in Pain Research and Management,
Vol. 16, edited by M. Devor, M.C. Rowbotham, and
Z. Wiesenfeld-Hallin, IASP Press, Seattle, © 2000.

66

Possible Causes of Pain in Repetitive Strain Injury[1]

Jane Greening and Bruce Lynn

*Department of Physiology, University College London,
London, United Kingdom*

Repetitive strain injury (RSI) is a chronic pain condition of the upper limb. Patients complain of diffuse regional arm pain with an apparent lack of objective physical signs. The condition does not conform to traditional medical models of musculoskeletal disease or injury. As such RSI has become a highly controversial subject among medical practitioners (e.g., Semple 1991; Hocking 1992; Hutson 1994; Mann 1994). Even more controversially, the condition appears to be associated with particular work practices and conditions. Occupation examples are office workers who spend long hours using display screen equipment, musicians, and production line workers. All have tasks that involve highly repetitive use of the hands and constrained and static postures that have been identified as risk factors for the condition (Latko 1999; Serina et al. 1999), although these risk factors also have been contested (Hadler 1997). Some authors regard RSI as a sociopolitical phenomenon (Lucire 1988; Miller 1988) and dispute its existence as a medical condition (Brooks 1993). Others regard it as just normal aches and pains associated with everyday life (Hadler 1990). Needless to say, this controversy has provoked fierce debate among members of the medical and legal professions and patients.

Since coming into widespread use in the early 1980s (see Arksey 1998, Chapter 7), "repetitive strain injury" has been a contentious term because it implies etiology and pathology. Many alternative terms describe this same chronic pain condition (see Table I). Confusingly, RSI is frequently used as an umbrella term for many specific work-related musculoskeletal conditions

[1] Mini-review based on a congress workshop.

Table I
Common terms for repetitive strain injury

Common Term	Acronym	Region(s) Used
Work-related upper limb disorder	WRULD	Europe
Occupational overuse syndrome	OOS	New Zealand, Australia
Occupational cervicobrachial disorder	OCB	Japan
Repetitive strain injury	RSI	United Kingdom, Australia
Nonspecific arm pain	NSAP	United Kingdom
Cumulative trauma disorder	CTD	United States

such as tenosynovitis and carpal tunnel syndrome (Yassi 1997). We should be clear at the outset that these specific disease entities with clear diagnostic criteria are are not the subject of this chapter.

SOCIAL AND ECONOMIC COSTS

Patients with the condition complain that their hand function becomes extremely limited, and many have difficulties both with everyday and work activities. RSI has a significant effect not only on individual sufferers and their families, but also on employers due to prolonged sickness, payment for treatment, cost of ergonomic interventions, and, where workplace conditions caused the condition, compensation settlements. Figures for economic cost or even prevalence are difficult to find, partly because terminology varies in different countries. However, Jayaraaman (1994) reported that in the United Kingdom, RSI was responsible for a loss of £400 million in lost working days/year. The United Kingdom recently identified surveillance case definitions for work-related upper limb pain syndromes (Harrington 1998) and named specific subjective criteria for RSI (termed in Harrington's report "nonspecific forearm pain"). These criteria should allow a more accurate estimation of the problem and comparability between research studies. In the United States, cumulative trauma disorders (CTDs), a designation that covers all work-related musculoskeletal conditions of the upper limb including carpal tunnel syndrome (CTS), account for 50% of all occupational injuries (Melhorn 1998).

RELATION OF RSI TO FIBROMYALGIA

The lack of obvious clinical signs has led some authors to diagnose diffuse RSI as a feature of fibromyalgia (Reilly 1993). Fibromyalgia is a condition of widespread musculoskeletal pain associated with specific muscle and bone tender points, fatigue, and emotional distress (Wolfe 1996; Littlejohn 1998). The inclusion of RSI into the fibromyalgia category, itself a contentious condition (Cohen 1998; Quinter and Cohen 1999), is interesting. Wigley (1998) proposes that many RSI patients later develop fibromyalgia. However, our experience is that many RSI patients present with a stable condition clearly limited to the upper limb(s). Even over a period of years, the problem does not usually spread to involve other body regions. The location and number of tender points, but little else, distinguish fibromyalgia sufferers from the general population. This criterion, combined with the lack of association with work activities (although see Wigley 1999), makes it tempting to reclassify RSI as regional fibromyalgia, thereby giving it a more "respectable profile." However tempting this possibility, a diagnosis of fibromyalgia (a functional state of lowered pain threshold) does not address problems of causation or pathology. In general, the relationship between RSI and fibromyalgia must still be considered uncertain.

KEY SIGNS AND SYMPTOMS OF RSI

The symptoms of diffuse RSI have been described many times (e.g., Elvey et al. 1986; Cohen 1992). The patient complains of diffuse wrist and forearm pain, sometimes accompanied by nondermatomal or single peripheral nerve paresthesia. Symptoms may be unilateral or bilateral and usually are more severe on the dominant side. When severe, symptoms may spread to the upper arm and shoulder girdle and are associated with muscle tenderness, loss of grip strength, and mechanical allodynia (Harrington 1998). Signs of tissue injury or inflammation are not apparent. Neck and upper back stiffness may occur but are not associated with radiculopathy. Standard neurological examination is normal and nerve conduction velocities are within normal limits. Clinicians who examine these patients using tests of upper limb peripheral nerve mobility (Butler 1991) invariably report positive tests, i.e., restricted movement and reproduction of symptoms (Byng 1997). Palpation of peripheral nerve trunks may also be painful and produce paresthesia in some patients (Hall and Elvey 1999).

Approximately one-third of patients describe marked temperature and color changes in their hands, while a minority have clear signs of autonomic dysfunction (Cohen 1992). Patients do not demonstrate signs of classical peripheral nerve entrapment; for instance, they do not exhibit the discrete pain referral of CTS or nerve conduction abnormalities.

POSSIBLE CAUSES OF RSI

Chronic arm pain may arise in three ways: nociceptive, psychogenic, or neuropathic. We will consider each in turn below.

DIRECT NOCICEPTIVE CAUSES

Possible chronic activation of muscle nociceptors could occur either through tissue pathology (Dennett and Fry 1988) or ischemia (Pritchard et al. 1999). However, independent evidence for local activation of nociceptors in joint and muscle is lacking. Low-force muscle activity sustained for long periods involves the continuous recruitment of low-threshold motor units. Such activity may possibly lead to necrotic changes in the affected muscles (Sjogaard and Sogaard 1998). However, the typical clinical picture in RSI is not the same as seen in inflammatory conditions of joint, tendons, or muscle. Symptoms of myofascial origin have been proposed as a component of the clinical picture seen in RSI. Myofascial pain is based largely on the presence of "trigger points" within muscle, which produce a characteristic aching (Simons and Travell 1984). Quinter and Cohen (1994) dispute that pain produced by trigger points is due to muscle C-fiber afferent input and argue that symptoms are due to "secondary hyperalgesia of peripheral nerve origin." Certainly, a comparison between the course of cutaneous peripheral nerves in the cervical spine, shoulder girdle, and arm (Williams et al. 1989) show a similar distribution to maps of trigger points and their pain referral patterns. These factors suggest a degree of convergence with the possibility of a peripheral nerve origin for the pain in RSI, as discussed in more detail below. On the general question of how far nociceptive input from musculoskeletal tissues is directly responsible for RSI, none of the evidence is compelling, although a role for such inputs certainly cannot be ruled out.

PSYCHOLOGICAL CAUSES

No definitive study has described a purely psychological cause for RSI (Estlander 1998), although factors such as high work load and time pressure, leading to stress, may contribute to the disorder (Helliwell 1992; Hales and Bernard 1996). Helme et al. (1992) measured psychological profiles in these patients and concluded that RSI was due to altered nociceptive mechanisms that involve somatic pathophysiology and that higher levels of anxiety and depression were secondary to the presence of chronic pain.

NEUROPATHIC CAUSES

RSI and entrapment neuropathies clearly share some similarities. For example, symptoms of CTS include wrist and forearm pain, paresthesia, and difficulties with gripping activities. However, as discussed earlier, RSI has features that do not match those of single-entrapment neuropathies. Multiple levels of minor nerve injury, in which fascicular loss is not sufficient to show up on electro-neurophysiological tests (Spindler et al. 1990), is another possibility.

The evidence for peripheral nerve involvement in RSI comes from several sources. As already mentioned, upper limb neural dynamic tests, e.g., upper limb tension test 1 (ULTT1), are positive in RSI patients (Elvey et al. 1986; Byng 1997). Additional evidence for neuropathy comes from quantitative sensory testing with vibration. Greening and Lynn (1998a) found elevated vibration perception thresholds, particularly affecting the median nerve distribution, indicating changed Aβ-fiber function. Patients also demonstrated an allodynic response to suprathreshold stimulation, which indicates changes to central sensory processing. Helme et al. (1992) measured flare responses as an indication of afferent C-fiber function. This study demonstrated a reduction in flare size, which was greater in the more severely affected limb. This pattern of reduced vibration sensitivity, a reduction in flare size, and painful responses to nonpainful stimuli, is the same pattern seen in patients with well-established painful neuropathic conditions such as postherpetic neuralgia (Rowbotham and Fields 1996).

Given the evidence for peripheral nerve involvement, we felt that a magnetic resonance imaging (MRI) study of the mobility of the median nerve at the carpal tunnel would be of interest. In patients with RSI we measured the change in position of the median nerve between 30° of wrist extension and 30° of flexion (Greening et al. 1999). The results showed a significant loss of neural mobility in RSI patients, as shown in Fig. 1. Patients with the most marked restriction of nerve movement on MRI also showed a clear trend for more severely restricted arm movement with the ULTT1 test. If supported by a larger study, this work promises to be the most objective evidence yet for peripheral neuropathy as a cause of pain in RSI. Previous MRI studies with CTS (Allman et al. 1997) have described a qualitative loss of nerve movement during wrist flexion and extension. However, minor median nerve entrapment at the carpal tunnel does not explain the diffuse nature of RSI. Also, if RSI were just a manifestation of early CTS, patients would respond to rest and splinting. Other sites of possible nerve entrapment and loss of neural mobility in the upper limb, including the thoracic inlet and outlet, need investigating.

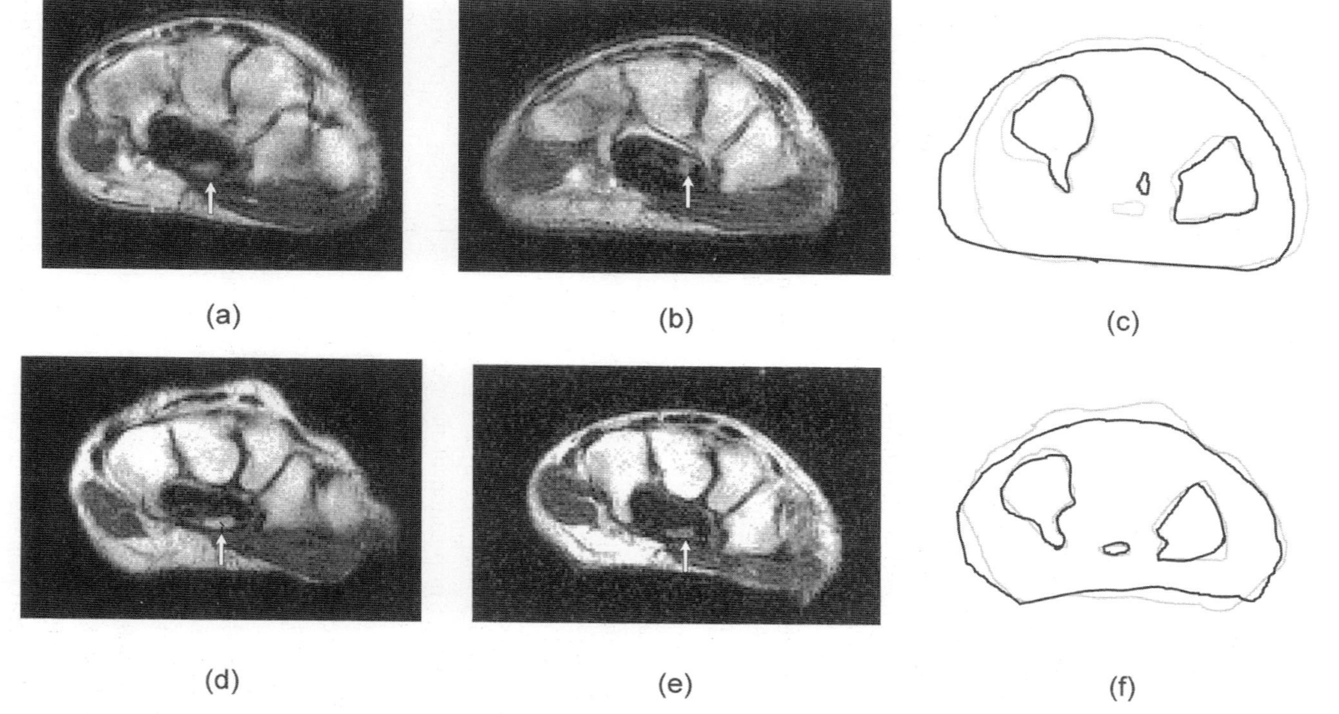

Fig 1. MR scans of the carpal tunnel, at the level of the hook of hamate, during (a) wrist extension and (b) flexion in a control subject and (d) wrist extension and (e) flexion in an RSI patient. Image overlays (c) and (f) are drawn from scans of the control subject and patient. The median nerve, indicated by white arrows, appears as a light gray structure next to the black tendons. Overlays show the position of the median nerve during extension (gray line) and flexion (black line). Modified from Greening et al. (1999), with permission.

CAN MODEST CHANGES IN THE NERVE ENVIRONMENT PRODUCE SEVERE CHRONIC PAIN?

Recent behavioral studies in animal models have revealed that minor treatments of various sorts applied to peripheral nerves can produce pain behavior where little or no axonal degeneration occurs. An example is experimental neuritis (Maves et al. 1993; Bennett 1999). Physiological studies have shown that the development of sensitivity to sympathetic manipulation, a feature of some neuropathic pain states, occurs after minor nerve stretching (Sato and Perl 1991). Human studies offer some evidence. Mackinnon (1986) reported a few cases where pain in the distribution of the superficial radial nerve was abolished by resection of nerve branches that, on histological examination, showed no sign of fiber degeneration, but did demonstrate changes in the perineurium and endoneurial microvessels.

A site of localized irritation along a peripheral nerve could generate abnormal input to the CNS in two ways, either through abnormal spontaneous activity from injured nerve fibers or from "normal" activation of nociceptors in the nerve sheath (the "nervi nervorum"). Recent studies have provided evidence for both possibilities.

NERVI NERVORUM

The evidence for involvement of the nervi nervorum in painful symptoms and abnormal sensory phenomena in RSI is indirect. These C fibers innervate the nerve sheath (Thomas 1963) and would be involved in the response of the nerve to friction or compression injury (Bove 1997). Mechanical irritation, inflammation, and longitudinal stretch will sensitize these sensory endings (Zochodne 1992; Sauer et al. 1999) and thus contribute to nociceptive input reaching the dorsal horn. Another consistent feature of RSI and many other neuropathic conditions is nerve trunk pain on palpation. This feature plus the restriction of limb movement during neural mobility tests, could be a result of primary sensitization of nociceptor afferents in the nervi nervorum.

ABNORMAL ECTOPIC ACTIVITY

Abnormal spontaneous activity has been observed in several partial nerve injury models in the rat, including firing of C fibers (Koltzenburg et al. 1994; Tal and Eliav 1996). The minimum lesion necessary to cause such activation is not clear (Greening and Lynn 1998b). Mechanical stress, changes in nerve fiber diameter, and ischemia can reduce the amount of growth factors available to the nerve cell body, for example by interfering with retrograde axonal transport (e.g., Dahlin et al. 1986; Tanoue et al. 1996). Loss of growth factors can in turn lead to several effects on sensory neurons, including changes to dorsal root ganglion neurochemistry and in the viability of synaptic terminals in the spinal cord (McMahon et al. 1997; McMahon and Bennett 1997).

AMPLIFICATION OF ABNORMAL INPUTS BY CENTRAL SENSITIZATION

The chronic pain associated with RSI may be the result of abnormal C-fiber input due to the factors described above. These changes can in turn lead to changes in CNS sensitivity ("central sensitization") (e.g., McMahon 1993; Devor 1988). The marked, widespread allodynia seen in RSI is consistent with central sensitization. Symptom presentation and subject responses to electrical stimulation led Arroyo and Cohen (1992) to conclude that RSI is largely a central sensitization phenomenon with secondary hyperalgesia related to abnormal C-fiber function. This conclusion may overstate the situation a little, but, as in many other chronic pain states, central sensitization is likely to play an important role.

DOES KEYBOARD USE ADVERSELY AFFECT THE NEURAL ENVIRONMENT?

Multilevel minor nerve compression caused by muscle imbalance and postural abnormalities, combined with direct pressure, traction, and irritation of nerves at sites of entrapment, has been proposed as a cause of RSI (Higgs and Mackinnon 1995; Novak and Mackinnon 1998). Fig. 2 depicts a common posture adopted by office workers. This posture, assumed for many hours, is associated with prolonged changes in muscle tension particularly around the neck, shoulder girdle region, and forearm musculature. Sustained or repetitive contraction of muscles, where they are anatomically closely associated with peripheral nerves, may cause an increase in local pressure or friction. Pressure around the ulnar nerve at the cubital fossa increases with elbow flexion, and around the median nerve at the carpal tunnel with wrist flexion and extension (Pechan and Julis 1975; Gellman et al. 1981). Increased pressure may lead to minor but chronic irritation of peripheral nerves and neurovascular bundles (Novak et al. 1998). Fibrosis surrounding nerves is apparent following minor irritation (Sommer et al. 1993). Fibrosis is a normal consequence of nerve injury and will have detrimental conse-

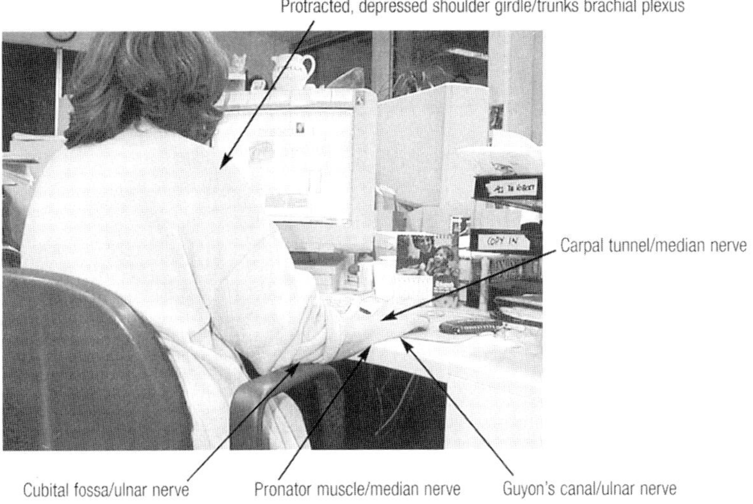

Fig 2. Typical office working posture. The main anatomical sites of possible peripheral nerve compression are indicated.

quences for normal neural gliding. During keyboard use, the carpal tunnel is a lively place when viewed with ultrasound imaging (Lynn et al., in press). The flexor tendons are in rapid motion and the median nerve makes repeated rapid position adjustments to accommodate these tendon movements. It is easy to see that any restriction of the ability of the nerve to move would lead to increased stresses. In susceptible persons, e.g., those with slightly narrower than average carpal tunnels (Greening et al. 1999), these stresses would in turn lead to minor nerve injury or to excitation of the nervi nervorum. Also of note is that the inherent susceptibility of nerves to injury appears to be partly genetically determined (Shir et al. 1991; Mogil et al. 1996).

TREATMENT AND PREVENTION OF RSI

Treatment. A comprehensive musculoskeletal examination is of primary importance to exclude conditions with clear pathology, e.g., tenosynovitis, epicondylitis, or CTS. Note that these conditions may co-exist with RSI. Treatment outcomes for RSI have not been evaluated systematically. On the whole these patients do not respond to rest, nonsteroidal anti-inflammatory drugs, or splinting. In a diffuse condition like RSI, surgery is seldom attempted and outcomes are not reported to be very satisfactory (e.g., see Terrono and Millender 1996). The recent findings of reduced median nerve mobility in the wrist (Greening et al. 1999) might appear at first glance to imply that carpal tunnel release operations should be effective. However, as mentioned above, the reduced mobility at the wrist may be due to restrictions on nerve movement at proximal sites, and the symptoms of RSI differ from those expected from localized entrapment restricted to the median nerve at the carpal tunnel. Response to expert physiotherapy has been successful (Arksey 1995), but is not always advocated (Hagberg 1996). Many authors (Keller et al. 1998; Melhorn 1998; Nainzadeh 1999) advise a multidisciplinary approach that includes physiotherapy, acupuncture, modification of work tasks, ergonomic intervention, and participation in chronic pain management programs. Patient education that explains the postural mechanisms that produce symptoms, and self-help methods for avoiding symptom aggravation, are essential. Unless early intervention is possible, treatment tends to be prolonged and patients rarely return full time to occupations that involve intensive hand use.

Prevention. It is possible, maybe even probable, that RSI is an entirely preventable disease (Melhorn 1999). Careful attention to working conditions should largely eliminate the risks. Thus, those regularly using a keyboard or mouse should have ergonomically sound workstations and take regular breaks (Health and Safety Executive, UK 1993). Maintaining flexibility with regular exercise also appears worthwhile in those with occupations that are mainly sedentary. This approach needs to be linked to an effective program to detect problems early, when they are most easily treated. Limb pain, numbness, or tingling are signs to look for, and should not be ignored. Clearly, while it is important not to incite exaggerated responses to minor aches, a working environment that encourages the early reporting of symptoms is an advantage.

CONCLUSION

The consequences of minor nerve injury appear to be underestimated. Patients with RSI, when examined in a more extensive fashion than the standard medical models, demonstrate clear signs of peripheral and central neural functional change. Early treatment that addresses the problems provoked by sustained poor posture and repetitive hand activities should lead to a more favorable prognosis. As with any condition that has the potential to develop into a chronic pain problem, prevention is the most desirable course of action.

ACKNOWLEDGMENTS

Grant support for Jane Greening from Action Research, Health and Safety Executive (UK), and the British Occupational Health Research Foundation.

REFERENCES

Allman KH, Horch R, Uhl M, et al. MR imaging of the carpal tunnel. *Eur J Rad* 1997; 25:141–145.

Arksey H. *The Sufferers Story. An Empirical Study into RSI Sufferers and Their Dealings with Doctors*. London: Trades Union Congress, 1995.

Arksey H. *RSI and the Experts*. London: UCL Press, 1998.

Arroyo JF, Cohen ML. Unusual responses to electrocutaneous stimulation in refractory cervicobrachial pain: clues to a neuropathic pathogenesis. *Clin Exp Rheumatol* 1992; 10:475–482.

Bennett GJ. Does a neuroimmune interaction contribute to the genesis of pain peripheral neuropathies? *Proc Natl Acad Sci USA* 1999; 96:7737–7738.

Bove GM, Light AR. The nervi nervorum: missing link for neuropathic pain? *Pain Forum* 1997; 6:181–190.

Brooks P. Repetitive strain injury. *BMJ* 1993; 307:1298.

Butler DS. *Mobilisation of the Nervous System*. London: Churchill Livingstone, 1991.

Byng J. Overuse syndromes of the upper limb and the upper limb tension test: a comparison between patients, asymptomatic keyboard workers and asymptomatic non-keyboard workers. *Manual Ther* 1997; 2:157–156.

Cohen ML, Quinter JL. Fibromyalgia syndrome and disability: a failed construct fails those in pain. *Med J Aust* 1998; 168:402–404.

Cohen ML, Arroyo HF, Champion GD, Browne C. In search of the pathogenesis of refractory cervicobrachial pain syndrome. *Med J Aust* 1992; 156:432–437.

Dahlin LB, et al. Graded inhibition of retrograde axonal transport by compression of rabbit vagus nerve. *J Neurol Sci* 1986; 76:221–230.

Devor M. Central changes mediating neuropathic pain. In: Dubner G, Gebhart GF, Bond MR (Eds). *Proceedings of the 5th World Congress on Pain*. Amsterdam: Elsevier, 1988; pp 114–128.

Dennett X, Fry HJ. Overuse syndrome: a muscle biopsy study. *Lancet* 1988; 1:905–908.

Estlander AM, Takala EP, Viikari-Juntura E. Do psychological factors predict changes in musculoskeletal pain? *J Occup Environ Med* 1998; 40:445–453.

Elvey R, Quinter JL, Thomas AN. A clinical study of RSI. *Aust Fam Physician* 1986; 15:1314–1322.

Gellman RH, Hergenroder PT, Hargens AR, Lundborg G, Akeson WH. The carpal tunnel syndrome: a study of carpal tunnel pressures. *J Bone Joint Surg* 1981; 63A:380–383.

Greening J, Lynn B. Vibration sense in the upper limb in patients with repetitive strain injury and a group of at-risk office workers. *Int Arch Occup Environ Health* 1998a; 71:29–34.

Greening J, Lynn B. Minor peripheral nerve injuries: an underestimated source of pain? *Manual Therapy* 1998b; 3:187–194.

Greening J, Smart S, Leary R, et al. Reduced movement of the median nerve in the carpal tunnel during wrist flexion in patients with non-specific arm pain. *Lancet* 1999; 354:217–218.

Hadler NM. Cumulative trauma disorders: an iatrogenic concept. *J Occup Med* 1990; 32(1):38–40.

Hadler NM. Repetitive upper-extremity motions in the workplace are not hazardous. *J Hand Surg (Am)* 1997; 22:1.

Hagberg M. ABC of work related disorders: neck and arm disorders. *BMJ* 1996; 313:419–422.

Hales TR, Bernard BP. Epidemiology of work related musculoskeletal disorders. *Orthop Clin North Am* 1996; 27:679–709.

Hall TM, Elvey RL. Nerve trunk pain: physical diagnosis and treatment. *Manual Therapy* 1999; 4:63–73.

Harrington JM, Carter JT, Birrell L, Gompertz D. Surveillance case definition for work related upper limb pain syndromes. *Occup Environ Med* 1998; 55:264–271.

Health and Safety Executive, UK. *The Health and Safety (Display Screen Equipment) Regulations.* London: HMSO, 1992.

Helliwell PS, Mumford DB, Smeathers JE, Wright V. Work related upper limb disorder: the relationship between pain, cumulative load, disability, and psychological factors. *Ann Rheum Dis* 1992; 51:1325–1329.

Helme RD, LeVasseur SA, Gibson, SJ. RSI revisited. Evidence for psychological and physiological differences from an aged matched control group. *Aust NZ Med J* 1992; 22:23–29.

Higgs PE, Mackinnon SE. Repetitive motion injuries. *Annu Rev Med* 1995; 46:1–16.

Hocking B. Comment. *Med J Aust* 1992; 156:670.

Hutson M. Comment. *BMJ* 1994; 308:269.

Ireland D. The Australian experience with cumulative trauma disorders. In: Millender LH, Louis DS (Eds). *Occupational Disorders of the Upper Extremity.* New York: Churchill Livingstone, 1992.

Jayaraaman KS. Lack of political will, clinical precision, stalls RSI research. *Nature* 1994; 371:8.

Keller K, Corbett J, Nichols D. Repetitive strain injury in computer keyboard users: pathomechanics and treatment principles in individual and group intervention. *J Hand Ther* 1998; 11:9–26.

Koltzenburg M, Kees S, Budweiser S, Ochs G, Toyka K. The properties of unmyelinated nociceptive afferents change in painful chronic constrictive injury. In: Gebhart GF, Hammond DL, Jensen TS. (Eds). *Proceedings of the 7th World Congress on Pain*, Progress in Pain Research and Management, Vol. 2. Seattle: IASP Press, 1994, pp 511–522.

Latko WA, Armstrong TJ, Franzblau A, et al. Cross-sectional study of the relationship between repetitive work and the prevalence of upper limb musculoskeletal disorders. *Am J Ind Med* 1999; 36:248–259.

Littlejohn GO. Fibromyalgia syndrome and disability: the neurogenic model. *Med J Aust* 1998; 168:398–401.

Lucire Y. Social iatrogenesis of the Australian disease 'RSI'. *Community Health Stud* 1988; 12:146–150.

Lynn B, Greening J, Leary R, et al. The use of high-frequency ultrasound imaging to measure nerve movements that occur during limb movements in healthy volunteers and in patients with non-specific arm pain. *J Physiol* 2000; in press.

Mann A. Comment in *BMJ* 1994; 308:269.

Mackinnon SE, Dellon AL, Hudson AR, Hunter DA. Chronic human nerve compression—a histological assessment. *Neuropath Appl Neurobiol* 1986; 126:547–565.

McMahon S. Central hyperexcitability triggered by noxious input. *Curr Opin Neurobiol* 1993; 3:602–610.

McMahon SB, Bennett DLH. Growth factors and pain. In: Dickenson A, Besson JM (Eds). The pharmacology of pain. *Handbook Exp Pharmacol* 1997; 130:135–165.

McMahon SB, Bennett DL, Michael GJ, Priestley. Neurotrophic factors and pain. In: Jensen TS, Turner JA, Wiesenfeld-Hallin Z (Eds). *Proceedings of the 8th World Congress on Pain,* Progress in Pain Research and Management, Vol. 8. Seattle: IASP Press, 1997, pp 353–379.

Maves TJ, Patty SP, Gebhart GF, Meller ST. Possible chemical contribution from chromic gut sutures produces disorders of pain sensation like those seen in man. *Pain* 1993; 54:57–69.

Melhorn JM. Cumulative trauma disorders and repetitive strain injuries. The future. *Clin Orthop* 1998; 351:107–126.

Melhorn JM. The impact of workplace screening on the occurrence of cumulative trauma disorders and workers' compensation claims. *J Occup Environ Med* 1999; 41:84–91.

Miller MH, Topliss D. Chronic upper limb pain syndrome (repetitive strain injury) in the Australian workforce: a systematic cross sectional rheumatological study of 299 patients. *J Rheumatol* 1988; 15:1705–1712.

Mogil JS, Sternberg WF, Marek P, et al. The genetics of pain and pain inhibition. *Proc Natl Acad Sci USA* 1996; 93:3048–3055.

Nainzadeh N, Malantic-Lin A, Alvarez M, Loeser AC. Repetitive strain injury (cumulative trauma disorder): causes and treatment. *Mt Sinai J Med* 1999; 66:192–196.

Novak CB, Mackinnon SE. Nerve injury in repetitive motion disorders. *Clin Orthop* 1998; 351:10–20.

Novak CB, Mackinnon SE. Repetitive use and static postures: a source of nerve compression and pain. *J Hand Ther* 1997; 10:151–159.

Pechan J, Julis I. The pressure measurement in the ulnar nerve. A contribution to the pathophysiology of the cubital tunnel syndrome. *J Biomech* 1975; 8:75–79.

Pritchard MH, Pugh N, Wright I, Brownlee M. A vascular basis for repetitive strain injury. *Rheumatology* 1999; 38:636–639.

Quinter JL, Cohen ML. Referred pain of peripheral nerve origin: an alternative to the "Myofascial Pain" construct. *Clin J Pain* 1994; 10:243–250.

Quinter JL, Cohen ML. Fibromyalgia falls foul of a fallacy. *Lancet* 1999; 353:1092–1094.

Reilly PA. Fibromyalgia in the workplace: a "management" problem. *Ann Rheum Dis* 1993; 52:249–251.

Rowbotham M, Fields H. The relationship of pain, allodynia and thermal sensation in post herpetic neuralgia. *Brain* 1996; 119:347–354.

Sato J, Perl ER. Adrenergic excitation of cutaneous pain receptors induced by peripheral nerve injury. *Science* 1991; 25:1608–1610.

Sauer SK, Bove GM, Averbeck B, Reeh PW. Rat peripheral nerve components release calcitonin gene-related peptide and prostaglandin E2 in response to noxious stimuli: evidence that nervi nervorum are nociceptors. *Neuroscience* 1999; 92:319–325.

Semple JC. Tenosynovitis, repetitive strain injury, cumulative trauma disorder, and overuse, et cetera. *J Bone J Surg* 1991; 73-B:536–568.

Serina ER, Tal R, Remplel D. Wrist and forearm postures and motion during typing. *Ergonomics* 1999; 42:938–951.

Shir Y, Devor M, Seltzer Z. Mechano- and thermal- sensitivity in rats genetically prone to developing neuropathic pain. *Neuroreport* 1991 2:313–316.

Simons DG, Travell JG. Myofascial pain syndromes. In: Wall P, Melzack R. (Eds) *Textbook of Pain*. Edinburgh: Churchill Livingstone, 1984; pp 263–276.

Sommer C, Galbraith J, Heckman H, Myers R. Pathology of experimental compression neuropathy producing hyperalgesia. *J Neuropath Exp Neur* 1993; 52:223–233.

Spindler HA, Dellon LA. Nerve conduction studies in the superficial radial nerve entrapment syndrome. *Muscle Nerve* 1990; 13:1–5.

Sjogaard G, Sogaard K. Muscle injury in repetitive motion disorders. *Clin Orthop* 1998; 351:21–31.

Tal M, Eliav E. Abnormal discharge originates at the site of nerve injury in experimental chronic constriction injury (CCI) in the rat. *Pain* 1996; 64:511–518.

Tanoue M, Yamaga M, Ide J, Takagi K. Acute stretching of peripheral nerves inhibits retrograde axonal transport. *J Hand Surg (Br)* 1996; 21:358–363.

Terrono AL, Millender LH. Management of work-related upper-extremity nerve entrapments. *Orthop Clin North Am* 1996; 27:783–793.

Thomas PK. The connective tissue of peripheral nerve: an electron microscope study. *J Anat* 1963; 97:35–44.

Wigley R. Can fibromyalgia be separated from regional pain syndrome affecting the arm? *J Rheumatol* 1999; 26:515–516.

Wigley RD. Can accident or occupation cause fibromyalgia? *N Z Med J* 1998; 111:60.

Williams P, Warwick R, Dyson M, Bannister L. *Grays Anatomy,* 37th ed. Edinburgh: Churchill Livingstone, 1989, pp 1129–1132.

Wolfe F, Vancouver Fibromyalgia Consensus Group (University of Kansas). 1996. The fibromyalgia syndrome: a consensus report on fibromyalgia and disability. *J Rheumatol* 1996; 23:534–539.

Yassi A. Repetitive strain injuries. *Lancet* 1997; 349:943–947.

Zochodne DW, Ho LT. Hyperemia of injured peripheral nerve: sensitivity to CGRP antagonism. *Brain Res* 1992; 598:59–66.

Correspondence to: Jane Greening, Physiology Department, University College London, Gower Street, London WC1E 6BT, United Kingdom. Tel: 44 (0)171-419-3230; Fax: 44 (0)171-383-7005; email: j.greening@ucl.ac.uk.

Proceedings of the 9th World Congress on Pain,
Progress in Pain Research and Management,
Vol. 16, edited by M. Devor, M.C. Rowbotham, and
Z. Wiesenfeld-Hallin, IASP Press, Seattle, © 2000.

67

SNS/PN3 and NaN/SNS2 Sodium Channel Immunoreactivity in Human Pain States

K. Coward,[a] G. Saldanha,[a] R. Birch,[b]
T. Carlstedt,[b] and P. Anand[a]

[a]*Peripheral Neuropathy Unit, Department of Neurology, Imperial College of Science, Technology and Medicine, Hammersmith Hospital, London, United Kingdom;* [b]*Peripheral Nerve Injury Unit, Royal National Orthopaedic Hospital, Stanmore, Middlesex, United Kingdom*

Several drugs that block sodium channels may relieve neuropathic pain (Devor et al. 1994), but they lack specificity and produce side effects. Two sensory-neuron-specific, tetrodotoxin-resistant (TTX-r) sodium channels, SNS/PN3 and NaN/SNS2, have been cloned from rat dorsal root ganglia (DRG) (Akopian et al. 1996; Sangameswaran et al. 1996; Dib-Hajj et al. 1998; Tate et al. 1998). The biophysical and pharmacological properties of these channels, particularly those of SNS/PN3, suggest that they may play a significant role in pain states. The aim of the present study was to localize and compare the distribution of SNS/PN3 and NaN/SNS2 sodium channels in injured and intact human DRG and peripheral nerve tissue, and in tissues from patients with chronic neurogenic pain.

MATERIALS AND METHODS

Avulsed cervical DRG were obtained from 12 patients (age range 20–46 years), all with trauma to the brachial plexus, 17 hours to 12 months after injury. Control DRG were obtained postmortem. Nerves injured distal to the DRG were collected from nine patients (age range 13–46 years), 3 days to 12 months after injury. Control peripheral nerves were collected from five patients undergoing amputation of a limb for a non-neurological indication, and were obtained from three other surgical patients when nerves were trimmed for grafting.

One neuroma was excised from the plantar nerve of a 46-year-old woman, 6 months after glass injury to the foot. The patient suffered exquisite local pain and hypersensitivity. A second neuroma was excised from the right radial nerve of a 26-year-old woman, 15 months after fracture of the right humerus. The patient suffered marked tenderness over the site of the nerve lesion.

Biopsies of sural nerve were studied from eight patients with peripheral neuropathy. One patient, aged 13 months, had hereditary sensory and autonomic neuropathy, type V (HSAN V), with congenital insensitivity to pain. The remaining patients, all adults, had sensory neuropathy with loss of sensory fibers, with or without motor and autonomic involvement. Three patients had spontaneous pain in both feet, and one patient had marked mechanical and thermal allodynia and hyperalgesia. Two patients had inflammatory changes on nerve histology, with demyelination. Normal sural nerves (obtained when trimmed for grafting) were also obtained from three patients.

A heel skin biopsy was studied from a 28-year-old man who developed marked persistent focal allodynia and hyperalgesia following trivial local trauma while playing football 5 years earlier. Normal skin was obtained from several patients undergoing cosmetic plastic surgery.

All tissues were removed as a necessary part of surgical repair, with the permission of the patients and of the local ethics committee.

Tissue specimens were snap frozen, with the exception of skin biopsies, which were fixed in Zamboni's fixative (2% w/v formalin; 0.1 M phosphate; 15% v/v saturated picric acid) for 4 hours. Frozen tissue sections (8μm) were post-fixed in 4% paraformaldehyde and immunostained with specific affinity-purified antibodies to SNS/PN3 or NaN/SNS2 (provided by GlaxoWellcome). Antibodies were detected using nickel-enhanced immunoperoxidase (ABC), and nuclei were visualized with neutral red (0.1% w/v). Negative controls included pre-incubation of antibodies with homologous antigen and replacement of primary antibody with normal rabbit serum.

RESULTS AND DISCUSSION

SNS/PN3 and NaN/SNS2 sodium channels were demonstrated for the first time in human peripheral nerve and dorsal root ganglia. All small neuronal cell bodies (15–30 μm) appeared to be immunoreactive to SNS/PN3 and NaN/SNS2 in postmortem ganglia (Fig. 1a,b) compared to 60–80% of

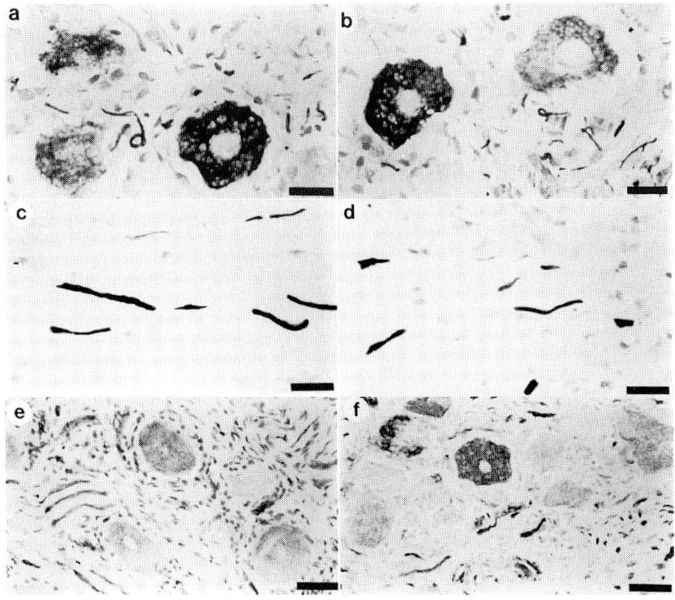

Fig. 1. SNS/PN3-like (a,c,e) and NaN/SNS2-like (b,d,f) immunoreactivity in postmortem cervical DRG (a,b), avulsed cervical DRG 4 days after injury (c,d) and avulsed cervical DRG 3 months after injury (e,f). Scale bar at lower right of each panel = 25 μm in panels a–d and 50 μm in panels e–f.

medium-sized (35–55 μm) and large neurons (60–80 μm). These ganglia contained numerous immunoreactive nerve fibers of strong staining intensity. Avulsed DRG collected within 20 hours of injury exhibited a pattern of immunostaining similar to control DRG. Soon thereafter (4–8 days after injury), however, there was only weak SNS/PN3-like and NaN/SNS2-like immunoreactivity in the avulsed DRG neuronal soma of all sizes; in tissues from three patients there was no immunoreactivity in the soma at all, but strong immunoreactivity in a small number of nerve fibers within the DRG (Fig. 1c,d). Some weeks (3 weeks to 3 months) after injury, there was moderate SNS/PN3 and NaN/SNS2-like immunoreactivity in both nerve fibers proximal to injury and in neuronal soma (Fig. 1e,f). Increased intensity of SNS/PN3-like and NaN/SNS2-like immunostaining was seen in some peripheral nerve fibers proximal to sites of injury (i.e., in injury distal to the DRG) (Fig. 2a,b), when compared to healthy nerves (Fig. 2c,d). In tissues obtained 12 months after injury, immunostaining of SNS/PN3 and NaN/SNS2 in avulsed DRG and injured nerve resembled that of postmortem DRG and healthy nerve, respectively. These findings suggest that the expression of these so-

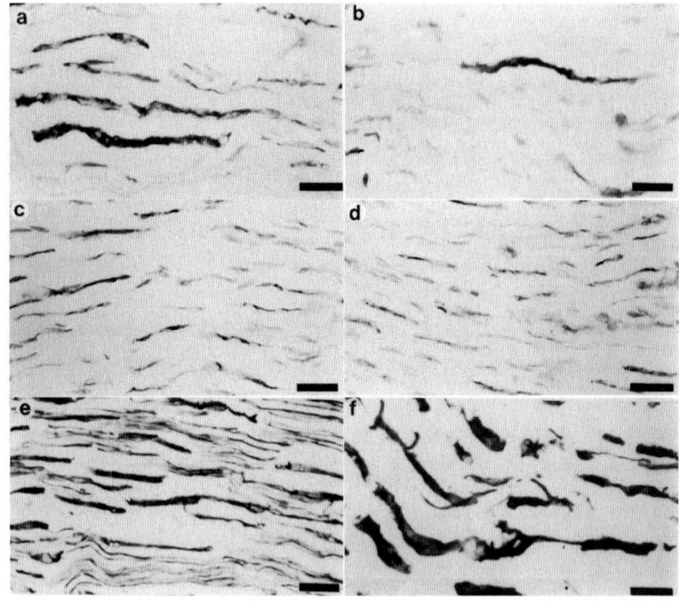

Fig. 2. SNS/PN3-like (a,c) and NaN/SNS2-like (b,d) immunoreactivity in injured peripheral nerve 4 days after injury (a,b) and in normal control peripheral nerve (c,d). Immunostaining with anti-neurofilament antibody in normal peripheral nerve and injured peripheral nerve (4 days after injury) is given in Fig. 1e and 1f, respectively. Scale bar = 25 μm.

dium channels is reduced after avulsion injury in humans, as in animal models of peripheral axotomy (Novakovic et al. 1998). Pre-synthesized, intracellularly located channel protein appears to be translocated to peripheral nerves following injury, with subsequent accumulation at the site of injury, which may contribute to pain phenomena.

Our present studies have also demonstrated, in peripheral tissues from patients with chronic local hypersensitivity, an apparent differential change in SNS/PN3-like and NaN/SNS2-like immunoreactivity. Distal limb neuromas exhibited intense immunoreactivity to SNS/PN3 in numerous nerve fibers (Fig. 3a), but no immunoreactivity to NaN/SNS2 (Fig. 3b). Moreover, hypersensitive heel skin biopsied from a patient also exhibited very intense SNS/PN3-like immunoreactivity (Fig. 3e) but no immunoreactivity to NaN/SNS2 (Fig. 3f).

All biopsies of sural nerves from patients with neuropathy exhibited immunoreactivity to both SNS/PN3 and NaN/SNS2 in axons, which presumably included small and large fibers. Interestingly, the sural nerve biopsied from a patient with idiopathic neuropathy and hypersensitivity exhibited

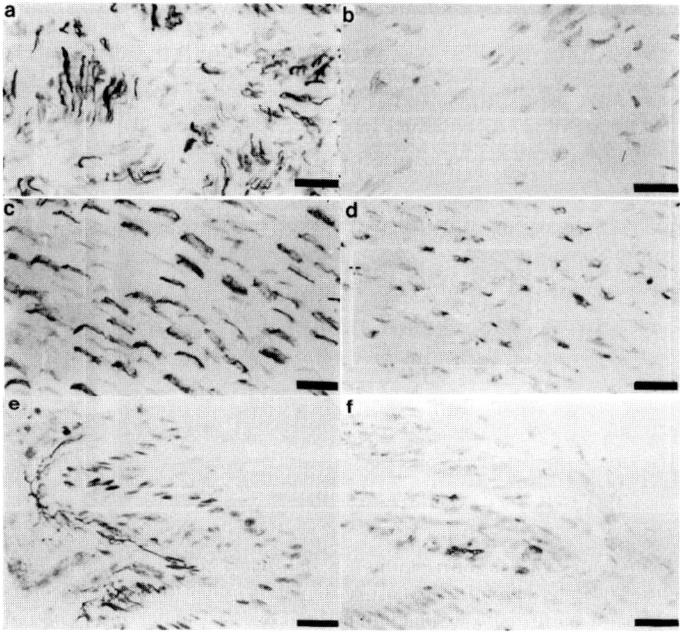

Fig. 3. SNS/PN3-like (a,c,e) and NaN/SNS2-like (b,d,f) immunoreactivity in a painful neuroma (a,b), in sural nerve from a patient with target hypersensitivity (c,d), and in a skin biopsy taken from a hypersensitive heel (e,f). Scale bar = 25 μm.

intense SNS/PN3-like immunoreactivity (Fig. 3c) but only weak NaN/SNS2-like immunoreactivity (Fig. 3d). Tissue from the infant with congenital insensitivity to pain (HSAN V) showed excellent axonal immunostaining for both channels. Both channels were also present at similar levels in axons of all sural nerve biopsies, irrespective of pain, inflammation, or demyelination. A combination of nerve injury and chronic inflammation may be most likely to lead to upregulation/maintenance of one sodium channel (SNS/PN3); density of this channel in subsets of axons may contribute to pain phenomena.

Our results suggest that local hypersensitivity may be the best initial target for SNS/PN3-blocking agents.

ACKNOWLEDGMENT

This work was supported by research funding from Imperial College School of Medicine, London University.

REFERENCES

Akopian AN, Sivilotti L, Wood JN. A tetrodotoxin-resistant voltage-gated sodium channel expressed by sensory neurons. *Nature* 1996; 379:257–262.

Devor M, Lomazov P, Matzner O. Sodium channel accumulation in injured axons as a substrate for neuropathic pain. In: Boivie J, Hansson P, Lindblom U (Eds). *Touch, Temperature and Pain in Health and Disease: Mechanisms and Assessments,* Progress in Pain Research and Management, Vol. 3. Seattle: IASP Press, 1994, pp 207–230.

Dib-Hajj SD, Tyrrell L, Black JA, Waxman SG. NaN, a novel voltage-gated Na channel, is expressed preferentially in peripheral sensory neurons and down-regulated after axotomy. *Proc Natl Acad Sci USA* 1998; 95:8963–8968.

Novakovic SD, Tzoumaka E, McGiven J, et al. Distribution of the tetrodotoxin-resistant sodium channel PN3 in rat sensory neurons in normal and neuropathic conditions. *J Neurosci* 1998; 88:2174–2187.

Sangameswaran L, Delgado SG, Fish LM, et al. Structure and function of a novel voltage-gated tetrodotoxin resistant sodium channel specific to sensory neurons. *J Biol Chem* 1996; 271:5953–5956.

Tate S, Benn S, Hick C, et al. Two sodium channels contribute to the TTX-R sodium current in primary sensory neurons. *Nat Neurosci* 1998; 1:653–655.

Correspondence to: Professor P. Anand, MA, MD, FRCP, Peripheral Neuropathy Unit, Department of Neurology, Imperial College School of Medicine, Area A, Ground Floor, Hammersmith Hospital, Du Cane Road, London, W12 ONN, United Kingdom. Tel: 0181-383-3309/3319; Fax: 0181-383-3363/3364; email: p.anand@ic.ac.uk.

Proceedings of the 9th World Congress on Pain,
Progress in Pain Research and Management,
Vol. 16, edited by M. Devor, M.C. Rowbotham, and
Z. Wiesenfeld-Hallin, IASP Press, Seattle, © 2000.

68

Chronic Neuropathic Pain in Leprosy

Aki Hietaharju,[a] Richard Croft,[b] Rezaul Alam,[b]
and Maija Haanpää[a]

[a]*Department of Neurology and Rehabilitation, Tampere University Hospital, Tampere, Finland;* [b]*Danish Bangladesh Leprosy Mission, Nilphamari, Bangladesh*

Leprosy, also known as Hansen's disease, is a chronic infectious disease caused by *Mycobacterium leprae*. It produces damage primarily in peripheral nerves and skin. Although the overall prevalence of the disease is decreasing, it still forms the most common treatable neuropathy in the world (Nations et al. 1998). The registered global prevalence of leprosy is around 1.4 per 10,000 population (WHO statistics, July 1999), and about 4 million people suffer from leprosy disability (Leprosy Mission 1999). Leprosy is divided into five subtypes based on histological and immunological features: tuberculoid, borderline tuberculoid, midborderline, borderline lepromatous, and lepromatous leprosy (Ridley and Jopling 1966). These subtypes have been consolidated into two groups, paucibacillary and multibacillary, for assignment to treatment regimens. According to World Health Organization (WHO) guidelines, the former is treated with dapsone 100 mg daily and rifampicin 600 mg monthly for 6 months. Multibacillary leprosy requires a minimum of 2 years of treatment, and clofazimine 50 mg daily is added to the paucibacillary regimen (WHO Study Group 1982).

The term "superficial neuropathy" has been used to describe the unique clinical pattern of peripheral nerve involvement in leprosy (Sabin et al. 1993). *M. leprae* infiltrates dermal nerves and superficial segments of peripheral nerve trunks at well-known sites of predilection, leaving the nerves in deeper tissues intact. Each form of leprosy is associated with specific patterns of neuropathy. The most devastating clinical consequence of intracutaneous nerve damage in leprosy is the total sensory loss in the extremities (Brand and Fritschi 1985). Pain and temperature sensation are most strikingly decreased in early cases; later, tactile and pressure sense are also lost. Anesthesia of the extremities predisposes the patient to chronic ulcers and severe secondary deformities, and therefore leprosy remains a significant cause of neurological disability worldwide. Considering this, it would be natural to believe that pain relief is hardly needed in the treatment of leprosy. However, we encountered a number of leprosy patients, most of whom had already completed their treatment, who came to the outpatient clinics to complain of stimulus-independent ongoing pain and ask for relief. The following report encompasses the detailed clinical findings on 16 patients with multibacillary leprosy and chronic neuropathic pain.

METHODS

The study area was Nilphamari District, located in the northwestern corner of Bangladesh. This area is highly endemic for leprosy (Richardus and Croft 1995): during the years 1979–1996, a total of 11,771 leprosy patients were registered there (5222 with multibacillary and 6549 with paucibacillary leprosy). Clinical diagnosis of leprosy and its classification was based on the Ridley-Jopling system (Ridley and Jopling 1966) and on national leprosy control program guidelines (TB and Leprosy Control Services 1995). This study was conducted on patients with multibacillary leprosy who had completed their therapy and had a history of moderate or severe chronic neuropathic pain problems that were causing sleep disturbances or were troublesome most of the time and had lasted more than 6 months. The patients were recruited for this study in spring 1997 with the help of local leprosy workers from four outpatient clinics. The workers were instructed to ask for the following symptoms: burning feet, formication, pricking, biting, or squeezing pain. Altogether, 38 patients were recruited. Nine referred patients canceled their appointment for unknown reasons, and 13 patients were excluded from the study either because their leprosy was paucibacillary or because their pain was purely nociceptive. None of the 16 patients included had a history of alcohol abuse, and all had normal levels of blood glucose.

The clinical neurological examination, performed by one of the authors (A. Hietaharju), included assessment of tactile, pinprick, thermal, and joint position sensation and tendon reflexes. Tactile sensation was tested with a piece of cotton wool and sensation to pinprick with a sharp plastic stick. Thermal sensation was assessed with the Thermal Sensation Tester, specifically designed for developing countries (B.S. Tech, Switzerland). The hot tip of this battery-run device can be heated up to 60°C. Dynamic allodynia was tested with a toothbrush, and static allodynia by gentle compression of the skin and by stretching the skin manually. Location of pain was recorded by using pain drawings. Quantitative sensory testing was performed at standard peripheral testing sites (dorsum of both hands in the middle of the anatomical snuff box and dorsum of both feet in the proximal part of the first intermetatarsal space) to evaluate the peripheral sensory loss that is typical of fully developed leprosy (Sabin et al 1993). Thresholds for pinprick sensation were measured by using the weighted needle apparatus (Chan et al 1992), and thresholds for tactile sensation by using Semmes-Weinstein monofilaments (Gillis W. Long, Hansen's Disease Center, Hansen's Disease Foundation, Inc., Filament Project Building 18, Carville, LA 70721 USA). Quantitative sensory testing was also performed on 21 healthy Bangladeshi controls (12 males, 9 females, age range 21–54 years, mean 34 years). The 95th percentiles of data of the healthy controls were used as reference values for the quantitative sensory testing results.

RESULTS

Relevant clinical and demographic data are summarized in Tables I and II. The mean age of the 16 patients was 49 years (range 32–75 years). The mean time elapsed from the completion of therapy, i.e., date released from leprosy treatment, was 44 months (range 4–107 months). In quantitative sensory testing at the standard testing sites in hands and feet, pinprick sensation was normal in 41% of measurements in hands and in 22% of measurements in feet, and tactile sensation was normal in 44% of measurements in hands and in 22% of measurements in feet.

The distribution of pain and sensory loss was equal in 11 of the 16 patients (69%), whereas we found inconsistencies between distribution of pain and sensory abnormalities in five cases. Patients 2 and 15 had total sensory loss in hands and feet, but pain was located more proximally. Patients 3 and 10 had widespread pain but very limited sensory loss. Patient 4 had recovered from glove- and stocking-like sensory loss during the antimicrobial treatment and had normal sensory findings at the time of the present study. However, her pain persisted in spite of the treatment.

DISCUSSION

Medical reports on neuropathic pain associated with leprosy are scarce and are mostly limited to premonitory symptoms or acute complications of the disease. Pain in one or several nerves may be the presenting feature in leprosy and is typical of neuritis, in which pain is usually a consequence of sudden entrapment of the grossly swollen inflamed nerve at the sites of predilection (Pfaltzgraff and Bryceson 1985, Bryceson and Pfaltzgraff 1990).

Table I
Summary of the demographics and characteristics of pain in 16 patients with leprosy

Patient Number	Age, Sex	Type of Leprosy	RFT	Duration of Pain (y)	Quality of Pain	Severity of Pain	Distribution of Pain	Occurrence of Pain
1	75, F	BT	5/94	10	Burning	Severe	Glove and stocking	Continuous
2	36, F	LL	1/95	3	Burning	Severe	Glove and stocking, feet spared	Periodic
3	60, F	BB	3/94	5	Burning	Moderate	Upper and lower extremities	Daytime
4	40, F	BL	9/96	9	Tingling, burning	Severe	Glove and stocking	Continuous
5	40, F	BT	2/95	4	Burning	Moderate	Right leg below knee	Periodic
6	37, F	BT	1/94	5	Burning, pricking	Severe	Left foot, lateral border	Continuous
7	50, F	BT	6/93	>5	Burning, pricking	Severe	Glove and stocking	Continuous
8	70, F	LL	12/92	3	Freezing, electric-shock-like	Severe	Glove and stocking	Nocturnal
9	52, F	BT	4/94	8	Burning	Moderate	Glove and stocking	Continuous
10	37, M	LL	8/92	5	Cutting, electric-shock-like	Severe	Right foot, sural nerve	Periodic
11	70, M	BL	7/88	4	Burning, biting	Severe	Glove and stocking	Periodic
12	45, M	BT	5/95	4	Tingling	Moderate	Both legs, below mid-thigh	Daytime
13	53, M	BT	10/88	>20	Cutting, pricking	Severe	Glove and stocking	Continuous
14	45, M	BT	5/94	5	Biting, electric-shock-like	Severe	Glove and stocking	Continuous
15	48, M	BL	4/94	3	Tingling, biting	Moderate	Glove and stocking, hands and feet spared	Evening
16	32, M	BT	2/97	>2	Tingling	Moderate	Left leg, medial femoral cutaneous nerve	Continuous

Abbreviations: RFT = date released from treatment (month/year); BT = borderline tuberculous leprosy; LL = lepromatous leprosy; BB = midborderline leprosy; BL = borderline lepromatous leprosy.

Neuritic pain was the main reason for the consumption of analgesic preparations in a study of 235 leprosy patients, of whom 46 (19.5%) admitted to having consumed more than 2 kg of analgesics (Segasothy et al. 1986). We found no published studies describing the clinical spectrum of chronic neuropathic pain in leprosy patients who have completed their antimicrobial therapy.

Our results indicate that there are leprosy patients who suffer from neuropathic pain, i.e., have pain combined with altered sensory function. The most typical sensory abnormalities seem to be severely impaired perception of tactile stimuli and mechanical and thermal pain, indicating damage of Aβ, Aδ, and C fibers at the painful site. In lepromatous leprosy, the cutaneous nerve branches that are most superficial, and hence coolest, are the predilection sites for mycobacterial colonization and subsequent nerve damage, which results first in patchy localization (patients 2 and 8 in Tables I and II) and later in glove- and stocking-like distribution of sensory loss (Nations et al. 1998). This temperature-linked nerve damage clarifies why the palms and soles are usually spared in the early phase of the disease, and explains the long-lasting preservation of long tendon reflexes and joint position sense. Patients with borderline leprosy develop multiple mononeuropathies with motor and sensory involvement in addition to the involvement of dermal nerves (Sabin et al. 1993). Typical representatives of borderline leprosy with local enlargement and tenderness of peripheral nerves in our series are patients 1, 5, 9, and 14 in Tables I and II. Interestingly, two patients (numbers 6 and 16) had mechanical allodynia of both the dynamic and static type, and both of them had well-preserved sensory functions.

In leprosy, different pathogenic mechanisms of pain can be suggested. In ongoing neuritis and subsequent entrapment of the nerve, firing of the nervi nervorum may be the main contributor to pain. Additionally, inflammation in the nerve and skin may excite and sensitize nociceptors. Following axonal damage and regeneration, peripheral functional changes such as spontaneous discharges, lowered activation thresholds, and exaggerated responses of the nociceptors can be postulated. The excessive peripheral activity may lead to central sensitization. Patients with repeated episodes of neuritis and immunological reactions (Negesse 1995) may be especially at risk. Patients with severe sensory loss may also represent the deafferentation type of neuropathic pain, although the preservation of sensory function in a considerable proportion of our patients suggests that deafferentation does not explain their pain.

Further epidemiological studies are necessary to determine the magnitude of the neuropathic pain problem among leprosy patients. If neuropathic pain is as common as our results indicate, new therapeutic avenues need to

Table II
Summary of the clinical findings in 16 patients with leprosy

Patient Number	Tendon Reflexes	Position Sense	Location of Sensory Loss (Qualitative Testing)	Allo-dynia	Thermal Loss*	Enlargement and/or Tenderness of Nerves
1	Normal	Normal	Glove and stocking, patchy in hands	No	Yes	Both ulnar, common peroneal, posterior tibial
2	Normal	Normal	Both feet; patchy in legs, arms, and face	No	Yes	No
3	P and A lost	Normal	Right foot	No	Yes	No
4	Normal	Normal	No sensory loss	No	No	No
5	Normal	Normal	Right foot, patchy in right leg	No	Yes	Right sural, posterior tibial
6	Normal	Normal	Left foot	Yes	Yes	Left common peroneal, posterior tibial
7	P and A lost	Lost	Glove and stocking	No	Yes	No
8	Normal	Normal	Both legs below knee, patchy in left leg and both arms	No	Yes	No
9	A lost	Normal	Both feet, patchy in arms and legs	No	Yes	Left popliteal, right cutaneous radial
10	Normal	Normal	Both feet, patchy in legs and hands	No	Yes	No
11	P and A lost	Not done	Glove and stocking	No	Yes	No
12	Normal	Normal	Anterior surface of both legs below mid-thigh	No	Yes	No
13	P and A lost	Normal	Both legs and arms, patchy in face	No	Yes	No
14	Normal	Lost	Patchy in right hand and both legs and feet	No	Yes	Both common peroneal nerves
15	P and A lost	Normal	Anterior surface of both legs below knee, patchy in hands	No	Yes	No
16	P lost	Normal	Left cutaneous femoral nerve distribution	Yes	Yes	Left cutaneous femoral

Abbreviations: P = patellar; A = achilles.
* Location identical with sensory loss in qualitative testing.

be opened in the future programs to provide "care after cure" for leprosy patients who have been released from treatment. Current pharmacological treatment regimens for neuropathic pain involve tricyclic antidepressants and anticonvulsant drugs (Koltzenburg 1998), both of which would be cost-effective in developing countries.

ACKNOWLEDGMENTS

The authors thank the field staff of the Danish Bangladesh Leprosy Mission for their help in identifying suitable patients, and the medical and nursing staff for their help while the subjects were in hospital for their examinations.

REFERENCES

Brand PW, Fritschi EP. Rehabilitation in leprosy. In: Hastings RC (Ed). *Leprosy*, 1st ed. Edinburgh: Churchill Livingstone, 1985, pp 287–319.

Bryceson A, Pfaltzgraff RE. *Leprosy*, 3rd edition. Edinburgh: Churchill Livingstone, 1990.

Chan AW, MacFarlane IA, Bowsher D, Campbell JA. Weighted needle pinprick sensory thresholds: a simple test of sensory function in diabetic peripheral neuropathy. *J Neurol Neurosurg Psychiatry* 1992; 55:56–59.

Koltzenburg M. Painful neuropathies. *Curr Opin Neurol* 1998; 11:515–521.

Leprosy Mission. Available via the Internet: http://www.leprosymission.org.au/challenge.htm. Accessed September 1999.

Nations SP, Katz JS, Lyde CB, Barohn RJ. Leprous neuropathy: an American perspective. *Semin Neurol* 1998; 18:113–124.

Negesse Y. Comment: "silently arising clinical neuropathy" and extended indication of steroid therapy in leprosy neuropathy. *Lepr Rev* 1996; 67:230–231.

Pfaltzgraff RE, Bryceson A. Clinical leprosy. In: Hastings RC (Ed). *Leprosy*, 1st ed. Edinburgh: Churchill Livingstone, 1985, pp 134–176.

Richardus JH, Croft RP. Estimating the size of the leprosy problem: the Bangladesh experience. *Lepr Rev* 1995; 66:158–164.

Ridley DS, Jopling WH. Classification of leprosy according to immunity: a five-group system. *Int J Lepr* 1966; 54:255–273.

Sabin TD, Swift TR, Jacobsen RR. Leprosy. In: Dyck PJ, Thomas PK, Griffin JW, Low PA, Podusco JF (Eds). *Peripheral Neuropathy*. Philadelphia: Saunders, 1993; 2:1354–1379.

Segasothy M, Muhaya HM, Musa A, et al. Analgesic use by leprosy patients. *Int J Lepr Other Mycobact Dis* 1986; 54:399–402.

TB and Leprosy Control Services. *Technical Guide and Operational Manual for Leprosy Control in Bangladesh*. Dhaka: Government of Bangladesh, 1995.

WHO Statistics. July 19991. Available via the Internet: http://www.who.int/lep/latest%20statistics.htm. Accessed September 1999.

WHO Study Group. *Chemotherapy of Leprosy for Control Programmes*, Technical Report Series 675. Geneva: World Health Organization, 1982.

Correspondence to: Aki Hietaharju, MD, Department of Neurology and Rehabilitation, Tampere University Hospital, PO Box 2000, 33521 Tampere, Finland. Tel: 358-3-247-5111; Fax: 358-3-247-4351; email: hietahar@koti.tpo.fi.

Proceedings of the 9th World Congress on Pain, Progress in Pain Research and Management, Vol. 16, edited by M. Devor, M.C. Rowbotham, and Z. Wiesenfeld-Hallin, IASP Press, Seattle, © 2000.

69

Acute Pain in Herpes Zoster

Robert H. Dworkin,[a] Robert W. Johnson,[b] and David R.J. Griffin[c]

[a]*Department of Anesthesiology, University of Rochester School of Medicine and Dentistry, Rochester, New York, USA;* [b]*Department of Anesthesiology, Bristol Royal Infirmary and University of Bristol, Bristol, United Kingdom;* [c]*SmithKline Beecham Pharmaceuticals, Harlow, Essex, United Kingdom*

The onset of herpes zoster is marked by a prodrome of dermatomal pain in most patients. The characteristic rash that typically appears several days later is usually accompanied by continued pain. Although the rash heals within 2–4 weeks, pain in the affected dermatome persists in a percentage of patients. This persisting pain is termed postherpetic neuralgia (PHN), a well-known chronic pain syndrome that is often refractory to treatment and that can last for years, causing disability, psychological distress, and increased use of the health care system (Watson 1993; Kost and Straus 1996; Wallace and Oxman 1997; Cluff and Rowbotham 1998; Dworkin and Johnson 1999).

Until recently, older age has been the only factor consistently associated with an increased risk of PHN in herpes zoster patients. Four additional risk factors for PHN have now been identified by independent groups of investigators—greater acute pain severity, greater rash severity, presence of a painful prodrome preceding the rash, and sensory deficits in the affected dermatome during acute zoster (Dworkin and Portenoy 1996; Dworkin and Banks 1999). Of these risk factors, the most well established is greater acute pain severity. The results of a considerable number of recent prospective studies have demonstrated that patients with more severe acute pain during herpes zoster are at greater risk for PHN, however it is defined.

Unfortunately, few of these studies provide a detailed examination of acute pain in herpes zoster. Little is therefore known regarding the associations between acute pain and other characteristics of herpes zoster patients, including demographic and clinical risk factors for PHN. For example, it has been hypothesized that age is a risk factor for PHN because older patients have more severe acute herpes zoster infections (Higa et al. 1988, 1992, 1997). This hypothesis suggests that older herpes zoster patients have more severe acute pain as well as a more severe rash. However, the results of several studies have not provided uniform support for these predictions. Older age has not been found to be associated with greater acute pain severity (Bamford and Boundy 1968; Harding et al. 1987; Haanpää et al. 1999) or longer acute pain duration (Boon and Griffin 1996). Moreover, older age is not consistently associated with either greater lesion severity (Harding et al. 1987; Higa et al. 1988, 1992, 1997) or longer rash duration (Burgoon et al. 1957; Wildenhoff et al. 1979, 1981; Harding et al. 1987; Bean 1993).

Knowledge of the extent to which acute pain severity is associated with rash severity and presence of a prodrome would be valuable in interpreting the findings that all three of these aspects of the acute herpes zoster infection are risk factors for PHN. Although two studies have reported that greater acute pain was associated with longer rash duration (Molin 1969; Harrison et al. 1999), two others reported that acute pain was not significantly associated with lesion severity (Bruxelle 1995; Haanpää et al. 1999). However, one of these studies did find that more severe acute herpes zoster pain was associated with the presence of a prodrome (Haanpää et al. 1999).

To clarify the relationships between acute pain and age, sex, rash severity, and presence of a prodrome in herpes zoster, we examined the data from two large samples of herpes zoster patients who were studied within 72 hours of rash onset.

METHODS

We examined the baseline data from two samples of herpes zoster patients who participated in two separate, previously published clinical trials of the antiviral agent famciclovir. In the first trial, famciclovir was compared with acyclovir in 545 immunocompetent patients (15–93 years of age) with herpes zoster in a randomized, multicenter, double-blind trial (DeGreef 1994). Treatment with famciclovir (250, 500, or 750 mg, three times daily) for 7 days, beginning within 72 hours of rash onset, was compared with acyclovir (800 mg, five times daily). The second study assessed the efficacy and safety of famciclovir in 419 immunocompetent patients (18–91 years of age) with herpes zoster in a randomized, multicenter, double-blind, placebo-controlled trial (Tyring et al. 1995; Dworkin et al. 1998). Treatment with famciclovir (500 mg or 750 mg, three times daily) for 7 days, beginning within 72 hours of rash onset, was compared with placebo. The methodological features of these clinical trials and the results of their analyses have been presented in detail elsewhere (DeGreef 1994; Tyring et al. 1995; Dworkin et al. 1998). In these trials, famciclovir had a significant beneficial effect on viral shedding, rash healing, acute pain, and PHN.

We examined data collected during these trials at the initial visit, which occurred within 72 hours of rash onset and before any treatment was begun. We analyzed the following data: age, sex, presence of a prodrome (defined as pain and/or abnormal sensations), rash severity (mild, <25 vesicles; moderate, 25–50 vesicles; or severe, >50 vesicles), and acute pain (none, mild, moderate, or severe).

RESULTS

The distributions of acute pain severity in each of the two samples are presented in Fig. 1. Within 72 hours of the onset of their rash, most patients rated the intensity of their pain as moderate or severe.

We examined the relationships between these ratings of acute pain severity and the other variables in a series of analyses of variance and chi-square tests, summarized in Table I. Greater acute pain severity was significantly associated with greater age, greater rash severity, and the presence of a prodrome in each of the two samples. In addition, women reported significantly more acute pain than did men in the placebo-controlled trial, but not in the famciclovir vs. acyclovir trial (Table I).

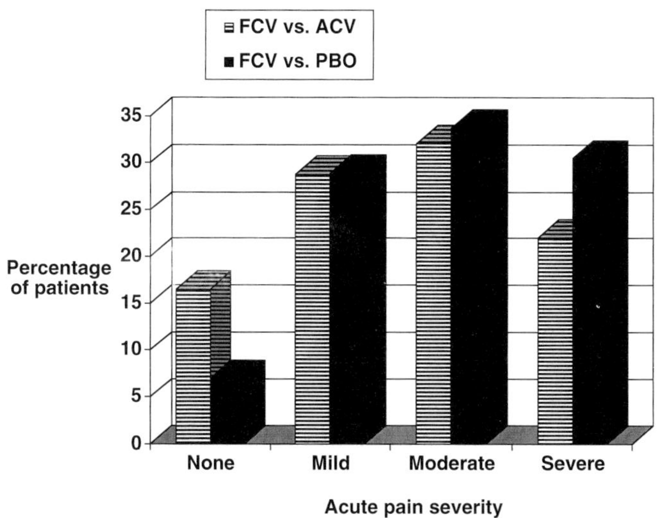

Fig. 1. Distribution of ratings of acute pain severity in two famciclovir trials. FCV = famciclovir; ACV = acyclovir; PBO = placebo.

Table I
Relationships between acute pain severity and age, sex, presence of a prodrome, and rash severity in herpes zoster

	Acute Pain Severity			
Variable	None	Mild	Moderate	Severe
Famciclovir vs. Acyclovir Trial				
Mean age (years)	48.4	52.4	52.8	60.4***
Sex (% female)	57.8	51.0	56.6	61.7
Prodrome present (%)	75.6	84.1	93.1	99.2***
Severe rash (%)	28.9	40.8	45.1	50.8*
Famciclovir vs. Placebo Trial				
Mean age (years)	47.1	47.6	47.9	54.3**
Sex (% female)	27.6	42.1	53.2	50.0*
Prodrome present (%)	51.7	88.4	94.3	93.0***
Severe rash (%)	41.4	40.5	54.3	68.8***

Note. Top rows of data are from the famciclovir vs. acyclovir trial ($n = 545$; Degreef 1994); bottom rows of data are from the famciclovir vs. placebo trial ($n = 419$; Tyring et al. 1995; Dworkin et al. 1998). Statistical significance levels in the rightmost column reflect the results of analyses of variance and chi-square tests: * $P < 0.05$; ** $P < 0.01$; *** $P < 0.001$.

In separate stepwise multiple regression analyses for each of the two samples, age, rash severity, and the presence of a prodrome were independently associated with greater acute pain severity. Sex was also independently associated with acute pain severity in the placebo-controlled trial but not in the famciclovir vs. acyclovir trial.

DISCUSSION

Previous studies have demonstrated that greater age, greater rash severity, and presence of a prodrome in acute herpes zoster patients are risk factors for PHN (Dworkin and Portenoy 1996; Dworkin and Banks 1999). The results of our analyses demonstrate that these three risk factors for PHN are also associated with greater acute pain severity at the very beginning of the herpes zoster infection. It is important to recognize, however, that the strength of these relationships does not appear to be great (in the two multiple regressions, the R^2 values for the full models were 0.11 and 0.13; see also Fig. 2). This may explain why previous studies investigating the relationships between acute pain and other characteristics of herpes zoster pa-

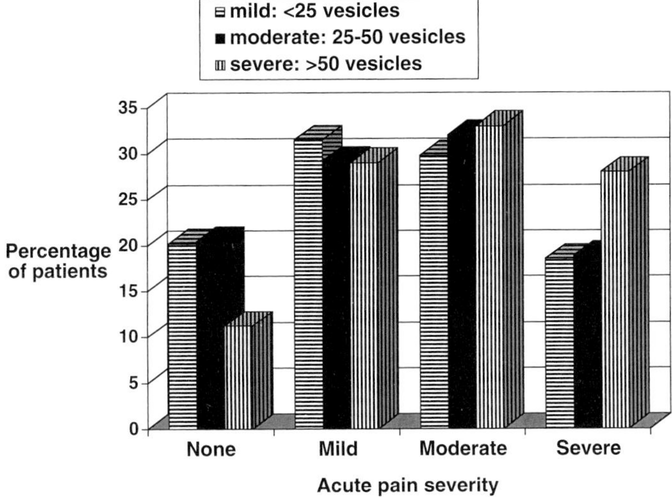

Fig. 2. Distribution of ratings of rash severity as a function of acute pain severity in the famciclovir vs. acyclovir trial (n = 545).

tients have yielded results that were inconsistent with one another and with the results of the present analyses. If we had not used relatively large samples of patients, our pattern of findings may well have been quite different. Nevertheless, the results provide additional support for the recommendation that herpes zoster patients who are older, who have had a prodrome, or who have a more severe rash should be targeted for treatment of their acute pain as well as for interventions designed to prevent PHN (Bennett 1994; Dworkin 1997, 1999).

In future research, it will be important to examine the relationships among acute pain, rash severity, presence of a prodrome, age, sex, and other aspects of the acute herpes zoster infection not investigated in the present analyses—for example, affected dermatome, prodrome duration, and cutaneous dissemination. It will also be important to examine the relationships between acute pain severity and other established and putative risk factors for PHN, including sensory deficits in the affected dermatome, more pronounced humoral and cell-mediated immune responses, generalized impairment of large-fiber afferents, and psychosocial distress. The results of such research on acute herpes zoster will be important in evaluating single-factor (e.g., Higa et al. 1997), multifactorial (Dworkin and Banks 1999), and multiple-mechanism (Rowbotham et al. 1998) approaches to understanding the pathogenesis of PHN.

ACKNOWLEDGMENT

Data collection was sponsored by SmithKline Beecham Pharmaceuticals.

REFERENCES

Bamford JAC, Boundy CAP. The natural history of herpes zoster (shingles). *Med J Aust* 1968; 13:524–528.

Bean B, Deamant C, Aeppli D. Acute zoster: course, complications and treatment in the immunocompetent host. In: Watson CPN (Ed). *Herpes Zoster and Postherpetic Neuralgia.* Amsterdam: Elsevier, 1993, pp 37–58.

Bennett GJ. Hypotheses on the pathogenesis of herpes zoster-associated pain. *Ann Neurol* 1994; 35(Suppl):S38–S41.

Boon RJ, Griffin DRG. Famciclovir: efficacy in zoster and issues in the assessment of pain. In: Mills J, Volberding PA, Corey L (Eds). *Antiviral Chemotherapy 4: New Directions for Clinical Application and Research.* New York: Plenum Press, 1996, pp 17–31.

Bruxelle J. Prospective epidemiologic study of painful and neurologic sequelae induced by herpes zoster in patients treated early with oral acyclovir. *Neurology* 1995; 45(Suppl 8):S78–S79.

Burgoon CF, Burgoon JS, Baldridge GD. The natural history of herpes zoster. *JAMA* 1957; 164:265–269.

Cluff RS, Rowbotham MC. Pain caused by herpes zoster infection. *Neurol Clin* 1998; 16:813–832.

DeGreef H. Famciclovir, a new oral antiherpes drug: results of the first controlled clinical study demonstrating its efficacy and safety in the treatment of uncomplicated herpes zoster in immunocompetent patients. *Int J Antimicrob Agents* 1994; 4:241–246.

Dworkin RH. Which individuals with acute pain are most likely to develop a chronic pain syndrome? *Pain Forum* 1997; 6:127–136.

Dworkin RH. Prevention of postherpetic neuralgia. *Lancet* 1999; 353:1636–1637.

Dworkin RH, Banks SM. A vulnerability-diathesis-stress model of chronic pain: herpes zoster and the development of postherpetic neuralgia. In: Gatchel RJ, Turk DC (Eds). *Psychosocial Factors in Pain: Critical Perspectives.* New York: Guilford Press, 1999, pp 247–269.

Dworkin RH, Johnson RW. A belt of roses from hell: pain in herpes zoster and postherpetic neuralgia. In: Block AR, Kremer EF, Fernandez E (Eds). *Handbook of Pain Syndromes: Biopsychosocial Perspectives.* Hillsdale, New Jersey: Erlbaum, 1999, pp 371–402.

Dworkin RH, Portenoy RK. Pain and its persistence in herpes zoster. *Pain* 1996; 67:241–251.

Dworkin RH, Boon RJ, Griffin DRG, Phung D. Postherpetic neuralgia: impact of famciclovir, age, rash severity, and acute pain in herpes zoster patients. *J Infect Dis* 1998; 178(Suppl 1):S76–S80.

Haanpää M, Laippala P, Nurmikko T. Pain and somatosensory dysfunction in acute herpes zoster. *Clin J Pain* 1999; 15:78–84.

Harding SP, Lipton JR, Wells JCD. Natural history of herpes zoster ophthalmicus: predictors of postherpetic neuralgia and ocular involvement. *Br J Opthalmol* 1987; 71:353–358.

Harrison RA, Soong S, Weiss HL, Gnann JW, Whitley RJ. A mixed model for factors predictive of pain in AIDS patients with herpes zoster. *J Pain Symptom Manage* 1999; 17:410–417.

Higa K, Dan K, Manabe H, Noda B. Factors influencing the duration of treatment of acute herpetic pain with sympathetic nerve block: importance of severity of herpes zoster assessed by the maximum antibody titers to varicella-zoster virus in otherwise healthy patients. *Pain* 1988; 32:147–157.

Higa K, Noda B, Manabe H, Sato S, Dan K. T-lymphocyte subsets in otherwise healthy patients with herpes zoster and relationships to the duration of acute herpetic pain. *Pain* 1992; 51:111–118.

Higa K, Mori M, Hirata K, et al. Severity of skin lesions of herpes zoster at the worst phase rather than age and involved region most influences the duration of acute herpetic pain. *Pain* 1997; 69:245–253.

Kost RG, Straus SE. Postherpetic neuralgia: pathogenesis, treatment, and prevention. *N Engl J Med* 1996; 335:32–42.

Molin L. Aspects of the natural history of herpes zoster. *Acta Derm Venereol* 1969; 49:569–583.

Rowbotham MC, Petersen KL, Fields HL. Is postherpetic neuralgia more than one disorder? *Pain Forum* 1998; 7:231–237.

Tyring S, Barbarash RA, Nahlik JE, et al. Famciclovir for the treatment of acute herpes zoster: effects on acute disease and postherpetic neuralgia: a randomized, double-blind, placebo-controlled trial. *Ann Intern Med* 1995; 123:89–96.

Wallace MS, Oxman MN. Acute herpes zoster and postherpetic neuralgia. *Anesth Clin North Am* 1997; 15:371–405.

Watson CPN (Ed). *Herpes Zoster and Postherpetic Neuralgia.* Amsterdam: Elsevier, 1993.

Wildenhoff KE, Ipsen J, Esmann V, Ingemann-Jensen J, Poulsen JH. Treatment of herpes zoster with idoxuridine ointment, including a multivariate analysis of symptoms and signs. *Scand J Infect Dis* 1979; 11:1–9.

Wildenhoff KE, Esmann V, Ipsen J, et al. Treatment of trigeminal and thoracic zoster with idoxuridine. *Scand J Infect Dis* 1981; 13:257–262.

Correspondence to: Robert H. Dworkin, PhD, Department of Anesthesiology, University of Rochester School of Medicine and Dentistry, 601 Elmwood Avenue, Box 604, Rochester, NY 14642, USA. Tel: 716-275-3524; Fax: 716-473-5007; email: robrt_dworkin@urmc.rochester.edu.

Proceedings of the 9th World Congress on Pain,
Progress in Pain Research and Management,
Vol. 16, edited by M. Devor, M.C. Rowbotham, and
Z. Wiesenfeld-Hallin, IASP Press, Seattle, © 2000.

70

Trigeminal Postherpetic Neuralgia Postmortem: Clinically Unilateral, Pathologically Bilateral

C. Peter N. Watson,[a] Rajiv Midha,[a] Marshall Devor,[b]
Sukriti Nag,[a] Catherine Munro,[a]
and Jonathan O. Dostrovsky[a]

[a]University of Toronto, Toronto, Ontario, Canada; [b]Department of Cell and Animal Biology, Institute of Life Sciences, Hebrew University of Jerusalem, Jerusalem, Israel

No patients have been autopsied who had ophthalmic (V_1) herpes zoster (HZ) and subsequently developed unequivocal postherpetic neuralgia (PHN). However, postmortem examinations have been done on a few patients with long survival who either did not have pain or in whom pain was not clearly documented. Autopsied spinal cases of PHN have shown dramatic pathology in the peripheral nerve, dorsal root ganglion, sensory root, and spinal cord (Watson et al. 1991; Watson and Deck 1993). This chapter reviews historical postmortem cases of V_1 HZ in patients who clearly did not experience pain, presents an autopsied case of a patient with severe PHN, and contrasts the findings with the pathology of spinal cases of this disorder (Watson and Deckser 1993).

Previous autopsied cases (Head and Campbell 1900; Reske-Nielsen et al. 1986) have not confirmed that patients clearly suffered PHN. Lesions have been found in the Gasserian ganglion and peripheral nerve. Reske-Nielsen and colleagues (1986) have described changes in the mesencephalic nucleus. Evidence is accumulating that a contralateral and a more generalized disorder may exist in PHN. We have published autopsy evidence of this disorder (Watson et al. 1991). Baron et al. (1997) have described electrophysiological studies indicating a bilateral multisegmental neuropathy in cases of PHN. Oaklander et al. (1998) found axonal loss in skin biopsies in the segment contralateral to the affected dermatome. The case we describe provides further evidence of contralateral abnormalities based on light and electron microscopic observations of myelinated and unmyelinated fibers in V_1 PHN.

CASE HISTORY

An 81-year-old woman with intractable left ophthalmic PHN of 10 years' duration was initially seen 4 years prior to death. The pain had steady burning, shock-like, and skin sensitivity components. The patient had scarring, sensory loss, and allodynia over the left V_1 territory. A variety of therapies, including several antidepressants, failed to provide relief. Ultimately, only opioids in a sustained-released oxycodone preparation at a dose of 20 mg every 12 hours relieved her pain or left her with only mild pain. She maintained this regimen for over 3 years prior to her death from heart disease in September 1998.

METHODS

About 24 hours postmortem, segments of the supra-orbital and ophthalmic nerves, the trigeminal roots, the Gasserian ganglia, and the trigeminal brain stem were removed bilaterally into a solution of mixed aldehydes. Nerve samples were taken at separate areas along a 2-cm section of the nerves. Nerve tissue was then rinsed, osmicated, dehydrated, and embedded in resin. Semithin transverse nerve sections stained with toluidine blue were used to measure the myelinated nerve fiber spectrum. A blinded observer (C. Munro) calculated myelinated fibers. Thin transverse sections of the peripheral nerves were stained with uranyl/lead for electron microscopic examination. The Gasserian ganglia and samples of the trigeminal brainstem were embedded in paraffin and stained with hematoxylin, eosin, and luxol-fast blue. For comparison with the V_1 PHN case, we used age-matched control autopsy material from individuals with no evidence of V_1 pathology or PHN.

RESULTS

PATHOLOGICAL FEATURES

Light microscopy (Fig. 1). Severe fibrosis and loss of myelinated fibers were features of the affected supra-orbital and ophthalmic nerves. We found no obvious abnormalities in the Gasserian ganglion or any part of the trigemi-

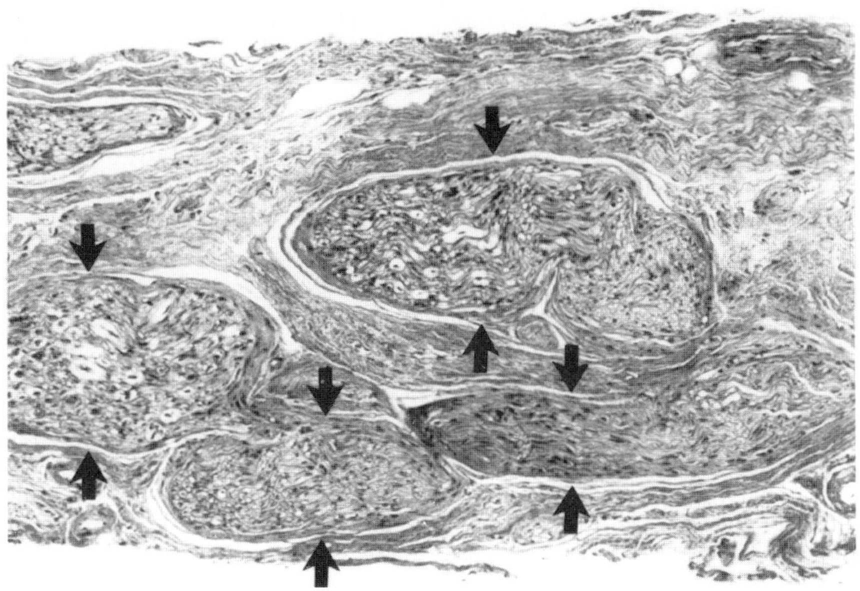

Fig. 1. Severe loss of myelinated axons in the affected ophthalmic nerve (arrows) in a case of V_1 PHN.

nal root, trigeminal spinal tract, or trigeminal nuclear complex, including the nucleus caudalis, the mesencephalic nucleus of the fifth cranial nerve, and the cervicomedullary junction.

Toluidine blue and myelinated nerve fiber spectrum (Fig. 2). The toluidine blue sections used for counting myelinated fibers showed greatly reduced numbers of myelinated fibers in the affected ophthalmic and supra-orbital nerves. In addition, on the contralateral clinically nonaffected side, peripheral areas of demyelination and large, thinly myelinated axons suggested demyelination or early remyelination of regenerating axons.

Supra-orbital nerve (Fig. 2). The studies showed a marked reduction in the number of myelinated axons of all diameters on the affected and nonaffected sides compared to the age-matched control (Fig. 2). Marked loss of larger axons of 6 μm or greater was evident on the affected side and with the contralateral control. Expressed as a percentage of total fibers seen, 90% of the fibers in the clinically affected supra-orbital nerve were 5 μm or smaller, whereas the figure for the clinically non-affected side was 76% and for the age-matched control 80%.

Ophthalmic nerve. A severe reduction of all fiber diameters in the myelinated axons in this nerve was evident on the affected side. As a percentage of total fibers, 80% of myelinated fibers were 5 μm in diameter or less compared to 76% for the nonaffected side and 64% for the age-matched control.

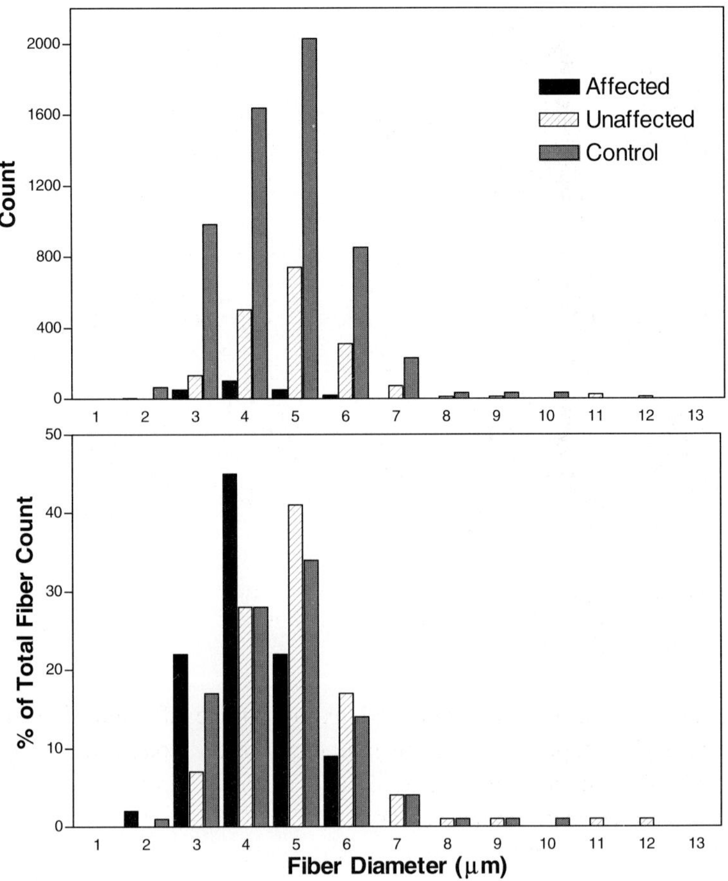

Fig. 2. Myelinated nerve fiber spectrum of the supra-orbital nerve in a case of V_1 PHN. There is marked overall loss of fibers and an increase in the percentage of small-diameter fibers on the affected (right) side compared to age-matched control.

These morphometric data support a marked loss of all fiber diameters and a shift in the myelinated spectrum to smaller fibers that could be pain transmitting on the affected side relative to age-matched controls. In addition, abnormalities were evident in the clinically nonaffected ophthalmic and supra-orbital nerves, specifically more smaller fibers, loss of larger fibers, demyelination, and thinly myelinated (regenerating) fibers.

Electron microscopy (Fig. 3). As in the light microscopic material, at the electron microscopic level the supra-orbital nerve had a low density of myelinated axons on both affected (left) and clinically nonaffected (right) sides, but with fiber loss much more prominent on the affected side. Both sides showed a large amount of endoneurial collagen and high densities of

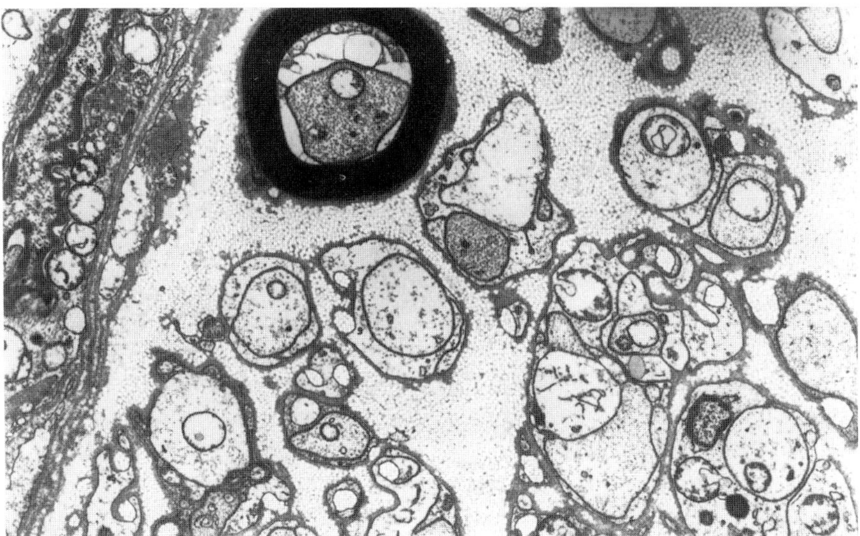

Fig. 3. Electron micrograph of the clinically affected (right) supra-orbital nerve showing a low density of myelinated axons, plentiful collagen, and many unmyelinated fibers, many presumably outgrowing sprouts.

unmyelinated axons. The unmyelinated axons on the affected side had a lucent, "watery" cytoplasm and axon diameters nearly double those on the nonaffected side, which suggests cytoplasmic swelling. On the affected side, occasional large-diameter nonmyelinated axons had an attached Schwann cell. These axons probably had been demyelinated.

The available samples of ophthalmic nerve on the affected side contained no identifiable axons but was nearly pure collagen. The clinically nonaffected side had few myelinated axons. but was densely packed with disorganized (nonaligned) unmyelinated axons and resembled a neuroma or a nerve filled with regenerating sprouts.

CONCLUSIONS

We have not been able to find any previous autopsied cases of V_1 PHN. The case we describe presented several features that were surprising in light of the literature on segmental (spinal) PHN. First, despite documented shingles, residual V_1 cutaneous scarring, and severe pain for more than 10 years, the central nervous system showed no significant morphological abnormalities. Second, severe pathological involvement of the ophthalmic and supra-orbital nerves included fibrosis, demyelination, significant myelinated fiber loss, and a shift in the fiber diameter spectrum toward small-diameter axons. This occurred without prominent pathology in the Gasserian ganglion or the trigeminal root, which suggests a dying-back type of pathology expressed mostly in the periphery. The lack of prominent findings in the ganglion, root, and central nervous system is strikingly different from cases of spinal PHN that show severe cell loss in the DRG and atrophy of the dorsal horn of the spinal cord (Watson et al. 1991).

The third outstanding finding in this case was the obvious pathological involvement of the contralateral ophthalmic and supra-orbital nerves, despite the lack of obvious clinical contralateral symptoms and signs. This finding supports other recently published information on bilateral involvement as noted in the introduction. Previous spinal cases we have autopsied also suggested that the myelinated fiber spectrum of the patient's contralateral ("nonaffected") side differs from that of age-matched controls (Cases 1 and 2; Watson 1991) and that an imbalance of myelinated fibers may favor fibers of small diameter. Furthermore, one of our previous cases (Case 5; Watson 1991) had contralateral inflammatory changes in nerves of the affected segment and also bilaterally in segments above and below. V_1 cases are of particular interest with regard to PHN because V_1 is purely sensory whereas the spinal nerves also have a motor component.

Although it is clearly inappropriate to draw firm conclusions from a single case that might not be representative of V_1 PHN in general, our observations suggest a particular pathophysiology. Specifically, they indicate that the pathology is primarily peripheral. Pain mechanisms could include an imbalance of small-diameter versus large-diameter input as predicted by the gate control theory. Alternatively, pain may be due to ectopic firing of peripherally injured axons, in association with central sensitization (Devor and Seltzer 1999). Finally, pain could result from abnormal response properties of residual, uninjured fibers. Each of these mechanisms, which are not mutually exclusive, may have a threshold below which symptoms and signs do not manifest clinically. This situation would account for the observation of neural pathology on the right side in our patient despite the absence of obvious pain. It is not unlikely that sensory abnormalities could have been detected on the right side through detailed, quantitative sensory testing methods.

REFERENCES

Baron R, Haendler G, Schulte H. Afferent large fiber polyneuropathy predicts the development of postherpetic neuralgia. *Pain* 1997; 73:231–238.

Devor M, Seltzer Z. Pathophysiology of damaged nerves in relation to chronic pain. Chapter 5. In: Wall PD, Melzack R (Eds). *Textbook of Pain,* 4th ed. London: Churchill Livingstone, 1999, pp 129–164.

Head H, Campbell AW. The pathology of herpes zoster and its bearing on sensory localization. *Brain* 1900; 23:353–523.

Oaklander AL, Romans K, Horasek S, et al. Unilateral postherpetic neuralgia is associated with bilateral sensory damage. *Ann Neurol* 1998; 44:789–795.

Reske-Nielsen E, Oster S, Pedersen B. Herpes zoster ophthalmicus and the mesencephalic nucleus. *Acta Pat Microbiol Scand* 1986; 94:263–269.

Watson CPN, Deck JH. The neuropathology of herpes zoster with particular reference to postherpetic neuralgia and its pathogenesis. In: Watson CPN (Ed). *Herpes Zoster and Postherpetic Neuralgia,* Pain Research and Clinical Management, Vol. 8. Amsterdam: Elsevier, 1993, pp 139–157.

Watson CPN, Deck JH, Morshead C, et al. Postherpetic neuralgia: further postmortem studies of cases with and without pain. *Pain* 1991; 44:105–117.

Correspondence to: C. Peter N. Watson, MD, FRCP, 1 Sir Williams Lane, Toronto, Ontario, Canada M9A 1T8.

Proceedings of the 9th World Congress on Pain, Progress in Pain Research and Management, Vol. 16, edited by M. Devor, M.C. Rowbotham, and Z. Wiesenfeld-Hallin, IASP Press, Seattle, © 2000.

71

Changes in Sodium Channel SNS/PN3 and Ankyrin$_G$ mRNAs in the Rat Trigeminal Ganglion following Inferior Alveolar Nerve Injury

Ulf Bongenhielm,[a,b] Christopher Nosrat,[a] Irina Nosrat,[a] Jonas Eriksson,[a] and Kaj Fried[a]

[a]*Department of Neuroscience, Karolinska Institute, Stockholm, Sweden;* [b]*Department of Oral and Maxillofacial Surgery, Huddinge Hospital, Karolinska Institute, Huddinge, Sweden*

A proportion of patients who sustain damage to the inferior alveolar nerve, a lower-jaw branch of the trigeminal nerve, develop persistent orofacial paresthesia and dysesthesia. Extensive studies on ectopic hyperexcitability in injured spinal nerves have suggested that membrane remodeling of voltage-gated sodium channels contributes to the pathophysiology of pain (see Devor and Seltzer 1999; Waxman et al. 1999). Given structural and functional differences in the outcome of nerve injury between trigeminal and spinal segmental nerves (Tal and Devor 1992; Bongenhielm and Robinson 1996; Bongenhielm et al. 1999), we have used in situ hybridization techniques to investigate the mRNA expression of the sodium channel α subtype SNS/PN3 in the trigeminal ganglion after neuroma formation of the inferior alveolar nerve. Sodium channels bind to ankyrins, which link ion channels to the membrane skeleton. Ankyrin$_G$, which is necessary for normal neuronal sodium channel function, is localized in the initial segments and nodes of Ranvier (Zhou et al 1998). After nerve injury, ankyrin$_G$ could be important in the assembly of the axonal membrane regions that emit ectopic electrical activity. For this reason, we have also studied the ankyrin$_G$ gene expression in the trigeminal ganglion and the protein localization in the inferior alveolar nerve after injury.

METHODS

Thirty adult male Sprague-Dawley rats were used in this study. Experiments were approved by the Animal Experiment Ethics Committee of N. Stockholm (N24/96). In 26 adult animals, under general anesthesia (chloral hydrate; 350 mg/kg, i.p.), the left inferior alveolar nerve was exposed, ligated, and cut. Recovery periods ranged from 3 days to 19 weeks. Four adult animals served as unoperated controls. All animals were then deeply anesthetized and decapitated, and the trigeminal ganglion on the left side was removed and cut in serial sections. Oligonucleotide probes complementary to the rat sodium channel SNS/PN3 (50-mer probes from bases 304 and 6386) and rat ankyrin$_G$ (50-mer probes from bases 4901 and 6902) were synthesized and labeled with ^{35}S-dATP. Sections were hybridized, exposed, developed, and counterstained with cresyl violet. In some animals the injured inferior alveolar nerve was removed, cut, and incubated with antibodies against ankyrin$_G$ (Oncogene, USA).

RESULTS

SNS/PN3. α-SNS/PN3 mRNA was expressed in the adult control trigeminal ganglion at all levels and in all three divisions (Fig. 1A). Within the mandibular division, SNS/PN3 mRNA-expressing small neurons constituted 28% of the total number of neurons, medium 17%, and large 1%. At the shortest post-injury period (3 days) following inferior alveolar nerve injury, the proportion of small SNS/PN3-expressing neurons within the mandibular division was reduced to 18% of all small neurons. At longer survival stages, normal levels were reestablished (Fig. 1B). No significant changes appeared within the medium- or large-sized neuron groups.

Ankyrin$_G$. In both normal and injured trigeminal ganglia, ankyrin$_G$ mRNA was expressed at all levels and in virtually all neurons, independent of size (Fig. 2A). However, measurements of the intensity of neuronal ankyrin$_G$ mRNA expression in the mandibular division indicated a marked overall decrease at 3 days post-injury. Subnormal intensity levels persisted up to 13 weeks post-injury (Fig. 2B–D). There was no indication of a specific correlation between the reduction in intensity and neuronal size. Immunolabeling showed ankyrin$_G$ immunoreactivity at nodes of Ranvier and in unmyelinated axons in the normal inferior alveolar nerve. After injury, the ankyrin$_G$ labeling was markedly reduced in the distal regions of the neuromas (data not shown).

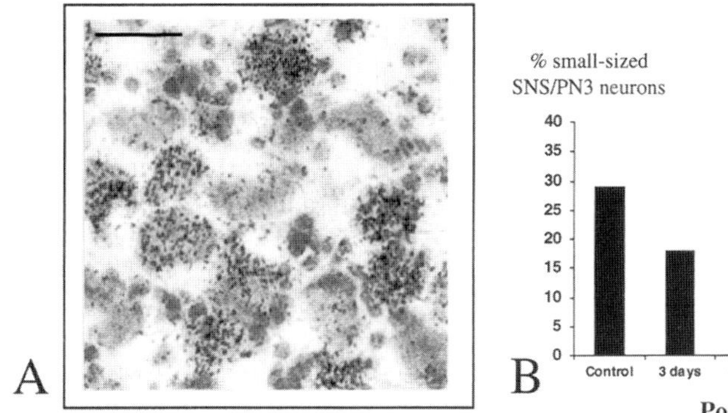

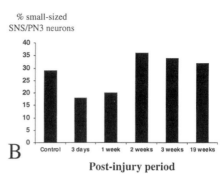

Fig. 1. (A) Section from the mandibular division of a normal rat trigeminal ganglion, labeled by in situ hybridization with a ^{35}S-labeled SNS/PN3-mRNA probe. Labeling is seen predominantly in small and medium neurons. Scale bar: 50 μm. (B) Diagram showing the proportion of small (<600 μm^2) SNS/PN3 mRNA expressing neurons within the trigeminal ganglion's mandibular division after inferior alveolar nerve injury. Note the early proportional decrease of small neurons at 3 days post-injury.

DISCUSSION

Inappropriate electrical activity in injured primary sensory neurons could be caused by changes in the expression of sodium channel subtypes. This process may be the source of pain and dysesthesia after peripheral nerve injury (see Devor and Seltzer 1999; Eglen et al. 1999; Waxman et al. 1999). Our results show a proportional decrease of small neurons expressing SNS/PN3 mRNA within the trigeminal ganglion's mandibular division at the shortest post-injury periods, followed by a normalization to control levels by 2 weeks after nerve lesion. Axotomy or chronic constriction injury of the sciatic nerve caused a similar downregulation of SNS/PN3 mRNA in the dorsal root ganglion (DRG) (Dib-Hajj et al. 1996; Okuse et al. 1997). However, the axotomy-induced reduction of SNS/PN3 levels was much more prolonged in the DRG. The normalization of primary sensory neuron SNS/PN3 mRNA following a peripheral trigeminal injury is of interest in view of earlier functional studies of injured trigeminal nerves. Thus, the time course for SNS/PN3 depletion in the trigeminal ganglion after peripheral nerve injury is similar to that seen for abnormal discharge from injured trigeminal nerve endings. Damage to the inferior alveolar nerve induced ectopic afferent electrical activity (Bongenhielm et al. 1996, 1998). However, the peak appeared earlier and the decline was more rapid than after sciatic nerve injuries (for review, see Devor and Seltzer 1999). Furthermore, trigeminal infraorbital injury produced no acute injury discharge, less ongoing discharge,

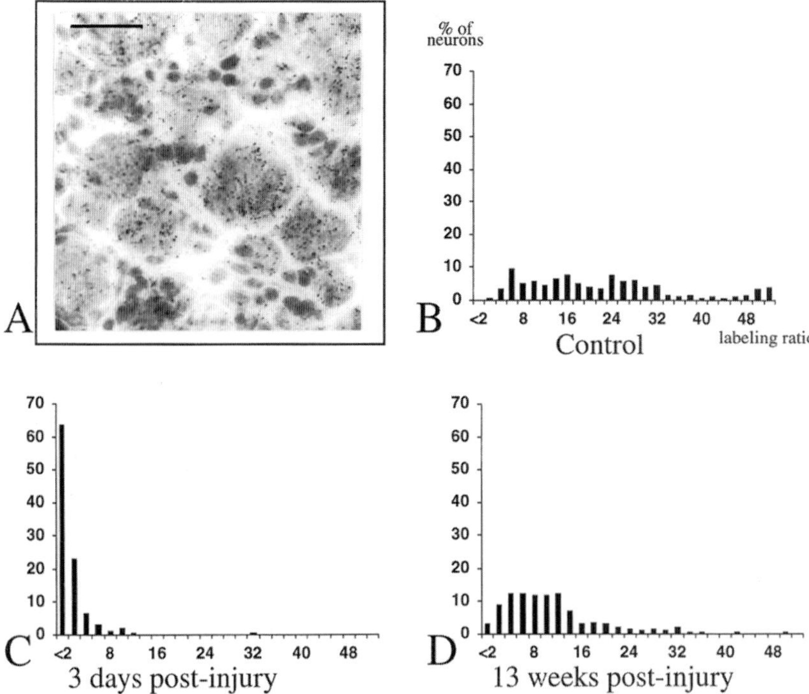

Fig. 2. (A) Section from the mandibular division of an operated rat trigeminal ganglion (13 weeks post-injury), labeled by in situ hybridization with a ^{35}S-labeled ankyrin$_G$-mRNA probe. Labeling is seen in virtually all neurons, independent of size. Scale bar: 50 µm. (B–D) Diagrams showing the ankyrin$_G$ mRNA labeling ratio (ratio between pixels/µm^2 in neuronal cell somata and pixels/µm^2 in background) in the mandibular division of the rat trigeminal ganglion. (B) Control; (C) 3 days after inferior alveolar nerve injury; (D) 13 weeks after inferior alveolar nerve injury. The labeling ratios show that intensity levels of ankyrin$_G$ mRNA are reduced from 3 days post-injury onwards.

and less mechanosensitivity than did sciatic nerve neuromas (Tal and Devor 1992). These differences could be related to differences in the injury-induced regulation of sodium channel transcripts in the trigeminal ganglion compared to the DRG.

Ankyrin$_G$ is necessary for the normal physiological function of sodium channels in myelinated nerve fibers, and also could be important in unmyelinated or demyelinated peripheral nerve axons (Kordeli et al. 1995; Lambert et al. 1997; Zhou et al. 1998). Ankyrin$_G$ mRNA levels were rapidly downregulated in trigeminal ganglion neurons after an inferior alveolar nerve lesion. This response also was evident on the protein level. This reduction of available ankyrin$_G$ may affect the assembly of sodium channel clusters in the axolemma of injured axons. The downregulation of ankyrin$_G$ may not impair sodium channel function in general, but it could influence the neuronal targeting of the various sodium channel isoforms, with a consequent change in electrical properties.

SUMMARY

We have used in situ hybridization techniques to investigate changes in the mRNA expression of the sodium channel SNS/PN3 and the membrane sodium channel-binding protein ankyrin$_G$ in the trigeminal ganglion after neuroma formation of the inferior alveolar nerve. Our results show an injury-induced downregulation of SNS/PN3 mRNA in small trigeminal ganglion neurons. In contrast to the downregulation of SNS/PN3 transcripts previously observed in DRG after spinal nerve injury, our results showed a rapid return to normal levels following downregulation. Ankyrin$_G$ mRNA expression was downregulated after nerve damage, and remained at low levels. The changes in trigeminal ganglion SNS/PN3 mRNA may contribute to the inappropriate firing associated with sensory dysfunction in the orofacial region. Changes in ankyrin$_G$ mRNA expression could also play a role in this process.

ACKNOWLEDGMENTS

This study was supported by grants from the Swedish MRC (project 8654).

REFERENCES

Bongenhielm U, Robinson PP. Spontaneous and mechanically evoked afferent activity originating from myelinated fibres in ferret inferior alveolar nerve neuromas. *Pain* 1996; 67:399–406.

Bongenhielm U, Boissonade FM, Westermark A, Robinson PP, Fried K. Sympathetic nerve sprouting fails to occur in the trigeminal ganglion after injury to the inferior alveolar nerve in the rat. *Pain* 1999; 82:283–288.

Devor M, Seltzer Z. Pathophysiology of damaged nerves in relation to chronic pain. In: Wall PD, Melzack R (Eds). *Textbook of Pain,* 4th ed. London: Churchill and Livingstone, 1999, pp 129–164.

Dib-Hajj S, Black, JA, Felts P, Waxman SG. Down-regulation of transcripts for Na channel alpha-SNS in spinal sensory neurons following axotomy. *Proc Natl Acad Sci USA* 1996; 93:14950–14954.

Eglen RM, Hunter JC, Dray A. Ions in the fire: recent ion-channel research and approaches to pain therapy. *Trends Pharmacol* 1999; 20:337–342.

Kordeli E, Lambert S, Bennett V, Ankyrin$_G$. A new ankyrin gene with neural-specific isoforms localized at the axonal initial segment and the node of Ranvier. *J Biol Chem* 1995; 270:2352–2359.

Lambert S, Davis, JQ, Bennett V. Morphogenesis of the node of Ranvier: co-clusters of ankyrin and ankyrin-binding integral proteins define early developmental intermediates. *J Neurosci* 1997; 17:7025–7036.

Okuse K, Chaplan SR, McMahon SB, et al. Regulation of expression of the sensory neuron-specific sodium channel SNS in inflammatory and neuropathic pain. *Mol Cell Neurosci* 1997; 10:196–207.

Tal M, Devor M. Ectopic discharge in injured nerves: comparison of trigeminal and somatic afferents. *Brain Res* 1992; 579:148–151.

Waxman SG, Cummins TR, Dib-Hajj S, Fjell J, Black JA. Sodium channels, excitability of primary sensory neurons, and the molecular basis of pain. *Muscle Nerve* 1999; 22:1177–1187.

Zhou D, Lambert S, Malen PL, et al. Ankyrin_G is required for clustering of voltage-gated Na channels at axon initial segments and for normal action potential firing. *J Cell Biol* 1998; 143:1295–1304.

Correspondence to: K. Fried, DDS, PhD, Department of Neuroscience, Karolinska Institutet, S-171 77, Stockholm, Sweden. Fax: 46-8-32-09-88; email: Kaj.Fried@neuro.ki.se.

Proceedings of the 9th World Congress on Pain,
Progress in Pain Research and Management,
Vol. 16, edited by M. Devor, M.C. Rowbotham, and
Z. Wiesenfeld-Hallin, IASP Press, Seattle, © 2000.

72

Neurogenic Vasodilatation in Trigeminal Neuralgia

Turo Nurmikko, Carol Haggett, and John Miles

Pain Research Institute, The Walton Centre for Neurology and Neurosurgery, NHS Trust, Liverpool, United Kingdom

Despite extensive research, there is no firm consensus on the mechanisms that initiate and maintain pain in trigeminal neuralgia (TGN). The clinical course of this condition and the unique characteristics of the pain suggest different pathophysiological mechanisms from those seen in other forms of neuropathic pain. Typically patients with TGN report intense, unilateral pain, which comes in paroxysms, is triggered by innocuous stimuli, starts and stops abruptly, and has a sharp, electric-shock-like quality. Pain in TGN is usually caused by vascular compression, but may be associated with tumor, bony anomalies, multiple sclerosis, or no known abnormality. The quality of pain remains the same, irrespective of cause.

Some authors believe that though the etiology of TGN is likely to be peripheral, pain itself is caused by aberrant barrages or abnormal processing of afferent neural impulses in the central nervous system (Pagni 1993; Bowsher 1997; Eide and Stubhaug 1998). Others suggest that ephaptic transmission at the site of pathology allows touch-evoked impulses to cross over to the afferent pain pathways (Hilton et al. 1994). Recent work suggests that pain in TGN results from a discharge in a cluster of neurons in the Gasserian ganglion, made hyperexcitable by compression or some other process involving the nerve root. This discharge is then thought to spread to neighboring neurons, triggering them to fire in turn, a phenomenon referred to as "crossed after-discharge" (Rappaport and Devor 1994). In indirect support of this theory, somatosensory evoked responses normalize immediately after microvascular decompression (Leandri et al. 1998).

Low-intensity electrical stimulation of the trigeminal nerve is known to cause peripheral vasodilatation (Lambert et al. 1984; Izumi 1999). We hypothesized that—if intense enough—spontaneous hyperactivity of the cells of the Gasserian ganglion could produce peripheral neurogenic inflammation by the same mechanism. Previous studies have suggested this is not the case (Hardy and Bowsher 1989; Hampf et al. 1990), but the authors did not specify whether the patients involved had persisting pain at the time of measurement, and the techniques used were relatively insensitive. In this chapter, we present a detailed case study of a patient with severe TGN who showed evidence of neurogenic inflammation in the affected dermatome, which disappeared following successful surgery. We also present results from three further patients with TGN associated with vasomotor changes.

CASE HISTORY

The patient was a 65-year-old woman with a 9-year history of TGN of the first and second divisions on the left. Prior to the recent exacerbation of her pain, the situation had remained completely under control with carbamazepine (CBZ; 600 mg/day). Within a short time she developed painful paroxysms confined to the first and second trigeminal divisions, which steadily worsened despite an increase in her CBZ dose. On her first visit to our clinic she described three components to her pain: (1) shooting from the left eye up to the forehead, provoked by talking, eating, and touching the face; (2) paroxysms of machine-gun-like pain inside the left eye; and (3) burning pain around the eye, made worse by heat. She had noted occasional lacrimation on the ipsilateral side. Clinical examination showed prominent periorbital redness and swelling in both the left upper and lower eyelid. We found no conjunctival injection (Fig. 1; left) and observed no lacrimation.

METHODS

Cutaneous blood flow was assessed by laser Doppler flowmetry with a dual Moor probe laser (MBI, 3D, Moor Instruments, United Kingdom). Probes were placed in the affected second division laterally under the ipsilateral eye and at the corresponding contralateral site. The measurement was done with the patient in a semi-sitting position in our climate-controlled physiology laboratory at an ambient temperature of 22°C.

RESULTS

Prior to surgery the sides showed substantial asymmetry. Blood flow was greatly increased on the affected side (Fig. 2). This asymmetry remained

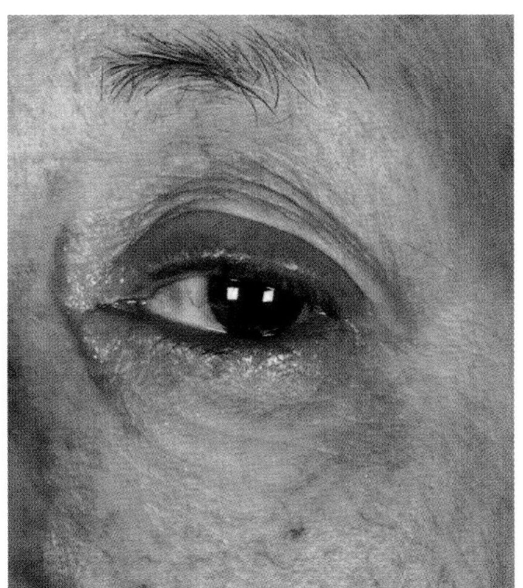
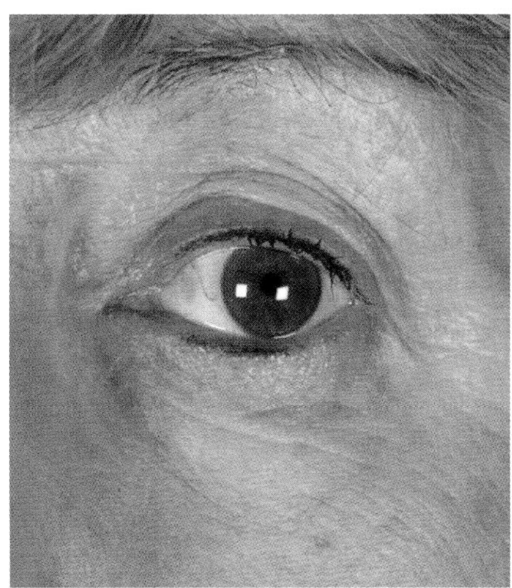

Fig. 1. Patient 1 during an episode of severe trigeminal neuralgia (left). Note periorbital redness and swelling of the eyelids. Narrowing of the palpebral fissure is caused by swelling. There is no miosis or conjunctival injection. The changes are likely to be due to neurogenic inflammation. These changes have disappeared 1 month after surgery (right).

constant during the measurement period of at least 20 minutes (a 10-minute recording is shown in Fig. 2). Magnetic resonance tomoangiography was negative. Pharmacotherapy with CBZ, phenytoin, and lamotrigine proved ineffective. The patient had partial trigeminal rhizotomy 6 weeks after her first admission; this procedure completely abolished all three components of her pain. All vasomotor changes disappeared in the ensuing month (Fig. 1B). During the 12-month follow-up period she developed occasional shooting sensations on the left side of her face and opted to remain on a low dose of CBZ. No erythema or swelling was noted postoperatively at any stage.

Repeat testing showed that the skin blood flow on the affected side had normalized at 1 month, and it remained normal during the follow-up (Fig. 2). Quantitative sensory testing performed postoperatively showed increased thresholds in three divisions, which returned to normal or near normal over 12 months.

Three other patients (all female, aged 57–67 years) with severe persistent pain in the first or second division have since had similar assessment of cutaneous blood flow. All described classical features of TGN, and had shown an unequivocal response to CBZ or lamotrigine in the past. They all either had a history of redness of the ipsilateral eye or showed signs of at least moderate eyelid swelling during their clinic visits. Two showed conjunctival injection on examination. One patient (No. 2) reported occasional

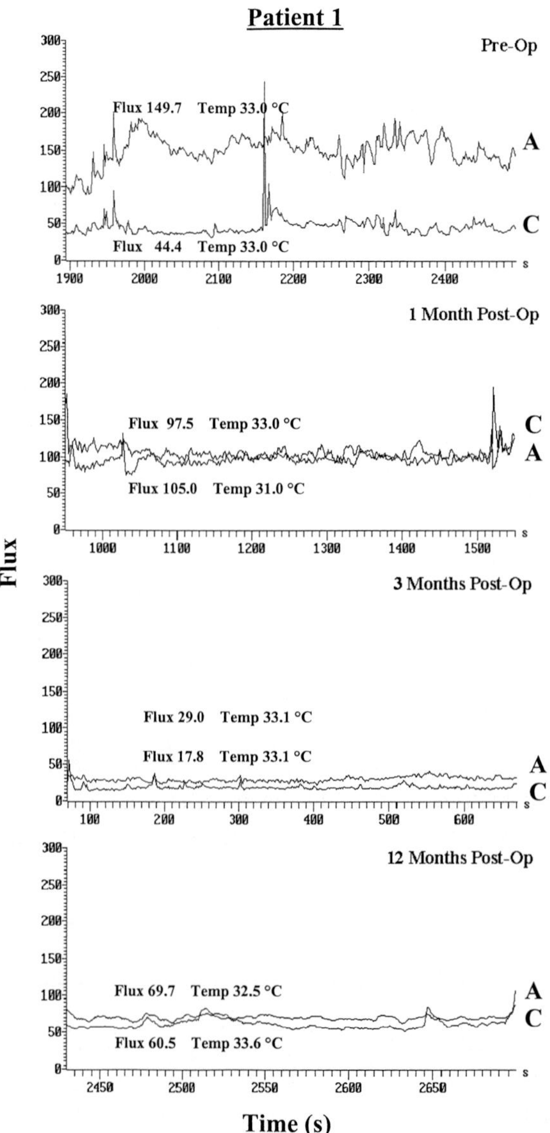

Fig. 2. Laser Doppler flowmeter traces recorded in Patient 1 before and repeatedly after partial rhizotomy. Recordings up to ten minutes shown for illustrative purposes. Probes were positioned within (A) the affected division and (C) the contralateral homologous site, and recordings were carried out simultaneously. Flux is expressed as arbitrary units. Note increased blood flow on the painful affected side preoperatively, decreasing to a normal level postoperatively.

watering of the ipsilateral eye, which was never witnessed during her visits. None had any nasal symptoms. On follow-up, they all reported recent or persistent pain, which tended to be less severe than during their first assessment.

Each of the three patients had laser Doppler flowmetry in the affected and contralateral dermatomes. Measurements were taken twice, at an interval of 2–3 months, in our laboratory under identical conditions (ambient temperature 22°C, same time of day). As indicated in Fig. 3, all three patients consistently showed increased blood flow on the affected compared to the contralateral side. This asymmetry, however, appeared to attenuate in all patients, coinciding with improved pain control.

DISCUSSION

The four patients with typical TGN of the first and second division showed evidence of neurogenic inflammation in the distribution of the pain. Two patients reported a burning quality to their pain in addition to tic douloureux. We suggest that this phenomenon represents a hitherto unrecognized feature of trigeminal neuralgia and hypothesize that it is caused by antidromic or reflex vasodilatation induced by abnormal ectopic activity in the Gasserian ganglion or in the trigeminal root at the site of the lesion (vascular compression or other pathology).

All patients were diagnosed years earlier with trigeminal neuralgia based on their clinical features and exclusion of other diagnoses. However, given the explicit vasomotor findings in our patients, we must consider other facial pain conditions. Pain and vasomotor changes are hallmark signs of trigeminal autonomic cephalgias (Goadsby and Lipton 1997). Two of these, cluster headache (CH) and chronic paroxysmal hemicrania (CPH), can be ruled out by their distinct clinical features not shown by our patients. In none of our patients was the pain description remotely similar to that seen in CH, and the associated clinical symptoms fall far short of the constellation of autonomic signs associated with it (ptosis, profuse lacrimation, and rhinorrhea). Similarly, pain description, number and duration of attacks, and excellent initial response to anticonvulsants distinguish our patients from those with CPH.

It could be argued that our patients had concomitant TGN and CH or CPH, as has been reported previously (Caminero et al. 1997); however, their clinical features including the pain description were very different from those reported in the literature.

A further condition, SUNCT (short-lasting, unilateral, neuralgiform headache with conjunctival injection and tearing), poses an interesting diagnos-

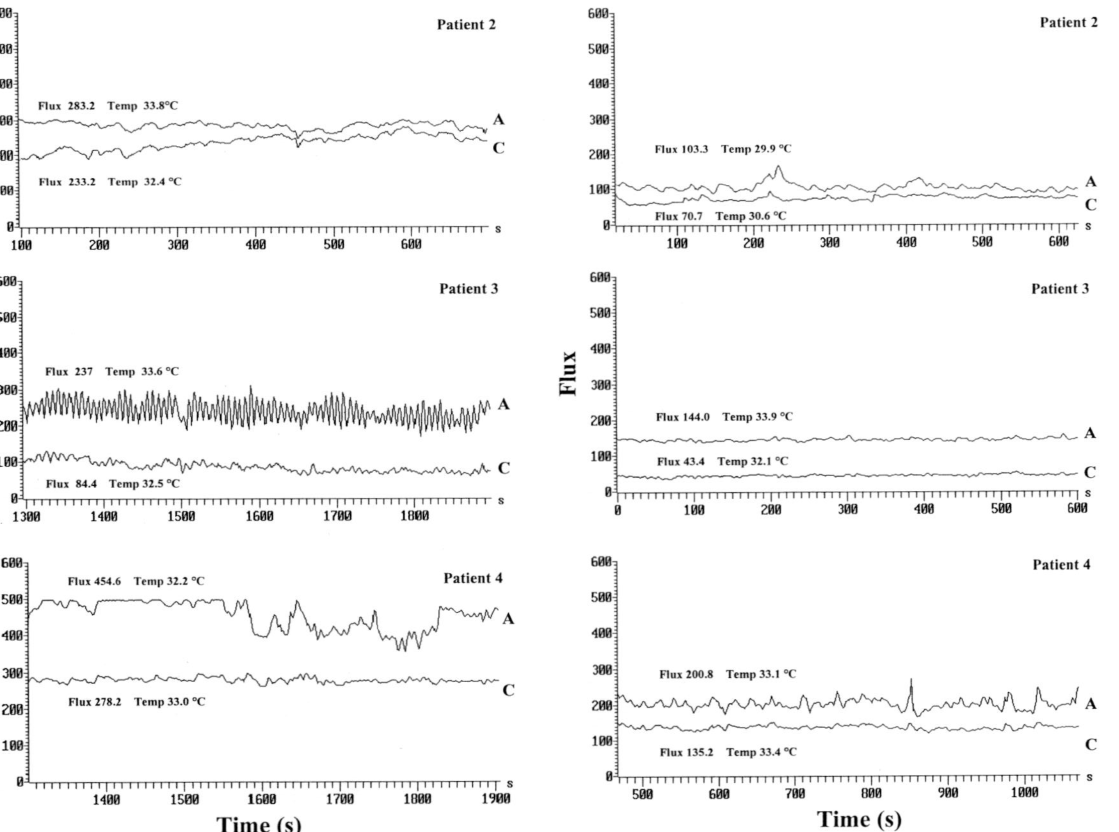

Fig 3. Laser Doppler flowmeter traces in three further patients with TGN who presented with poorly controlled pain. 10-minute recordings shown only. Probes were positioned within the affected (A) and contralateral (C) divisions and blood flow monitored simultaneously. Results are expressed as arbitrary units. Measurements were carried out on two occasions, prior to (left) and following pharmacotherapy (right). Note increased cutaneous blood flow in each case on the side of the pain.

tic challenge. The similarities between this condition and TGN of the first division are well recognized (Pareja and Sjaastad 1997; Sjaastad et al. 1997). The differences relate to duration of paroxysms (in TGN 1–2 seconds, in SUNCT >20 seconds), male preponderance in SUNCT (whereas all our patients were female), and full-blown autonomic symptoms in SUNCT (and not in our patients). The excellent effects of anticonvulsants in our patients would also speak against SUNCT, which is usually considered refractory to any medical treatment (Goadsby and Lipton1997). However, other investigators have commented on "forme frustes of SUNCT," with less marked autonomic symptoms, and have suggested that one condition might evolve into another (Pareja and Sjaastad 1997). The etiology of SUNCT is unknown (Goadsby and Lipton 1997), but from the point of view of pathophysiology it may represent part of the same spectrum of neuralgic pain that includes TGN (but not necessarily CH and CPH).

The four patients all showed local hyperemia (i.e., increase in skin blood flow due to vasodilatation) and swelling (conceivably due to plasma extravasation), which are key traits of neurogenic inflammation. Neurogenic inflammation forms part of the tissue response to injury; a well-known example is axon-reflex-mediated vasodilatation around cutaneous injuries. However, neurogenic inflammation can also be induced by stimulation of the dorsal root ganglion fibers via antidromic release of vasoactive neuropeptides from their distal terminals. Electrical stimulation of the dorsal root and trigeminal ganglia has been routinely employed to study conditions as diverse as asthma, arthritis, and migraine (Holzer and Maggi 1998). Some researchers suggest that antidromic vasodilatation is mediated by a subset of heat nociceptors only, and that there may be important differences between species (Lynn et al. 1996).

Patients undergoing radiofrequency lesioning of the Gasserian ganglion sometimes show increased skin blood flow within the stimulated division, but not outside it (Goadsby and Lipton 1997). Studying this effect in cats, Lambert et al. (1984) suggested that 20% of vasodilatation is due to antidromic vasodilatation and 80% due to parasympathetic reflex vasodilatation via a centrally mediated loop involving the ipsilateral greater superficial petrosal nerve. Their experiments involved stimulating an intact trigeminal nerve on one side and the stump of the cut nerve on the other, and it is not clear how well this model correlates with the clinical situation. Activation of the parasympathetic reflex mechanism explains lacrimation and swelling of the nasal mucosa in patients with cluster headache (Goadsby and Lipton 1997). As discussed above, these autonomic features were only seen to a limited extent in our patients, which suggests a less important role for parasympathetic reflex activation.

Neurogenic plasma extravasation is linked to both antidromic and axon-reflex mechanisms; in our cases axon-reflex can be ruled out as it would imply repeated cutaneous injury (such as rubbing or stroking the skin, which the patients tended to avoid). Prominent swelling in our patients was unlikely to be caused by any local mechanical or chemical factor, and hence its presence supports a role for antidromic release of vasoactive substances. A recent study, however, suggests that the parasympathetic nervous system can trigger neurogenic inflammation, at least in the dura (Delepine and Aupineau 1997).

We propose that the likely explanation for the four patients described is increased ectopic firing in the trigeminal ganglion or at the site of local nerve root pathology, leading to antidromic release of vasoactive substances in the skin and subsequent neurogenic inflammation. The burning component could be explained by secondary sensitization of C fibers (Reeh et al. 1986). A further contribution to the observed vasodilatation may come from a parasympathetic reflex induced by trigeminal activation. Our observations are compatible with the hypothesis by Rappaport and Devor (1994) of ectopic paroxysmal crossed interganglionic discharge, and favor a peripherally oriented explanation for the cause of pain in TGN. Further studies are needed to evaluate how common this phenomenon is, whether it has any diagnostic value, and whether a simple measurement of cutaneous skin blood flow can be used to assess neural activity in TGN to assist in clinical decision-making.

REFERENCES

Bowsher D. Trigeminal neuralgia: an anatomically oriented review. *Clin Anat* 1997; 10:409–415.

Caminero AB, Pareja JA, Dobato JL. Chronic paroxysmal hemicraniatic syndrome. *Cephalalgia* 1998; 18:159–161.

Delepine L, Aupineau P. Plasma protein extravasation in the rat dura mater by stimulation of the parasympathetic sphenopalatine ganglion. *Exp Neurol* 1997; 147:389–400.

Eide PK, Stubhaug A. Relief of trigeminal neuralgia after percutaneous retrogasserian glycerol rhizolysis is dependent on normalization of abnormal temporal summation of pain, without general impairment of sensory perception. *Neurosurgery* 1998; 43:462–472.

Goadsby PJ, Lipton RB. A review of paroxysmal hemicranias, SUNCT and other short-lasting headaches with autonomic feature, including new cases. *Brain* 1997; 120:193–209.

Hampf G, Bowsher D, Wells C, Miles J. Sensory and autonomic measurements in idiopathic trigeminal neuralgia before and after radiofrequency thermocoagulation: differentiation from some other causes of facial pain. *Pain* 1990; 40:241–248.

Hardy PA, Bowsher DR. Contact thermography in idiopathic neuralgia and other facial pains. *Br J Neurosurg* 1989; 3:399–402.

Hilton DA, Love S, Gradidge T, Coakham HB. Pathological findings associated with trigeminal neuralgia caused by vascular compression. *Neurosurgery* 1994; 35(2):299–303.

Holzer P, Maggi CA. Dissociation of dorsal root ganglion neurons into afferent and efferent like neurones. *Neuroscience* 1998; 86:398–396.

Izumi H. Nervous control of blood flow in the orofacial region. *Pharmacol Ther* 1999; 81:141–161.
Lambert GA, Bogduk N, Goadsby PJ, Duckworth JW, Lance JW. Decreased carotid arterial resistance in cats in response to trigeminal stimulation. *J Neurosurg* 1984; 61:307–315.
Leandri M, Eldridge P, Miles J. Recovery of nerve conduction following microvascular compression for trigeminal neuralgia. *Neurology* 1998; 51:1641–1646.
Lynn B, Schutterle S, Pierau F-K. The vasodilator component of neurogenic inflammation is caused by a special subclass of heat-sensitive nociceptors in the skin of the pig. *J Physiol* 1996; 494:587–593.
Pagni CA. The origin of tic douloureux: a unified view. *J Neurol Sci* 1993; 37:185–194.
Pareja JA, Sjaastad O. SUNCT syndrome. A clinical review. *Headache* 1997; 37:195–202.
Rappaport ZH, Devor M. Trigeminal neuralgia: the role of self-sustaining discharge in the trigeminal ganglion (TRG). *Pain* 1994; 56:127–138.
Reeh PW, Kocher L, Jung S. Does neurogenic inflammation alter sensitivity of unmyelinated nociceptors in the rat? *Brain Res* 1986; 384:42–50.
Sjaastad O, Pareja JA, Zukerman E, Jansen J, Kruszewski P. Trigeminal neuralgia. Clinical manifestations of the first division involvement. *Headache* 1997; 37:346–357.

Correspondence to: Dr. Turo Nurmikko, MD, PhD, Pain Research Institute, The Walton Centre for Neurology and Neurosurgery, NHS Trust, Lower Lane, Liverpool L9 7LJ, United Kingdom. Tel: 44-151-529-5750; Fax: 44-151-529-5486; email: tjn@liv.ac.uk.

Proceedings of the 9th World Congress on Pain,
Progress in Pain Research and Management,
Vol. 16, edited by M. Devor, M.C. Rowbotham, and
Z. Wiesenfeld-Hallin, IASP Press, Seattle, © 2000.

73

Understanding Clinical Trials: What Have We Learned from Systematic Reviews?

R. Andrew Moore

Pain Research and Nuffield Department of Anaesthetics, University of Oxford, Oxford Radcliffe Hospitals, The Churchill, Oxford, United Kingdom

Evidence-based medicine has been described as the "conscientious, explicit and judicious use of current best evidence in making decisions about the care of individual patients" (Sackett et al. 1996). But what constitutes "current best evidence"? Because of the vast array of biomedical journals (perhaps as many as 30,000), the chance of any practitioner being aware of all the developments of interest is vanishingly small.

Most clinicians depend on reading reviews, but even these can be biased if the authors have chosen selectively from available literature or failed to use overt quality standards in making an overall judgment. The ideal review systematically finds all the relevant information on a topic, applies criteria to ensure the quality of studies included in the review, and then integrates the information available to help clinicians in their everyday practice.

SYSTEMATIC REVIEWS

Reviews are called systematic when they include a thorough search for all published (and sometimes unpublished) information on a topic. This used to be a task of heroic proportions. Now it is relatively easy, thanks to the wider availability of electronic databases. The Cochrane Library, available quarterly on CD-ROM, not only has good systematic reviews, but includes references for over 200,000 controlled trials, including pain trials found by hand-searching the scientific literature (Jadad et al. 1996). The systematic review sifts through the mass of information that may be available and distills it through quality filters, integrating different sorts of knowledge. Clinicians can further refine such information by taking into account each patient's unique biology and the circumstances in which they live and work (Fig. 1). If a systematic review pools numerical information from trials, it may be called a meta-analysis.

The systematic review process, because it is so thorough, lends itself to evaluating features that might affect the outcome of a trial, such as the study design, the types of patients, and the severity of disease. Systematic reviews provide information on how we can improve clinical trials, though not all such reviews are equally helpful (Jadad and McQuay 1996).

BIAS IN CLINICAL TRIALS

Bias has a dictionary definition of "a one-sided inclination of the mind." In clinical trials, bias refers to features of trial design or conduct that favor one of the treatment groups. Several sources of bias may occur in systematic reviews of treatment efficacy.

Placebo control group. In trials that directly compare two active drugs, we need to know that either or both treatments were effective. Only if we know the extent of the placebo response, and that it does not vary, can this criterion be fulfilled (McQuay and Moore 1996). Performing studies of drug A versus drug B when the extent and variability of the placebo response are unknown can be misleading. Results showing no difference between A and B could mean that both A and B were effective or that neither A nor B was effective. The only current defense is to have a placebo group. Designs of

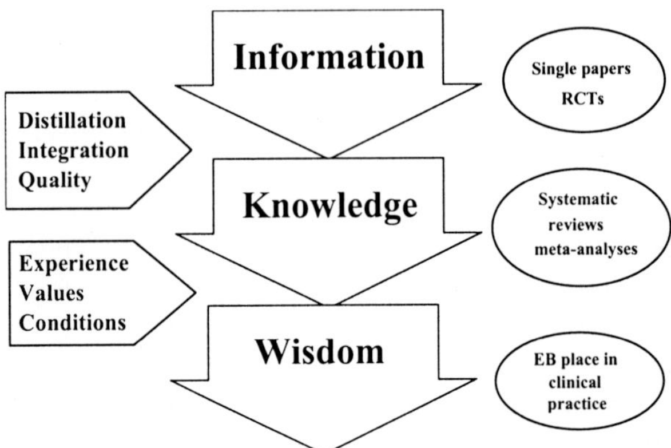

Fig. 1. The process of systematic review distills information through quality filters and integrates different types of information to form knowledge, which can be used according to the unique biology of the patient, the values of society, and the conditions of the time. RCTs = randomized clinical trials; EB = evidence-based research.

trials of analgesics 30 years ago understood this and included both standard active and placebo groups. Only in trials in which sensitivity is proved (that is, standard treatment beats placebo) can correct conclusions of equivalence be made. What constitutes an appropriate placebo depends upon circumstances: it may be necessary to use "active" placebos (Max et al. 1987).

Randomization. Studies that are not randomized can overestimate treatment effects by up to 40% (Schulz et al. 1995). A classic example is the use of transcutaneous electrical nerve stimulation (TENS) in postoperative pain relief: randomized studies overwhelmingly show that it does not work, while nonrandomized studies say that it does (Carroll et al. 1996). Reviews of treatment efficacy should thus include only randomized studies.

Blinding. Where possible, studies should be double-blind, as nonblinded studies overestimate treatment effects by about 17% (Schulz et al. 1995).

Quality. Several reviews have used a scoring system for methodological quality to show that studies of lower quality are likely to overestimate treatment effects (Khan et al. 1996; Moher et al. 1998).

Duplication. Trials may be reported more than once. While this may be legitimate, duplicate publication often occurs without cross-referencing. Up to 30% of all patients reported in the literature appear in duplicate publications, and this can lead to an overestimation in treatment effect by 20% or more (Tramèr et al. 1997b).

Not all of these sources of bias will occur every time, but some will, and there may be others still to be recognized. What the systematic review process teaches us about trials of effectiveness is that there are many sources of potential bias, all of which tend to *overestimate* the effects of treatment.

BIAS IN CLINICAL PAIN TRIALS

For decades we have recognized the need for randomization to overcome selection bias, and for double-blinding to overcome observer bias in trials of pain treatments. Nevertheless, many studies still are not randomized (or are inadequately randomized), are not double-blind, or break fundamental tenets of clinical trial design.

In a systematic review of aspirin in acute pain (Edwards et al. 1999b), out of 175 papers considered for inclusion after an initial search, 2 were not double-blind, 8 were not randomized, and 16 included patients whose pain was not of moderate or severe intensity. Consequently, 18% of possible trials had to be discarded. Only 17 of 36 (47%) trials of TENS for acute postoperative pain were adequately randomized (Carroll et al. 1996). A review of TENS in chronic pain (Carroll 1999) revealed that half of the studies included had used only a single application of TENS to judge its effectiveness.

Almost any systematic review in pain mentions significant numbers of trials that were omitted because they were not randomized or were not double-blind, or because of some methodological defect. Although some of this represents the legacy of times when the quality issues were less well understood, contemporary publications and planned trials still too often suffer from the same defects. This represents a massive loss to human knowledge, and a significant challenge to the ethical base of clinical trials.

DESCRIBING TRIAL RESULTS

Clinical trials are often criticized for measuring only what is measurable rather than what is meaningful. A summed pain intensity difference (SPID), or a percentage of total pain relief (TOTPAR), or the outcome of a particular statistical test may be meaningful in the context of a single trial, but beyond that may have little relevance. Systematic reviews often force the issue of whether a particular outcome is worthwhile to our patients, their caregivers, or to society as a whole. This sometimes means imposing *our* values on a group of studies, rather than taking the outcomes that authors have considered adequate.

One of the most useful tools that systematic reviews use to describe results is the "number needed to treat" (NNT) (Cook and Sackett 1995; McQuay and Moore 1997). Using NNTs forces decisions about what is a useful clinical outcome. This can be particularly relevant when trial result data are highly skewed, as occurs in acute pain trials. There is huge variability in the responses of individual patients to interventions. In acute pain, patients given placebo or analgesic can get complete pain relief, or none at all (Fig. 2). The mean is an inadequate way to describe TOTPAR, or the percentage of maximum pain relief that patients achieve (%maxTOTPAR). It is possible to define a point on the horizontal scale of Fig. 2 that represents a judgment about what is a useful result. Half pain relief (or at least 50% maxTOTPAR) is a judgment commonly made. It has the benefit of being fairly easily understood by patients and their caregivers, and produces robust estimates for NNTs (Moore and McQuay 1997).

A concern is that by dichotomizing pain outcomes into less than or at least 50% pain relief, we may lose much other useful data. Another criticism is that we have not sought the judgment of patients themselves, either for this outcome, or indeed any pain intensity or relief outcome on any of the myriad of measurement scales that have been used. Both these concerns are legitimate. However, as we begin this journey of discovery, we have to work with what is available now. Systematic reviews tell us that we have no better

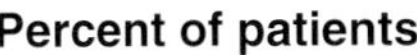

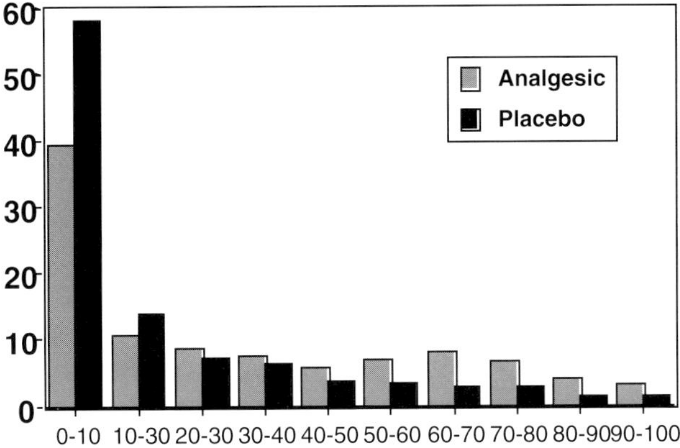

Fig. 2. Percentage of maximum pain relief obtained by 826 patients receiving placebo and 3157 patients receiving an analgesic in randomized, double-blind, single-dose studies with moderate or severe initial pain intensity. Patients given a placebo or analgesic can have 0% or 100% pain relief, and the distribution is highly skewed.

way of judging what outcomes are important to patients, and that a huge number of different pain scales have been used in research (A. Jadad, personal communication), and there are lessons here for clinical trials to be carried out in the future.

The NNT is a description of the therapeutic effort needed to achieve a desired outcome in one patient. It is easily calculated. The NNT for treatment is given by 1/([proportion benefiting from experimental intervention] – [proportion benefiting from control intervention]) (Cook and Sackett 1995):

$$NNT = \frac{1}{(IMP_{act} / TOT_{act}) - (IMP_{con} / TOT_{con})}$$

where IMP_{act} = number of patients given active treatment achieving the target, TOT_{act} = total number of patients given the active treatment, IMP_{con} = number of patients given a control treatment achieving the target, and TOT_{con} = total number of patients given the control treatment.

If 75% (or 0.75 as a proportion) of patients benefit from treatment and 25% (0.25) benefit with control, the NNT is 1/(0.75 – 0.25), or 2. NNT is treatment specific; it describes the *difference* between active treatment and control in achieving a particular clinical outcome (McQuay and Moore 1997). An NNT of 1 means that a favorable outcome occurs in every patient given the treatment but in no patient in a comparison group, the "perfect" result in, say, a therapeutic trial of an antibiotic compared with placebo. Studies of treatments usually involve large effects in small numbers of patients. NNTs of 2 or 3 indicate effective treatments. The 95% confidence intervals of the NNT are an indication that 19 times out of 20 the "true" value will be in the specified range.

The same arguments can be used for adverse effects, or harm, when NNT becomes NNH (number needed to harm). However they are used, the NNT or NNH should mention the comparison condition (placebo or other treatment), the intensity of treatment (dose and duration of drug), the outcome, and time when the outcome is achieved.

SIZE OF TRIALS

Fig. 3 shows the enormous variation between individual trials. The implication is that random chance might play an important role in trial outcomes. The challenge is to tease apart variability among trials that derives from systematic issues in trial design and conduct from that which derives from the random play of chance. Only substantial amounts of information can help us do this.

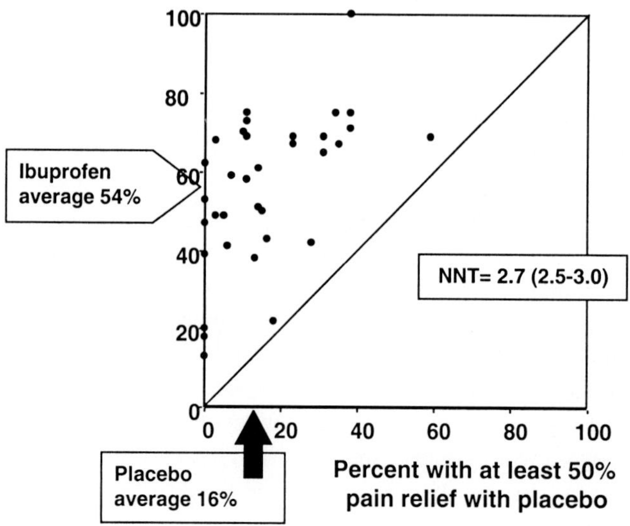

Fig. 3. Systematic review of randomized, double-blind, single-dose studies comparing 400 mg ibuprofen with placebo. Each symbol is a single trial.

SYSTEMATIC ISSUES

A recent systematic review of aspirin trials in acute pain (Edwards et al. 1999b) has the largest set of trials for a single intervention, with 68 trials and 5061 patients (2499 given 600–650 mg aspirin and 2562 given placebo). All of these trials were randomized and double-blind, included only patients with moderate or severe pain intensity, and used the same outcome of at least 50% maxTOTPAR to calculate the NNT. Thus, they were studies of the highest methodological quality, clear of known sources of bias. These studies allowed us to draw several conclusions about acute pain trials: (1) within this high-quality data set, the quality of reporting of the trials had no effect on trial outcome; (2) the pain model (third molar extraction, post-surgical, or episiotomy) had no effect on trial outcome; (3) the pain measurement (categorical or visual analogue scales to measure SPID or TOTPAR) had no effect on trial outcome; and (4) the difference in time for trials conducted over 4, 5, or 6 hours had no effect on outcome.

Systematic reviews confirm, therefore, that the design of trials in acute pain is robust. Despite this, and despite the homogeneous nature of the studies included for analysis, the variation in measured NNT for 600–650 mg aspirin was large, and ranged from 2 to 10 (Edwards et al. 1999b). NNTs of about 2 are excellent, while those of 10 are very poor. The extremes represent a therapeutic benefit of 10–50% of patients achieving at least half pain relief with this dose of aspirin.

RANDOM CHANCE

Why is there such an enormous difference between individual high-quality studies? It is not confined to aspirin, but occurs commonly in acute pain studies, both in patients receiving placebo and those receiving an analgesic. Fig. 3 shows a plot of the percentage of patients achieving at least 50% pain relief with placebo and with 400 mg ibuprofen, in which each symbol is a comparison in similar high-quality trials. Can the spread of results be explained by random chance?

If we have a large box of balls, half of which are red and half blue, how many balls do we need to sample out of the box to be 99% sure that the proportion of blue balls is between 49% and 51%? The answer is about 16,000 balls. If we wanted to be only 95% certain, the answer would be about 10,000 balls. At their simplest, clinical trials could be regarded as a number of different boxes with different proportions of blue and red balls. But the number of patients included in clinical trials is often quite small, about 40 individuals per treatment group (Moore et al. 1998). If we were using this number as the sample for our box of balls, because of random sampling errors we could only be about 35% sure that the actual proportion was between 49% and 51%.

We know the distribution of individual patient responses to analgesics and placebo in acute pain trials from information on over 5000 patients (Fig. 2). It is therefore possible to use mathematical models to see how the amount of available information affects the reliability of results we obtain (Moore et al. 1998). These modeling exercises tell us that that the range of responses seen for ibuprofen (Fig. 3) and for aspirin are entirely explicable by the random play of chance.

Size is everything. Results of a single trial of conventional size to test ibuprofen in acute pain are unlikely to be correct. A trial with group sizes of 40 could have NNT values between 1 and 9 just by chance, when the true value was 3. The variability in the response rates of both placebo and active treatments means that we must study many more than the conventional 40 patients per group if we want to be sure of getting clinically credible results. Conventional trials are sized according to a different criterion—that of being reasonably sure not to miss a statistical difference.

To measure the effectiveness (defined as an NNT value ± 0.5) of an analgesic such as ibuprofen, we need not 40 patients per group, but 500 (Table I). Acute pain trials with 1000 patients are rare, so that credible estimates of clinical efficacy are only likely to come from large trials or from pooling multiple trials of conventional (small) size. Only when analgesics are particularly efficacious, with NNTs of about 2, will comparisons with a few hundred patients provide accurate estimates.

The corollary is that single small trials are unlikely to be correct in terms of the *magnitude* of an analgesic's effectiveness, and may even be incorrect in showing that it is an analgesic. Systematic reviews show that the

Table I
Percentage of clinical trials with number-needed-to-treat (NNT) value within ± 0.5 of true value according to group size

	Percentage of Trials		
Group Size	NNT = 4.00	NNT = 3.00	NNT = 2.30
25	26	37	57
50	28	51	73
100	38	61	88
200	55	81	96
300	63	89	99
400	71	93	99
500	74	95	100

Note: Calculated by simulating 10,000 trials, with "true" NNTs of 2.3, 3.0, and 4.0 (Moore et al. 1998).

variability in trials of conventional size just because of random chance is enormous. It follows that, for some purposes, we may have to find ways to conduct trials that include many more patients than is conventional today.

The problem of trial size is especially relevant in chronic pain conditions, where outcomes may be measured over months, and where trial conduct and patient recruitment are much more difficult than in single-dose acute pain trials. For instance, in postherpetic neuralgia and diabetic neuropathy, 10 studies recruited fewer than 25 patients per treatment, nine recruited between 50 and 100, and only one had more than 100 patients per treatment (McQuay et al. 1995, 1996; Backonja et al. 1998; Rowbotham et al. 1998).

PLACEBO RESPONSES

Trial size and variability because of random chance influences judgments we may wish to make about other aspects of clinical trials. One is the placebo response. Patients given placebo may have significant pain relief in both acute (Fig. 2) and chronic painful conditions (McQuay et al. 1995, 1996). Individual studies show that the placebo response rate may be variable (Fig. 3). Is it possible for us to define what the placebo response rate may be in a standard clinical setting?

For single-dose analgesic trials in acute pain we may now be able to provide an answer. Fig. 4 shows the overall response rate to placebo in about 50 systematic reviews of randomized, double-blind trials with patients with initial pain of moderate or severe intensity—studies in which all other known influences have been eradicated. Across all trials, with over 10,000 patients given placebo, 18% had at least 50% pain relief. The figure shows that a relatively accurate estimate was given in all systematic reviews where the total number of patients given placebo was 500 or more. Below 500 patients the placebo response rate varied widely, with an absolute rate of 0–56%. This demonstrates how difficult it is likely to be to investigate subtle influences on patients' responses to any intervention.

ADVERSE EFFECTS

Interventions may benefit patients, but they also carry a risk of harm. The balance of benefit and harm is a difficult judgment, because harm (adverse effects) can be common or rare, mild or severe, reversible or irreversible. Mostly, adverse effects occur less frequently than the good outcomes we desire, and the potential that single randomized trials will be adequate to assess their frequency is limited by size. Systematic reviews can help by giving us an insight into the quality (or otherwise) of adverse effect reporting.

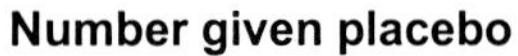

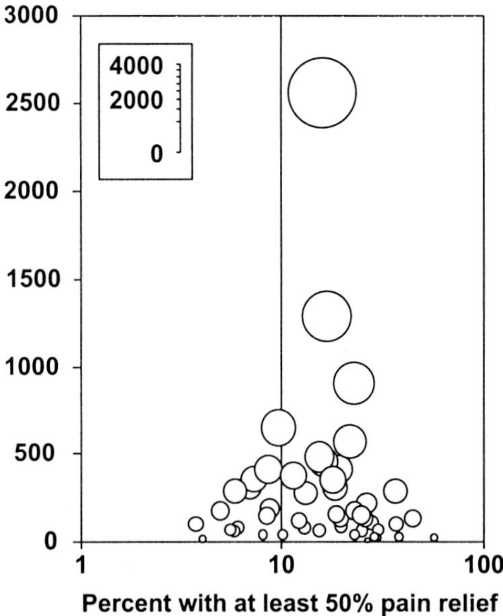

Fig. 4. Placebo responses in randomized, double-blind, single-dose studies in acute pain. Each symbol shows the percentage with at least 50% pain relief with placebo in a systematic review. The overall average was 18%. The diameter of each symbol is related to the number of patients given placebo, as is indicated by the scale.

In an analysis of 52 randomized, double-blind trials of ibuprofen and paracetamol with over 4500 patients, Edwards and colleagues (1999a) examined adverse effect reporting. Reporting methods were categorized and reported as: adverse effects not mentioned in the report (4% of trials); statement that no adverse effects occurred (12% of trials); statement that there was no difference between active treatment and placebo (4% of trials); statement that adverse effects occurred but with no detail of frequency or type (15% of trials); full description of type and frequency of the individual adverse effects (65% of trials).

In effect, 35% of potential information on adverse effects was lost because of inadequate reporting. Edwards et al. (1998a) made several recommendations on how to report adverse effects in clinical trials, in an extension of the current CONSORT guidelines (Anonymous 1997). Suggestions include providing details of the type of anesthetic used (if relevant); a description of the format of questions and/or checklists used to assess adverse effects; details of the severity of adverse effects and how this was assessed; full details of the type and frequency of adverse effects reported for active drug and for placebo; full details of patient withdrawals related to adverse effects; and, where possible, the likely relationship between adverse effects and the study drug.

No single clinical trial is likely to provide adequate information about adverse effects unless it is very large. Yet collecting high-quality information is crucial to understanding the benefit/harm relationships of different treatments. Using the large amounts of information from systematic reviews, we can derive a treatment-specific estimate for the number of patients who benefit for every one harmed (Edwards 1999) using NNT and NNH. For oral opioids, the ratio of NNH to NNT is of the order of 1–2. For oral paracetamol and intramuscular morphine the ratio is 3–5, and for oral aspirin and NSAIDs it is 10 or more. For the latter, therefore, 10 patients benefit for every one suffering minor harm. This sort of information can be useful to clinicians making informed choices about treatments based on systematic reviews and meta-analyses. Yet the quality of the meta-analyses are only as good as the individual trials. Better reporting of adverse effects in individual trials is clearly essential.

Rare, but more serious, adverse effects are sometimes ignored in reporting clinical trials. This is a mistake. Again, the accumulation of evidence from clinical studies can lead to associations between treatment and rare adverse effects, which with time can become causal. Considerable epidemiological evidence links gastrointestinal bleeding with NSAIDs, for example, but the evidence could have been gleaned from randomized trials. Two Cochrane reviews of NSAIDs in the hip and knee report on just over 3000 patients using NSAIDs (Towheed et al. 1999; Watson et al. 1999). Careful examination of the original reports shows that gastrointestinal bleeding events, covering positive stool tests to frank bleeding, occurred on about 0.7% of all patients in the studies, despite their median length being only 6 weeks. Another example is the association between the use of propofol and bradycardia, asystole, and cardiac death (Tramèr et al. 1997a), which was only possible because the events had been recorded in the original trial reports.

COMMENT

Each particular topic has its own complexities, but a checklist of features that contribute to the quality of studies in systematic reviews will often include some or all of the following: *Randomization:* Nonrandomized trials overestimate the effect of treatment; unless there is a compelling reason, nonrandomized trials of treatments should be ignored. *Blinding:* Nonblinded studies overestimate the effect of treatment, and should likewise be ignored or treated with caution. *Withdrawals:* Studies in which large numbers of patients have dropped out may be unsatisfactory. *Size:* Large studies done well should carry particular weight. *Statistics:* Were good statistical tests performed, such as analysis if variance? Any study where the authors choose a single positive statistical answer out of many that are negative can be downgraded. *Statistical significance:* $P < 0.05$ isn't *that* clever. It is only 1 in 20, and you can roll two sixes with a couple of dice quite often. Weight trials with $P < 0.001$ much more highly. *Credible patient enrollment:* Are the patients at entry into the trial representative of typical patients with a particular complaint? *Outcomes:* Were the outcomes used at all valuable to doctors or patients, or were they just unsubstantiated surrogate measures?

Large randomized trials appear to be the prerogative of the pharmaceutical industry. Clinical trials of sumatriptan for migraine have enrolled over 7500 patients (Tfelt-Hansen 1998), and some of the newer drugs in this class will have data on similar numbers of patients. The new COX-2 selective inhibitors, rofecoxib and celecoxib, have similarly been tested on many thousands of patients, in studies as long as a year and with individual enrollments of over 1000 patients in a single trial. Gabapentin has been studied in postherpetic neuralgia and diabetic neuropathy in somewhat smaller studies (Backonja et al. 1998; Rowbotham et al. 1998) that still dwarf previous efforts (McQuay et al. 1995, 1996). Replicating the gathering of evidence in the requisite amounts will pose a challenge for noncommercial research.

The process of gathering evidence in systematic reviews and meta-analysis is changing the way we think about clinical trials. The fact that we now have

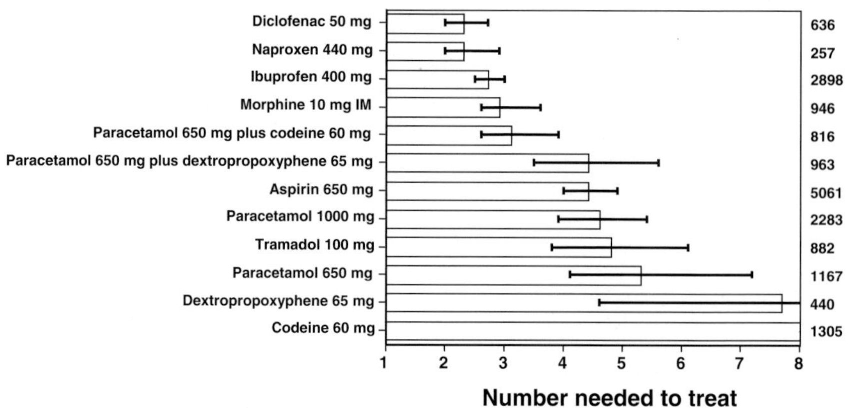

Fig. 5. League figure of analgesics in randomized, double-blind, single-dose studies in acute pain (after McQuay and Moore 1998). Each bar is a systematic review that demonstrated at least 50% pain relief and included comparison with placebo. Numbers at right are total numbers of patients in the comparison.

league tables of relative analgesic effectiveness in acute pain (Fig. 5) demonstrates that benchmarks are being set for the future (McQuay and Moore 1998). The results of systematic reviews are being made increasingly available, for instance at the Oxford Pain Internet Site (www.ebando.com/painres/painpag/index.html). This site provides an evidence-based collection of systematic review summaries and other evidence. Another useful site is www.cochrane.org. At the Oxford site, league tables are available for treatments for migraine and dysmenorrhea. Those planning, designing, and conducting clinical trials have a firm base on which to work, and benchmarks against which their efforts will be judged.

ACKNOWLEDGMENTS

It is a pleasure to acknowledge the many people in Oxford and around the world who have contributed so much to understanding the evidence base of pain, including Henry McQuay, Alex Jadad, Martin Tramèr, Dawn Carroll, Phil Wiffen, David Gavaghan, Jayne Edwards, Sally Collins, Lesley Smith, Anna Oldman, Eija Kalso, and many others.

REFERENCES

Anonymous. Working Group on Recommendations for Reporting of Clinical Trials in the Biomedical Literature. Call for comments on a proposal to improve reporting of clinical trials in the biomedical literature. *Ann Intern Med* 1994; 121:894–895.

Backonja M, Beydoun A, Edwards KR, et al. Gabapentin for the symptomatic treatment of painful neuropathy in patients with diabetes mellitus: a randomized controlled trial. *JAMA* 1998; 280:1831–1836.

Carroll D. A systematic review to evaluate the effectiveness of TENS in chronic pain. MSc Dissertation, University of Oxford, 1999.

Carroll D, Tramèr MR, McQuay HJ, Nye B, Moore RA. Randomization is important in studies with pain outcomes: systematic review of transcutaneous electrical nerve stimulation in acute postoperative pain. *Br J Anaesth* 1996; 77:798–803.

Cook RJ, Sackett DL. The number needed to treat: a clinically useful measure of treatment effect. *BMJ* 1995; 310:452–454.

Edwards JE. Determining risk and benefit in systematic reviews. DPhil Thesis, University of Oxford, 1999.

Edwards JE, McQuay HJ, Moore RA, Collins SL. Reporting of adverse effects in clinical trials should be improved: lessons from acute postoperative pain. *J Pain Symptom Manage* 1999a, in press.

Edwards JE, Oldman A, Smith L, et al. Oral aspirin in postoperative pain: a quantitative systematic review. *Pain* 1999b; 81:289–297.

Jadad AR, McQuay HJ. Meta-analyses to evaluate analgesic interventions: a systematic qualitative review of their methodology. *J Clin Epidemiol* 1996; 49:235–243.

Jadad AR, Carroll D, Moore RA, McQuay HJ. Developing a database of published reports of randomised clinical trials in pain research. *Pain* 1996; 66:39–46.

Khan KS, Daya S, Jadad AR. The importance of quality of primary studies in producing unbiased systematic reviews. *Arch Intern Med* 1996; 156:661–666.

Max MB, Culnane M, Schafer SC, et al. Amitriptyline relieves diabetic neuropathy pain in patients with normal or depressed mood. *Neurology* 1987; 37:589–596.

McQuay HJ, Moore RA. Placebo mania. Placebos are essential when extent and variability of placebo responses are unknown. *BMJ* 1996: 313:1008.

McQuay HJ, Moore RA. Using numerical results from systematic reviews in clinical practice. *Ann Intern Med* 1997; 126:712–720.

McQuay HJ, Moore RA. *An Evidence-Based Resource For Pain Relief.* Oxford: Oxford University Press, 1998.

McQuay HJ, Carroll D, Jadad AR, Wiffen P, Moore RA. Anticonvulsants for the management of pain—a systematic review. *BMJ* 1995; 311:1047–1052.

McQuay HJ, Tramèr MR, Nye BA, et al. A systematic review of antidepressants in neuropathic pain. *Pain* 1996; 68:217–227.

Moher D, Pham B, Jones A, et al. Does quality of reports of randomised trials affect estimates of intervention efficacy reported in meta-analyses? *Lancet* 1998; 352:609–613.

Moore RA, McQuay HJ. Single-patient data meta-analysis of 3,453 postoperative patients: oral tramadol versus placebo, codeine and combination analgesics. *Pain* 1997; 69:287–294.

Moore RA, Gavaghan D, Tramèr MR, Collins SL, McQuay HJ. Size is everything: large amounts of information are needed to overcome random effects in estimating direction and magnitude of treatment effects. *Pain* 1998; 78:217–220.

Rowbotham M, Harden N, Stacey B, Bernstein P, Magnus-Miller L. Gabapentin for the treatment of postherpetic neuralgia: a randomized controlled trial. *JAMA* 1998; 280:1837–1842.

Sackett DL, Rosenberg WMC, Muir Gray JA, Haynes RB, Richardson WS. Evidence-based medicine: what it is and what it isn't. *BMJ* 1996; 312:71–72.

Schulz KF, Chalmers I, Hayes RJ, Altman DG. Empirical evidence of bias: dimensions of methodological quality associated with estimates of treatment effects in controlled trials. *JAMA* 1995; 273:408–412.

Tfelt-Hansen P. Efficacy and adverse events of subcutaneous, oral, and intranasal sumatriptan used for migraine treatment: a systematic review based on number needed to treat. *Cephalaglia* 1998; 18:532–538.

Towheed T, Shea B, Wells G, Hochberg M. Analgesia and non-aspirin, non-steroidal anti-inflammatory drugs for osteoarthritis of the hip. *Cochrane Library* 1999, issue 2.

Tramèr MR, Moore RA, McQuay HJ. Propofol and bradycardia: causation, frequency and severity. *Br J Anaesth* 1997a; 78:642–651.

Tramèr M, Reynolds DJM, Moore RA, McQuay HJ. Effect of covert duplicate publication on meta-analysis: a case study. *BMJ* 1997b; 315:635–640.

Watson MC, Brookes ST, Kirwan JR, Faulkner A. Non-aspirin, non-steroidal anti-inflammatory drugs (NSAIDs) for osteoarthritis of the knee. *Cochrane Library* 1999, issue 2.

Correspondence to: R. Andrew Moore, DSc, Pain Research and Nuffield Department of Anaesthetics, University of Oxford, Oxford Radcliffe Hospitals, The Churchill, Oxford OX3 7LJ, United Kingdom. Tel: 44-1865-226132; Fax: 44-1865-226978; email: andrew.moore@pru.ox.ac.uk.

Proceedings of the 9th World Congress on Pain,
Progress in Pain Research and Management,
Vol. 16, edited by M. Devor, M.C. Rowbotham, and
Z. Wiesenfeld-Hallin, IASP Press, Seattle, © 2000.

74

Spinal Actions of Cyclooxygenase Isozyme Inhibitors[1]

Gerd Geisslinger[a] and Tony L. Yaksh[b]

[a]*Center of Pharmacology, Johann Wolfgang Goethe-University, Frankfurt am Main, Germany;* [b]*Departments of Anesthesiology and Pharmacology, University of California, San Diego, La Jolla, California, USA*

Aspirin-like drugs, now referred to as nonsteroidal anti-inflammatory drugs (NSAIDs) and originally as the non-narcotic, peripherally acting analgesics, are among the most widely used therapeutic classes of compounds (see Lewis and Furst 1987). The efficacy of these agents in reducing pain is widely recognized not only in the popular lore of our time, but in the many clinical trials that focus on the management of postsurgical pain (see, for example, Reasbeck et al. 1982; Gillies et al. 1987) and persistent pain states, such as in arthritis and cancer (Foley 1985; Takeda 1991). McQuay and Moore (1999) reviewed the analgesic efficacy of NSAIDs as compiled from randomized trials with various pain conditions. Considering efficacy in terms of "numbers-needed-to-treat" (NNT, which describes the difference between active treatment and control) to establish clinically significant effects, they noted that at clinical doses of agents such as ibuprofen (400 mg) and diclofenac (25–50 mg), NNT values were about 2–3. This means that of every two to three patients who receive the drug, one patient will report at least 50% relief. In contrast, the NNTs for codeine (60 mg) or tramadol (100 mg) were 16.7 and 4.8, respectively.

ANTIHYPERALGESIC VERSUS ANALGESIC ACTIONS OF NSAIDS

Although NSAIDs have long been used to treat mild or moderate pain following injury, disease, or minor surgery (Smith 1949), their mechanism

[1] Mini-review based on a congress workshop.

of analgesic action remains a controversial subject. Preclinical studies (Table I) have emphasized that these agents do not elevate the pain threshold (as measured by acute escape models, i.e., thermally evoked hot-plate and tail-flick or mechanical pressure), but that they usually normalize the exaggerated pain behavior (hyperalgesia) that is observed after tissue injury or inflammation (Fig. 1).

An explanation of how NSAIDs exert their action must consider their relatively selective antihyperalgesic effect versus an analgesic effect. Two broad sites of action, peripheral and central, have been postulated for the hyperalgesic state. First, after tissue injury, an increase occurs in the local extracellular levels of serotonin, kinins, ions (H^+/K^+), cytokines, and metabolites of the arachidonic acid cascade (e.g., prostaglandins [PGs]). These products jointly activate small peripheral afferents and sensitize the free nerve endings (nociceptors), with the result that their stimulus-response curve is shifted to the left, i.e., a greater response is evoked by a given or lesser stimulus. Injection of these products into the paw, for example, will cause an animal to display an escape response at lower intensities or with shorter latencies, typical of hyperalgesia, as shown in Fig. 1.

Second, following tissue injury, repetitive activity is generated in small primary afferents, produced in part by the injury-induced changes in the peripheral chemical milieu. Persistent small afferent input will initiate a spinal cascade that facilitates dorsal horn sensory processing (Mendell and Wall 1965). This spinal sensitization is characterized by an increase in the peripheral receptive fields and in the response of dorsal horn neurons to small afferent input (Woolf and King 1990; Owens et al. 1992). These elec-

Table I
The relative effect (0 = no effect) of spinally delivered COX-2-selective or mixed COX-1/COX-2 inhibitors or μ-opioid receptor agonists on different pain models in rats

Assay	Stimulus	COX-1/2 Inhibitor	COX-2 Inhibitor	μ-Opioid Agonist
Hot-plate test	thermal	0	0	+ +
Tail-flick test	thermal	0	0	+ +
Writhing test	chemical	+ +	+ +	+ +
Formalin phase 1	chemical	+	+/0	+ +
Formalin phase 2	chemical	+ +	+/0	+ +
Normal paw	mechanical	0	0	+ +
Inflamed paw	mechanical	+ +	+ +	+ +
Inflamed paw	thermal	+ +	+ +	+ +
Intrathecal SP	thermal	+ +	+ +	+ +
Intrathecal NMDA	thermal	+ +	+ +	+ +

Note: For details see Yaksh (1999).

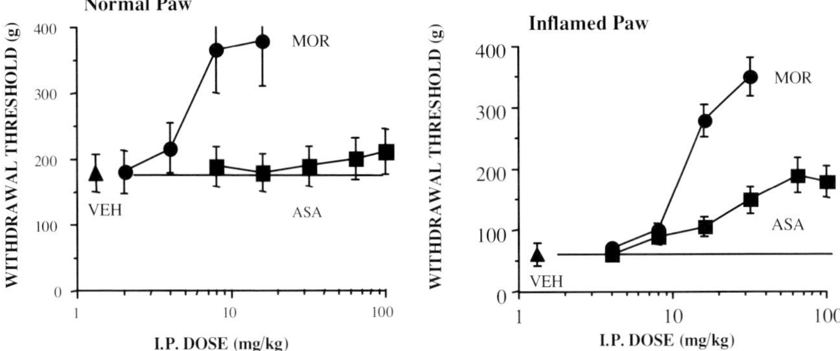

Fig. 1. Dose-response curves for intraperitoneal morphine (MOR), acetylsalicylic acid (ASA), and vehicle (VEH) on the mechanical paw withdrawal threshold in normal rats (left) or in rats with a single inflamed hindpaw (right). Each point presents the mean and SEM of 4–6 rats.

trophysiological properties are behaviorally manifested by an enhanced response to small afferent input generated by mechanical, thermal, and chemical stimuli applied to the receptive field (see Dickenson et al. 1997). Studies on the spinal pharmacology of this cascade suggest that it begins in part with the release of peptides such as substance P (SP) and excitatory amino acids such as glutamate, which activate neurokinin-1 and N-methyl-D-aspartate (NMDA) receptors, respectively. Thus, intrathecal (i.t.) injection of these agents alone produces thermal and mechanical hyperalgesia, while i.t. injection of the corresponding antagonists attenuates the injury-evoked hyperalgesic state without altering normal baseline thresholds (Yaksh et al. 1999).

PERIPHERAL ACTIONS OF NSAIDS

Several early observations provided convergent evidence that NSAIDs may exert a direct peripheral effect. First, the non-narcotic, nonsteroidal antipyretic agents, despite their structural variations, were shown to share the ability to inhibit cyclooxygenase-mediated synthesis of prostaglandins (Smith and Willis 1971; Vane 1971). Second, these prostaglandins, locally elaborated following tissue injury, served to sensitize peripheral nerve endings and to facilitate pain behavior in animal models (Lim 1970). These properties were viewed as support for the unifying and inviting hypothesis that NSAIDs act in models of peripheral inflammation where the hallmark of nociception is a "hyperalgesic state" (Ferreira 1972; Moncada et al. 1975). It was appreciated, however, that the anti-inflammatory and analgesic actions of these agents could be dissociated (McCormack and Brune 1991).

Such dissociations suggested that actions other than those involved with peripheral inflammation might account for the observed antihyperalgesic effects. Significant emphasis has been placed on the role of spinal cyclooxygenase (COX) systems in spinal nociceptive processing.

SPINAL ACTIONS OF NSAIDS

Substantial data support the hypothesis that spinal prostaglandins play an important role in the nociceptive processing that leads to hyperalgesia and that conversely, agents that inhibit prostaglandin synthesis can reverse such hyperalgesic states by a spinal action. Hence, NSAIDs may exert a potent antihyperalgesic effect at the spinal level, as follows.

1) Prostaglandins are released from the spinal cord following stimulation of small sensory afferents (Ramwell et al. 1966). Following peripheral noxious stimulation, PGE_2 is released in the spinal cord or the cerebrospinal fluid, as has been determined by spinal superperfusion and microdialysis (Yaksh 1992; Malmberg and Yaksh 1995a,b; Yang et al. 1996; Scheuren et al. 1997; Muth-Selbach et al. 1999). The release appears secondary to the activation of small afferents. Thus, in vitro spinal cord superperfusion demonstrates PGE_2 release following stimulation with capsaicin (Malmberg and Yaksh 1994; Dirig and Yaksh 1999). In vivo, i.t. SP results in NK1-receptor-mediated PGE_2 release from the spinal cord. The release of PGE_2 from the spinal cord that is evoked by intraplantar formalin is blocked by analgesic doses of morphine (Malmberg and Yaksh 1995c).

2) Intrathecal injections of a variety of cyclooxygenase products, including PGE_2, result in a dose-dependent hyperalgesia (Ferreira et al. 1978; Yaksh 1982; Taiwo and Levine 1986; Uda et al. 1990; Minami et al. 1994a,b; Ferreira and Lorenzetti 1996), while i.t. PGE_2 antagonists can diminish hyperalgesic states (Malmberg et al. 1994). Prostaglandins such as PGE_2 act via prostanoid receptors, for example of the EP type, to enhance calcium conductance or to block the increase in an inwardly rectifying K^+ current, which leads to a net enhancement of excitability of the dorsal root ganglia and thereby increases terminal release of primary afferent transmitters (Nicol et al. 1992; Vasko et al. 1994).

3) The spinal delivery of structurally diverse NSAIDs results in a dose-dependent suppression of the hyperalgesic state induced by local tissue injury or inflammation, although the drugs have no effect on acute nociceptive thresholds (Yaksh 1982; Malmberg and Yaksh 1992a,b; Dirig et al. 1998a,b). The i.t. effect is not mediated by systemic redistribution; doses required to produce an equal antinociception after systemic delivery were

100–900 times greater than those required after spinal delivery, and the peak achievable effect after either route was the same (Malmberg and Yaksh 1992a; Dirig et al. 1998a). While the ordering of potency among NSAIDs displayed considerable variation, the maximum achievable effect was the same, which suggests a common mechanism. The antihyperalgesic effects of these agents appear to reflect a role for COX inhibition, as the relative antihyperalgesic potency of each drug was comparable to its respective potency for COX inhibition. Moreover, with i.t. ibuprofen, the COX-inhibiting S(+)-enantiomer alone was active (Malmberg and Yaksh 1992a; Dirig et al. 1998a).

4) Finally, additional evidence supporting a relation between antinociception of spinal or systemic NSAIDs and spinal COX activity was observed using spinal perfusion and microdialysis in rats. Formalin injection into the rat paw produces a biphasic pain behavior (flinching and licking of the injected paw) and a spinal release of PGE_2 (Malmberg and Yaksh 1995a,b; Muth-Selbach et al. 1999). Importantly, antinociceptive i.t. doses of S(+)-ibuprofen, but not the R(–)-enantiomer, abolished the increased spinal PGE_2 release, while lower, inactive doses were without effect. In addition, systemic doses of ibuprofen that were effective in reducing the behavioral response were similarly effective in diminishing the formalin-evoked spinal PGE_2 release (Malmberg and Yaksh 1995a). In contrast, the antinociceptive agent R(–)-flurbiprofen, which is not a COX inhibitor in vitro, inhibited spinal PGE_2 release (G. Geisslinger et al., unpublished manuscript). Thus, at least some nonopioid analgesics may have COX-independent but PG-dependent spinal mechanisms.

Given the structural diversity of the NSAIDs, additional pharmacological mechanisms independent of COX inhibition may play a role. Thus, the spinal effects of ketorolac are antagonized by a κ-opioid receptor antagonist (Uphouse et al. 1993). The central effect of diclofenac can be suppressed by the opioid antagonist naloxone (Bjorkman et al. 1990), and a recent study has suggested that acetaminophen produces central antinociception by interfering with the nitric oxide system (Bjorkman et al. 1994). Antinociceptive doses of acetaminophen, which is only a weak COX inhibitor in vitro, dose-dependently inhibited spinal PGE_2 release following systemic administration. Interestingly, the same doses of acetaminophen did not affect urinary excretion of prostaglandins (Muth-Selbach et al. 1999). Salicylate may act by blocking the activation of the transcription factor known as nuclear factor κB (NFκB) (Frantz and O'Neill 1995), although this effect may occur at doses that are not systemically relevant. R-ibuprofenoyl-CoA thioester, a metabolite of R(–)-ibuprofen formed during the inversion process, did not inhibit COX but prevented COX-2 induction in LPS-stimulated monocytes

(Neupert et al. 1997). Last, but not least, NSAIDs may block inflammation-evoked intraspinal release of SP (Schaible et al. 1998).

DISCOVERY OF TWO CYCLOOXYGENASES

An important advance from a scientific and therapeutic perspective has been the discovery of two COX isoforms. COX-1 demonstrates a high level of stable constitutive expression in both the central nervous system (CNS) and the periphery. This molecule has the characteristic of a housekeeping enzyme whose activity depends solely on availability of its substrate, arachidonic acid. By contrast, COX-2, which bears 60% overall identity with COX-1 at the amino acid level, behaves as an immediate early gene and is subject to rapid regulation at the transcription/translation level (DuBois et al. 1998). Its messenger RNA (mRNA) displays several consensus sequences for transcription factors such as NFκB (D'Acquisto et al. 1997). While the original work on peripheral COX showed a pattern of constitutive COX-1 and revealed expression of COX-2 only after induction, central expression of the isoforms has been less clear. As in the periphery, COX-1 is expressed constitutively in the brain and spinal cord. Surprisingly, however, COX-2 was also found to be constitutively expressed in the spinal cord (Beiche et al. 1996, 1998b; Willingale et al. 1997). Moreover, research suggests that under control conditions (before any noxious stimulation), COX-2 is the predominating COX isoform in the spinal cord (Beiche et al. 1996).

As the conventional NSAIDs (e.g., ibuprofen, ketorolac, diclofenac) are mixed inhibitors of COX-1 and COX-2, the respective contribution of PGs produced by the COX isozymes to the hyperalgesic states induced by tissue injury have been uncertain. Studies using selective COX-inhibitors have shown that the i.t. or systemic delivery of COX-2-specific agents at the time of injury is as efficacious as that of nonspecific (COX-1 and COX-2) inhibitors in blocking the thermal hyperalgesia that is produced by inflammation of the rat paw (Dirig et al. 1998a; H. Gühring et al., unpublished manuscript). In contrast, a COX-1-selective agent had no effect (D.M. Dirig, P.C. Isakson, and T.L. Yaksh, unpublished observations; see Fig. 2). This finding argues that under such conditions, a constitutive presence of spinal COX-2 is important for the development of thermal hyperalgesia. Given the apparent absence of constitutive COX-2 in the periphery, these observations suggest that the ability of systemic COX-2 inhibitors to block the hyperalgesia shortly after the induction of the irritant must also be reflected by an effect upon a constitutive COX-2 within the spinal cord or brain. Further confirmation of the role played by a constitutive COX-2 comes from the observation

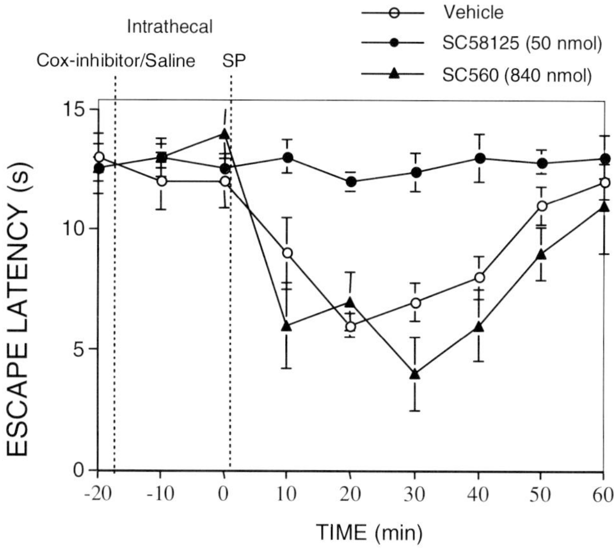

Fig. 2. Time effect curve for thermal escape latency observed following the intrathecal injection time 0 of substance P (20 nmol) in animals pretreated at –15 minutes with vehicle, SC58125 (50 nmol; COX-2 inhibitor), or SC560 (840 nmol; COX-1 inhibitor). Each point presents the mean and SEM of 6–8 rats. (D.M. Dirig, P.C. Isakson, and T.L. Yaksh, unpublished observations.)

that the thermal hyperalgesia induced by i.t. injections of NMDA and SP is reversed by nonspecific COX inhibitors (Malmberg and Yaksh 1992b) and by COX-2, but not COX-1 inhibitors (Dirig et al. 1998b).

The absence of any apparent difference in the activity of nonspecific COX-1 inhibitors and COX-2-selective agents, along with the lack of effect of a COX-1-preferring inhibitor, would suggest that in some models spinal COX-1, though constitutively expressed, does not contribute to the facilitatory effects. Importantly, and consistent with the effect of spinal COX-1 and COX-2 inhibition on several models of hyperalgesia, the spinal release of PGE_2 evoked by i.t. SP was blocked by COX-2 but not COX-1 inhibitors (Fig. 3).

Other data, however, lead us to question the importance of constitutive spinal COX-2 in at least some aspects of nociceptive processing. In the formalin assay, selective COX-2 inhibitors failed to reduce flinching behavior at doses that were COX-2 selective after both i.t. (Dirig et al. 1997) and systemic administration (Euchenhofer et al. 1998). In the latter study, the nonselective COX inhibitor diclofenac showed a dose-dependent antihyperalgesic effect as expected. As diclofenac works just 20 minutes after formalin paw injection, and as expression of the induced COX-2 protein needs at least one to several hours (Beiche et al. 1996), COX-1 may play an early

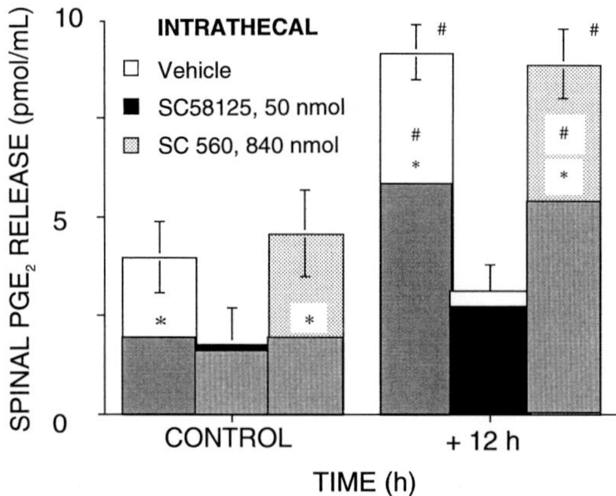

Fig. 3. Histograms present the release of PGE_2 into the dialysate before (lower shaded section) and after the intrathecal (i.t.) injection of SP (20 nmol) in rats with chronic loop dialysis catheters measured before and 12 hours after the injection of kaolin and carrageenan into the left knee joint. Rats in each survival category (each histogram bar) received i.t. injections of vehicle (left bar), SC58125 (50 nmol; COX-2 inhibitor: middle bar), or SC560 (840 nmol; COX-1 inhibitor: right bar). Each histogram point presents the mean and SEM of 6–8 rats. Asterisks (*) indicate that SP-evoked release is greater than preinjection baseline. # $P < 0.05$ as compared to comparable treatment under control conditions. Note that COX-2, but not COX-1, inhibition reduced the SP-evoked release at both the control and the 12 hours post-inflammation time point. (T.L. Yaksh, D.M. Dirig, C. Conway, and L. Marsala, unpublished observations.)

role in nociception. Moreover, in some animal models, COX-1 mediates at least some inflammation (Wallace et al. 1998). Another line of evidence suggesting that spinal COX-1 contributes to nociception is presented by Watkins et al. (1997), who showed that formalin-induced hyperalgesia can be inhibited by i.t. administration of substances that disrupt glial function or the action of glial products. Glial cells exclusively express the COX-1 isoform (C. Maihöfner et al., unpublished manuscript). Thus, PGs derived from glial COX-1 may be involved in synaptic processing. Although much is known about localization and regulation of COX isozymes in the spinal cord, more information is needed to clearly distinguish between the roles of the different COX isoforms in spinal nociceptive processing.

REGULATION AND CELLULAR LOCALIZATION OF SPINAL COX ISOZYMES

Regulation of COX isozymes in the spinal cord has been a subject of interest over the last few years (Kaufmann et al. 1997). COX-1 is expressed constitutively in the spinal cord in both in the ventral and dorsal horns (Beiche et al. 1996, 1998b). In the mouse, immunostaining techniques revealed COX-1 immunoreactivity (ir) predominantly in glial cells. Following peripheral noxious stimulation (zymosan injection into the paw), COX-1 was not regulated at the mRNA or protein level (C. Maihöfner et al., unpublished manuscript). In contrast, a recent study reported that COX-1 mRNA was rapidly induced in rat cerebral cortex in a model of ischemia (Holtz et al. 1996). Unexpectedly, COX-2 mRNA and protein are also constitutively expressed in the spinal cord of rats and mice, as shown by reverse transcription polymerase chain reaction (RT-PCR), immunohistochemistry, and Northern and Western blot techniques. Within the spinal cord, there is no doubt that COX-2 is constitutively expressed in the ventral horn. However, the question of dorsal horn presence under normal conditions is controversial. Nevertheless, there is little doubt that COX-2 displays a significant augmentation after peripheral inflammation. Zymosan injection into the paw leads to a dramatic increase of COX-2-ir in neurons of laminae I–IV and X of the dorsal horn. Most interestingly, COX-2 is colocalized with neuronal nitric oxide synthase (nNOS) in individual dorsal neurons that are most numerous in laminae II–III; this arrangement allows for a possible crosstalk between COX-2/PGs and nNOS/NO systems (C. Maihöfner et al., unpublished manuscript). Most likely, spinal COX-2 upregulation is mediated via activation of NFκB, as has been shown in other cellular systems. Electronmicroscopy now provides evidence that COX-2 protein is mainly expressed within the nucleus of spinal neurons, where it is bound to the nuclear membrane and rough endoplasmic reticulum (C. Maihöfner et al., unpublished manuscript). In this study, nNOS was detected in the cytoplasm of neurons. Double staining of COX-2 and GFAP, an immunohistochemical marker for astrocytes, revealed that COX-2 is also present in some astrocytes.

Prostaglandins act via EP receptors. A recent study showed that the EP3 receptor is expressed in the spinal cord (Beiche et al. 1998a). It is not yet clear whether the EP3 receptor is expressed presynaptically or postsynaptically or at both sites. Experiments in which nociceptive behavior challenged by i.t. administration of PGE_2 was blocked by pretreatment with an NMDA antagonist would suggest that the EP3 receptor is localized presynaptically. Stimulation of EP3 receptors would then lead to glutamate release, which can be antagonized by NMDA-receptor antagonists (Ferreira and Lorenzetti 1996).

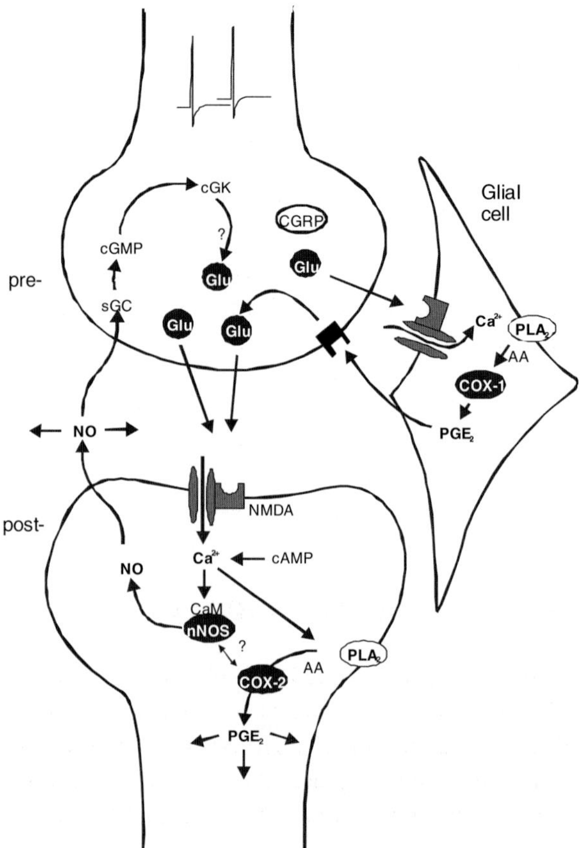

Fig. 4. Schematic illustration of the dorsal horn presenting potential structures that may produce prostaglandins and mechanisms whereby cyclooxygenase (COX) products may alter spinal nociceptive processing. C-fiber activation releases various excitatory neurotransmitters, including substance P (SP) and glutamate (Glu). This process results in increased intracellular calcium (Ca^{2+}), which in turn activates several intracellular enzymes, including phospholipase A_2 (PLA_2). This results in an increase in free arachidonic acid (AA), which then enters the COX cascade to stimulate the formation of various prostaglandins (PGs) that gain access to the extracellular space. Several of these prostanoids increase intracellular calcium in sensory afferents and thus could facilitate afferent transmitter release. Although the spinal prostanoids may act only on the sensory C fiber, it is suspected that many terminals in the dorsal horn are similarly affected. Histochemistry has shown that COX-2 is expressed in the neurons while COX-1 is present in glial cells. This system is not static. Thus, an enhanced expression of mRNA and protein for COX-2 is initiated by persistent afferent input generated by peripheral tissue injury and inflammation. It is important to note that several structures within the dorsal horn may account for the expression of COX-2, including non-neuronal elements that may be activated secondary to activity in adjacent synaptically coupled systems (e.g., via glutamate) (C. Maihöfner et al., unpublished manuscript.).

ORGANIZATION OF SPINAL COX SYSTEMS

Given the evidence outlined above, it appears certain that prostaglandins play an important role as a volume-transmitting system that through specific receptors can regulate the excitability of dorsal horn systems that process sensory information. In brief, current thinking suggests that activation of second-order neurons by the release of glutamate or SP through the NMDA or NK1 receptors, respectively, increases intracellular calcium, which in turn activates phospholipase A_2 and leads to increased cytosolic levels of arachidonic acid. This provides the substrate for the COX isoenzymes and results in production of prostaglandins. The current data assessing the enhanced expression of COX-2 in the spinal dorsal horn in the face of repetitive afferent activity, in concert with the behavioral data, emphasize that this neurocrine system can be rapidly upregulated by input generated by tissue injury and inflammation. Fig. 4 presents a schematic summary of several mechanisms outlined in this brief review.

ACTIONS OF COX INHIBITORS IN HUMANS

Clinical trials have demonstrated that NSAIDs specific for COX-2 relieve pain and inflammation in patients with osteoarthritis and rheumatoid arthritis as effectively as do nonselective NSAIDs (Lefkowith 1999). However, we still lack data showing activity of COX-2-specific agents in the treatment of acute crystal-induced arthritis, i.e., gout (Mandell 1999).

As outlined above, various preclinical approaches suggest that COX inhibitors, and COX-2 inhibitors specifically, have a central action even when administered systemically. Two lines of inquiry also support a CNS action of COX inhibitors in humans: (1) Certain nociceptive reflexes evoked by direct electrical activation of peripheral sensory nerves are diminished by systemically delivered ketoprofen, diflunisal, indomethacin, acetylsalicylic acid, zomepirac, or acetaminophen (Schady and Torebjörk 1984; Willer et al. 1989; Piletta et al. 1991; Fabbri et al. 1992; Guieu et al. 1992). These results reflect the direct activation of small afferent input and provide strong support for a central component of the antinociceptive actions of these agents. (2) Intrathecal delivery of lysine acetylsalicylate produced a significant degree of pain relief in cancer patients (Devoghel 1983; Pellerin et al. 1987). So far, it is clear that nonselective NSAIDs, administered systemically, can penetrate into the spinal cord in patients (Bannwarth et al. 1995), a pathway not yet demonstrated for selective COX-2 inhibitors.

Current thinking emphasizes the importance of spinal cyclooxygenase in upregulating the processing of nociceptive input after peripheral tissue injury. The ability of COX-2 inhibitors to acutely diminish hyperalgesia in noninjurious states of hyperalgesia (as after i.t. substance P) suggests that COX-2 plays a constitutive role in at least some forms of nociceptive processing. Given the immediacy of the effects of COX-2 inhibitors in humans, we suggest that the rapidity of onset of activity reflects a role for constitutively expressed COX-2. Accordingly, it appears probable that an important action of these new inhibitors is at sites where there is some constitutive expression. This observation in turn emphasizes the importance of the CNS as a site of NSAID action in altering hyperalgesia following tissue injury.

REFERENCES

Bannwarth B, Lapicque F, Rehourcq F, et al. Stereoselective disposition of ibuprofen enantiomers in human cerebrospinal fluid. *Br J Clin Pharmacol* 1995; 40:266–269.

Beiche F, Scheuerer S, Brune K, Geisslinger G, Goppelt-Struebe M. Up-regulation of cyclooxygenase-2 mRNA in the rat spinal cord following peripheral inflammation. *FEBS Lett* 1996; 390:165–169.

Beiche F, Klein T, Nusing R, Neuhuber W, Goppelt-Struebe M. Localization of cyclooxygenase-2 and prostaglandin E2 receptor EP3 in the rat lumbar spinal cord. *J Neuroimmunol* 1998a; 89:26–34.

Beiche F, Brune K, Geisslinger G, Goppelt-Struebe M. Expression of cyclooxygenase isoforms in the rat spinal cord and their regulation during adjuvant-induced arthritis. *Inflamm Res* 1998b; 47:482–487.

Bjorkman R, Hedner J, Hedner T, Henning M. Central, naloxone-reversible antinociception by diclofenac in the rat. *Naunyn Schmiedebergs Arch Pharmacol* 1990; 342:171–176.

Bjorkman R, Hallman KM, Hedner J, Hedner T, Henning M. Acetaminophen blocks spinal hyperalgesia induced by NMDA and substance P. *Pain* 1994; 57:259–264.

D'Acquisto F, Iuvone T, Rombola L, et al. Involvement of NF-kappaB in the regulation of cyclooxygenase-2 protein expression in LPS-stimulated J774 macrophages. *FEBS Lett* 1997; 418:175–178.

Devoghel JC. Small intrathecal doses of lysine-acetylsalicylate relieve intractable pain in man. *J Int Med Res* 1983; 11:90–91.

Dickenson AH, Stanfa LC, Chapman V, Yaksh TL. Response properties of dorsal horn neurons: Pharmacology of the dorsal horn. In: Yaksh TL, Lynch III C, Zapol WM, et al. (Eds). *Anesthesia: Biologic Foundations*. Philadelphia: Lippincott-Raven, 1997, pp 611–624.

Dirig DM, Konin GP, Isakson PC, Yaksh TK. Effect of spinal cyclooxygenase inhibitors in rat using the formalin test and in vitro prostaglandin E2 release. *Eur J Pharmacol* 1997; 331:155–160.

Dirig DM, Isakson PC, Yaksh TL. Effect of COX-1 and COX-2 inhibition on induction and maintenance of carrageenan-evoked thermal hyperalgesia in rats. *J Pharmacol Exper Ther* 1998a; 285:1031–1037.

Dirig DM, Wagner R, Isakson PC, Myers RR, Yaksh TL. Spinal cyclooxygenase-2 (COX-2) inhibition blocks intrathecal substance P-evoked thermal hyperalgesia in rats. *Soc Neurosci Abstr* 1998b; 24.

DuBois RN, Abramson SB, Crofford L, et al. Cyclooxygenase in biology and disease. *FASEB J* 1998; 12:1063–1073.

Euchenhofer C, Maihöfner C, Brune K, Tegeder I, Geisslinger G. Differential effect of selective cyclooxygenase-2 (COX-2) inhibitor NS 398 and diclofenac on formalin-induced nociception in the rat. *Neurosci Lett* 1998; 248:25–28.

Fabbri A, Cruccu G, Sperti P, et al. Piroxicam-induced analgesia: evidence for a central component which is not opioid mediated. *Experientia* 1992; 48:1139–1142.

Ferreira SH. Prostaglandins, aspirin-like drugs and analgesia. *Nature New Biol* 1972; 240:200–203.

Ferreira SH, Lorenzetti BB. Intrathecal administration of prostaglandin E2 causes sensitization of the primary afferent neuron via the spinal release of glutamate. *Inflamm Res* 1996; 45:499–502.

Ferreira SH, Lorenzetti BB, Correa FM. Central and peripheral antialgesic action of aspirin-like drugs. *Eur J Pharmacol* 1978; 53:39–48.

Foley KM. The treatment of cancer pain. *N Engl J Med* 1985; 313:84–95.

Frantz B, O'Neill EA. The effect of sodium salicylate and aspirin on NF-kappa B. *Science* 1995; 270:2017–2019.

Gillies GW, Kenny GN, Bullingham RE, McArdle CS. The morphine sparing effect of ketorolac tromethamine. A study of a new, parenteral non-steroidal anti-inflammatory agent after abdominal surgery. *Anaesthesia* 1987; 42:727–731.

Guieu R, Blin O, Pouget J, Serratrice G. Analgesic effect of indomethacin shown using the nociceptive flexion reflex in humans. *Ann Rheum Dis* 1992; 51:391–393.

Kaufmann WE, Andreasson KI, Isakson PC, Worley PF. Cyclooxygenases and the central nervous system. *Prostaglandins* 1997; 54:601–624.

Lefkowith JB. Cyclooxygenase-2 specificity and 1st clinical implications. *Am J Med* 1999; 106:43S–50S.

Lewis AJ, Furst DW. *Steroid Anti-Inflammatory Drugs, Mechanism and Clinical Use*. New York: Marcel Dekker, 1987.

Lim RK. Pain. *Annu Rev Physiol* 1970; 32:269–288.

Malmberg AB, Yaksh TL. Antinociceptive actions of spinal nonsteroidal anti-inflammatory agents on the formalin test in the rat. *J Pharmacol Exp Ther* 1992a; 263:136–146.

Malmberg AB, Yaksh TL. Hyperalgesia mediated by spinal glutamate or substance P receptor blocked by spinal cyclooxygenase inhibition. *Science* 1992b; 257:1276–1279.

Malmberg AB, Yaksh TL. Capsaicin-evoked prostaglandin E_2 release in spinal cord slices: relative effect of cyclooxygenase inhibitors. *Eur J Pharmacol* 1994; 271:293–299.

Malmberg AB, Yaksh TL. Cyclooxygenase inhibition and the spinal release of prostaglandin E2 and amino acids evoked by paw formalin injection: a microdialysis study in unanesthetized rats. *J Neurosci* 1995a; 15:2768–2776.

Malmberg AB, Yaksh TL. The effect of morphine on formalin-evoked behavior and spinal release of excitatory amino acids and prostaglandin E_2 using microdialysis in conscious rats. *Br J Pharmacol* 1995b; 114:1069–1075.

Mandell BF. COX-2 selective NSAIDs: biology, promises, and concerns. *Cleveland Clin J Med* 1999; 66:285–292.

McCormack K, Brune K. Dissociation between the antinociceptive and anti-inflammatory effects of the nonsteroidal anti-inflammatory drugs. A survey of their analgesic efficacy. *Drugs* 1991; 41:533–547.

McQuay H, Moore A (Eds). *An Evidence-Based Resource for Pain Relief*. Oxford: Oxford University Press, 1999.

Mendell LM, Wall PD. Response of single dorsal cord cells to peripheral cutaneous unmyelinated fibres. *Nature* 1965; 206:97–99.

Minami T, Nishihara I, Uda R, et al. Involvement of glutamate receptors in allodynia induced by prostaglandins E2 and F2 alpha injected into conscious mice. *Pain* 1994a; 57:225–231.

Minami T, Uda R, Horiguchi S, et al. Allodynia evoked by intrathecal administration of prostaglandin E2 to conscious mice. *Pain* 1994b; 57:217–223.

Moncada S, Ferreira SH, Vane JR. Inhibition of prostaglandin biosynthesis as the mechanism of analgesia of aspirin-like drugs in the dog knee joint. *Eur J Pharmacol* 1975; 31:250–260.

Muth-Selbach U, Tegeder I, Brune K, Geisslinger G. Acetaminophen inhibits spinal prostaglandin E2 release after peripheral noxious stimulation. *Anesthesiology* 1999; 91:231–239.

Neupert W, Brugger R, Euchenhofer C, Brune K, Geisslinger G. Effects of ibuprofen enantiomers and its coenzyme A thioesters on human prostaglandin endoperoxide synthases. *Br J Pharm* 1997; 122:487-492.

Nicol GD, Klingberg D, Vasko MR. Prostaglandin E2 increases calcium conductance and stimulates release of substance P in avian sensory neurons. *J Neurosci* 1992; 12:1917–1927.

Owens CM, Zhang D, Willis WD. Changes in the response states of primate spinothalamic tract cells caused by mechanical damage of the skin or activation of descending controls. *J Neurophysiol* 1992; 67:1509–1527.

Pellerin M, Hardy F, Abergel A, et al. Chronic refractory pain in cancer patients. Value of the spinal injection of lysine acetylsalicylate. 60 cases. *Presse Med* 1987; 16:1465–1468.

Piletta P, Porchet HC, Dayer P. Central analgesic effect of acetaminophen but not of aspirin. *Clin Pharmacol Ther* 1991; 49:350–354.

Ramwell PW, Shaw JE, Jessup R. Spontaneous and evoked release of prostaglandins from frog spinal cord. *Am J Physiol* 1966; 211:998–1004.

Reasbeck PG, Rice ML, Reasbeck JC. Double-blind controlled trial of indomethacin as an adjunct to narcotic analgesia after major abdominal surgery. *Lancet* 1982; 2:115–118.

Schady W, Torebjörk E. Central effects of zomepirac on pain evoked by intraneural stimulation in man. *J Clin Pharmacol* 1984; 24:429–435.

Schaible H-G, Neugebauer V, Geisslinger G, Beck U. The effects of S- and R-flurbiprofen on the inflammation-evoked intraspinal release of immunoreactive substance P—a study with antibody microprobes. *Brain Res* 1998; 798:287–293.

Scheuren N, Neupert W, Ionac M, et al. Peripheral noxious stimulation releases spinal PGE2 during the first phase in the formalin assay of the rat. *Life Sci* 1997; 60:PL 295–300.

Smith JB, Willis AL. Aspirin selectively inhibits prostaglandin production in human platelets. *Nature New Biol* 1971; 231:235–237.

Smith P. Certain aspects of the pharmacology of the salicylates. *Pharmacol Rev* 1949; 1:353–382.

Taiwo YO, Levine JD. Indomethacin blocks central nociceptive effects of PGF2 alpha. *Brain Res* 1986; 373:81–84.

Takeda F. WHO cancer pain relief programme. *Pain Res Clin Manage* 1991; 4:467–474.

Uda R, Horiguchi S, Ito S, Hyodo M, Hayaishi O. Nociceptive effects induced by intrathecal administration of prostaglandin D2, E2, or F2 alpha to conscious mice. *Brain Res* 1990; 510:26–32.

Uphouse LA, Welch SP, Ward CR, Ellis EF, Embrey JP. Antinociceptive activity of intrathecal ketorolac is blocked by the kappa-opioid receptor antagonist, nor-binaltorphimine. *Eur J Pharmacol* 1993; 242:53–58.

Vane JR. Inhibition of prostaglandin synthesis as a mechanism of action for aspirin-like drugs. *Nature New Biol* 1971; 231:232–235.

Vasko MR, Campbell WB, Waite KJ. Prostaglandin E2 enhances bradykinin-stimulated release of neuropeptides from rat sensory neurons in culture. *J Neurosci* 1994; 14:4987–4997.

Watkins LR, Martin D, Ulrich P, Tracey KJ, Maier SF. Evidence for involvement of spinal cord glia in subcutaneous formalin induced hyperalgesia in the rat. *Pain* 1997; 71:225–235.

Willer JC, De Broucker T, Bussel B, Roby-Brami A, Harrewyn JM. Central analgesic effect of ketoprofen in humans: electrophysiological evidence for a supraspinal mechanism in a double-blind and cross-over study. *Pain* 1989; 38:1–7.

Willingale HL, Gardiner NJ, McLymont N, Giblett S, Grubb BD. Prostanoids synthesized by cyclo-oxygenase isoforms in rat spinal cord and their contribution to the development of neuronal hyperexcitability. *Br J Pharmacol* 1997; 122:1593–1604.

Woolf CJ, King AE. Dynamic alterations in the cutaneous mechanoreceptive fields of dorsal horn neurons in the rat spinal cord. *J Neurosci* 1990; 10:2717–2726.

Yaksh TL. Central and peripheral mechanism for the antialgesic action of acetylsalicylic acid. In: Barnet JM, Hirsh J, Mustard JF (Eds). *Acetylsalicylic Acid: New Uses for an Old Drug*. New York: Raven Press, 1982, pp 137–152.

Yaksh TL. Preclinical models of nociception. In: Yaksh TL, Lynch III C, Zapol WM, et al. (Eds). *Anesthesia: Biologic Foundations*. Philadelphia: Lippincott-Raven, 1997, pp 685–718.

Yaksh TL. Central pharmacology of nociceptive processing. In: Wall, PD, Melzack R (Eds). *Textbook of Pain*. Edinburgh: Churchill Livingstone, 1999, pp 253–308.

Yaksh TL, Hua X-Y, Kalcheva I, Nozaki-Taguchi N, Marsala M. The spinal biology in humans and animals of pain states generated by persistent small afferent input. *Proc Natl Acad Sci USA* 1999; 96:7680–7686.

Yang LC, Marsala M, Yaksh TL. Characterization of time course of spinal amino acids, citrulline and PGE_2 release after carrageenan/kaolin-induced knee joint inflammation: a chronic microdialysis study. *Pain* 1996; 67:345–354.

Correspondence to: Gerd Geisslinger, PhD, MD, Institut für Klinische Pharmakologie, Klinikum der Johann Wolfgang Goethe Universität, Theodor-Stern-Kai 7, 60590 Frankfurt am Main, Germany. email: geisslinger@em.uni-frankfurt.de.

Proceedings of the 9th World Congress on Pain,
Progress in Pain Research and Management,
Vol. 16, edited by M. Devor, M.C. Rowbotham, and
Z. Wiesenfeld-Hallin, IASP Press, Seattle, © 2000.

75

High-Tech Versus Low-Tech Approaches to Postoperative Pain Management

Harald Breivik

Department of Anesthesiology, The National Hospital,
University of Oslo, Norway

The last decade has seen tremendous advances in the management of postoperative pain (Breivik 1995; Smith et al. 1999). In addition, there is a new understanding of the importance of prevention and relief of pain after surgery. Optimal postoperative pain management not only improves the comfort and well-being of patients, but more importantly, beneficially influences the outcome of surgery by reducing complications such as pulmonary infections (Ballantyne et al. 1998) and chronic postoperative pain (Kalso et al. 1992; Richardson et al. 1994; Katz et al. 1996; Katz 1997; Perttunen et al. 1999). Nursing care is facilitated, allowing early mobilization and feeding, and thus enhancing rehabilitation of body functions after surgery (Kehlet 1998).

Increased interest in postoperative pain management is due in part to new, high-technology methods for delivering pain relief. Evidence indicates that only epidural analgesia and blocks of major peripheral nerves can reduce complications and improve rehabilitation after major surgery by decreasing dynamic pain, i.e., pain when the patient is moving, coughing, and breathing deeply (Balantyne et al. 1998; Capdevila et al. 1999). However, since most patients must rely on low-tech, low-cost postoperative pain management, even in affluent countries, we must focus on how to improve these forms of pain control and make them available to the majority of patients.

Any of the more aggressive approaches to postoperative pain management can involve risks to the patients. It is mandatory that we minimize these risks. This can be accomplished by an educational program for all personnel involved in care of surgical patients and by exploiting the analgesic synergy between two or more drugs with different side-effect profiles to reduce the needed doses and adverse effects. These are basic principles of effective and safe postoperative pain management, whether we are using low-tech or high-tech approaches. Improving postoperative pain management also has a price tag: each hospital requires a dedicated pain nurse and anesthesiologist. However, the cost-benefit ratio can be good because surgical patients are more satisfied with their postoperative course and have fewer complications from surgery and reduced adverse effects from pain management, resulting in more rapid and successful rehabilitation and decreasing the overall costs to the health care system (Breivik 1995).

OPTIMIZING LOW-TECH, CONVENTIONAL PAIN RELIEF AFTER SURGERY

Low-tech, conventional pain treatment for postoperative pain has a bad reputation, with about one-third of patients having moderate to severe pain and fewer than one-third of patients being satisfied with pain relief after surgery. In conventional treatment, analgesics are administered on demand as subcutaneous injections of opioid drugs and oral or rectal non-opioid drugs (Bonica 1990). Outcome can be improved if clinicians pay attention to dosing and choice of drugs and exploit positive interactions among the available drugs.

THE BASICS: APPROPRIATE ADMINISTRATION OF ACETAMINOPHEN

Any approach to improved postoperative pain control should include the optimal use of acetaminophen (paracetamol). It can be given by mouth, rectally, and in many countries intravenously as well (as propacetamol). But all too often clinicians use doses of acetaminophen that are much too low, especially with rectal administration (Korpela and Olkkola 1999). We should use at least 1 g orally every 6 hours for adult patients, and if we are using acetaminophen as the only non-opioid analgesic, we should increase the dose to 1 g every 4 hours, i.e., 6 g per 24 hours, to obtain optimal analgesic effects (Acute Pain Management Guideline Panel 1992; Schug et al. 1998). As even 1.5 g of acetaminophen rectally is ineffective (Montgomery et al. 1996), the initial rectal dose to adult patients should be 2 g, followed by 1 g every 4–6 hours. Note that this dose is safe for the liver of otherwise healthy patients who require relief of acute pain for up to a week after surgery (Schug et al. 1998). For more prolonged pain relief, in patients with hepatic dysfunction, and in patients on enzyme P-450-inducing agents (anticonvulsants, ethanol), the dose probably should not exceed 4 g/day (Schug et al. 1998). If acetaminophen is combined with a traditional NSAID, 4 g/day will suffice for adult patients (see section below on synergy between non-opioid analgesics).

Children, even more frequently than adult patients, tend to be underdosed with acetaminophen after surgery. In a recently published study from Helsinki (Korpela et al. 1999), rectal acetaminophen was given in increasing doses up to 60 mg/kg to children having outpatient surgery. This double-blind, placebo-controlled study revealed that with no acetaminophen, 90% of patients required morphine for rescue analgesia during the first 24 hours after surgery. The need for rescue analgesia decreased as the dose of acetaminophen increased; only 20% of children given 60 mg/kg acetaminophen rectally as lipophilic suppositories (after induction of anesthesia) needed rescue analgesia. The authors demonstrated a good dose-response curve and a median effective dose (ED_{50}) of about 35 mg/kg, which means that even with 35 mg/kg of acetaminophen rectally, 50% of the patients required morphine for rescue analgesia (Fig. 1). More than one-third of patients not receiving acetaminophen had nausea after surgery, whereas none of the patients receiving 60 mg/kg of acetaminophen rectally had nausea.

If the ED_{50} is 35 mg/kg rectally for children and the maximal safe dose of acetaminophen to children is 120 mg/kg per 24 hours (Gaukroger 1991), we should give at least 40 mg/kg as the initial rectal dose (Birmingham et al. 1997), even in neonates (Hansen et al. 1999). For outpatient or day-case surgery, Korpela et al. (1999) recommend an initial, single dose of 60 mg/kg acetaminophen, with ibuprofen 10 mg/kg as a rescue analgesic thereafter. Even if the initial dose is followed by 20 mg/kg acetaminophen given every 6 hours, the amount will not exceed the maximal safe dose of 120 mg/kg on the day of surgery (when surgery is started early in the day) and 80 mg/kg

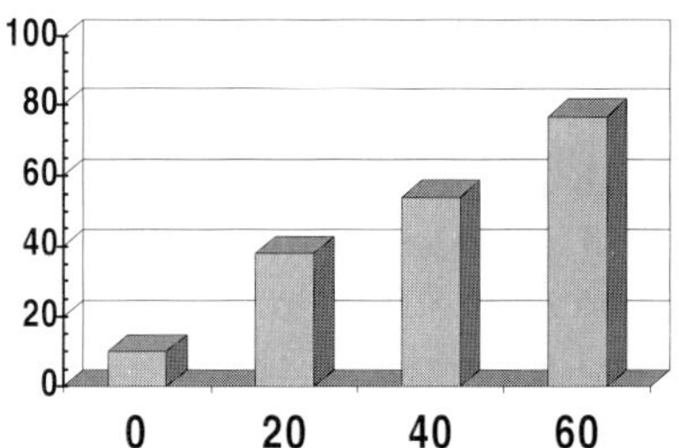

Fig. 1. Dose response (percentage of children not needing morphine rescue analgesia) with rectal acetaminophen for pain after day-case surgery in children. ED_{50} for need of rescue analgesic (morphine) is about 35 mg/kg. Redrawn from Korpela et al. (1999).

per 24 hours thereafter. For postoperative pain lasting up to 2–3 days, this dose is safe for otherwise healthy children (Gaukroger 1991). Acute hepatotoxicity appears to be less common and less likely to be fatal in children than in adults (Birmingham et al. 1997). For prolonged use (more than 3 days), a dose of 60 mg/kg of acetaminophen should not be exceeded in 24 hours (Korpela et al. 1999). Absorption is more rapid and complete when acetaminophen is given orally, which is another reason for reducing the dose when children can take the drug orally in the later postoperative phase.

As mentioned above, Korpela et al. (1999) used ibuprofen 10 mg/kg as a rescue analgesic if acetaminophen alone was not sufficient. Opioids, especially in day-case surgical patients, may cause nausea and vomiting. Ibuprofen, like diclofenac and ketoprofen, is likely to have an additive analgesic effect when given with acetaminophen. This is not well known, perhaps due to the widespread misconception that acetaminophen and the NSAIDs have similar mechanisms of analgesia with a common ceiling effect on the dose-response curve. Their mechanisms of analgesia differ, however, so it makes sense to use acetaminophen and NSAIDs together.

EXPLOITING THE SYNERGY BETWEEN NON-OPIOID ANALGESICS

Whenever we coadminister drugs that affect the same process via different mechanisms of action, we are likely to obtain additive or even supra-additive or synergistic effects (Berenbaum 1991). Acetaminophen and NSAIDs have different analgesic effects in that the NSAIDs inhibit the cyclooxygenases in the periphery and in the CNS, and acetaminophen inhibits the release of prostaglandin in the spinal cord and affects the serotonin mechanisms for spinal pain inhibition; both drugs seem to reduce nitric oxide production in the CNS (Malmberg and Yaksh 1992; Tjölsen et al. 1992; Björkman et al. 1994; Björkman 1995; Muth-Selbach et al. 1999). Only acetaminophen inhibits COX-3 (Willoughby et al. 2000).

In animal studies the supra-additive effect between acetaminophen and NSAIDs has been well documented. Peak effect, duration of analgesia, and anti-inflammatory effect were increased and prolonged when acetaminophen and the NSAID tolmetin were coadministered to arthritic animals (Wong and Gardocki 1983). Similarly, acetaminophen and diclofenac showed synergy in rats (Fletcher et al. 1997a). Acetaminophen and NSAIDs are increasingly coadministered to patients, and many clinicians are convinced from what they see in their daily practice that this combination improves the quality of analgesia. However, few clinical studies have addressed this important issue. Fletcher et al. (1997b) documented additive analgesic effects between propacetamol (an i.v. pro-drug for acetaminophen) and i.v. ketoprofen. A recent controlled, double-blind, pragmatically oriented study on postoperative pain relief after surgical removal of impacted third molars provides good evidence that it makes sense to coadminister acetaminophen and diclofenac (Breivik et al. 1999). When acetaminophen 1 g and diclofenac 100 mg were given simultaneously, pain relief occurred rapidly and was more pronounced and significantly longer lasting than for each individual drug given alone (Fig. 2). Of particular clinical significance are the findings that coadministration of acetaminophen and diclofenac caused superior and longer lasting pain relief with less severe side effects than did acetaminophen and codeine. Opioid side effects such as sedation, nausea, and dizziness thus can be avoided or significantly reduced when acetaminophen and an NSAID are coadministered (Korpela et al. 1999), as compared with adding an opioid to acetaminophen or an NSAID. Reduced side effects are especially valued by day-case patients who can go home early after surgery (Korpela et al. 1999).

Evidence is sufficient to recommend that an NSAID should be added to acetaminophen for postoperative pain relief. The dose of acetaminophen can be kept within a definitely safe range (1 g every 6 hours for adults; 20

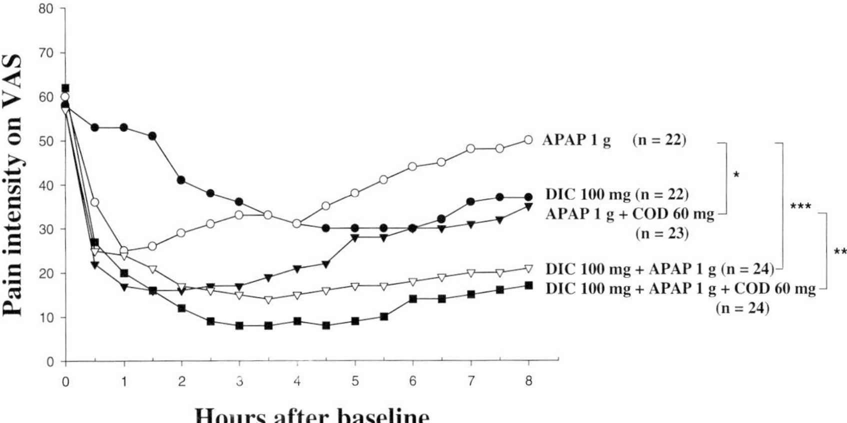

Fig. 2. Comparison of pain intensity recorded for 8 hours on a visual analogue scale (VAS) when various analgesic combinations are taken following surgery. In a randomized, double-blind study, 120 patients with moderate to strong pain after surgical removal of wisdom teeth received in single oral doses combinations of diclofenac (DIC; enteric-coated tablets), acetaminophen (APAP), and codeine (COD). Adding 60 mg of codeine increased side effects. These results support the clinical practice of combining diclofenac plus acetaminophen for acute pain. Of special clinical importance are superior and prolonged analgesia and minimal side effects after diclofenac enteric-coated tablets plus acetaminophen compared with acetaminophen plus codeine. Reproduced with permission from Breivik et al. (1999).

mg/kg every 6 hours for children after an initial loading dose of 40 mg/kg when rectal administration is necessary). Several alternatives to diclofenac are available in various countries for oral, rectal, or i.v. administration: indomethacin, ketoprofen, tenoxicam, and ketorolac. Ibuprofen is one of the cheapest and safest NSAIDs, but it cannot be given by injection. However, most patients can take their drugs orally or rectally. (See below for dosing of NSAIDs.)

Thus, the basis for any low-tech, low-cost approach to pain management after surgery is to give acetaminophen reinforced with an NSAID when there is no contraindication to the cyclooxygenase-inhibiting effect of the NSAIDs. NSAIDs should be avoided when patients have renal impairment, are hypovolemic, are taking loop diuretics, or have circulatory failure. In elderly patients, who quite often have significant renal impairment, one should be careful with dose or avoid the NSAIDs. The same is true when a patient has a known risk of increased bleeding. Known allergy or bronchospastic reaction to aspirin must be excluded before NSAIDs are administered.

OPTIMAL ADMINISTRATION REGIME FOR OPIOID ANALGESICS

Many patients will require an opioid in addition to acetaminophen and an NSAID. Although they can be given by mouth or rectally, opioids are more effective by injection. Harmer and Davis (1998) have published a study in which nurses were taught to observe pain regularly using a simple verbal categorical pain intensity scale and given standing orders to give morphine by intramuscular (i.m.) injection:

- if the patient has moderate or severe pain in spite of acetaminophen,
- and the patient is awake or only dozing intermittently,
- and respiratory rate is above 8 per minute,
- and systolic blood pressure is above 100 mm Hg,
- and if more than 60 minutes have elapsed since the last i.m. dose of morphine or pethidine,

  the nurse has standing orders to give an i.m. injection of:
- morphine 5 mg (or pethidine 75 mg) to patients weighing 40–65 kg,
- morphine 10 mg (or pethidine 100 mg) to patients weighing 66–100 kg.

If respiratory rate slows to less than 8 breaths per minute and the patient is difficult to awaken, the nurse has standing orders to give naloxone 0.1 mg i.v., repeated until the respiratory rate recovers to 12 breaths per minute and the patient can easily be awakened.

Harmer and Davis (1998) documented that this regimen including standardized prescription, education of all clinical staff, and assessment of pain with a simple verbal categorical scale, markedly improved pain relief: the percentage of patients with moderate to severe pain at rest decreased from 32% to 12%, and on movement from 37% to 13%. About 75% of the patients in their study were treated with these simple techniques for the management of postoperative pain.

In many hospitals in Scandinavia, ward nurses are trained to give morphine (or ketobemidone) i.v. according to an algorithm similar to that of Harmer and Davis (1998), except that only 10 minutes are required between the last intravenous opioid injection and the next dose, and the doses are smaller: 1 mg morphine (or 1 mg ketobemidone) intravenously to patients weighing 40–65 kg, 2 mg to those 66–100 kg. A similar approach was demonstrated to be both effective and safe by Borchgrevink et al. (1999).

HIGH-TECH APPROACHES TO POSTOPERATIVE PAIN MANAGEMENT

PATIENT-CONTROLLED ANALGESIA (PCA) WITH INTRAVENOUS OPIOIDS

Patients can take control of their own pain relief when given the opportunity to administer analgesic drugs to themselves when they experience pain that they cannot tolerate. For moderate postoperative pain, patients can simply control their own intake of tablets, but for more severe pain a bolus injection of i.v. opioids is more suitable. This technique gives patients fast relief when they push the analgesic-demand button, and makes them feel in control of their pain (Breivik et al. 1995). Fast-onset patient-controlled relief of severe pain can also be obtained with an epidural bolus infusion of a local anesthetic with a lipophilic opioid.

Several disposable, relatively low-tech, nonelectronic mechanical devices appear to function with reasonable safety. Several microprocessor-controlled programmable and electronically driven pumps are also available. These pumps are designed to be tamper-resistant (for patients and unauthorized persons) and fool-proof (for nurses and doctors), and the complexity and price of these pumps vary. Several different pumps were evaluated at our university hospitals (Rikshospitalet in Oslo, Norway and Inselspital in Berne, Switzerland), and we have used the same pump for i.v. PCA and for continuous infusion and patient-controlled bolus infusion of epidural analgesic mixtures over the last decade with a minimum of equipment-generated adverse events (Breivik et al. 1995). From early 1992 until the end of 1999, close to 6000 patients were followed prospectively for about 25,000 days with i.v. opioid PCA and 10,000 patients for about 50,000 days with epidural analgesia after surgery (H. Breivik, H. Högström, M. Curatolo, and G. Kvarstein, personal communications).

After this extensive experience with PCA, we agree with the conclusions of a meta-analysis of published studies comparing PCA with conventional analgesia (Ballantyne et al. 1993): most patients are satisfied with having control of administering their own analgesics. Analgesic efficacy is improved, but PCA and conventional analgesic administration do not differ in occurrence or severity of postoperative complications and side effects. This is a pity, because PCA is a simple and relatively inexpensive technique that can be used with low-tech equipment. Several strategies could improve the effectiveness and reduce the adverse effects of PCA.

HOW CAN THE EFFECTIVENESS OF PCA BE IMPROVED?

The principle described above, of coadministering two or more drugs with different mechanisms of analgesia so as to exploit synergistic analgesic effects of drugs with different side-effect profiles, can improve i.v. patient-controlled analgesia. Two effective options will be discussed: acetaminophen and an NSAID and mini-doses of the NMDA antagonist ketamine.

Morphine-sparing effect of acetaminophen and NSAIDs. Oral acetaminophen at 6 g per 24 hours reduces morphine consumption and improves analgesia, providing an overall increase in patient satisfaction (Schug et al. 1998). Intravenous propacetamol at 1 g, 4 times/24 hours similarly reduced PCA morphine consumption by almost 40% after orthopedic surgery (Delbos and Boccard 1995). Various NSAIDs also have morphine-sparing effects and improve analgesia when coadministered with PCA morphine (Etches et al. 1995; Fredman et al. 1995; Liaw et al. 1995; Kostamovaara et al. 1996; Plummer et al. 1996; Perttunen et al. 1999).

For NSAIDs, this may be a pharmacokinetic as much as a pharmacodynamic interaction: NSAIDs transiently decrease renal function (Irwin et al. 1995), and coadministration of morphine and NSAIDs impedes renal excretion of active morphine metabolites, increasing plasma concentrations and intensifying opioid effects and side effects if doses of morphine are not markedly reduced (Hobbs et al. 1997; Tighe et al. 1999).

Many surgical patients have relative contraindications for NSAIDs, such as reduced renal function, hypovolemia, age above 65–70 years, and risks of increased bleeding from high-dose, low-molecular-weight heparin (LMWH) thromboembolic prophylaxis. An example of an unfortunate combination of patient and drug interactions would be an elderly woman of light body weight with 75% reduced renal function, receiving routine high-dose LMWH in connection with orthopedic surgery. Not only will she have almost the full heparinizing effect of the "standard" dose of LMWH, but her reduced kidney function will cause accumulation of the LMWH (which is excreted by the kidneys only). If she is given a full, routine dose of ketorolac, her kidneys will reduce further excretion of LMWH and the risk of bleeding may become critical.

Therefore, full-dose NSAIDs cannot be recommended as the routine non-opioid for coadministration with opioid PCA. Most patients without these obvious relative contraindications, however, tolerate and benefit from short-term NSAIDs and have a minimal risk of adverse effects when NSAIDs are used for 2–3 days.

The additive analgesic effects of acetaminophen and diclofenac described above are now documented (Breivik et al. 1999). This combination is already appreciated and widely used by clinicians, and reduces morphine consumption more than when either agent is used alone (Montgomery et al. 1996). Fletcher et al. (1997) documented a clear additive effect of acetaminophen 1 g (given as i.v. propacetamol) and ketoprofen 50 mg i.v. every 6 hours on pain relief at rest and during movement, and showed that the combination reduced morphine consumption.

Optimum non-opioid analgesic regimens for i.v., oral, or rectal coadministration with i.v. opioid PCA are as follows:

- acetaminophen 1 g every 4 hours
  or, when no contraindications to NSAIDs exist:
- acetaminophen 1 g every 6 hours, reinforced and prolonged (during the first 2–3 days after surgery) by one of the NSAIDs with infrequent adverse effects, such as:
- diclofenac (50 mg every 8 hours)
- ketoprofen (100 mg every 8 hours)
- ketorolac (10–30 mg every 8 hours)
- ibuprofen (400 mg every 8 hours) when oral/rectal administration suffices.

Coadministration of an NMDA antagonist with morphine i.v. PCA. Another way to exploit the principle of coadministering synergistic analgesic drugs with different side-effect profiles is to administer 1 mg morphine with a very small dose of a completely different drug such as ketamine (1 mg) (an NMDA-receptor antagonist) via i.v. PCA (Javery et al. 1995). This regimen decreased morphine consumption by 50%, improved pain relief, and reduced side effects. These findings were confirmed by Stubhaug et al. (1997): a small dose of ketamine reduced the consumption of morphine and lessened side effects, and patients gave significantly higher ratings to the global effects of morphine with ketamine compared with morphine with placebo.

However, Stubhaug et al. (1997) demonstrated one potentially very important additional beneficial effect of adding a very small ketamine i.v. infusion to morphine PCA. Living kidney donors have a large painful wound in the dorsolateral abdominal wall, around which develops a large area of secondary hyperalgesia. A small dose of ketamine, 2 $\mu g \cdot kg^{-1} \cdot min^{-1}$ on the day of surgery, reduced to an even smaller dose, 1 $\mu g \cdot kg^{-1} \cdot min^{-1}$, for another 2 days markedly reduced the area of secondary hyperalgesia (Fig. 3). This effect was still present on the seventh day after surgery, i.e., 4 days after the ketamine infusion was stopped.

This finding is important because the neuronal mechanisms behind secondary hyperalgesia are likely to be involved in the phenomenon of persistent postoperative pain (Woolf and Thompson 1991). Two-thirds (64%) of patients having thoracic surgery suffer from persistent discomfort and pain, severe enough to interfere with normal daily life in more than 50% of patients (Kalso et al. 1999). Some develop severe postoperative neuropathic pain, which is difficult to treat. It is important to find ways to prevent this normal hyper-phenomenon after surgery from developing into a chronic pain problem.

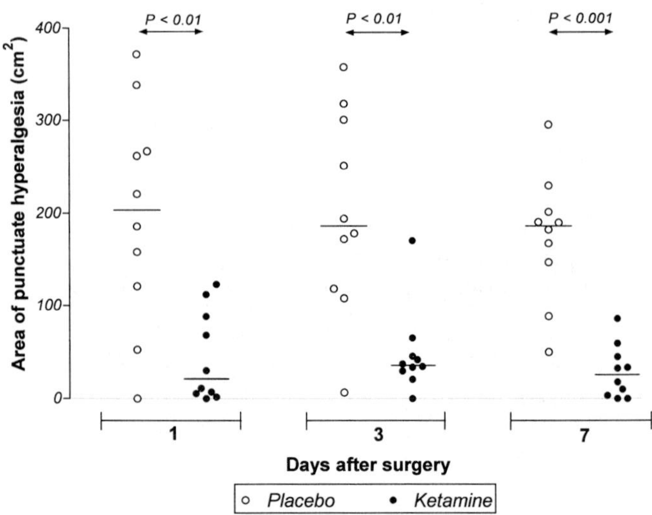

Fig. 3. Area of punctate mechanical hyperalgesia surrounding the surgical incision 1, 3, and 7 days after living kidney nephrectomy. Values for each patient are displayed as open circles (placebo) or filled circles (ketamine). A horizontal line represents the median for each group. Statistical differences between the groups (Mann-Whitney U-test) are displayed above. Reproduced with permission from Stubhaug et al. (1997).

Patients who received this mini-dose of ketamine had some hyperalgesia around the wound on the first day after surgery, but on the seventh day after surgery it had disappeared (Fig. 4). Thus, Stubhaug et al. (1997) have shown that by giving a very low dose of ketamine in addition to morphine, secondary hyperalgesia around the wound almost disappears. This must mean that the NMDA-glutamate receptor antagonistic effect of ketamine inhibits the central sensitization in the spinal cord. We hope that ketamine used in this way will prevent development of chronic pain after surgery, although we do not yet have definitive evidence that this is true (see Schmid et al. 1999).

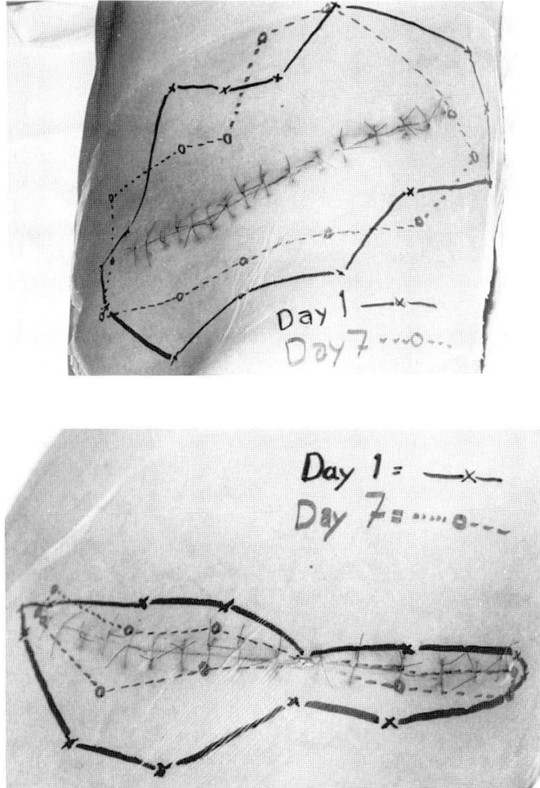

Fig. 4. Area of punctate hyperalgesia around kidney donor nephrectomy wound on day 1 and day 7 after surgery in a typical patient from the placebo group (upper panel) and from a typical patient given an infusion of ketamine 2 $\mu g \cdot kg^{-1} \cdot min^{-1}$ on the day of surgery and ketamine 1 $\mu g \cdot kg^{-1} \cdot min^{-1}$ for 48 hours thereafter (lower panel) (Stubhaug et al. 1997). Ketamine patients consumed less morphine early after surgery and had fewer side effects and better pain relief, as documented with a superior global evaluation score.

IMPROVING OUTCOME AFTER SURGERY BY RELIEVING DYNAMIC PAIN

The intense pain provoked by deep breathing, coughing, or moving a body part affected by the surgery can be effectively relieved only with neuraxial or peripheral nerve blocks. Such procedures enable patients to breathe deeply and cough, thereby preventing the development of atelectasis, pneumonia, and sepsis. Reducing dynamic pain also enables patients to perform active movements of limbs after orthopedic surgery, hastening rehabilitation of normal function.

Continuous peripheral nerve blocks. Continuous cervical/brachial plexus blockade with catheter techniques and infusions of local anesthetics provides excellent analgesia and improves circulation and mobility of the upper extremity after shoulder, arm, or hand surgery (Brown and Bridenbaugh 1998; see Niv et al., this volume). In patients recovering from major knee surgery, Capdevila et al. (1999) showed that patients who received either femoral nerve block or epidural block were able to move their knees more during the early days after surgery. This resulted in a more rapid rehabilitation compared with morphine i.v. PCA. Intercostal nerve blockade tends to improve pulmonary function and reduce pulmonary complications (Ballantyne et al. 1998).

Epidural analgesia. According to a recent meta-analysis, epidural local anesthetics, with or without opioids, decrease the risk of developing postoperative pulmonary complications such as atelectasis and pneumonia by 50–70% compared with systemic opioids (Ballantyne et al. 1998). Another important finding in that meta-analysis was that epidural opioids alone do not reduce significantly the risk of postoperative pulmonary complications. Thus, it is important to realize that a local anesthetic is needed in an epidural infusion for the patient to receive these benefits on pulmonary functions after major surgery. This is also true for gastrointestinal motility after abdominal surgery: an epidural local anesthetic and an epidural local anesthetic combined with an opioid shorten the time of intestinal paralysis after surgery compared with morphine i.v. PCA or morphine alone epidurally (Wattwill et al. 1989; Lui et al. 1995a,b; Steinbrook 1998).

Thoracic or lumbar epidural catheter? Anesthesiologists have long debated whether to use thoracic epidural or lumbar epidural for postoperative pain relief. It is now well established that thoracic epidural is more beneficial for patients who are at high risk of cardiac or pulmonary complications after thoracic or major abdominal surgery (Liu et al. 1995a; Van Aken et al. 1999).

Thoracic epidural analgesia with a local anesthetic dilates stenotic coronary arteries and increases myocardial oxygen supply; decreases myocardial oxygen consumption, decreases myocardial ischemic events and postoperative myocardial infarction, improves lung function and oxygenation, and improves gastrointestinal motility. *Lumbar epidural analgesia* with a local anesthetic, on the other hand, dilates the arteries of lower part of body, constricts the coronary arteries, decreases myocardial oxygen supply, causes leg weakness and urinary retention, and does not improve gastrointestinal motility (Steinbrook 1998). Thus, a lumbar epidural may even increase the cardiac risk and does not improve pulmonary functions or gastrointestinal motility. Lack of awareness of these important differences between thoracic/thoracolumbar and lumbar epidural analgesia is one important reason for the confusion and conflicting opinions on the effects of epidural analgesia on outcome after surgery (Breivik 1998a).

Risks to the patient from epidural analgesia. If too high a dose of a local anesthetic is administered epidurally, the patient may develop orthostatic hypotension, motor blockade, and urinary retention, even if the catheter is in a low thoracic or thoracolumbar area. If too high a dose of an opioid is administered epidurally, respiratory depression may occur, and the incidence and severity of the less dangerous, but bothersome, itching and nausea may increase. Epidural bleeding and epidural infection are rare, but potentially catastrophic complications: early warning symptoms (leg weakness and back pain) are easily missed if excessive doses of local anesthetics are used, especially if lumbar epidural catheters are employed and monitoring routines are inadequate for detecting changes in leg weakness (Breivik 1998b, 1999).

Optimizing the efficacy and safety of epidural analgesia. The efficacy and safety of epidural analgesia can be optimized by combining two or more drugs with different mechanisms of analgesia and different side-effect profiles. Over the last decade we have used low concentrations of a local anesthetic (bupivacaine 1 mg/mL), an opioid (fentanyl 2 μg/mL), and an adrenergic agonist (epinephrine 2 μg/mL). These three drugs elicit spinal cord analgesia by different mechanisms that act on the pain-impulse transmission process in the spinal cord: fentanyl and epinephrine (like clonidine) act on pre- and postsynaptic opioid receptors and α_2 receptors, respectively, to increase inhibition of pain impulse transmission from the primary afferent nociceptive neurons to the interneurons and transmission neurons in the dorsal horn of the spinal cord. Subanesthetic doses of bupivacaine inhibit excitatory synaptic mechanisms in the same area of the spinal cord.

Exploiting these three pain-inhibiting mechanisms concurrently allows dose reduction because of their additive or synergistic antinociceptive effects (Niemi and Breivik 1998; G. Niemi and H. Breivik, unpublished manuscript). These three drugs have different side effects, and so overall risks are lower for adverse effects such as respiratory depression, nausea, itching, gastrointestinal immobility, sedation, hypotension, urinary retention, motor blockade, and leg weakness (Breivik et al. 1995). Nurses on the surgical wards titrate the infusion rate of the epidural analgesic mixture, and when it is appropriate, patients are allowed to use the dose-control button to give themselves boluses when needed.

Epinephrine increases effectiveness of the epidural analgesic infusion. Epinephrine (adrenaline) has been used with opioids and local anesthetics for epidural analgesia for vaginal deliveries and pain after C-section (Cohen et al. 1992, 1993). Over the last decade, we have regularly used epinephrine in order to be able to reduce the dose of local anesthetics and opioids for postoperative epidural analgesia (Breivik 1993). In a randomized, double-blind, cross-over study we documented the powerful effects of epinephrine (Niemi and Breivik 1998). Pain intensity was practically zero at rest after major abdominal or thoracic surgery with an epidural mixture of bupivacaine, fentanyl, and epinephrine (Fig. 5). When epinephrine was removed from the mixture, pain increased, in spite of increasing infusion rate and morphine rescue i.v. When the standard mixture with epinephrine was reintroduced, pain relief again became optimal. Pain during coughing was only mild after major thoracic and upper abdominal surgery when the triple-component mixture was infused (Fig. 5). When epinephrine was removed from the mixture, pain became quite severe, but adding epinephrine again reduced cough-provoked pain to mild intensity.

Epinephrine increases the safety of bupivacaine and fentanyl epidural analgesia. Epinephrine, in addition to its importance for the analgesic effect of the epidural infusion, also has an important effect on safety because it reduces absorption of fentanyl into the systemic circulation. Serum concentration of fentanyl is significantly lower when epinephrine is added to the epidural infusion. With epinephrine 2 μg/mL, fentanyl is almost not measurable. When epinephrine is removed from the epidural infusion, serum fentanyl concentration increases and the patients experience adverse effects from systemic absorption: sedation, nausea, and pruritis (Niemi and Breivik 1998).

In summary, at least two positive interactions occur between epinephrine and the two other components. First, epinephrine reduces systemic absorption and systemic side effects of fentanyl and bupivacaine so that more of these to drugs can diffuse through the meninges and into the CSF and spinal cord, where they exert their analgesic action. Second, epinephrine, an α_2 agonist, has an analgesic effect of its own in the spinal cord (Collins et al. 1984).

PRESCRIPTION FOR SAFE EPIDURAL ANALGESIA AND PCA FOR POSTOPERATIVE PAIN RELIEF

Our prescription for a safe and effective epidural and patient controlled i.v. analgesia, which have been practiced for almost a decade at the Pain Services of Rikshospitalet, Oslo, Norway, and at the Inselspital, Berne, Switzerland (since my sabbatical there in 1992) are briefly summarized as follows (for details see Breivik 1993, 1999; Breivik et al. 1995).

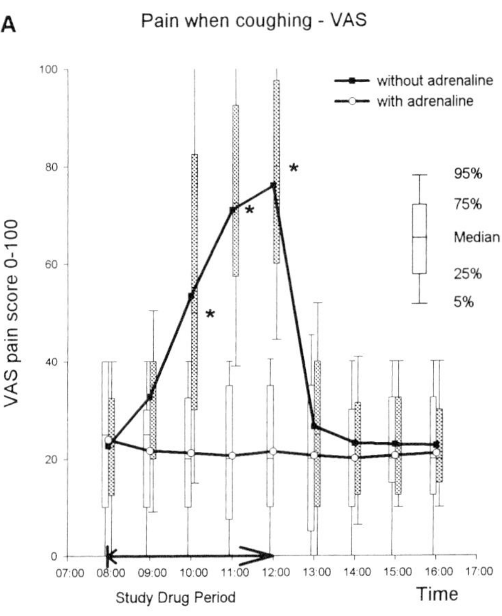

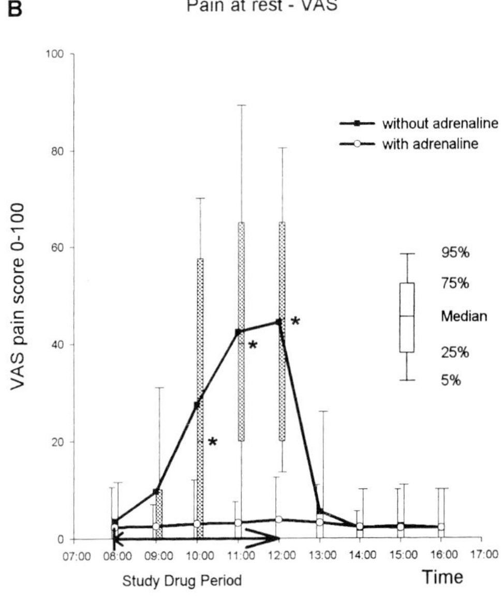

Fig. 5. VAS scores of pain when coughing and at rest after major thoracic or abdominal surgery during infusion of epidural analgesic mixture containing bupivacaine 1 mg/mL and fentanyl 2 μg/mL with or without epinephrine 2 μg/mL. This double-blind, crossover study documented the marked potentiation of epidural analgesia from bupivacaine and fentanyl when epinephrine was present. Reproduced with permission from Niemi and Breivik (1998).

Epidural analgesic

- Use a thoracic or thoraco-lumbar epidural catheter for major thoracic and abdominal surgery.
- Use a triple-component analgesic mixture with low doses of a local anesthetic, an opioid, and epinephrine for nurse-adjusted infusion of epidural analgesia and patient-controlled rescue bolus injections. With a reliable, closed infusion pump system, adverse effects such as major respiratory depression, hypotension (in normovolemic patients) are practically eliminated. There is only minimal motor block in a few patients with low thoracic or high-lumbar catheters.
- Nurses on the surgical wards must monitor sensory level (using cold stimuli, e.g., an ice-cube in a plastic glove) and motor function (Bromage score for leg weakness). They also should measure pain intensity at rest and on movement (using a simple 5-point verbal categorical rating scale), and record sedation, respiratory rate, systolic blood pressure, drug consumption, and occurrence of any side effects. Recordings should be made every 4 hours.
- Nurses must pay strict attention to hygienic standards in caring for epidural catheters and line connections.
- Staff involved in the care of these patients must look for early signs of infection or hematoma in the epidural space and be prepared for urgent MRI or CT scans to verify diagnosis and expedite appropriate interventions.

Intravenous PCA/opioid analgesia

- Use the same pump for i.v. PCA and for epidural analgesia (Breivik et al. 1995). Staff involved in the care of postoperative patients will become familiar with this pump so that human errors and technical problems are minimized.
- It is important to use acetaminophen and an NSAID (when not contraindicated) for basic analgesia to reduce the need for opioids.
- Our standard prescription is for 1 mg morphine (or 1 mg ketobemidone) on patient demand, lockout time 8 minutes, maximum dose 7 mg/hour.
- Nurses should record observations of pain intensity at rest (5-point verbal categorical rating scale) and during provoking movement, respiratory rate, systolic blood pressure, any adverse effects, and total drug consumption, every 4 hours.

OUTCOME

By the end of 1999, at Rikshospitalet, Oslo and Inselspital, Berne, we had prospectively followed close to 10,000 patients having epidural analgesia after major surgery for more than 50,000 postoperative patient days and 6000 patients having i.v. opioid PCA, mostly morphine or ketobemidone, for about 25,000 postoperative days. Approximately 90% of the patients having epidural analgesia, and a somewhat smaller percentage with PCA, were satisfied with the pain relief they received. Side effects (e.g., nausea, dizziness) during i.v. PCA and technical epidural catheter problems are the common reasons for unsatisfactory results in 10–15% of patients. We have had three cases of severe respiratory depression in the i.v. morphine PCA group, all caused by human errors, all discovered early and treated successfully with naloxone. In the epidural group we have had nine potentially serious complications, i.e., less than one per 1000 patients and less than one per 5000 patient days. These involved bleeding in one patient in whom the epidural catheter was removed about 2 hours after LMWH was given subcutaneously, epidural abscess in one, a paravertebral abscess in one, and epidural infections without abscess formation in six patients.

All complications were discovered early and treated successfully, and none of the patients had permanent neurological complications. We have had no patients with severe respiratory depression in the epidural group. However, one patient had the morphine PCA line erroneously connected to an epidural catheter and another patient was erroneously prescribed fentanyl at 100 μg epidural bolus doses by a junior doctor. These two developed respiratory depression from human errors, which were both discovered early and successfully treated with repeated naloxone injections.

Thus, it is possible to successfully monitor patients having epidural or i.v. PCA on busy surgical wards, and our regimen appears to enhance patient safety (Breivik 1992, 1995, 1999; H. Breivik, H. Högström, M. Curatolo, and G. Kvarstein, personal communications).

COST OF A PAIN SERVICE OFFERING HIGH-TECH PATIENT-CONTROLLED AND EPIDURAL ANALGESIA

Counting capital costs, depreciation, wages, drugs, and disposables, the cost per day is between U.S.$25 and $50 for a patient to receive i.v. PCA or epidural analgesia in our department (Breivik 1995). This may seem expensive. However, our acute pain team not only offers high-tech approaches to pain control after surgery, but also has improved low-tech, low-cost approaches through an extensive educational program and by emphasizing better nursing care of all patients in pain on surgical wards. And this means that most of our surgical patients now receive improved postoperative pain management, not only the 10% who directly benefit from epidural analgesia or i.v. PCA. This brings the medication cost per patient (averaged across all patients receiving low and high-tech approaches) down to about U.S.$5 per day.

Our surgeons are as convinced as we are that by using optimal epidural analgesia, we reduce the postoperative complications in high-risk patients after thoracic and upper abdominal surgery. Therefore, the hospital is most likely saving money by providing high-quality postoperative pain management (Breivik 1995).

REQUIREMENTS FOR A SUCCESSFUL POSTOPERATIVE PAIN MANAGEMENT PROGRAM

Requirements for an improved postoperative pain management program, using any combination of high-tech or low-tech approaches, are as follows.

- A minimum of dedicated pain personnel—at least a pain nurse and an anesthesiologist who are able to use most of their time for postoperative pain management.
- An ongoing educational program in which the nurses on the surgical wards learn and relearn how to monitor and record pain, pain management, and any side effects at least every 4 hours. This will help to "make pain visible" (Rawal and Berggren 1994), focus attention on inadequate pain relief, and attract resources for improved pain relief.

The regimen we describe can be an instrument for continuous quality improvement, so that all patients will have better pain control—not only those who benefit from high-skill, high-tech postoperative pain management, but also those who only require low-tech approaches.

REFERENCES

Acute Pain Management Guideline Panel. *Acute Pain Management: Operative or Medical Procedures and Trauma. Clinical Practice Guideline.* AHCPR Publication No. 92-0032. Rockville, MD: Agency for Health Care Policy and Research, Public Health Service, U.S. Department of Health and Human Services, February, 1992.

Ballantyne JC, Carr DB, Chalmers TC, et al. Postoperative patient-controlled analgesia: meta-analyses of initial randomized controlled trials. *J Clin Anesth* 1993; 5:182–193.

Ballantyne JC, Carr DB, deFerranti S, et al. The comparative effects of postoperative analgesic therapies on pulmonary outcome: cumulative meta-analyses of randomized, controlled trials. *Anaesth Analg* 1998; 86:598–612

Berenbaum MC. What is synergy? *Pharmacol Rev* 1989; 41:93–141.

Birmingham PK, Tobin MJ, Henthorn TK, et al. Twenty-four-hour pharmacokinetics of rectal acetaminophen in children. An old drug with new recommendations. *Anesthesiology* 1997; 87:244–252.

Björkman R. Central antinociceptive effects of non-steroidal anti-inflammatory drugs and paracetamol. Experimental studies in the rat. *Acta Anaesthesiol Scand* 1995; 39:103S.

Björkman R, Hallman KM, Hedner T, Henning M. Acetaminophen blocks spinal hyperalgesia induced by NMDA and substance P. *Pain* 1994; 57:259–264.

Bonica JJ. Management of postoperative pain. In: Bonica JJ (Ed). *The Management of Pain*. Philadelphia: Lea & Febiger, 1990, pp 461–480.

Borchgrevink P, Hval B, Jystad Å, Kleppestad P. Changing from i.m. to nurse controlled i.v. morphine on ward—is it dangerous? *Abstracts: 9th World Congress on Pain*. Seattle: IASP Press, 1999.

Breivik EK, Barkvoll P, Skovlund E. Combining diclofenac with acetaminophen or acetaminophen-codeine after oral surgery: a randomized, double-blind single-dose study. *Clin Pharmacol Ther* 1999; 66:625–635.

Breivik H. Recommendations for foundation of a hospital-wide postoperative pain service—a European view. *Pain Digest* 1993; 3:27–30.

Breivik H. Benefits, risks and economics of post-operative pain management programmes. *Baillieres Clin Anaesthesiol* 1995; 9:403–422.

Breivik H. Postoperative pain management: why is it difficult to show that it improves outcome? *Eur J Anaesthesiol* 1998a; 15:748–751.

Breivik H. Neurological complications in association with spinal and epidural analgesia—again. *Acta Anaesthesiol Scand* 1998b; 42:609–613.

Breivik H. Infectious complications of epidural anaesthesia and analgesia. *Curr Opin Anaesthesiol* 1999; 12:573–577.

Breivik H, Högström H, Niemi G, et al. Safe and effective post-operative pain-relief: introduction and continuous quality-improvement of comprehensive post-operative pain management programmes. *Baillieres Clin Anaesthesiol* 1995; 9:423–460.

Brown DL, Bridenbaugh LD. The upper extremity. Somatic block. In: Cousins MJ, Bridenbaugh PO (Eds). *Neural Blockade in Clinical Anesthesia and Management of Pain*, 3rd ed. Philadelphia: Lippincott-Raven, 1998, pp 345–371.

Capdevila X, Barthelet Y, Biboulet P, et al. Effects of perioperative analgesic technique on the surgical outcome and duration of rehabilitation after major knee surgery. *Anesthesiology* 1999; 91:8–15.

Cohen S, Armar D, Pantuck CB, et al. Epidural patient-controlled analgesia after cesarean section buprenorphine-0.015% bupivacaine with epinephrine versus fentanyl-0.015% bupivacaine with and without epinephrine. *Anesth Analg* 1992; 74:226–230.

Cohen S, Armar D, Pantuck CB, et al. Postcesarean delivery epidural patient-controlled analgesia. Fentanyl or sufentanil? *Anesthesiology* 1993; 78:486–491.

Collins JG, Kitahata LM, Suzukawa M. Spinally administered epinephrine suppresses noxiously evoked activity of WDR neurons in the dorsal horn of the spinal cord. *Anesthesiology* 1984; 60:269–275.

Delbos A, Boccard E. The morphine-sparing effect of propacetamol in orthopedic postoperative pain. *J Pain Symptom Manage* 1995; 10:279–286.

Etches RC, Warriner CB, Badner N, et al. Continuous intravenous administration of ketorolac reduces pain and morphine consumption after total hip or knee arthroplasty. *Anesth Analg* 1995; 81:1175–1180.

Fletcher D, Benoist JM, Gautron M, Guilbaud G. Isobolographic analysis of interactions between intravenous morphine, propacetamol, and diclofenac in carrageenin-injected rats. *Anesthesiology* 1997a; 87:317–326.

Fletcher D, Nègre I, Barbin C, et al. Postoperative analgesia with iv propacetamol and ketoprofen combination after disc surgery. *Can J Anaesth* 1997b; 44:479–485.

Fredman B, Olsfanger D, Jedeikin R. A comparative study of ketorolac and diclofenac on post-laparoscopic cholecystectomy pain. *Eur J Anaesthesiol* 1995; 12:501–504.

Gaukroger PB. Paediatric analgesia: Which drug? Which dose? *Drugs* 1991; 41:52–59.

Hansen TG, O'Brien K, Morton NS, Rasmussen SN. Plasma paracetamol concentrations and pharmacokinetics following rectal administration in neonates and young infants. *Acta Anaesthesiol Scand* 1999; 43:855–859.

Harmer M, Davies KA. The effect of education, assessment and a standardised prescription on postoperative pain management. *Anaesthesia* 1998; 53:424–430.

Hobbs GJ. Ketorolac alters the kinetics of morphine metabolites. *Br J Anaesthesiol* 1997; 78:95.

Irwin MG, Roulseon CJ, Jones RDM. Peri-operative administration of rectal diclofenac sodium. The effect on renal function in patients undergoing minor orthopedic surgery. *Eur J Anaesthesiol* 1995; 12: 403–405.

Javery KB, Ussery TW, Steger HG, Colclough GW. Comparison of morphine and morphine with ketamine for postoperative analgesia. *Anesth Analg* 1996; 43:212–215.

Kalso E, Perttunen K, Kaasinen S. Pain after thoracic surgery. *Acta Anaesth Scand* 1992; 36:96–100.

Katz J. Perioperative predictors of long-term pain following surgery. In: Jensen TS, Turner JA, Wiesenfeld-Hallin Z (Eds). *Proceedings of the 8th World Congress on Pain,* Progress in Pain Research and Management, Vol. 8. Seattle: IASP Press, 1997, pp 231–240.

Katz J, Jackson M, Kavanagh BP, Sandler AN. Acute pain after thoracic surgery predicts long-term post-thoracotomy pain. *Clin J Pain* 1996; 12:50–55.

Kehlet H. Modification of responses to surgery by neural blockade: clinical implications. In: Cousins MJ, Bridenbough PO. *Neural Blockade in Clinical Anesthesia and Management of Pain,* 3rd ed. Philadelphia: Lippincott-Raven. 1998, pp 129–175.

Korpela R, Olkkola KT. Paracetamol—misused good old drug? *Acta Anaesthesiol Scand* 1999; 43:245–247.

Korpela R, Korvenoja P, Meretoja OA. Morphine-sparing effect of acetaminophen in pediatric day-case surgery. *Anesthesiology* 1999; 91:442–447.

Kostamovaara PA, Laitinen JO, Nuutinen LS, Koivuranta MK. Intravenous ketoprofen for pain relief after total hip or knee replacement. *Acta Anaesthesiol Scand* 1996; 40:697–703.

Liaw WJ, Day YJ, Wang JJ, Ho ST. Intravenous tenoxicam reduces dose and side effects of PCA morphine in patients after thoracic endoscopic sympathectomy. *Acta Anaesthesiol Sin* 1995; 33:73–77.

Liu SS, Carpenter RL, Meal JM. Epidural anesthesia and analgesia: their role in postoperative outcome. *Anesthesiology* 1995a; 82:1474–1506.

Liu SS, Carpenter RL, Mackey DC, et al. Effects of perioperative analgesic technique on rate of recovery after colon surgery. *Anesthesiology* 1995b; 83:757–765.

Malmberg AB, Yaksh TL. Antinociceptive actions of spinal nonsteroidal anti-inflammatory agents on the formalin test in the rat. *J Pharmacol Exp Ther* 1992; 263:136–146.

Montgomery JE, Sutherland CJ, Kestin IG, Sneyd JR. Morphine consumption in patients receiving rectal paracetamol and diclofenac alone and in combination. *Br J Anaesth* 1996; 77:445–447.

Muth-Selbach US, Tegeder I, Brune K, Geisslinger G. Acetaminophen inhibits spinal prostaglandin E_2 release after peripheral noxious stimulation. *Anesthesiology* 1999; 91:231–239.

Niemi G, Breivik H. Adrenaline markedly improves thoracic epidural analgesia produced by a low-dose infusion of bupivacaine, fentanyl and adrenaline after major surgery. *Acta Anaesthesiol Scand* 1998; 42:897–909.

Perttunen K, Nilsson E, Kalso E. I.V. diclofenac and ketorolac for pain after thoracoscopic surgery. *Br J Anaesth* 1999; 82:221–227.

Perttunen K, Tasmuth T, Kalso E. Chronic pain after thoracic surgery. *Acta Anaesthesiol Scand* 1999; 43:563–567.

Plummer JL, Owen H, Ilsley AH, Tordoff K. Sustained-release ibuprofen as an adjunct to morphine patient-controlled analgesia. *Anesth Analg* 1996; 83:92–96.

Rawal N, Berggren L. Organization of acute pain services: a low cost model. *Pain* 1994; 57:117–123.

Richardson J, Sabanathan S, Mearns AJ, Sides C, Goulden CP. Post-thoracotomy neuralgia. *Pain Clin* 1994; 7:87–97.

Schug SA, Sidebotham DA, McGuinnety M, Thomas J, Fox L. Acetaminophen as an adjunct to morphine by patient-controlled analgesia in the management of acute postoperative pain. *Anesth Analg* 1998; 87:368–372.

Schmid RL, Sandler AN, Katz J. Use and efficacy of low-dose ketamine in the management of acute postoperative pain: a review of current techniques and outcomes. *Pain* 1999; 82:111–125.

Smith G, Power I, Cousins MJ. Acute pain—is there scientific evidence on which to base treatment? *Br J Anaesth* 1999; 82:817–819.

Steinbrook RA. Epidural anesthesia and gastrointestinal motility. *Anesth Analg* 1998; 86:837–844.

Stubhaug A, Breivik H, Eide PK, Kreunen M, Foss A. Mapping of punctate hyperalgesia surrounding a surgical incision demonstrates that ketamine is a powerful suppressor of central sensitisation to pain following surgery. *Acta Anaesthesiol Scand* 1997; 41:1124–1132.

Tighe KE, Webb AM, Hobbs GI. Persistently high plasma morphine-6-glucuronide levels despite decreased hourly patient-controlled analgesia morphine use after single-dose diclofenac: potential for opioid related toxicity. *Anesth Analg* 1999; 88:1137–1142.

Tjölsen A, Lund A, Hole K. Antinociceptive effect of paracetamol in rats is partly dependent on spinal serotonergic systems. *Eur J Pharmacol* 1991; 193:193–201.

Van Aken H, Gogarten W, Rolf N. Epidural anesthesia in cardiac risk patients. *Anesth Analg* 1999; Review Course (Suppl) 89:104–110.

Wattwil M, Thoren T, Hennerdal S, Garvill J-E. Epidural analgesia with bupivacaine reduces postoperative paralytic ileus after hysterectomy. *Anesth Analg* 1989; 68:353–358.

Willoughby DA, Moore AR, Colville-Nash PR. COX-1, COX-2, and COX-3 and the future treatment of chronic inflammatory disease. *Lancet* 2000; 355:646–648.

Wong S, Gardocki JF. Anti-inflammatory and antiarthritic evaluation of acetaminophen and its potentiation of tolmetin. *J Pharmacol Exp Ther* 1983; 226:625–632.

Woolf CJ, Thompson SWN. The induction and maintenance of central sensitization is dependent on N-methyl-D-aspartic acid receptor activation; implications for the treatment of post-injury pain hypersensitivity states. *Pain* 1994; 158:347–354.

Correspondence to: Harald Breivik, MD, Department of Anesthesiology, University of Oslo, Rikshospitalet, 0027 Oslo, Norway. Tel: 47-22-867-111; Fax: 47-22-360-355; email: harald.breivik@klinmed.uio.no.

Proceedings of the 9th World Congress on Pain,
Progress in Pain Research and Management,
Vol. 16, edited by M. Devor, M.C. Rowbotham, and
Z. Wiesenfeld-Hallin, IASP Press, Seattle, © 2000.

76

A Comparison of the Tolerability of Ibuprofen, Acetaminophen, and Aspirin for Short-Term Analgesia

Nicholas Moore,[a] Eric Van Ganse,[b]
Jean-Marie Le Parc,[c] Richard Wall,[d] Hélène Schneid,[e]
Mahdi Farhan,[d] François Verrière,[e]
and François Pelen[e]

[a]*Department of Pharmacology, Victor Segalen University, Bordeaux, France;* [b]*Clinical Pharmacology Department, University of Lyon, Lyon, France;* [c]*Rheumatology Department, Ambroise Paré Hospital, Boulogne-Billancourt, France;* [d]*Boots Healthcare International, Nottingham, United Kingdom;* [e]*Boots Healthcare, Courbevoie, France*

Aspirin, ibuprofen, and acetaminophen (paracetamol) are widely used first-line analgesic agents, generally available over the counter (OTC). Endoscopic studies (Lanza 1984; Misra 1990), single-dose clinical trials (Furey 1992), anti-inflammatory dose trials (Haase 1991), retrospective case-control studies of gastrointestinal (GI) bleeding (Henry 1996), and a meta-analysis (Rainsford 1997) indicate that ibuprofen is as well tolerated as acetaminophen, and better tolerated than aspirin, even at low doses, but this finding has not been established by prospective comparative studies.

Because these drugs are widely used, small differences in adverse event rates affecting hundreds of thousands of patients will result in significant morbidity and health care costs. Only direct comparison can provide definite answers. We conducted a clinical trial (Moore 1999) with the hypothesis that ibuprofen would have a tolerability equivalent to that of acetaminophen and better than that of aspirin. To ensure applicability to the OTC situation, this study, conducted in general practice and relying mainly on patient data, was designed to parallel as much as possible the doses and durations of everyday OTC use for various common pain indications.

METHODS

Procedures and medication. The PAIN study (Paracetamol, Aspirin, Ibuprofen New Tolerability Study) was a randomized, multicenter, double-blind, parallel group study (Moore 1999). All patients gave written informed consent for the study, which had been previously approved by the Committee for the Protection of Persons Participating in Biomedical Research (Ambroise Paré Hospital, Boulogne-Billancourt, France). The study was conducted according to Good Clinical Practices (FDA 1997) and the Declaration of Helsinki.

Inclusion criteria were concordant with the approved indications of the drugs: patients aged 18–75 with a need (actual or expected within a few days) for analgesic treatment for more than 1 day and not more than 7 days, for relief of mild to moderate pain. Non-inclusion criteria included the contra-indications for the three drugs from their summary of product characteristics and methodological or legal requirements. Patients started treatment within 24 hours of consultation unless the general practitioner (GP) recommended otherwise, e.g., for dysmenorrhea, and used a diary to record adverse events and their severity, medication taken (trial and concomitant medication), a global treatment opinion, and any comments.

Aspirin and acetaminophen (paracetamol) 500-mg tablets and ibuprofen 200-mg tablets were repackaged identically (Creapharm) and identified only by treatment number. The maximal dose allowed was aspirin or acetaminophen 3 g/day, and ibuprofen 1200 mg/day, as approved for analgesic use in France. Treatment allocation to patients was randomized through a central telephone service to ensure continuously balanced group distribution The investigator prescribed the exact dosage of the allocated treatment, but the prescription did not exceed two tablets three times a day for up to 7 days.

The diary instructed patients how to report adverse effects (AEs) and their severity. Patients were not required to see their physician again. Physicians called the patients the day after the expected start of treatment to ensure that medication had been started, to record or qualify any early AEs, and to verify that the patients understood and would complete the diary. They called again 6–8 days later to ensure the diary would be returned, and to record any AEs. Any second consultation and its reason were also recorded.

AEs were identified and graded from the patient diary, from the telephone calls, and from further visits. Events were graded as serious, severe, moderate, or mild, according to the usual definitions. If severity was not recorded, it was classified as "missing." A study safety committee checked consistency of grading and coding (COSTART; FDA 1989) of events before unblinding.

The primary outcome measure was the number of patients with at least one significant AE, defined as an event that was serious, severe, or moderate, resulted in a second physician consultation, led to cessation of treatment, or where severity was classified as "missing." The secondary outcome measures were AEs by COSTART body systems and terms, and especially GI events; the distribution of serious, severe, moderate, and other categories of events; the reasons for premature discontinuation; prognostic factors such as indication and duration of treatment, number of tablets taken, concomitant disorders and medication; all AEs (including mild ones); and patient's global opinion of treatment.

Statistical analysis. The study analysis tested two primary hypotheses: equivalence between ibuprofen and acetaminophen, and difference between ibuprofen and aspirin. The difference between acetaminophen and aspirin was not tested. The expected incidence rates for significant events were 9% for acetaminophen and ibuprofen, and 12% for aspirin. Aspirin and ibuprofen were compared using a χ-square test to establish any difference. Ibuprofen and acetaminophen were compared to establish equivalence, which was considered to occur when the incidence of significant AEs with ibuprofen was within 30 percentage points of the expected rate for acetaminophen, i.e., if the one-sided 96.5% upper limit of the confidence interval (CI) of the difference was less than 2.7% (30% of 9%). The test was one-sided, with the null hypothesis that ibuprofen had more AEs than acetaminophen. To account for multiple testing, and to achieve an overall 5% level of significance, we used Dunnett's correction (Dunnett 1981) to hold both comparisons to 3.5%. Considering the expected incidence of significant AEs for aspirin, ibuprofen, and acetaminophen, 2583 patients per group were sufficient to achieve 90% power. Assuming a 10% dropout rate, we set the recruitment target at 8610 subjects.

RESULTS

The study included 1108 GPs and 8677 patients between September 1997 and March 1998; 2900 were randomized to aspirin, 2886 to ibuprofen, and 2888 to acetaminophen. In three patients, it was not possible to ascertain which treatment had been taken. Forty-four patients (0.5%) were not evaluable, mostly because of lack of data; 8633 patients (99.5%) were evaluable (Intention-to-Treat population, ITT), of which 8233 had followed the protocol (95%). The main protocol deviations were GP failure to use the central telephone service to allocate treatment (177 patients) and the use of prohibited medications (215 patients), and were equally distributed. The baseline characteristics of the treatment groups were similar, and factors that could affect tolerance such as age and indication were similarly distributed (Table I), as were duration of treatment and number of tablets used.

The study was completed by 7456 patients, of whom 3771 used the drug to the end of prescription; 3685 stopped early because of cessation of pain (aspirin 1235, ibuprofen 1246, acetaminophen 1204). A total of 1177 patients withdrew early from the study, 541 because of adverse events (aspirin 7.6%, ibuprofen 5.1%, acetaminophen 6.1%), and 576 because of lack of treatment effect (aspirin 7.0 %, ibuprofen 6.1 %, acetaminophen 6.9%).

There were six serious AEs, none considered to be treatment related. These events were: gardening accident, pneumothorax, neck of right humerus fracture, cerebral neoplasm, renal colic, and bronchitis. Three occurred in the aspirin group, three in the ibuprofen group.

Significant AEs were reported by 18.7% of evaluable patients on aspirin, 13.7% on ibuprofen, and 14.5% on acetaminophen (Table II). The one-sided 96.5% CL for the difference between acetaminophen and ibuprofen was below 2.7, thus fulfilling the requirements for equivalence. Significantly fewer patients on ibuprofen had significant AEs than did patients on aspirin.

Each category of significant AEs had significantly more patients in the aspirin than in the ibuprofen or acetaminophen groups. Equivalence be-

Table I
Baseline characteristics of the evaluable population, and number (percentage in parentheses) of patients with the indications for treatment listed

	Treatment Group		
Criteria	Aspirin (n = 2890)	Ibuprofen (n = 2869)	Acetaminophen (n = 2874)
Baseline Characteristics			
Age (years, mean and SD)	43.6 (14.7)	43.3 (14.7)	43.6 (14.8)
Gender (no. female, % female)	1672 (57.9)	1673 (58.4)	1664 (58.0)
Indications for Treatment			
Musculoskeletal condition	925 (32.0)	954 (33.3)	907 (31.6)
Cold/flu	586 (20.3)	571 (19.9)	548 (19.1)
Backache	461 (16.0)	431 (15.0)	476 (16.6)
Sore throat	317 (11.0)	332 (11.6)	341 (11.9)
Headache	304 (10.5)	297 (10.4)	291 (10.1)
Other	126 (4.4)	105 (3.7)	123 (4.3)
Toothache	112 (3.9)	116 (4.0)	113 (3.9)
Menstrual cramps	55 (1.9)	59 (2.1)	65 (2.3)

Note: All tests for differences between groups were nonsignificant.

Table II
Number (percentage) of patients with significant adverse events (evaluable population)

Aspirin	Ibuprofen	Acetaminophen
539 (18.7%)	392 (13.7%)	416 (14.5%)

Note: One-sided 96.5% confidence limit for difference between ibuprofen and acetaminophen = 0.85; equivalence is concluded if upper CL is < 2.7. $P < 0.001$ for aspirin vs. ibuprofen.

tween ibuprofen and acetaminophen was confirmed for all categories of significant AEs (data not shown).

More patients reported significant events concerning the body as a whole (which includes abdominal pain) with aspirin (10.1%) than with ibuprofen (7.0%) ($P < 0.001$) or acetaminophen (7.8%). More patients reported significant digestive events with aspirin (7.1%) than with ibuprofen (4.0%) ($P < 0.001$) or acetaminophen (5.3%), and more with acetaminophen than ibuprofen ($P = 0.025$). This finding was also true for dyspepsia and for abdominal pain (Table III). The other system organ classes and other individual reaction terms showed no differences. Two rectal hemorrhages and two hematemeses occurred with acetaminophen (0.14%), two rectal hemorrhages and one peptic ulcer with aspirin (0.1%), and none with ibuprofen (upper limit of 95% CI = 0.1%). None were considered serious. Analysis of all AEs (including mild-intensity ones) gave similar results (data not shown). On global evaluation, 74.2% of patients on ibuprofen rated the treatment as excellent or good, a significantly higher rating than for acetaminophen (69.2%) or aspirin (68.6%) (both $P < 0.001$).

Table III
Percentage of most frequent significant adverse events in the evaluable population by COSTART body system and terms (with 95% CI* in parentheses)

	Aspirin	Ibuprofen	Acetaminophen
Systems			
Body as a whole	10.1 (9.0–11.2)	7.0 (6.1–7.9)	7.8 (6.8–8.8)
Digestive	7.1 (6.2–8.0)	4.0 (3.3–4.7)	5.3 (4.4–6.1)
Terms			
Abdominal pain	6.8 (5.9–7.7)	2.8 (2.2–3.4)	3.9 (3.2–4.6)
Dyspepsia	3.1 (2.5–3.7)	1.4 (1.0–1.8)	2.2 (1.7–2.7)
Nausea	2.5 (1.9–3.1)	1.5 (1.1–1.9)	1.5 (1.1–1.9)

* Normal approximation; computed only when overall frequency >1%.

DISCUSSION

This blinded, randomized, parallel group study in general practice showed that the tolerability of ibuprofen at OTC analgesic doses was equivalent to that of acetaminophen and better than that of aspirin. Overall, the AEs were of the same nature for the three drugs, though those observed with aspirin tended to be more severe and more frequent. Contrary to common opinion, minor GI events were not more frequent with ibuprofen than with acetaminophen. This finding had already been established for serious events in children (Lesko 1995).

The study was designed to assess the tolerability of these drugs as used commonly for analgesia, i.e., short-term use at OTC doses. The indications, doses, and durations of treatment, and the non-inclusion criteria, were consistent with those approved in France, to ensure maximal applicability of the results to current prescription practice as well as everyday OTC use. We found no indication of differences in treatment effectiveness.

The primary source of information for AEs was the patient diary card. When only the data from the diary cards were considered, the results were the same as when physician data were also included (data not shown). The results from the primary outcome were those anticipated, i.e., equivalence of significant AE rates between ibuprofen and acetaminophen, and a lower rate than aspirin, but the observed rates were higher than expected (observed 13.7%, 14.5%, and 18.7% vs. expected 9%, 9%, and 12% for ibuprofen, acetaminophen, and aspirin, respectively). This discrepancy could be related to patient- rather than physician-based recording of data, or to the evaluation options, which were designed to maximize event recognition and severity attribution. The distribution of event rates between aspirin, ibuprofen, and acetaminophen was consistent over the entire event range, whether they were significant or nonsignificant, and for most organ systems or reaction terms. This was also true in patients with previous history of GI disorders, and in patients above 65 years old (data not shown).

In conclusion, this study is the first to directly compare the three most commonly used first-line analgesics at their approved OTC doses, and confirms that ibuprofen had equivalent tolerability to acetaminophen and was better tolerated than aspirin. These findings could lead to a reassessment of the use of first-line analgesics for painful conditions in general practice, possibly to recommending ibuprofen before aspirin or acetaminophen, because of the poor tolerability of aspirin and the potential risks of acetaminophen overdose.

REFERENCES

Dunnett C, Goldsmith C. When and how to do multiple comparisons. In: Buncher C, Tsay J (Eds). *Statistics in the Pharmaceutical Industry*. New York: Dekker, 1981, pp 397–433.

FDA. *Coding Symbol Thesaurus for Adverse Reaction Terms*, 3rd ed. Rockville, MD: Center for Drugs and Biologics, Division of Drugs and Biological Products Experience, 1989.

FDA. *Federal Register* 1997; 62(90):25,691–25,709.

Furey SA, Waksman JA, Dash BH. Nonprescription ibuprofen: side effect profile. *Pharmacotherapy* 1992; 12(5):403–407.

Haase W, Fischer M. Statistische Metaanalyse von multizentrischen klinischen Studien mit Ibuprofen in Hinblick auf die Kohortengröße [Statistical meta-analysis of multicenter clinical studies with ibuprofen with regard to cohort size]. *Z Rheumatol* 1991; 50(Suppl 1):77–83.

Henry D, Lim LL, Garcia Rodriguez LA, et al. Variability in risk of gastrointestinal complications with individual non-steroidal anti-inflammatory drugs: results of a collaborative meta-analysis. *BMJ* 1996; 312(7046):1563–1566.

Lanza FL. Endoscopic studies of gastric and duodenal injury after the use of ibuprofen, aspirin, and other nonsteroidal anti-inflammatory agents. *Am J Med* 1984; 77(1A):19–24.

Lesko SM, Mitchell AA. An assessment of the safety of pediatric ibuprofen. A practitioner-based randomized clinical trial. *JAMA* 1995; 273(12):929–933.

Misra R, Pandey H, Chandra M, Agarwal PK, Pandeya SN. Effects of commonly used NSAID's on gastric mucosa. A clinico- endoscopic and histopathological study. *J Assoc Physicians India* 1990; 38(12):913–915.

Moore N, Van Ganse E, Le Parc J-M, et al. The PAIN Study: paracetamol, aspirin and ibuprofen new tolerability study. *Clin Drug Invest* 1999; 18(2):89–98.

Rainsford KD, Roberts SC, Brown S. Ibuprofen and paracetamol: relative safety in non-prescription doses. *J Pharm Pharmacol* 1997; 49(4):345–376.

Correspondence to: Nicholas Moore, MD, PhD, Department of Pharmacology, University Hospital Bordeaux-Pellegrin, 33076 Bordeaux, France. email: nicholas.moore@pharmaco.u-bordeaux2.fr.

Proceedings of the 9th World Congress on Pain,
Progress in Pain Research and Management,
Vol. 16, edited by M. Devor, M.C. Rowbotham, and
Z. Wiesenfeld-Hallin, IASP Press, Seattle, © 2000.

77

Clinical Trials of NMDA-Receptor Antagonists as Analgesics

Per Kristian Eide

Department of Neurosurgery, The National Hospital, University of Oslo, Oslo, Norway

THE ROLE OF NMDA RECEPTORS IN PAIN PERCEPTION

Chronic pain may involve various characteristics: spontaneous ongoing pain, spontaneous intermittent pain, allodynia (static or dynamic), hyperalgesia, abnormal radiation of pain outside the site of nerve or tissue injury, abnormal temporal summation of pain, and long-lasting aftersensations. These characteristics involve different pathophysiological mechanisms, both peripheral and central. Pain therapy designed to interfere with these mechanisms could specifically target various manifestations of chronic pain.

During the last decade, major attention has been given to the role of central sensitization in the development of chronic pain (Dubner 1997). Animal studies suggest that the N-methyl-D-aspartate (NMDA) receptor, a receptor subtype of the excitatory amino acid glutamate, has an important role in mechanisms underlying central sensitization (Coderre et al. 1993; Dickenson et al. 1997). NMDA-receptor antagonists lessen the hyperactivity of dorsal horn neurons following prolonged activation of primary afferent neurons and inhibit nociceptive behavior induced by peripheral tissue or nerve injury. Clinical trials of NMDA-receptor antagonists were made possible by such research on central sensitization.

NMDA-receptor mechanisms play an important role in the pathophysiology of numerous central nervous system (CNS) diseases, including acute excitotoxic neurodegeneration (e.g., cerebral ischemia and stroke), epilepsy, and chronic neurodegenerative diseases (e.g., dementia of the Alzheimer type, Parkinsonism, and Huntington's disease) (Meldrum 1991). The receptor subtype also has a crucial role in the synaptic plasticity underlying learning and memory (Morris 1994).

Glutamate is the most abundant excitatory neurotransmitter in the CNS, with three main receptor subtypes (metabotropic, non-NMDA, and NMDA-receptor subtypes). The NMDA-receptor channel is a ligand-gated calcium (Ca^{2+}) channel that mediates excitatory and modulatory actions of glutamate. Activation of the channel occurs when the membrane of the cell is partly depolarized by activation of other (non-NMDA) receptors. At normal resting membrane potential, the channel is blocked by Mg^{2+}. When sufficient depolarization is generated to remove Mg^{2+} from the channel, the NMDA receptor is activated and Ca^{2+} ions flow through the channel into the cell. Calcium triggers several biochemical processes, including phosphorylation of membrane (receptor) proteins, activation of nitric oxide synthase, and activation of immediate early genes coding for factors that regulate protein synthesis. The outcome of these biochemical alterations may be persistent changes in neuronal excitability. The NMDA receptors may become sensitized by prolonged activation, which can enhance synaptic function in that particular synapse. Regulatory sites other than the Mg^{2+} binding site include the phencyclidine (PCP), glycine, and Zn^{2+} binding sites.

CLINICALLY AVAILABLE NMDA-RECEPTOR ANTAGONISTS

Several NMDA-receptor antagonists have been developed and used in animals, although safety and toxicity testing has not been brought up to clinical standards. The need for NMDA-receptor antagonists has led to the rediscovery of old, well-known drugs, including ketamine, dextromethorphan/dextrorphan, and amantadine/memantine.

Ketamine. Ketamine has been available for clinical use as an anesthetic for more than 30 years (Domino et al. 1965). It was recognized early on that this compound exhibits analgesic properties when given in subanesthetic doses (Sadove et al. 1971). Ketamine is a noncompetitive NMDA-receptor antagonist that acts at the phencyclidine (PCP) binding site in the NMDA-receptor channel (Anis et al. 1983). Ketamine's interaction with other receptor subtypes is dose-dependent. Öye and coworkers (1991) have shown that both the optical isomers of ketamine (R- and S-ketamine) have markedly higher affinity for the NMDA channel (the PCP recognition site) than for opioid-binding sites. For S-ketamine and R-ketamine the affinity for the PCP site was 0.9 and 2.5 μmol/L, respectively. At higher concentrations S- and R-ketamine interact with μ-opioid receptors (K_i = 11 and 28 μmol/L for S- and R-ketamine, respectively), σ-opioid receptors (K_i = 131 and 19 μmol/L, respectively), κ-opioid receptors (K_i = 24 and 100 μmol/L, respectively), and δ-opioid receptors (K_i values 130 and 130 μmol/L, respectively). For the binding of racemic ketamine to PCP sites in the human brain, a K_i value of 0.6 μmol/L was calculated (Tam and Zhang 1988).

We have observed inhibition of the various characteristics of pain by ketamine at serum concentrations below 1 μmol/L (Eide et al. 1995a,b, Stubhaug et al. 1997, in press). We have found a highly significant correlation between pain relief and serum concentrations of ketamine. Analgesia is obtained by 1/10 to 1/5 of an anesthetic dose. Surgical anesthesia is obtained at serum concentrations above 4–5 μmol/L racemic ketamine. In humans the local anesthetic effect of ketamine occurs at concentrations above 50–100 μmol/L. Ketamine affected voltage-operated membrane channels at concentrations above 100 μmol/L (Kress 1994) and depressed sodium channels at concentrations above 50 μmol/L (Frenkel and Urban 1992). Therefore, the analgesic effects of ketamine shown in humans in subanesthetic doses are likely to occur at concentrations sufficient to block a substantial fraction of the NMDA receptors.

Dextromethorphan. Dextromethorphan (dextrorphan) was found to be an effective cough suppressant more than 40 years ago (Benson et al. 1953). The compound has NMDA-receptor antagonist properties (Choi et al. 1987).

Memantine (amantadine). The closely related drugs 1-amino-3,5-dimethyladamantane (memantine) and 1-amino-adamantane (amantadine) have been used as antiviral and anti-Parkinsonian drugs. Recently, memantine was shown to be a noncompetitive NMDA-receptor antagonist (Parsons et al. 1993).

CLINICAL STUDIES ON EXPERIMENTALLY INDUCED PAIN

An overview of randomized, double-blind, placebo-controlled studies concerning effects of NMDA-receptor antagonists on experimentally induced pain is given in Table I.

Several controlled studies have shown that ketamine inhibits acute pain caused by different noxious stimuli, including ischemic (Maurset et al. 1989), chemical (Park et al. 1995), heat (Ilkjaer et al. 1996) and electrical stimuli (Arendt-Nielsen et al. 1995). The R- and S-enantiomers of ketamine also reduced ischemic pain with an analgesic potency of the enantiomers that correlated positively with their relative affinity for PCP sites (Klepstad et al. 1990). Dextromethorphan, on the other hand, does not inhibit the intensity of acute painful stimuli (Kauppila et al. 1995; Ilkjaer et al. 1997; Kinnman et al. 1997).

Table I
Results of randomized, double-blind, placebo-controlled studies on the analgesic effect of NMDA-receptor antagonists on experimentally induced acute pain

Drug	Dose/Administration Route	*N*	Type of Noxious Stimulation	Pain Characteristics Inhibited	Reference
Ketamine	0.3 mg/kg, i.v.	6	Ischemia	↓ Intensity of spontaneous pain	Maurset et al. 1989
Ketamine	10 μg·kg^{-1}·min^{-1} after 0.07 mg/kg bolus, i.v.	12	Intradermal capsaicin	↓ Intensity of spontaneous pain ↓ Area/magnitude of secondary hyperalgesia (pinprick stimuli) ÷ Allodynia	Park et al. 1995
Ketamine	0.15 mg/kg, i.v.	12	Local burn injury	↓ Area of secondary hyperalgesia (punctuate and brush stimuli) ↓ Temporal summation (mechanical stimuli)	Warncke et al. 1997
Ketamine	0.30 mg/kg, i.v.	19	Local burn injury	↓ Intensity of spontaneous pain ↓ Area of secondary hyperalgesia (punctuate and stroke stimuli)	Ilkjaer et al. 1996
Dextromethorphan	120 mg, p.o.	24	Local burn injury	÷ Intensity of spontaneous pain ↓ Area of secondary hyperalgesia (pinprick stimuli)	Ilkjaer et al. 1997
Dextromethorphan	90 mg, p.o.	10	Intradermal capsaicin	÷ Intensity of spontaneous pain ÷ Area of secondary hyperalgesia	Kinnman et al. 1997
Dextromethorphan	100 mg, p.o.	8	Topical capsaicin	÷ Intensity of spontaneous pain	Kauppila et al. 1995
Ketamine	9 μg·kg^{-1}·min^{-1} after 0.5 mg/kg bolus, i.v.	12	Electrical	↓ Intensity of spontaneous pain ↓ Temporal summation (electrical stimuli)	Arendt-Nielsen et al. 1995
Ketamine	5 μg·kg^{-1}·min^{-1} after 0.2 mg/kg bolus, i.v.	17	Topical capsaicin	↓ Temporal summation (electrical stimuli)	Andersen et al. 1996
Dextromethorphan	30–45 mg, p.o.	6	Heat	↓ Temporal summation (heat stimuli)	Price et al. 1994

Symbols: ↓ (significantly reduced); ÷ (not significantly changed).

SECONDARY HYPERALGESIA

Central sensitization may be an important mechanism underlying secondary hyperalgesia (Bennett 1994). As indicated in Table I, NMDA-receptor antagonists inhibit secondary hyperalgesia. Randomized, double-blind, placebo-controlled studies have shown that ketamine inhibits the area of secondary hyperalgesia induced by chemical (Park et al. 1995) or heat stimuli (Ilkjaer et al. 1996; Warncke et al. 1997). Dextromethorphan reduced the area of secondary hyperalgesia induced by heat (Ilkjaer et al. 1997), but not chemical stimuli (Kinnman et al. 1997).

TEMPORAL SUMMATION OF PAIN

Temporal summation of pain describes progressive enhancement of pain intensity following repeated noxious stimuli of constant stimulus intensity. This phenomenon is considered a psychophysical correlate of the wind-up response recorded electrophysiologically in dorsal horn neurons of animals following repetitive C-fiber stimulation. Wind-up is considered to reflect at least some characteristics of central sensitization (Eide et al. 1999).

As presented in Table I, controlled studies in healthy volunteers have shown that ketamine-induced NMDA-receptor blockade inhibits temporal summation of repeated mechanical (Warncke et al. 1997) and electrical stimuli (Arendt-Nielsen et al. 1995; Andersen et al. 1996). Dextromethorphan inhibits temporal summation of repetitive heat stimuli (Price et al. 1994).

Taken together, different controlled studies provide consistent data that NMDA-receptor antagonists inhibit both temporal summation and secondary hyperalgesia. Clinical evidence demonstrates that NMDA-receptor antagonists inhibit central sensitization.

CLINICAL STUDIES ON ACUTE POSTOPERATIVE PAIN

Several controlled studies have examined different characteristics of postoperative pain after pre- and perioperative treatment with NMDA-receptor antagonists (Table II). Pre- and perioperative treatment with low-dose ketamine reduced postoperative morphine consumption, although the intensity of ongoing postoperative pain was less affected (Roytblat et al. 1993) or was not significantly reduced (Fu et al. 1997; Ngan-Kee et al. 1997). Treatment with dextromethorphan before elective bilateral tonsillectomy significantly reduced the intensity of spontaneous pain and pain evoked by swallowing, and reduced the analgesic requirements for the first seven postoperative days (Kawamata et al. 1998).

Table II
Results of randomized, double-blind, placebo-controlled studies on the "pre-emptive" effect of NMDA-receptor antagonists

Drug	Dose/Administration Route	*N*	Type of Noxious Stimulation	Pain Characteristics Inhibited	Reference
Ketamine	0.15 mg/kg, i.v. (preop.)	11	Cholecystectomy	↓ Intensity of ongoing pain (4 h) ↓ Morphine consumption (24 h)	Roytblat et al. 1993
Ketamine	2 mg/kg, i.v. (preop.) 20 μg·kg^{-1}·min^{-1} (periop.)	9	Transabdominal hysterectomy	÷ Intensity of ongoing pain (48 h) ↓ Wound hyperalgesia (48 h) ÷ Intensity of movement-associated pain (48 h)	Tverskoy et al. 1994
Ketamine	0.5 mg/kg, i.v. (preop.) 10 μg·kg^{-1}·min^{-1} (periop.)	20	Abdominal surgery	÷ Intensity of ongoing pain (48 h) ↓ Morphine consumption (48 h)	Fu et al. 1997
Ketamine	1 mg/kg (preop.)	20	Cesarean section	÷ Intensity of ongoing pain (24 h) ↓ Morphine consumption (24 h)	Ngan-Kee et al. 1997
Dextromethorphan	45 mg, p.o. (preop.)	12	Tonsillectomy	↓ Intensity of ongoing pain (7 d) ↓ Swallowing evoked pain (7 d) ↓ Analgesic requirements (7 d)	Kawamata et al. 1998
Ketamine	0.5 mg/kg (preop.) 2 μg·kg^{-1}·min^{-1} (periop.) 2 μg·kg^{-1}·min^{-1} (1st day postop.) 1 μg·kg^{-1}·min^{-1} (2nd–3rd days postop.)	10	Nephrectomy	↓ Intensity of ongoing pain (1 h) ↓ Wind-up-like pain (3 d) ↓ Area of wound hyperalgesia (7 d) ↓ Morphine consumption (6 h)	Stubhaug et al. 1997

Symbols: ↓ (significantly reduced); ÷ (not significantly changed).

Two studies found that inhibition of wound hyperalgesia was a more sensitive measure of pain relief than was assessment of postoperative pain intensity. Wound hyperalgesia was reduced for 48 hours, without change in ongoing pain, after termination of ketamine treatment (Tverskoy et al. 1994). Stubhaug et al. (1997) demonstrated that the area of wound hyperalgesia was reduced for 4 days after termination of low-dose ketamine infusion, whereas ongoing pain was reduced for only 1 hour; most serum concentrations of ketamine measured 24 and 72 hours after the bolus injection were below 0.36 μmol/L.

Assuming that wound hyperalgesia results from central sensitization, the observations that ongoing pain was not reduced suggest that central sensitization represents only one of several mechanisms behind postoperative pain. Therefore, NMDA-receptor antagonists might be useful in combination with other drugs.

In a double-blind study of 91 patients undergoing major surgery, the addition of ketamine (0.4 mg/mL) to postoperative epidural infusion (0.02 mg/mL morphine, 0.8 mg/mL bupivacaine, 4 μg/mL epinephrine) enhanced postoperative pain relief and reduced analgesic requirements (Chia et al. 1998). Another study examined postoperative pain in patients undergoing total knee replacement with epidural lidocaine anesthesia (Wong et al. 1997). Co-administration of epidural ketamine/morphine with lidocaine 30 minutes before skin incision enhanced postoperative analgesia and reduced analgesic requirements for 72 hours postoperatively. These clinical studies confirm the usefulness of combining NMDA-receptor antagonists with other drugs.

CLINICAL STUDIES ON CHRONIC PAIN

A number of controlled studies have shown that NMDA-receptor antagonists modulate different characteristics of chronic pain (Table III). The clinical trials include patients with peripheral and central neuropathic pain, muscular pain, ischemic pain, and cancer pain.

SPONTANEOUS ONGOING PAIN

After healing of the tissue or nerve injury, spontaneous ongoing pain may persist independently of noxious stimulation. Case reports have shown that NMDA-receptor antagonists, in particular ketamine, may inhibit spontaneous ongoing pain in patients with chronic pain. Ketamine given via various administration routes (intravenously, intramuscularly, subcutaneously,

Table III
Results of randomized, double-blind, placebo-controlled studies on the analgesic effect of NMDA-receptor antagonists in chronic pain syndromes

Drug	Dose/Administration Route	*N*	Pain Syndrome	Pain Characteristics Inhibited	Reference
Ketamine	0.15 mg/kg, i.v.	8	Postherpetic neuralgia	↓ Intensity of ongoing pain ↓ Wind-up-like pain ↓ Allodynia	Eide et al. 1994
Ketamine	6 $\mu g \cdot kg^{-1} \cdot min^{-1}$ after 60 μg/kg bolus, i.v.	9	Central neuropathic pain after spinal cord injury	↓ Intensity of ongoing pain ÷ Wind-up like pain ↓ Allodynia	Eide et al. 1995b
Ketamine	5 $\mu g \cdot kg^{-1} \cdot min^{-1}$ after 0.2 mg/kg bolus, i.v.	10	Peripheral neuropathic pain	↓ Intensity of ongoing pain ↓ Area of allodynia	Felsby et al. 1995
Ketamine	7 $\mu g \cdot kg^{-1} \cdot min^{-1}$ after 0.1 mg/kg bolus, i.v.	11	Stump and phantom limb pain	↓ Intensity of ongoing pain ↓ Wind-up like pain	Nikolajsen et al. 1996
Dextromethorphan	40.5 or 81 mg/day, p.o.	19	Peripheral or central neuropathic pain	÷ Intensity of ongoing pain	McQuay et al. 1994
Dextromethorphan	~381 mg/d, p.o.	14	Diabetic neuropathy	↓ Intensity of ongoing pain	Nelson et al. 1997
Dextromethorphan	~381 mg/d, p.o.	18	Postherpetic neuralgia	÷ Intensity of ongoing pain	Nelson et al. 1997
Amantadine	200 mg/3 h, i.v.	15	Neuropathic cancer pain	↓ Intensity of ongoing pain	Pud et al. 1998
Ketamine	0.3 mg/kg, i.v.	18	Fibromyalgia	↓ Intensity of ongoing pain ↓ Hyperalgesia, tender points	Sörensen et al. 1997
Ketamine	0.3-0.45 mg/kg, i.v.	8	Ischemic pain	↓ Intensity of ongoing pain	Persson et al. 1998
Ketamine	0.75 $\mu g \cdot kg^{-1} \cdot (2\ h)^{-1}$, i.v.	8	Post-traumatic pain	↓ Intensity of ongoing pain ↓ Allodynia	Max et al. 1995
Ketamine	2 and 4 $\mu g \cdot kg^{-1} \cdot d^{-1}$, p.o.	12	Postherpetic neuralgia	÷ Intensity of ongoing pain ÷ Allodynia ↓ Wind-up-like pain	Stubhaug et al. 1999

Symbols: ↓ (significantly reduced); ÷ (not significantly changed).

and orally) inhibited ongoing pain in patients with peripheral and central neuropathic pain (Stannard and Porter 1993; Backonja et al. 1994; Hoffmann et al. 1994; Eide et al. 1995a; Mathisen et al. 1995; Klepstad and Borchgrevink 1997; Nikolajsen et al. 1997). Several case reports also found that ketamine was effective in relieving cancer pain (Clark and Kalan 1995; Mercadante et al. 1995). A double-blind "*n* of 1" trial, including one patient with glossopharyngeal neuralgia, examined the effect of randomized treatment with oral ketamine (60 mg, 6 times daily) or placebo. Oral ketamine significantly reduced the intensity of spontaneous ongoing pain and of pain caused by swallowing, with an acceptable side-effect profile (Eide and Stubhaug 1997).

In a case study of a patient with neuropathic pain, intrathecal injection of the NMDA-receptor antagonist CPP (3-(2-carboxypiperazin-4-yl) propyl-1-phosphoric acid) failed to affect spontaneous ongoing pain or allodynia, but inhibited the spread of pain outside the territory of nerve injury and reduced pain that lasted after the end of mechanical stimulation (Kristensen et al. 1992).

Recent case studies have reported long-lasting effects of short trials of NMDA-receptor antagonists. Takahashi et al. (1998) reported a case with neuropathic pain (complex regional pain syndrome, type II) after sciatic nerve injury that had lasted for several weeks. Epidural infusion of a low dose of ketamine (25 $\mu g \cdot kg^{-1} \cdot h^{-1}$) for 10 days completely abolished pain for the observation period of 8 months. Eisenberg and Pud (1998) reported that three patients with peripheral neuropathic pain became pain free for several months after a short course of amantadine treatment.

As shown in Table III, several controlled studies have demonstrated that ketamine significantly inhibits spontaneous ongoing pain in patients with different types of chronic pain, including peripheral neuropathic pain (Eide et al. 1994; Felsby et al. 1995; Max et al. 1995; Nikolajsen et al. 1996), central neuropathic pain (Eide et al. 1995b), fibromyalgia (Sörensen et al. 1997), and chronic ischemic pain (Persson et al. 1998). Dextromethorphan appears to be less effective in relieving spontaneous ongoing neuropathic pain (McQuay et al. 1994; Nelson et al. 1997). One controlled study has shown that amantadine inhibits spontaneous ongoing pain in patients with neuropathic cancer pain (Pud et al. 1998). Another controlled study showed that ketamine inhibited hyperalgesia at tender points in patients with fibromyalgia (Sörensen et al. 1997).

In one recent controlled study, ketamine was given in a low oral dose that by itself failed to inhibit the intensity of spontaneous ongoing pain (Stubhaug et al., in press). However, ketamine combined with oral morphine synergistically inhibited ongoing pain. Furthermore, in patients with terminal cancer pain, a double-blind crossover study revealed that analgesia induced by intrathecal morphine was enhanced by co-administration of ketamine (Yang et al. 1996). These studies are useful in demonstrating the possible benefit of applying NMDA-receptor antagonists in a multi-drug regimen.

ALLODYNIA

Central sensitization may be an important mechanism underlying certain types of allodynia (i.e., pain caused by normally nonpainful stimuli) (Bennett 1994). Several case studies reported that ketamine reduced allodynia in patients with neuropathic pain (Backonja et al. 1994; Eide et al. 1995a; Nikolajsen et al. 1997).

The effect of NMDA-receptor antagonists on allodynia may last longer than the pharmacological action. In a case with mechanical allodynia surrounding an infected surgical wound, intravenous (i.v.) administration of ketamine at 0.2–0.5 $mg \cdot kg^{-1} \cdot (2\ min)^{-1}$ during wound dressing produced acute short-term pain relief that was not obtained with opioids (Persson et al. 1995). In this case, mechanical allodynia diminished considerably during the 3-month period of intermittent ketamine administration 1–2 times daily.

As indicated in Table III, several controlled studies have shown that the effect of i.v. ketamine in inhibiting allodynia in patients with central or peripheral neuropathic pain was associated with inhibition of spontaneous ongoing pain (Eide et al. 1994, 1995b; Felsby et al. 1995; Max et al. 1995). An oral dose of ketamine that did not relieve spontaneous pain also failed to affect allodynia (Stubhaug et al., in press). These studies assessed dynamic mechanical allodynia, evoked by applying an electric tooth brush (Eide et al. 1994, 1995b; Stubhaug et al., in press) or a cotton swab (Felsby et al. 1995; Max et al. 1995) to the skin.

ABNORMAL TEMPORAL SUMMATION OF PAIN (WIND-UP-LIKE PAIN)

Like dynamic tactile allodynia, wind-up-like pain may also result from central sensitization. Wind-up-like pain was described in patients with postherpetic neuralgia (PHN) (Eide et al. 1994). Repetitive pricking of the skin with a von Frey filament (2741 mN) at a rate of 3 pricks/second was initially painless but after a few seconds led to markedly enhanced pain, with radiation of pain outside the stimulated area and aftersensation. This abnormal response was different from temporal summation found in normal individuals or in skin areas without persistent pain. As indicated in Table

III, controlled studies have shown that ketamine inhibits wind-up-like pain in patients with peripheral neuropathic pain (Eide et al. 1994; Nikolajsen et al. 1996; Stubhaug et al., in press), which may be associated with inhibition of ongoing pain (Eide et al. 1994; Nikolajsen et al. 1996). Wind-up-like pain in patients with neuropathic cancer pain also was inhibited by amantadine (Pud et al. 1998). In patients with central neuropathic pain, the effect of ketamine on wind-up-like pain did not reach significance (Eide et al. 1995b), probably due to low serum concentrations in three of nine patients. There was a significant correlation between serum concentrations of ketamine and the inhibition of wind-up like pain.

The controlled clinical trials presented here indicate that NMDA-receptor antagonists inhibit central sensitization, and that this effect may be associated with their inhibition of spontaneous ongoing pain.

SIDE EFFECTS OF NMDA-RECEPTOR ANTAGONISTS

NMDA receptors are ubiquitous in the human CNS. Therefore, NMDA-receptor antagonists at analgesic doses interfere not only with pain perception, but with sensory perception in general. The main problem with NMDA-receptor antagonists as analgesics is their psychotomimetic side effects. The psychomimetic and psychotogenic effects of NMDA-receptor antagonists are well known (Olney and Farber 1995). Dextromethorphan and amantadine have better side-effect profiles than ketamine.

Psychic disturbances on awakening from ketamine anesthesia include pleasant or unpleasant dreams, hallucinations, excitation, and "emergence delirium." In subanesthetic doses, ketamine dose-dependently produces psychotomimetic side effects including visual disturbances (altered color perception, reduced visual acuity), auditory disturbances, cognitive impairment, disturbed proprioception (dizziness, feelings of detachment from the body), feelings of unreality, hallucinations, mental disturbances (anxiety, aggression), and discomfort (illness and nausea) (Öye et al. 1992). The psychic side effects are reduced when ketamine is given in combination with benzodiazepines or other sedative drugs. Among other observed side effects of ketamine, daily oral doses of 900–1500 mg produced liver failure (Kato et al. 1995).

Öye et al. (1992) examined the relative potencies of the enantiomers S- and R-ketamine for inhibition of sensory perception. The relative potencies of S- and R-ketamine in both producing analgesia as well as disturbed sensory perception (visual and auditory disturbance, disturbed proprioception, and impairment of short-term memory) corresponded with their relative affinities for the PCP sites. Therefore, psychotomimetic side effects of subanesthetic doses of ketamine are related to PCP-site-mediated blockade of channels operated by NMDA receptors. Ketamine and other PCP-like drugs are "open channel" blockers, i.e., they block NMDA channels that are already activated.

Dextromethorphan has a better side-effect profile than ketamine (Bem and Peck 1992). Amantadine may have an even better side-effect profile. The most severe side effect of i.v. amantadine (200 mg/3 hours) given to relieve neuropathic pain was dryness in the mouth in 3 of 15 cancer patients (Pud et al. 1998).

STRATEGIES TO REDUCE SIDE EFFECTS

The main limitation in clinical use of NMDA-receptor antagonists is the frequency and severity of side effects. Strategies to reduce the side-effect profile of NMDA-receptor antagonists are required. One important strategy would be the development of drugs that interact with other regulatory sites in the NMDA-receptor-operated channel (e.g., Mg^{2+}, Zn^{2+}, and glycine binding sites) (Dickenson 1997). Another strategy would be to deliver the drug by routes other than systemic administration. With regard to intrathecal (i.t.) administration of NMDA-receptor antagonists, detailed toxicological analysis is required. It should be noted that i.t. infusion of an NMDA-receptor antagonist has caused severe psychotomimetic side effects, including anxiety, uneasiness, hyperacusis, and nightmares, due to rostral spread of the drug (Kristensen et al. 1992).

The most interesting strategy is the combination of low doses of NMDA-receptor antagonists with other drugs. Data from animal studies suggest that NMDA-receptor antagonists and opioids may synergistically enhance antinociception (Chapman and Dickenson 1992). As mentioned above, clinical studies have indicated synergistic analgesic interactions between ketamine and morphine (Yang et al. 1996; Wong et al. 1997; Chia et al. 1998). In a recent randomized, double-blind study of 12 patients with PHN, combined oral treatment using ketamine and morphine significantly enhanced pain relief compared to either drug alone (Stubhaug et al., in press).

CONCLUSIONS

Controlled clinical trials in healthy volunteers show that NMDA-receptor antagonists inhibit experimentally induced pain, including secondary hyperalgesia and temporal summation. Controlled trials have demonstrated that NMDA-receptor antagonists also inhibit characteristics of pathological pain perception (in particular allodynia and abnormal temporal summation). The results suggest a role of NMDA receptors in pain mechanisms involving central sensitization, and may represent a step toward mechanism-based pain therapy. NMDA-receptor antagonists may become useful in a multi-drug regimen to treat certain pain characteristics (secondary hyperalgesia, allodynia, abnormal summation, and spread of pain). Strategies to reduce the frequency and severity of side effects of NMDA-receptor antagonists are urgently needed, however. Presently, treatment with selected NMDA-receptor antagonists (ketamine, dextrorphan, or amantadine) requires close follow-up and can only be recommended in selected patients who can tolerate the side effects.

REFERENCES

Andersen OK, Felsby S, Nicolaisen L, et al. The effect of ketamine on stimulation of primary and secondary hyperalgesic areas induced by capsaicin—a double-blind, placebo-controlled, human experimental study. *Pain* 1996; 66:51–62.

Anis NA, Berry SC, Burton NR, Lodge D. The dissociative anaesthetics, ketamine and phencyclidine, selectively reduce excitation of central mammalian neurones by N-methyl-aspartate. *Br J Pharmacol* 1983; 79:565–575.

Arendt-Nielsen L, Petersen-Felix S, Fischer M, et al. The effect of N-methyl-D-aspartate antagonist (ketamine) on single and repeated nociceptive stimuli: a placebo-controlled experimental human study. *Anesth Analg* 1995; 81:63–68.

Backonja M, Arndt G, Gombar KA, Check B, Zimmermann M. Response of chronic neuropathic pain syndromes to ketamine: a preliminary study. *Pain* 1994; 56:51–57.

Bem JL, Peck R. Dextromethorphan: an overview of safety issues. *Drug Saf* 1992; 7:190–199.

Bennett GJ. Neuropathic pain. In: Wall PD, Melzack RM (Eds). *Textbook of Pain*. Edinburgh: Churchill Livingstone, 1994, pp 201–224.

Benson WM, Stefko PL, Randall LO. Comparative pharmacology of levorphan, racemorphan and dextrorphan and related methyl ethers. *J Pharmacol Exp Ther* 1953; 109:189–200.

Chapman V, Dickenson AH. The combination of NMDA antagonism and morphine produces profound antinociception in the rat dorsal horn. *Brain Res* 1992; 573:321–323.

Chia YY, Liu K, Liu YC, Chang HC, Wong CS. Adding ketamine in a multimodal patient-controlled epidural regimen reduces postoperative pain and analgesic consumption. *Anesth Analg* 1998; 86:1245–1249.

Choi DW, Peter S, Viseskul V. Dextrorphan and levorphenol selectively block N-methyl-D-aspartate receptor-mediated neurotoxicity on cortical neurons. *J Pharmacol Exp Ther* 1987; 242:713–720.

Clark JL, Kalan GE. Effective treatment of severe cancer pain of the head using low-dose ketamine in an opioid-tolerant patient. *J Pain Symptom Manage* 1995; 10:310–314.

Coderre TJ, Katz J, Vaccarino AL, Melzack R. Contribution of central neuroplasticity to pathological pain: review of clinical and experimental evidence. *Pain* 1993; 52:259–285.

Dickenson A. Mechanisms of central hypersensitivity: excitatory amino acid mechanisms and their control. In: Dickenson A, Besson JM (Eds). *The Pharmacology of Pain*. Berlin: Springer Verlag, 1997, pp 167–210.

Domino EF, Chodoff P, Corssen G. Pharmacologic effects of CI-581, a new dissociative anesthetic, in man. *Clin Pharmacol Ther* 1965; 6:279–291.

Dubner R. Neural basis of persistent pain: sensory specialization, sensory modulation, and neuronal plasticity. In: Jensen TS, Turner JA, Wiesenfeld-Hallin Z (Eds). *Proceedings of the 8th World Congress on Pain,* Progress in Pain Research and Management, Vol. 8. Seattle: IASP Press, 1997, pp 243–257.

Eide PK. Wind-up and the NMDA receptor complex from a clinical perspective. *Eur J Pain* 1999; in press.

Eide PK, Stubhaug A. Relief of glossopharyngeal neuralgia by ketamine-induced N-methyl-aspartate receptor blockade. *Neurosurgery* 1997; 41:505–508.

Eide PK, Jørum E, Stubhaug A, Bremnes J, Breivik H. Relief of post-herpetic neuralgia with the N-methyl-D-aspartic acid receptor antagonist ketamine: a double-blind, cross-over comparison with morphine and placebo. *Pain* 1994; 58:347–354.

Eide PK, Stubhaug A, Øye I, Breivik H. Continuous subcutaneous administration of the N-methyl-D-aspartic acid (NMDA) receptor antagonist ketamine in the treatment of post-herpetic neuralgia. *Pain* 1995a; 61:221–228.

Eide PK, Stubhaug A, Stenehjem AE. Central dysesthesia pain after traumatic spinal cord injury is dependent on N-methyl-D-aspartate receptor activation. *Neurosurgery* 1995b; 37:1080–1087.

Eisenberg E, Pud D. Can patients with chronic neuropathic pain be cured by acute administration of the NMDA receptor antagonist amantadine? *Pain* 1998; 74:337–339.

Felsby S, Nielsen J, Arendt-Nielsen L, Jensen TS. NMDA receptor blockade in chronic neuropathic pain: a comparison of ketamine and magnesium chloride. *Pain* 1995; 64:283–291.

Frenkel C, Urban BW. Molecular actions of racemic ketamine on human CNS sodium channels. *Br J Anaesth* 1992; 69:292–297.

Fu ES, Miguel R, Scharf JE. Preemptive ketamine decreases postoperative narcotic requirements in patients undergoing abdominal surgery. *Anesth Analg* 1997; 84:1086–1090.

Hoffmann V, Coppejans H, Vercauteren M, Adriaensen H. Successful treatment of postherpetic neuralgia with oral ketamine. *Clin J Pain* 1994; 10:240–242.

Ilkjaer S, Petersen KL, Brennum J, Wernberg M, Dahl JB. Effect of systemic N-methyl-D-aspartate receptor antagonist (ketamine) on primary and secondary hyperalgesia in humans. *Br J Anaesth* 1996; 76:829–834.

Ilkjaer S, Dirks J, Brennum J, Wernberg M, Dahl JB. Effect of systemic N-methyl-D-aspartate receptor antagonist (dextromethorphan) on primary and secondary hyperalgesia in humans. *Br J Anaesth* 1997; 79:600–605.

Kato Y, Homma I, Ichiyanagi K. Postherpetic neuralgia [letter]. *Clin J Pain* 1995; 11:336–337.

Kauppila T, Grönroos M, Pertovaara A. An attempt to attenuate experimental pain in humans by dextromethorphan, an NMDA receptor antagonist. *Pharmacol Biochem Behav* 1995; 52:641–644.

Kawamata T, Omote K, Kawamata M, Namiki A. Premedication with oral dextromethorphan reduces postoperative pain after tonsillectomy. *Anesth Analg* 1998; 86:594–597.

Kinnman E, Nygårds EB, Hansson P. Effects of dextromethorphan in clinical doses on capsaicin-induced ongoing pain and mechanical hypersensitivity. *J Pain Symptom Manage* 1997; 14:195–201.

Klepstad P, Maurset A, Moberg ER, Øye I. Evidence of a role for NMDA receptors in pain perception. *Eur J Pharmacol* 1990; 187:513–518.

Klepstad P, Borchgrevink PC. Four years' treatment with ketamine and a trial of dextromethorphan in a patient with severe post-herpetic neuralgia. *Acta Anaesthesiol Scand* 1997; 41:422–426.

Kress HG. NMDA- und opiatrezeptoren-unabhängige Wirkungen von Ketamin. *Anaesthesist* 1994; 43(Suppl 2): S15–S24.

Kristensen JD, Svensson B, Gordh T. The NMDA-receptor antagonist CPP abolishes neurogenic "wind-up pain" after intrathecal administration in humans. *Pain* 1992; 51:249–253.

Mathisen LC, Skjelbred P, Skoglund LA, Øye I. Effect of ketamine, an NMDA receptor inhibitor, in acute and chronic orofacial pain. *Pain* 1995; 61:215–220.

Maurset A, Skoglund LA, Hustveit O, Øye I. Comparison of ketamine and pethidine in experimental and postoperative pain. *Pain* 1989; 36:37–41.

Max MB, Byas-Smith MG, Gracely RH, Bennett GJ. Intravenous infusion of the NMDA antagonist, ketamine, in chronic posttraumatic pain with allodynia: a double-blind comparison to alfentanil and placebo. *Clin Neuropharmacol* 1995; 18:360–368.

McQuay HJ, Carroll D, Jadad AR, et al. Dextromethorphan for the treatment of neuropathic pain: a double-blind randomised controlled crossover trial with integral n-of-1 design. *Pain* 1994; 59:127–133.

Meldrum BS (Ed). *Excitatory Amino Acid Antagonists*. Oxford: Blackwell Scientific, 1991.

Mercadante S, Lodi F, Sapio M, Calligara M, Serretta R. Long-term ketamine subcutaneous continuous infusion in neuropathic cancer pain. *J Pain Symptom Manage* 1995; 10:564–568.

Morris RGM, Davis M. The role of NMDA receptors in learning and memory. In: Collingridge GL, Watkins JC (Eds). *The NMDA Receptor*, 2nd ed. Oxford: Oxford University Press, 1994, pp 340–375.

Nelson KA, Park KM, Robinovitz E, Tsigos C, Max MB. High-dose oral dextromethorphan versus placebo in painful diabetic neuropathy and postherpetic neuralgia. *Neurology* 1997; 48:1212–1218.

Ngan Kee WD, Khaw KS, Ma ML, Mainland PA, Gin T. Postoperative analgesic requirement after cesarean section: a comparison of anesthetic induction with ketamine or thiopental. *Anesth Analg* 1997; 85:1294–1298.

Nikolajsen L, Hansen CL, Nielsen J, et al. The effect of ketamine on phantom pain: a central neuropathic disorder maintained by peripheral input. *Pain* 1996; 67:69–77.

Nikolajsen L, Hansen PO, Jensen TS. Oral ketamine therapy in the treatment of postamputation stump pain. *Acta Anaesthesiol Scand* 1997; 41:427–429.

Olney JW, Farber NB. NMDA antagonists as neurotherapeutic drugs, psychotogens, neurotoxins, and research tools for studying schizophrenia. *Neuropsychopharmacology* 1995; 13:335–345.

Öye I, Hustveit O, Maurset A, et al. The chiral forms of ketamine as probes for NMDA receptor functions in humans. In: Kameyama T, Nabeshima T, Domino EF (Eds). *NMDA Receptor Related Agents: Biochemistry, Pharmacology and Behavior*. Ann Arbor: NPP Books, 1991, pp 381–389.

Öye I, Paulsen O, Maurset A. Effects of ketamine on sensory perception: evidence for a role of N-methyl-D-aspartate receptors. *J Pharmacol Exp Ther* 1992; 260:1209–1213.

Park KM, Max MB, Robinovitz E, Gracely RH, Bennett GJ. Effects of intravenous ketamine, alfentanil, or placebo on pain, pinprick hyperalgesia, and allodynia produced by intradermal capsaicin in human subjects. *Pain* 1995; 63:163–172.

Parsons CG, Gruner R, Rozental J, Millar J, Lodge D. Patch clamp studies on the kinetics and selectivity of N-Methyl-D-Aspartate receptor antagonism by memantine (1-amino-3,5-dimethyladamantan). *Neuropharmacology* 1993; 32:1337–1350.

Persson J, Axelsson G, Hallin RG, Gustafsson LL. Beneficial effects of ketamine in a chronic pain state with allodynia, possibly due to central sensitization. *Pain* 1995; 60:217–222.

Persson J, Hasselström J, Wiklund B, et al. The analgesic effect of racemic ketamine in patients with chronic ischemic pain due to lower extremity arteriosclerosis obliterans. *Acta Anaesthesiol Scand* 1998; 42:750–758.

Price DD, Mao J, Frenk H, Mayer DJ. The N-methyl-D-aspartate receptor antagonist dextromethorphan selectively reduces temporal summation of second pain in man. *Pain* 1994; 59:165–174.

Pud D, Eisenberg E, Spitzer A, et al. The NMDA receptor antagonist amantadine reduces surgical neuropathic pain in cancer patients: a double blind, randomized, placebo controlled trial. *Pain* 1998; 75:349–354.

Roytblat L, Korotkoruchko A, Katz J, et al. Postoperative pain: the effect of low-dose ketamine in addition to general anesthesia. *Anesth Analg* 1993; 77:1161–1165.

Sadove MS, Shulman M, Hatano S, Fevold N. Analgesic effects of ketamine administered in subdissociative doses. *Anesth Analg* 1971; 50:452–457.

Sörensen J, Bengtsson A, Ahlner J, et al. Fibromyalgia—are there different mechanisms in the processing of pain? A double blind crossover comparison of analgesic drugs. *J Rheumatol* 1997; 24:1615–1621.

Stannard CF, Porter GE. Ketamine hydrochloride in the treatment of phantom limb pain. *Pain* 1993; 54:227–230.

Stubhaug A, Breivik H, Eide PK, Kreunen M, Foss A. Mapping of punctuate hyperalgesia around a surgical incision demonstrates that ketamine is a powerful suppresser of central sensitization to pain following surgery. *Acta Anaesthesiol Scand* 1997; 41:1124–1132.

Stubhaug A, Eide PK, Øye I, Breivik H. The combination of oral morphine and ketamine improves pain relief in postherpetic neuralgia compared with morphine or ketamine alone: a randomised, double-blind, placebo-controlled crossover comparison. *Pain;* in press.

Takahashi H, Miyazaki M, Nanbu T, Yanagida H, Morita S. The NMDA-receptor antagonist ketamine abolishes neuropathic pain after epidural administration in a clinical case. *Pain* 1998; 75:391–394.

Tam SW, Zhang AZ. σ and PCP receptors in human frontal cortex membranes. *Eur J Pharmacol* 1988; 154:343–344.

Tverskoy M, Oz Y, Isakson A, et al. Preemptive effect of fentanyl and ketamine on postoperative pain and wound hyperalgesia. *Anesth Analg* 1994; 78:205–209.

Warncke T, Stubhaug A, Jørum E. Ketamine, an NMDA receptor antagonist, suppresses spatial and temporal properties of burn-induced secondary hyperalgesia in man: a double-blind, cross-over comparison with morphine and placebo. *Pain* 1997; 72:99–106.

Wong CS, Lu CC, Cherng CH, Ho ST. Pre-emptive analgesia with ketamine, morphine and epidural lidocaine prior to total knee replacement. *Can J Anaesth* 1997; 44:31–37.

Yang CY, Wong CS, Chang JY, Ho ST. Intrathecal ketamine reduces morphine requirements in patients with terminal cancer pain. *Can J Anaesth* 1996; 43:379–383.

Correspondence to: Per Kristian Eide, MD, PhD, Department of Neurosurgery, The National Hospital, Pilestredet 32, 0027 Oslo, Norway. Tel: 47-228-67190; Fax: 47-228-67189; email: p.k.eide@labmed.uio.no.

Proceedings of the 9th World Congress on Pain,
Progress in Pain Research and Management,
Vol. 16, edited by M. Devor, M.C. Rowbotham, and
Z. Wiesenfeld-Hallin, IASP Press, Seattle, © 2000.

78

Recent Developments in the Treatment of Neuropathic Pain

Michael C. Rowbotham, Karin L. Petersen,
Pamela S. Davies, Erika K. Friedman,
and Howard L. Fields

*UCSF Pain Clinical Research Center, University of California,
San Francisco, California, USA*

Pain states associated with injury or disease affecting the peripheral or central nervous system remain among the most difficult to treat of the chronic pain syndromes. Well-designed and appropriately controlled clinical trials conducted since 1990 have expanded the list of proven treatment options. Four medication categories can be considered "first-line" treatment for neuropathic pain: antidepressants, anticonvulsants, opioids, and topical agents. Only topical lidocaine patches (for postherpetic neuralgia) and the anticonvulsant gabapentin are "new" within the last decade. The available treatments in the four categories have limitations, and none provide "moderate" or better relief in more than about 60% of treated patients. There is ample room for future improvement in each category and a continuing need for innovative treatments.

ANTIDEPRESSANTS: ARE NON-TRICYCLICS AS GOOD AS TRICYCLICS?

Why would a patient with chronic pain want to take a medication with numerous side effects that is described in drug package inserts and patient information leaflets as treatment for psychiatric disorders only? Although no medication in any category has been proven unequivocally superior to tricyclic antidepressants (TCAs) as an analgesic for chronic neuropathic pain, nearly all patients experience the anticholinergic side effects of dry mouth and constipation. Many also experience urinary hesitancy and blurred vision. Cognitive impairment, sedation, orthostatic hypotension, and sexual dysfunction are also common and poorly tolerated. TCAs can be lethal in an accidental or intentional overdose; the likelihood of successful suicide is 8–16-fold higher for TCAs compared to non-tricyclic antidepressants (non-TCAs) such as trazodone and fluoxetine (Kapur et al. 1992). Current treatment of depression favors the many newer, non-TCAs because the differences in efficacy are small compared to the benefits of greater safety and reduced side effects. The serotonin-selective reuptake inhibitors (SSRIs) and the antidepressants that alter both serotonergic (5HT) and noradrenergic (NE) neurotransmission would become the first-choice antidepressants *if* their analgesic efficacy were proven equivalent to TCAs.

TCAs were the first medication category proven effective for chronic neuropathic pain in double-blind placebo-controlled trials (Watson et al. 1982). Contrary to the assumptions of the initial trials, pain relief and relief of depression are independent effects (Max et al. 1987; Sindrup et al. 1992a). Essentially every blinded clinical trial of TCAs has found them efficacious (McQuay et al. 1996; Kingery 1997). How strong is the evidence for analgesic efficacy with the newer antidepressants? The crossover trial by Sindrup and colleagues comparing the TCA imipramine and the SSRI paroxetine for diabetic neuropathy pain is instructive (Sindrup et al. 1992b). Paroxetine was equal to imipramine in most subjects, inferior in 30-40%, and essentially never superior. For postherpetic neuralgia, Watson and colleagues found the SSRI zimelidine to be far inferior to amitriptyline (Watson and Evans 1985). The randomized controlled trial of the SSRI fluoxetine by Max and co-workers failed to find the non-tricyclic superior even to placebo (Max et al. 1992). In a separate study, Watson and colleagues found the relatively NE-selective antidepressant maprotiline to have good efficacy, but still less effective overall than a TCA (Watson et al. 1992). Clinical trials of newer non-TCAs that affect both 5HT and NE reuptake, such as venlafaxine and nefazodone, are needed.

What is the reason for the apparent analgesic superiority of TCAs? The presumed mechanisms underlying antidepressant analgesia, facilitation of descending serotonergic and noradrenergic pain modulatory pathways, may not be the only mechanisms. TCAs, in addition to blocking serotonin and norepinephrine reuptake, are relatively potent sodium channel blockers, may act as NMDA receptor blockers, and some have significant sympatholytic effects (Deffois et al. 1996). With the introduction of many non-TCAs in the past decade, it is possible that a series of adequately powered clinical trials could find one or more drugs that are safer and equal to or better than tricyclics from an analgesic efficacy perspective. In the meantime, the following general treatment recommendations can be made. (1) If a TCA is tried at doses producing blood levels in the "therapeutic range" (for depression) without pain relief, the available literature would suggest that other TCAs, SSRIs, and MRIs are also likely to fail (Watson et al. 1988; Sindrup et al. 1992b; Watson et al. 1998). (2) If a TCA relieves the patient's pain but the side effects prove intolerable, the non-TCAs should be tried in the hope of finding one that is analgesic with fewer side effects. (3) Starting with the newer non-TCAs and switching to a TCA only if pain is not relieved is a valid approach. (4) Patients with safety contraindications to TCAs or intolerable side effects at subtherapeutic doses of a TCA should be given a trial of a non-tricyclic before abandoning this drug category.

ANTICONVULSANTS AND ANTIARRHYTHMICS

Anticonvulsants are a broad category tied together only by their ability to suppress epileptic seizures. Anticonvulsants and related local anesthetic drugs have been used for decades to treat chronic pain. Systemic administration of procaine, and later lidocaine, have been in use since at least the 1930s to treat a variety of acute and chronic pain states. In his 1953 textbook Bonica noted anecdotal evidence for an analgesic effect of i.v. procaine in disorders as diverse as postoperative pain, burn pain, acute traumatic pain (such as fractures and sprains), chronic musculoskeletal pain and arthritis, acute herpes zoster, postherpetic neuralgia, various neuralgias, and causalgia/reflex dystrophies (Bonica 1953). Of the oral anticonvulsants, carbamazepine has shown dramatic efficacy in the treatment of trigeminal neuralgia (Dunsker and Mayfield 1976). Evidence is sufficient to firmly establish anticonvulsants and local anesthetic drugs as specialized analgesics for neuropathic pain (Swerdlow and Cundill 1981; McQuay et al. 1995; Fields et al. 1997). Neither anticonvulsants nor local anesthetics have clearly established analgesic efficacy for musculoskeletal or nociceptive pain, but anticonvulsant drugs such as valproic acid and gabapentin are effective in migraine prophylaxis (Magnus-Miller et al. 1998).

Anticonvulsants differ in their mechanism of action (McQuay et al. 1995; Fields et al. 1997). Many drugs have in common an ability to block sodium channels in a use-dependent manner, but also exert their effect through non-sodium-channel mechanisms. Other anticonvulsant drugs are highly effective in controlling pain, but seem to do so without blocking sodium channels. Proposed mechanisms of analgesic actions for non-sodium–channel-blocking drugs revolve around effects on sensitized central neurons, such as direct or indirect inhibition of the release of excitatory amino acids, blockade of neuronal calcium channels, and augmentation of CNS inhibitory pathways by increasing GABAergic transmission.

SODIUM CHANNELS AND ECTOPIC IMPULSE GENERATION

Recent research in animals with experimental nerve injury and humans with chronic neuropathic pain has highlighted one clinically important mechanism for the production of neuropathic pain: ectopic impulse generation by damaged, dysfunctional, primary sensory neurons and their axons (Devor and Seltzer 1999). In teased axon recordings from dorsal roots in rats and rabbits with chronic nerve injury, Wall and Gutnick and Kirk demonstrated an increased level of persisting discharge in afferent A and C fibers compared to normal intact dorsal root and dorsal root just after acute nerve section (Kirk 1974; Wall and Gutnick 1974). Subsequent studies identified two principal sources of this activity: the nerve injury site (e.g., neuroma or nerve compression zone) and the associated dorsal root ganglia (DRG) (Wall and Devor 1983; Kajander et al. 1992). The development of ectopic hyperexcitability may be due in part to remodeling of the electrical properties of the axon membrane via local increases in sodium channel density and changes in their distribution. In addition to spontaneous firing, ectopic discharge can be produced by gentle tapping and by a range of chemical stimuli. Abnormal afferent barrages that propagate into the CNS will directly elicit paraesthesias, dysesthesias, and pain. For example, continuous discharge in C fibers produces continuous sensations of burning pain, and intermittent spontaneous bursts in Aδ or Aβ fibers produce lancinating dysesthesias or paresthesias (Nordin et al. 1984; Cline et al. 1989). Abnormally increased afferent input via nociceptors can also trigger and maintain "central sensitization" (LaMotte et al. 1991; Torebjörk et al. 1992). Central neurons become sensitized in response to a brief but intense barrage of nociceptor input or sustained low-level nociceptor input. Once central neurons are sensitized, even innocuous mechanoreceptor stimulation from an area around the nerve injury is perceived as painful (Campbell et al. 1988; Woolf 1992).

A variety of anticonvulsant and local anesthetic drugs suppress abnormal discharge originating at nerve injury sites and associated DRGs via sodium channel blockade. These drugs include the anticonvulsants carbamazepine, phenytoin, and lamotrigine, the antiarrhythmics mexiletine and tocainide, and lidocaine-like local anesthetics (Catterall 1987). Each prevents the generation of spontaneous ectopic impulses at concentrations 2–3 orders of magnitude lower than are required to block normal impulse propagation. Because the process of ectopic impulse generation is so sensitive to sodium channel blockade, these drugs can be given systemically or regionally without fatal toxicity from failure of normal nerve conduction.

CLINICAL USE OF SODIUM CHANNEL BLOCKING ANTICONVULSANTS

Carbamazepine is the first-line drug treatment of trigeminal neuralgia and is the only anticonvulsant approved by the U.S. Food and Drug Administration (FDA) for treatment of any neuropathic pain disorder. Like the local anesthetics lidocaine, mexiletine, and tocainide, carbamazepine reduces spontaneous activity in experimental neuromas (Burchiel 1988). Controlled clinical trials with carbamazepine have produced mixed results. Success has been documented in trigeminal neuralgia and diabetic neuropathy, but not in postherpetic neuralgia and central pain (Campbell et al. 1966; Rockliff and Davis 1966; Nicol 1969; Rull et al. 1969; Leijon and Boivie 1989). Carbamazepine appears effective in a variety of neuropathic pain disorders, but the studies are either small or uncontrolled. The main drawbacks to carbamazepine are sedation, ataxia, the need for regular monitoring of hematological and hepatic function, drug interactions, and the rare occurrence of irreversible aplastic anemia.

By blocking voltage-dependent sodium channels and suppressing peripherally generated ectopic impulse activity, lamotrigine has reduced central release of the excitatory transmitters glutamate and aspartate (Cheung et al. 1992; Teoh et al. 1995). Animal studies have demonstrated analgesic effects of lamotrigine (Nakamura-Craig and Follenfant 1995; Hunter et al. 1997). In a study of postoperative pain, 200-mg single doses of lamotrigine reduced both postoperative pain and analgesic requirements (Bonicalzi et al. 1997). Two double-blind, placebo-controlled studies of the analgesic effect of lamotrigine for neuropathic pain have been published. A placebo-controlled study of 100 patients with a variety of neuropathic pain complaints showed no reduction in pain from a daily dose of 200 mg (McCleane 1999). In contrast, a maintenance dose of 400 mg lamotrigine was superior to placebo as an add-on therapy for trigeminal neuralgia (Zakrzewska et al. 1997). Doses up to 300–400 mg/day have been used anecdotally and in open trials with success in central pain, trigeminal neuralgia, and diabetic neuropathy (Canavero and Bonicalzi 1996; Eisenberg and Alon 1996; Harbison et al. 1997; Lunardi et al. 1997). Drawbacks specific to lamotrigine are relatively high frequencies of rash (including rare fatalities from Stevens-Johnson syndrome), and drug-drug interactions.

Among the drugs marketed as antiarrhythmics, mexiletine has received the most study. Structurally similar to lidocaine, mexiletine is a local anesthetic and a class IB antiarrhythmic. Pain, dysesthesias, and parasthesias were reduced in patients with chronic painful diabetic neuropathy in a randomized, double-blind, placebo-controlled crossover study by Dejgard and colleagues (1988). Relatively high doses of mexiletine were administered based on the subject's weight. In studies of diabetic neuropathy and various nerve injuries using lower doses of 450 mg to 750 mg/day, the analgesic effect has been modest (Chabal et al. 1992; Stracke et al. 1992; Oskarsson et al. 1997; Wright et al. 1997). Two recent studies of patients with HIV-related neuropathy failed to demonstrate an analgesic effect with a relatively low dose of 600 mg/day of mexiletine (Kemper et al. 1998; Kieburtz et al. 1998). Specific drawbacks to mexiletine are cardiac contraindications, worsening of arrhythmias, drug-drug interactions, upper GI distress (common and frequently treatment limiting), and tremor. The antiarrhythmic flecainide is occasionally used as an alternative therapy for neuropathic pain if the use of mexiletine is limited by side effects (Sinnott et al. 1991). A third oral local-anesthetic type antiarrhythmic, tocainide, had accumulated evidence for efficacy in animal studies and in a double-blind clinical trial in trigeminal neuralgia (Lindstrom and Lindblom 1987). However, its use has been severely restricted because of a higher than expected incidence of aplastic anemia.

Phenytoin was the first anticonvulsant to be specifically tried in pain management, but is now little used. Uncontrolled studies reported phenytoin to be effective in the treatment of trigeminal neuralgia (Iannone et al. 1958). Double-blind, placebo-controlled studies have demonstrated analgesia with phenytoin in diabetic neuropathy and Fabry's disease (a small-fiber neuropathy) (Lockman et al. 1973; Chadda and Mathur 1978). Phenytoin (like lidocaine) can be given parenterally and is sometimes used to provide immediate relief for patients who are having severe and frequent attacks of trigeminal neuralgia (Albert 1978). Specific drawbacks to phenytoin are its complex kinetics, drug-drug interactions, and combined signs of neurotoxicity and cardiac conduction effects at very high blood levels.

Topiramate has been used for seizure disorders since 1996, but until recently had not been reported as an analgesic agent (Bajwa et al. 1999). Topiramate reduces neuronal activity by voltage-dependent blockade of Na^+ channels, enhances GABA at $GABA_A$ receptors, and antagonizes the kainate subtype of the glutamate receptors. Based on the mechanism of action, some analgesic efficacy seems probable and topiramate is occasionally used to treat chronic pain. Specific drawbacks to topiramate are a higher incidence of sedation and psychomotor slowing, carbonic-anhydrase inhibition, renal stones, and drug-drug interactions. Topiramate also has the unusual side effect of producing weight loss in 10–20% of patients (Perucca 1997; Jones 1998).

ANTICONVULSANTS THAT DO NOT BLOCK SODIUM CHANNELS: GABAPENTIN AND VALPROIC ACID

Gabapentin was approved for marketing in the United States in 1995 as adjunctive therapy in the treatment of seizures. Gabapentin was developed as an analogue to the neurotransmitter GABA, but new evidence shows that it does not interact with either $GABA_A$ or $GABA_B$ receptors (Taylor et al. 1998). Gabapentin is excreted unmetabolized, so active metabolites can not explain the analgesic effect in humans. GABAergic function could be potentiated without direct interaction with GABA sites by increasing the concentration of GABA in neuronal tissue through release of GABA from nerve terminals, enzyme effects, or decreased GABA breakdown (Upton 1994; Honmou et al. 1995; Taylor et al. 1998). Another possible mechanism is mobilization of intracellular GABA via gabapentin-sensitive transporters. However, the best evidence to date comes from studies that rank order effects of gabapentin and related drugs on a specific gabapentin binding protein found in brain and spinal cord. The binding site, called $\alpha_2\delta$, is a subunit of a voltage-gated calcium channel found in high density in the cerebral cortex, superficial dorsal horn, cerebellum, and hippocampus (Gee et al. 1996). Gabapentin binding is primarily postsynaptic and is resistant to neonatal capsaicin treatment and rhizotomy. GABA itself has no activity at this binding site, but gabapentin analogues that bind to the $\alpha_2\delta$ subunit do appear to have analgesic activity. At present, it is not certain which, if any, of the suggested mechanisms may be relevant to the analgesic efficacy of gabapentin.

In the United States, gabapentin is probably used more frequently than any other anticonvulsant for chronic pain. This popularity appears due to ease of monitoring, a relatively low incidence of serious adverse events, and a perception of efficacy bolstered by evidence from placebo-controlled trials. Case-reports, chart reviews, and open-label clinical trials reported analgesic efficacy of gabapentin in a variety of painful conditions (Mellick et al. 1995; Rosner et al. 1996; Rosenberg et al. 1997). Recently, two multicenter, double-blind, placebo-controlled clinical trials demonstrated that gabapentin at a target dose of 3600 mg/day reduced pain from postherpetic neuralgia (PHN) and from diabetic neuropathy (Backonja et al. 1998; Rowbotham et al. 1998a). Together, these two trials of nearly identical design totalled more than 400 subjects, making them larger than any other randomized controlled trial of a pharmacological therapy for neuropathic pain. Both were analyzed using a conservative intent-to-treat analysis. In the study of PHN, pain was reduced by 33%, compared to a reduction of 8% with placebo (Rowbotham et al. 1998a). In the diabetic neuropathy study, pain was reduced by 39% with gabapentin, compared to 22% with placebo (Backonja et al.

1998). Based on a calculation of the NNT (number needed to treat), a measure of efficacy, gabapentin is comparable to tricyclic antidepressants.

Gabapentin has a short half-life and is absorbed via a saturable active transport mechanism. As with nearly all anticonvulsants, the most common side effects are related to CNS depression, such as dizziness, ataxia, and somnolence. Compared to other anticonvulsants, drug-drug interactions are not a problem. The dose must be adjusted in patients with renal failure, but no adjustment is necessary in patients with hepatic disorders because the drug is excreted unmetabolized.

Valproic acid is structurally unrelated to any of the other anticonvulsants. Its analgesic mechanism of action is unknown, but valproic acid increases GABAergic neurotransmission, increases brain GABA, and alters brain levels of excitatory amino acids (Cutrer et al. 1997). Valproic acid has proved useful in the prophylaxis of migraine in controlled clinical trials (Silberstein 1996). Although one study found no effect of valproate in central pain compared to placebo, only amitriptyline has been reported effective in a controlled trial for this condition (Drewes et al. 1994). In an open-label study, Peiris et al. reported partial or complete control of trigeminal neuralgia in 9 of 20 patients with valproic acid in doses of up to 1200 mg/day (Peiris et al. 1980). No plasma level therapeutic range has been established for pain control with valproic acid. Side effects and potentially serious toxicity have greatly limited its use for chronic pain. The combination of sedation, GI side effects, hair loss (usually reversible), abnormal liver function tests, potentially fatal hepatotoxicity, inhibition of platelet aggregation, drug-drug interactions, and numerous other potential hematologic and nonhematologic effects make pretreatment screening and close follow-up mandatory.

OPIOIDS

Beginning in the early 1980s, the long-held view that opioids were useless for chronic neuropathic pain was challenged by uncontrolled and mostly retrospective reports that opioids were effective as long-term therapy for nonmalignant pain (including neuropathic pain) with a low risk of addiction (Maruta et al. 1979; Porter and Jick 1980; Taub 1982; France et al. 1984; Portenoy and Foley 1986; Urban et al. 1986; Watson CPN 1988; Wall 1990).

STUDIES OF INTRAVENOUS OPIOID ADMINISTRATION

In 1988, Arnér and Meyerson set off a lively debate with an article entitled "Lack of analgesic effect of opioids on neuropathic and idiopathic forms of pain." In it they presented the results of a complex, randomized, double-blind, placebo-controlled trial of i.v. opioids in patients with nociceptive visceral pain (n = 15), neuropathic pain (n = 12), and "idiopathic" pain (pain of unknown etiology, n = 21). The 12 patients with neuropathic pain had long histories of "severely incapacitating pain which had resisted all previous treatments," including opioids, and were scheduled for placement of electrodes for deep brain stimulation. The nociceptive group reported dramatic pain reduction with opioid infusion (87% reduction in VAS) compared to saline placebo (17% reduction). The neuropathic and idiopathic pain groups did not experience pain relief from opioids. In 1990, Portenoy and colleagues published a comprehensive review of the concept of opioid responsiveness supported by data from uncontrolled infusions of various opioids in patients with neuropathic pain, primarily of malignant origin. They proposed a continuum of opioid responsiveness in which patients with neuropathic pain may simply require higher drug doses to experience analgesia.

Controlled evidence showing that neuropathic pain is responsive to i.v. opioid administration first appeared in 1991 and now includes four studies. In the first, we performed a three-session, double-blind, crossover study comparing 1-hour i.v. infusions of 0.3 mg/kg of morphine (average total dose of 19.2 mg), lidocaine 5 mg/kg (average total dose of 316 mg), and saline placebo in 19 patients with established PHN (Rowbotham et al. 1991). Pre-infusion pain intensity VAS ratings declined by 33% during the morphine sessions, compared to a 13% decline during the placebo sessions. Subsequently, Kupers and colleagues reported the effect of i.v. morphine 0.3 mg/kg and saline placebo in a two-session crossover study of patients with pain of central and peripheral neuropathic origin and a small group of idiopathic pain patients (Kupers et al. 1991). They hypothesized that the primary reason patients with pain consumed opioids long term was for their mood-changing effects. Therefore, they used a modification of the McGill Pain Questionnaire to train subjects to separately rate the affective (unpleasantness) and sensory (intensity) components of persistent pain. Affective pain ratings decreased significantly in both groups of neuropathic pain patients, but sensory pain ratings were unchanged. The group with idiopathic pain demonstrated no change in either aspect of pain. We have reported preliminary results of a two-session, random-order, double-blind, placebo-controlled study of intravenous fentanyl (total dose 5.4 μg/kg) in patients with PHN (Wilsey et al. 1997). Pain intensity, allodynia severity, and skin surface area demonstrating allodynia were all reduced by fentanyl independent of side-effect severity. The largest study to date is the two-session crossover trial reported by Dellemijn and Vanneste (1997). In 50 patients with different types of pain, they compared the analgesic effect of i.v. fentanyl with either saline placebo or the benzodiazepine diazepam. Diazepam was included as a control agent in the belief that it would modulate the subject's emotional experience of pain without producing intrinsic analgesic effects. Each infusion lasted a total of 5 hours, fentanyl at a rate of 5 $\mu g \cdot kg^{-1} \cdot h^{-1}$ and diazepam at a rate of 0.2 $mg \cdot kg^{-1} \cdot h^{-1}$. Fentanyl reduced both the affective and sensory dimensions of pain, with a maximum 65% pain reduction with fentanyl compared to 15–20% for control infusions. Diazepam produced sedation that was nearly as great as with fentanyl, but was no more effective in relieving pain than was saline placebo. Dellemijn and Vanneste's study is especially important because they specifically controlled for the sedating effects of opioids by including a benzodiazepine. Together, these four studies provide compelling evidence in favor of a specific analgesic effect of opioids on both the intensity and the unpleasantness of neuropathic pain.

CONTROLLED STUDIES OF ORAL OPIOID ADMINISTRATION

The three prospective, placebo-controlled trials of oral opioids for neuropathic pain that have been published in full form during the last 2 years have all shown benefit (Harati et al. 1998; Watson and Babul 1998; Sindrup et al. 1999). The drugs studied, oxycodone and tramadol, together comprise a significant percentage of the oral opioid market in the United States. Oxycodone is a typical μ-opioid agonist of moderate potency. Tramadol is an atypical drug that shows low-affinity binding to μ-opioid receptors and weak inhibition of norepinephrine and serotonin reuptake. Tramadol is FDA-approved for use in the United States for "moderate to moderately severe" pain. It remains unsettled how much mechanisms other than μ-opioid receptor binding contribute to overall pain reduction with tramadol.

Watson and Babul (1998) described a random-order, crossover trial of twice-daily controlled-release oxycodone in 50 patients with PHN. Treatment periods were 4 weeks. The 45% of subjects with prior opioid experience (typically acetaminophen-codeine or acetaminophen-oxycodone combinations) abstained from all opioid use for at least 7 days before study entry. At randomization, subjects began with either placebo or 10 mg oxycodone twice a day and titrated at weekly intervals up to a maximum of 30 mg twice a day. A total of 38 subjects completed the trial (dropout rate = 24%). Outcomes in the 12 dropouts were not reported, and only data from completing subjects were analyzed. Completing subjects achieved a mean total daily oxycodone intake of 45 mg. Overall pain intensity VAS during the last week of treatment was 54 mm during treatment with placebo and 35 mm during treatment with oxycodone. Mean pain relief ratings on a six-point scale were "moderate" with oxycodone compared to "slight" with placebo. Not surprisingly, significantly more adverse events were reported during oxycodone therapy, particularly constipation, nausea, and sedation. Despite the greater reduction of pain during oxycodone therapy, no treatment differences were seen on the Beck Depression Inventory or on any of the six scales of the Profile of Mood States. Given the planned dose escalation during a treatment period of only 4 weeks, tolerance was not expected and was not evident.

Two randomized, placebo-controlled trials have examined use of the atypical opioid tramadol for neuropathic pain. Harati and co-workers (1998) reported the results of a 6–week, multicenter, parallel design study in 131 subjects with chronic neuropathic pain due to distal symmetric diabetic neuropathy. A total of 82 subjects completed the study (dropout rate = 37%), and took a mean dose of 210 mg/day of tramadol. More "adverse event" drops occurred in the tramadol group, and more "lack of efficacy" drops in the placebo group. In contrast to the Watson and Babul study, this one used an intent-to-treat data analysis. Subjects treated with tramadol had significantly less pain and greater pain relief at all time points from day 14 of treatment to day 42 at the end of the treatment period. Pain intensity on a 5-point Likert scale was reduced from 2.5 to 1.4, compared to a change from 2.6 to 2.2 for those subjects assigned to placebo. Tramadol produced "moderate" relief, compared to "slight" relief with placebo. Tramadol therapy did not improve sleep, current health perception, psychological distress, and overall role functioning scales. Sindrup and co-workers recently reported a crossover study in 45 patients with polyneuropathy of diverse etiologies (Sindrup et al. 1999). The total noncompletion rate was 25%, with seven of nine adverse event drop-outs during tramadol treatment. Data analysis on the 34 subjects completing the trial showed that tramadol reduced pain by approximately 33% (compared to no change in pain during placebo) at a mean dose of 347 mg/day. Reductions in spontaneous and touch-evoked pain were both significant and correlated with each other during tramadol treatment.

As tolerance is a major concern of clinicians, more data need to be gathered prospectively on the importance of this issue in clinical practice. Except for a study of chronic musculoskeletal pain by Moulin et al., the blinded trials have either used short treatment periods of 4–6 weeks or did not search for evidence of tolerance development (Moulin et al. 1996). Although animal studies can demonstrate near complete loss of antinociceptive effects in as little as 24–48 hours during continuous opioid administration, the clinical implications are uncertain. If humans with chronic pain showed loss of analgesia comparable to that seen in the animal studies, opioids would be useless as chronic therapy. The studies of i.v. and oral opioids for neuropathic pain provide persuasive evidence that neuropathic pain of peripheral nervous system origin *is* opioid responsive. For pain of CNS origin, more study is needed. It is surprising that we have so little evidence from controlled studies to support opioid therapy for chronic nonmalignant pain that is non-neuropathic in origin. Although opioids are likely to remain a controversial therapy for chronic neuropathic pain, the evidence accumulated thus far suggests opioids have efficacy comparable to the best available antidepressants and anticonvulsants (Dellemijn 1999; Rowbotham 1999).

TOPICAL AGENTS

A thorough review of all the topical agents tested for treatment of neuropathic pain is beyond the scope of this paper (Kingery 1997). PHN has received far more study than any other neuropathic pain disorder. Topical capsaicin has been intensively studied, albeit with conflicting results (Watson et al. 1993; Rowbotham 1994; Watson 1994). Topical aspirin and nonsteroidal anti-inflammatory drugs (NSAIDs) have undergone limited study, with encouraging initial results but little in the way of long-term controlled treatment studies (DeBenedittis et al. 1992; King 1993). Topical lidocaine for the problem of PHN has received substantial study since the first uncontrolled trial by Rowbotham and Fields (1989a) showed benefit. In 1999, the FDA approved lidocaine patches for the specific indication of PHN.

The evidence in favor of topical lidocaine for PHN comes from four double-blind, randomized, vehicle-controlled trials. The first study was a three-session crossover evaluation of 10% topical lidocaine gel in 39 patients with established PHN (Rowbotham et al. 1995) In all three sessions, subjects had gel applied under an occlusive dressing on both the painful area and the contralateral mirror-image skin. Sessions consisted of lidocaine application on PHN skin + vehicle on mirror-image skin; vehicle on PHN skin + lidocaine on mirror-image skin (a control for systemic absorption of lidocaine as the basis for pain relief); and a session of vehicle application bilaterally. Pain reduction was significantly greater when lidocaine was applied directly on painful skin. The second study was a four-session crossover trial of lidocaine patches in 35 PHN patients (Rowbotham et al. 1996a). In two sessions, subjects wore lidocaine patches on the painful skin area for 12 hours. In one session subjects wore the vehicle patch on their painful area. One session was a "no treatment" reference session. Active lidocaine patches were superior to vehicle patches at all time points beyond 4 hours. Vehicle alone had a significant pain-reducing effect compared with "no treatment," presumably due to protection of painfully sensitive skin from contact with clothing and gentle touch.

The third study was a longer term trial in 150 subjects treated for 3 weeks with either lidocaine (n = 100) or vehicle (n = 50) patches after two full-day laboratory sessions in which acute pain-reducing effects, blood levels, and sensory effects of patch application were assessed (Rowbotham et al. 1996b). A multivariate analysis demonstrated the superiority of active patches to vehicle patches; more than 60% of subjects assigned to the lidocaine patch group achieved "moderate" or better pain relief. Lidocaine blood levels were well below the minimum concentration needed for systemic antiarrhythmic effects in all three studies. The fourth study used an "enriched enrollment" design to determine the value of the lidocaine component of the patch formulation in a group of 32 PHN patients with "moderate" or better pain relief during long-term, open-label patch use (Galer et al. 1999) The crossover two-period design used "time to exit" as the primary efficacy variable. Subjects exited the treatment period if pain control significantly deteriorated for two consecutive days. Subjects continued blinded lidocaine patch application for the full 14 days of planned treatment, but exited vehicle patch treatment after a mean of only 3.8 days. Collectively, these studies indicate lidocaine patches are an effective treatment strategy for PHN through a direct effect of the local anesthetic and a "protective" effect of the patch vehicle on painfully sensitive skin.

FROM CLINICAL TRIALS TO CLINICAL PRACTICE

Clinical trials recruit patients who are motivated to try new therapies and can meet strict medical, psychological, and diagnostic entry criteria. The highly artificial setting of the clinical trial can serve to sharpen the distinction between active and inactive drugs. For example, clinical trials typically require study participants to withdraw from most or all of their other analgesics before they receive either the study drug or placebo. Response rates in clinical trials can also be misleadingly high when the data analysis scheme does not include subjects not completing the trial. In clinical trials, subjects who voluntarily discontinue participation usually do so because of a lack of relief, unpleasant side effects, or both; i.e., they failed to achieve meaningful benefit. The more conservative intent-to-treat (ITT) data analysis is preferred because it includes *all* drug-exposed subjects in the outcome analysis. ITT analyses were rare in the analgesic trials of the 1980s and early 1990s, including those involving tricyclic antidepressants. ITT analyses are now common, especially in pharmaceutical company-sponsored multicenter trials of new analgesics.

Few studies have directly compared the different medication classes. Instead, meta-analyses have rated the quality of clinical trials and used standardized calculations to estimate efficacy and risk. Calculations that consider the observed effects of the control (placebo) therapy on pain and in producing adverse effects, such as number needed to treat (NNT) and number needed to harm (NNH), are important advances (McQuay et al. 1995, 1996; Kingery 1997). However, estimates of NNT and NNH may still overstate benefit and minimize the impact of unpleasant but nonhazardous side effects because they cannot be readily adjusted if the trial report does not include results in noncompleting subjects. What is also difficult to evaluate in a meta-analysis are aspects of the individual research designs that could have subtly "enriched" the subject population toward likely treatment responders or inadvertently biased the study against showing benefit of the experimental treatment.

The best medications in each of the four categories discussed above provided satisfactory pain relief (defined as a 50% or greater reduction in pain intensity or "moderate" pain relief) in 50–60% of clinical trial subjects. In practice, response rates are likely to be lower. The probability of "complete" relief with a single drug is on the order of only 10–20%. This undoubtedly explains why polypharmacy is the rule rather than the exception in the clinic. Few prospective data address the overall success of polypharmacy regimens. As new compounds with highly selective mechanisms of action are proven effective, multidrug regimens may be even more necessary to maximize pain control.

In clinical practice, the physician must choose which medication category to try first in a particular patient and, if necessary, construct a polypharmacy regimen. Topical lidocaine patches for PHN represents a special case because the drug delivery vehicle is itself therapeutic and this treatment has a low likelihood of systemic side effects. For the oral medications, no compelling reason favors one medication category over the others. Opioids, tricyclic antidepressants, and gabapentin have comparable response rates. Unfortunately, all three also pose a significant possibility of producing sedation or other untoward effects on cognition.

THE FUTURE: MATCHING PATIENTS WITH THERAPIES

Three strategies can be pursued to expand the range of therapeutic options and better match patients with therapies: (1) use human experimental pain models that mimic clinical phenomena, (2) use i.v. infusion regimens to test potential therapies in patients prior to longer term trials of the analogous oral agents, and (3) develop a pain mechanism-based approach to therapy as an alternative to the current diagnosis-based treatment approach.

Human experimental pain models can play an important role in the study of pain mechanisms and in the testing of new analgesic drugs (Petersen 1997). The current path of testing new analgesic drugs moves from animal experimental pain models to pharmacokinetic and tolerability studies in healthy volunteers. Costly clinical trials in pain patients are then initiated without proof in healthy volunteers that the drug to be tested has analgesic activity. Therefore, a reliable noninvasive human experimental pain model that shares features with clinical pains could bridge the gap between experimental pain in animals and acute and chronic pain in humans. Some models focus on pain detection and pain tolerance thresholds to ascending stimuli. Others focus on perceived painfulness of short-duration repetitive stimulation near or above the pain threshold produced by thermal probes, pressure algometry, lasers, or electrical stimulation. Both methods provide information about neural processing of an acute noxious input. Although production of cutaneous secondary hyperalgesia may occur, it is not an intended effect.

A third category of human experimental models simulates clinical pain conditions by intentionally inducing temporary cutaneous hyperalgesia with either thermal or chemical stimulation or a combination of both. Such models offer information about temporary inflammatory changes and sensitization of both the peripheral and the central nervous system (Raja et al. 1988; LaMotte et al. 1992; Treede et al. 1992). The capsaicin injection, burn injury, and heat/capsaicin sensitization models are examples of skin-based models, and to a limited extent each has been used to assess the analgesic activity of a variety of drugs in clinical use. (LaMotte et al. 1991; Dahl et al. 1993; Petersen et al. 1997; Petersen and Rowbotham 1999). Other models focus on of muscle and visceral hyperalgesia (Arendt-Nielsen 1997; Arendt-Nielsen et al. 1998). For obvious ethical reasons there are no human models of experimental nerve injury. Thus far, human models have been little used to test experimental compounds that are still in the early phases of development.

An i.v. drug infusion of a highly selective drug may be a useful way to predict the long-term therapeutic response to the analogous oral agent. The response to intravenous lidocaine partially predicts response to oral local anesthetics for arrhythmia control (Murray et al. 1989). However, the evidence that the lidocaine infusion test is useful in predicting analgesic response to analogous oral medications is limited to one small blinded prospective study (Galer et al. 1996). In this study, patients with peripheral neuropathy pain received high and low-dose lidocaine infusions followed by open-label treatment with oral mexiletine titrated to a maximum dose of

1200 mg/day or to side effects. Pain relief with lidocaine and pain relief with mexiletine were positively correlated. As only nine subjects were studied, the results need to be confirmed in a large-scale, randomized, double-blind study. As lidocaine is also a potent anticonvulsant medication when given systemically, central actions independent of modulation of ectopic impulse generation in dysfunctional peripheral nerve fibers need to be considered. The applicability of this general approach remains limited by the number of available pairs of selective i.v. drugs that have closely analogous oral compounds.

As proposed by Woolf, Bennett, Koltzenburg, and others, a change from the current classifications of pain based on disease, duration, and location, to a mechanism-based classification is overdue (Woolf et al. 1998; Woolf and Decosterd 1999). By identifying in individual patients the neural mechanisms responsible for their pain, we can employ treatment specifically targeting those mechanisms. This shift in paradigm will require knowing the mechanisms involved in a patient's pain. Substantial research will be needed to develop and validate new pain assessment tools.

The greatest progress along this line has come from the study and treatment of PHN. The clinical mechanisms underlying PHN pain have been evaluated using every available method (thermal/mechanical quantitative sensory testing, EMG, allodynia assessment, infrared thermography, response to provocative tests of epinephrine/histamine injection and capsaicin application, response to inactivation of cutaneous nociceptors with local anesthetic skin infiltration, and skin biopsy) except microneurography (Rowbotham and Fields 1989b, 1996; Baron and Saguer 1993; Rowbotham et al. 1996c, 1999; Baron et al. 1997; Choi and Rowbotham 1997; Haanpää et al. 1998, 1999; Oaklander et al. 1998). Based on the results of these studies, we have proposed that the pain in a person with PHN derives to varying degrees from at least two different mechanisms (Fields et al. 1998; Rowbotham et al. 1998b). These mechanisms are not mutually exclusive and likely co-exist in most PHN patients. At one end are "irritable nociceptors," dysfunctional primary afferents connected to both peripheral and central targets, with abnormal afferent input maintaining a sensitized CNS. Patients with this type of PHN have little or no sensory loss, prominent allodynia, and achieve relief with local anesthetic skin infiltration. At the other end are the results of deafferentation profound enough to result in anatomical reorganization of the CNS. Patients with this type of PHN have marked sensory loss, variable allodynia, and no response to local anesthetic skin infiltration. In 17 patients with PHN we have tested the hypothesis that input from preserved, but "irritable" nociceptors maintains pain, allodynia, and a chronic state of sensitization of central pain-transmitting neurons (Rowbotham et al. 1999). We characterized subjects by assessment of pain, allodynia, thermal sensory function, cutaneous innervation, and response to controlled application of 0.075% capsaicin. Capsaicin application resulted in increased PHN pain and allodynia in 11 subjects. At baseline, the "capsaicin responders" were characterized by higher average daily pain, preserved sensory function, and higher allodynia ratings than were nonresponders. In three of the "capsaicin responders" the area of allodynia expanded into skin that had normal sensory function and cutaneous innervation. These observations are evidence that the allodynia in some PHN patients is a form of chronic cutaneous secondary hyperalgesia maintained by "irritable nociceptors."

Evidence of "irritable nociceptors" and the effects of deafferentation have been inferred from clinical examination and provocative tests in individual pain patients with other types of neuropathic pain. If clinical practice is to change from disease-based treatment to mechanism-based treatment, it will be necessary to show that the mechanism-based approach produces better results. We need clinical trials using target-selective drugs in subject cohorts who have had their pain "dissected" into its component mechanisms. No clinical drug trials reported to date have used detailed testing of this scope in the subject screening phase.

In conclusion, our understanding of the neurobiology of pain, the mechanisms underlying neuropathic pain, and the clinical management of neuropathic pain disorders has greatly improved in the past decade. The efficacy of several medication classes has been confirmed in randomized controlled trials. Much work remains to be done to expand the list of treatments proven through controlled trials, determine "first-choice" treatments through head-to-head comparison studies, and test the value of polypharmacy regimens. Tools (such as i.v. infusion tests and mechanism-based pain classifications) that can improve treatment by effectively matching individual patients with therapies need validation through prospective studies.

ACKNOWLEDGMENTS

This work was supported by NINDS 21445. Dr. Petersen is supported by the VZV Education and Research Foundation. Dr. Rowbotham's current or past pharmaceutical industry support for research or consulting includes Algos, Asta-Medica, Astra Zeneca, Bristol Myers Squibb, Endo, Glaxo Wellcome, Hind Health Care, Merck, Parke-Davis, and Wyeth-Ayerst.

REFERENCES

Albert HH. Infusion therapy of acute trigeminal neuralgia using phenytoin i.v., MMW. *Muench Med Wochenschr* 1978; 120:529–530.

Arendt-Nielsen L. Induction and assessment of experimental pain from human skin, muscle, and viscera. In: Jensen TS, Turner JA, Wiesenfeld-Hallin Z (Eds). *Proceedings of the 8th World Congress on Pain,* Progress in Pain Research and Management, Vol. 8. Seattle: IASP Press, 1997, pp 393–425.

Arendt-Nielsen, L, Graven-Nielsen T, Drewes AD. Referred pain and hyperalgesia related to muscle and visceral pain. *IASP Newsletter*, Technical Corner (Jan/Feb) 1998, 3–6.

Arnér S, Meyerson BA. Lack of analgesic effect of opioids on neuropathic and idiopathic forms of pain. *Pain* 1988; 33:11–23.

Backonja M, Beydoun A, Edwards KR, et al. Gabapentin for the symptomatic treatment of painful neuropathy in patients with diabetes mellitus: a randomized controlled trial. *JAMA* 1998; 280:1831–1836.

Bajwa ZH, Sami N, Warfield CA, Wootton J. Topiramate relieves refractory intercostal neuralgia. *Neurology* 1999; 52:1917.

Baron R, Saguer M. Postherpetic neuralgia. Are C-nociceptors involved in signalling and maintenance of tactile allodynia? *Brain* 1993; 116:1477–1496.

Baron R, Haendler G, Schulte H. Afferent large fiber polyneuropathy predicts the development of postherpetic neuralgia. *Pain* 1997; 73:231–238.

Bonica JJ. *The Management of Pain, with Special Emphasis on the Use of Analgesic Block in Diagnosis, Prognosis, and Therapy.* Philadelphia: Lea & Febiger, 1953, p 1533.

Bonicalzi V. Canavero S. Cerutti F, et al. Lamotrigine reduces total postoperative analgesic requirement: a randomized double-blind, placebo-controlled pilot study. *Surgery* 1997; 122:567–670.

Burchiel KJ. Carbamazepine inhibits spontaneous activity in experimental neuromas. *Exp Neurol* 1988; 102:249–253.

Campbell FG, Graham JG, Zilkha KJ. Clinical trial of carbazepine (tegretol) in trigeminal neuralgia. *J Neurol Neurosurg Psychiatry* 1966; 29:265–267.

Campbell JN, Raja SN, Meyer RA, Mackinnon SE. Myelinated afferents signal the hyperalgesia associated with nerve injury. *Pain* 1988; 32:89–94.

Canavero S, Bonicalzi V. Lamotrigine control of central pain. *Pain* 1996; 68:179–181.

Catterall WA. Common modes of drug action on Na+ channels: local anaesthetics, antiarrhythmics, and anti-convulsants. *Trends Pharmacol Sci* 1987; 57–65.

Chabal C, Jacobson L, Mariano A, Chaney E, Britell CW. The use of oral mexiletine for the treatment of pain after peripheral nerve injury. *Anesthesiology* 1992; 76:513–517.

Chadda VS, Mathur MS. Double blind study of the effects of diphenylhydantoin sodium on diabetic neuropathy. *J Assoc Physicians India* 1978; 26:403–406.

Cheung H, Kamp D, Harris E. An in vitro investigation of the action of lamotrigine on neuronal voltage-activated sodium channels. *Epilepsy Res* 1992; 13:107–112.

Choi B, Rowbotham MC. Effect of adrenergic receptor activation on post-herpetic neuralgia pain and sensory disturbances. *Pain* 1997; 69:55–63.

Cline MA, Ochoa J, Torebjörk HE. Chronic hyperalgesia and skin warming caused by sensitized C nociceptors. *Brain* 1989; 112:621–647.

Cutrer FM, Limmroth V, Moskowitz MA. Possible mechanisms of valproate in migraine prophylaxis. *Cephalalgia* 1997; 17:93–100.

Dahl JB, Brennum J, Arendt-Nielsen L, Jensen TS, Kehlet H. The effect of pre- versus postinjury infiltration with lidocaine on thermal and mechanical hyperalgesia after heat injury to the skin. *Pain* 1993; 53:43–51.

DeBenedittis G, Besana F, Lorenzetti A. A new topical treatment for acute herpetic neuralgia and postherpetic neuralgia: the aspirin/diethyl ether mixture. An open-label study plus a double-blind controlled clinical trial. *Pain* 1992; 48:383–390.

Deffois A, Fage D, Carter C. Inhibition of synaptosomal veratridine-induced sodium influx by antidepressants and neuroleptics used in chronic pain. *Neurosci Lett* 1996; 220:117–120.

Dejgard A, Petersen P, Kastrup J. Mexiletine for treatment of chronic painful diabetic neuropathy. *Lancet* 1988; 1:9–11.

Dellemijn P. Randomized double-blind active-placebo-controlled crossover trial of intravenous fentanyl in neuropathic pain. *Lancet* 1997; 349:753–758.

Dellemijn P. Are opioids effective in relieving neuropathic pain? *Pain* 1999; 80:453–462.

Devor M, Seltzer Z. Pathophysiology of damaged nerves in relation to chronic pain. In: Wall PD, Melzack R (Eds). *Textbook of Pain,* 4th ed. Edinburgh: Churchill Livingstone, 1999, pp 129–164.

Drewes AM, Andreasen A, Poulsen LH. Valproate for treatment of chronic central pain after spinal cord injury. A double-blind cross-over study. *Paraplegia* 1994; 32:565–569.

Dunsker SB, Mayfield FH. Carbamazepine in the treatment of the flashing pain syndrome. *J Neurosurg* 1976; 45:49–51.

Eisenberg E, Alon N. Lamotrigine in the treatment of painful diabetic neuropathy. *Abstracts: 8th World Congress on Pain.* Seattle: IASP Press, 1996, p 372.

Fields HL, Rowbotham MC, Devor M. Excitability blockers: anticonvulsants and low concentration local anesthetics in the treatment of chronic pain. In: Dickenson A, Besson JM (Eds). *Handbook of Experimental Pharmacology.* Berlin: Springer-Verlag, 1997, pp 93–116.

Fields HL, Rowbotham M, Baron R. Postherpetic neuralgia: irritable nociceptors and deafferentation. *Neurobiol Dis* 1998; 5:209–227.

France RD, Urban BJ, Keefe FJ. Long-term use of narcotic analgesics in chronic pain. *Soc Sci Med* 1984; 19:1379–1382.

Galer BS, Harle J, Rowbotham MC. Response to intravenous lidocaine infusion predicts subsequent response to oral mexiletine: a prospective study. *J Pain Symptom Manage* 1996; 12:161–167.

Galer BS, Rowbotham MC, Perander J, Friedman E. Topical lidocaine patch relieves postherpetic neuralgia more effectively than a vehicle topical patch: results of an enriched enrollment study. *Pain* 1999; 80:533–538.

Gee NS, Brown JP, Dissanayake VU. The novel anticonvulsant drug, gabapentin (Neurontin), binds to the alpha$_2$delta subunit of a calcium channel. *J Biol Chem* 1996; 271:5768–5776.

Haanpää M, Dastidar P, Weinberg A. CSF and MRI findings in patients with acute herpes zoster. *Neurology* 1998; 51:1405–1411.

Haanpää M, Laippala P, Nurmikko T. Pain and somatosensory dysfunction in acute herpes zoster. *Clin J Pain* 1999; 15:78–84.

Harati Y, Gooch C, Swenson M, et al. Double-blind randomized trial of tramadol for the treatment of the pain of diabetic neuropathy. *Neurology* 1998; 50:1842–1846.

Harbison J, Dennehy F, Keating D. Lamotrigine for pain with hyperalgesia. *Ir Med J* 1997; 90:56.

Honmou O, Kocsis JD, Richerson GB. Gabapentin potentiates the conductance increase induced by nipecotic acid in CA1 pyramidal neurons in vitro. *Epilepsy Res* 1995; 20:193–202.

Hunter JC, Gogas KR, Hedley LR. The effect of novel anti-epileptic drugs in rat experimental models of acute and chronic pain. *Eur J Pharmacol* 1997; 324:153–160.

Iannone A, Baker AB, Morrell F. Dilantin in the treatment of trigeminal neuralgia. *Neurology* 1958; 126–128.

Jones MW. Topiramate—safety and tolerability. *Can J Neurol Sci* 1998; 25:S13–S15.

Kajander KC. Wakisaka S, Bennett GJ. Spontaneous discharge originates in the dorsal root ganglion at the onset of a painful peripheral neuropathy in the rat. *Neurosci Lett* 1992; 138:225–228.

Kapur S, Mieczkowski T, Mann JJ. Antidepressant medications and the relative risk of suicide attempt and suicide. *JAMA* 1992; 268:3441–3445.

Kemper CA, Kent G, Burton S, Deresinski SC. Mexiletine for HIV-infected patients with painful peripheral neuropathy: a double-blind, placebo-controlled, crossover treatment trial. *J Acquir Immune Defic Syndr Hum Retrovirol* 1998; 19:367–372.

Kieburtz K, Simpson D, Yiannoutsos C, et al. A randomized trial of amitriptyline and mexiletine for painful neuropathy in HIV infection. AIDS Clinical Trial Group 242 Protocol Team. *Neurology* 1998; 51:1682–1688.

King RB. Topical aspirin in chloroform and the relief of pain due to herpes zoster and postherpetic neuralgia. *Arch Neurol* 1993; 50:1046–1053.

Kingery WS. A critical review of controlled clinical trials for peripheral neuropathic pain and complex regional pain syndromes. *Pain* 1997; 73:123–139.

Kirk EJ. Impulses in dorsal spinal nerve rootlets in cats and rabbits arising from dorsal root ganglia isolated from the periphery. *J Comp Neurol* 1974; 155:165–175.

Kupers RC, Konings H, Adriaensen H, Gybels JM. Morphine differentially affects the sensory and affective pain ratings in neurogenic and idiopathic forms of pain. *Pain* 1991; 47:5–12.

LaMotte RH, Shain CN, Simone DA, Tsai EF. Neurogenic hyperalgesia: psychophysical studies of underlying mechanisms. *J Neurophysiol* 1991; 66:190–211.

LaMotte RH, Lundberg LE, Torebjörk HE. Pain, hyperalgesia and activity in nociceptive C units in humans after intradermal injection of capsaicin. *J Physiol* 1992; 448:749–764.

Leijon G, Boivie J. Central post-stroke pain—a controlled trial of amitriptyline and carbamazepine. *Pain* 1989; 36:27–36.

Lindstrom P, Lindblom U. The analgesic effect of tocainide in trigeminal neuralgia. *Pain* 1987; 28:45–50.

Lockman LA, Hunninghake DB, Krivit W, Desnick RJ. Relief of pain of Fabry's disease by diphenylhydantoin. *Neurology* 1973; 23:871–875.

Lunardi G, Leandri M, Albano C, et al. Clinical effectiveness of lamotrigine and plasma levels in essential and symptomatic trigeminal neuralgia. *Neurology* 1997; 48:1714–1717.

Magnus-Miller L, Podolnick P, Mathew NT. Efficacy and safety of gabapentin (neurontin) in migraine prophylaxis. 17th Annual Scientific Meeting of the American Pain Society, Houston Headache Clinic, 1998.

Maruta T, Swanson D, Finlayson R. Drug abuse and dependency in patients with chronic pain. *Mayo Clin Proc* 1979; 54:241–244.

Max MB, Culnane M, Schafer SC, et al. Amitriptyline relieves diabetic neuropathy pain in patients with normal or depressed mood. *Neurology* 1987; 37:589–596.

Max MB, Lynch SA, Muir J, et al. Effects of desipramine, amitriptyline, and fluoxetine on pain in diabetic neuropathy. *N Engl J Med* 1992; 326:1250–1256.

McCleane G. 200 mg daily of lamotrigine has no analgesic effect in neuropathic pain: a randomised, double-blind, placebo controlled trial. *Pain* 1999; 83:105–107.

McQuay H, Carroll D, Jadad AR, Wiffen P, Moore A. Anticonvulsant drugs for management of pain: a systematic review. *BMJ* 1995; 311:1047–1052.

McQuay HJ, Tramer M, Nye BA, et al. A systematic review of antidepressants in neuropathic pain. *Pain* 1996; 68:217–227.

Mellick GA, Mellicy LB, Mellick LB. Gabapentin in the management of reflex sympathetic dystrophy. *J Pain Symptom Manage* 1995; 10:265–266.

Moulin DE, Iezzi A, Amireh R, et al. Randomised trial of oral morphine for chronic non-cancer pain. *Lancet* 1996; 347:143–147.

Murray KT, Barbey JT, Kopelman HA, et al. Mexiletine and tocainide: a comparison of antiarrhythmic efficacy, adverse effects, and predictive value of lidocaine testing. *Clin Pharmacol Ther* 1989; 45:553–561.

Nakamura-Craig M, Follenfant RL. Effect of lamotrigine in the acute and chronic hyperalgesia induced by PGE2 and in the chronic hyperalgesia in rats with streptozotocin-induced diabetes. *Pain* 1995; 63:33–37.

Nicol CF. A four year double-blind study of tegretol in facial pain. *Headache* 1969; 9:54–57.

Nordin M, Nystrom B, Wallin U, Hagbarth KE. Ectopic sensory discharges and paresthesiae in patients with disorders of peripheral nerves, dorsal roots and dorsal columns. *Pain* 1984; 20:231–245.

Oaklander AL, Romans K, Horasek S, et al. Unilateral postherpetic neuralgia is associated with bilateral sensory neuron damage. *Ann Neurol* 1998; 44:789–795.

Oskarsson P, Ljunggren JG, Lins PE. Efficacy and safety of mexiletine in the treatment of painful diabetic neuropathy. The Mexiletine Study Group. *Diabetes Care* 1997; 20:1594–1597.

Peiris JB, Perera GL, Devendra SV, Lionel ND. Sodium valproate in trigeminal neuralgia. *Med J Aust* 1980; 2:278.

Perucca E. A pharmacological and clinical review on topiramate, a new antiepileptic drug. *Pharmacol Res* 1997; 35:241–256.

Petersen KL. Experimental cutaneous hyperalgesia in humans. *IASP Newsletter,* Technical Corner (Nov/Dec) 1997; 4–8.

Petersen KL, Rowbotham MC. A new human experimental pain model: the heat/capsaicin sensitization model. *Neuroreport* 1999; 10:1511–1516.

Petersen KL, Brennum J, Dahl JB. Experimental evaluation of the analgesic effect of ibuprofen on primary and secondary hyperalgesia. *Pain* 1997; 70:167–174.

Portenoy RK, Foley KM. Chronic use of opioid analgesics in non-malignant pain: report of 38 cases. *Pain* 1986; 25:171–186.

Portenoy RK, Foley KM, Inturrisi CE. The nature of opioid responsiveness and its implications for neuropathic pain: new hypotheses derived from studies of opioid infusions. *Pain* 1990; 43:273–286.

Porter J, Jick H. Addiction rare in patients treated with narcotics. *N Engl J Med* 1980; 302:123.

Raja SN, Meyer RA, Campbell JN. Peripheral mechanisms of somatic pain. *Anesthesiology* 1988; 68:571–590.

Rockliff BW, Davis EH. Controlled sequential trials of carbamazepine in trigeminal neuralgia. *Arch Neurol* 1966; 15:129–136.

Rosenberg JM, Harrell C, Ristic H, Werner RA, de Rosayro AM. The effect of gabapentin on neuropathic pain. *Clin J Pain* 1997; 13:251–255.

Rosner H, Rubin L, Kestenbaum A. Gabapentin adjunctive therapy in neuropathic pain states. *Clin J Pain* 1996; 12:56–58.

Rowbotham MC. Postherpetic neuralgia. *Semin Neurol* 1994; 14:247–254.

Rowbotham MC. The debate over opioids and neuropathic pain. In: Kalso E, Wiesenfeld-Hallin Z, McQuay H (Eds). *Opioid Sensitivity of Chronic Noncancer Pain,* Progress in Pain Research and Management, Vol. 14. Seattle: IASP Press, 1999, pp 307–318.

Rowbotham MC, Fields HL. Topical lidocaine reduces pain in post-herpetic neuralgia. *Pain* 1989a; 38:297–301.

Rowbotham MC, Fields HL. Post-herpetic neuralgia: the relation of pain complaint, sensory disturbance, and skin temperature. *Pain* 1989b; 39:129–144.

Rowbotham MC, Fields HL. The relationship of pain, allodynia and thermal sensation in post-herpetic neuralgia. *Brain* 1996; 119:347–354.

Rowbotham MC, Reisner-Keller LA, Fields HL. Both intravenous lidocaine and morphine reduce the pain of postherpetic neuralgia. *Neurology* 1991; 41:1024–1028.

Rowbotham MC, Davies PS, Fields HL. Topical lidocaine gel relieves postherpetic neuralgia. *Ann Neurol* 1995; 37:246–253.

Rowbotham MC, Davies PS, Verkempinck C, Galer BS. Lidocaine patch: double-blind controlled study of a new treatment method for post-herpetic neuralgia. *Pain* 1996a; 65:39–44.

Rowbotham MC, Davies PS, Galer BS. Multicenter, double-blind, vehicle-controlled trial of long term use of lidocaine patches for postherpetic neuralgia. *Abstracts: 8th World Congress on Pain.* Seattle: IASP Press, 1996b.

Rowbotham MC, Yosipovitch G, Connolly MK, et al. Cutaneous innervation density in the allodynic form of postherpetic neuralgia. *Neurobiol Dis* 1996c; 3:205–214.

Rowbotham M, Harden N, Stacey B, Bernstein P, Magnus-Miller L. Gabapentin for the treatment of postherpetic neuralgia: a randomized controlled trial. *JAMA* 1998a; 280:1837–1842.

Rowbotham MC, Petersen KL, Fields HL. Is postherpetic neuralgia more than one disorder? *Pain Forum* 1998b; 7:231–237.

Rowbotham MC, Petersen KL, Sandroni P, et al. Chronic secondary hyperalgesia in some PHN patients: results of capsaicin application verified by skin biopsy. *Abstracts: 9th World Congress on Pain.* Seattle: IASP Press, 1999, p 438.

Rull JA, Quibrera R, Gonzalez-Millan H, Lozano Castaneda O. Symptomatic treatment of peripheral diabetic neuropathy with carbamazepine (Tegretol): double blind crossover trial. *Diabetologia* 1969; 5:215–218.

Silberstein SD. Divalproex sodium in headache: literature review and clinical guidelines. *Headache* 1996; 36:547–555.

Sindrup SH, Brosen K, Gram LF. Antidepressants in pain treatment: antidepressant or analgesic effect? *Clin Neuropharmacol* 1992a; 15:636A–637A.

Sindrup SH, Brosen K, Gram LF. The mechanism of action of antidepressants in pain treatment: controlled cross-over studies in diabetic neuropathy. *Clin Neuropharmacol* 1992b; 15:380A–381A.

Sindrup SH, Andersen G, Madsen C, et al. Tramadol relieves pain and allodynia in polyneuropathy: a randomised, double-blind, controlled trial. *Pain* 1999; 83:85–90.

Sinnott C, Edmonds P, Cropley I, Hanks G. Flecainide in cancer nerve pain. *Lancet* 1991; 337:1347.

Stracke H, Meyer UE, Schumacher HE, Federlin K. Mexiletine in the treatment of diabetic neuropathy. *Diabetes Care* 1992; 15:1550–1555.

Swerdlow M, Cundill JG. Anticonvulsant drugs used in the treatment of lancinating pain. A comparison. *Anaesthesia* 1981; 36:1129–1132.

Taub A. Opioid analgesics in the treatment of chronic intractable pain of non-neoplastic origin. Kitihata LM, Collins JD (Eds). *Narcotic Analgesics in Anesthesiology*. Baltimore: Williams & Wilkins, 1982; pp 199–208.

Taylor CP, Gee NS, Su TZ, et al. A summary of mechanistic hypotheses of gabapentin pharmacology. *Epilepsy Res* 1998; 29:233–249.

Teoh H, Fowler LJ, Bowery NG. Effect of lamotrigine on the electrically-evoked release of endogenous amino acids from slices of dorsal horn of the rat spinal cord. *Neuropharmacology* 1995; 34:1273–1278.

Torebjörk HE, Lundberg LE, LaMotte RH. Central changes in processing of mechanoreceptive input in capsaicin-induced secondary hyperalgesia in humans. *J Physiol (Lond)* 1992; 448:765–780.

Treede RD, Meyer RA, Raja SN, Campbell JN. Peripheral and central mechanisms of cutaneous hyperalgesia. *Prog Neurobiol* 1992; 38:397–421.

Upton N. Mechanisms of action of new antiepileptic drugs: rational design and serendipitous findings. *Trends Pharmacol Sci* 1994; 15:456–463.

Urban BJ, France RD, Steinberger EK, Scott DL, Maltbie AA. Long-term use of narcotic/antidepressant medication in the management of phantom limb pain. *Pain* 1986; 24:191–196.

Wall PD. Neuropathic pain. *Pain* 1990; 43:267–268.

Wall PD, Devor M. Sensory afferent impulses originate from dorsal root ganglia as well as from the periphery in normal and nerve injured rats. *Pain* 1983; 17:321–339.

Wall PD, Gutnick M. Properties of afferent nerve impulses originating from a neuroma. *Nature* 1974; 248:740–743.

Watson CPN. Topical capsaicin as an adjuvant analgesic. *J Pain Symptom Manage* 1994; 9:425–433.

Watson CP, Babul N. Efficacy of oxycodone in neuropathic pain: a randomized trial in postherpetic neuralgia. *Neurology* 1998; 50:1837–1841.

Watson CP, Evans RJ. A comparative trial of amitriptyline and zimelidine in post-herpetic neuralgia. *Pain* 1985; 23:387–394.

Watson CP, Evans RJ, Reed K, et al. Amitriptyline versus placebo in postherpetic neuralgia. *Neurology* 1982; 32:671–673.

Watson CP, Evans RJ, Watt VR, Birkett N. Postherpetic neuralgia: 208 cases. *Pain* 1988; 35:289–297.

Watson CP, Chipman M, Reed K, Evans RJ, Birkett N. Amitriptyline versus maprotiline in postherpetic neuralgia: a randomized, double-blind, crossover trial. *Pain* 1992; 48:29–36.

Watson CP, Tyler KL, Bickers DR, et al. A randomized vehicle-controlled trial of topical capsaicin in the treatment of postherpetic neuralgia. *Clin Ther* 1993; 15:510–526.

Watson CP, Vernich L, Chipman M, Reed K. Nortriptyline versus amitriptyline in postherpetic neuralgia: a randomized trial. *Neurology* 1998; 51:1166–1171.

Wilsey BL, Davies PS, Rowbotham MC. Changes in pain, mood, and sensation from i.v. fentanyl in patients with PHN. *Abstracts, 16th Annual Scientific Meeting,* American Pain Society, 1997, p 205.

Woolf CJ. Excitability changes in central neurons following peripheral damage. In: Willis WDJ (Ed). *Hyperalgesia and Allodynia: the Bristol-Myers-Squibb Symposium on Pain Research.* New York: Raven Press, 1992, pp 221–243.

Woolf CJ, Decosterd I. Implications of recent advances in the understanding of pain pathophysiology for the assessment of pain in patients. *Pain* 1999; (Suppl 6):S141–S147.

Woolf CJ, Bennett GJ, Doherty M. Towards a mechanism-based classification of pain? *Pain* 1998; 77:227–229.

Wright JM, Oki JC, Graves L III. Mexiletine in the symptomatic treatment of diabetic peripheral neuropathy. *Ann Pharmacother* 1997; 31:29–34.

Zakrzewska JM, Chaudhry Z, Nurmikko TJ, Patton DW, Mullens EL. Lamotrigine (lamictal) in refractory trigeminal neuralgia: results from a double-blind placebo controlled crossover trial. *Pain* 1997; 73:223–230.

Correspondence to: Michael C. Rowbotham, MD, UCSF Pain Clinical Research Center, 1701 Divisadero Street, Suite 480, San Francisco, CA 94115, USA. Tel: 415-885-7899; Fax: 415-885-7855; email: mcrwind@itsa.ucsf.edu.

Proceedings of the 9th World Congress on Pain,
Progress in Pain Research and Management,
Vol. 16, edited by M. Devor, M.C. Rowbotham, and
Z. Wiesenfeld-Hallin, IASP Press, Seattle, © 2000.

79

Lamotrigine in the Treatment of Painful Diabetic Neuropathy: A Randomized, Placebo-Controlled Study

Yael Luria,[a] Clara Brecker,[a,b] Dib Daoud,[c]
Avraham Ishay,[d] and Elon Eisenberg[a,b]

[a]*Pain Relief Unit,* [b]*Haifa Pain Research Group, and* [c]*Endocrine Institute, Rambam Medical Center, The Technion-Israel Institute of Technology, Haifa, Israel;* [d]*Endocrine Institute, Central Emek Hospital, Afula, Israel*

Abundant evidence accumulating over the past several years indicates that abnormal neural firing is a principle cause of neuropathic pain (Devor 1995). Spontaneous activity of primary afferent neurons was found in diabetic rats (Burchiel et al. 1985) and in the dorsal horn of rats with experimental peripheral neuropathy (Laired and Bennett 1993). Furthermore, evidence now shows that excitatory amino acids, particularly glutamate, play a key role in dorsal horn spinal hyperexcitability by acting at the N-methyl D-aspartate (NMDA) receptor (Dickenson and Sullivan 1987; Dubner and Ruda 1992). Lamotrigine is a novel antiepileptic agent that inhibits the release of glutamate, possibly by stabilizing the neural membrane through blocking activation of voltage-sensitive sodium channels (Cheung et al. 1992). At least two studies have demonstrated the ability of lamotrigine to reduce hyperalgesia in rats with streptozotocin-induced diabetes (Makamura-Craig and Follenfant 1994, 1995). A recent open study in humans has suggested that lamotrigine may reduce clinical painful diabetic neuropathy (Eisenberg et al. 1998). The present study was designed as a randomized, placebo-controlled trial aimed at establishing the analgesic effect of lamotrigine in painful diabetic neuropathy.

METHODS

Patients. Patients with painful diabetic neuropathy were enrolled in the study only if they met all the following criteria: (I) established clinical diabetes; (II) evidence of peripheral neuropathy indicated by at least two of the three following criteria: (1) medical history suggestive of peripheral neuropathy, (2) abnormal neurological examination, and (3) abnormal nerve conduction tests; (III) pain intensity of at least 4 on a numerical scale of 0–10; (IV) they provided written consent to participate in the study, which was approved by the hospital's Ethics Committee.

Design. Once found eligible for the study, each patient was randomly assigned to receive either lamotrigine or a placebo. Subsequent to a one-week washout period from previous analgesics, lamotrigine treatment was initiated at a dose of 25 mg daily for 2 weeks. The dose was increased to 50 mg/day for a further 2 weeks, and to 100, 200, 300, and 400 mg/day, each dose for 1 week. Patients in the placebo group received identical-looking tablets of placebo according to the same schedule. The last part of the study consisted of a 2-week post-treatment period. During the entire study period, patients were allowed to use rescue doses of simple analgesics (paracetamol, dipyrone), or a nonsteroidal anti-inflammatory drug. Both the lamotrigine and the identical-looking placebo tablets were supplied by Glaxo-Wellcome, USA.

Pain measurement. Pain measurements included self-record of pain levels on a 0–10 numerical pain scale (NPS) twice daily and daily rescue analgesic consumption. Seven office visits primarily focused on assessing adverse effects. In addition, each patient completed the McGill Pain Questionnaire (MPQ) (Melzack 1975), the Beck Depression Inventory (BDI) (Beck et al. 1961), and the Pain Disability Index (PDI) (Pollard 1984); plasma glucose and HbA1C levels were measured before and at the end of the treatment period.

Statistical analysis. SAS (SAS Institute, North Carolina, USA) was used for statistical analysis. We used repeated-measures ANOVA to analyze weekly visit measurements and Dunnett's test to compare the baseline visit (visit 2) to each subsequent visit. Daily NPS scores were averaged across weeks and analyzed in a similar way. In this case the baseline week (week 0) was compared to all subsequent weeks. MPQ, BDI, and PDI questionnaires, and glucose and HbA1C levels, were evaluated by paired t test, which compared baseline to end-of-treatment scores. Gender differences were compared by χ-square. P was considered significant at the 0.05 level. Data are presented as means ± SEM.

RESULTS

We performed an interim analysis of the first 40 patients who entered the study. Data from 34 patients who completed the study (18 in the treatment group and 16 in the placebo group) were available for analysis. Table I presents demographic data.

Spontaneous pain. A gradual drop in mean pain intensity (measured by NPS) from 6.5 ± 0.5 at the pretreatment week to a minimum of 3.8 ± 0.7 at week 8 (–46%) was found in the lamotrigine group, and a drop from 6.6 ± 0.3 to a minimum of 5.2 ± 0.5 (–22%) in the placebo group (Fig. 1). Differences in pain intensity between the two groups were significant at lamotrigine doses of 50, 200, 300, and 400 mg. A reduction of 50% or more in pain intensity was found in nine patients from the lamotrigine group and only in three from the placebo group during the last 4 weeks of treatment. Most patients did not use rescue analgesics, so we did not formally analyze their use.

Additional parameters. The MPQ, BDI, and PDI scores and the results of the laboratory tests remained unchanged in both groups (data not shown). A trend of improvement in the PDI score was noted in the lamotrigine group (a drop of 3.6 points compared to only 1.4 in the placebo group; $P = 0.07$).

Adverse events. A total of 16 and 11 adverse events were recorded in the lamotrigine and in the placebo groups, respectively (Table II). Two patients in the lamotrigine group developed allergic skin responses (rash), and one was dropped from the study during the first week of treatment. The rash in the second patient was noted at the end of the last week of treatment, so

Table I
Demographic data (mean ± SEM)

	Lamotrigine (n = 18)	Placebo (n = 16)	P	Statistics
Age (years)	53 ± 3	55 ± 2	0.3	t test (two-tailed)
Gender:				
Male	13	9	0.3	χ^2
Female	5	7		
Weight (kg)	85 ± 4	84 ± 4	0.7	t test (two-tailed)
Diabetes type:				
Non-insulin-dependent	16	15	1.0	χ^2
Insulin-dependent	2	1		
Duration of diabetes (years)	15 ± 2	9 ± 1	0.03	t test (two-tailed)
Fasting glucose (mg/dL)	202 ± 18	185 + 16	0.49	t test (two-tailed)
HbA1C (%)	7.8 ± 0.4	8.4 ± 0.5	0.01	Contrast within ANOVA

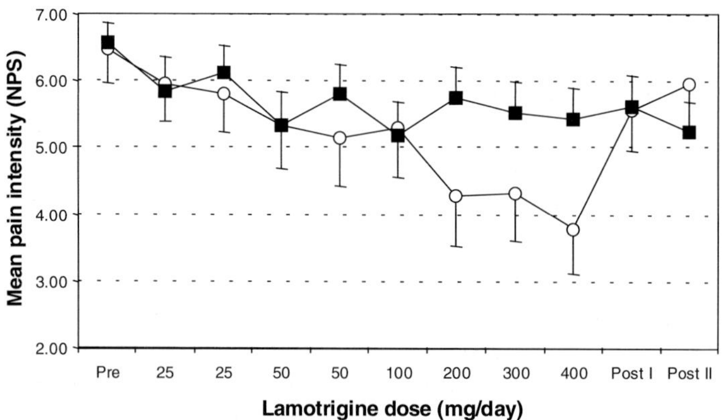

Fig. 1. Weekly pain intensity (mean ± SEM) in the lamotrigine (open labels) and placebo (dark labels) groups. $^{*}P < 0.05$.

he was able to complete the study. In both cases the rash completely resolved within a few days following the discontinuation of treatment. Altogether six patients were withdrawn from the study: two in the treatment group (one due to rash and the other for lack of compliance), and four in the placebo group (two for protocol violation, one who complained of impotence subsequent to randomization but prior to treatment, and one who asked to withdraw for "personal reasons").

DISCUSSION

The results of this study clearly show that lamotrigine offers dose-related analgesia that is significantly superior to placebo for patients with refractory painful diabetic neuropathy. Spontaneous pain rather than evoked pain was chosen to be the primary outcome measurement, as it seems to be the most troublesome symptom for these patients (Thomas and Tomlinson 1993). Evoked pain (hyperalgesia and allodynia) is not a common feature of

Table II
Adverse effects

Adverse Event	Lamotrigine	Placebo
Rash	2	0
Gastrointestinal	7	4
Headache	3	1
Drowsiness	2	3
Other	2	3
Total	16	11

diabetic neuropathy (Brown and Asbury 1984), and indeed, was only found in a few patients.

It is true that other parameters such as depression and the MPQ scores have not improved as a result of lamotrigine treatment. However, these patients have had long-lasting intractable pain, and the treatment period, at an effective dose, was relatively short. It is likely that a longer treatment period with the highest dose used in this study (400 mg), or perhaps even a higher dose, may also lead to an improvement in those parameters. No changes in the biochemical parameters (glucose and HbA1C levels) could be detected during the study period. This result further supports the working hypothesis that lamotrigine exerts its analgesic effect via neural rather than biochemical mechanisms. Finally, if slowly titrated, lamotrigine is safe and well tolerated.

ACKNOWLEDGMENTS

The study was supported by Glaxo-Wellcome, USA.

REFERENCES

Beck AT, Ward CH, Mendelson MM, Mock J, Erbaugh J. An inventory for measuring depression. *Arch General Psych* 1961; 4:561–571.

Brown MJ, Asbury AK. Diabetic neuropathy. *Ann Neurol* 1984; 15:2–12.

Burchiel KJ, Russell LC, Lee RC, Sima AFF. Spontaneous activity of primary afferent neurons in diabetic BB/Wistar rats. *Diabetes* 1985; 34:1210–1213.

Cheung H, Kamp D, Harris E. An in vitro investigation of the action of lamotrigine on neural voltage-activated sodium channels. *Epilepsy Res* 1992; 13:107–112.

Devor M. Neurobiological basis for selectivity of Na^+ channel blockers in neuropathic pain. *Pain Forum* 1995; 4:83–86.

Dickenson AH, Sullivan AF. Evidence for a role of the NMDA receptor in frequency dependent potentiation of deep dorsal horn neurons following c-fiber stimulation. *Neuropharmacology* 1987; 26:1235–1238.

Dubner R, Ruda MA. Activity dependent neural plasticity following tissue injury and inflammation. *Trends Neurosci* 1992; 14:96–103.

Eisenberg E, Alon N, Avraham I, Daud D, Yarnitski D. Lamotrigine in the treatment of diabetic neuropathy. *Eur J Neurol* 1998; 5:167–173.

Laired JMA, Bennett GJ. An electrophysiological study of dorsal horn neurons in the spinal cord of rats with an experimental peripheral neuropathy. *J Neurophysiol* 1993; 69:2072–2085.

Makamura-Craig M, Follenfant RL. Effect of lamotrigine in the acute and chronic hyperalgesia induced by PGE2 and in the chronic hyperalgesia in rats with streptozotocin-induced diabetes. *Pain* 1995; 63:33–37.

Melzack R. The McGill Pain Questionnaire. *Pain* 1975; 1:272–299.

Makamura-Craig M, Follenfant RL. Lamotrigine and analogs: a new treatment for chronic pain? In: Gebhart GF, Hammond DL, Jensen TS (Eds). *Proceedings of the 7th World Congress on Pain,* Progress in Pain Research and Management, Vol. 2. Seattle: IASP Press, 1994, pp 725–730.

Pollard CA. Preliminary validity study of the Pain Disability Index. *Percept Mot Skills* 1984; 59:974.

Thomas PK, Tomlinson DR. Diabetic and hypoglycemic neuropathy. In: Dyck PJ, Thomas PK, Griffin JW, Low PA, Poduslo JF (Eds). *Peripheral Neuropathy*, 3rd ed. Philadelphia: W.B. Saunders, 1993, pp 1219–1250.

Correspondence to: Elon Eisenberg, MD, Pain Relief Unit, Rambam Medical Center, P.O.B. 9602, Haifa 31096, Israel. Tel: 972-4-8542578; Fax: 972-4-8542880; email: L_eisenberg@rambam.health.gov.il.

Proceedings of the 9th World Congress on Pain,
Progress in Pain Research and Management,
Vol. 16, edited by M. Devor, M.C. Rowbotham, and
Z. Wiesenfeld-Hallin, IASP Press, Seattle, © 2000.

80

Effects of Intravenous Lidocaine on Spontaneous and Evoked Pains in Patients with CNS Injury

Nadine Attal,[a] Louis Brasseur,[a] Frédéric Guirimand,[a] Martine Dupuy,[a] Fabrice Parker,[b] Valérie Gaude,[a] and Didier Bouhassira[a,c]

[a]Pain Evaluation and Treatment Unit, Ambroise Paré Hospital, Boulogne, France; [b]Neurosurgery Department, Kremlin-Bicêtre Hospital, le Kremlin-Bicêtre, France; [c]INSERM U-161, Paris, France

Central pain can occur after a primary lesion or dysfunction of the central nervous system (CNS). It may have various qualities, including spontaneous pain, most often described as a burning or dysesthetic sensations. In addition to spontaneous pain, mechanical and thermal (notably cold-induced) allodynia and hyperalgesia are frequent (Casey 1991; Gonzales 1995). Treatment for such pains is usually particularly difficult, as few effective treatments are available. Some patients seem to benefit from tricyclic antidepressants and anticonvulsants (Leijon and Boivie 1989; Gonzales 1995). Systemic local anesthetics, notably lidocaine and its oral analogue mexiletine, are sometimes used for such conditions, based on results of open or single-blind trials (Awerbuch and Sandyk 1990; Backonja et al. 1992; Edmonson et al. 1993), but no placebo-controlled study has been conducted for lidocaine in relation to central pain.

Quantitative sensory tests represent a method of choice in assessing allodynia and hyperalgesia in patients with various neuropathic pain syndromes (Hansson and Lindblom 1992). This approach has been rarely used to assess the efficacy of pharmacological agents against evoked pains in such patients (see however, Eide et al. 1995; Felsby et al. 1995; Attal et al. 1998, 1999). This method is now considered one of the most appropriate for determining the usefulness of analgesic agents (Woolf and Decosterd 1999).

It allows a symptom-based treatment of neuropathic pain, and can provide information about the mechanisms of action of the drugs.

Our study used a cross-over, double-blind placebo-controlled design to examine the efficacy of intravenous lidocaine on spontaneous and evoked pains in patients with central neuropathic pain due to stroke or spinal cord injury.

METHODS

STUDY POPULATION

The inclusion criteria were: daily pain of at least moderate severity (40 or more at baseline on a 100-mm visual analogue scale [VAS]) for more than 6 months, clearly attributable to a CNS injury. Patients were excluded for any of the following reasons: pains other than the neuropathic pain, previous treatment with lidocaine or mexiletine, severe depression or psychosis, severe nephropathy, pregnancy, chronic alcoholism or substance abuse, mental disorders preventing an accurate understanding of the tests, and contraindications to the use of lidocaine. Patients who were receiving other pharmacological treatment for their pain at the time of screening continued this medication with stable dosages throughout the study.

Sixteen patients (6 men and 10 women; mean age 55 ± 12 years) suffering from persistent pain due to post-stroke or spinal cord injury (median duration of pain 47 months) were randomized and completed the study. Post-stroke pain was due to hemorrhagic (three patients), ischemic (two patients), or lacunar (one patient) stroke. Spinal cord injuries included syringomyelia (five patients), post-traumatic myelomalacia (three patients), and cervical spondylosis with myelopathy (two patients). All the patients had continuous pain, most commonly burning in quality. Thirteen had intermittent attacks of pain (lancinating, electric-shock type pain).

PROCEDURE

The study used a double-blind, placebo-controlled design. After giving their written informed consent, patients were randomized to receive lidocaine then placebo or placebo then lidocaine, in two separate study sessions 3 weeks apart. The treatment (lidocaine 5 mg/kg [ASTRA] or equal volumes of 0.9% NaCl) was administered intravenously over a 30-minute period by an anesthesiologist unaware of the treatment, and prepared by a study nurse, who maintained the blind nature of the study. The infusion was stopped if unacceptable side effects occurred (e.g., convulsions, vomiting, cardiac arrhythmia). Three-lead ECG, heart rate, and blood pressure were monitored throughout the study.

STUDY MEASURES

We used a 100-mm VAS graduated from 0 (no pain) to 100 (worst possible pain) to assess pain intensity just before injection, every 15 minutes up to 60 minutes postinjection, then 90 and 120 minutes postinjection, and finally 6 hours after the injection. Patients also reported on a diary their mean and maximal continuous pain over a 24-hour period at the same time each day (8 pm), starting in the week preceding the first injection, and during 3 consecutive weeks after each injection.

In those patients who suffered from attacks of pain (lancinating, shooting pains), the daily number of painful attacks (mean number of attacks over the previous 24 hours) was assessed starting in the week prior to the first injection and continuing up to 3 weeks after the second injection. This criterion was not considered in those patients who had only infrequent attacks of pain (less than one per day). In patients suffering innumerable attacks, the cut-off was fixed at 20 attacks.

We used a brush (three movements) to investigate tactile allodynia (dynamic) before injection, then every 15 minutes for up to 2 hours postinjection. A clear sensation of pain evoked by stroking the skin constituted a positive test. The intensity of allodynia within the area of maximal pain was marked on a VAS (as the mean of two consecutive VAS scores).

Before and immediately after each injection the same experienced investigator systematically administered psychophysical tests in a quiet room maintained at a constant temperature (22°C). Measurements were taken in the area of maximal pain and in a normal, nonpainful, area. The order of testing was randomized. The detection and pain thresholds for mechanical stimuli were assessed with calibrated von Frey hairs as described previously (Attal et al. 1998). The detection threshold was defined as the lowest pressure perceived by the subject within 3 seconds of the stimulus. The pain threshold was defined as the lowest pressure that the patient considered to be painful. The force required to bend the filaments (0.057–140 g) was converted into logarithmic units. After the pain thresholds had been determined, the investigator used selected von Frey filaments to apply suprathreshold stimuli in a pseudo-random order. After each stimulus had been applied for 2 seconds, the patients were asked to quantify the pain intensity on a VAS. This method allowed the construction of mean stimulus/response curves for pain intensity as a function of graded nociceptive mechanical stimuli.

Thermal sensations were assessed with a Somedic thermotest according to the Marstock method (Fruhstorfer et al. 1976). A contact thermode of Peltier elements measuring 25 × 50 mm was applied to the skin. The baseline temperature of the thermode was adjusted to the patient's skin temperature. Thresholds were measured according to the method of limits described previously by Fruhstorfer et al. (1976). The maximum and minimum temperatures were set at 50°C and 4°C. All thresholds were calculated as the average of five successive determinations. The sequence of testing was the same for all the patients, i.e., determination of the cold then the warm detection thresholds followed by measurements of hot pain and cold pain thresholds on alternate sides; this sequence allowed test-free intervals of at least 2 minutes on each side.

After the determination of the pain thresholds, a series of suprathreshold cold and hot thermal stimuli was applied in pseudo-random order, according to a previously described method (Hansson and Lindblom 1992; Attal et al. 1998, 1999). Each stimulus had a duration of 2 seconds and an intensity that was increased in steps of 4°C for hot stimuli (between 40° and 48°C) and 5°C for cold stimuli (between 5° and 20°C). After each stimulus, the patients were asked to rate the pain intensity on a VAS. This method allowed the construction of mean stimulus/response curves for pain intensity against graded thermal stimuli.

Confirmation of allodynia to static mechanical or thermal stimuli required a decrease in pain thresholds of at least 20% on the painful side compared with the control side. Confirmation of hyperalgesia required increased responses to suprathreshold mechanical, hot, or cold stimuli were elicited on the painful side compared with the normal side (Attal et al. 1998).

SIDE EFFECTS, BLINDING, AND STATISTICAL ANALYSIS

During each injection and for up to 2 hours thereafter, the patients were asked to report any undesirable side effect, regardless of the relationship with the treatment. After completion of the two phases of the study, the patients also blindly chose the treatment they thought they had received at each test session, and explained the main reason for their choice.

Group data are expressed as means ± 1 SD. Wilcoxon's signed rank test and the Mann-Whitney test were used for comparison of paired and unpaired data, respectively. Two-way analysis of variance (ANOVA) with the Fisher's post hoc least significant difference tests were used for comparisons of intensity/response curves. In all instances, $P < 0.05$ was regarded as significant.

RESULTS

EFFECTS OF LIDOCAINE INFUSION ON SPONTANEOUS PAIN AND DYNAMIC MECHANICAL ALLODYNIA

The effects of lidocaine were significantly greater than those observed with the placebo, starting at the end of injection and for up to 45 minutes (the mean VAS scores for lidocaine and placebo were 61 ± 18 and 61 ± 17 before the injection and dropped to 31 ± 28 and 46 ± 24 immediately after the injection) (Fig. 1A). The daily VAS scores collected from the pain diaries were stable for the week preceding the injection and remained constant for 3 weeks postinjection, with no significant difference between lidocaine and the placebo. This finding confirmed that the drug had no significant prolonged efficacy. However, in two patients, long-term relief of pain (with a decrease by 30% to 50% in the VAS scores for 2 days in one case and for 10 days in another) was observed after lidocaine, but not after the placebo.

The daily number of attacks could be evaluated in 7 of the 13 patients with paroxysmal lancinating pain. In these patients, the daily average number of attacks did not decline significantly in the days following the injection of lidocaine.

Prior to the injections, eight patients had brush-induced allodynia. Lidocaine, but not saline, produced a significant reduction in the intensity of allodynia, starting 15 minutes postinjection and lasting for up to 30 minutes after the end of the injection (Fig. 1B).

EFFECTS OF LIDOCAINE ON DETECTION AND PAIN THRESHOLDS

The mean baseline (preinjection) mechanical and thermal, detection and pain thresholds on the painful and the control sides, did not differ significantly between the two test sessions. Detection and pain thresholds were not significantly altered on the normal side after the injection of lidocaine or placebo. Eight patients showed a decreased mechanical pain threshold to von Frey hairs on the painful side, indicative of a static (punctate) mechanical allodynia. Lidocaine was not significantly better than the placebo against this subtype of mechanical allodynia: the mean mechanical pain thresholds on the painful side (measured in milligrams, then logarithmically converted) were 4.4 ± 0.6 and 4.2 ± 0.5 after lidocaine and placebo injections compared to preinjection measurements of 4.2 ± 0.4 and 4.1 ± 0.5. Similarly, lidocaine and the placebo showed no significant difference in effects on cold allodynia (i.e., decreased cold pain thresholds on the painful side), which was evident in six patients. In this subgroup of patients, the mean cold pain thresholds

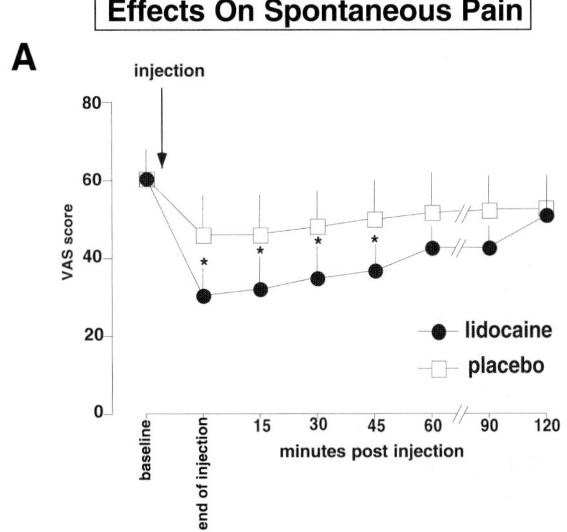

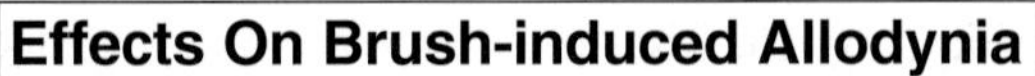

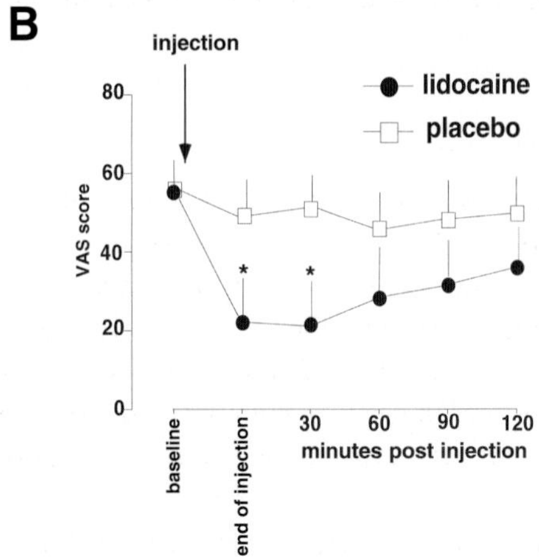

Fig. 1. (A) Comparison of the effects of lidocaine and placebo on spontaneous persistent pain (VAS score) measured every 15 minutes for 120 minutes after the injection. In comparison with the placebo, lidocaine induced a significant reduction in spontaneous persistent pain lasting for 45 minutes after the infusion. (B) Comparison of the effects of lidocaine and placebo on the intensity of brush-induced allodynia for 120 minutes after the injection. In comparison with the placebo, lidocaine induced a significant reduction of brush-induced allodynia for 30 minutes after the infusion. Data are expressed as means ± 1 SD; * $P < 0.05$.

on the painful side were 14.6° ± 8.4°C and 17.0° ± 5.4°C after lidocaine and placebo injection compared to preinjection measurements of 18.7° ± 5.0°C and 19.5° ± 6.5°C. Only two patients had allodynia to heat, which remained unchanged after lidocaine or the placebo.

EFFECTS OF LIDOCAINE ON PAIN DUE TO SUPRATHRESHOLD STIMULI

At baseline, the intensity-response curves for suprathreshold mechanical, hot, and cold stimuli were not significantly different between the two test sessions (Fig. 2A,C). Seven patients presented increased responses to suprathreshold mechanical stimuli on the painful side, suggestive of a static (punctate) mechanical hyperalgesia (Fig. 2A,C). Lidocaine induced a significant reduction in the responses to suprathreshold mechanical stimuli on the painful side (when compared to the placebo). In contrast, the responses obtained on the control side were not affected (Fig. 2B,D). Six patients had hyperalgesia to cold, and three patients had hyperalgesia to heat. The effects of lidocaine and the placebo on the intensity-response curves in patients with cold hyperalgesia were not significantly different on the painful and the control side (Fig. 3). The three patients with heat hyperalgesia showed no significant differences in the stimulus-response curves after either treatment (not shown).

SIDE EFFECTS AND BLINDING

Lidocaine produced side effects in 68% of the patients whereas the placebo produced side effects in 31%. The side effects were generally mild to moderate and essentially consisted of lightheadedness (seven patients with lidocaine versus no patient with placebo). Two patients had nausea and vomiting immediately after the infusion of lidocaine and one patient presented with muscle twitching and nausea at the end of the placebo infusion (possibly vagal malaise). These side effects were rapidly reversible, and did not disturb the evaluation.

Nine patients (56%) identified the active treatment, six thought that the placebo was the active treatment, and one patient was unable to identify which was which. Among the patients who correctly identified their active treatment, four did so because they felt a significant improvement in their pain and five did so essentially because of their side effects. These five patients tended to show a slightly, but not significantly, better analgesic response to lidocaine than did the other patients at the end of the injection.

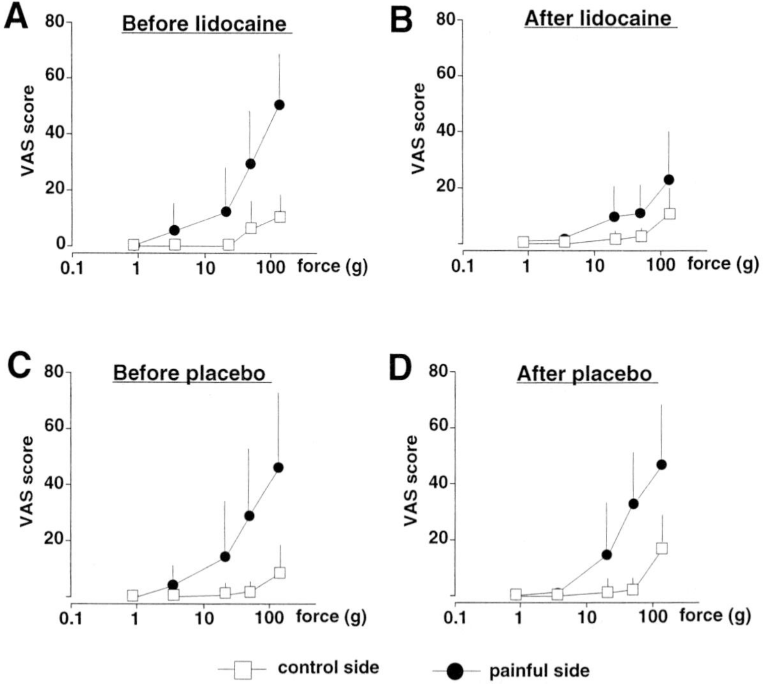

Fig. 2. Intensity-response curves for suprathreshold mechanical stimuli. These curves were obtained on both the painful side and the control side, before and after the administration of lidocaine (A,B) or placebo (C,D) in seven patients with static mechanical hyperalgesia (i.e., increased responses to suprathreshold mechanical stimuli on the painful side prior to the injections). Values are expressed as means ± 1 SD. These intensity/response curves were reduced after lidocaine injections ($P < 0.05$ for the comparison of the areas under the curves) on the painful side, but not on the normal side. No significant alterations were observed after the placebo administration.

DISCUSSION

This double-blind, placebo-controlled study shows that intravenous lidocaine can produce significant analgesic effects on several measurements of pain in a group of patients with central neuropathic pain due to stroke or spinal cord injury.

The clinical analgesic effects of intravenous lidocaine are well documented for various types of pain , most notably peripheral neuropathic pain (see references in Kalso et al. 1998). By contrast, its efficacy on central pain has been observed only in two open or single–blind, small prospective studies (Backonja et al. 1992; Edmonson et al. 1993) and in one retrospective survey (Galer et al. 1993). In our study, lidocaine significantly decreased the intensity of spontaneous persistent pain, although the difference be-

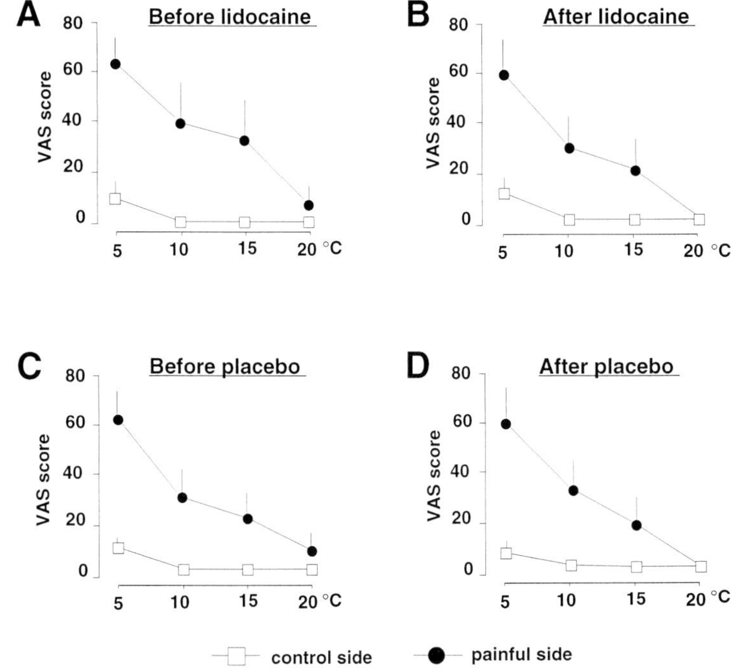

Fig. 3. Intensity-response curves for suprathreshold cold stimuli obtained on both the painful and the control sides, before and after the administration of lidocaine (A,B) or placebo (C,D), in six patients with cold hyperalgesia (i.e., patients with increased responses to suprathreshold cold stimuli on the painful side prior to the injections). Values are expressed as means ± 1 SD. These intensity/response curves were not significantly altered after the administration of lidocaine or the placebo.

tween the effects of lidocaine and of the placebo was moderate and the duration of the analgesic effects of lidocaine was particularly short, not exceeding 45 minutes. However, two patients reported long-term analgesic effects with lidocaine. These findings seem to indicate that at least in patients with central pain, long-term analgesic effects of lidocaine are uncommon, contrasting with previously reported observations in patients with neuropathic pain (Kastrup et al. 1987; Backonja et al. 1992).

No study has used psychophysical measurements to address the question of the efficacy of lidocaine on evoked pains in patients suffering from central pain. Interestingly, however, experimental data have been obtained from animals. In a model of chronic spinal cord ischemia in the rat, other local anesthetics or analogues such as tocainide and oral mexiletine have alleviated allodynia-like symptoms (Hao et al. 1992; Xu et al. 1992). In our study, lidocaine was significantly effective on brush-induced allodynia and relieved mechanical (static) hyperalgesia, as evidenced by the intensity/response curves, although it did not modify the mechanical pain thresholds, even in patients with allodynia. By contrast, lidocaine did not significantly alleviate cold hyperalgesia or allodynia (the effects on heat allodynia and hyperalgesia were difficult to assess due to the low number of patients with such symptoms). This lack of significant effect on pain due to thermal cold stimuli contrasts with the observed dramatic attenuation of mechanical allodynia and hyperalgesia. This finding may suggest that the analgesic effects of lidocaine are modality specific, and that the thermal and mechanical hyperalgesias in central pain patients are sustained by distinct mechanisms.

Lidocaine did not modify pain thresholds or the stimulus/response curves on the normal side, which suggests that the drug has specific anti-allodynic/hyperalgesic properties and that our results are not related to general analgesic effects. A lack of effect of lidocaine on thermal sensations and heat-pain thresholds has also been reported in patients with diabetic neuropathy (Bach et al. 1990).

The mechanisms of the analgesic action of intravenous lidocaine remain poorly understood. Lidocaine has the ability to suppress the ectopic neural discharges originating from injured primary afferent fibers (Devor et al. 1992), due to its properties of blocking voltage-gated sodium channels. However, the analgesic effects of lidocaine observed in our study appear to be mediated centrally, because the painful symptoms were related to spinal or supraspinal lesions. In fact, several investigators have proposed a predominant central site of action for systemic lidocaine. In healthy humans, a single i.v. bolus injection of lidocaine results in sustained and constant concentrations in the CSF, whereas the plasma levels show a faster decay (Usubiaga et al. 1967). In patients with diabetic neuropathy, an increase in the threshold for a nociceptive flexion reflex, which is mediated at the spinal level, has been observed with doses that do not modify the peripheral conduction (Bach et al. 1990). Electrophysiological studies in animals have indicated that systemic lidocaine produces a selective depression of C-fiber- but not of A-fiber-evoked activity in wide-dynamic-range neurons in the spinal cord (Woolf and Wiesenfeld-Hallin 1985; Nagy and Woolf 1996).

In summary, our results demonstrate that intravenous lidocaine can induce a significant and selective reduction of several components of pain due to CNS injuries. The observed preferential anti-hyperalgesic and anti-allodynic effects of this drug suggest a selective central action on the mechanisms underlying these evoked pains and support the need to perform a specific evaluation of evoked pains, notably by using suprathreshold stimuli. The lack of a prolonged analgesic effect renders its administration difficult in the clinical setting, unless the duration of efficacy increases with repeated injections as has been suggested for its use after peripheral nerve lesions (Edwards et al. 1985). However, some authors advocate the use of lidocaine as a screening test to predict the analgesic effect of oral analogues such as mexiletine (Galer et al. 1996). Most of our patients subsequently received oral mexiletine, titrated according to the efficacy and side effects (data not shown). However, most of the patients reported troublesome side effects, and only a minority (25%) gained pain relief, even among those who had previously responded to lidocaine.

ACKNOWLEDGMENTS

The authors thank Dr. S.W. Cadden for advice in the preparation and correction of the manuscript. This work was supported by l'Institut UPSA de la Douleur.

REFERENCES

Attal N, Brasseur B, Parker F, Chauvin M, Bouhassira D. Effects of the anticonvulsant gabapentin on neuropathic peripheral and central pain: a pilot study. *Eur Neurol* 1998; 40:191–200.

Attal N, Brasseur L, Chauvin M, Bouhassira D. Effects of single and repeated applications of eutectic mixture of local anesthetics (EMLA®) cream on spontaneous and evoked pains in patients with postherpetic neuralgia. *Pain* 1999; 81:203–210.

Awerbuch GI, Sandyk R. Mexiletine for thalamic pain syndrome. *Int J Neurosci* 1990; 55:129–133.

Bach FW, Jensen TS, Kastrup J, Sitgsby B, Dejgard A. The effect of intravenous lidocaine on nociceptive processing in diabetic neuropathy. *Pain* 1990; 40:29–34.

Backonja M, Gombar K. Response of central pain syndromes of intravenous lidocaine. *J Pain Symptom Manage* 1992; 7:172–178.

Casey KL (Ed). *Pain and Central Nervous System Disease. The Central Pain Syndromes.* New York: Raven Press, 1991.

Devor M, Wall PD, Catalan N. Systemic lidocaine silences ectopic neuroma and DRG discharge without blocking nerve conduction. *Pain* 1992; 48:261–268.

Edmonson EA, Simpson RK, Stubler DK, Beric A. Systemic lidocaine therapy for poststroke pain. *South Med J* 1993; 86:1093–1096.

Edwards WT, Habib F, Burney RG, Begin G. Intravenous lidocaine in the management of various chronic pain states. *Reg Anesth* 1985; 10:1–6.

Eide PK, Stubhaug A, Stenehjem AE. Central dysesthesia pain after traumatic spinal cord injury is dependent on N-methyl-D-aspartate receptor activation. *Neurosurgery* 1995; 37:1080–1087.

Felsby S, Nielsen J, Arendt-Nielsen L, Jensen TS. NMDA receptor blockade in chronic neuropathic pain: a comparison of ketamine and magnesium chloride. *Pain* 1995; 64:283–291.

Fruhstorfer H, Lindblom U, Schmidt WG. Method for quantitative estimation of thermal thresholds in patients. *J Neurol Neurosurg Psychiatry* 1976; 39:1071–1075.

Galer BS, Miller KV, Rowbotham MC. Response to intravenous lidocaine infusion differs based on clinical diagnosis and site of nervous system injury. *Neurology* 1993; 43:1233–1235.

Galer BS, Harle J, Rowbotham M. Response to intravenous lidocaine infusion predicts subsequent response to oral mexiletine. A prospective study. *J Pain Symptom Manage* 1996; 12:161–167.

Gonzales GR. Central pain: diagnosis and treatment strategies. *Neurology* 1995; 45(Suppl 9):S11–S16.

Hansson P, Lindblom U. Hyperalgesia assessed with quantitative sensory testing in patients with neurogenic pain. In: Willis WD (Ed). *Hyperalgesia and Allodynia.* New York: Raven Press, 1992, pp 335–343.

Hao JX, Yu YX, Seiger A, Wiesenfeld-Hallin Z. Systemic tocainide relieves mechanical hypersensitivity and normalizes the responses of hypersensitive dorsal horn wide dynamic range neurons after transient spinal cord ischemia in rats. *Exp Brain Res* 1992; 229–235.

Kalso E, Tramer MR, McQuay HJ, Moore RA. Systemic local-anaesthetic-type drugs in chronic pain: a systematic review. *Eur J Pain* 1998; 2:3–14.

Kastrup J, Petersen P, Dejgard A, Angelo H, Hilsted J. Intravenous lidocaine infusion. A new treatment of chronic painful diabetic neuropathy? *Pain* 1987; 28:69–75.

Leijon G, Boivie J. Central post-stroke pain—a controlled trial of amitriptyline and carbamazepine. *Pain* 1989; 36:27–36.

Nagy I, Woolf CJ. Lignocaine selectively reduces C fiber-evoked neuronal activity in rat spinal cord in vitro by decreasing N-methyl-D-aspartate and neurokinin receptor-mediated postsynaptic depolarizations: implications for the development of novel centrally acting analgesics. *Pain* 1996; 64:59–70.

Usubiaga J, Moya F, Wikinski J. Relationship between the passage of local anaesthetic across the blood brain barrier and their effects on the central nervous system. *Br J Anaesth* 1967; 39:943–947.

Woolf CJ, Decosterd I. Implications of recent advances in the understanding of pain pathophysiology for the assessment of pain in patients. *Pain* 1999; (Suppl 6):S141–S148.

Woolf CJ, Wiesenfeld-Hallin Z. The systemic administration of local anesthetics produces a selective depression of C-afferent fiber evoked activity in the spinal cord. *Pain* 1985; 23:361–374.

Xu XJ, Hao JX, Seiger A, Arner S, Lindblom U, Wiesenfeld-Hallin Z. Systemic mexiletine relieves chronic allodynia-like symptoms in rats with ischemic spinal cord injury. *Anesthes Analg* 1992; 74:649–652.

Correspondence to: Didier Bouhassira, MD, PhD, INSERM U-161, 2, rue d'Alésia, 75014 Paris, France. Tel: 33-1-40-78-93-50; Fax: 33-1-45-88-13-04; email: bouhassira@broca.inserm.fr.

Proceedings of the 9th World Congress on Pain, Progress in Pain Research and Management, Vol. 16, edited by M. Devor, M.C. Rowbotham, and Z. Wiesenfeld-Hallin, IASP Press, Seattle, © 2000.

81

New and Old Anticonvulsants as Analgesics[1]

Anthony H. Dickenson[a] and Victoria Chapman[b]

[a]*Department of Pharmacology, University College, London, United Kingdom;* [b]*School of Biomedical Sciences, University of Nottingham, Nottingham, United Kingdom*

Epilepsy and neuropathic pain arise from excess activity in the nervous system. Neuropathic pain syndromes are sensory disorders that result from damage or dysfunction of neuronal pathways, peripheral or central. Neuropathic symptoms can arise from injury, trauma, surgery, or disease (postherpetic neuralgia, diabetes, AIDS, etc.). Patients with cancer also commonly have neuropathic symptoms, caused by a tumor invading nerve tissue or compression of a nerve by an adjacent neoplasm. It is a paradox that after damage to a nerve or neurons, neuropathic pain is often characterized by both positive (abnormal spontaneous or evoked sensations) and negative symptoms (sensory deficits); intuitively, we might expect only the latter. Pain can be persistent in areas of sensory loss, and a range of natural stimuli may evoke painful or unpleasant sensations (Fields and Rowbotham 1994), including dysesthesia, allodynia, and hyperalgesia. Counterparts of these sensations can be studied in animal models (Bennett 1994; Zeltser and Seltzer 1994). An important issue is that despite the high prevalence of behaviors indicative of pain in the animal models (ca. 80%), chronic pain occurs in only about 10–50% of patients with neuropathies. The presence of marked genetic variability in animal strains, and the huge range of human phenotypes, may indicate important individual differences in susceptibility to neuropathic pain.

[1] Mini-review based on a congress workshop.

WHY ANTICONVULSANTS FOR PAIN?

Anticonvulsant drugs were developed without any rationale based on defined pharmacological actions (Upton 1994), but they have proved efficacious in the treatment of epilepsy. Epilepsy and neuropathic pain have several parallels beyond the usefulness of anticonvulsant drugs for some pain symptoms following nerve injury (Kingery 1997). Epileptic seizures are triggered by the hyperexcitability of neurons in the brain and can be spontaneous, recurrent, or paroxysmal, similar to nerve injury pains. Epilepsy also can be idiopathic or symptomatic, yet can be categorized according to symptoms and also by electroencephalogram findings, a diagnostic tool that is lacking for many neuropathic syndromes. The neuronal discharges in epilepsy can be restricted or spread across the brain. As pain and epilepsy result from excess neuronal activity, both disorders can be treated by either blocking excitability or increasing inhibitions to balance the hyperexcitability. The association between opioid systems and sensory pathways subserving pain provides a key inhibitory target for pain control, yet, as discussed later,

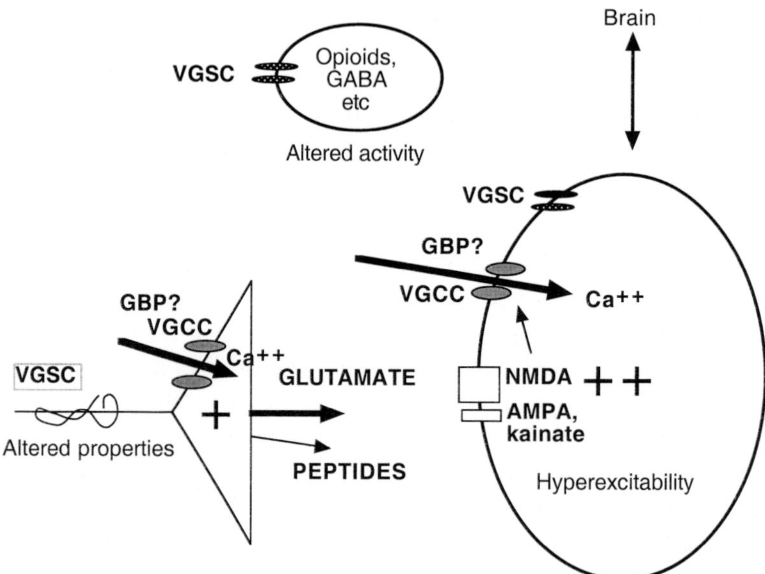

Fig. 1. The diagram presents some possible substrates for the actions of anticonvulsants described in this chapter. Voltage-gated sodium channels (VGSC), voltage-gated calcium channels (VGCC), and altered properties of primary afferents will contribute to primary afferent activity and transmitter release. In the spinal cord, changes in local inhibitory interneuronal activity and spinal neurons will also be critical in determining the level of activity through the spinal cord. The gabapentin-binding protein (GBP) may be associated with the VGCC, which when located postsynaptically, will also contribute to neuronal activity.

the effectiveness of opioid therapy may be compromised after nerve injury. We mention the symptoms and classifications of epilepsy to point out the similarities with neuropathic pain and because the type of epilepsy guides the use of particular classes of antiepileptic drugs used for convulsions.

It is becoming clear that the grouping of neuropathic pains into one category is too simplistic. Recategorization may be critical, not only for assessment of current therapies, but also for new drug treatments of neuropathic pain. The basic mechanistic studies in animals suggest that different pain states and symptoms may have different underlying mechanisms. Although difficult, an attempt to distinguish and quantify different pain symptoms in human clinical studies and trials could be fruitful. Clinical approaches to this issue have been widely discussed, and some suggest that quantitative somatosensory testing may also reveal underlying mechanistic differences (Hansson and Kinnman 1996). This approach may prevent the discarding of drugs with relevant mechanisms if their specific actions on selected symptoms were masked in studies that only monitored general estimates of pain. In a recent clinical study, gabapentin controlled ongoing spontaneous pain and paroxysmal pain and also brush and cold allodynia, but did not influence static mechanical or heat pain (Attal et al. 1998).

MECHANISMS OF PAIN AFTER NERVE INJURY

PERIPHERAL EVENTS

This chapter surveys the use of anticonvulsants, both old and new, in the context of what is known regarding the consequences of nerve injury. Considerable evidence supports the concept that the mechanisms of pain and the ability to control pain may differ in different pain states (Dickenson 1995). This concept is of great importance in considering a rational basis for the treatment of neuropathic pain, where the pathology leads to alterations in both peripheral and central pain systems, for example, changes in the effectiveness of opioids. In some cases, neuropathic pain requires other analgesic approaches, including anticonvulsants. The exact neurobiological basis for both understanding the causes and improving the treatment of this major pain state remain somewhat unclear, but animal models of nerve injury produced by manipulating peripheral nerves in the rat (Bennett 1994; Zeltser and Seltzer 1994) can help expand our knowledge. The recent explosion of information about novel sodium channels and their expression in different pain models will shed much light on the factors that govern the effectiveness of agents such as carbamazepine, mexiletine, and local anesthetics that act on these substrates (see Waxman 1999).

Early animal studies of neuropathic pain used complete nerve section. More recent animal models are based on a restricted partial denervation of the hindlimb following sciatic nerve injury. Several animal models of neuropathic pain have replicated various components of the syndrome (Zeltser and Seltzer 1994). Two models that involve sciatic nerve ligation distal to the spinal cord have been widely studied with behavioral approaches. These models are chronic constriction injury (CCI) and partial spinal nerve ligation (SNL); both result in a restricted partial denervation of the hindlimb. A more recent model of sciatic nerve injury involves selective tight ligation of two (L5 and L6) of the three spinal nerves that form the sciatic nerve (Kim and Chung 1992). Many studies have clearly demonstrated reproducible behavioral consequences of these various peripheral lesions, including mechanical and cooling allodynia, and mechanical and thermal hyperalgesia. These behaviors mimic some aspects of human symptoms of neuropathic pain. Techniques will inherently vary from laboratory to laboratory because different fiber types may differ in extent of degeneration. Given the variability in the extent of peripheral nerve damage in patients, an important point is that the similar behavioral results reported by many groups suggest that common consequences can result from potentially variable peripheral and central changes.

Evidence suggests that the aberrations in somatosensory processing that follow partial nerve injury are the culmination of several changes in the peripheral nervous system (Gracely et al. 1993). Studies after nerve section suggest that the generation of ectopic discharges within the neuroma and the dorsal root ganglia (DRG) contributes to these changes (Devor et al. 1992). After partial denervation (CCI model), high-frequency spontaneous activity originating in the DRG targets the spinal neurons via injured A fibers. Both A fibers and DRG contribute to the behavioral responses, including allodynia, associated with the SNL model. A structural reorganization of large-fiber (Aβ) termination in the spinal cord has also been reported, so it is possible that low-threshold inputs can gain access to spinal nociceptive transmission circuits following nerve injury (Woolf and Mannion 1999).

CENTRAL EVENTS

Few electrophysiological studies have examined spinal neurons in nerve injury models. In the CCI model, a high percentage of spinal neurons exhibited abnormal levels of spontaneous activity, although many neurons had absent somatic receptive fields. Spinal neurons had increased afterdischarges and were sensitive to tapping of the nerve injury site. The number of neurons sensitive to low-intensity mechanical stimuli and the magnitude of mechanical evoked responses of the neurons also were reduced. Subtle changes in spinal neuronal responses have been reported after partial ligation. After selective SNL, neurons have shown spontaneous activity, lowered thresholds to thermal and mechanical stimuli (with decreased magnitudes of responses), and finally, enlarged mechanical receptive fields (see Chapman et al. 1998a). It is still unclear how these changed peripheral and central neuronal responses contribute to the resultant pain states, although the combination of both increased and decreased responses fits well with the clinical profile of pain/allodynia and sensory deficits after nerve injury. However, what tends to be overlooked is that neuropathic pain arises from damage to nervous system pathways. Thus, the sensory deficits are to be expected. In the Seltzer and Bennett models, the partial section of the nerve and the loose ligation restrict afferent input. In the Chung model, ligation of L5 and L6 results in a loss of input into these segments, but even in L4 afferent input could be decreased by about 35%, the estimated contribution of adjacent nerves to a segment (Besse et al. 1991). The findings of no dramatic increases in spinal neuronal activity in all three models may still represent central compensations for the loss of input.

Thus, we cannot underestimate the contribution of central mechanisms to neuropathic pains. The NMDA receptor for glutamate appears to be of great importance in the induction and maintenance of spinal nociceptive events leading to hyperalgesia following tissue damage, nerve dysfunction, and surgery. A C-fiber stimulus of constant intensity induces NMDA-receptor-mediated wind-up, whereby the responses of certain dorsal horn nociceptive neurons increase in magnitude and duration, despite the constant input into the spinal cord (Dickenson 1995). A similar situation may exist with regard to epilepsy. Other causal factors likely include changes in phenotype and anatomy (Woolf and Mannion 1999), which will decrease neuronal thresholds and allow access of different afferent inputs to central nociceptive transmission. We have good reason to suspect that NMDA-mediated events are relevant to nerve-injury-evoked pain. Behavioral studies have shown that NMDA-receptor activation is required for both the induction and maintenance of pain-related behaviors (Bennett 1994; Dickenson 1997). Thus, aberrant peripheral activity is probably amplified and enhanced by NMDA-receptor-mediated spinal mechanisms in neuropathic pain. The degree of hyperexcitability after peripheral nerve damage is hard to gauge because peripheral fibers, central neurons, and pharmacological systems may change their properties after injury. As the operation of the NMDA receptor/channel critically depends on the underlying level of excitability, spinal neurons are probably hyperactive and compensate for much of the peripheral nerve damage. Human evidence points to the effectiveness of agents acting at the

NMDA-receptor complex, especially ketamine (Eide et al. 1995), but it appears that although some patients obtain good pain relief, most cannot achieve complete pain control because dose escalation is compromised by the narrow therapeutic window. The same factor would apply to the potential use of glutamate receptor/channel antagonists in the treatment of epilepsy. Success of new therapies for pain and epilepsy, based on blocking the actions of glutamate on NMDA or other receptors, such as AMPA/kainate receptors, will depend on strategies that increase their therapeutic window over existing drugs.

Recent studies with agents that block neuronal voltage-sensitive calcium channels also suggest an increase in central neuronal excitability. N-type channels, blocked by ω-conotoxin, appear to be important in behavioral allodynia and play a major role in the neuronal responses to low- and high-threshold natural stimuli and in C-fiber-evoked central hyperexcitability. Blockers of this channel are considerably more effective after nerve injury (SNL), and because the channel is voltage operated, these results again suggest increased excitability of the spinal cord neurons after injury (Matthews and Dickenson 1999). SNX-111 is an example of a drug that blocks calcium channels, but its use is restricted to the spinal route (Mathur et al. 1998).

Allodynia is a good example of how central inhibitory neurons set the level of transmission. Blocking glycine or the $GABA_A$ receptors in normal animals produces NMDA-mediated allodynia. NMDA antagonists are effective against this tactile-evoked nociception, whereas morphine is not, probably because low-threshold pathways are minimally controlled by opioid receptors (Yaksh 1989). The benzodiazepines, drugs that enhance GABA-mediated inhibitions, are widely used in epilepsy, yet little evidence exists for their possible therapeutic role in nerve injury pains. Following peripheral noxious stimulation, spinal mechanisms that are also driven by NMDA-receptor-mediated activity limit further neuronal responses. Adenosine may be involved in this type of control and can be effective in humans with neuropathic pain (Belfrage et al. 1995). Thus, control of NMDA events has potential indirect targets.

One problem with assessment of opioids in both animal and clinical studies is that the type of neuropathy and the extent, duration, and intensity of symptoms may all be critical factors, as may the route of administration and type of opioid used. Thus, a series of clinical studies reporting on the efficacy of morphine in neuropathic pain states has produced no real consensus. Dose escalation produced good analgesia in one study (Portenoy et al. 1990), and others showed that in general, morphine could be effective in a group of patients with neuropathy (Rowbotham et al. 1991), although opioid analgesia was decreased in neuropathic pain patients compared to a group with nociceptive pain (Jadad et al. 1992). Resolution of this problem has important clinical implications, yet the animal literature also reveals a similar series of discrepant results (see Suzuki 1999).

OLD ANTICONVULSANTS

Evidence for increased excitability in many cases of neuropathic pain, which can be less responsive to conventional analgesic therapy, has prompted use of alternative agents. Evidence indicates that novel substrates contributing to the etiology of neuropathic pain states are sensitive to membrane-stabilizing drugs such as the anticonvulsant carbamazepine (Chabal 1994; McQuay et al. 1995; Fields et al. 1997). Reviews of clinical studies indicate that this drug is well established as the primary treatment for trigeminal neuralgia, but the drug may also be considered as a primary agent for other types of nerve injury pains (McQuay et al. 1995). In addition, local anaesthetics such as lignocaine (Tanelian and Brosse 1991; Ferrante et al. 1996) and the class Ib antiarrhythmic sodium channel blocker mexiletine (Chabal et al. 1992; Dejgard et al. 1988; Fields et al. 1997) are effective in neuropathic pain states. Recent evidence suggests that newer anticonvulsant drugs, such as gabapentin (Neurontin [Warner-Lambert]) and lamotrigine, another sodium channel blocker (Zakrzewska et al. 1997), may offer an alternative therapeutic approach.

The site and mechanism of action of anticonvulsant drugs in persistent pain states have been addressed with animal models of inflammatory and neuropathic pain states. Systemic administration of carbamazepine, a drug that blocks sodium channels, reduces spontaneous activity of saphenous neuromas (Burchiel 1988) and blocks spontaneous activity of spinal neurons of spinal nerve (L5 and L6) ligated rats (Chapman et al. 1998b). Furthermore, systemic carbamazepine inhibits innocuous and noxious evoked responses of spinal neurons of spinal-nerve-ligated, but not sham-operated, rats (Chapman et al. 1998b).

The actions of systemically administered sodium channel blockers such as carbamazepine, lignocaine, and mexiletine in relieving clinical neuropathic pain may include both peripheral and central sites. Systemic lidocaine inhibits spontaneous activity and ectopic activity at the neuroma, in the dorsal root ganglia, and in the dorsal horn (Devor et al. 1992; Sotgui et al. 1994; Omana-Zapata et al. 1997) in various models of neuropathic pain. Interestingly, acute rhizotomy does not alter the hyperactivity of spinal neurons of CCI rats, although systemic administration of lidocaine is effective (Sotgui et al. 1994). These findings suggest that a novel central pacemaker underlies the maintenance of this aberrant spinal neuronal activity, which is independent of the concurrent DRG hyperactivity. Behavioral studies have shown that intravenous lidocaine reduces both mechanical allodynia (Chaplan et al. 1995) and thermal hyperalgesia (Abram et al. 1994) in neuropathic pain models. Similarly, systemic mexiletine reduces touch-evoked pain behavior (Jett et al. 1997), mechanical hyperalgesia (Koch et al. 1996), and cold-induced allodynia (Hedley et al. 1995) in models of neuropathic pain. Although we did not investigate the site of drug action, we demonstrated a novel effect of spinal mexiletine on Aδ-fiber and C-fiber, but not Aβ-fiber-mediated somatosensory transmission following nerve injury (Chapman et al. 1998c), which agrees with the findings of behavioral studies. The efficacy of topical lignocaine applied to the painful area in patients would support the importance of peripheral actions in addition to central mechanisms (Rowbotham et al. 1996).

NEW ANTICONVULSANTS

Gabapentin is an antiepileptic drug that has analgesic activity in neuropathic pain states of varying origins. A randomized, controlled trial of gabapentin in patients with postherpetic neuralgia concluded that gabapentin was effective in treating this pain state and improving quality of life (Rowbotham et al. 1998). Further, another large-scale controlled trial showed clear effectiveness in patients with diabetic neuropathy (Backonja et al. 1998). These studies are landmarks due to the many patients enrolled. In addition, a study reported that gabapentin is effective in pain caused by peripheral nerve injury and central lesions, with particular effectiveness on paroxysmal pain and allodynia (Attal et al. 1998). In keeping with clinical reports, systemic and intrathecal gabapentin reduces heat hyperalgesia and mechano- and cold allodynia associated with the CCI model of neuropathy (Hunter et al. 1997). A recent behavioral study reported that systemic gabapentin blocks both static and dynamic mechanical allodynia in streptozocin-treated rats, a model of diabetic neuropathy (Field et al. 1999). In addition, we have demonstrated that gabapentin has inhibitory effects on innocuous and noxious evoked responses of spinal neurons of rats with SNL, effects comparable in magnitude to those of carbamazepine. In contrast to carbamazepine, gabapentin produced similar inhibitory effects on neuronal responses of sham-operated rats. These electrophysiological studies suggest that the effectiveness of gabapentin is not determined by direct consequences of spinal nerve ligation but by general invasive surgery or tissue damage (Chapman et al. 1998b).

One major outcome of the recent behavioral and electrophysiological studies is the growing evidence that anticonvulsant drugs are effective not only in models of neuropathic pain but also in inflammatory pain states. Carrageenan inflammation produced a selective and novel sensitivity of C-fiber-mediated responses to carbamazepine and gabapentin (Chapman and Dickenson 1997; Stanfa et al. 1997). Neither drug was effective in normal animals. Systemic gabapentin reduced formalin-evoked behavioral responses and blocks thermal and mechanical hyperalgesia in a rat model of postoperative pain (Field et al. 1997) and diminished secondary hyperalgesia following a mild burn injury (Jones and Sorkin 1998). Although other agents are used clinically to treat pains from tissue damage, these data indicate that the substrates for the mechanisms of action of both gabapentin and carbamazepine are not restricted to nerve injury. The novel effectiveness of carbamazepine after inflammation may relate to an upregulation of the novel SNS/PN3 sodium channel in DRG neurons projecting to the inflamed limb (Waxman 1999).

The exact mode of action of gabapentin is yet to be established, but indications are that the drug may interact with calcium channels in that the so-called gabapentin-binding protein is associated with a subunit of the calcium channel (Taylor et al. 1998). Thus, the $\alpha_2\delta$ subunit of the channel may be a target for gabapentin, and we must assume that it acts as an antagonist. This action would fit with the evidence that N-type calcium channel blockers are more effective in reducing behavioral and electrophysiological responses to sensory stimuli after both nerve injury and tissue damage (Matthews and Dickenson 1999). It appears that, at least after nerve damage, N-type calcium channels are upregulated (Cizkova et al. 1999).

FUTURE APPROACHES TO NEUROPATHIC PAIN

The use of preclinical models in animals and humans, and the application of sensory testing to patients, are worthwhile goals in the effort to produce a more rational approach for using anticonvulsants, both old and new, in the treatment of neuropathic pain. Various syndromes and symptoms may have differential neurobiological bases and so require different pharmacological approaches. Finally, similar to the use of adjunct drugs in epilepsy, neuropathic pain is often treated by polypharmacy; the most judicious combinations of drugs for neuropathic pain need to be clinically assessed.

Further consideration of many of the issues arising from the points made in this chapter can be found in the recent supplement to *Pain* (1999), which is a tribute to Patrick Wall. His impact on the field is undiminished.

REFERENCES

Abram SE, Yaksh TL. Systemic lidocaine blocks nerve injury induced hyperalgesia and nociceptor-driven spinal sensitization in the rat. *Anesthesiology* 1994; 80:383–391.

Attal N, Brasseur L, Parker F, Chauvin M, Bouhassira D. Effects of gabapentin on the different components of peripheral and central neuropathic pain syndromes: a pilot study. *Eur Neurol* 1998; 40:191–200.

Backonja M, Beydoun A, Edwards KR, et al. Gabapentin for the symptomatic treatment of painful neuropathy in patients with diabetes mellitus: a randomized controlled trial. *JAMA* 1998; 280(21):1831–1836.

Belfrage M, Sollevi A, Segerdahl M, Sjolund K-F, Hansson P. Systemic adenosine infusion alleviates spontaneous and stimulus evoked pain in patients with peripheral neuropathic pain. *Anesth Analg* 1995; 81:713–717.

Bennett GJ. Animal models of neuropathic pain. In: Gebhart GF, Hammond DL, Jensen T. *Proceedings of the 7th World Congress on Pain*, Progress in Pain Research and Management, Vol. 2. Seattle: IASP Press, 1994, pp 495–510.

Besse D, Lombard MC, Besson JM. The distribution of μ and δ opioid binding sites belonging to a single cervical dorsal root in the superficial dorsal horn of the spinal cord: a quantitative autoradiographic study. *Eur J Neurosci* 1991; 3:1343–1352.

Burchiel KJ. Carbamazepine inhibits spontaneous activity in experimental neuromas. *Exp Neurol* 1998; 102:249–253.

Chabal C. Membrane stabilizing agents and experimental neuromas. In: Fields HL, Liebeskind JC (Eds). *Pharmacological Approaches to the Treatment of Chronic Pain: New Concepts and Critical Issues*. Seattle: IASP Press, 1994, pp 205–210.

Chabal C, Jacobson L, Mariano A, Chaney E, Britell CW. The use of oral mexiletine for the treatment of pain after peripheral nerve injury. *Anaesthesiology* 1992; 76:513–517.

Chaplan SR, Bach FW, Shafer SL, Yaksh TL. Prolonged alleviation of tactile allodynia by intravenous lidocaine in neuropathic rats. *Anesthesiology* 1995; 83:775–785.

Chapman V, Dickenson AH. Inflammation reveals inhibition of noxious responses of rat spinal neurones by carbamezapine. *Neuroreport* 1997; 8:1399–1404.

Chapman V, Suzuki R, Dickenson AH. Electrophysiological characterisation of spinal neuronal response properties of anaesthetised rats after ligation of spinal nerves L5–6. *J Physiol* 1998a; 507.3:881–894.

Chapman V, Suzuki R, Chamarette HLC, Rygh LJ, Dickenson AH. An electrophysiological study of the inhibitory effects of systemic carbamazepine and gabapentin on spinal neuronal responses in spinal nerve ligated rats. *Pain* 1998b; 75:261–273.

Chapman V, Ng J, Dickenson AH. A novel spinal action of mexiletine in spinal somatosensory transmission of nerve injured rats. *Pain* 1998c; 77:289–296.

Cizkova D, Marsala M, Stauderman K, Yaksh TL. Calcium channel α1B subunit in spinal cord/DRG of normal and nerve-injured rats. *Abstracts: 9th World Congress on Pain*. Seattle: IASP Press, 1999, p 134.

Dejgard A, Petersen P, Kastrup J. Mexiletine for treatment of chronic painful diabetic neuropathy. *Lancet* 1988; 9–11.

Devor M, Wall PD, Catalan N. Systemic lidocaine silences ectopic neuroma and DRG discharge without blocking nerve conduction. *Pain* 1992; 48:261–268.

Dickenson AH. Spinal cord pharmacology of pain. *Br J Anaesth* 1995; 75:132–144.

Dickenson AH. Mechanisms of central hypersensitivity In: Dickenson AH, Besson JM (Eds). *The Pharmacology of Pain*, Handbook of Experimental Pharmacology, Vol. 130. Heidelberg: Springer-Verlag, 1997, pp 168–210.

Eide PK, Stubhaug A, Oye I, Breivik H. Continuous subcutaneous administration of the N-methyl-D-aspartic acid (NMDA) receptor antagonist ketamine in the treatment of post-herpetic neuralgia. *Pain* 1995; 61:221–228.

Ferrante FM, Paggioli J, Cherukuri S, Arthur GR. The analgesic response to intravenous lidocaine in the treatment of neuropathic pain. *Anesth Analg* 1996; 82:91–97.

Field MJ, Holloman EF, McCleary S, Hughes J, Singh L. Evaluation of gabapentin and S-(+)-isobutylgaba in a rat model of postoperative pain. *J Pharmacol Exp Ther* 1997; 282:1242–1246.

Field MJ, McCleary S, Hughes J, Singh L. Gabapentin and pregabalin, but not morphine and amitriptyline, block both static and dynamic components of mechanical allodynia induced by streptozocin in the rat. *Pain* 1999; 80:391–398.

Fields HL, Rowbotham MC. Multiple mechanisms of neuropathic pain: a clinical perspective. In: Gebhart GF, Hammond DL, Jensen TS (Eds). *Proceedings of the 7th World Congress on Pain*, Progress in Pain Research and Management, Vol. 2. Seattle: IASP Press, 1994, pp 437–454.

Fields HL, Rowbotham MC, Devor M. Excitability blockers: anticonvulsants and low concentration local anesthetics in the treatment of chronic pain. In: Dickenson AH, Besson JM (Eds). *The Pharmacology of Pain*, Handbook of Experimental Pharmacology, Vol. 130. Heidelberg: Springer, 1997, pp 93–116.

Gracely R, Lynch SA, Bennett GJ. Painful neuropathy: altered central processing maintained dynamically by peripheral input. *Pain* 1993; 52:251–253.

Hansson P, Kinnman E. Unmasking neuropathic pain mechanisms in a clinical perspective. *Pain Rev* 1996; 3:272–292.

Hedley LR, Martin B, Waterbury LD, Clarke DE, Hunter JC. A comparison of the action of mexiletine and morphine in rodent models of acute and chronic pain. *Proc West Pharmacol Soc* 1995; 38:103–104.

Hunter JC, Gogas KR, Hedley LR, et al. The effect of novel anti-epileptic drugs in rat experimental models of acute and chronic pain. *Eur J Pharm* 1997; 324:153–160.

Jadad AR, Carroll D, Glynn CJ, Moore RA, McQuay HJ. Morphine responsiveness of chronic pain: double-blind randomized crossover study with patient-controlled analgesia. *Lancet* 1992; 339:1367–1371.

Jett M-F, McGuirk J, Waligora D, Hunter JC. The effects of mexiletine, desipramine and fluoxetine in rat models involving central sensitization. *Pain* 1997; 69:161–169.

Jones DL, Sorkin LS. Systemic gabapentin and S-(+)-isobutylgamma-aminobutyric acid block secondary hyperalgesia. *Brain Res* 1998; 810:93–99.

Kim KJ, Yoon YW, Chung JM. Comparison of three rodent neuropathic pain models. *Exp Brain Res* 1997; 113:200–206.

Kim SH, Chung JM. An experimental model for peripheral neuropathy produced by segmental spinal nerve ligation in the rat. *Pain* 1992; 50:355–363.

Kingery WS. A critical review of controlled clinical trials for peripheral neuropathic pain and complex regional pain syndromes. *Pain* 1997; 73:123–139.

Koch BD, Faurot GF, McGuirk JR, Clarke DE, Hunter JC. Modulation of mechano-hyperalgesia by clinically effective analgesics in rats with a peripheral mononeuropathy. *Analgesia* 1996; 2:157–164.

Mathur VS, McGuire D, Bowersox SS, et al. *Pharm News* 1998; 5:25–29.

Matthews E, Dickenson AH. Plasticity in the effects of the N-type calcium channel blocker, ω-conotoxin GVIA on dorsal horn neuronal activity in normal and neuropathic rats. *Abstracts: 9th World Congress on Pain*. Seattle: IASP Press, 1999, p 203.

McQuay H, Carroll D, Jasdad AR, Wiffen P, Moore A. Anticonvulsant drugs for management of pain: a systematic review. *BMJ* 1995; 311:1047–1052.

Omana-Zapata I, Khabbaz MA, Hunter JC, Clarke DE, Bley KR. Tetrodotoxin inhibits neuropathic ectopic activity in neuromas, dorsal root ganglia and dorsal horn neurons. *Pain* 1997; 72:41–49.

Portenoy RK, Foley KM, Inturrisi CE. The nature of opioid responsiveness and its implications for neuropathic pain: new hypotheses derived from studies of opioid infusions. *Pain* 1990; 43:273–286.

Rowbotham MC, Reisner-Keller LA, Fields HL. Both intravenous lidocaine and morphine reduce the pain of postherpetic neuralgia. *Neurology* 1991; 41:1024–1028.

Rowbotham MC, Davies PS, Verkempinck CV, Galer BS. Lidocaine patch: double-blind controlled study of a new treatment method for post-herpetic neuralgia. *Pain* 1996; 65:39–44.

Rowbotham MC, Harden N, Stacey B, Bernstein P, Magnus-Miller L. Gabapentin for the treatment of postherpetic neuralgia. *JAMA* 1998; 280(21):1837–1842.

Sotgui ML, Biella G, Castagna A, Lacerenza M, Marchettini P. Different time-courses of i.v. lidocaine effect on ganglionic and spinal units in neuropathic rats. *Neuroreport* 1994; 5:873–876.

Stanfa LC, Singh L, Williams RG, Dickenson AH. Gabapentin, ineffective in normal rats, markedly reduces C-fibre evoked responses after inflammation. *Neuroreport* 1997; 8:587–590.

Suzuki R, Chapman V, Dickenson AH. The effectiveness of spinal and systemic morphine on rat dorsal horn neuronal responses in the spinal nerve ligation model of neuropathic pain. *Pain* 1999; 80:215–228.

Tanelian DL, Brosse WG. Neuropathic pain can be relieved by drugs that are use-dependent sodium channel blockers: lidocaine, carbamazepine, and mexiletine. *Anaesthesiology* 1991; 74:949–951.

Taylor CP, Gee NS, Su T, et al. A summary of mechanistic hypotheses of gabapentin pharmacology. *Epilepsy Res* 1998; 29:233–249.

Upton N. Mechanisms of action of new antiepileptic drugs: rational design and serendipitous findings. *Trends Pharmacol Sci* 1994; 12:456–463.

Waxman S. The molecular pathophysiology of pain: abnormal expression of sodium channel genes and its contribution to hyperexcitability of primary sensory neurons. *Pain* 1999; 6:S133–140.

Woolf CJ, Mannion RJ. Neuropathic pain: aetiology, symptoms, mechanisms, and management. *Lancet* 1999; 353:1959–1964.

Yaksh TL. Behavioral and autonomic correlates of the tactile evoked allodynia produced by spinal glycine inhibition: effects of modulatory receptor systems and excitatory amino acid antagonists. *Pain* 1989; 37:111–123.

Zakrzewska JM, Chaudhry Z, Nurimikko TJ, Patton DW, Mullens EL. Lamotrigine (Lamictal) in refractory trigeminal neuralgia: results from a double-blind placebo controlled crossover trial. *Pain* 1997; 73:223–230.

Zeltser R, Seltzer Z. A practical guide for the use of animal models in the study of neuropathic pain. In: Boivie J, Hansson P, Lindblom U (Eds). *Touch, Temperature, and Pain in Health and Disease: Mechanisms and Assessments,* Progress in Pain Research and Management, Vol. 3. Seattle: IASP Press, 1994, pp 295–338.

Correspondence to: Anthony H. Dickenson, PhD, Department of Pharmacology, University College, Gower Street, London WC1E 6BT, United Kingdom. Fax: 44-(0)171-419-3742; email: anthony.dickenson@ucl.ac.uk.

Proceedings of the 9th World Congress on Pain,
Progress in Pain Research and Management,
Vol. 16, edited by M. Devor, M.C. Rowbotham, and
Z. Wiesenfeld-Hallin, IASP Press, Seattle, © 2000.

82

Patient Information Leaflets and Antidepressant Prescription in Chronic Pain Patients

Christine Cedraschi,[a] Valérie Piguet,[a] Werner Fischer,[b]
Anne-Françoise Allaz,[a] Jules Desmeules,[a]
and Pierre Dayer[a]

*[a]Multidisciplinary Pain Center, and [b]Department of Psychiatry,
University Hospital, Geneva, Switzerland*

Inappropriate or excessive medication use is commonly observed among chronic pain patients. Some patients fail to take their prescribed medication regularly, and thus forfeit the possible benefits of treatment. However, patients do not think of taking drugs merely in terms of obeying the doctor's prescription. Instead, they weigh up the costs and benefits of taking particular medications within the contexts and constraints of their everyday lives and needs (Donovan and Blake 1992). This perspective implies that nonobservance may not simply be lack of compliance but a rational decision, based essentially on the patients' representations or beliefs as well as on previous experiences. Patients have various sources of information about medication, including health care professionals, patient information leaflets, family and friends, television, and newspapers. The information from these sources may or may not fit into the patients' representations or experiences of medication.

There is clear-cut evidence that antidepressants (ADs) can relieve both acute pain, as demonstrated in experimental pain studies, and chronic pain, as observed in patients suffering from diabetic neuropathy, postherpetic neuralgia, atypical facial pain, tension and migraine headache, fibromyalgia, and rheumatic pain (Onghena and van Handenhove 1992; Coquoz et al. 1993; Godfrey 1996). Analgesic effects can be dissociated from antidepressant or sedative effects (Max et al. 1988, 1992). However, ADs are associated with a relatively high number of adverse effects (AEs) in therapeutic usage. The incidence of AEs raises the issue of patients' observance with AD treatment. In a study in which chronic pain patients received 25 mg of amitriptyline or placebo, only 9 patients out of 14 preferred therapy over placebo, even if they had significantly greater relief when taking amitriptyline and could tolerate it (McQuay et al. 1992). Studies have shown that AEs and patients' representations of AEs are major determinants of nonobservance. For example, occurrence and severity of AEs decreased patient observance of migraine medication (MacGregor 1997), and fear of becoming addicted impaired observance in asthmatic patients (Adams et al. 1997) and in patients suffering from ankylosing spondylitis (de Klerk and van der Linden 1996). As for ADs, fear of AEs has been shown in depressive patients (Fawcett 1995) and in the general population (Benkert 1997).

The aim of this study was to investigate (1) the kind of information laypersons look for when taking medication and where they get it from; and (2) whether the nature of this information may explain some of the compliance problems with ADs prescribed for chronic refractory pain among patients referred to a pain clinic.

METHODS

INTERVIEW PROCEDURE AND ANALYSIS

The setting for this study was the Multidisciplinary Pain Center of the Geneva University Hospital. The center is an outpatient facility to which chronic refractory pain patients (CPPs) are referred by their physician for evaluation and treatment (Piguet et al. 1998). This study was part of a research project on representations of medication in general, and more specifically of ADs, among CPPs. A pain-free control group (Cs) was included to allow us to assess possible between-group differences. Controls were nonpatient subjects, matched a priori for age, sex, and education.

This study was conducted with 76 consecutive CPPs referred to the pain center and 54 Cs, who were investigated through semi-structured interviews. The interview included 21 open questions that explicitly referred to the individuals' definitions of medication and ADs, to their drug intake, and also to their access to information about medication. Four questions addressed this particular aspect: (1) When you take medication, what do you do to obtain information about it? (2) Which information do you find most useful? (3) Which is the easiest to understand? (4) Ideally, what information would you like to have before taking medication and how would you like to receive it? We chose to ask the individuals to give their own definitions instead of using multiple-choice questions, as the latter mainly call upon recognition memory. Furthermore, a multiple-choice format might deter alternative answers (Schwartz and Sudman 1992). As obtaining individuals' definitions was our main goal, the method of investigation had to provide an opportunity to assess patients' ways of thinking about medication and ADs. Free responses allowed a more thorough assessment of these representations.

The procedure used to examine the individuals' responses was qualitative. As is often the case in psychosocial studies investigating representations, various related dimensions were assessed by means of open questions (Moscovici 1976; Angermeyer and Matschinger 1994). The procedure then used was a content analysis (Blanchet et al. 1987). All responses were transcribed and categorized. Bivariate statistical procedures were used to evaluate within-group and between-group differences in CPPs and Cs. These analyses were performed using SPSS (1993). Prior written informed consent was obtained from all participants, and the protocol was approved by the local ethics committee. All interviews were conducted by two members of the research team trained in interview procedures.

POPULATION

The 76 CPPs were representative of the global population referred to the center regarding age, sex, and pain characteristics (Allaz et al. 1998). The two study groups were not significantly different in terms of their sociodemographic characteristics (Table I). Among the CPPs, 96% mentioned taking a prescription drug versus 44% among the Cs ($P < 0.001$). Drugs included ADs in 34% of CPPs and 7% of Cs ($P < 0.001$). To the question "Have you ever taken ADs?," reported intake increased to 68% in CPPs and 33% in Cs ($P < 0.001$).

REPORTED AND "IDEAL" SOURCES OF INFORMATION ABOUT MEDICATION

Reported sources of information. Patient information leaflets (PILs) were the most common source of information about medication, ahead of any other, including physicians (Table II): 88% of CPPs and 94% of Cs said they always or very often read the PILs. Up to 11% of CPPs and Cs even pointed out that their decision about taking a drug relied on the PIL only. Cross-examination of information was reported by 28% of CPPs and 30% of Cs. Both groups mainly looked for AE, dosage, and indications and contra-indications; an important proportion of individuals said they also checked the medication's mode of action and components (Table II). However, 21%

Table I
Sociodemographic characteristics of patients and controls

		CPPs	Cs
Age (years) (n.s.)	Mean (SD)	47.2 (14.7)	44.3 (16.6)
	Range	19–88	18–86
Sex (n.s.)	Percentage female	54%	54%
Educational status (n.s.)	Elementary school	34%	32%
	Qualified worker	38%	26%
	High school	12%	18%
	University	16%	24%
Origin (n.s.)	Swiss	51%	63%
	French	12%	20%
	Italian	7%	0%
	Spanish	8%	5%
	Portuguese	9%	6%
	Other	13%	6%
Patient's diagnosis	Neuropathic pain	18%	—
	Osteoarticular pain	41%	—
	Neuropathic and osteoarticular pain	15%	—
	Headache	5%	—
	Somatization pain	13%	—
	Other types of pain (chronic)	8%	—

Note: CPPs = chronic pain patients ($N = 76$); Cs = controls ($N = 54$); n.s. = not significant.

of CPPs and 13% of Cs described the PILs as difficult to understand, and 17% of CPPs and 11% of Cs sometimes considered them alarming. The pharmacist was more often mentioned in Cs ($P = 0.01$), which may be linked to more frequent use of over-the-counter drugs in this group.

"Ideal" information. The doctor-patient relationship was important to both groups (Table II). Emphasis was placed on information about medication indication and action, and to a lesser extent, about treatment adaptations. Expectations about information on AEs and contra-indications significantly differed between groups ($P = 0.003$ and 0.002, respectively), with Cs mentioning them more often than CPPs. Compared to contra-indications, however, AEs were a major concern. Cs significantly less often emphasized that information was difficult to provide or that they found it difficult to determine what information they would ideally like to receive and how they would like to receive it ($P = 0.009$). Dosage ($P < 0.001$), drug components ($P < 0.001$), contra-indications ($P < 0.001$), and even AEs in CPPs ($P < 0.001$) were significantly less often mentioned as part of an "ideal" information situation than as pertaining to the information individuals usually looked for.

Table II
Main reported sources of information about medication, and expected "ideal" information

	CPPs (%)	Cs (%)	*P*
Information Sources			
Physician	69.7	63.0	n.s.
Pharmacist	22.4	42.6	0.01
PIL, always	69.7	79.6	n.s.
PIL, very often	18.4	14.8	n.s.
PIL, never	6.6	3.7	n.s.
Information in PIL:			
Side effects	68.4	63.0	n.s.
Dosage	40.8	51.9	n.s.
Contra-indications	38.2	51.9	n.s.
Drug components	28.7	25.9	n.s.
Indications	46.1	40.7	n.s.
Mode of action	36.8	35.2	n.s.
Interactions	26.3	27.8	n.s.
Media	17.1	29.6	n.s.
Dictionary/guidebook	14.5	16.7	n.s.
Expected "Ideal" Information			
Doctor-patient interaction	51.3	57.4	n.s.
Pharmacist	1.3	9.3	0.03
Treatment adaptation	21.1	37.0	0.04
No information (the doctor decides)	11.8	11.1	n.s.
Difficult to determine	15.8	1.9	0.009
Information on:			
Side effects	36.8	63.0	0.003
Dosage	10.5	18.5	n.s.
Contra-indications	2.6	18.5	0.002
Drug components	1.3	7.4	n.s.
Drug indication and action	47.4	61.1	n.s.

Note: CPPs = chronic pain patients ($N = 76$); Cs = controls ($N = 54$); PIL = patient information leaflet; n.s. = not significant.

PATIENT INFORMATION LEAFLETS IN ANTIDEPRESSANT MEDICATION

Given the importance of PILs as a source of information, we analyzed the indications and AEs described in the Swiss version of PILs for 16 commonly prescribed ADs. Seven tricyclics, four SSRI, and five other ADs (venlafaxine, moclobemide, nefazodone, mianserin, and maprotiline) were included. Indications and AEs were analyzed on a lexical basis, taking into account AE frequency or severity (e.g., "urinary retention" was labeled as "possible," "occasional," "rare," or "severe").

Among the 16 PILs, 15 referred to the treatment of depression. Further indications included obsessive-compulsive disorders, bulimia, social phobia, and enuresis in children. Only 5 PILs mentioned pain as a possible indication, directly or indirectly. Physical symptoms linked to depression or with no organic cause were considered an indication in three of them. It should be noted that Swiss drug regulation authorities have accepted chronic refractory pain as a possible indication for three ADs where the manufacturers asked for this indication. Textual analysis confirmed that "pain" was negatively associated with AD indications ($V = -0.37$, $P < 0.001$), whereas "depression" and "mood" were strongly associated ($V = 0.62$, $P < 0.001$; and $V = 0.45$, $P < 0.001$, respectively). (The strength of the association was computed through Cramer's V, a χ-square measure of association for nominal variables [Norusis 1997].)

Analysis of AEs ($N = 66$) showed that 85% were somatic and 15% psychological. Mean number of AEs mentioned in the PILs was 18.5 (range: 6–49), with a mean of 16.1 (6–42) somatic AEs and 2.3 (0–7) psychological AEs. Five out of 16 PILs (31%) pointed out only frequent, possible, or occasional AEs that should not lead to treatment withdrawal or require medical consultation unless they persisted; 11 PILs (69%) also mentioned AEs that required treatment interruption and/or medical consultation, usually describing them as rare or severe.

DISCUSSION

PILs were the main reported source of information about medication in both groups. Physicians came second. Results regarding the proportion of patients who stated that they read the PILs are in accord with previous findings (Gibbs et al. 1989; Weinman 1990). Other studies have shown that pharmacists (Mottram and Reed 1997) and manufacturers (Bradley et al. 1995) may be largely underestimating the importance of PILs, with most pharmacists estimating that less than half of patients read them and manufacturers estimating that only about one-third of patients do so.

When asked to describe what information they would ideally like to receive before taking medication, both groups mentioned the role of physicians. They emphasized the doctor-patient relationship: the physician was expected to provide information and also to be available to discuss it as well as to adapt medication type and dosage in the course of treatment. Comparison between the main reported sources of information and "ideal" information showed a gap, mainly regarding the information content. Dosage, contra-indications, medication components, and even AEs in CPPs were reported significantly more often when individuals were asked about actual information than when asked to describe "ideal" information. This gap may suggest that the information they said they received was not congruent with their expectations. An alternative explanation is that "ideal" information as described in the interviews was not meant to replace other sources of information, mainly PILs, but to be combined with them, as one of the interviewees stated: "because the doctor knows what he has prescribed ... but also the leaflet, because it is down to earth" (36-year-old female; control). Both sources would then be used "as needed." From this perspective, PILs, considered as reference material, would—at least partly—achieve their goal of encouraging individuals to take an active part in their treatment and make better use of the doctor (Hermann et al. 1978). Some of our subjects stressed that they would like to discuss the leaflet with the doctor. For example, a woman who said she always reads the PIL noted: "I would like to have a week to read it and experience the effects of the medication and then ask the doctor all the questions I may have. In the leaflet, they say for example if you have headaches ... but if I have my period the day after, how can I know whether the headache is linked to my period or to the medication" (39-year-old; control). One patient indicated that he would like to have the opportunity to call the doctor "to check whether the side effects are normal or not, and also if the medication might be contra-indicated in my case because when you read the leaflet, you start to wonder ..." (43-year-old; chronic low back pain). A patient who described PILs as sometimes difficult to understand noted: "they are a bit ... cumbersome ... sometimes there are as many reasons to avoid taking the medication as there are to take it ... there seems to be an explanation for both good and bad, so that you can no longer tell if the medication is any good or not" (82-year-old female; chronic abdominal pain).

Content analysis of PILs also showed that AD leaflets point to indications that have a clear psychological, if not psychiatric, connotation. This is in line with both groups' representations of ADs (Piguet et al. 1999), such that they may consider such medication inappropriate for the treatment of pain. Asked whether he had ever taken ADs, one of the CPPs first answered no, and then "well, yes, I was prescribed something, but when I read the leaflet I saw it was an antidepressant ... I immediately stopped taking it because I'm not crazy"; but he never told his physician why he had stopped (41-year-old; chronic back pain). Another patient explained that her physician prescribed her ADs: "he told me it was not because of depression but because of my pain, but then I read the leaflet, and it was all clear ... I refused to take them; I said: Sorry, it is not depression!" (45-year-old; chronic palate pain).

These examples are characteristic, as these patients stated that they always thoroughly read the PIL; moreover, they also indicated that they made up their mind after reading it. The fact, however, that some patients clearly expressed that they stopped taking or refused to take ADs because of the leaflet emphasizes the gap between prescription and observance. These misunderstandings seem to mainly involve indications. Further analysis of interviews and PILs is underway in order to determine whether individuals remember only the elements that fit in with their own representations.

Studies on the mutual understanding between patients and their health care providers, in particular concerning the etiology of the disorder, demonstrate its importance: such accord is strongly associated with the resolution of symptoms or with a positive perception of changes in symptoms during treatment (Starfield et al. 1981; Cedraschi et al. 1996). In the context of chronic pain, where the causes of pain persistence often remain elusive, prescription of ADs may be seen as a "delegitimation," referring to a perceived denial of the patient's experience of pain and suffering (Kleinman 1992). Even when ADs are prescribed because of their analgesic effect, indications as described in the PILs may lead the patient to think that the physician does not truly believe he or she is in pain. Thus, noncongruence between PIL descriptions and the doctor's motive for prescribing ADs may account for some of the problems regarding patient observance of such medication.

REFERENCES

Adams S, Pill R, Jones A. Medication, chronic illness and identity: the perspective of people with asthma. *Soc Sci Med* 1997; 45:189–201.

Allaz AF, Vannotti M, Desmeules J, et al. Use of the label "litigation neurosis" in patients with somatoform pain disorder. *Gen Hosp Psychiatry* 1998; 20:91–97.

Angermeyer MC, Matschinger H. Lay beliefs about schizophrenic disorder: the results of a population survey in Germany. *Acta Psychiatr Scand* 1994; 89:39–45.

Benkert O, Graf-Morgenstern M, Hillert A, et al. Public opinion on psychotropic drugs: an analysis of the factors influencing acceptance or rejection. *J Nerv Ment Dis* 1997; 185:151–158.

Blanchet A, Ghiglione R, Massonnat J, Trognon A. *Les Techniques d'Enquête en Sciences Sociales* [Survey Techniques in Social Sciences]. Paris: Dunod, 1987.

Bradley B, McCusker E, Scott E, Li Wan Po A. Patient information leaflets on over-the-counter (OTC) medicines: the manufacturer's perspective. *J Clin Pharmacy Ther* 1995; 20:37–40.

Cedraschi C, Robert J, Perrin E, et al. The role of congruence between patient and therapist in chronic low back pain patients. *J Manipulative Physiol Ther* 1996; 19:244–249.

Coquoz D, Porchet HC, Dayer P. Central analgesic effects of desipramine, fluvoxamine, and moclobemide after single oral dosing: a study in healthy volunteers. *Clin Pharmacol Ther* 1993; 54:339–344.

De Klerk E, van der Linden SJ. Compliance monitoring of NSAID drug therapy in ankylosing spondylitis, experiences with an electronic monitoring device. *Br J Rheumatol* 1996; 35:60–65.

Donovan JL, Blake DR. Patient non-compliance: deviance or reasoned decision-making? *Soc Sci Med* 1992; 34:507–513.

Fawcett J. Compliance: definitions and key issues. *J Clin Psychiatry* 1995; 56:4–8.

Gibbs S, Waters WE, George CF. The benefits of prescription information leaflets. *Br J Clin Pharmacol* 1989; 27:723–739.

Godfrey RG. A guide to the understanding and use of tricyclic antidepressants in the overall management of fibromyalgia and other chronic pain syndromes. *Arch Intern Med* 1996; 156:1047–1052.

Hermann F, Herxheimer A, Lionel NDW. Package inserts for prescribed medicines: what minimum information do patients need? *BMJ* 1978; 2:1132–1135.

Kleinman A. Pain and resistance. The delegitimation and relegitimation of local worlds. In: Delvecchio-Good C, Brodwin PE, Good BJ, Kleinman A (Eds). *Pain as Human Experience*. Berkeley: University of California Press, 1992, pp 169–197.

MacGregor EA. The doctor and the migraine patient: improving compliance. *Neurology* 1997; 48(Suppl 3):S16–S20.

McQuay HJ, Carroll D, Glynn CJ. Low dose amitriptyline in the treatment of chronic pain. *Anaesthesia* 1992; 47:646–652.

Max MB, Schafer SC, Culnane M, et al. Amitriptyline, but not lorazepam, relieves postherpetic neuralgia. *Neurology* 1988; 38:1427–1432.

Max MB, Lynch SA, Muir J, et al. Effects of desipramine, amitriptyline, and fluoxetine on pain in diabetic neuropathy. *N Engl J Med* 1992; 326:1250–1256.

Moscovici S. *La Psychanalyse, son Image et son Public* [Psychoanalysis, Its Image, Its Public]. Paris: PUF, 1976.

Mottram DR, Reed C. Comparative evaluation of patient information leaflets by pharmacists, doctors and the general public. *J Clin Pharmacy Ther* 1997; 22:127–134.

Norusis MY. *SPSS 7.5 Guide to Data Analysis*. Upper Saddle River, New York: Prentice-Hall, 1997, pp 339–361.

Onghena P, van Handenhove B. Antidepressant-induced analgesia in chronic non-malignant pain: a meta-analysis of 39 placebo-controlled studies. *Pain* 1992; 49:205–219.

Piguet V, Allaz AF, Desmeules J, et al. Différences liées au sexe dans l'expression d'une douleur chronique. Expérience d'un centre d'évaluation et de traitement de la douleur [Gender differences in the expression of chronic pain. Experience of a pain center]. *Doul Anal* 1998; 11:101–105.

Piguet V, Cedraschi C, Fischer W, et al. Representations of antidepressants in chronic pain patients. *Abstracts: 9th World Congress on Pain*. Seattle: IASP Press, 1999.

Schwartz N, Sudman S (Eds). *Context Effects in Social and Psychological Research*. New York: Springer-Verlag, 1992.

SPSS (Statistical Package for Social Sciences). *Release 6.0, Base System User's Guide*. Chicago: SPSS Inc., 1993.

Starfield B, Wray C, Hess K, et al. The influence of patient-practitioner agreement on outcome of care. *Am J Public Health* 1981; 71:127–131.

Weinman J. Providing written information for patients: psychological considerations. *J R Soc Med* 1990; 83:303–305.

Correspondence to: C. Cedraschi, PhD, Multidisciplinary Pain Center, Division of Clinical Pharmacology, University Cantonal Hospital, 1211 Geneva 14, Switzerland. Tel: 41-22-382-36-79; Fax: 41-22-382-35-30; email: christine.cedraschi@hcuge.ch.

Proceedings of the 9th World Congress on Pain,
Progress in Pain Research and Management,
Vol. 16, edited by M. Devor, M.C. Rowbotham, and
Z. Wiesenfeld-Hallin, IASP Press, Seattle, © 2000.

83

The Role of Adenosine in the Treatment of Neuropathic Pain[1]

Rolf Karlsten and Torsten Gordh

Multidisciplinary Pain Treatment Center, University Hospital, Uppsala, Sweden

Neurogenic pain remains a burden for the patient and a challenge for the clinician. The current available treatments for patients with pain originating from injuries to the nervous system are not very effective and often have severe or disturbing side effects. Current drugs are mostly tricyclic antidepressants (TCAs), anticonvulsants, tramadol, or drugs with local anesthetic properties. The need for new pharmacological tools for treating patients with neurogenic pain is obvious, and several new pharmacological principles have been tried in the past few years including NMDA-receptor antagonists, somatostatin, and the anticonvulsant gabapentin (Karlsten and Gordh 1997). This chapter will discuss the potential of a new pharmacological approach that stimulates endogenous adenosine receptors. Experimental and clinical data are pointing at the adenosine system as an interesting target for hypersensitivity states, a common feature of neuropathic pain.

The endogenous compound adenosine is present in all cells. Adenosine may be released from cells directly or via degradation of adenosine triphosphate (ATP) and is involved in many regulatory mechanisms in both physiological and pathophysiological conditions (for reviews, see Pelleg and Porter 1990 and Abbracchio and Burnstock 1998). This chapter will consider aspects of the effects of adenosine on nociception and pain.

[1] Mini-review based on a congress workshop.

EXPERIMENTAL BACKGROUND

ADENOSINE AS A NEUROTRANSMITTER

Purines (adenosine, AMP, ADP, and ATP) mediate their effects by acting on a novel type of purine receptor. The two main subgroups of purine receptors, P1 and P2, differ in some characteristics (Table I). The endogenous compound adenosine is pharmacologically active on extracellular P1 receptors (Burnstock 1972).

Adenosine acts mainly via P1 receptors. It is now accepted that the P1 receptors can be further divided into A1, A2a, A2b, and A3 receptors (Fredholm et al. 1994). Activation of A1 receptors inhibits adenylate cyclase activity and thereby decreases the intracellular levels of cyclic adenosine monophosphate (cAMP), while activation of the A2 receptor stimulates adenylate cyclase and increases the intracellular level of cAMP (Van Calker et al. 1979). A1 and A2 receptors occur in the spinal cord, whereas A1 receptors occur predominantly in the substantia gelatinosa (Choca et al. 1987, 1988) and also in the brain (Goodman and Snyder 1982). Recently, an A3 receptor was classified based on the inhibition constant of antagonist binding. A3 receptors have not yet been found in the nervous system, but peripheral effects have been demonstrated. It is known that activation of A3 receptors on mast cells mediates a release of histamine and 5-hydroxytryptamine (serotonin) (Sawynok et al. 1997), which in turn act on histamine H1 and 5-HT2 receptors on the sensory nerve terminal to induce a pronociceptive action (Sawynok 1998).

Biochemical markers for adenosine activity in the spinal cord, such as enzymes for synthesis of adenosine, adenosine immunoactivity, receptors, uptake sites, and catabolic enzymes, show poor correlation in the central nervous system (CNS) (Fastbom 1988). This is not the case within the substantia gelatinosa, which contains a concentration of biochemical markers. Adenosine, perhaps originating from ATP, is released from spinal synapto-

Table I
Characteristics of the P1 and P2 purinergic receptors

Characteristic	P1	P2
Relative potency	ADO > AMP > ADP > ATP	ATP > ADP > AMP > ADO
Adenylate cyclase activity	↑/↓	No change
Methylxanthines	Antagonists	No effect
Induction of prostaglandin synthesis	No	Yes

Source: Burnstock (1972).

somes (Sawynok and Sweeney 1989). These findings indicate that adenosine may play a role in the modulation of nociceptive transmission.

INVOLVEMENT OF ADENOSINE IN NOCICEPTIVE TRANSMISSION

Animal studies in mice and rats that used escape reactions as endpoints for measuring nociceptive threshold provided early suggestions that adenosine and adenosine analogues have antinociceptive properties after systemic or intrathecal (i.t.) administration (Holmgren et al. 1983, 1986; Post 1984; Ahlijanian and Takemori 1985; DeLander and Hopkins 1986; Sawynok et al. 1986). Later studies, using adenosine analogues with different efficacy for the A1 and A2 adenosine receptors, indicated that spinal A1 receptors are involved in inducing the antinociceptive effects (Karlsten et al. 1990; Sawynok 1991; Lee and Yaksh 1996). The role of the A1 receptor in inhibiting spinal sensory transmission has been confirmed by the inhibitory effect of A1 analogues on the C-fiber-evoked responses, wind-up, and post-discharge of dorsal horn neurons (Reeve and Dickenson 1995). Recordings of evoked potentials from the spinal cord in rats support the findings of Reeve and Dickenson (Nakamura et al. 1997). Adenosine agonists dose-dependently inhibited the slow ventral root potential, which is the C-fiber-evoked excitatory response associated with nociceptive information. The rank order of agonist potency indicated that adenosine agonists inhibit spinal sensory transmission by acting on A1 receptors (Nakamura et al. 1997). It seems that adenosine modulates spinal nociceptive transmission by inhibition of intrinsic neurons through an increase in K^+ conductance and presynaptic inhibition of sensory nerve terminals to inhibit the release of substance P and perhaps glutamate (Sawynok 1998).

In 1989, Sosnowski and Yaksh demonstrated that the adenosine agonists R-phenylisopropyl-adenosine (R-PIA) and N-ethylcarboxamide-adenosine (NECA) induced a dose-dependent inhibition of the hypersensitivity evoked by intrathecal strychnine in rats. The response was seen in doses (0.3–1 nmol) that have only mild antinociceptive effects on thermal stimulation and withdrawal tests (hot-plate, tail-flick, and tail immersion) (Sosnowski and Yaksh 1989). This study was the first to suggest that adenosine might have be involved in the modulation of pathological pain as seen in many patients with neuropathic pain. In a later study, R-PIA inhibited the spontaneous and touch-evoked agitation seen after i.t. prostaglandin F_2 in mice (Minami et al. 1992). NECA was also tested in this study but it was not possible to separate the inhibitory effects on agitation from the motor impairment.

In new experimental methods in rodents, induced nerve injuries produced hypersensitive reactions to low-threshold mechanical stimulation and heat, similar to clinical findings often seen in neurogenic pain in humans. Bennett and Xie introduced a model where four loose ligatures are placed around the sciatic nerve (Bennett and Xie 1988), called the chronic constriction injury (CCI) model. Application of CCI revealed that the adenosine agonist NECA reduced the hypersensitive reaction to heat stimuli in doses that did not affect normal paw latencies in rats (Yamamoto and Yaksh 1991). Sjölund et al. demonstrated 1996 that R-PIA reduces the scratching behavior of rats with CCI, both after i.v. administration (30 nmol) and i.t. injection (3 nmol) (Sjölund et al. 1996). In rats subjected to CCI, Cui et al. (1998) demonstrated a dose-dependent reduction of hypersensitivity to tactile stimulation after i.t. R-PIA (1–10 nmol). The effect was abolished by i.t. injection of the A1-receptor antagonist cyclopentylxanthine. The same study revealed a potentiation of the effect of spinal cord stimulation after concomitant i.t. injection of a submaximal dose of R-PIA (3 nmol).

In studies with the animal model developed by Kim and Chung (1991) in which a tight ligation of the L4–S1 spinal nerves produces a state of tactile hypersensitivity, adenosine analogues dose-dependently diminished the hypersensitivity reaction to mechanical stimulation with von Frey filaments (Lee and Yaksh 1996). Comparing the effects of A1 and A2 adenosine receptor agonists and antagonists suggested that the "antiallodynic" effect of adenosine is mediated by activation of the A1 receptor and that motor dysfunction effects are mediated by activation of the A2 receptor (Lee and Yaksh 1996).

In a recently published study, Lavand'homme and Eisenach (1999) demonstrated that adenosine given i.t. induced a dose-dependent reduction of tactile hypersensitivity in rats following spinal nerve ligation. Interestingly, the response persisted more than 24 hours after a single i.t. injection of 30 μg of adenosine. The authors also observed a delay in onset, with a maximal effect after 2 hours and lasting at least 24 hours.

In a new model of photochemically induced ischemic spinal cord injury in rats, which causes hypersensitivity to cold and mechanical stimuli, i.t. R-PIA reduced the hypersensitivity to both mechanical and cold stimulation (Sjölund et al. 1998). Another study with the same model demonstrated that R-PIA injected repeatedly twice daily maintained the effect on hypersensitivity for 5–7 days (von Heijne et al. 1998).

STUDIES ON POTENTIAL SPINAL NEUROTOXICITY

The above indications that spinal administration of adenosine or adenosine agonists with selectivity for the A1 receptor might have potential use as analgesic drugs in humans have prompted several neurotoxicological studies. It is important to investigate potential noxious effects on the spinal cord in animals before performing studies in humans. Studies have used laser Doppler flowmetry technique (Karlsten et al. 1992) and the iodoantipurine method (Kristensen et al. 1993) to test the adenosine analogue R-PIA, selective for the A1 receptor, for effects on spinal cord blood flow in rats. In both studies, R-PIA induced a slight but significant increase in spinal cord blood flow. A neurotoxicological evaluation using morphologic and morphometric methods in rats showed that chronic i.t. administration of R-PIA once daily (5 and 25 nmol in two groups) for 14 days induced no changes (Karlsten et al. 1993). In a recent similar study using the same methods, i.t. adenosine at doses of 10 µg administered to rats twice daily for 14 days showed no neurotoxic effects (Rane et al. 1999)

GENERAL CONCLUSIONS OF RESULTS FROM ANIMAL STUDIES

EFFECTS ON NOCICEPTION IN RODENTS

The effects of adenosine on nociception in rodents can be summarized as follows: (1) A1-receptor activation induces an antinociceptive effect, both in the periphery and in the spinal cord. (2) A2-receptor activation in the spinal cord induces motor dysfunction, and peripheral A2-receptor activation induces a pronociceptive effect. (3) A3-receptor activation mediates release of 5-HT and serotonin from mast cells, which in turn may activate sensory nerve terminals. (4) Adenosine analogues are more potent in inhibiting the hypersensitivity reactions seen in animal models of nerve injury than in nociceptive tests. This indicates that adenosine and its analogues may interfere with pathological pain states such as neuropathic pain and other states characterized by hyperexcitability.

Animal studies have revealed that adenosine and its analogues may have a role in clinical treatment of pain. Most interesting is the potential to modulate pathological pain states, such as hyperexcitability associated with injuries to the peripheral and central nervous system. Several obvious difficulties arise in transferring animal data to humans. In humans a nerve lesion may result in hypo- or hypersensitive reactions, and sometimes neurological examination reveals both phenomena in the same patient. Most patients with injuries to the nervous system do not develop pain, a situation that contrasts with the findings in the Bennett and Chung models, where the rats as a rule seem to develop a hypersensitive reaction to mechanical stimulation. Neuropathic pain in humans is often longstanding and chronic, while the hyperphenomena seen in rodents after nerve ligation sometimes subside within weeks. Of course, it is not possible to know whether the reaction the rats show after nerve ligation is truly that of pain. A point to remember is that the pharmacological properties of the different adenosine receptors differ between species (Kennedy and Ijzerman 1994) and thus it might be difficult to extrapolate from animal experiments when considering potential effects of adenosine and its analogues in humans. We should use great care in interpreting animal data and try to avoid terms such as hyperalgesia and allodynia.

SYSTEMIC ADMINISTRATION OF ADENOSINE TO HUMANS

The effect of adenosine on pain in humans has mostly been studied using intravenous (i.v.) administration of adenosine. The first indication that adenosine might induce pain relief in humans was the demonstration that an adenosine infusion combined with isoflurane-nitrous oxide anesthesia abolished the need for additional analgesics during surgery (Sollevi 1992). A single-blinded study that used a tourniquet technique revealed that i.v. adenosine (70 $\mu g \cdot kg^{-1} \cdot min^{-1}$) reduced experimentally induced ischemic muscle pain in healthy volunteers (Segerdahl et al. 1994). Another single-blinded study in healthy volunteers found that i.v. infusion of adenosine at 50–80 $\mu g \cdot kg^{-1} \cdot min^{-1}$ increased the cutaneous heat pain threshold, but did not influence the perception thresholds for heat and cold (Ekblom et al. 1995).

Spontaneous pain was reduced and touch-evoked pain thresholds were increased, in a double-blind, placebo-controlled, crossover study in seven patients with neuropathic pain who received i.v. infusion of adenosine 50 $\mu g \cdot kg^{-1} \cdot min^{-1}$ during 45–60 minutes (Belfrage et al. 1995). Two patients with peripheral neuropathic pain received adenosine 50–70 $\mu g \cdot kg^{-1} \cdot min^{-1}$. Tactile allodynia and spontaneous pain were relieved in one, and hyperalgesia to pinprick was attenuated in the other (Sollevi et al. 1995). These two reports indicate that adenosine may play a role as a modulator of neuropathic pain in humans. Further support for this role comes from evidence that patients with neuropathic pain have reduced levels of adenosine in the blood and cerebrospinal fluid as compared to patients with nociceptive pain and patients with nervous system lesions without pain (Guieu et al. 1996). In a recent double-blind, placebo-controlled, multicenter study of patients with neuropathic pain, i.v. adenosine (50 $\mu g \cdot kg^{-1} \cdot min^{-1}$) significantly reduced the area of allodynia to touch (K.F. Sjölund et al., this volume).

INTRATHECAL ADMINISTRATION OF ADENOSINE TO HUMANS

Animal studies have shown that adenosine and adenosine analogues induce antinociception predominantly by a spinal site of action. This finding may indicate that the i.t. route of administration could be superior to systemic administration. In a single-case report, R-PIA 25 nmol was injected i.t. to a patient with chronic neuropathic pain with severe allodynia to light touch and vibration (Karlsten and Gordh 1995). Following administration of the A1-receptor agonist R-PIA, the allodynia to light touch and vibration was abolished completely and the spontaneous pain decreased. The detection thresholds for thermal stimuli and pain thresholds for heat and cold remained unchanged after i.t. R-PIA. Vital signs such as blood pressure, pulse, and respiratory status also were unaffected (Karlsten and Gordh 1995). In a study in which adenosine was injected i.t. to 12 healthy volunteers (500–2000 μg), the forearm ischemic pain rating decreased and the areas of secondary allodynia were reduced by adenosine after skin inflammation induced by mustard oil. One patient receiving 2000 μg i.t. experienced a transient lumbar pain following the injection; doses up to 1000 μg were tolerated without any side effects (Rane et al. 1998).

In an open study in 14 patients with chronic neuropathic pain of traumatic origin with tactile hyperalgesia or allodynia, i.t. adenosine (500 or 1000 μg) reduced spontaneous and evoked pain. An increase in tactile pain thresholds in the allodynic areas also occurred. In total, 12 patients experienced pain relief lasting a median 24 hours. Five patients had a transient lumbar pain after the i.t. injection of adenosine (Belfrage et al. 1999).

SUMMARY AND CONCLUSIONS

Evidence is now abundant that adenosine can modulate nociception. Behavioral and neurophysiological studies in animal models have indicated that A1 receptors are involved in the antinociceptive effect. In humans, almost all studies have been performed using systemic and i.t. administration of adenosine, which is unselective for the A1 and A2 receptor. Most studies in humans confirm the results from the animal studies, which indicate that adenosine and adenosine analogues may have a role in the future treatment of patients with pathological pain conditions with associated hyperexcitability. Even if small studies on potential neurotoxicity have not shown any signs of neuronal damage, future studies need to explain the transient pain on i.t. injection experienced by some patients. More controlled studies in patients with defined pain states are a prerequisite for establishing the effectiveness of adenosine in pain treatment.

ACKNOWLEDGMENTS

Supported by grants from the Swedish Medical Research Council No. 09077.

REFERENCES

Abbracchio MP, Burnstock G. Purinergic signalling: pathophysiological roles. *Jpn J Pharmacol* 1998; 78:113–145.

Ahlijanian MK, Takemori AE. Effects of (-)-N6-(R-phenylisopropyl)-adenosine (PIA) and caffeine on nociception and morphine-induced analgesia, tolerance and dependence in mice. *Eur J Pharmacol* 1985; 112:171–179.

Belfrage M, Sollevi A, Segerdahl M, Sjölund KF, Hansson P. Systemic adenosine infusion alleviates spontaneous and stimulus evoked pain in patients with peripheral neuropathic pain. *Anesth Analg* 1995; 81:713–717.

Belfrage M, Segerdahl M, Arner S, Sollevi A. The safety and efficacy of intrathecal adenosine in patients with chronic neuropathic pain. *Anesth Analg* 1999; 89:1136–1142.

Bennett GJ, Xie Y-K. A peripheral mononeuropathy in rat that produces disorders of pain sensation like those seen in man. *Pain* 1988; 33:87–107.

Burnstock G. Purinergic nerves. *Pharmacol Rev* 1972; 24:509–581.

Choca JI, Proudfit HK, Green RD. Identification of A1 and A2 adenosine receptors in the rat spinal cord. *J Pharmacol Exp Ther* 1987; 242:905–910.

Choca JI, Green RD, Proudfit HK. Adenosine A1 and A2 receptors in the substantia gelatinosa are located predominantly on intrinsic neurons: an autoradiography study. *J Pharmacol Exp Ther* 1988; 247:757–764.

Cui JG, Meyerson BA, Sollevi A, Linderoth B. Effect of spinal cord stimulation on tactile hypersensitivity in mononeuropathic rats is potentiated by simultaneous GABA(B) and adenosine receptor activation. *Neurosci Lett* 1998; 247:183–186.

DeLander GE, Hopkins CJ. Spinal adenosine modulates descending antinociceptive pathways stimulated by morphine. *J Pharmacol Exp Ther* 1986; 239:88–93.

Ekblom A, Segerdahl M, Sollevi A. Adenosine increases the cutaneous heat pain threshold in healthy volunteers. *Acta Anaesthesiol Scand* 1995; 39:717–722.

Fastbom J. Adenosine receptors in the central nervous system. Dissertation. Stockholm: Karolinska Institutet, 1988.

Fredholm BB, Abbracchio MP, Burnstock G, et al. VI. Nomenclature and classification of purinoreceptors. *Pharmacol Rev* 1994; 46:143–156.

Goodman RR, Snyder SH. Autoradiographic localization of adenosine receptors in rat brain using (H)cyclohexyladenosine. *J Neurosci* 1982; 2:1230–1241.

Guieu R, Peragut JC, Roussel P, et al. Adenosine and neuropathic pain. *Pain* 1996; 68:271–274.

Holmgren M, Hedner T, Nordberg G, Mellstrand T. Antinociceptive effects in the rat of an adenosine analogue, N-phenylisopropyladenosine. *J Pharm Pharmacol* 1983; 35:679–680.

Holmgren M, Hedner J, Mellstrand T, Nordberg G, Hedner T. Characterization of the antinociceptive effects of some adenosine analogues in the rat. *Naunyn Schmiedebergs Arch Pharmacol* 1986; 334:290–293.

Karlsten R, Gordh T Jr. An A1-selective adenosine agonist abolishes allodynia elicited by vibration and touch after intrathecal injection. *Anesth Analg* 1995; 80:844–847.

Karlsten R, Gordh T. How do drugs relieve neurogenic pain? *Drugs Aging* 1997; 11:398–412.

Karlsten R, Gordh T Jr, Hartvig P, Post C. Effects of intrathecal injection of the adenosine receptor agonists R-phenylisopropyl-adenosine and N-ethylcarboxamide-adenosine on nociception and motor function in the rat. *Anesth Analg* 1990; 71:60–64.

Karlsten R, Kristensen JD, Gordh T. R-phenylisopropyl-adenosine increases spinal cord blood flow after intrathecal injection in the rat. *Anesth Analg* 1992; 75:972–976.

Karlsten R, Gordh T, Svensson BA. A neurotoxicologic evaluation of the spinal cord after chronic intrathecal injection of R-phenylisopropyl adenosine in the rat. *Anesth Analg* 1993; 77:731–736.

Kennedy C, Ijzerman A. Adenosine and ATP: from receptor structure to clinical applications. *Trends Pharmacol Sci* 1994; 15:311–312.

Kim SH, Chung JM. Sympathectomy alleviates mechanical allodynia in an experimental animal model for neuropathy in the rat. *Neurosci Lett* 1991; 134:131–134.

Kristensen JD, Karlsten R, Gordh T, Holtz A. Spinal cord blood flow after intrathecal injection of a N-methyl-D-aspartate receptor antagonist or an adenosine receptor agonist in rats. *Anesth Analg* 1993; 76:1279–1283.

Lavand'homme PM, Eisenach JC. Exogenous and endogenous adenosine enhance the spinal antiallodynic effects of morphine in a rat model of neuropathic pain. *Pain* 1999; 80:31–36.

Lee YW, Yaksh TL. Pharmacology of the spinal adenosine receptor which mediates the antiallodynic action of intrathecal adenosine agonists. *J Pharmacol Exp Ther* 1996; 277:1642–1648.

Minami T, Uda R, Horiguchi S, et al. Allodynia evoked by intrathecal administration of prostaglandin F2 alpha to conscious mice. *Pain* 1992; 50:223–229.

Nakamura I, Ohta Y, Kemmotsu O. Characterization of adenosine receptors mediating spinal sensory transmission related to nociceptive information in the rat. *Anesthesiology* 1997; 87:577–584.

Pelleg A, Porter S. The pharmacology of adenosine. *Pharmacotherapy* 1990; 10:157–174.

Post C. Antinociceptive effects in mice after intrathecal injection of 5'-N-ethylcarboxamide adenosine. *Neurosci Lett* 1984; 51:325–330.

Rane K, Segerdahl M, Goiny M, Sollevi A. Intrathecal adenosine administration: a phase 1 clinical safety study in healthy volunteers, with additional evaluation of its influence on sensory thresholds and experimental pain. *Anesthesiology* 1998; 89:1108–1115.

Rane K, Karlsten R, Sollevi A, Gordh T, Svensson BA. Spinal cord morphology after chronic intrathecal administration of adenosine in the rat. *Acta Anaesthesiol Scand* 1999; 43:1035–1040.

Reeve AJ, Dickenson AH. The roles of spinal adenosine receptors in the control of acute and more persistent nociceptive responses of dorsal horn neurones in the anaesthetized rat. *Br J Pharmacol* 1995; 116:2221–2228.

Sawynok J. Adenosine and pain. In: Phillis JW (Ed). *Adenosine and Adenine Nucleotides as Regulators of Cell Function*. Boca Raton: CRC Press, 1991, pp 391–402.

Sawynok J. Adenosine receptor activation and nociception. *Eur J Pharmacol* 1998; 347:1–11.

Sawynok J, Sweeney MI. The role of purines in nociception. *Neuroscience* 1989; 32:557–569.

Sawynok J, Sweeney MI, White TD. Classification of adenosine receptors mediating antinociception in the rat spinal cord. *Br J Pharmacol* 1986; 88:923–930.

Sawynok J, Zarrindast MR, Reid AR, Doak GJ. Adenosine A3 receptor activation produces nociceptive behaviour and edema by release of histamine and 5-hydroxytryptamine. *Eur J Pharmacol* 1997; 333:1–7.

Segerdahl M, Ekblom A, Sollevi A. The influence of adenosine, ketamine, and morphine on experimentally induced ischemic pain in healthy volunteers. *Anesth Analg* 1994; 79:787–791.

Sjölund KF, Sollevi A, Segerdahl M, Hansson P, Lundeberg T. Intrathecal and systemic R-phenylisopropyl-adenosine reduces scratching behaviour in a rat mononeuropathy model. *Neuroreport* 1996; 7:1856–1860.

Sjölund KF, von Heijne M, Hao JX, et al. Intrathecal administration of the adenosine A1 receptor agonist R-phenylisopropyl adenosine reduces presumed pain behaviour in a rat model of central pain. *Neurosci Lett* 1998; 243:89–92.

Sollevi A. Adenosine infusion during isoflurane-nitrous oxide anaesthesia: indications of perioperative analgesic effect. *Acta Anaesthesiol Scand* 1992; 36:595–599.

Sollevi A, Belfrage M, Lundeberg T, Segerdahl M, Hansson P. Systemic adenosine infusion: a new treatment modality to alleviate neuropathic pain. *Pain* 1995; 61:155–158.

Sosnowski M, Yaksh TL. Role of spinal adenosine receptors in modulating the hyperesthesia produced by spinal glycine receptor antagonism. *Anesth Analg* 1989; 69:587–592.

Van Calker D, Müller M, Hamprecht B. Adenosine regulates via two different types of receptors, the accumulation of cyclic AMP in cultured brain cells. *J Neurochem* 1979; 33:999–1005.

von Heijne M, Hao JX, Yu W, et al. Reduced anti-allodynic effect of the adenosine A1-receptor agonist R-phenylisopropyladenosine on repeated intrathecal administration and lack of cross-tolerance with morphine in a rat model of central pain. *Anesth Analg* 1998; 87:1367–1371.

Yamamoto T, Yaksh TL. Spinal pharmacology of thermal hyperesthesia induced by incomplete ligation of sciatic nerve. I. Opioid and nonopioid receptors. *Anesthesiology* 1991; 75:817–826.

Correspondence to: Rolf Karlsten MD, PhD, Multidisciplinary Pain Treatment Center, University Hospital, S-75185 Uppsala, Sweden. Tel: 46-18-663740; Fax: 46-18-503539; email: rolf.karlsten@anestesi.uu.se.

Proceedings of the 9th World Congress on Pain,
Progress in Pain Research and Management,
Vol. 16, edited by M. Devor, M.C. Rowbotham, and
Z. Wiesenfeld-Hallin, IASP Press, Seattle, © 2000.

84

Systemic Adenosine Infusion Reduces the Area of Neuropathic Tactile Allodynia: A Multi-Center, Placebo-Controlled Study

Karl-Fredrik Sjölund,[a] Måns Belfrage,[b] Rolf Karlsten,[c] Märta Segerdahl,[d] Staffan Arnér,[a] Torsten Gordh,[c] and Alf Sollevi[d]

[a]Karolinska Institute, Departments of Anesthesiology and Intensive Care, Karolinska Hospital, Stockholm; [b]St Görans Hospital, Stockholm; [c]Uppsala University Hospital, Uppsala; and [d]Huddinge Hospital, Huddinge, Sweden

Adenosine receptor agonists reduce painlike behavior in animal models of acute (Sawynok and Sweeney 1989) and neuropathic pain (Yamamoto and Yaksh 1991). In humans, intravenous adenosine infusion shows analgesic properties in both experimental and clinical studies (Segerdahl et al. 1995a,b). Human data also show modulation of neuronal hyperexcitability following systemic adenosine administration (Segerdahl et al. 1995a). Further, intrathecal adenosine and adenosine agonists administered to patients suffering neuropathic pain produce analgesic effects (Karlsten and Gordh 1995; Lindblom et al. 1997; Belfrage et al. 1999). Our study further assesses the influence of systemic adenosine infusion (50 $\mu g \cdot kg^{-1} \cdot min^{-1}$) on pathological tactile somatosensory phenomena and spontaneous pain in peripheral neuropathic pain.

PATIENTS AND METHODS

The study was approved by the local research ethics committee. Twenty-six patients suffering a peripheral neuropathic pain condition following a surgical or traumatic injury, and showing cutaneous dynamic tactile allodynia (pain evoked by brush) were included after they gave informed consent (demographic data in Table I). We used a crossover, double-blind, placebo-

Table I
Demographic data

Patient No.	Gender/ Age	Duration (months)	Initial Injury
1	M/25	16	traumatic, finger amputation
2	F/40	20	surgical, n. infrapatellaris
3	F/61	60	surgical, mastectomy
4	F/71	23	surgical, mastectomy
5	F/52	21	surgical, mastectomy
6	F/82	6	traumatic, n. ulnaris
7	F/44	5	surgical, mastectomy
8	F/43	8	traumatic, ankle and foot
9	F/55	78	traumatic, n. radialis
10	F/25	56	traumatic, n. radialis
11	F/34	8	surgical, n. peroneus
12	F/52	14	surgical, thrombophlebitis
13	M/45	48	n. peroneus
14	F/62	6	n. cutaneous femoris lateralis
15	F/51	8	surgical, hallux valgus
16	F/22	10	n. ulnaris
17	M/46	50	surgical, n. suralis
18	F/40	10	surgical, n. infrapatellaris
19	F/48	85	surgical, n. saphenus
20	M/65	18	surgical, n. infrapatellaris
21	F/35	30	surgical, n. infrapatellaris + saphenus
22	F/22	25	surgical, n. saphenus
23	F/44	7	surgical, n. infrapatellaris
24	F/43	25	surgical, hallux valgus
25	M/43	96	traumatic, n. ulnaris
26	F/37	36	surgical, n. obturatorius

controlled design. Adenosine (Adenosin, 5 mg/mL in isotonic mannitol, Item Development AB) 50 $\mu g \cdot kg^{-1} \cdot min^{-1}$ and placebo (isotonic mannitol) were infused intravenously (i.v.) for 60 minutes on separate occasions. In most cases the interval between treatments was 1-2 weeks. In six cases, however, we decided in advance that the second treatment should immediately follow the evaluation of the first treatment if this had not produced changes in the tested sensory modalities. In a follow-up session, the patient stated the global subjective outcome for the clinical pain condition.

Sensory tests, as described below, were performed immediately before treatments and again, starting after 45 minute treatment. First, we assessed spontaneous pain with a visual analogue scale (VAS), graded from 0 to 100.

Second, we mapped the skin area where the light stroke of a soft brush produced pain (dynamic tactile allodynia). Third, we used calibrated graded von Frey filaments to assess the tactile thresholds to touch perception and pain in the affected skin area and in the contralateral corresponding unaffected skin area.

The statistical analysis used the Wilcoxon test for matched pairs to determine the percentage changes in spontaneous pain, the area of tactile allodynia, and tactile pain threshold over the two treatments, and also the duration of reported subjective global improvement. $P < 0.05$ was considered significant. Median values and quartiles are shown.

RESULTS

All 26 patients received adenosine treatment, and 24 patients received placebo treatment. No patient experienced long-lasting pain relief after placebo treatment.

Results from the evaluation of tactile threshold in the neuropathic and corresponding control areas are shown in Table II. The absolute difference in threshold between baseline measurements before treatment was 0.08 g (0.03–0.16 g) in the control area and 0.18 g (0.02–0.44 g) in the area of neuropathy. Spontaneous pain was perceived by 19 patients before placebo treatment and by 21 patients before adenosine. In these patients the VAS pain intensity rating was 43 (30–56)/100 before placebo and 38 (27–55)/100 before adenosine. Compared to the pre-infusion baseline, the intensity of spontaneous pain was reduced by adenosine ($P = 0.006$) but not significantly by placebo ($P = 0.10$). However, the effect of adenosine was not significantly different from placebo ($P = 0.18$).

The area of dynamic tactile allodynia before treatment ranged from 15 to 780 cm^2. The change following placebo treatment was a reduction by 0% (0–14% [median, quartile]), while adenosine treatment reduced the area by

Table II
Threshold of tactile perception as assessed with calibrated graded von Frey filaments in the neuropathic and corresponding contralateral skin areas

Tactile Threshold (g)	Placebo		Adenosine	
	Pretreatment	Post-treatment	Pretreatment	Post-treatment
Control area	0.26 (0.13–0.50)	0.30 (0.12–0.46)	0.27 (0.13–0.71)	0.28 (0.13–0.48)
Neuropathic area	0.29 (0.13–0.70)	0.48 (0.14–0.78)	0.40 (0.14–0.86)	0.48 (0.13–0.76)

Note: Medians (and quartiles) are given ($n = 24$ for placebo and 26 for adenosine).

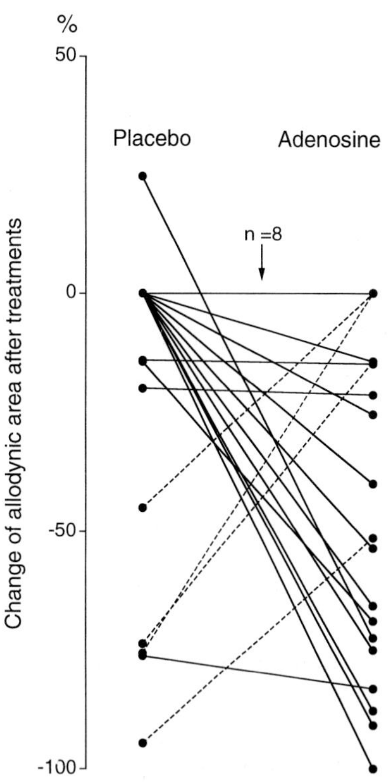

Fig. 1. Difference in individual response between the randomized study treatments, placebo and adenosine, on the size of the area of dynamic tactile (brush-evoked) allodynia. Data are expressed as percentage change from baseline measurements. Data points of individual patients (n = 26) are joined with lines; dashed lines indicate subjects in whom placebo treatment had better efficacy than adenosine.

18% (0–67%). Individual data are shown in Fig. 1. The area of tactile allodynia was significantly reduced by adenosine when compared to placebo treatment (P = 0.048). The tactile pain threshold in the allodynic area ranged from 0.008 to 29 g before placebo, and from 0.008 to 20 g before adenosine treatment. Median values were 4.0 g (0.7–8.3 g) and 2.1 g (0.4–7.1 g), respectively. The tactile pain threshold was increased by 15% (–22 to +141%) after placebo, and by 71% (0–334%) after adenosine treatment. The change from pre-infusion values was significant both for placebo (P = 0.045) and adenosine (P = 0.0005). Comparison of the effect of the two treatments revealed that the difference was not significant (P = 0.37). Three patients reported subjective improvement of the clinical pain condition after placebo, with a duration outlasting the test procedures by 2, 10, and 50 hours, respectively. Eleven patients reported subjective improvement after adenosine treatment. Two patients (numbers 2 and 9) reporting complete or near complete pain relief with a duration of more than 6 months were not given placebo treatment. Improvements after adenosine typically lasted for 10 hours. Compared to placebo, adenosine had significant positive subjective effects on the clinical condition (P = 0.028).

DISCUSSION

The results of this multicenter, double-blind, placebo-controlled study show that the area of dynamic tactile allodynia in patients with peripheral neuropathic pain is reduced by systemic adenosine infusion. Subjective global improvement of the clinical pain condition also occurred following adenosine treatment. Spontaneous pain and tactile pain threshold were not significantly improved when compared to placebo. A relatively high frequency of placebo responses occurred in this study. We observed reduced sensory dysfunction after placebo in 30–50% of the patients in each parameter. This finding is in line with earlier observations of frequent placebo responses in neuropathic pain (Verdugo and Ochoa 1991), although it is unclear whether this is a characteristic of neuropathic pain per se, or of the specific procedures used. Changes in psychophysical quantitative sensory tests during placebo treatment may result from activation of endogenous neuromodulatory systems due to resting, or other aspects of the test procedure.

Inclusion criteria for this study were the combination of a known traumatic injury and the occurrence of dynamic tactile allodynia. Despite the relatively homogeneous case histories and clinical findings of the patients studied, divergent mechanisms may well be involved. Specific effects on pathophysiological mechanisms of importance in a subgroup of patients may thus be difficult to detect in the presence of frequent placebo effects. We used psychophysical tests to evaluate tactile sensory dysfunction and pain. Each parameter analyzed may reflect one of many dimensions in the mosaic of long-lasting neuropathic pain (Arnér et al. 1990). Results in each parameter may reflect effects of a pharmacological intervention on specific pathophysiological mechanisms.

Adenosine administration has reduced spontaneous pain (Belfrage et al. 1995). However, in our study the reduction in spontaneous pain was not significant when compared to placebo treatment. We observed a reduction of the area of dynamic tactile allodynia after adenosine treatment. Dynamic tactile allodynia is likely to be mediated via activation of low-threshold mechanoreceptors activating central pain pathways via sensitized second-order neurons in the spinal cord dorsal horn (Koltzenburg et al. 1994). Antinociceptive effects of adenosine may be mediated primarily via adenosine A1 receptors in the spinal cord dorsal horn (Karlsten et al. 1995), where adenosine receptor activation hyperpolarizes the postsynaptic membrane of interneurons (Li and Perl 1994). This process could reduce the hyperexcitability of second-order neurons involved in tactile allodynia, and thus account for our observation. Also, the reduced area of dynamic tactile allodynia is in line with animal data (Sumida et al. 1998) and human experimental studies (Segerdahl et al. 1995a), where adenosine seems to induce modulatory effects on the mechanisms of central sensitization. The observations of stable tactile perception thresholds in normal skin and in the affected area (Table II) indicate unchanged function in normal low-threshold mechanosensory pathways. However, a spinal cord site of action is only one possibility; adenosine may modulate neurotransmission both in the periphery and supraspinally (Sawynok 1998). A low tactile pain threshold was found in most, but not all patients. This discrepancy between dynamic and static components of hyperalgesia confirms earlier results (Gottrup et al. 1998). We also observed a high variability in tactile pain threshold between individuals as well as between treatments within a single patient. The mechanisms of this phenomenon are probably different from those of dynamic tactile hyperalgesia, and may involve activation of sensitized nociceptors (LaMotte et al. 1991). The highly significant effect of adenosine on tactile pain threshold was not statistically different from changes after placebo treatment. Adenosine infusion in neuropathic pain has reduced static hyperalgesia, as demonstrated by use of a fixed suprathreshold stimulus (Belfrage et al. 1995).

The clinical relevance of changes in sensory dysfunction is limited unless accompanied by reduced pain and increased quality of life. Nevertheless, pain ratings and quality of life measurements will not provide information about effects on specific components of the pathophysiological mechanisms involved. Intrathecal administration of adenosine and an adenosine receptor agonist has produced long-lasting pain relief (Karlsten and Gordh 1995; Lindblom et al. 1997).

CONCLUSIONS

This study demonstrates that systemic adenosine treatment reduces the area of dynamic tactile allodynia associated with peripheral neuropathic pain, although not pain intensity, in parallel with subjective improvement of the clinical pain outlasting the infusion. Further studies should address the underlying mechanisms for this neuromodulatory effect of adenosine in states of neuronal hyperexcitability and evaluate the long-term clinical effects in neuropathic pain.

REFERENCES

Arnér S, Lindblom U, Meyerson B, Molander C. Prolonged relief of neuralgia after anaesthetic blocks: a call for further experimental and clinical studies. *Pain* 1990; 43:287–297.

Belfrage M, Sollevi A, Segerdahl M, et al. Systemic adenosine infusion alleviates spontaneous and stimulus evoked pain in patients with peripheral neuropathic pain. *Anesth Analg* 1995; 81:713–717.

Belfrage M, Segerdahl M, Arnér S, Sollevi A. The safety and efficacy of intrathecal adenosine in patients with chronic neuropathic pain. *Anesth Analg* 1999; 89:136–142.

Gottrup H, Nielsen J, Arendt-Nielsen L, Jensen TS. The relationship between sensory thresholds and mechanical hyperalgesia in nerve injury. *Pain* 1998; 75:321–329.

Karlsten R, Gordh T. An A1-selective adenosine agonist abolishes allodynia elicited by vibration and touch after intrathecal injection. *Anesth Analg* 1995; 80:844–847.

Koltzenburg M, Torebjörk HE, Wahren LK. Nociceptor modulated central sensitization causes mechanical hyperalgesia in acute chemogenic and chronic neuropathic pain. *Brain* 1994; 117:579–591.

LaMotte RH, Shain CN, Simone DA, Tsai EP. Neurogenic hyperalgesia: psychophysical studies of underlying mechanisms. *J Neurophysiol* 1991; 66:190–211.

Li J, Perl ER. Adenosine inhibition of synaptic transmission in the substantia gelatinosa. *J Neurophysiol* 1994; 72:1611–1621.

Lindblom U, Nordfors L-O, Sollevi A, Sydow O. Adenosine for pain relief in a patient with intractable secondary erythromelalgia. *Eur J Pain* 1997; 1:299–302.

Sawynok J. Adenosine receptor activation and nociception. *Eur J Pharmacol* 1998; 317:1–11.

Sawynok J, Sweeney MI. The role of purines in nociception. *Neuroscience* 1989; 32:557–569.

Segerdahl M, Ekblom A, Sjölund K-F, et al. Systemic adenosine attenuates touch evoked allodynia induced by mustard oil in humans. *Neuroreport* 1995a; 6:753–756.

Segerdahl M, Ekblom A, Sandelin K, et al. Perioperative adenosine infusion reduces the requirements for isoflurane and postoperative analgesics. *Anesth Analg* 1995b; 80:1145–1149.

Sumida T, Smith MA, Maehara JG, Kitahata LM. Spinal R-phenyl-isopropyl adenosine inhibits spinal dorsal horn neurons responding to noxious heat stimulation in the absence and presence of sensitization. *Pain* 1998; 74:307–313.

Verdugo R, Ochoa JL. High incidence of placebo responders among chronic neuropathic pain patients. *Ann Neurol* 1991; 30:294.

Yamamoto T, Yaksh TL. Spinal pharmacology of thermal hyperesthesia induced by incomplete ligation of sciatic nerve. *Anesthesiology* 1991; 75:817–826.

Correspondence to: Alf E. Sollevi, MD, PhD, Department of Anesthesiology, Huddinge Hospital, 14186 Huddinge, Sweden. Fax: 46-8-779-5424; email: alf.sollevi@anaesth.hs.sll.se.

Proceedings of the 9th World Congress on Pain,
Progress in Pain Research and Management,
Vol. 16, edited by M. Devor, M.C. Rowbotham, and
Z. Wiesenfeld-Hallin, IASP Press, Seattle, © 2000.

85

Cannabinoids and Pain Modulation in Animals and Humans[1]

Anita Holdcroft,[a] Kenneth M. Hargreaves,[b] Andrew S.C. Rice,[c] and Roger G. Pertwee[d]

[a]Department of Anaesthesia, Hammersmith Hospital, Imperial College School of Medicine, London, United Kingdom; [b]Departments of Endodontics and Pharmacology, Dental School, University of Texas Health Science Center, San Antonio, Texas, USA; [c]Imperial College School of Medicine, St Mary's Hospital Campus, London, United Kingdom; [d]Institute of Medical Sciences, University of Aberdeen, Aberdeen, Scotland, United Kingdom

Although preparations of cannabis have been used medically for pain relief for thousands of years, not until 1964 did Gaoni and Mechoulam characterize the exact structure of Δ-9-tetrahydrocannabinol (THC). THC is the main active constituent of cannabis plant material, which contains small quantities of about 60 other C_{21} compounds termed "cannabinoids." One such compound, cannabidiol (CBD), was synthesized before 1940. Although it has central nervous system (CNS) activity as an anticonvulsant (Dewey 1986), it lacks the psychotropic properties of THC. Factors such as genetics, method of preparation, and storage determine the amount of cannabinoids in a plant preparation. Standardization of plant material for medicinal use, either for total content of cannabinoids or proportions of individual cannabinoids, was not possible until analytical techniques became available in the 1970s, by which time legal restrictions on the use of cannabis had been internationally applied. More recently, cannabinoid research has led to the discovery that specific receptors mediate cannabinoid effects.

[1] Mini-review based on a congress workshop.

WHAT IS THE MOLECULAR BASIS FOR THE ROLE OF CANNABINOIDS IN PAIN?

The identification of endogenous cannabinoids (Devane et al. 1992; Di Marzo 1994), the cloning of CB1 (Matsuda et al. 1990) and CB2 (Munroe et al. 1993) cannabinoid receptors, and their localization in central and peripheral tissues involved in nociceptive processing (Herkenham et al. 1991; Galiegue et al. 1995) suggested that they may have a functional role in modulating pain. More recent studies have determined the chemistry and metabolism of endogenous cannabinoid receptor agonists such as anandamide and arachidonoyl glycerol (Mechoulam et al. 1995) and have investigated their mechanisms of action (Pertwee 1997). Cannabinoids are nonpeptide compounds and arachidonic acid derivatives with a diversity of structures and intracellular actions that are not wholly explained by cannabinoid receptor mechanisms. The four main groups of cannabinoid receptor agonists have disparate chemical structures. The groups are: (1) the dibenzopyran derivatives or "classical" cannabinoids; (2) analogues of THC lacking a pyran ring, e.g., CP 55,940; (3) aminoalkylindoles, e.g., WIN 55,212-2; and (4) eicosanoids discovered by Mechoulam and his team (Devane et al. 1992). These studies have developed the framework for advances in the therapeutic potential of the cannabinoids.

Cannabinoids may not just act through CB1 and CB2 receptors. For example, they are highly fat-soluble compounds and thus may also act through perturbation of membrane lipids. Anandamide and CBD can induce arachidonic acid mobilization. This process is not receptor mediated (Felder et al. 1992), and anandamide also acts at vanilloid receptors (Zygmunt et al. 1999). The molecular structures and pharmacological properties of the cloned cannabinoid receptors, CB1 and CB2, indicate that they are members of the superfamily of G-protein coupled receptors. Cannabinoid receptors resemble opioid receptors in that they are coupled to G_i/G_o proteins. Moreover, activation of cannabinoid CB1 receptors leads to decreased cyclic AMP production, closing of specific calcium channels, and opening of specific potassium channels (Fig. 1). Cannabinoid CB1-receptor agonists inhibit ongoing neural activity and in pain management may act as analgesics or antihyperalgesic agents. Development of clinical evidence for the analgesic effects of cannabis and individual cannabinoids has progressed more slowly, partly due to a lack of standardized plant material and of drug delivery systems that are efficient, reliable, and acceptable.

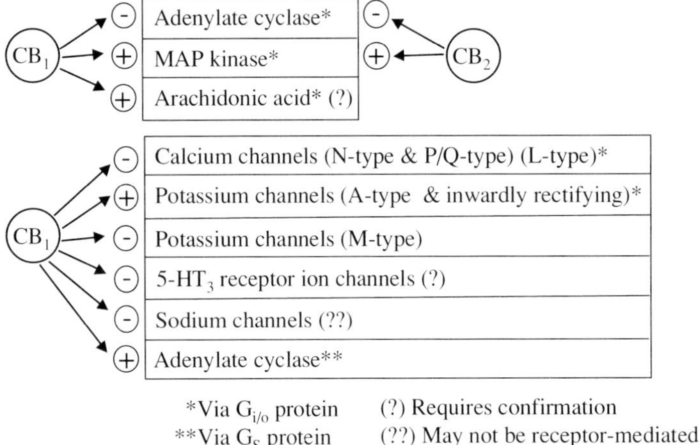

Fig. 1. Proposed effector systems for cannabinoid receptors. MAP = mitogen-activated protein.

WHAT IS THE EVIDENCE FOR CANNABINOID ACTIVITY IN NOCICEPTION? WHERE DO CANNABINOIDS ACT TO MODULATE PAIN?

The numerous sites at which cannabinoids can induce their analgesic and antihyperalgesic effects in rats and mice are shown in Fig. 2. They include the peripheral and central terminals of primary sensory neurons and their cellular environment, the dorsal horn of the spinal cord, and terminals of neurons projecting from supraspinal regions and pain centers within the brain (Hohmann et al. 1999; Hohmann and Herkenham 1999). The brain distribution of cannabinoid receptors was first studied autoradiographically and then with tissue homogenates from rat brain. CB1-receptor density in animals and humans is highest in the cerebral cortex, the basal ganglia, the cerebellum, and the hippocampus (Herkenham et al. 1991; Mailleux and Vanderhaeghen 1992), sites that correlate with the motor and cognitive effects of cannabinoids.

The techniques of immunohistochemistry and intracerebral microinjections of a cannabinoid agonist have highlighted the anatomical basis for antinociception with the identification of sites sensitive to cannabinoids (Tsou et al. 1998; Martin et al. 1999). These include the thalamus, amygdala, periaqueductal gray (PAG), and rostral ventromedial medulla (RVM). Modulation of nociception originates from supraspinal sites through projections from the PAG and RVM. In elegant experiments on the RVM in the brainstem, Meng et al. (1998) have distinguished the motor and sensory effects of

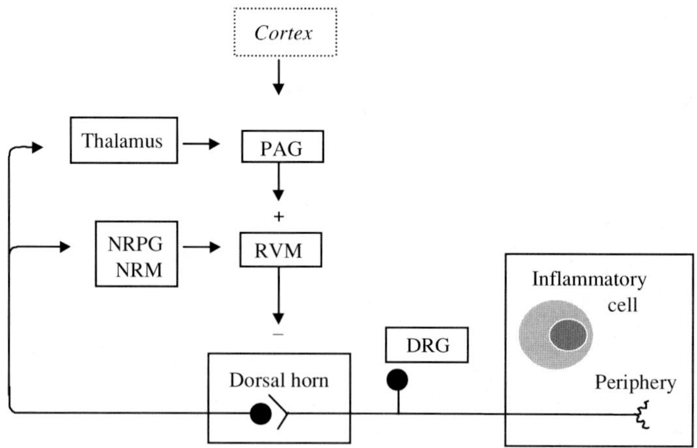

Fig. 2. Sites at which cannabinoids induce antinociception in rodents. PAG = periaqueductal gray; DRG = dorsal root ganglion; RVM = rostral ventromedial medulla; NRPG = nucleus reticularis paragigantocellularis; NRM = nucleus raphe magnus; + = stimulation; – = inhibition.

cannabinoids. Inactivation of the RVM by the γ-aminobutyric acid ($GABA_A$) receptor agonist muscimol prevented analgesia, but not motor deficits such as hypomotility produced by systemically administered cannabinoids, which can confound results from tail-flick experiments. In addition, the effects were pharmacologically distinguishable from opioids, which also modulate RVM neuronal activity. Other studies of the brain stem and spinal cord have revealed that antinociception induced by cannabinoid receptor activation may depend at least in part on the release of norepinephrine from descending neurons and its action on spinal α_2 adrenoceptors (Lichtmann and Martin 1991a).

Cannabinoids in the brain, spinal cord, and peripheral tissues modulate the release of neurotransmitters involved in nociceptive processing at nerve terminals. In the brain these include acetylcholine, norepinephrine, dopamine, GABA, and D-aspartate. Anatomical localization of cannabinoid receptor binding sites in lamina X and particularly the superficial dorsal horn of the spinal cord (Tsou et al. 1998) supports electrophysiological and behavioral studies demonstrating cannabinoid modulation of pain at the spinal cord level. Double-labeling techniques reveal that CB1 expression co-localizes in the same region of the spinal cord as the central terminals of nerve growth factor (NGF)-dependent peptidergic class of primary afferent neuron (Fig. 3). Furthermore, NGF-dependent dorsal root ganglion cells express the gene encoding the CB1 receptor (Friedel et al. 1997), and in vitro anandamide inhibits the capsaicin-evoked release of calcitonin gene-related peptide (CGRP) both from lumbar dorsal horn (Richardson et al. 1998a) and isolated

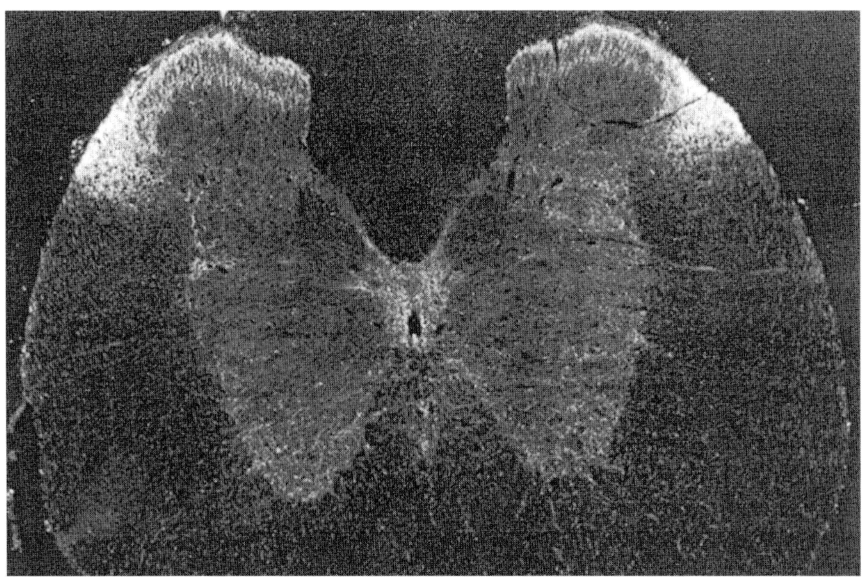

Fig. 3. CB1-like immunoreactivity in the spinal cord (W.P. Farquhar-Smith et al., unpublished data). A transverse section of rat lumbar spinal cord immunocytochemically stained with an antibody raised against the C-terminal of the CB1 receptor. The most intense CB1-like immunoreactivity is seen in the dorsolateral funiculus, the superficial dorsal horn, and lamina X. The expression in the dorsolateral funiculus is located on fibers that run rostrocaudally. In the superficial dorsal horn the CB1 staining appears as a bilayer located in lamina I and II and is located on intrinsic spinal neurons rather than primary afferent fibers. Double-labeling studies indicate laminar co-localization with markers of the NGF-dependent, peptidergic class of primary afferent nociceptor (Farquhar-Smith et al. 2000).

skin of rat paw (Richardson et al. 1998c). Additional evidence for the presence of CB1 receptors at peripheral and central terminals of primary afferent neurons comes from the recent finding that transport of these receptors from the dorsal root ganglion is bidirectional (Hohmann and Herkenham 1999).

CB1 mRNA has been identified in components of the immune system (Lynn and Herkenham 1994) and in cultured human endothelial cells (Randall and Kendall 1998). Recent evidence suggests that activation of vascular cannabinoid receptors induces cardiovascular changes in pathophysiological conditions (Wagner et al. 1997, 1998), and that macrophage and platelet-derived endogenous cannabinoids contribute to this effect. CB2 mRNA is also expressed in macrophages (Munroe et al. 1993), but elsewhere has a different peripheral and central distribution than CB1 receptors. The relevance to pain modulation of the presence of CB2 receptors on macrophages could be in controlling the release of nociceptive neurochemicals from inflammatory cells close to peripheral sensory nerves. Mast cells in particular express both CB2 and trkA receptors, and NGF-induced hyperalgesia may be modulated by cannabinoids (Rice 2000). Moreover, an agonist for putative CB2-like receptors, palmitoylethanolamide (PEA), accumulates in inflamed tissues (Natarajan et al. 1982) and reduces mast cell degranulation (Facci et al. 1995), thereby decreasing release of nociceptive/inflammatory agents such as histamine and release of serotonin (5HT). PEA also decreases plasma extravasation and hyperalgesia (Mazzari et al. 1996; Jaggar et al. 1998).

Some evidence points to the presence of CB2 receptors on microglial cells in rat brain (Kearn and Hillard 1999). These neuronal supporting structures are not inert during nociceptive processing, and research developments are clearly required to elucidate the functional role of microglial CB2 receptors.

WHAT IS THE IN VIVO RESPONSE TO CANNABINOIDS?

Cannabinoids demonstrate antinociceptive activity in acute, inflammatory, and neuropathic pain models. Systemic, intrathecal (i.t.), intraventricular, and intracerebral microdialysis administration of cannabinoid agonists or antagonists, respectively, inhibits acute behavioral responses or changes nociceptive thresholds to noxious heat, chemical, and mechanical stimuli (Lichtman and Martin 1991b; Martin et al. 1993; Richardson et al 1997; Jaggar et al 1998).

The interpretation of data from animal experiments requires consideration of the type of test, the route of administration, the time of events (because anandamide has a short duration of action), and the dosages used. For example, during hot-plate tests for antinociception in normal animals, a positive response was obtained to i.t. administration of anandamide at a dose of 100 μg (288 nmol) (Smith et al. 1994) compared with no change in response at doses ranging from 0.07 fmol to 70 pmol (Richardson et al. 1998a). In a double-blind, randomized study design, 1 fmol anandamide i.t. completely prevented thermal hyperalgesia when inflammatory changes were induced with carrageenan injection into a hindpaw. In normal animals, many primary afferent neurons are quiescent until stimulated by inflammation when both C-polymodal and Aδ fibers are activated. In the experiments conducted by Richardson and colleagues (1998a), anandamide induced potent antihyperalgesia but no antinociception at a spinal site, unlike studies using larger doses. The mechanism may be either by presynaptic inhibition of neurosecretion by closing calcium channels to prevent exocytosis or depolarization, or postsynaptic stabilization of cell membranes to prevent signal transduction or disinhibit an inhibitory circuit. The mechanism was further investigated in superfusion experiments on isolated lumbar spinal cord. Anandamide had little effect on basal release of CGRP but it had a detectable effect on capsaicin-stimulated release, which supports the hypothesis that cannabinoid presynaptic receptor activation inhibits neurosecretion from primary afferent neurons.

A potential criticism of behavioral antinociceptive tests is that they could be influenced by alterations in locomotor responses. However, as detailed elsewhere (Martin and Lichtman 1998), good evidence suggests the lack of a cause-and-effect relationship between cannabinoid-induced motor dysfunction and the antinociceptive properties of cannabinoids.

After i.t. administration of the CB1-selective antagonist, SR141716A, the hot-plate test demonstrated short-lasting hyperalgesia in mice (Richardson et al. 1998b). NMDA-receptor antagonists blocked this hyperalgesia. Other evidence for tonic activation of the endogenous spinal cannabinoid system in normal rodents comes from a recent study by Meng et al. (1998), who recorded from "on" and "off" cells in the rat RVM. Systemic SR 141716A decreased "off" activity that precedes tail withdrawal from noxious heat, thus decreasing nociceptive thresholds. These results may indicate an ongoing release of an endogenous cannabinoid. Alternatively, SR141716A may be acting as an inverse agonist. Thus, as shown in Fig. 4, it is possible that the CB1 receptor can fluctuate between two conformational states and that SR141716A binds preferentially to receptors in the uncoupled (off) state and shifts the equilibrium away from the precoupled (on) state. The possibilities of adjusting the proportion of receptors in the precoupled state and of modulating the synthesis and metabolism of endogenous cannabinoids broaden the options for the pharmacological development of analgesics.

The peripheral activity of cannabinoids in tissues and immune cells during inflammation has generated intense investigation. Concentrations of anandamide and PEA in rat paw skin are 5 to 10-fold higher than those measured in rat brain by gas chromatography/mass spectroscopy and can be considered sufficient to tonically activate cannabinoid receptors. Therapeutic use of anandamide is restricted by rapid metabolism but synthetic can-

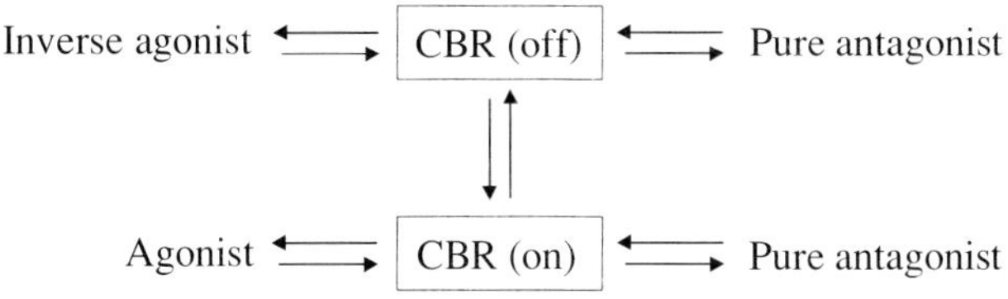

Fig. 4. Tonic activity in the endogenous cannabinoid system. CBR (off) = uncoupled cannabinoid receptors; CBR (on) = precoupled (constitutional) cannabinoid receptors.

nabinoids do not have this limitation. Thus, an approach awaiting exploration is the development of topical or locally applied cannabinoids to reduce pain and inflammation without CNS effects. Obviously, systemic absorption would negate such a therapeutic development so that studies have carefully limited dosages and assessed systemic effects. When injected locally rather than intravenously or intraperitoneally, anandamide was 100 times more potent in preventing the early phase of formalin-evoked pain behavior (Calignano et al. 1998). The simultaneous release into tissues of anandamide and PEA, which have a common precursor but different mechanisms of action (probably on CB1 and CB2-like receptors, respectively), prompted a further experiment to determine their combined effects. When injected in equal amounts, they inhibited the formalin-evoked response with a potency 100-fold greater than each of the cannabinoids did separately.

If basal thermal nociceptive thresholds are modulated by a tonically active endogenous cannabinoid system, then a reduction in the number of cannabinoid receptors might well produce hyperalgesia. This hypothesis has been studied in acute and chronic inactivation studies of the CB1 receptor using i.t. antisense oligonucleotide injections or CB1-receptor knockout mice, respectively. In the acute study (Richardson et al. 1997) a receptor knockdown technique decreased cannabinoid receptor density in the lumbar but not cervical spinal cord and resulted in hyperalgesia to heat. In contrast, one strain of CB1-receptor knockout mice had reduced pain sensitivity to hotplate test (Zimmer et al. 1999), but the response was unchanged in another strain (Ledent et al. 1999). One important observation was that measured antinociceptive effects of cannabinoids were not artifacts of motor or temperature effects. Further research using these techniques should identify which cannabinoid effects are CB1 mediated and which are CB1 independent.

WHAT ARE THE DIFFICULTIES OF CLINICAL TRIALS OF CANNABINOIDS FOR PAIN RELIEF?

Clinical trials of cannabinoids have either used a single cannabinoid, usually synthetic, or a mixture of cannabinoids from plant material. If plant extracts are not standardized they can vary in composition from one study to another, contain untested chemicals, and be subject to contamination with pesticides and other harmful residues. Anecdotal evidence indicates that users who have tried both cannabis and synthetic cannabinoids prefer cannabis (House of Lords 1998). This preference may result from numerous factors, including improved symptom control from additive effects of the several components of cannabis (e.g., CBD), altered mood, or from higher blood concentrations achieved by the inhalational rather than the oral route of administration.

Standardized cannabis plant material has only been used in one long-term, randomized, double-blind, placebo-controlled clinical trial for pain relief in a patient with familial Mediterranean fever who experienced acute and chronic pain (Holdcroft et al. 1997a). A preparation containing 1:0.8 THC:CBD was administered as oral capsules in a patient stabilized with regular oral morphine medication. Escape analgesia was provided with oral morphine and the amount was enumerated for the active and placebo weeks (Fig. 5). Both the amount of escape and total morphine consumed was significantly reduced ($P < 0.001$) during the active weeks when daily cannabis in five regular doses of 10 mg THC equivalent was prescribed. This morphine-sparing effect was achieved while patient compliance was demonstrated by biochemical tests for total urinary concentrations of opioids and cannabinoids.

The patient experienced mood symptoms during withdrawal, a lack of appetite stimulation, and a reduction in efficacy after continuous use for more than one week (Holdcroft et al. 1997b). The lack of CNS effects during the active weeks was encouraging. However, the patient was not naïve to cannabis and tolerance may have developed despite a preliminary washout period with biochemical screening for cannabinoids. Biochemical screening should be a requirement for clinical studies because cannabinoids are misused in the community, are highly lipid soluble, and can be detected in tissues for more than a week after use. Where studies have not used

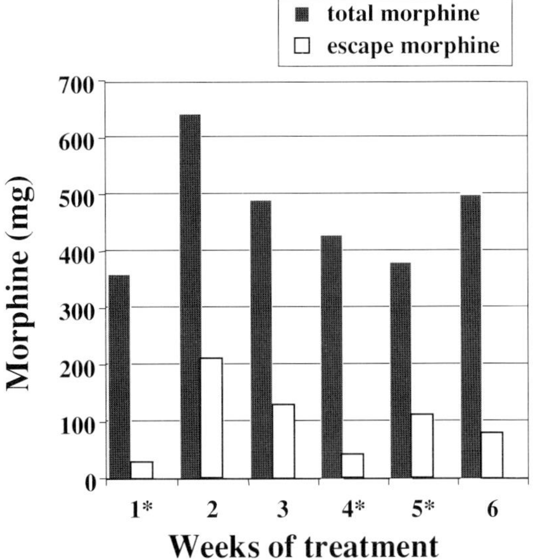

Fig. 5. The total and escape morphine taken during a randomized, placebo-controlled clinical trial of cannabis in a patient with familial Mediterranean fever (active weeks are denoted by asterisks).

cannabis-naïve subjects nor tested for cannabinoid concentrations, background cannabinoid activity may influence results.

A dose-response effect to the analgesic activity of oral capsules of THC has been reported in terminal cancer patients experiencing moderate pain. THC in doses from 5 to 20 mg was given to cannabis-naive patients in a randomized, placebo-controlled, crossover study design that used a standardized protocol with withdrawal of other analgesic medication. Measurements of pain relief showed significant differences between 15 and 20 mg THC and placebo, and the effects persisted for up to 6 hours (Noyes et al. 1975a,b).

These preliminary clinical trials will be the basis for future studies. The present formulations of cannabinoids target cannabinoid receptors and other effector mechanisms. The endogenous cannabinoid system also can be manipulated through agonist and antagonist activity and by affecting the processes of endogenous cannabinoid production, tissue uptake, and metabolism. Presently, concerns about the quality, efficacy, and safety of plant-derived cannabinoids and the unwanted central effects from systemic synthetic cannabinoids prevent clinical use. It is anticipated that developments in pharmaceutical agents and formulations should overcome these clinical difficulties.

REFERENCES

Calignano A, LaRana G, Giuffrida A, Piomelli D. Control of pain initiation by endogenous cannabinoids. *Nature* 1998; 394:277–281.

Devane WA, Hanus L, Breuer A, et al. Isolation and structure of a brain constituent that binds to the cannabinoid receptor. *Science* 1992; 258:1946–1949.

Dewey WL. Cannabinoid pharmacology. *Pharm Rev* 1986; 38:151–178.

Di Marzo V, Fontana A, Cadas H, et al. Formation and inactivation of endogenous cannabinoid anandamide in central neurones. *Nature* 1994; 372:686–691.

Facci L, DalToso R, Romanello S, et al. Mast cells express a peripheral cannabinoid receptor with differential sensitivity to anandamide and palmitoylethanolamide. *Proc Natl Acad Sci USA* 1995; 92:3376–3380.

Farquhar-Smith WP, Egertova M, Bradbury EJ, et al. Cannabinoid CB1 receptor expression in rat spinal cord. *Mol Cell Neurosci* 2000; in press.

Felder CC, Veluz JS, Williams HL, Briley EM, Marsuda LA. Cannabinoid agonists stimulate both receptor- and non-receptor-mediated signal transduction pathways in cells transfected with and expressing cannabinoid receptor clones. *Mol Pharmacol* 1992; 42:838–845.

Friedel RH, Schnurch H, Stubbusch J, Barde Y. Identification of genes differentially expressed by nerve growth factor and neurotrophin-3 dependent sensory neurones. *Proc Natl Acad Sci USA* 1997; 94:12670–12675.

Galiegue S, Mary S, Marchand J, et al. Expression of central and peripheral cannabinoid receptors in human immune tissues and leucocyte subpopulations. *Eur J Biochem* 1995; 232:54–61.

Gaoni Y, Mechoulam R. Isolation, structure and partial synthesis of an active constituent of hashish. *J Am Chem Soc* 1964; 86:1646–1647.

Herkenham M, Lynn AB, Johnson MR, et al. Characterisation and localisation of cannabinoid receptors in rat brain: a quantitative in vitro autoradiographic study. *J Neurosci* 1991; 11:563–583.

Hohmann AG, Herkenham M. L Cannabinoid receptors undergo axonal flow in sensory nerves. *Neuroscience* 1999; 92:1171–1175.

Hohmann AG, Briley EM, Herkenham M. Pre-and postsynaptic distribution of cannabinoid and mu opioid receptors in rat spinal cord. *Brain Res* 1999; 822:17–25.

Holdcroft A, Smith M, Jacklin A, et al. Pain relief with oral cannabinoids in familial Mediterranean fever. *Anaesthesia* 1997a; 52:483–488.

Holdcroft A, Smith M, Smith B, Hodgson H, Evans FJ. Clinical trial experience with cannabinoids. *Pharm Sci* 1997b; 3:546–550.

House of Lords. *Cannabis: the Scientific and Medical Evidence.* Ninth Report from the Select Committee on Science and Technology. London: The Stationery Office, 1998.

Jaggar SI, Hasnie FS, Sellaturay S, Rice ASC. The anti-hyperalgesic actions of the cannabinoid anandamide and the putative CB_2 agonist palmitoylethanolamide, investigated in models of visceral and somatic inflammatory pain. *Pain* 1998; 76:189–199.

Kearn CS, Hillard C. A model for the study of cannabinoid actions in microglia. In: *Symposium on the Cannabinoids.* Burlington, VT: International Cannabinoid Research Society, 1999, p 44.

Ledent C, Valverde O, Cossu G, et al. Unresponsiveness to cannabinoids and reduced addictive effects of opiates in CB_1 receptor knockout mice. *Science* 1999; 283:401–404.

Lichtmann AH, Martin BR. Cannabinoid-induced antinociception is mediated by a spinal $alpha_2$-noradrenergic mechanism. *Brain Res* 1991a; 559:309–314.

Lichtman AH, Martin BR. Spinal and supraspinal components of cannabinoid-induced antinociception. *J Pharmacol Exp Ther* 1991b; 258:517–523.

Lynn AB, Herkenham M. Localization of cannabinoid receptors and nonsaturable high-density cannabinoid binding sites in peripheral tissues of the rat: implications for receptor-mediated immune modulation by cannabinoids. *J Pharmacol Exp Ther* 1994; 268:1612–1623.

Mailleux P, Vanderhaeghen J-J. Localisation of cannabinoid receptor in the human developing and adult basal ganglia: higher levels in the striatonigral neurons. *Neurosci Lett* 1992; 148:173–176.

Martin BR, Lichtman AH. Cannabinoid transmission and pain perception. *Neurobiol Dis* 1998; 5:447–461.

Martin WJ, Coffin PO, Attias E, et al. Anatomical basis for cannabinoid-induced antinociception as revealed by intracerebral microinjections. *Brain Res* 1999; 822:237–242.

Matsuda LA, Lolait SJ, Brownstein MJ, Young AC, Bonner TI. Structure of a cannabinoid receptor and functional expression of the cloned cDNA. *Nature* 1990; 346:561–564.

Mazzari S, Canella R, Petrelli L, Marcolongo G, Leon A. N-(2-Hydroxyethyl) hexadecanamide is orally active in reducing edema formation and inflammatory hyperalgesia by down-modulating mast cell activation. *Eur J Pharmacol* 1996; 300:227–236.

Mechoulam R, Ben-Shabat S, Hanus L, et al. Identification of an endogenous 2-monoglyceride, present in canine gut, that binds to cannabinoid receptors. *Biochem Pharmacol* 1995; 50:83–90.

Meng ID, Manning BH, Martin WJ, Fields HL. An analgesic circuit activated by cannabinoids. *Nature* 1998; 395:381–383.

Munroe S, Thomas KL, Abu-Shaar M. Molecular characterisation of a peripheral receptor for cannabinoids. *Nature* 1993; 365:61–65.

Natarajan V, Reddy PV, Schmid PC, Schmid HHO. N-acylation of ethanolamine phospholipids in canine myocardium. *Biochim Biophys Acta* 1982; 712:342–355.

Noyes R, Brunk SF, Avery DH, Canter A. The analgesic properties of delta-9-tetrahydrocannabinol and codeine. *Clin Pharm Ther* 1975a:18:84–89.

Noyes R, Brunk SF, Baram DA, Canter A. Analgesic effect of delta-9-tetrahydrocannabinol. *J Clin Pharmacol* 1975b; 15:139–143.

Pertwee RG. Pharmacology of cannabinoid CB_1 and CB_2 receptors. *Pharmacol Ther* 1997; 74:129–180.

Randall MD, Kendall DA. Endocannabinoids: a new class of vasoactive substances. *Trends Pharmacol Sci* 1998; 19:55–58.
Rice ASC. Local neuro-immune interactions in visceral hyperalgesia: bradykinin, neurotrophins and cannabinoids. In: Bountra C, Schmidt W, Munglani R (Eds). *Pain: Current Understanding, Emerging Therapies and Novel Approaches to Drug Discovery.* New York: Marcel Dekker, 2000, in press.
Richardson JD, Aanonsen L, Hargreaves KM. SR 141716A, a cannabinoid receptor antagonist, produces hyperalgesia in untreated mice. *Eur J Pharmacol* 1997; 319:R3–R4.
Richardson JD, Aanonsen L, Hargreaves KM. Antihyperalgesic effects of spinal cannabinoids. *Eur J Pharmacol* 1998a; 345:145–153.
Richardson JD, Aanonsen L, Hargreaves KM. Hypoactivity of the spinal cannabinoid system results in NMDA-dependent hyperalgesia. *J Neurosci* 1998b; 18:451–457.
Richardson JD, Kilo S, Hargreaves KM. Cannabinoids reduce hyperalgesia and inflammation via interaction with peripheral CB_1 receptors. *Pain* 1998c; 75:1111–1119.
Smith PB, Compton DR, Welch SP, et al. The pharmacological activity of anandamide, a putative endogenous cannabinoid in mice. *J Pharmacol Exp Ther* 1994; 270:219–227.
Tsou K, Brown S, Sanudo-Pena MC, Mackie K, Walker JM. Immunohistochemical distribution of cannabinoid CB_1 receptors in the rat central nervous system. *Neuroscience* 1998; 83:393–411.
Wagner JA, Varga K, Ellis EF, et al. Activation of peripheral CB_1 cannabinoid receptors in haemorrhagic shock. *Nature* 1997; 390:518–521.
Wagner JA, Varga K, Kunos G. Cardiovascular actions of cannabinoids and their generation during shock. *Mol Med* 1998; 76:824–836.
Zimmer A, Zimmer AM, Hohmann AG, Herkenham M, Bonner TI. Increased mortality, hypoactivity, and hypoalgesia in cannabinoid CB_1 receptor knockout mice. *Proc Natl Acad Sci USA* 1999; 96:5780–5785.
Zygmunt PM, Petersson J, Andersson DA, et al. Vanilloid receptors on sensory nerves mediate the vasodilator action of anandamide. *Nature* 1999; 400:452–457.

Correspondence to: Anita Holdcroft, MB ChB, MD, FRCA, Department of Anaesthesia, Hammersmith Hospital, Imperial College School of Medicine, London W12 0HS, United Kingdom. Tel: 0181-383-3290; Fax: 0181-749-9974; email: aholdcro@ic.ac.uk.

Proceedings of the 9th World Congress on Pain, Progress in Pain Research and Management, Vol. 16, edited by M. Devor, M.C. Rowbotham, and Z. Wiesenfeld-Hallin, IASP Press, Seattle, © 2000.

86

The Contribution of the Cannabinoid CB1 Receptor to Spinal Nociceptive Processing

Victoria Chapman

School of Biomedical Sciences, University of Nottingham Medical School, Queen's Medical Centre, Nottingham, United Kingdom

Currently there is a heightened interest in the analgesic potential of cannabinoid receptor agonists such as Δ-9-tetrahydrocannabinol (Δ-9-THC) and synthetic agonists. Thus, there is a need for an improved understanding of the sites of cannabinoid receptors and mechanisms by which cannabinoids affect central nervous system (CNS) function. Behavioral (Smith and Martin 1992) and electrophysiological (Hohmann et al. 1998) studies indicate a role of spinal cannabinoid (CB) receptors in the modulation of acute nociceptive transmission. Spinal cannabinoid receptors have been identified (Tsou et al. 1998), and studies with SR141716A, a potent and selective CB1-receptor antagonist, suggest that the antinociceptive effects of spinally administered cannabinoids are mediated by CB1 receptors (Welch et al. 1998).

There is increasing evidence for a tonic control of spinal nociceptive processing by endogenous cannabinoids acting at the CB1 receptor. Spinal administration of SR141716A results in thermal hyperalgesia in mice (Richardson et al. 1998) and facilitates formalin-evoked pain behavior in rats (Strangman et al. 1998). In contrast, the nociceptive thresholds of CB1-receptor knockout mice are similar to those of wild-type mice (Ledent et al. 1999). Thus, the importance of a tonic control of nociceptive thresholds and responses by the endogenous cannabinoids is unclear.

This chapter presents the results of recent in vivo electrophysiological studies of the tonic role of endogenous cannabinoids in modulating nociceptive activity at the level of the spinal cord. The second part of this chapter presents evidence that a spinally administered cannabinoid agonist reduces noxious evoked responses of dorsal horn neurons, in particular facilitated responses, via the activation of CB1 receptors.

METHODS

Extracellular recordings of convergent dorsal horn neurons (depth 500–1000 μm) were made in anesthetized (1.5% halothane in 66% N_2O/33% O_2) Sprague-Dawley rats (200–250 g). Neuronal responses to transcutaneous electrical stimulation (three times the C-fiber threshold, trains of 16 stimuli at 0.5 Hz) of the peripheral receptive field were recorded, and post-stimulus histograms were constructed. Evoked responses were separated and quantified on the basis of latencies: Aβ fiber, 0–20 ms post-stimulus; C fiber, 90–300 ms post-stimulus; and post-discharge, 300–800 ms post-stimulus. The nonpotentiated C-fiber-evoked neuronal response was calculated as the number of action potentials evoked by the first stimulus multiplied by the total number of stimuli (16). The nonpotentiated component of the C-fiber-evoked response reflects the C-fiber input into the dorsal horn prior to the activation of post-synaptic NMDA-receptor-mediated events and the facilitation of C-fiber-evoked responses.

Control responses (<10% variance) were established. We measured the effects of spinal administration of the selective CB1-receptor antagonist SR141716A (0.001–1 ng/50 μL [0.042–42 nM]; n = 6 rats) and the selective CB2-receptor antagonist SR144528 (0.001–1 ng/50 μL; n = 5 rats) on evoked neuronal responses (n = 6 and 5 neurons, respectively). SR141716A and SR144528 were dissolved in distilled H_2O and ethanol (final concentration for highest dose studied < 0.1% ethanol). Drugs were given cumulatively, and their effects were measured at 5, 10, 20, 30, and 40 minutes post-administration. Statistical analysis was performed with repeated-measures ANOVA and Dunnett's multiple comparisons test.

In another group of rats (n = 7), we studied the effect of spinal administration of the potent cannabinoid agonist HU210 (0.5, 5, 50, and 500 ng/50 μL, from Tocris, U.K.) on electrically evoked responses of dorsal horn neurons (n = 5–7 neurons per dose, mean depth 650 ± 20 μm). HU210 was dissolved in distilled H_2O and ethanol (final concentration for the highest concentration of HU210 studied < 0.3% ethanol). Effects of HU210 were measured for 60 minutes at 10-minute intervals.

The site of action of spinally administered HU210 was addressed by applying specific cannabinoid CB1- and CB2-receptor antagonists. The effect of spinally administered HU210 (500 ng/50 μL) on dorsal horn neurons (n = 7) following a 60-minute pre-administration with the CB1-receptor antagonist SR141716A (0.01 μg/50 μL; spinal route of administration) was studied over a 60-minute period in a separate group of rats (n = 7). The effect of spinally administered HU210 (500 ng/50 μL) on dorsal horn neurons (n = 8) following a 60-minute pre-administration with the CB2-receptor antagonist SR144528 (0.01 μg/50 μL; spinal route of administration) was studied over a 60-minute period in another group of rats ($n = 8$). SR141716A and SR144528 were dissolved in distilled H_2O and ethanol (final concentration of ethanol < 0.1%). Statistical analysis was performed with a one-way analysis of variance (ANOVA) with Fisher's protected least significant difference test or Kruskal-Wallis test where appropriate.

RESULTS

CB1-RECEPTOR ANTAGONISM FACILITATES NOXIOUS EVOKED RESPONSES OF DORSAL HORN NEURONS

Spinal administration of SR141716A significantly facilitated the nonpotentiated component of the C-fiber-evoked neuronal responses in a dose-related manner (Fig. 1). Maximal effect of SR141716A (1 ng/50 μL) was observed at 18 ± 5 minutes post-administration. SR141716A produced a nonsignificant facilitation of the post-discharge response of neurons (Fig. 1).

A minor facilitation of the overall C-fiber-evoked neuronal response was produced by the highest concentration of SR141716A studied (126 ± 11%; mean maximal percentage of the pre-drug control value ± SEM). SR141716A (1 ng/50 μL) did not influence the Aβ-fiber-evoked responses of the dorsal horn neurons (100 ± 15% of control).

Spinal administration of SR144528 (0.001–1 ng/50 μL) did not influence the evoked responses of dorsal horn neurons. The mean maximal effect

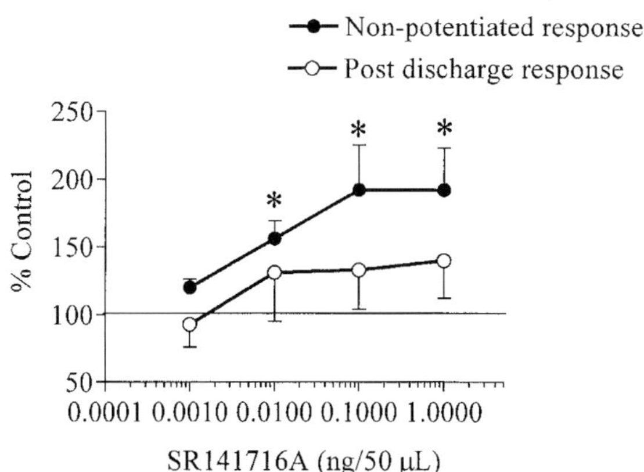

Fig. 1. Spinal administration of SR141716A significantly facilitated the nonpotentiated component of the C-fiber-evoked response of dorsal horn neurons. A minor facilitation of the post-discharge response is evident. Note logarithmic scale on x-axis. Statistical analysis: repeated-measures (ANOVA) and Dunnett's multiple comparisons test, $*P \leq 0.01$.

of 1 ng/50 μL of SR144528 on the nonpotentiated component of the C-fiber-evoked neuronal responses and the post-discharge was 93 ± 18% of control and 103 ± 17% of control, respectively. The mean maximal effect of SR144528 (1 ng/50 μL) on the overall C-fiber- and Aβ-fiber-evoked neuronal response was 82 ± 7% and 85 ± 9% of control, respectively.

HU210 DIFFERENTIALLY INHIBITS NOXIOUS VERSUS INNOCUOUS EVOKED RESPONSES OF DORSAL HORN NEURONS

The cannabinoid agonist HU210 (at 0.5, 5, 50, and 500 ng/50 μL) dose-relatedly and significantly reduced post-discharge responses of dorsal horn neurons (Fig. 2). The nonpotentiated component of the C-fiber-evoked neuronal response also was attenuated by HU210, although statistical significance was not reached (Fig. 2). HU210 dose-relatedly reduced both the overall C-fiber (94 ± 9%, 93 ± 11%, 71 ± 7%, and 68 ± 7% of control) and Aδ-fiber (92 ± 9%, 92 ± 11%, 78 ± 15%, and 64 ± 19% of control) evoked responses of the dorsal horn neurons, although significance was not reached. Only the highest concentration of HU210 studied (500 ng/50 μL) produced some inhibition of Aβ-fiber-evoked neuronal responses of dorsal horn neurons (79 ± 10% of control).

CB1-RECEPTOR, BUT NOT CB2-RECEPTOR, ANTAGONISM BLOCKS THE ANTINOCICEPTIVE EFFECT OF HU210

We studied the ability of a single concentration of 0.01 μg/50 μL of SR141716A or SR144528 to block the inhibitory effect of the highest concentration of HU210 (500 ng/50 μL) on evoked responses of dorsal horn

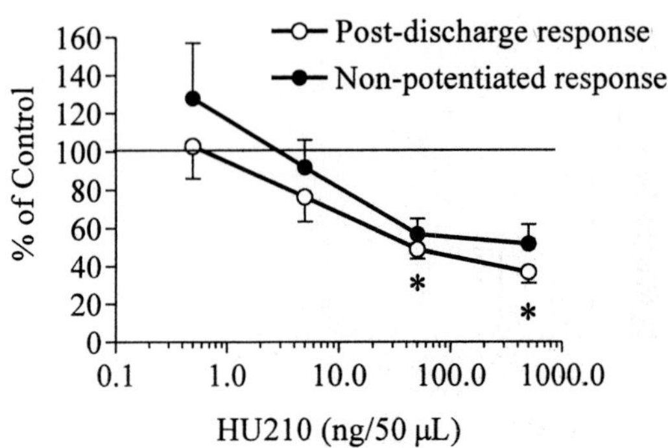

Fig. 2. HU210 dose-relatedly attenuated the post-discharge response and nonpotentiated component of the C-fiber response of dorsal horn neurons; effects of HU210 on the post-discharge response were significant. Note logarithmic scale on *x*-axis. Statistical analysis: one-way ANOVA as compared to control, $^*P \leq 0.05$.

neurons. Pre-administration of spinal SR141716A consistently blocked the inhibitory effect of spinal HU210 on C-fiber-evoked neuronal responses (Fig. 3). Significant differences were observed between the effect of HU210 alone and HU210 following pre-administration of SR141716A for both the overall C-fiber-evoked response and the post-discharge response ($P < 0.05$, one-way ANOVA, Kruskal-Wallis post hoc test for both). In addition, SR141716A blocked the minor effect of HU210 on Aβ-fiber-evoked neuronal responses (95 ± 13% of control), but not the Aδ-fiber-evoked response (66 ± 6% of control). When given alone at this concentration, SR141716A had no effect on electrically evoked responses of dorsal horn neurons. Spinal pre-administration of SR144528 (0.01 μg/50 μL) had little influence on the inhibitory effect of HU210 (Fig. 3). These data suggest that the antinociceptive effect of spinal HU210 results, at least in part, from an action at spinal CB1 receptors.

DISCUSSION

Our findings, showing that CB1-receptor antagonism facilitates noxious evoked (C-fiber-mediated) responses of spinal neurons, indicate a tonic control of nociceptive evoked activity of spinal neurons by endogenous inhibitory cannabinoids acting at the CB1 receptor. Innocuous evoked neuronal

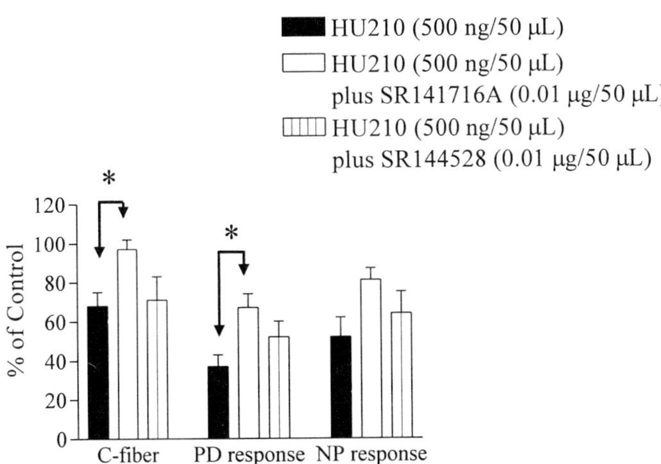

Fig. 3. The CB1-receptor antagonist SR141716A (0.01 μg/50 μL, spinal administration) reduced the inhibitory effect of spinal HU210 (500 ng/50 μL) on the overall C-fiber-evoked response, post-discharge (PD) response, and nonpotentiated (NP) response of dorsal horn neurons. The CB2-receptor antagonist SR144528 (0.01 μg/50 μL) did not influence the inhibitory effect of spinal HU210 on evoked neuronal responses. Statistical analysis: Kruskal-Wallis test and Dunnett's multiple comparisons test, $^{*}P \leq 0.05$.

(Aβ-fiber-mediated) responses were not influenced by SR141716A. These results are in keeping with previous behavioral studies (Richardson 1998; Strangman 1998) of the effects of SR141716A and CB1 receptor antisense oligonucleotides. Collectively, our findings suggest that following noxious stimulation there is a release or formation of endogenous cannabinoids, which then serves to reduce nociceptive transmission. Spinal release of endogenous cannabinoids following noxious stimulation has yet to be demonstrated. However, the endogenous cannabinoid anandamide is released in the periaqueductal gray following noxious stimulation (Walker et al. 1999).

Spinal administration of the cannabinoid agonist HU210 dose-relatedly reduced noxious evoked responses of dorsal horn neurons, in particular the C-fiber-mediated post-discharge response, a measure of neuronal hyperexcitability following repetitive C-fiber stimulation. In addition, Aδ-fiber-evoked neuronal responses were subject to dose-related cannabinoid-mediated inhibitions, although only minor inhibitions of Aβ-fiber-evoked responses were observed with the highest concentration of HU210 studied. The CB1 receptor antagonist (SR141716A), but not the CB2 receptor antagonist (SR144528), markedly diminished the antinociceptive effect of HU210. These data demonstrate that the spinal CB receptor system does not solely influence C-fiber-mediated events and that the antinociceptive effects of spinally HU210 result from CB1-receptor activation.

Our findings confirm and extend earlier reports that a spinally administered cannabinoid agonist inhibits nociceptive transmission (Hohmann et al. 1998) and agree with a recent report that a systemic cannabinoid agonist predominantly inhibits C-fiber-mediated wind-up, a measure of neuronal hyperexcitability, of spinal neurons (Strangman and Walker 1999). Demonstration of a direct spinal action of the cannabinoid receptor agonists is important because the effect of systemic cannabinoids on spinal neurons (Hohmann et al. 1999b; Strangman and Walker 1999) depends, at least in part, on descending antinociceptive mechanisms (Hohmann et al. 1999b).

Our findings and those of Strangman and Walker (1999) show a dominant effect of the cannabinoid agonist HU210 on C-fiber-driven hyperexcitability of dorsal horn neurons. These facilitated responses develop following repetitive nociceptive stimulation and are mediated by activation of the N-methyl-D-aspartate receptor (see references in Dickenson 1997). The mechanism is still unknown by which cannabinoid receptors, which are both pre- and post-synaptic to the primary afferent fibers (Hohmann et al. 1999a), inhibit facilitated responses of dorsal horn neurons. A functional role of CB1 receptors located pre-synaptically on C-fiber afferents has been demonstrated in that anandamide inhibits capsaicin-evoked CGRP release from the dorsal half of the spinal cord (Richardson et al. 1998). Cannabinoid receptors mediate inhibition of N- and P/Q-type calcium channels in cultured rat hippocampal neurons (Twitchell et al. 1997), and blockade of N- and P-type calcium channels attenuates formalin evoked hyperexcitability of dorsal horn neurons (Diaz and Dickenson 1997). Thus it is feasible that cannabinoid-receptor-mediated inhibition of calcium channels may contribute to the effect of spinal cannabinoid agonists on facilitated C-fiber-driven neuronal responses reported here.

ACKNOWLEDGMENTS

SR141716A was provided by Research Biochemicals International as part of the chemical synthesis program of the National Institute of Mental Health, Contract N01MH30003. SR144528 was a gift from Sanofi (Montpellier, France). The Royal Society, Wellcome Trust, and the Research Opportunity Fund (Nottingham University) supported this study.

REFERENCES

Diaz A, Dickenson AH. Blockade of spinal N- and P-type, but not L-type, calcium channels inhibits the excitability of rat dorsal horn neurones produced by subcutaneous formalin inflammation. *Pain* 1997; 69:93–100.

Dickenson AH. Mechanisms of central hypersensitivity: excitatory amino acid mechanisms and their control. In: Dickenson AH, Besson JM (Eds). *The Pharmacology of Pain:* Handbook of Experimental Pharmacology, Vol. 130. Heidelberg: Springer-Verlag, 1997, pp 167–196.

Hohmann AG, Tsou K, Walker JM. Cannabinoid modulation of wide dynamic range neurones in the lumbar dorsal horn of the rat by spinally administered WIN55,212-2. *Neurosci Letts* 1998; 257:119–122.

Hohmann AG, Briley EM, Herkenham M. Pre-and postsynaptic distribution of cannabinoid and mu opioid receptors in rat spinal cord. *Brain Res* 1999a; 822:17–25.

Hohmann AG, Tsou K, Walker JM. Cannabinoid suppression of noxious heat-evoked activity in wide dynamic range neurones in the lumbar dorsal horn of the rat. *J Neurophysiol* 1999b; 81:575–583.

Ledent C, Valverde O, Cossu G, et al. Unresponsiveness to cannabinoids and reduced addictive effects of opiates in CB_1 receptor knockout mice. *Science* 1999; 283:401–404.

Richardson JD, Aanonsen L, Hargreaves KM. Antihyperalgesic effects of spinal cannabinoids. *E J Pharmacol* 1998; 345:145–153.

Smith PB, Martin BR. Spinal mechanisms of Δ9-tetrahydrocannabinol-induced analgesia. *Brain Res* 1992; 578:8–12.

Strangman NM, Walker JM. Cannabinoid WIN55, 212-2 inhibits the activity-dependent facilitation of spinal nociceptive responses. *J Neurophysiol* 1999; 81:472–477.

Strangman NM, Patrick SL, Hohmann AG, Tsou K, Walker JM. Evidence for a role of endogenous cannabinoids in the modulation of acute and tonic pain sensitivity. *Brain Res* 1998; 813:323–328.

Tsou K, Brown S, Sanudo-Pena MC, Mackie K, Walker JM. Immunohistochemical distribution of cannabinoid CB_1 receptors in the rat central nervous system. *Neuroscience* 1998; 83:393–411.

Twitchell W, Brown S, Mackie K. Cannabinoids inhibit N- and P/Q-type calcium channels in cultured rat hippocampal neurons. *J Neurophysiol* 1997; 78:43–50.

Walker JM, Huang SM, Strangman NM, Tsou K, Sanudo-Pena MC. Pain modulation by release of the endogenous cannabinoid anandamide. *International Cannabinoid Research Society Symposium* [Abstract], 1999.

Welch SP, Huffman JW, Lowe J. Differential blockade of the antinociceptive effects of centrally administered cannabinoids by SR141716A. *J Pharmacol Exp Ther* 1998; 286:1301–1308.

Correspondence to: Victoria Chapman, PhD, School of Biomedical Sciences, E Floor, University of Nottingham Medical School, Queen's Medical Centre, Nottingham, NG7 2UH, United Kingdom. Tel: 01159-709-459; Fax: 01159-709-259; email: victoria.chapman@nottingham.ac.uk.

Proceedings of the 9th World Congress on Pain,
Progress in Pain Research and Management,
Vol. 16, edited by M. Devor, M.C. Rowbotham, and
Z. Wiesenfeld-Hallin, IASP Press, Seattle, © 2000.

87

Efficacy of Permanent Indwelling Catheters Used for Regional Analgesia[1]

David Niv,[a] P. Prithvi Raj,[b] and Serdar Erdine[c]

[a]Center for Pain Medicine, Tel-Aviv Sourasky Medical Center, Sackler Faculty of Medicine, Tel-Aviv University, Tel-Aviv, Israel; [b]Department of Anesthesiology, Texas Tech University, Health Sciences Center, Lubbock, Texas, USA; [c]Department of Algology, Medical Faculty of Istanbul, Istanbul University, Istanbul, Turkey

Infusion techniques with catheters located epineurally, epidurally, intrathecally, or subcutaneously are now commonly used to manage acute and chronic pain patients. For patients who are suffering from acute pain, continuous infusion has been beneficial for trauma, postsurgery, and acute medical diseases. Similarly, for chronic pain sufferers the technique has been useful for rehabilitation of patients with chronic low back pain, complex regional pain syndromes (CRPS), peripheral neuropathy, and cancer pain. If a sensory, motor, or sympathetic blockade is needed for considerably longer than that provided by long-acting local anesthetics, then continuous regional analgesia is indicated. The goal is to provide prolonged pain relief to a portion of the body, using the smallest possible dose of the drugs infused, and thus minimizing side effects. It is also indicated for facilitating early mobilization, increased distal limb vascularity, and improved nutrition.

Common sites of continuous regional analgesia are epidural regions (cervical, thoracic, and lumbar), the subarachnoid space, and peripheral nerves (brachial plexus, lumbar plexus, femoral, and sciatic). Less common sites for indwelling catheters are subcutaneous and sympathetic nerves and plexuses. In addition to local anesthetics, some pain management techniques involve administration of opioids and other drugs (e.g., clonidine, steroids) via indwelling catheters.

---

[1] Mini-review based on a congress workshop.

This chapter describes the most common sites for indwelling catheters, techniques for drug administration, efficacy, and side effects. For more detailed descriptions of indications, contraindications, equipment and drugs used, adjuvant techniques for localization of catheter, complications, cost-effectiveness, long-term outcome, and effect on quality of life, the reader is referred to Raj (1991), Brown (1996), and Cousins and Bridenbaugh (1998).

EPINEURAL INDWELLING CATHETERS

Peripheral continuous techniques are usually carried out exactly like single-injection techniques (Raj 1996). A variety of catheter/needle systems are available for providing continuous blockade. Previously, catheters were inserted through needles. While this method protected the catheter during insertion, the needle hole in the nerve sheath was often larger than the catheter and resulted in leakage of local anesthetic after removal of the needle. The use of thin-bore needles with catheters over the needle has improved the success of continuous techniques. When the sheath has been penetrated, as indicated either by paresthesia or use of nerve-stimulator, the catheter is advanced slightly as the needle is withdrawn. Sometimes it is best to first inject a test dose of local anesthetic through the needle to expand the perineural space. If the catheter is to be used for several days, or if movement is a problem, a second smaller catheter, similar to a nylon epidural catheter, can be advanced through the first catheter further into the perineural compartment.

BRACHIAL PLEXUS CATHETERIZATION

Indications. For two decades prolonged brachial plexus blocks have been used perioperatively for trauma and postoperative pain (Fisher and Meller 1991). Prolonged sympathetic blocks have also been administered to patients with vascular compromise (Matsuda et al. 1982). Catheters placed on the brachial plexus after surgery may provide up to 48 hours of pain relief. Experience with acute perioperative patients has prompted attempts to use prolonged brachial plexus analgesia for patients with difficult, intractable conditions such CRPS-I and -II and phantom pain (Hartrick 1992).

Site. The brachial plexus is an ideal location for a continuous regional technique because of its well-defined perineural compartment and the close proximity of the many nerves supplying the upper extremity. All techniques of brachial plexus blockade have been described as continuous, but some are easier to achieve than others. An axillary approach is easy to perform, and the technique is familiar to many clinicians. Unfortunately, movement of the upper extremity, either passive or active, can dislodge the catheter. Hair and moisture in the axilla also can make it difficult, if not impossible, to maintain a sterile environment. The interscalene technique can be challenging because the catheter is difficult to thread when the approach is 90° to the skin. A subclavian perineural approach allows easy threading of the catheter, and head or neck movements do not affect its position. Likewise, the infraclavicular approach to the brachial plexus allows easy threading, and patient movement does not affect the catheter (Raj 1973).

All four approaches to the brachial plexus have been tried for continuous infusion (Tuominen et al. 1989; Pham-Dang et al. 1995). The technique performed most often is at the axillary site, perhaps due to the familiarity of anesthesiologists with insertion of intra-arterial catheters, which was the impetus for trying this technique initially. It has remained popular ever since. Some clinicians use an interscalene approach. Once mastered, it is technically simple to perform, but catheters placed in this way usually do not stay at the target site for more than about 48 hours. Many clinicians prefer the infraclavicular approach and use this block routinely. It has the advantage of maintaining the catheter in a fixed position for long durations, sometimes as long as 3 weeks.

Drugs and technique. Even though lidocaine and mepivacaine have been used for continuous infusion, bupivacaine is the most commonly chosen local anesthetic. In a typical case, after the catheter is placed on the brachial plexus, a bolus of 20–30 mL of 0.5% bupivacaine or a 1:1 mixture of 2% lidocaine and 0.5% bupivacaine is administered. Monitoring is mandatory for at least 45 minutes, during which time the onset of block is tested. If the block is adequate, then up to 10 mL/hour of either 0.25% or 0.125% bupivacaine is administered via an infusion pump. A steady state is reached in five drug half-lives, i.e., approximately 18 hours. The infusion should be started at least 2 hours before the bolus effect wears off, which usually occurs well before 18 hours, and most commonly after 6 hours. The infusion of 0.25% bupivacaine would not be effective to maintain analgesia for another 12 hours. If pain is intolerable at 6 hours, then it is imperative to provide another bolus of 20 mL of 0.5% bupivacaine. Monitoring is required for 45 minutes, as with the initial bolus.

In the last decade, adjuvant drugs have been tried in brachial plexus infusions. Drugs that have been administered with bupivacaine include narcotics and clonidine. Their efficacy is yet to be determined.

Plasma concentration and pharmacokinetics of brachial plexus infusion are similar to those seen with epidural infusion. Once steady state is reached, the drugs infused do not accumulate if infused at a constant rate. Drug metabolites also remain at an insignificant level without causing deleterious effects. However, brachial plexus infusion should be used with caution in patients with liver and kidney disease.

EFFICACY AND SIDE EFFECTS OF INDWELLING BRACHIAL CATHETERS

Continuous brachial plexus analgesia is reliably efficacious for periods up to 48 hours, after which efficacy drops precipitously. Sympathetic block can be maintained for up to 2 or 3 weeks with 0.125% or 0.25% bupivacaine, quite reliably if catheters are well anchored. The best site for catheter insertion seems to be at the infraclavicular region, while the second-best site is at the axilla. The interscalene site is too superficial for reliable anchoring for prolonged periods. In a recent study, phrenic nerve block was observed in all patients at 3 hours after an interscalene brachial plexus block with continuous infusion (Pere et al. 1992). Between 3 and 24 hours after initiation of the continuous infusion, the motility of the diaphragm improved as the motor block caused by the bolus dose (0.5–0.75% bupivacaine) wore off. The 0.25% bupivacaine commonly infused into the interscalene space has a milder motor-blocking effect on the diaphragm than does the 0.75% solution used for the initial block. Urmey and colleagues (Urmey et al. 1991; Urmey and McDonald 1992) noted a 100% incidence of phrenic nerve block when examining diaphragm motion with ultrasound 5 minutes after injection of a local anesthetic.

Various frequencies of phrenic nerve block have been reported with different approaches to the brachial plexus. Knoblanche (1979) reported a 67% incidence of phrenic nerve block with supraclavicular access. Dhuner et al. (1955) reported a 28% incidence with the supraclavicular technique. Farrar et al. (1981) had frequencies of 36–38% of phrenic nerve block after interscalene, subclavian perineural, and Kulenkampff's (1911) technique to access the brachial plexus. The variations in frequency of phrenic nerve block may depend on the technique used and the time of examination of diaphragmatic function. With administration of short-acting local anesthetics, the phrenic nerve block may disappear before the motility of the diaphragm is examined. Respiratory stress following phrenic nerve block, as observed with spirometry, is related to reduced mobility of the diaphragm and is clearly seen in double-exposure chest radiographs. Measurements of maximal inspiratory and expiratory pressures indicate that premedication also can cause a significant decrease in respiratory muscle power. These pressures, which may be correlated with respiratory muscle power, should be independent of the patient's position.

LUMBOSACRAL PLEXUS CATHETERIZATION

Vaghadia et al. (1992) have reported placement of a lumbosacral catheter with an epidural needle. They achieved successful blockade of the lumbar and sacral plexuses for unilateral lower extremity surgery. The catheter is placed between the quadratus lumborum and psoas muscles between the transverse processes of L4 and L5. The main disadvantage is the large volume of local anesthetic needed, 40–70 mL.

SCIATIC NERVE CATHETERIZATION

Many of the nerves innervating the lower extremity can be blocked using continuous techniques. Smith et al. (1984) have described techniques for continually blocking the sciatic nerve. Continuous regional anesthesia can be obtained anywhere along the course of the nerve. A 16-gauge intravenous infusion needle and catheter or Tuohy needle with an epidural catheter can be used. The catheter is usually advanced 4–6 cm into the perineural space. The lateral approach described by Guardini et al. (1985) can be useful for obtaining a continuous block. The catheter is placed along the nerve just posterior to the quadratus femoris muscle in the subgluteal space.

FEMORAL NERVE CATHETERIZATION

Continuous techniques for the femoral nerve have been used for a variety of surgeries. Edwards and Wright (1992) recently reported significantly lower postoperative pain scores and reduced opioid requirements in patients undergoing total knee replacement with continuous infusion of 0.125% bupivacaine at 6 mL/hour within the femoral sheath as compared to analgesia from conventional i.m. injections of opioids.

EFFICACY OF LOWER EXTREMITY EPINEURAL INDWELLING CATHETERS

Lower extremity infusion is technically difficult and unreliable. However, it is an alternative when lumbar epidural infusion is not possible, such as with infection or coagulation abnormality. Postoperative knee pain, CRPS-I, and CRPS-II may be the best indications for these procedures.

The drugs administered for lower extremity infusions follow the same principles as for brachial plexus infusions. The concentration of drug infusion is dependent upon the need to block the motor or sensory fibers, and the rate of infusion is usually at 10–15 mL/hour. Complications include peripheral neuropathy, motor weakness, dysesthesias, and decubitus ulcers secondary to sensory loss.

INTRASPINAL INDWELLING CATHETERS

Continuous epidural and continuous subarachnoid analgesia are the most common methods for prolonged use of an indwelling catheter (hours to years). The potential to administer long-term analgesia prompted development of many drug delivery systems to facilitate accurate and safe administration. The intraspinal drug delivery systems are classified in Table I.

Percutaneous epidural catheters are generally used in acute intraoperative, postoperative, and obstetric pain. Percutaneously inserted epidural catheters are also used during the preimplantation trial period to observe the efficacy of the method and the route of administration. They may be used for patients with a life expectancy of days. However, prolonged use of a percutaneous catheter has also been reported to be reliable and safe (Coombs 1990). For longer-term application, the subcutaneous, epidural, or intrathecal catheter has the advantage of being minimally invasive for patients with poor general status and short life expectancy. The catheter can be attached to an external infusion pump, and it can easily be placed and removed, which is both an advantage and disadvantage. Even though this method carries a higher risk of infection, clinicians should consider the advantages of low cost and ease of implantation. If the percutaneous catheter is planned for a preimplantation trial, it should be inserted under fluoroscopy.

Totally implanted epidural or intrathecal catheters connected to access ports are stable for longer periods, and the risk of infection is relatively low. However, they have the disadvantages of multiple punctures of the skin, kinking, and obstruction of the catheter. A recent advance is the mechanical pump, activated by pushing a button. It has several advantages over the port systems. Skin punctures are required only for filling the reservoir, so the infection risk is low. The patient or the caregiver can activate mechanical pumps. However, bolus injection is not possible through these pumps, and if

Table I
Intraspinal drug delivery systems

Percutaneous epidural catheters*
Subcutaneously tunneled epidural and intrathecal catheters*
Implanted epidural or intrathecal catheters connected to access ports*
Implanted intrathecal manual pumps
Implanted intrathecal or epidural infusion pumps

*Can be activated by external pumps.

a dosage increase is required, the reservoir capacity might not be large enough to accommodate the patient's needs. Mechanical pumps are suitable for intrathecal, but not epidural use, as the volume delivered is only 1–1.5 mL/day. For this reason also, their use is confined to patients who respond to opioids. Mechanical failure with the buttons is the main cause of surgical removal.

Totally implanted continuous infusion pumps have the advantage over mechanical pumps of avoiding repeated peaks in cerebrospinal fluid and plasma morphine levels due to repeated bolus injections. Implanted infusion pumps help achieve a steady state, so they can be used for very long periods and are suitable for patients with noncancer pain. Implanted infusion systems vary from fixed rate to programmable pumps, which are favored for noncancer patients as infusion rate can be adjusted easily. They may be considered too expensive for cancer patients with limited life expectancy, although some studies claim cost-effectiveness even in cancer patients after 3 months (Hassenbush et al. 1997).

EPIDURAL INDWELLING CATHETERS

Indwelling catheterization for epidural analgesia is not a new concept but was first described in 1949 as a method for long-lasting postoperative pain relief of up to 5 days (Cleland 1949). Although bolus injections of local anesthetics produced effective analgesia, significant sympathetic blockade accompanied the pain relief, and levels of analgesia fluctuated with the repeated bolus injections. In addition, continuous analgesia with intermittent bolus injections is labor intensive and requires skilled personnel to reassess the patient and administer injections every few hours. Because of these shortcomings, continuous epidural infusion has now become commonplace.

The primary advantage of continuous epidural infusion over intermittent bolus injection is that it provides continuous analgesia. Although single boluses of opioids such as epidural morphine may provide 12 hours of pain relief, wide variability is reported in the duration of effective analgesia, ranging from 4 to 24 hours (Bromage et al. 1980; Akerman et al. 1988). Thus, it is difficult to titrate uniform levels of pain relief. Continuous infusion allows easier titration, particularly with shorter-acting opioids such as fentanyl or sufentanil. For the intermittent bolus technique to be successful, longer-acting agents such as morphine and hydromorphone must be administered to provide a reasonable duration of analgesia. These opioids are associated with a higher risk of delayed-onset respiratory depression (Bromage et al. 1980).

Catheter location. Segmental limitation of epidural analgesia mandates placing an epidural catheter at sites adjacent to dermatomes covering the painful field. This placement reduces dose requirements while increasing the specificity of spinal analgesia (Lubenow et al. 1988; Rosseel et al. 1988). Interspaces for catheter placement for epidural infusion of analgesic solutions are: for thoracic surgery, T2–T8; for upper abdominal surgery, T4–L1; for lower abdominal surgery, T10–L3; for upper extremity surgery, C2–C8; and for lower extremity surgery, T12–L3.

Local anesthetics. Local anesthetic agents are best used to provide analgesia and anesthesia for surgical patients and to maintain postoperative pain relief. Both lidocaine and bupivacaine are effective for achieving and maintaining adequate analgesia (Raj et al. 1982; Scott et al. 1989). In general, lidocaine use is limited to bolus form to establish or rescue a block, whereas bupivacaine can be used as an infusion. Development of tachyphylaxis is a problem inherent with bolus administration of a local anesthetic through the epidural catheter. Tachyphylaxis rarely develops when bupivacaine is administered as an infusion. Continuous infusion of dilute local anesthetic solutions has simplified maintenance and improved analgesic uniformity. However, concentrations sufficient to produce pain relief usually result in progressive sensorimotor blockade. Such deficits are undesirable because they compromise the ability to ambulate.

Limitations of continuous epidural local anesthetics. Epidural infusion analgesia does have limitations. First, it cannot independently control pain originating at multiple sites. Epidural analgesia normally can only provide analgesia for 5–7 continuous dermatomal regions such as L4–S5 or T2–T8. Patients with multiple injuries may require other forms of pain control.

Opiate–local anesthetic combinations. Extremely dilute concentrations of local anesthetics (e.g., 0.03% bupivacaine) plus opioids may produce profound analgesia. In general, patients receiving epidural injections of low-concentration local anesthetics plus opioids report more rapid onset of analgesia, more profound and long-lasting pain relief, and less motor blockade than when each drug is used alone.

In an effort to combine the desirable analgesic properties of local anesthetics and epidural opioids, several investigators have described the concomitant use of opioid-bupivacaine epidural infusions for pain relief (Cullen et al. 1985; Logas et al. 1987; Chestnut et al. 1988; Fisher et al. 1988). These studies demonstrate either additive or synergistic analgesic activity among a variety of opioids and dilute concentrations of bupivacaine (Hjortsø et al. 1986; Fisher et al. 1988; Lubenow et al. 1988). The incidence and severity of side effects are minimal.

Specific concentrations of drugs and rates of infusion should be tailored to the individual patient. For example, it is possible to treat or prevent significant hypotension by decreasing the concentration of local anesthetic, decreasing the rate of a combined local anesthetic/opioid infusion, or infusing intravenous fluids. Sedation or carbon dioxide retention due to respiratory depression can be treated by changing the specific epidurally administered opioid.

SUBARACHNOID (INTRATHECAL) INDWELLING CATHETERS

In acute pain. Continuous spinal anesthesia may be an option when regional anesthesia is desirable and epidural anesthesia proves inadequate. In patients with severe kyphoscoliosis, or otherwise altered spinal anatomy where continuous spinal anesthesia with hyperbaric local anesthetics has resulted in an inadequate or patchy block, the addition of isobaric local anesthetic may provide adequate anesthesia (Penn et al. 1984). Hyper-, hypo-, and isobaric technique refers to the use of drug formulations heavier, lighter, or equal in density to cerebrospinal fluid, with postural arrangement of the patient used to guide the movement of the drug.

In chronic and cancer pain. Intraspinal infusion of opioids is commonly used to manage intractable cancer pain (Auld et al. 1985; Coombs et al. 1985). These infusions have been maintained with implanted pumps connected to intrathecal catheters. The treatment of patients with severe, chronic noncancer pain in the lower body has been a difficult problem. Included among the possible causes of this pain are arachnoiditis, epidural scarring, vertebral body compression fracture, CRPS-I (reflex sympathetic dystrophy), and phantom limb pain. Intraspinal infusions are increasingly being used with minimal complications and limited instances of drug tolerance in such noncancer patients (Coombs et al. 1982; Carl et al. 1986; Murphy et al. 1987; Penn and Paice 1987; Glynn et at. 1988). Programmable pumps allow clinicians to adjust the infusion rates at any time to meet the patient's needs. Extensive testing has shown that these pumps are quite reliable and cost-effective (Coombs et al. 1982).

Analgesic agents. Morphine is the usual agent for these infusions. In resistant cases requiring temporary or prolonged intraspinal infusions, the addition of dilute bupivacaine to the morphine infusion improves pain relief (Nitescu et al. 1990; Richard and Kanoff 1994).

Efficacy. A study of 15 patients with intractable pain from CRPS-I and arachnoiditis and a follow-up of 2–44 months reported excellent pain relief for eight patients, good for three, and fair for four (Richard and Kanoff 1994). Six patients returned to work. Few complications occurred, but most patients needed increasingly larger doses over time to maintain pain relief. The authors concluded that intraspinal infusion of morphine sulfate via implanted, externally programmable pump is safe and effective in selected patients with intractable pain of nonmalignant origin.

An important point is that spinal morphine dose requirements will increase over time. All patients need to be started at the lowest dose possible to avoid early toxicity, overdosing, or overtreating. Most patients need greater doses over time to maintain adequate pain relief. Each patient will reach pain relief at a different level, as evidenced by the effective therapeutic range of morphine seen in various studies. Most patients respond fairly well with a continuous infusion at the onset of therapy. As their pain decreases and they become active, they become aware that the pain is more intense at certain times of day. As a result, individual dose patterns need to be established. Such individualization can be done efficiently only with an externally programmable infusion system. Most patients tolerate the medication well and without significant side effects, but increasingly larger doses may be necessary over time. The system may allow return to a more normal lifestyle, including improved ability to perform activities of daily living and, for many patients, resumption of vocational activities. The best results occur among well-motivated patients who have realistic goals and a clear understanding of spinal morphine therapy and who have demonstrated appropriate responses during a screening trial. Meticulous attention to detail in the care and maintenance of the system, and a willingness of the clinician to devote ample time to the patient, will maximize the effectiveness of this modality.

COMPLICATIONS, ADVANTAGES, AND DISADVANTAGES OF INTRASPINAL DRUG DELIVERY SYSTEMS

Complications of the drug delivery systems. Complications may be due to several factors independent of the choice of the system, route, and application. Complications of the drug delivery systems may be categorized as related to time, the site of the catheter, parts of the system, and rare complications. Time-related complications are either immediate or late. Immediate complications are bleeding at the site of surgery, hematoma along the course of the subcutaneous tunneling device, epidural hematoma, early infection, cerebrospinal fluid leakage, postspinal headache, edema, pump pocket seroma, and improper placement of the system. Late complications are obstruction of the catheter, obstruction of the port or the pump, catheter kinking, catheter dislodgment, pump malfunction or failure, late infection, fibrosis, and injection-related burning pain. Complications related to the site of the catheter are either epidural or intrathecal. Complications related to the epidural space are fibrosis in the epidural space, injection-related burning pain, epidural hematoma, epidural abscess, and fibrous sheath formation around the catheter. Complications related to the intrathecal space are leakage of cerebrospinal fluid, fistula of the dura, cerebrospinal hygroma, spinal headache, and meningitis.

Complications with parts of the system are related to the catheter, the port, or the pump. Complications related to the catheter are clot formation, kinking, curling, and knotting; misplacement, displacement, occlusion, or migration of the catheter; and difficulties associated with removal. Complications related to the port or pump are obstruction of the port, leakage from the port membrane, mechanical pump failure, pump malfunction, disconnection of the catheter, and seroma formation around the port or the pump. Rare complications are skin necrosis and skin reaction to the percutaneous or subcutaneously tunneled devices (Coombs 1990, Erdine 1998).

Advantages and disadvantages. In summary, the potential advantages of the epidural route are as follows: placement at the desired dermatomal level, no risk of spinal fluid leakage and related spinal headache, the ability of the dura to act as a barrier, and reduced risk of infection at the site of the tip of the catheter, with infection generally limited to the reservoir pocket. Clinicians have greater flexibility in choice of drugs, and can use nonopioids either together with opioids or alone to potentiate the analgesia. However, in numerous patients, fibrosis develops in the epidural space around the tip of the catheter that may occlude the catheter. Burning pain on epidural injection may occur in patients receiving prolonged treatment.

The advantages of the intrathecal route are less risk of catheter obstruction, no risk of fibrosis obstructing the catheter, less burning pain, less risk of catheter migration, longer and stronger analgesia, and reduced opioid requirement. Among the disadvantages of intrathecal delivery are frequent occurrence of cerebrospinal fluid leakage and postspinal headache.

No controlled studies in patients with intractable pain have compared the epidural and intrathecal routes of administration for dosage and analgesic efficacy. Agreement is still needed on guidelines for the selection of the route, but the following points may be considered. For cancer patients with short life expectancy, the epidural route and the less expensive drug delivery systems may be preferable. Pain management can be started rapidly with percutaneous or subcutaneously implanted catheters or ports. As already noted, internalized pumps are not feasible for the epidural route as the volumes that can be delivered are generally too small. With the intrathecal route, lower doses and volume of drugs may be sufficient for extensive pain relief. In noncancer pain, intrathecal spinal opioid therapy may be continued for years with the use of infusion pumps (Erdine 1998).

SYMPATHETIC INDWELLING CATHETERS

Some clinicians routinely perform continuous sympathetic infusions (Knoblanche 1979) such as continuous stellate ganglion and continuous lumbar sympathetic infusions. The stellate ganglion infusion is often unreliable due to catheter dislodgment. In contrast, continuous celiac and lumbar sympathetic infusions are often successful, and for patients with no significant problems can even be administered in outpatient units. These techniques are most useful in treating visceral pain, pain secondary to cancer, CRPS-I, and sympathetically maintained pain (Dhuner et al. 1955).

Drugs. The drugs administered for sympathetic infusions follow the same principles as for brachial plexus infusion. The drug of choice has been bupivacaine (0.125–0.25%), usually without a narcotic. Morphine, fentanyl, and sufentanil have been mixed with the local anesthetic to prolong the analgesia.

Efficacy. Stellate ganglion infusion is unreliable due to catheter dislodgment. Lumbar sympathetic infusion is quite reliable even though access to the lumbar plexus will eventually be blocked, with diversion of local anesthetic solution into the psoas muscle. Hypotension and nausea are rare complications of bilateral celiac plexus infusion. Insufficient data are available to state that continuous sympathetic infusion is a safe, reliable, and efficacious technique (Niv and Chayen 1995).

SUBCUTANEOUS INDWELLING CATHETERS

Unlike previously described techniques of regional analgesia, the subcutaneous indwelling catheter technique is used to obtain pain relief via the systemic route. Subcutaneous infusion of opioids is the most effective technique in patients who cannot be treated effectively with oral medications due to side effects such as nausea and xerostomia, by the rectal route due to local irritation, or sublingually due to the bitter taste of opioids. This method has been used for both adults (Russell 1979) and children (Miser et al. 1983), and especially for patients with terminal diseases (Bruera et al. 1988; Storey et al. 1990; Moulin et al. 1991). A small-gauge butterfly needle is inserted under the skin of the thigh, abdomen, or upper arm, and is connected to a portable pump or syringe that administers bolus doses. The volume of infusion usually ranges from 1 to 2 mL/hour. The opioids used most often are morphine and hydromorphone (Bruera et al. 1988). Serum concentrations achieved by subcutaneous administration are similar to those achieved with the intravenous route (Waldmann et al. 1984; Moulin et al.

1991). The method is efficacious in the home setting (Ohlsson et al. 1995), and the main complication is local irritation at the infusion site. This complication is treated by removing the needle to a new site, and if problems persist by the addition of 25 mg of hydrocortisone (Shvartzman and Bonneh 1994). Large infusion volumes are associated with a more frequent need to change the infusion site (Bruera et al. 1993). Biopsies taken from irritated subcutaneous sites have revealed lobular subcutaneous inflammation with subdermal signs of necrosis (Adams et al. 1989); the author believed that plaque formation was related to hydraulic irritation at the infusion site.

REFERENCES

Adams F, Cruz L, Deachman MJ, Zamora E. Focal subdermal toxicity with subcutaneous opioid infusion in patients with cancer pain. *J Pain Symptom Manage* 1989; 4:31–33.

Akerman B, Arwenstrom E, Post C. Local anesthetics potentiate spinal morphine antinociception. *Anesth Analg* 1988; 67:913–943.

Auld AW, Maki-Jokela A, Murdoch DM. Intraspinal narcotic analgesia in the treatment of chronic pain. *Spine* 1985; 10:777–781.

Bromage PR, Camporesi E, Chestnut D. Epidural narcotics for postoperative analgesia. *Anesth Anal* 1980; 59:473–480.

Brown DC. *Regional Anesthesia and Analgesia.* Philadelphia: W.B. Saunders, 1996.

Bruera E, Brenneis C, Michaud M, et al. Use of subcutaneous route for administration of narcotics in patients with cancer pain. *Cancer* 1988: 62:407–411.

Bruera E, MacEachern T, Macmillan K, Miller MJ, Hanson J. Local tolerance to subcutaneous infusions of high concentrations of hydromorphone: a prospective study. *J Pain Symptom Manage* 1993; 8:201–204.

Carl P, Crawford ME, Ravlo O, et al. Long term treatment with epidural opioids: a retrospective study comprising 150 patients with morphine chloride and buprenorphine. *Anaesthesia* 1986; 41:32–38.

Chestnut DH, Owen CLL, Bates JN, et al. Continuous infusion epidural analgesia during labor: a randomized double-blind comparison of 0.0625% bupivacaine/0.0002% fentanyl versus 0.125% bupivacaine. *Anesthesiology* 1988; 68:754–759.

Cleland JG. Continuous peridural caudal analgesia in surgery and early ambulation. *Northwest Med* 1949; 48:266.

Coombs DW. Delivery systems for chronic spinal analgesia. In: N. Rawal and W. Coombs (Eds). *Current Management of Pain Series.* Kluwer Academic, 1990, pp 115–128.

Coombs DW, Pageau MG, Saunders RL, et al. Intraspinal narcotic tolerance: preliminary experience with continuous bupivacaine HC1 infusion via implanted infusion device. *Int J Artif Organs* 1982; 5:379–382.

Coombs DW, Saunders RL, Lachance D, et al. Intrathecal morphine tolerance. Use of intrathecal clonidine, DADLE, and intraventricular morphine. *Anesthesiology* 1985; 62:358–363.

Cousins MJ, Bridenbaugh PO. *Neural Blockade in Clinical Anesthesia and Management of Pain,* 3rd ed. Philadelphia: J.B. Lippincott, 1998.

Cullen M, Staren E, Ganzouri A, et al. Continuous thoracic epidural analgesia after major abdominal operations: a randomized prospective double-blind study. *Surgery* 1985; 98:718.

Dhuner K-G, Moberg E, Omne L. Paresis of the phrenic nerve during brachial plexus analgesia and its importance. *Acta Chir Scand* 1955; 109:53–57.

Edwards ND, Wright EM. Continuous low-dose 3-in-1 nerve blockade for postoperative pain relief after total knee replacement. *Anesth Analg* 1992; 75:265.

Erdine S. Intraspinal drug delivery systems for pain treatment: when are they appropriate? In: Aronoff GM (Ed). *Evaluation and Treatment of Chronic Pain.* Baltimore: Williams and Wilkins, 1998; pp 543–553.

Farrar MD, Scheybani M, Nolte H: Upper extremity block. Effectiveness and complications. *Reg Anesth* 1981; 6:133–134.

Fisher A, Meller Y. Continuous postoperative regional anesthesia by nerve sheath block for amputation surgery——a pilot study. *Anesth Analg* 1991; 72:300–303.

Fisher R, Lubenow TR, Liceaga A, et al. Comparison of continuous epidural infusion of fentanyl-bupivacaine and morphine-bupivacaine in the management of postoperative pain. *Anesth Analg* 1988; 67:559–563.

Glynn C, Dawson D, Sanders R. A double-blind comparison between epidural morphine and epidural clonidine in patients with chronic non-cancer pain. *Pain* 1988; 34:123–128.

Guardini R, Waldron, BA, Wallace WA. Sciatic nerve block: a new lateral approach. *Acta Anesthesiol Scand* 1985; 29:515.

Hartrick, C. Pain due to trauma including sports injuries. In: Raj PP (Ed). *Practical Management of Pain,* 2nd ed. St. Louis: Mosby Yearbook, 1992, pp 409–433.

Hassenbush SJ, Paice JA, Patt RB, Bedder MD, Bell GK. Clinical realities and economic considerations: economics of intrathecal therapy. *J Pain Symptom Manage* 1997; 14:536–548.

Hjorts NC, Lunc C, Mogensen T, et al. Epidural morphine improves pain relief and maintains sensory analgesia during continuous epidural bupivacaine after abdominal surgery. *Anesth Analg* 1986; 65:1033–1036.

Kanoff RBS. Intraspinal delivery of opiates by all implantable, programmable pump in patients with chronic intractable pain of nonmalignant origin. *J Am Osteopath Assoc* 1994; 94:487–493.

Knoblanche GE. The incidence and aetiology of phrenic nerve blockade associated with supraclavicular brachial plexus block. *Anesth Intensive Care* 1979; 7:346–349.

Kulenkampff D. Die anesthesie des plexus brachialis. *Zentralbl Chir* 1911; 38:1337–1340.

Logas WG, El-Baz NM, El-Ganzouri A, et al. Continuous thoracic epidural analgesia for postoperative pain relief following thoracotomy: a randomized prospective study. *Anesthesiology* 1987; 67:787–791.

Lubenow TR, Durrani Z, Ivanovich AD. Evaluation of continuous epidural fentanyl/butorphanol infusion for postoperative pain. *Anesthesiology* 1988; 69(3A):381; *Anesthesiology* 1990; 73:A800.

Matsuda M, Kato N, Hosoi M. Continuous brachial plexus block for replantation in the upper extremity. *Hand* 1982; 14:129–134.

Miser AW, Davis DM, Hughes CS, Muline LAF, Miser JS. Continuous subcutaneous infusion of morphine in children with cancer. *Am J Dis Child* 1983; 137:383–385.

Moulin DE, Kreeft JH, Murray-Parsons N, Bouquillon AI. Comparison of continuous subcutaneous and intravenous hydromorphone infusions for management of cancer pain. *Lancet* 1991; 337:465–468.

Murphy TM, Hinds S, Cherry D. Intraspinal narcotics: nonmalignant pain. *Acta Anesthesiol Scand Suppl* 1987; 85:75–76.

Niv D, Chayen M. Sympathetic block and sympathectomy. In: Korczyn AD (Ed). *Handbook of Autonomic Nervous System Dysfunction.* New York: Marcel Dekker, 1995, pp. 399–411.

Nitescu P, Applegren L, Linder LE, et al. Epidural versus intrathecal morphine-bupivacaine: assessment of consecutive treatments in advanced cancer pain. *J Pain Symptom Manage* 1990; 5:18–26.

Ohlsson LJ, Rydberg TS, Eden T, Grimhall BAK, Thulin LA. Microbiologic and economic evaluation of multi-day infusion pumps for control of cancer pain. *Ann Pharmacother* 1995; 29:972–976.

Penn RD, Paice JA. Chronic intrathecal morphine for intractable pain. *J Neurosurg* 1987; 67:182–186.

Penn RD, Paice JA, Gottschalk W, et al. Cancer pain relief using chronic morphine infusion. Early experience with a programmable implanted drug pump. *J Neurosurg* 1984; 61:302–306.

Pere P, Pitkanen M, Rosenberg PH, et al. Effect of continuous interscalene brachial plexus block on diaphragm motion and on ventilatory function. *Acta Anaesthesiol Scand* 1992; 36:53–57.

Pham-Dang C, Meunier JF, Poirier P, et al. A new axillary approach for continuous brachial plexus block. A clinical and anatomic study. *Anesth Analg* 1995: 81(4):686–693.

Raj PP. *Clinical Practice of Regional Anesthesia.* St. Louis: Churchill Livingstone, 1991.

Raj PP. Continuous brachial plexus analgesia. *Abstracts: 21st Annual Meeting, American Society of Regional Anesthesia.* 1996, pp 501–502.

Raj PP, Denson D, Finnason R. Prolonged epidural analgesia: intermittent or continuous? In: Meyer J, Nolte H (Eds). *Die Kontinuerliche Peridural Anesthesia.* 7th International Symposium über die Regionale Anesthesia, January 7, 1982, Minden, Germany.

Raj PP, Montgomery SJ, Nettles D, et al. Infraclavicular brachial plexus—a new approach. *Anesth Analg* 1973; 52:897.

Richard B, Kanoff DO. Intraspinal delivery of opiates by implantable, programmable pump in patients with chronic, intractable pain of non-malignant origin. *J Am Osteopath Assoc* 1994; 94:487–493.

Rosseel PMJ, Van Der Broeck J, Boer EC, et al. Epidural sufentanil for intraoperative and postoperative analgesia in thoracic surgery: a comparative study with intravenous sufentanil. *Acta Anesthesiol Scand* 1988; 32:193–198.

Russell PSB. Analgesia in terminal malignant disease. *BMJ* 1979; 1:1561.

Shvartzman P, Bonneh D. Local skin irritation in the course of subcutaneous morphine infusion: a challenge (case report). *J Palliat Care* 1994; 10:44–45.

Smith BE, Fischer ABJ, Scott PU. Continuous sciatic nerve block. *Anaesthesia* 1984; 39:155.

Storey P, Hill HH Jr, St. Louis RH, Tarver EE. Subcutaneous infusions for control of cancer symptoms. *J Pain Symptom Manage* 1990; 5:33–41.

Tuominen M, Haasio J, Hekali R, et al. Continuous interscalene brachial plexus block: clinical efficacy, technical problems and bupivacaine plasma concentrations. *Acta Anaesthesiol Scand* 1989; 33:84–88.

Urmey WF, McDonald M. Reductions in pulmonary function resulting from interscalene brachial plexus block. *Reg Anesth* 1990; 15:A17.

Urmey WF, McDonald M. Hemidiaphragmatic paresis during interscalene brachial plexus block: effects on pulmonary function and chest wall mechanics. *Anesth Analg* 1992; 44:352–357.

Urmey WF, Talts KH, Schraft S, et al. Ipsilateral hemidiaphragm paresis associated with interscalene brachial plexus anesthesia. *Anesthesiology* 1988; 71:A728.

Urmey WF, Talts KH, Sharrock NE. One hundred percent incidence of hemidiaphragmatic paresis associated with interscalene brachial plexus anesthesia as diagnosed by ultrasonography. *Anesth Analg* 1991; 72:498–503.

Vaghadia H, Kapnoudhis P, Jenkins LC, et al. Continuous lumbosacral block using a Tuohy needle and catheter technique. *Can J Anesth* 1992; 39:75.

Waldmann CS, Bason JR, Rambohul E, et al: Serum morphine levels: a comparison between continuous subcutaneous infusion and continuous intravenous infusion in postoperative patients. *Anaesthesia* 1984; 39: 768–771.

Correspondence to: David Niv, MD, Center for Pain Medicine, Tel-Aviv Sourasky Medical Center, Sackler Faculty of Medicine, Tel-Aviv University, Tel-Aviv, Israel. Email: davidniv@tasmc.health.il.

Proceedings of the 9th World Congress on Pain,
Progress in Pain Research and Management,
Vol. 16, edited by M. Devor, M.C. Rowbotham, and
Z. Wiesenfeld-Hallin, IASP Press, Seattle, © 2000.

88

Infection Rates in Patients with Long-Term Intrathecal Infusion of Opioids and Bupivacaine

Peter Dahm, Christopher Lundborg, Magnus Jansson, Cecilia Olegård, Petre Nitescu, Ioan Curelaru, and Lennart Appelgren

Department of Anesthesiology, Pain Section, Sahlgren's University Hospital, Göteborg, Sweden

Following the introduction of intrathecal (i.t.) opioids for the treatment of pain in cancer patients, clinicians considered that this method might also be useful for "refractory" nonmalignant pain conditions such as ischemic pain, phantom pain, postherpetic neuralgia, complex regional pain syndromes, avulsion of nerve plexus, and failed back surgery. However, i.t. administration of morphine in these patients proved to be unreliable, with lack of optimal analgesic control in up to 81% of patients treated (Krames and Lanning 1993). In an attempt to increase the analgesic control obtainable with this method, we added bupivacaine to the i.t. opioid, or even replaced morphine with bupivacaine. We had previously obtained good results with a low incidence of bacterial infections in cancer patients using open, externalized i.t. pump systems. This experience encouraged us to try the method in nonmalignant pain syndromes (Nitescu et al. 1992). Between 1987 and 1995 we used the method to treat 90 consecutive patients with nonmalignant pain and carefully followed treatment efficacy, failure, and infection rates.

PATIENTS AND METHODS

Between February 11, 1987 and December 31, 1995, 90 patients entered a prospective, cohort, nonrandomized, consecutive trial (40 men and 50 women, 20–96 years old, median age 70 years). Ethical committee approval was obtained.

Of the 90 patients, 9 suffered from nociceptive pain, 17 from neuropathic pain, and 64 from mixed nociceptive-neuropathic pain (Table I). The patients were treated for refractory pain conditions lasting for 0.3–50 years (median 3 years) with continuous i.t. infusions of bupivacaine (n = 49) or of bupivacaine combined with an opioid (morphine, n = 11; or buprenorphine, n = 30). At the end of the study 85 patients had terminated the i.t. treatment and 5 patients were still receiving treatment.

The patients entered the study after a comprehensive evaluation and assessment and after fulfilling the following criteria: (a) the pain totally dominated the patient's life, (b) other methods failed to provide acceptable pain relief, and (c) the patients refused, were intolerant to, or had experienced unacceptable side effects from opioids. We found a wide variety of pathological findings before the start of the i.t. pain treatment, including 43 local infections (42 in the lower extremities), 7 urinary infections, and 7 cases of sepsis. In accordance with the admission criteria, we included these patients in the study despite their prior infection and the possible risk of spinal infection. All patients provided written consent.

After evaluation and assessment, we performed an i.t. bupivacaine test by injecting 2.5–15 mg (median 8 mg) of 0.5% isotonic bupivacaine solution. If the test provided acceptable pain relief, we inserted an 18-g nylon catheter into the subarachnoidal space under sterile conditions in the operating room, as previously reported (Nitescu et al. 1991). The tip of the catheter was placed with the help of C-arm fluoroscopy at the level corresponding to maximal pain intensity. The catheter was then tunneled from the insertion site (usually paravertebrally), over the shoulder, and further parasternally until the tunnel exit was at the level of the third chondrocostal junction. A 0.22-μm micropore antibacterial filter was connected to the exiting

Table I
Type of pain (number of patients in parentheses)

Nociceptive Pain (n = 9)	Neuropathic Pain (n = 17)	Mixed Nociceptive/ Neuropathic Pain (n = 64)
Complications of hip prosthesis (2)	Acute herpes zoster (2)	Chronic venous insufficiency (1)
Unstable femur fracture (2)	Amyloidosis polyneuropathy (2)	Collagen disease (3)
Chronic pancreatitis (1)	Postherpetic neuralgia (2)	Arterial insufficiency (32)
Portal vein thrombosis (1)	Lumbosacral radiation plexopathy (1)	CRPS-I (3)
Endometriosis (1)	Ischemic myelopathy (5)	Postamputation pain (10)
Unstable angina pectoris (2)	Multiple sclerosis (2)	Failed spinal surgery (3)
	Post-traumatic myelopathy (3)	Spinal spondylosis (4)
		Vertebral compression (6)
		Idiopathic coccygodynia (1)
		Double heart transplantation (1)

catheter luer lock and the other end to the pump system. In the operating room we began an infusion of plain bupivacaine 5.0 mg/mL or of bupivacaine 4.75 mg/mL combined with an opioid (morphine 0.5 mg/mL or buprenorphine 0.015 mg/mL) from an external electronic programmable pump. We have found that a starting dose of 4–5 mL/day provides acceptable pain relief for most patients (0–2 out of 10 on a visual analogue scale [VAS]). When necessary, we adjusted the pump delivery system to provide acceptable pain relief. Before a patient left the operating theater, we applied a gauze compress between the filter and the skin. The tunnel exit and the catheter hub were covered with a split, 9 × 15 cm self-adhesive, absorbent compress, and a label indicating "intrathecal catheter" was pasted on it to warn against accidental injection of other substances. Finally, the whole tunnel exit, including catheter hub, filter, and the last 6–8 cm of the extension tubing of the pump, was covered and fixed to the skin with a 12.7 × 17.8 cm self-adhesive, sterile, transparent polyurethane film.

The patients were supervised for 24 hours in the postoperative ward. Heart rate, blood pressure, electrocardiogram, pulse oxymetry, respiration rate, temperature, and 24-hour diuresis were recorded. Patients received prophylactic i.v. administration of antibiotics (cloxacillin) for 3 days beginning on the day of catheter insertion. Some patients needed further institutional care for somatic pathological conditions (longer hospital stays were unrelated to the i.t. pain treatment). Due to the potential risk of contamination on "opening" the closed system (catheter hub, catheter, subarachnoidal space), specially trained pain nurses changed the antibacterial filter under sterile conditions approximately once a month or every other month for patients released to home care (Nitescu et al. 1991). Regular staff nurses were trained in the procedure for changing pump cassettes for hospitalized patients. Timing of change of cassettes (which contained 100 mL solution) depended on the infusion rate. Most patients had infusion volumes of 4–10 mL/day, and the cassettes were changed every 1–2 weeks.

RESULTS

The i.t. treatment lasted for 3–1706 days (median 60 days), with a cumulative total of 14,686 days, of which 7460 (50%) were spent at home. The great range of the treatment periods in this study is explained by the wide variety of the nonmalignant pain conditions included, and by the fact that treatment sometimes failed, leading to early termination. Treatment was discontinued if pain relief was unsatisfactory (<40% reduction of the initial pain intensity), if the patient refused to continue, or when adverse effects made the treatment uncontrollable (e.g., epidural fibrosis, adhesive arachnoiditis, lack of compliance by the patient).

Mean VAS scores decreased from 3–9 (median 7) before the treatment to 0–7 (median 1.5) afterwards. Most patients (86 of 90) reported a decrease in pain intensity to a level considered acceptable (VAS mean < 4). This result represents pain relief of 60–100% (median 85%). Catheters sometimes required reinsertion due to complications such as dislodgment, obstruction, and accidental withdrawal: 101 catheters were needed for 90 patients. Throughout the entire treatment period we carefully noted signs of infection and other complications. The following infection rates were recorded (number of complications/number of patients [n = 90] or number of catheters [n = 101]): catheter entry site infection 0/90 (0%), skin suture entry site infection 5/90 (5%), tunnel exit infection 0/90 (0%), deep catheter track infection 1/90 (1%), fascitis 0/90 (0%), localized cellulitis 0/90 (0%), epidural abscess 0/90 (0%), meningism 0/90 (0%), meningitis 4/90 patients (4%) or 4/101 catheters (a rate of 0.27 cases of meningitis per 1000 treatment days). Overall, 11 of the 90 patients (12%) contracted infections, and infections occurred with 11 of the 101 catheters (10%) for an infection rate of 0.76 per 1000 catheterization days. All infections were successfully treated with antibiotics during i.t. pain treatment. We consulted an infection specialist regarding antibiotic choice for patients with meningitis.

At the end of the study, five patients continued to receive treatment for periods ranging from 30 to 1706 days (median 206 days). In the remaining 85 patients the i.t. treatment was terminated for the following reasons: 23 patients died (no death could be attributed to the i.t. pain treatment); 33 patients no longer needed the treatment (pain resolved for 32 and 1 patient switched to dorsal column stimulation); and 19 patients refused to continue after treatment ranging from 3 to 286 days (median 15 days) even though 16 had acceptable pain relief. Another 8 patients would not cooperate, and for 2 patients, the i.t. treatment lost its effectiveness.

DISCUSSION

Long-term i.t. infusion of opioid and bupivacaine with externalized systems and a programmable pump initially provided satisfactory (>60–100%) pain relief in 95% of the patients. In the long run the system failed in 34% of the patients (median time to failure = 60 days, longest effective case = 6 years). It seems that this "open" externalized system does not lead to more infections (spinal or otherwise) when compared to other studies on long-term intraspinal (epidural/intrathecal) pain treatment (Dahm et al. 1998).

We consider this open, externalized system to be acceptably safe. We believe that certain procedures are important during insertion and treatment to reduce risk of infection: (a) The insertion should be made in the operating theater under sterile conditions; (b) the patients should receive prophylactic antibiotics before the insertion procedure and for 3 days following; (c) the antibacterial filter should be changed only once a month, or every other month, by specially trained pain nurses; (d) dressings and cassettes should be changed under sterile conditions (usually every 1–2 weeks); (e) all personnel involved with the i.t. pain treatment should be instructed in the treatment regime and informed of early symptoms of infection, especially meningitis; and (f) close contact should be maintained with patients or their families (initially every day, and in the long run every week).

ACKNOWLEDGMENTS

This study was supported by grants from families and friends of the patients with "refractory" pain treatment with intrathecal morphine-bupivacaine in Göteborg (5753-24 955 02), by grant 8190 30 from the Research Council of the Faculty of Medicine of Göteborg University, and by a grant from Inga-Britt and Arne Lundberg's Research Foundation for acquisition of modern X-ray and physiological monitoring equipment for the study.

REFERENCES

Dahm P, Nitescu P, Appelgren L, Curelaru I. Efficacy and technical complications of long term continuous intraspinal infusions of opioid and/or bupivacaine in refractory nonmalignant pain: a comparison between the epidural and the intrathecal approach with externalized or implanted catheters and infusion pumps. *Clin J Pain* 1998; 14:4–16.

Krames ES, Lanning RM. Intrathecal infusional analgesia for nonmalignant pain: analgesic efficacy of intrathecal opioid with or without bupivacaine. *J Pain Symptom Manage* 1993, 8:539–558.

Nitescu P, Appelgren L, Hultman LE. Long term, open catheterization of the spinal subarachnoid space for continuous infusion of narcotic and bupivacaine in patients with refractory cancer pain: a technique of catheterization and its problems and complications. *Clin J Pain* 1991; 7:143–161.

Nitescu P, Appelgren L, Linder LE, et al. Long term intrathecal (IT) narcotic (buprenorphine or morphine) and bupivacaine in "refractory" benign pain (results from the first series of 27 patients). *Reg Anesth* 1992; 17:3S–145.

Correspondence to: Peter Dahm, MD, Department of Anesthesiology, Sahlgren's University Hospital, 413 45 Göteborg, Sweden. Tel: 46-31-3421000; Fax: 46-31-413862; e-mail: peterdahm@yahoo.com.

Proceedings of the 9th World Congress on Pain,
Progress in Pain Research and Management,
Vol. 16, edited by M. Devor, M.C. Rowbotham, and
Z. Wiesenfeld-Hallin, IASP Press, Seattle, © 2000.

89

A Prospective, Open Study of Oral Methadone in the Treatment of Cancer Pain

Eduardo Bruera,[a] Maria Antonieta Rico,[b] Mariela Bertolino,[c] Jairo R. Moyano,[d] Silvia R. Allende,[e] Roberto Wenk,[c] Catherine M. Neumann,[f] and John Hanson[g]

[a]Department of Symptom Control and Palliative Care, University of Texas, and M.D. Anderson Cancer Center, Houston, Texas, USA; [b]Dr. C. Pardo Correa Oncology Institute, Santiago, Chile; [c]Hospital Tornu, FEMEBA, Buenos Aires, Argentina; [d]National Cancer Institute, Bogota, Colombia; [e]National Cancer Institute, Mexico City, Mexico; [f]Division of Palliative Care Medicine, University of Alberta, Edmonton, Alberta, Canada; [g]Cross Cancer Institute, Edmonton, Alberta, Canada

In recent years, it has become apparent that prolonged administration of high doses of opioids can cause a number of side effects, such as delirium, myoclonus, and hyperalgesia, that are at least partially caused by the accumulation of active metabolites (Bruera and Pereira 1997; Ripamonti and Bruera 1997). This opioid-induced neurotoxicity can improve with a change in the type of opioid agonist prescribed (Bruera and Pereira 1997; Ripamonti and Bruera 1997). Studies by our group and others have found that methadone, a synthetic opioid agonist, can be an effective alternative in patients requiring chronic opioids (Bruera et al. 1996; De Conno et al. 1996; Lawlor et al. 1998; Ripamonti et al. 1998). However, these studies have found that methadone is much more potent than previously estimated, probably because only partial tolerance occurs between methadone and other opioid agonists. Therefore, opioid rotation to methadone in ambulatory patients requires frequent observation and personalized titration.

We performed a prospective, multi-center, open study to assess the analgesic and side effects of methadone in a population of advanced cancer patients.

METHODS

SUBJECTS

Consecutive patients with pain due to advanced cancer were admitted to this study at the National Cancer Institute, Bogota, Colombia; National Institute of Cancer, Mexico City, Mexico; Hospital Tornu, FEMEBA, Buenos Aires, Argentina; and Dr. C. Pardo Correa Oncological Institute, Santiago, Chile. All patients were followed up at the cancer pain and palliative care programs in the respective participating institutions.

All patients fulfilled the following criteria for admission: (1) pain due to cancer; (2) no contra-indications to oral methadone (history of allergies or severe toxicity to methadone); (3) normal cognitive status (defined as a score on a short mental state questionnaire of 24 or more out of 30 in patients at a grade 8 or higher level of education, or evaluated by the clinical impression of the main treating physician in other cases); (4) ability to complete the assessment forms; (5) ability to attend assessments daily for 7 days and weekly for 2 months; and (6) written informed consent.

PROCEDURES

All patients were changed from their previous opioid dose to methadone, or were started on methadone if they were not previously receiving opioids. The following guidelines were used: (1) Patients not receiving opioids were started on methadone at 5 mg every 8 hours regularly and 5 mg every 2 hours as needed for extra pain. (2) For patients on previous opioids, the equianalgesic dose of morphine was calculated following standard equianalgesic dose tables from the clinical practice guidelines on cancer pain (U.S. Department of Health and Human Services 1994). If the equivalent daily dose of morphine was less than 100 mg/day, the previous opioid was discontinued and patients were started on methadone at 5 mg every 8 hours regularly and 5 mg every 2 hours as needed for extra pain.

If the morphine equivalent dose was more than 100 mg/day, the switchover took place over 3 days. On day 1, the previous opioid was reduced by 30–50% and replaced with methadone using a 10:1 morphine/methadone conversion rate. On days 2 and 3, the previous opioid was further decreased by another 30–50% so that by day 3, the patient was receiving only methadone.

During the daily assessment required in the first week, the investigators were able to increase or decrease the dose according to side effects, analgesia, and number of rescue doses during the previous 24 hours. Adjustments after the first week were made on a weekly basis. If sedation occurred, the dose of the previous opioid was reduced first. If sedation continued, or was severe, the dose of methadone was withheld until this side effect disappeared.

On admission to the study, patients underwent the following assessments: (1) A demographic assessment, including age, gender, primary tumor, and pain location and mechanism. (2) The Edmonton staging system for cancer pain (Bruera et al. 1989, 1995). (3) Determination of the type, dose, and route of all previous opioids. (4) Pain intensity assessment. Every day, patients were asked to rate their pain on a numerical scale (0 = no pain, 10 = worst possible pain) and a 5-item verbal descriptor between none and excruciating pain during the last 24 hours. (5) In addition, patients were asked to complete a numerical assessment (0 = no symptoms, 10 = worst possible symptoms) of sedation and nausea during the last 24 hours. (6) After the beginning of the opioid rotation the daily regular and extra doses of methadone and the interval of administration were recorded. These assessments took place daily for the first 7 days of the study and weekly thereafter for the remainder of the patient's life, or up to a maximum of 8 weeks.

STATISTICAL ANALYSIS

The median dose ratio between the previous opioid and methadone was calculated, as well as the difference in median pain intensity before and after the completion of the rotation. Dose ratios and symptom assessment were calculated 24 hours after the completion of the opioid rotation to methadone, to ensure complete elimination of the previous opioid. Because of the long half-life of methadone, values were also calculated for 3 days after completion of the rotation. These results, as well as the intensity of sedation and nausea before and after the rotation, were analyzed using analysis of variance. The correlation between the previous opioid dose and the methadone dose ratio was established using Pearson's correlation coefficient. Data were analyzed using the SAS system for personal computers.

RESULTS

A total of 108 patients met the study criteria. All patients were on oral opioids except for one patient receiving intravenous and one receiving subcutaneous administration. Table I summarizes the results after the opioid

Table I
Results after the opioid rotation to methadone

	N	Mean ± SD	Median (quartile)
MEDD (mg/day)	108	165.9 ± 457.6	48 (30–90)
Methadone (mg/day) 1 day after opioid rotation	99	36.6 ± 123.7	15 (15–22.5)
Methadone (mg/day) 3 days after opioid rotation	91	35.6 ± 124.9	15 (15–22.5)
MEDD/ME dose ratio 1 day after opioid rotation	99	4.84 ± 6.04	2.67 (1.6–6)
MEDD/ME dose ratio 3 days after opioid rotation	93	4.35 ± 4.34	3 (1.6–5.4)
Number of days to completion of opioid rotation	108	1.44 ± 1.04	1 (1–2)

Note: MEDD = morphine equivalent daily dose prior to rotation; ME = methadone.

rotation to methadone. The rotation was completed in 103 patients (95%). The reasons for noncompletion of the rotation were death due to cancer (n = 1), noncompliance (n = 1), loss to follow-up (n = 2), and refusal to continue on study because of fear of potential side effects (n = 1).

Table II summarizes the symptom assessment before and one and three days after after the completion of the methadone rotation. Both the numerical (visual analogue scale) and verbal pain scores were significantly lower after the methadone rotation. There was no significant difference in the intensity of nausea, and a small trend toward an increase in sedation in patients after the methadone rotation (P = 0.11). Fig. 1 shows the high correlation between the log of the previous opioid dose and the log of the day 3 methadone ratio. This finding suggests that the opioid/methadone ratio is not fixed over a range of opioid dosages, but rather that methadone becomes progressively more potent relative to other opioids as the dose increases (partial cross-tolerance).

Table II
Symptom measurement before and after methadone rotation

	Day 0	Day 1	Day 3	P
Pain VAS score	6.33 ± 2.6	3.6 ± 2.7	3.2 ± 2.4	0.0001
Verbal pain score	2.5 ± 1.1	1.4 ± 1.1	1.2 ± 0.9	0.0001
Nausea	1.2 ± 2.4	1.7 ± 2.9	1.4 ± 2.3	n.s.
Sedation	2.3 ± 2.8	3.0 ± 3.1	3.1 ± 3.1	0.1076
No. patients	108	102	94	

Note: Day 0 = day before methadone rotation; day 1 = 1 day after rotation; day 3 = 3 days after rotation.

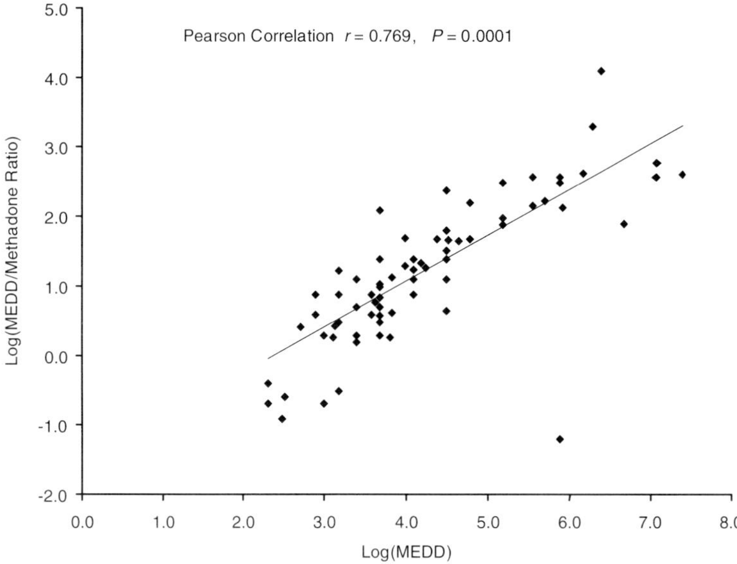

Fig. 1. The correlation between the previous morphine equivalent daily dose before methadone rotation (MEDD) (x-axis) and the ratio of MEDD to day 3 methadone dose (y-axis).

DISCUSSION

Our results agree with previous studies (Bruera et al. 1996; Lawlor et al. 1998; Ripamonti et al. 1998) regarding the much higher potency of methadone compared to other opioid agonists, and confirm the correlation between methadone dose and the previous dose of opioids. These findings suggest that methadone becomes relatively more potent in patients who have developed previous tolerance to other opioids. The relatively higher effectiveness of methadone in these tolerant patients may be related to its ability to block NMDA receptors (Clark and Kalan 1995; Ebert et al. 1995; Gorman et al. 1997).

The results of both our initial rotation and long-term follow-up suggest that methadone was well tolerated by this very ill population, as shown in the numerical ratings for nausea and sedation (Table II).

Our findings in ambulatory patients in public hospitals in different regions in Latin America suggest that a regime of oral methadone every 8 hours is safe and effective for the management of cancer pain.

As the frequency of cancer increases dramatically in Latin America (World Health Organization 1990), and opioids are used earlier in the trajectory of illness (World Health Organization 1996; World Health Organization Collaborating Centre for Palliative Cancer Care 1997), spending on opioid analgesics is likely to escalate in the region. Methadone appears to be well tolerated and can result in decreased dose escalation as well as increased interval of administration in these patients. One important additional advantage of this drug in developing countries is the fact that it is 10–20 times less expensive than morphine.

Over the last 15 years the World Health Organization has proposed morphine as the first-choice opioid for the management of cancer pain. Our findings and several recent reports (Bruera et al. 1996; De Conno et al. 1996; Lawlor et al. 1998; Ripamonti et al. 1998) strongly suggest that randomized, controlled trials should be conducted to compare methadone with morphine as a first-line opioid in patients with cancer pain.

ACKNOWLEDGMENT

Funding for this research project was generously provided by Mallinckrodt Incorporated.

REFERENCES

Bruera E, Pereira J. Neuropsychiatric toxicity of opioids. In: Jensen T, Turner J, Wiesenfeld-Hallin Z (Eds). *Proceedings of the 8th World Congress on Pain,* Progress in Pain Research and Management, Vol. 8. Seattle: IASP Press, 1997, pp 717–738.

Bruera E, MacMillan K, Hanson J, MacDonald RN. The Edmonton staging system for cancer pain: preliminary report. *Pain* 1989; 37:203–209.

Bruera E, Schoeller T, Wenk R, et al. A prospective multicenter assessment of the Edmonton staging system for cancer pain. *J Pain Symptom Manage* 1995; 10:348–355.

Bruera E, Pereira J, Watanabe S, et al. Opioid rotation in patients with cancer pain. A retrospective comparison of dose ratios between methadone, hydromorphone, and morphine. *Cancer* 1996; 78:852–857.

Clark JL, Kalan GE. Effective treatment of severe cancer pain of the head using low-dose ketamine in an opioid-tolerant patient. *J Pain Symptom Manage* 1995; 10:310–314.

De Conno F, Groff L, Brunelli C, et al. Clinical experience with oral methadone administration in the treatment of pain in 196 advanced cancer patients. *J Clin Oncol* 1996; 14:2836–2842.

Ebert B, Andersen S, Krogsgaard-Larsen P. Ketobemidone, methadone and pethidine are non-competitive N-methyl-D-aspartate (NMDA) antagonists in the rat cortex and spinal cord. *Neurosci Lett* 1995; 187:165–168.

Gorman AL, Elliott KJ, Inturrisi CE. The d- and l-isomers of methadone bind to the non-competitive site on the N-methyl-D-aspartate (NMDA) receptor in rat forebrain and spinal cord. *Neurosci Lett* 1997; 223:5–8.

Lawlor PG, Turner KS, Hanson J, Bruera ED. Dose ratio between morphine and methadone in patients with cancer pain: a retrospective study. *Cancer* 1998; 82:1167–1173.

Ripamonti C, Bruera E. CNS adverse effects of opioids in cancer patients. Guidelines for treatment. *CNS Drugs* 1997; 8:21–37.

Ripamonti C, De Conno F, Groff L, et al. Equianalgesic dose/ratio between methadone and other opioid agonists in cancer pain: comparison of two clinical experiences. *Ann Oncol* 1998; 9:79–83.

U.S. Department of Health and Human Services. *Management of Cancer Pain.* Clinical Practice Guidelines, No. 94-0592. Rockville, MD: AHCPR Publications, 1994.

World Health Organization. *Cancer Pain Relief and Palliative Care,* Technical Series 804, Geneva, Switzerland: World Health Organization, 1990.

World Health Organization. *Cancer Pain Relief*, 2nd ed. Geneva, Switzerland: World Health Organization, 1996.

World Health Organization Collaborating Centre for Palliative Cancer Care. *Looking Forward to Cancer Pain Relief for All.* Oxford: CBC Oxford, 1997.

Correspondence to: Eduardo Bruera, MD, Director, Department of Symptom Control and Palliative Care, University of Texas, M.D. Anderson Cancer Center, 1515 Holcombe Boulevard, Room P12.2911, Houston, TX 77030, USA. Tel: 713-792-6085; Fax: 713-792-6092; email: ebruera@notes.mdacc.tmc.edu.

Proceedings of the 9th World Congress on Pain, Progress in Pain Research and Management, Vol. 16, edited by M. Devor, M.C. Rowbotham, and Z. Wiesenfeld-Hallin, IASP Press, Seattle, © 2000.

90

Opioids in Chronic Nonmalignant Pain: A Criteria-Based Review of the Literature

Sandy Graven,[a] Henrica C.W. de Vet,[a,b] Maarten van Kleef,[a] and Wilhelm E.J. Weber[a]

[a]*Pain Management and Research Center, Departments of Anesthesiology and Neurology, and* [b]*Department of Epidemiology, Maastricht University Hospital, Maastricht, The Netherlands*

Long-term opioid analgesic therapy is traditionally reserved for patients suffering cancer-related pain syndromes. Withholding such treatment from patients with chronic nonmalignant pain has been justified by the perceived likelihood of tolerance, side effects, increased disability, addiction, and limited efficacy (Rayport 1954; Buckley et al. 1986; Turk 1996). In the last decade this conventional thinking has been challenged by the experience with opioids in the cancer population (Anonymous 1990). Long-term opioid therapy in cancer patients is seldom associated with neuropsychological problems (Portenoy 1994). Moreover, tolerance or physical dependence does not cause management problems, and addiction, even in noncancer populations, is rare (Graeven and Folmer 1977; Medina and Diamond 1977; Perry and Heidrich 1982; Chapman and Hill 1989).

These observations have prompted a critical reconsideration of the role of opioids in managing chronic nonmalignant pain syndromes (Taub 1982), a development reflected in a growing literature, including editorials, trials, and reviews (McQuay 1989; Zenz et al. 1992; Clark and Sees 1993; Portenoy 1994; Moulin 1996). These publications vary in quality, so the issue remains controversial.

In an attempt to critically evaluate the available scientific data, we performed a criteria-based meta-analysis of the literature on opioids in chronic nonmalignant pain (Jadad 1996; Vet et al. 1997).

MATERIALS AND METHODS

We identified relevant publications through computerized searches and citation tracking. The search included MEDLINE (Index Medicus 1/1966–1/1997) and EMBASE (Excerpta Medica 1/1986–1/1997). We used the keywords chronic pain, opioids, opiates, morphine, narcotics, benign, nonmalignant, and noncancer. We identified the publications that discuss chronic benign pain and its treatment with opioids. The references of all retrieved articles were screened for additional relevant publications. We divided the publications into editorials, case reports, uncontrolled trials (both retrospective and prospective), and randomized controlled trials.

The authors independently assessed the randomized clinical trials (RCTs) for quality of study methods. We used a criteria list for methodological assessment of the RCTs (Vet et al. 1997). The assessment was based on four categories: study population, interventions, measurement of effect, and data presentation. These categories are divided into 14 criteria. For each we assigned a weight, relative to its putative importance for validity, precision, or clinical relevance. The information in the papers was judged by each criterion. If sufficient information was reported, we evaluated the likelihood of potential bias. If bias was unlikely, the criterion was rated as positive. For each study, we calculated a method score by summing the weights for all criteria that were positive. The studies were subsequently ranked according to this sum score. The theoretical sum score of 100 points could be obtained when the design, conduct, and results of a study were adequately reported and bias was considered to be unlikely in all criteria.

In all studies (except the editorial commentaries) we tried to distinguish three types of pain: nociceptive pain (with a clear visceral or somatic activation of nociceptors), neuropathic pain (or neurogenic pain, associated with functional abnormalities of the nervous system), or idiopathic pain (cannot be accounted for by any demonstrable organic pathology). We then compared the effect of opioid therapy on these different types of pain.

RESULTS

STUDY SELECTIONS

Sixty possibly relevant papers were found. We excluded patients' and health care workers' questionnaire surveys (Novy et al. 1994; Poyhia 1994; Rapp et al. 1994; Turk 1996) and papers in which outcome parameters were not reported separately for benign versus malignant pain (Behar et al. 1979; Jadad et al. 1992). One publication was excluded because it gave undifferentiated data on both controlled and uncontrolled studies (Bapat et al. 1980). Papers predominantly reporting on the adverse effects on long-term opioid therapy were also excluded (Medina and Diamond 1977; Maruta et al. 1979; Hendler et al. 1980; Evans 1981; Tennant and Rawson 1982; Turner et al. 1982; McNairy et al. 1984; Doleys et al. 1986). The 45 remaining publications were divided into 20 editorials, 5 case reports, 12 uncontrolled trials (5 retrospective, 7 prospective), and 8 RCTs. The RCTs, considered to give the best evidence for efficacy of the opioid therapy, were studied in detail (Mays et al. 1987; Arnér and Meyerson 1988; Kupers et al. 1991; Rowbotham et al. 1991; Arkinstall et al. 1995; Moulin et al. 1996; Dellemijn and Vanneste 1997).

QUALITY ASSESSMENT OF RCTS

Initial disagreement between the three independent reviewers on the methodological criteria was easily resolved during a consensus discussion, so the method scores are based on full agreement. Table I presents the results of the assessment, and for each study shows the points assigned to each criterion and the method score. The range of the method scores is wide (average = 55 points; range = 34–82). This difference between the studies is mostly due to the treatment allocation, the study size, and the number, reasons, and handling of dropouts.

Table I
Method scores of the RCTs

Reference	A 4	B 15	C 12	D 8	E 12	F 10	G 4	H 6	I 6	J 6	K 5	L 2	M 5	N 5	Sum 100
Mays et al. 1987				6		10		4		4	1	2	5	2	34
Moulin et al. 1996	4		8	6	2	8		4		4	4	2	5	2	49
Kupers et al. 1991	2			8	12	9	4	4		4	1	2		5	51
Arnér and Meyerson 1988	2			8	12	7	4	4	4	4	1	2		5	53
Arkinstall et al. 1995		15	4	7	4	6		4		4	3	2	5	2	56
Rowbotham et al. 1991	4			8	12	10		4		4	2	2	5	5	56
Kjaersgaard-Andersen et al. 1990	4		12	7	4	8		4	4	4	2	2	5	2	58
Dellemijn and Vanneste 1997	4	15	4	8	12	10		6	6	6	2	2	5	2	82

Note: Letters A–N represent 14 categories of methodological quality (see text); the sum of the scores from each category is the total method score. Numbers directly below each letter represent the maximum possible score for each category.

TREATMENT EFFICACY

Table II show the effect of opioids on the different types of pain as studied in the RCTs. In general, patients suffering nociceptive pain syndromes respond well to long-term opioid therapy (Arnér and Meyerson 1988; Kjaersgaard-Andersen et al. 1990). Patients with neuropathic pain syndromes respond slightly less favorably, although in general still reasonably well (Arnér and Meyerson 1988; Kupers et al. 1991; Rowbotham et al. 1991; Dellemijn and Vanneste 1997). Patients with so-called idiopathic pain tend to show no response at all to long-term opioid therapy (Arnér and Meyerson 1988; Kupers et al. 1991; Moulin et al. 1996). In the two studies not specifying the diagnosis of the chronic pain syndromes, patients tend to report favorable results on long-term opiate therapy (Mays et al. 1987; Arkinstall et al. 1995). Although the information from the uncontrolled trials is less valid, these studies do reveal the same trend. Table III presents the results in the prospective uncontrolled trials (Gillman and Lichtigfeld 1981; Auld et al. 1985; Urban et al. 1986; Penn and Paice 1987; Plummer et al. 1991; McQuay et al. 1992; Fenollosa et al. 1993).

DISCUSSION

The traditional view that long-term opiate therapy should be reserved for cancer pain patients, excluding patients with nonmalignant chronic pain syndromes, has been challenged since 1982 (Taub 1982). Since then, numerous papers have been published on the subject. Nevertheless, the long-

Table II
Overall outcome of RCTs on opioid therapy for different chronic noncancer pain syndromes

Pain Type	Reference	Control	Results
Nociceptive	Arnér and Meyerson 1988	placebo	+
	Kjaersgaard-Andersen et al. 1990	paracetamol	+ *
Neuropathic	Arnér and Meyerson 1988	placebo	–
	Dellemijn and Vanneste 1997	placebo/diazepam	+
	Kupers et al. 1991	placebo	+
	Rowbotham et al. 1991	placebo	+
Idiopathic	Arnér and Meyerson 1988	placebo	–
	Kupers et al. 1991	placebo	–
	Moulin et al. 1996	benztropine	+ *
Not specified	Arkinstall et al. 1995	placebo	+ *
	Mays et al. 1987	bupivacaine/placebo	+

Note: + = positive effect; – = no effect; * = significant adverse effects.

Table III
Overall efficacy of opiates on different pain syndromes
(prospective uncontrolled studies)

Pain Type	Reference	Results
Nociceptive	McQuay et al. 1992	+
Neuropathic	Fenollosa et al. 1993	+
	McQuay et al. 1992	±
	Urban et al. 1986	+
Idiopathic	McQuay et al. 1992	–
Not specified or mixed	Auld et al. 1985	+
	Gilmann and Lichtigfeld 1981	+
	Penn and Paice 1987	+
	Plummer et al. 1991	±

Note: + = positive effect; – = no effect; ± = mixed effects.

term use of opiates in the chronic noncancer pain patient population is still controversial. This lack of consensus is well illustrated in Tables II and III, which summarize the opinions of experts. In an effort to systematically summarize the published evidence on this controversy, we conducted a criteria-based meta-analysis (Jadad 1996; Vet et al. 1997). As we hypothesized that differences in diagnoses of the chronic pain syndromes studied contributed to the lack of consensus, we divided the published evidence into three subcategories: nociceptive, neuropathic, and idiopathic chronic pain syndromes (Arnér and Meyerson 1988; Kupers and Gybels 1992).

The results support the conclusion that long-term opiate therapy may benefit patients with chronic pain syndromes from nociceptive and neuropathic origin. In general, patients with nociceptive chronic pain tend to respond more favorably than do patients with neuropathic pain. It is also evident that positive effects from long-term opiate therapy reported in uncontrolled trials are larger and more frequent than in prospective controlled studies. This finding accords with other scientific issues and once more underlines the importance of controlled clinical studies. Patients with so-called idiopathic chronic pain syndromes tend to respond less well to long-term opiate therapy. One study observed a decrease in pain complaints; however, this did not coincide with improvement in functional status (Moulin et al. 1996). These findings underscore the importance of categorizing chronic nonmalignant pain syndromes.

Taken together, the data support the clinical impression that patients with nociceptive and neuropathic chronic pain syndromes may benefit from long-term opiate therapy, while this positive effect is less clear in the population with idiopathic chronic pain syndromes.

When generalizing these conclusions we must consider that none of the controlled trials answer questions regarding long-term side effects of opiate intake. This is an important issue, as the average life expectancy of chronic nonmalignant pain patients will be considerably longer than for the cancer pain population. This issue also stresses the importance of including functional status and quality of life parameters as outcome measures in future trials.

Our literature review decreases the doubt about the efficacy of opioids for some types of chronic noncancer pain syndromes. Reaching a correct diagnosis appears to be essential when considering long-term opioid therapy for chronic nonmalignant pain syndromes (Portenoy 1994; Moulin 1996; Portenoy 1996; Anonymous 1997).

ACKNOWLEDGMENTS

We thank Sandra Reinders for helpful secretarial assistance.

REFERENCES

Anonymous. *Cancer Pain Relief And Palliative Care.* Geneva: World Health Organization, 1990.

Anonymous. The use of opioids for the treatment of chronic pain. A consensus statement from the American Academy for Pain Medicine and the American Pain Society. *Clin J Pain* 1997; 13:6–8.

Arkinstall W, Sandler A, Goughnour B, et al. Efficacy of controlled-release codeine in chronic non-malignant pain: a randomized, placebo-controlled clinical trial. *Pain* 1995; 62:169–178.

Arnér S, Meyerson BA. Lack of analgesic effect of opioids on neuropathic and idiopathic forms of pain. *Pain* 1988; 33:11–23.

Auld AW, Maki Jokela A, Murdoch DM. Intraspinal narcotic analgesia in the treatment of chronic pain. *Spine* 1985; 10:777–781.

Bapat AR, Kshirsagar NA, Bapat RD. Epidural morphine in the treatment of chronic pain. *J Postgrad Med* 1980; 26:242–245.

Behar M, Magora F, Olshwang D, Davidson JT. Epidural morphine in treatment of pain. *Lancet* 1979; 1:527–529.

Buckley FP, Sizemore WA, Charlton JE. Medication management in patients with chronic non-malignant pain. A review of the use of a drug withdrawal protocol. *Pain* 1986; 26:153–166.

Chapman CR, Hill HF. Prolonged morphine self-administration and addiction liability: evaluation of two theories in a bone marrow transplant unit. *Cancer* 1989; 63:1636–1644.

Clark HW, Sees KL. Opioids, chronic pain, and the law. *J Pain Symptom Manage* 1993; 8:297–305.

Dellemijn PLI, Vanneste JAL. Randomised double-blind active-placebo-controlled crossover trial of intravenous fentanyl in neuropathic pain. *Lancet* 1997; 349:753–758.

Doleys DM, Dolce JJ, Doleys AL, Crocker M, Wolfe SE. Evaluation, narcotics and behavioral treatment influences on pain ratings in chronic pain patients. *Arch Phys Med Rehabil* 1986; 67:456–458.

Evans PJD. Narcotic addiction in patients with chronic pain. *Anaesthesia* 1981; 36:597–602.

Fenollosa P, Pallares J, Cervera J, et al. Chronic pain in the spinal cord injured: statistical approach and pharmacological treatment. *Paraplegia* 1993; 31:722–729.

Gillman MA, Lichtigfeld FJ. A comparison of the effects of morphine sulphate and nitrous oxide analgesia on chronic pain states in man. *J Neurol Sci* 1981; 49:41–45.

Graeven DB, Folmer W. Experimental heroin users: an epidemiological and psychosocial approach. *Am J Drug Alcohol Abuse* 1977; 4:365–375.

Hendler N, Cimini C, Ma T, Long D. A comparison of cognitive impairment due to benzodiazepines and to narcotics. *Am J Psychiatry* 1980; 137:828–830.

Jadad AR. Systematic reviews and meta-analyses in pain relief research: what can (and cannot) they do for us? In: Campbell JN (Ed). *Pain 1996: An Updated Review*. Seattle: IASP Press, 1996, pp 445–452.

Jadad AR, Carroll D, Glynn CJ, Moore RA, McQuay HJ. Morphine responsiveness of chronic pain: double-blind randomised crossover study with patient-controlled analgesia. *Lancet* 1992; 339:1367–1371.

Kjaersgaard-Andersen P, Nafei A, Skov O, et al. Codeine plus paracetamol versus paracetamol in longer-term treatment of chronic pain due to osteoarthritis of the hip. A randomised, double-blind, multi-centered study. *Pain* 1990; 43:309–318.

Kupers R, Gybels J. Responsiveness of chronic pain to morphine. *Lancet* 1992; 340:310–311.

Kupers RC, Konings H, Adriaensen H, Gybels JM. Morphine differentially affects the sensory and affective pain ratings in neurogenic and idiopathic forms of pain. *Pain* 1991; 47:5–12.

Maruta T, Swanson DW, Finlayson RE. Drug abuse and dependency in patients with chronic pain. *Mayo Clin Proc* 1979; 54:341–244.

Mays KS, Lipman JJ, Schnapp M. Local analgesia without anesthesia using peripheral perineural morphine injections. *Anesthes Analg* 1987; 66:417–420.

McNairy SL, Maruta T, Ivnik RJ, Swanson DW, Ilstrup DM. Prescription medication dependence and neuropsychologic function. *Pain* 1984; 18:169–177.

McQuay HJ. Opioids in chronic pain. *Br J Anaesth* 1989; 63:213–226.

McQuay H, Jadad AR, Carroll D, et al. Opioid sensitivity of chronic pain: a patient-controlled analgesia method. *Anaesthesia* 1992; 47:757–767.

Medina JL, Diamond S. Drug dependency in patients with chronic headache. *Headache* 1977; 17:12–14.

Moulin DE. Medical management of chronic nonmalignant pain. In: Campbell JN (Ed). *Pain 1996: An Updated Overview*. Seattle: IASP Press, 1996, pp 485–492.

Moulin DE, Iezzi A, Amireh R, et al. Randomised trial of oral morphine for chronic non-cancer pain. *Lancet* 1996; 347:143–147.

Novy DM, Nelson DV, Hays JR. Attitudes of chronic pain patients to the use of narcotics. Differences within and across sub-populations. *Pain Clin* 1994; 7:267–274.

Penn RD, Paice JA. Chronic intrathecal morphine for intractable pain. *J Neurosurg* 1987; 67:182–186.

Perry S, Heidrich G. Management of pain during debridement: a survey of U.S. burn units. *Pain* 1982; 13:267–280.

Plummer JL, Cherry DA, Cousins MJ, et al. Long-term spinal administration of morphine in cancer and non-cancer pain: a retrospective study. *Pain* 1991; 44:215–220.

Portenoy RK. Opioid therapy for chronic nonmalignant pain: current status. In: Fields HL, Liebeskind JC (Eds). *Pharmacological Approaches to the Treatment of Chronic Pain: New Concepts and Critical Issues,* Progress in Pain Research and Management, Vol. 1. Seattle: IASP Press, 1994, pp 247–287.

Portenoy RK. Opioids in the management of chronic non-malignant pain. In: Portenoy RK, Kanner RM (Eds). *Pain Management: Theory and Practice.* Philadelphia: FA Davis, 1996, pp 264–269.

Poyhia R. Opioids in anaesthesia: a questionnaire survey in Finland. *Eur J Anaesthesiol* 1994; 11:221–230.

Rapp SE, Wild LM, Egan KJ, Ready LB. Acute pain management of the chronic pain patient on opiates: a survey of caregivers at University of Washington Medical Center. *Clin J Pain* 1994; 10:133–138.

Rayport M. Experience in the management of patients medically addicted to narcotics. *JAMA* 1954; 156:684–691.

Rowbotham MC, Reisner-Keller LA, Fields HL. Both intravenous lidocaine and morphine reduce the pain of postherpetic neuralgia. *Neurology* 1991; 41:1024–1028.

Taub A. Opioid analgesics in the treatment of chronic intractable pain of non-neoplastic origin. In: Kihata LM, Collins D (Eds). *Narcotic Analgesics in Anesthesiology.* Baltimore: Williams & Wilkins, 1982, pp 199–208.

Tennant FS Jr, Rawson RA. Outpatient treatment of prescription opioid dependence: comparison of two methods. *Arch Intern Med* 1982; 142:1845–1847.

Turk DC. Clinicians' attitudes about prolonged use of opioids and the issue of patient heterogeneity. *J Pain Symptom Manage* 1996; 11:218–230.

Turner JA, Calsyn DA, Fordyce WE, Ready LB. Drug utilization patterns in chronic pain patients. *Pain* 1982; 12:357–363.

Urban BJ, France RD, Steinberger EK, Scott DL, Maltbie AA. Long-term use of narcotic/antidepressant medication in the management of phantom limb pain. *Pain* 1986; 24:191–196.

Vet HCWD, Bie RAD, van der Heijden GJMG, et al. Systematic reviews on the basis of methodological criteria. *Physiotherapy* 1997; 83:284–289.

Zenz M, Strumpf M, Tryba M. Long-term opioid therapy in patients with chronic nonmalignant pain. *J Pain Symptom Manage* 1992; 7:69–77.

Correspondence to: Wilhelm E.J. Weber, MD, PhD, Pain Management and Research Center, University Hospital Maastricht, P.O. Box 5800, 6202 AZ Maastricht, The Netherlands. Tel: 31-43-3877455; Fax: 31-43-3875457; email: pijn@sane.azm.nl.

Proceedings of the 9th World Congress on Pain,
Progress in Pain Research and Management,
Vol. 16, edited by M. Devor, M.C. Rowbotham, and
Z. Wiesenfeld-Hallin, IASP Press, Seattle, © 2000.

91

Preemptive Analgesia: How Can We Make It Work?[1]

Igor Kissin

Department of Anesthesiology, Perioperative and Pain Medicine, Brigham & Women's Hospital, Harvard Medical School, Boston, Massachusetts

Preemptive analgesia is an antinociceptive treatment that prevents establishment of altered central processing of afferent input, which amplifies postoperative pain. Several years ago, views on the concept of preemptive analgesia were summarized by a statement that positive evidence obtained in experimental studies was overwhelmingly convincing; however, results of clinical studies regarding the value of preemptive analgesia were not unanimous (Kissin 1996). Five recent reviews (Pasqualucci 1998; Grass 1998; Niv et al. 1999; Kehlet 1999; Schmid et al. 1999) summarize many new studies on preemptive analgesia. Although new clinical studies have not altered the balance of negative versus positive conclusions on the clinical value of preemptive analgesia, opinions have clearly changed on the approach to this concept. This chapter will briefly discuss the most important new developments in this area.

NEW EVIDENCE FROM EXPERIMENTAL STUDIES

Several findings from recent basic science studies are important for the correct assessment of the potential clinical value of preemptive analgesia. Perhaps most important are studies attempting to answer the question of how long central sensitization can persist after the primary source that led to its establishment is removed. If central sensitization is a short-lived effect, its prevention might be of little clinical relevance. A study by Vatine et al. (1999) demonstrated that a 10-minute electrical stimulation supramaximally

[1] Mini-review based on a congress workshop.

activating C fibers in the sciatic nerve of the rat is sufficient to produce hyperalgesia lasting up to 3 weeks. In addition to the initial studies on central sensitization and its persistent nature (Woolf 1983; Coderre and Melzack 1987), Vatine's study is a convincing demonstration of a sensory alteration that can continue long after the end of injury discharge. In addition, Cleland et al. (1999) reported that pain sensitivity in young rats can be permanently altered by brief injury during critical development periods.

However, other evidence indicates that, even for short periods of time, both central mechanisms and afferent input are required to maintain pain hypersensitivity (Dickenson et al. 1997). Contrary to previous studies with the formalin model of pain hypersensitivity in rats, Taylor et al. (1995) found that if the paw is anesthetized with a local anesthetic 15 minutes after formalin injection, the signs of hypersensitivity rapidly disappear. The authors concluded that ongoing activity in peripheral afferent fibers is required for the persistent pain evoked by formalin. This finding compares well with that by Puig and Sorkin (1996) of an ongoing peripheral nerve activity during the phase 2 response to formalin (the phase that seems to reflect central sensitization). If the peripheral afferent input is responsible for maintenance of central sensitization, the established postoperative pain hypersensitivity can be reversed by the blockade of afferent input. This response was demonstrated in a study with carrageenan-induced inflammation in rats: hyperalgesia (usually lasting >5 days) was permanently reversed by a prolonged (>12 hour) nerve block but not with a block lasting <1 hour (Kissin et al. 1998).

While previous experimental studies almost without exception reported positive evidence regarding preemptive analgesia, results of more recent studies sometimes are as equivocal as those obtained in clinical studies. Most interesting in this respect is the study by Brennan et al. (1997), involving a brief incision at the plantar hindpaw of the rat. The authors found no difference between preincisional and postincisional treatment with intrathecal bupivacaine or intrathecal morphine. Yashpal et al. (1996) demonstrated that the difference between the effects of intrathecal lidocaine given 5 minutes before versus 5 minutes after hindpaw injection of formalin depends on the degree of injury. The preemptive effect of lidocaine was observed only with 2.5%, not with 3.75% or 5% formalin.

All the above-mentioned experimental studies indicate the following: (1) Central sensitization caused by noxious stimulation is a complex phenomenon that depends on many factors; it may fade rapidly or very slowly or become permanent. Accordingly, the clinical significance of central sensitization prevention may be negligible or very profound. (2) Surgery-induced central sensitization has two phases: incisional and inflammatory.

The first phase may be brief relative to the second phase. In this case, inflammatory injury could play the dominant role in central sensitization. Therefore, antinociceptive protection provided by preemptive treatment should extend well into the postoperative period, or it can be ineffective, as evident in the rat paw incisional model (Brennan et al. 1997). (3) Prolonged blockade of afferent input after establishment of central sensitization has a potential to reverse it. Benefits of reversal versus prevention may depend on the persistency of the particular postoperative sensitization and the availability of long-lasting blockade required for reversal.

CLINICAL STUDIES

PREINCISIONAL VERSUS POSTINCISIONAL TREATMENT

Comparing preincisional versus postincisional administration of antinociceptive treatment modalities failed to provide convincing evidence of the clinical value of preemptive analgesia. Multiple studies demonstrated no difference between treatments. Reported positive clinical effects, although statistically significant, were of relatively small magnitude. The conclusions of the recent reviews based on the comparison of preincisional versus postincisional treatments are presented in Table I.

One of the most important factors in the failure to demonstrate clinical significance of preemptive anesthesia with these treatment trials is the exclusion of the results of central sensitization caused by inflammatory injury that occurs after surgery (Woolf and Chong 1993; Katz 1995). A partial preemptive effect in the postincisional group, such as that caused by intraoperative opioids, could also be a factor in reducing the difference between the treatment groups. Another factor could be suppression of already established central sensitization in the postincisional group due to intensive antinociceptive treatment that starts immediately following incision (e.g., prolonged antinociceptive blockade; Kissin 1998). The role of all these factors might be so significant that the overall antinociceptive effect in the control group is anything but perfect. For example, in a study of pain after tonsillectomy, Ørntoft et al. (1994) compared the effect of preoperative tonsillar infiltration with bupivacaine to that of preoperative infiltration with saline or postoperative infiltration with bupivacaine. The authors did not observe any preemptive analgesia. The spontaneous pain intensity scores in the saline group on the first postoperative day (measured on a 100-mm visual analogue scale [VAS]) was 14 mm. Reductions of the VAS pain intensity score to ≤15 mm could be regarded as complete pain relief because direct questioning of patients with this score indicated that they had no pain

Table I
Recent reviews of clinical studies of preincisional vs. postincisional treatments

Reference	Topic of Review	Conclusions
Grass 1998	Local anesthetic infiltration or nerve blocks, neuraxial local anesthetics, neuraxial opioids, systemic NSAIDs, intravenous or epidural ketamine	Inconsistent findings from one study to the next, without any dramatic clinical advantages demonstrated in any study with any preemptive analgesic modality, including a multimodal approach. Preemptive administration of neuraxial opioids alone or with ketamine appears to offer some clinically significant advantages over postincisional administration.
Kehlet 1999	Local anesthetic blocks, neuraxial and intravenous opioids, NSAIDs, NMDA-receptor antagonists (dextromethorphan and ketamine)	More than 40 controlled clinical studies comparing preoperative vs. postoperative administration of identical doses of different drugs are reported, but most have been negative. Any positive clinical effects were usually small and without important clinical implications.
Niv et al. 1999	Local anesthetic blockade, epidural analgesia using local anesthetics or opioids, intravenous opioids, systemic NSAIDs, epidural and systemic ketamine	While many studies found no difference in postoperative pain between preincisional and postincisional patient groups, some found a modest but statistically significant benefit to preincisional analgesia. No clear answer can be given as to whether preemptive analgesia does or does not work.
Pasqualucci 1998	Epidural blocks, nerve blocks, local anesthetic infiltrations	Four of the 11 studies examined seem to confirm the validity of preemptive analgesia, and an equal number deny it.
Schmid et al. 1999	Intravenous and epidural ketamine	Results of the studies evaluating efficacy of preemptive ketamine are promising. The role of ketamine in the treatment of postoperative pain remains controversial.

(Gourlay et al. 1984; Tverskoy et al. 1996). Another study (Jebeles et al. 1991) of the effect of preincisional infiltration of tonsils with bupivacaine reported that the spontaneous pain intensity score on the first day following tonsillectomy was 20 mm (VAS) with bupivacaine and 70 mm with saline; the difference between groups was significant for 5 days. The comparison of these two studies indicates that with "perfect" treatment in the nonpreemptive (control) group (as in the Ørntoft et al. 1994 study), low-intensity nociceptive stimuli may not trigger the long-lasting central sensitization. We might argue that preemptive analgesia can be observed only when a control group demonstrated that the surgery was painful enough to have a preemptive effect.

BLOCKADE VERSUS NO BLOCKADE

One way to eliminate some of the problems associated with preincisional versus postincisional trials is to compare preincisional antinociceptive blockade versus no blockade. Table II summarizes studies that used this approach; they were selected according to both general quality criteria (randomization and double-blinding) and criteria specific to preemptive analgesia (verification of block sufficiency and degree of initial difference in nociceptive response between control and preemptive groups). Quality of study methods varied. A clinically significant outcome was observed in five of six studies. Three studies had a higher specific quality score (see columns 4 and 5 in Table II), and the difference in clinical significance of the effects was especially evident in all of them. In two of the six studies, a possible anti-inflammatory action of a local anesthetic could not be excluded because of tissue infiltration (field block). Nevertheless, the table demonstrates that clinically meaningful effects could be observed when the degree of nociceptive blockade was confirmed and the block was extended into the initial postoperative period.

The important role of sufficiency in the degree of afferent blockade was evident in the studies on preemptive analgesia with epidural anesthesia. Shir et al. (1994) compared three groups of patients having radical prostatectomy with general, epidural, or combined epidural and general anesthesia. Preemptive analgesia was observed only with epidural anesthesia, which allows for even minor discomfort to be noticed and treated during surgery. The authors concluded that complete intraoperative blockade is fundamental for observing a preemptive effect.

Another study with well-controlled sufficiency of epidural anesthesia in patients having radical prostatectomy also reported positive results. Gottschalk et al. (1998) administered epidural bupivacaine or epidural fentanyl prior to induction of general anesthesia and throughout the surgery, and compared the pain outcomes with those of similar treatment initiated at the fascial closure. Sufficiency of epidural blockade was verified by measurement of the sensory level (at least the fourth thoracic dermatome) before induction of general anesthesia and also in the postanesthesia care unit. Patients who did not have a T4 sensory level were excluded from the study; in addition, the patient's response to injury was assessed by measuring plasma cortisol levels. The patients who received epidural bupivacaine or fentanyl prior to surgical incision (preemptive analgesia group) experienced 33% less pain while hospitalized. At 9.5 weeks, 86% of the patients who received preemptive analgesia were pain-free compared with only 47% of the control group. Patients receiving preemptive analgesia were also more active at 3.5

Table II
Studies comparing verified preoperative nerve block with no block

Reference*	Procedure	Block	Block Assessment	Difference in Response†	Difference in Pain Outcome†		Additional Conditions
					Pain Intensity	Analgesic Use	
Langer et al. 1987	Herniorrhaphy in children under general anesthesia	Ilioinguinal/ iliohypogastric block, 0.5% bupivacaine	Statistically signif. difference in analgesic requirement 1–4 h postop.	Not assessed	Not assessed	Statistically and clinically signif. decrease for 48 h	
Tverskoy et al. 1990	Herniorrhaphy under general anesthesia	Inguinal field block, 0.25% bupivacaine	Time to first analgesic 9 h vs. 1 h in control	Pain at rest 8 vs. 44 mm (VAS) at 24 h	Statistically and clinically signif. decrease for >48 h	Standard postop. analgesic regimen, insignif. difference between groups	
Bugedo et al. 1990	Herniorrhaphy under spinal anesthesia	Ilioinguinal/ iliohypogastric block, 0.5% bupivacaine	Patients who did not have inguinal hypoesthesia at 3 h postop. were excluded	Pain at rest ~32 vs. 62 mm (VAS) at 3 h	Statistically and clinically signif. decrease for 48 h	Statistically and clinically signif. decrease for 24 h	Spinal anesthesia in both groups
Ding and White 1995	Herniorrhaphy under infiltration anesthesia	Ilioinguinal/ iliohypogastric block, 0.25% bupivacaine	Statistically signif. difference in pain score at 30 min postop.	Pain at rest ~15 vs. 35 mm (VAS) at 30 min	No difference beyond 30 min	Statistically and clinically signif. decrease for 24 h after discharge	Infiltration anesthesia and intraoperative fentanyl in both groups
Gordon et al. 1997	Third molar extractions under general anesthesia	Mandibular block, 0.5% bupivacaine	Block efficacy assessed before general anesthesia (if block not complete, bupivacaine was readministered)	Beta-endorphin increase from ~40 to 90 pg/mL in control, no change in treatment group	Statistically signif. difference at 24–48 h	Statistically and clinically signif. difference at 24–48 h	
Johansson et al. 1997	Herniorrhaphy under general anesthesia	Inguinal field block, 0.5% ropivacaine	Statistically signif. difference in pain score at 3 h. Time to first analgesic ~6 h vs. 2.5 h in control	Pain at rest ~20 vs. 35 mm (VAS) at 3 h	No difference beyond 3 h	Statistically signif. difference for 24 h	Multicenter study. Intraoperative alfentanil in all groups

* Only randomized, double-blind studies are included.
† Treatment versus control.

weeks after surgery. The authors concluded that even with aggressive postoperative pain management, preemptive epidural analgesia decreases postoperative pain during hospitalization and long after discharge. Moller et al. (1982) demonstrated that only an extensive epidural blockade from T4 to S5 prevents the cortisol response to lower abdominal surgery. Conflicting results reported in the literature about the preemptive effect of epidural blockade are probably attributable to the insufficient density of the blockade.

Block of sufficient duration is another requirement for positive clinical outcome of preemptive treatment. Kehlet stated recently (1999) that a key question is whether the term "preemptive analgesia" has been used correctly, because it ideally implies a prevention of the development of central hyperexcitability, even if it occurs after surgery. A local anesthetic should be given both preoperatively and as a continuous postoperative administration. Møiniche et al. (1994) compared the effects of epidural bupivacaine and morphine anesthesia followed by continuous epidural analgesia postoperatively to those of general anesthesia followed by a conventional intramuscular opioid and acetaminophen regimen in patients having knee or hip arthroplasty. The knee patients in the epidural analgesia group, once they had completed the epidural regimen, received less morphine than did the conventional treatment group for another 4 days. However, important improvements in convalescence and hospital stay were not observed in this study. In a study by Capdevila et al. (1999), patients having major knee surgery followed by continuous 72-hour epidural analgesia (lidocaine-morphine-clonidine combination) or continuous femoral block had earlier functional recuperation compared to the group with intravenous patient-controlled analgesia (morphine). Similar findings regarding the reduction of convalescence time with prolonged epidural bupivacaine had been reported earlier (Pflug et al. 1974; William-Russo et al. 1996).

NARROWING THE SCOPE OF PREEMPTIVE ANALGESIA LEADS TO EQUIVOCAL CLINICAL RESULTS

Studies on preventing postoperative pain hypersensitivity have been limited by the inappropriate narrowing of the scope of their approach. A clinically irrelevant definition of preemptive analgesia has played an important role. Preemptive analgesia can be a misleading term because it creates an impression that the secondary feature associated with the phenomenon represents its basis. The term *preemptive analgesia* suggests that an antinociceptive intervention provided preoperatively prevents or reduces pain after surgery. (This is only partially true.) With this definition, the difference in the outcome measure of antinociceptive interventions made before and at the end of surgery is evidence of a preemptive effect. However, the emphasis should not be on the timing of treatment initiation but on the pathophysiological phenomenon it should prevent—central sensitization. Table III presents several definitions of preemptive analgesia that were used as the basis for the recent clinical trials. The first one (A) is an erroneous definition that can lead to a false conclusion in a clinical trial. A warning regarding this "semantic confusion" was best presented by Carr (1996). He indicated that preemptive means "preventive," not simply "before" incision. There should be proof that an intervention provides at least its direct effect. An insufficient afferent block cannot be preemptive, even if it is administered before the incision. The second definition (B) represents preemptive analgesia only in a narrow sense because it excludes central sensitization caused by inflammatory injury that occurs in the initial postoperative period. The balance between incisional injury and inflammatory injury depends on the nature of surgery; with certain conditions, inflammatory injury can be a dominant factor. The third definition (C) represents the phenomenon of preemptive analgesia in its broadest sense.

COMBINED APPROACHES TO PREVENTING POSTOPERATIVE PAIN HYPERSENSITIVITY

The goal of preventing postoperative pain hypersensitivity should not be narrowed by focusing exclusively on the preemptive effect. The approach should be wider and centered on central sensitization in general. Preemptive treatment, although essential, should be only one part of the combined approach to preventing postoperative pain hypersensitivity. The reversal of previously established central sensitization is another part of this approach. The reversal of central hypersensitivity is determined by two factors: persistency of central sensitization and continuance of the afferent input that can initiate, reinitiate, and maintain pain hypersensitivity (in accordance with

Table III
Definitions of preemptive analgesia used as the basis for recent clinical trials

Preemptive analgesia is a treatment that:

A) starts before surgery;

B) prevents the establishment of central sensitization caused by incisional injury (covers only the period of surgery);

C) prevents the establishment of central sensitization caused by incisional and inflammatory injuries (covers the period of surgery and the initial postoperative period).

the declining level of the input intensity). The blockade should last until central sensitization subsides and the intensity of the afferent input is below the level that could potentially reinitiate central hypersensitivity (Kissin et al. 1998). Because the intensity of afferent input for reinitiation of central hypersensitivity is lower than that for its initiation, blockade for a successful reversal of pain hypersensitivity should be longer (to permit greater input fading) than that for preemptive effect. The hypothetical relationships between the preemptive effect and reversal of pain hypersensitivity versus block duration are presented in Fig. 1, which indicates that the longer the block duration, the less the difference in the analgesic outcome of the block administered before or after establishment of central hypersensitivity.

Preempting central sensitization, maintenance of the obtained effect, or reversal of the sensitization all can decrease the intensity and duration of postoperative pain by targeting pain-induced changes in the central nervous system. Prevention or reversal of central sensitization is directed at the mechanisms responsible for pathological pain. In contrast, conventional perioperative analgesia targets physiological pain. How prolonged could the preventive effect be after the block resolution? This is the critical factor. If the pain hypersensitivity does not last well beyond block resolution, the treatment would not be different from simple perioperative analgesia directed at physiological pain. Studies with continuous neural blockade (Pflug et al. 1974; Møiniche et al. 1994; Williams-Russo et al. 1996; Capdevila et al. 1999) indicate that this period may be clinically meaningful, at least with some surgeries.

Combining various approaches to attenuate central sensitization increases the probability of meaningful clinical benefits. Preemptive effect, maintenance of the obtained effect, and reversal of central sensitization (in the case of an incomplete preemptive effect) could be part of the treatment regimen directed at pain hypersensitivity (Fig. 2). Several experimental studies have reported reversal of the established hyperalgesia with the use of

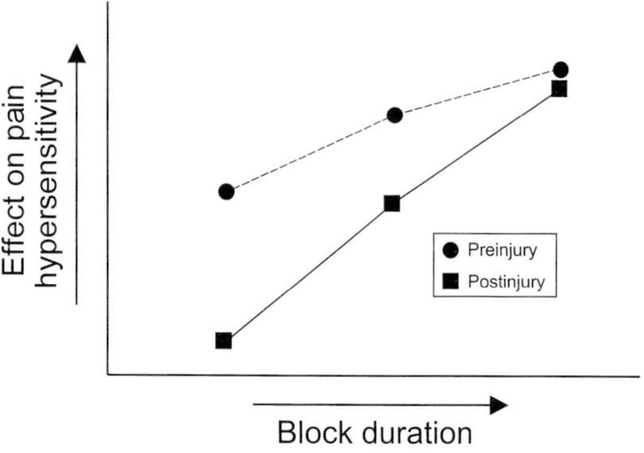

Fig. 1. Preemptive effect versus reversal of hypersensitivity: role of the duration of nerve blockade. Hypothetical conditions indicate that with the increase in block duration, the potential advantage of the preemptive effect over the reversal declines.

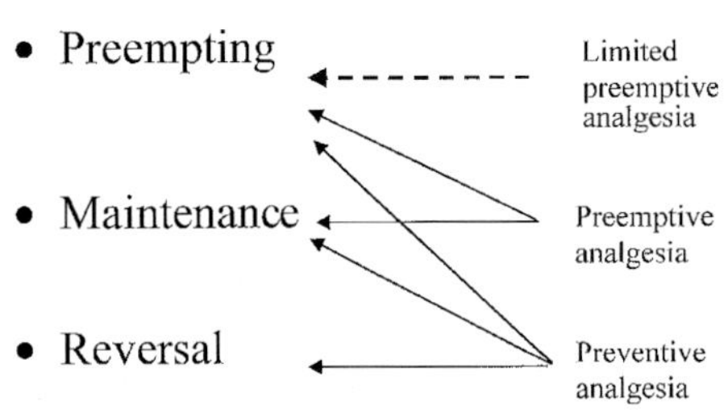

Fig. 2. Different scope of the approaches for prevention of postoperative pain by targeting central sensitization.

glutamate receptor antagonists (Coderre and Melzack 1991; Mao et al. 1992; Ren et al. 1992; Yamamoto and Yaksh 1992; Ma and Woolf 1995; Zahn and Brennan 1998; Zahn et al. 1998). The observed effects of NMDA and non-NMDA receptor antagonists differed, as did the outcomes in various experimental models of hyperalgesia. Thus, only clinical studies can validate the usefulness of this class of pharmacological agents for the reversal of pain hypersensitivity. Many novel agents can affect the facilitated states of central processing of afferent input after tissue and nerve injury. Along with NMDA and non-NMDA receptor antagonists, they may include adenosine A1-receptor agonists, α_2-adrenoceptor agonists, N-type Ca^{2+} channel blockers, and many enzyme inhibitors such as COX-2, acetylcholinesterase, adenosine kinase, and protein kinases. (For a recent review of the effects of these agents in the preclinical models of nociception, see Yaksh 1999). Some of these agents (which are not always active in acute pain) may change the course of central sensitization.

CONCLUSIONS

When preemptive analgesia was studied by comparing preincisional versus postincisional patient groups, many authors found no difference in the pain outcome, while some reported statistically significant but modest benefits with preincisional analgesia. It is clear that the above approach is too simple to overcome the multiple problems posed by the complexities of central sensitization and the technical difficulties of clinical studies. Comparison of preincisional versus postincisional treatment, with strict requirements confirming that certain conditions are met, can probably produce a greater proportion of positive results. However, some of the previous clinical studies in combination with basic science results are probably enough to indicate that preemptive analgesia is a valid phenomenon. A different approach is required to assess the clinical value of this phenomenon. Two conditions are especially important: (1) treatment should be continued long enough to effectively suppress the afferent input; and (2) different treatment approaches aimed at reducing central sensitization should be used in combination: preemptive treatment, maintenance of the obtained effect, and reversal of central sensitization (in the case of an incomplete preemptive effect). A narrow and clinically irrelevant definition of preemptive analgesia leads to a belief that this concept is clinically meaningless. Preemptive analgesia continues to have promise for the effective treatment of postoperative pain. Evaluation of the true importance of preemptive analgesia must await further research with new, more comprehensive approaches.

REFERENCES

Brennan TJ, Umali EF, Zahn PK. Comparison of pre- versus post-incision administration of intrathecal bupivacaine and intrathecal morphine in a rat model of postoperative pain. *Anesthesiology* 1997; 87:1517–1528.

Bugedo GJ, Cárcamo CR, Mertens RA, Dagnino JA, Muñoz HR. Preoperative percutaneous ilioinguinal and iliohypogastric nerve block with 0.5% bupivacaine for post-herniorrhaphy pain management in adults. *Reg Anesth* 1990; 15:130–133.

Capdevila X, Barthelet Y, Biboulet P, et al. Effects of perioperative analgesic technique on the surgical outcome and duration of rehabilitation after major knee surgery. *Anesthesiology* 1999; 91:8–15.

Carr DB. Preemptive analgesia implies prevention. *Anesthesiology* 1996; 85:1498.

Cleland CL, Ritter SM, Hawkins AR, Broghammer M, Gebhart GF. Neonatal inflammation causes permanent, dose-dependent changes in thermal pain sensitivity in rats. In: *Abstracts: 9th World Congress on Pain.* Seattle: IASP Press, 1999, p 413.

Coderre TJ, Melzack R. Cutaneous hyperalgesia: contributions of the peripheral and central nervous systems to the increase in pain sensitivity after injury. *Brain Res* 1987; 404:95–106.

Coderre TJ, Melzack R. Central neural mediators of secondary hyperalgesia following heat injury in rats: neuropeptides and excitatory amino acids. *Neurosci Lett* 1991; 131:71–74.

Dickenson AH, Chapman V, Green GM. The pharmacology of excitatory and inhibitory amino acid-mediated events in the transmission and modulation of pain in the spinal cord. *Gen Pharmacol* 1997; 28:633–638.

Ding Y, White PF. Post-herniorrhaphy pain in outpatients after pre-incision ilioinguinal-hypogastric nerve block during monitored anaesthesia care. *Can J Anaesth* 1995; 42:12–15.

Gordon SM, Dionne RA, Brahim J, Jabir F, Dubner R. Blockade of peripheral neuronal barrage reduces postoperative pain. *Pain* 1997; 70:209–215.

Gottschalk A, Smith DS, Jobes DR, et al. Preemptive epidural analgesia and recovery from radical prostatectomy: a randomized controlled trial. *JAMA* 1998; 279:1076–1082.

Gourlay GK, Willis RJ, Wilson PR. Postoperative pain control with methadone: influence of supplementary methadone doses and blood concentration-response relationships. *Anesthesiology* 1984; 61:19–26.

Grass JA. Preemptive analgesia. In: Grass JA (Ed.). *Problems in Anesthesia,* Vol. 10. Philadelphia: Lippincott-Raven, 1998, pp 107–121.

Jebeles JA, Reilly JS, Gutierrez J, Bradley EL, Kissin I. The effect of pre-incisional infiltration of tonsils with bupivacaine on the pain following tonsillectomy under general anesthesia. *Pain* 1991; 47:305–308.

Johansson B, Hallerbäck B, Stubberöd A, et al. Preoperative local infiltration with ropivacaine for postoperative pain relief after inguinal hernia repair. *Eur J Surg* 1997; 163:372–377.

Katz J. Pre-emptive analgesia: evidence, current status and future directions. *Eur J Anaesth* 1995; 12(Suppl 10):8–13.

Kehlet H. Controlling acute pain—role of pre-emptive analgesia, peripheral treatment, balanced analgesia, and effects on outcome. In: Max M (Ed). *Pain 1999—An Updated Review*. Seattle: IASP Press, 1999, pp 459–462.

Kissin I. Pre-emptive analgesia. Why its effect is not always obvious. *Anesthesiology* 1996; 84:1015–1019.

Kissin I, Lee SS, Bradley EL Jr. Effect of prolonged nerve block on inflammatory hyperalgesia in rats: prevention of late hyperalgesia. *Anesthesiology* 1998; 88:224–232.

Langer JC, Shandling B, Rosenberg M. Intraoperative bupivacaine during outpatient hernia repair in children: a randomized double blind trial. *J Pediatr Surg* 1987; 22:267–270.

Ma Q-P, Woolf CJ. Noxious stimuli induce an N-methyl-D-aspartate receptor dependent hypersensitivity of the flexion withdrawal reflex to touch—implications for the treatment of mechanical allodynia. *Pain* 1995; 61:383–390.

Mao J, Price DD, Mayer DJ, Lu J, Hayes RL. Intrathecal MK-801 and local nerve anesthesia synergistically reduce nociceptive behaviors in rats with experimental peripheral mononeuropathy. *Brain Res* 1992; 576:254–262.

Møiniche S, Hjortsø N-C, Hansen BL, et al. The effect of balanced analgesia on early convalescence after major orthopaedic surgery. *Acta Anaesthesiol Scand* 1994; 38:328–335.

Moller IW, Rem J, Brandt MR, Kehlet H. Effect of posttraumatic epidural analgesia on the cortisol and hyperglycemic response to surgery. *Acta Anaesthesiol Scand* 1982; 26:56–58.

Niv D, Lang DE, Devor M. The effect of preemptive analgesia on subacute postoperative pain. *Minerva Anestesiol* 1999; 65:127–140.

Ørntoft S, Løngren A, Møiniche S, Dahl JB. A comparison of pre- and postoperative tonsillar infiltration with bupivacaine on pain after tonsillectomy. *Anaesthesia* 1994; 94:151–154.

Pasqualucci A. Experimental and clinical studies about the preemptive analgesia with local anesthetics. *Minerva Anestesiol* 1998; 64:445–457.

Pflug AE, Murphy TM, Butler SH, Tucker GT. The effects of postoperative peridural analgesia on pulmonary therapy and pulmonary complications. *Anesthesiology* 1974; 41:8–18.

Puig S, Sorkin LS. Formalin-evoked activity in identified primary afferent fibers: systemic lidocaine suppresses phase-2 activity. *Pain* 1996; 64:345–355.

Ren K, Hylden JLK, Williams GM, Ruda MA, Dubner R. The effects of a non-competitive NMDA receptor antagonist, MK-801, on behavioural hyperalgesia and dorsal horn neuronal activity in rats with unilateral inflammation. *Pain* 1992; 50:331–344.

Schmid RL, Sandler AN, Katz J. Use and efficacy of low-dose ketamine in the management of acute postoperative pain: a review of current techniques and outcomes. *Pain* 1999; 82:111–125.

Shir Y, Raja SN, Frank SM. The effect of epidural versus general anesthesia on postoperative pain and analgesia requirements in patients undergoing radical prostatectomy. *Anesthesiology* 1994; 80:49–56.

Taylor BK, Peterson MA, Basbaum AI. Persistent cardiovascular and behavioral nociceptive responses to subcutaneous formalin require peripheral nerve input. *J Neurosci* 1995; 15:7575–7584.

Tverskoy M, Cozacov C, Ayache M, Bradley EL Jr, Kissin I. Postoperative pain after inguinal herniorrhaphy with different types of anesthesia. *Anesth Analg* 1990; 70:29–35.

Tverskoy M, Oren M, Dashkovsky I, Kissin I. Alfentanil dose-response relationship for relief of postoperative pain. *Anesth Analg* 1996; 83:387–393.

Vatine JJ, Tsenter J, Argov R, Seltzer Z. Long lasting sensory alterations induced by a brief electrical stimulation of C-fibers in the rat. In: *Abstracts: 9th World Congress on Pain*. Seattle: IASP Press, 1999, p 385.

Williams-Russo P, Sharrock NE, Haas SB, et al. Randomized trial of epidural versus general anesthesia: outcomes after primary total knee replacement. *Clin Orthop* 1996; 331:199–208.

Woolf CJ. Evidence for a central component of postinjury pain hypersensitivity. *Nature* 1983; 308:686–688.

Woolf CJ, Chong M-S. Preemptive analgesia—treating postoperative pain by preventing the establishment of central sensitization. *Anesth Analg* 1993; 77:362–379.

Yaksh TL. Spinal systems and pain processing: development of novel analgesic drugs with mechanistically defined models. *Trends Pharmacol Sci* 1999; 20:329–336.

Yamamoto T, Yaksh TL. Spinal pharmacology of thermal hyperaesthesia induced by constriction injury of sciatic nerve. Excitatory amino acid antagonists. *Pain* 1992; 49:121–128.

Yashpal K, Katz J, Coderre TJ. Effects of preemptive or postinjury intrathecal local anesthesia on persistent nociceptive responses in rats: Confounding influences of peripheral inflammation and the general anesthetic regimen. *Anesthesiology* 1996; 84:1119–1128.

Zahn PK, Brannan TJ. Lack of effect of intrathecal NMDA receptor antagonists in a rat model for postoperative pain. *Anesthesiology* 1998; 88:143–156.

Zahn PK, Umali E, Brannan TJ. Intrathecal non-NMDA excitatory amino acid receptor antagonists inhibit pain behaviors in a rat model of postoperative pain. *Pain* 1998; 74:213–223.

Correspondence to: Igor Kissin, MD, PhD, Department of Anesthesiology, Perioperative and Pain Medicine, Brigham & Women's Hospital, 75 Francis Street, Boston, MA 02115, USA. email: kissin@zeus.bwh.harvard.edu.

Proceedings of the 9th World Congress on Pain,
Progress in Pain Research and Management,
Vol. 16, edited by M. Devor, M.C. Rowbotham, and
Z. Wiesenfeld-Hallin, IASP Press, Seattle, © 2000.

92

Development of an Active Placebo for Studies of TENS Treatment

Mary-Christine Chakour, Stephen J. Gibson, Maxwell Neufeld, Zeinab Khalil, and Robert D. Helme

National Ageing Research Institute, Parkville, Victoria, Australia

A suitable sham procedure is of vital importance in assessing the efficacy of any physical treatment, and transcutaneous electrical nerve stimulation (TENS) is no exception. However, due to a lack of well-circumscribed optimal TENS parameters for effecting analgesia, and the problems in reproducing the distinct physical sensations associated with TENS treatment, it has been difficult to implement a suitable placebo for this treatment modality. Inactive or "dead battery" TENS (e.g., Deyo et al. 1990; Marchand et al. 1993) has become the placebo treatment of necessity. This involves using a seemingly functional TENS unit to give the impression of active treatment when no current is actually delivered. Such treatment is usually reinforced by instructions that stimulation may or may not be perceptible. TENS-naive subjects are usually recruited to such studies. The validity of this approach, however, has often been questioned.

One of the aims of the present experiment was to investigate the possibility of a more appropriate placebo TENS treatment. This required us to identify TENS parameters that consistently do and do not alter pain perception in normal skin. Many TENS parameter combinations have been explored with respect to their ability to alter pain perception, including high-frequency/low-intensity (conventional) TENS, low-frequency/high-intensity (acupuncture-like) TENS, and high-frequency/high-intensity (brief, intense) TENS. Recently, 2000-Hz sinusoidal stimulation has been suggested to be Aβ-specific (Chado 1995), and thus may represent an alternative TENS treatment. However, little consensus exists regarding which frequency and intensity parameters are best suited for the consistent alleviation of pain. In terms of intensity, maximal as opposed to "strong but comfortable" stimulation protocols appear to be more effective in producing robust, clinically significant levels of pain relief (Woolf 1979). We investigated the effect of TENS treatment over a wide range of frequencies and intensities, using pain threshold as an index of pain sensitivity, to identify parameters that are "clinically relevant" as well as those that may constitute a perceptible, yet essentially neutral TENS placebo treatment.

METHODS

We recruited 80 healthy volunteers ranging in age between 21 and 51 years (mean age = 33.0 years) from the local area surrounding the National Ageing Research Institute (NARI) and screened them for entry into the study. Exclusion resulted from (1) the use of analgesic medications, (2) the presence of clinical pain at the time of testing, and (3) recent trauma at the proposed site of stimulation. Although prior experience with TENS treatment was not an automatic exclusion criterion, all subjects involved in the present experiment were naive. Eligible subjects were asked to complete an informed consent form (approved by the North West Hospital Ethics Committee) and were then randomly assigned to eight TENS frequency/intensity groups: 2-Hz (the lowest frequency setting of the commercially available TENS device used in the study), 5-Hz, 80-Hz, and 2000-Hz (sinusoidal) stimulation at either submaximal or maximal intensity. Each test session followed the same protocol. First, laser pain thresholds were determined over the distribution of the superficial radial nerve. Then, an initial 5 minutes of TENS treatment was applied and continued until repeat pain threshold measures were completed. This relatively short duration of TENS treatment was selected because we have previously demonstrated no difference in TENS treatment effects between a 5- and 30-minute stimulation period (Chakour 1998). Pain threshold was measured using computer-controlled CO_2 laser stimuli (10.6 μm wavelength, 1–100 W power, 5 mm beam diameter, 50 ms) applied using a guiding He/Ne sighting beam to determine the exact site of stimulation on the hand and to prevent multiple stimulations at one site. A double random staircase (DRS) technique, as fully described by Gracely (1988), was used as the threshold algorithm. For 2-Hz/submaximal, 5-Hz/submaximal, and 80-Hz submaximal and maximal TENS, a commercially available Model E2 TENS device (Biostim, Japan) was employed featuring continuous stimulation, constant current, 200-μs pulse duration with biphasic square wave output. Frequency was precalibrated using an oscilloscope by a third party, and the dial was taped over so that both investigator and subjects remained blinded to frequency output. A Grass S48 Stimulator

(Quincy, MA, USA) was set at the same output parameters as the commercially available TENS device and was used for the 2- and 5-Hz maximal intensity group to ensure adequate current delivery. Care was taken to precisely emulate the waveform emitted by the commercial stimulator, and subjects were not made aware of the stimulation frequency. A custom-designed, battery-operated Sine Wave Stimulator capable of delivering an alternating current at a constant level independent of electrode/tissue impedance was used for 2000-Hz sinusoidal stimulation. The unit was AC coupled to the subject to avoid sudden fluctuations when switching the power on or off. Frequency was set using a standard commercially available function generator (GW-GFG-8019, Radio Parts, Korea) and the current manipulated by adjustment of amplitude. In all cases, TENS treatment was applied via 1 × 1 cm carbon rubber electrodes treated with a coating of conductive gel (MediTrace, USA). The electrodes were applied to skin pretreated with alcohol and a colloidal abrasive (Omniprep, DO Weaver and Co., USA) to enhance electrical conductivity. Once applied 2 cm apart, electrodes were held in place with strips of close-fitting surgical plastic film (Tegaderm, 3M, USA) and covered with tape (Micropore, 3M, USA) to ensure immobility and close contact with the skin. In all cases, electrodes were positioned with the cathode proximal on the nondominant hand, and CO_2 laser thresholds were measured between the TENS electrodes. All current intensities were determined by instructing subjects to induce a "strong but comfortable" (SBC; see Fig. 1), nonpainful paresthesia, or a sensation subjectively "high enough to perceive distinct noxious pricking under the electrodes." Subjects were allowed to adjust intensity levels at random throughout the stimulation periods to maintain the levels required by each condition of the experiment, and were asked to report the quality of sensations arising from the treatment.

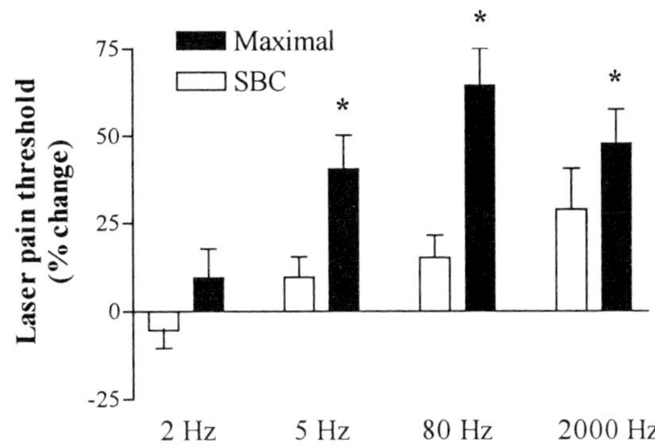

Fig. 1. Laser pain threshold (± SEM, in watts) expressed as a percentage of baseline pain sensation following maximal and submaximal ("strong but comfortable," SBC) TENS treatment for the four frequency groups tested (n = 80). Asterisks (*) denote a significant difference from all other groups, except for 2000-Hz SBC ($P < 0.05$; post hoc Student-Newman-Keuls).

RESULTS

The quality of maximal stimulation at all frequencies was required to induce noxious pricking, whereas the quality of submaximal stimulation differed at each frequency, as indicated by subjective report. Most subjects reported a "twitching" sensation arising from both 2- and 5-Hz stimulation. In contrast, 80-Hz stimulation elicited a "buzzing" sensation in a majority of subjects, while the 2000-Hz treatment was primarily described as "vibrating."

Mean (± SEM) laser pain thresholds before and during submaximal and maximal TENS treatment delivered at 2, 5, 80, and 2000 Hz are shown in Table I. A three-way, repeated-measures ANOVA revealed no significant main effects for TENS intensity ($F_{1,72} = 1.93$, $P = 0.169$), or TENS frequency ($F_{3,72} = 1.42$, $P = 0.244$), but showed a significant increase in laser pain threshold during the period of TENS treatment ($F_{1,72} = 69.73$, $P = 0.0001$) (see Table I). Analysis showed a significant TENS frequency by TENS treatment interaction ($F_{3,72} = 7.67$, $P = 0.0001$), a TENS intensity by TENS treatment interaction ($F_{1,72} = 21.3$, $P = 0.0001$), and a three-way interaction effect ($F_{3,72} = 3.11$, $P = 0.032$), suggesting that the magnitude of change in laser pain threshold is dependent on both the intensity and frequency of TENS stimulation. In order to further characterize these interaction effects, we performed post hoc Student-Newman-Keuls pairwise comparisons on the pre- and post-TENS treatment difference scores for each intensity/frequency combination. As illustrated in Fig. 1, maximal intensity TENS at 5, 80, or 2000 Hz was equally effective in raising laser pain thresholds by approximately 50%, whereas TENS of strong but comfortable intensity was without significant effect except at the highest (sinusoidal) frequency. TENS of 2 Hz, on the other hand, although perceptible, did not alter laser pain thresholds, regardless of perceived intensity.

Table I
Mean (± SEM) laser pain threshold in response to submaximal and maximal TENS for the frequency groups tested (*n* = 80*)

	Laser Pain Threshold (watts)			
	Submaximal TENS		Maximal TENS	
Frequency	Pre-TENS	TENS	Pre-TENS	TENS
2 Hz	21.7 ± 3.0	20.9 ± 3.3	19.0 ± 2.8	20.1 ± 2.9
5 Hz	22.8 ± 2.5	25.2 ± 3.1	21.2 ± 2.8	29.4 ± 3.7
80 Hz	18.2 ± 2.4	20.0 ± 2.0	18.7 ± 2.4	30.6 ± 1.3
2000 Hz	19.9 ± 2.3	24.8 ± 2.8	21.5 ± 2.0	30.7 ± 2.8

Note: For each frequency there were two intensity conditions, for a total of eight conditions (*n* = 10 subjects per group).

DISCUSSION

Two major problems have hampered efforts to definitively assess the efficacy of TENS treatment: the lack of well-circumscribed, optimal pain-relieving stimulation parameters, and the absence of an appropriate positive TENS placebo. The present work yielded some interesting findings related to the frequency and intensity of TENS-induced alterations in experimental pain perception. With respect to TENS intensity, maximal stimulation was significantly more effective in raising laser pain thresholds at 5, 80, and 2000 Hz than at 2 Hz. This is consistent with a limited body of past work on the influence of TENS intensity on pain relief (Andersson et al. 1977; Woolf 1979), but little is known about the underlying mechanism. Explanations based on diffuse noxious inhibitory control (DNIC) and counterirritation principles are considered most likely. However, much work is still required to substantiate these ideas.

In contrast, the majority of heuristic interest has focused on frequency as the primary determinant of TENS success (Johnson et al. 1989). It is noteworthy that with maximal intensity treatment, the influence of stimulation frequency was almost negligible; 5-Hz, 80-Hz, and 2000-Hz maximal stimulation protocols were all significantly and equally effective in elevating laser pain thresholds. The influence of TENS frequency was more noticeable with submaximal intensity stimulation. The only form of stimulation that was useful at this intensity was 2000-Hz sinusoidal TENS. It has recently been proposed that such stimulation is neuroselective for the Aβ fibers (Chado 1995), which have been identified as central to the gate control mechanism of pain modulation (Melzack and Wall 1965). The present findings suggest that further investigation of this mode of TENS treatment may yield a viable alternative to high-intensity protocols.

The problem of devising a neutral placebo TENS treatment that mimics the physical sensations induced by active stimulation is one of the most difficult problems facing TENS research. Past attempts to devise physical placebo treatments have largely arisen from incidental findings based on a failure to produce expected positive results at stimulation sites (Melzack 1975). In the current study, 2-Hz submaximal stimulation produced the most subtle alteration in pain threshold over the treatment period. The relative inefficiency of 2-Hz submaximal stimulation in influencing experimental pain has been reported previously (Andersson et al. 1977; Jette 1986). It has also been suggested that the intensity required to produce strong sensations at this frequency lies beyond the capabilities of most commercially available stimulators. This inadequacy provides an inbuilt safeguard against achieving a real physiological effect during low-frequency TENS treatment. Admittedly, the slower stimulation rate produces periodic, pulsing twitches, which, though clearly perceived, are somewhat different in character to those induced by faster stimulation rates. Nevertheless, it may be argued that placebo treatments should mirror as closely as possible the active treatment and that any physical, non-active sensation represents an improvement over current "dead battery" techniques. Future studies should refine this procedure and examine placebo stimulation in patients with prolonged experimental and clinical pain conditions. In light of the present findings, the three modes of TENS treatment, currently classified according to their characteristic operating parameters, may need to be reconsidered. Rather than being considered as distinct modes of treatment, conventional, acupuncture-like, and brief intense TENS may need to be viewed as part of a continuum, with stimulation intensity as the central consideration.

ACKNOWLEDGMENTS

We gratefully acknowledge the valuable contribution of Mr. Michael Gorman, who devised the Sine Wave Stimulator for use in this experiment.

REFERENCES

Andersson SA, Holmgren MD, Roos MB. Analgesic effects of peripheral conditioning stimulation. II. Importance of certain stimulation parameters. *Acupunct Electrotherapeut Res Int J* 1977; 2:237–246.

Chado HN. The current perception threshold evaluation of sensory nerve function in pain management. *Pain Digest* 1995; 5:127–134.

Chakour MC. An examination of different modes of TENS treatment upon experimental pain perception. PhD Thesis, University of Melbourne, 1998.

Deyo RA, Walsh NE, Martin DC, Schoenfeld LS, Ramamurthy S. A controlled trial of transcutaneous electrical nerve stimulation (TENS) and exercise for chronic low back pain. *N Engl J Med* 1990; 322:1627–1634.

Gracely RH. Multiple-random staircase assessment of thermal pain sensation. In: Dubner R, Gebhart G, Bond M (Eds). *Proceedings of the Vth World Congress on Pain.* Amsterdam: Elsevier, 1988, pp 391–395.

Jette DU. Effect of different forms of transcutaneous electrical nerve stimulation on experimental pain. *Phys Ther* 1986; 66:87–190.

Johnson MI, Ashton CH, Bousfield DR, Thompson JW. Analgesic effects of different frequencies of transcutaneous electrical nerve stimulation on cold-induced pain in normal subjects. *Pain* 1989; 39:231–236.

Marchand S, Charest J, Li J, et al. Is TENS purely a placebo effect? A controlled study on chronic low back pain. *Pain* 1993; 54:99–106.

Melzack R. Prolonged relief of pain by brief intense transcutaneous somatic stimulation. *Pain* 1975; 1:357–373.

Melzack R, Wall PD. Pain mechanisms: a new theory. *Science* 1965; 150:971–979.

Woolf CJ. Transcutaneous electrical nerve stimulation and the reaction to experimental pain in human subjects. *Pain* 1979; 7:115–127.

Correspondence to: Mary-Christine Chakour, PhD, National Ageing Research Institute, Poplar Road, Parkville, Victoria 3052, Australia. Tel: 61-3-9864 4205; Fax: 61-3-9804 5233; email: christine.chakour@australia.ppdi.com.

Proceedings of the 9th World Congress on Pain,
Progress in Pain Research and Management,
Vol. 16, edited by M. Devor, M.C. Rowbotham, and
Z. Wiesenfeld-Hallin, IASP Press, Seattle, © 2000.

93

Epidural Spinal Cord Stimulation for Treatment of Chronic Pain: Some Predictors of Success

Cesare Bonezzi, Massimo Barbieri, Laura Demartini, Danilo Miotti, Livio Paulin, Raffaella Bettaglio, and Massimo Allegri

Pain Management Unit, Salvatore Maugeri Foundation, I.R.C.C.S., Pavia, Italy

Spinal cord stimulation (SCS) has been used for almost 30 years to manage different chronic pain syndromes. The procedure offers several potential benefits, including reversibility, a relatively simple implantation technique, and control of stimulation parameters by patients. Nevertheless, reports of SCS efficacy vary considerably, with success rates ranging from 18% to 86% (De la Porte 1993). A complicating factor in the treatment of neuropathic pain is the heterogeneity of pain mechanisms that may be operant within the same individual and even within the same neuropathic disorder (Fields 1994; Galer 1995). The term "deafferentation pain" is applied to some neuropathic pains that are inferred to have sensory deficits, evidence of destruction of dorsal root ganglion cells, and a sustained central mechanism (Portenoy 1996). The label "peripheral neuropathic pain" is applied to painful diseases due to peripheral nerve injury, but this term does not imply that central mechanisms are absent or unimportant (Portenoy 1996). If we consider that different mechanisms may coexist within the same clinical picture, it is difficult to evaluate the success and efficacy of SCS by comparing different pain syndromes.

In clinical practice we often see mixed pain conditions in which different neuropathic pain types might be present or in which neuropathic and nociceptive pain coexist, for example, "failed back surgery syndrome" and vascular pain. The former mixed pain syndrome is the most common indication for SCS, especially in the United States. SCS is known to relieve pain associated with disturbed peripheral circulation due to arteriosclerosis or diabetic vasculopathy. In vascular pain conditions the pain due to tissue ischemia may be either neuropathic (ischemic neuropathy) or nociceptive, and thus can be effectively influenced, either directly or indirectly, by SCS. Many factors can influence the outcome in clinical practice, including not only psychological factors, but also electrode positioning, choice of stimulation parameters, and surgical technique.

We attempted to clarify the role of some of these factors in a prospective study of success and efficacy in 100 patients screened for implantation with SCS pulse generators during 1996–1999. We analyzed type of pain, patient motivation and affect, and paresthesia coverage.

MATERIALS AND METHODS

PATIENTS AND PAIN TYPE

The study population was drawn from a series of consecutive patients with chronic pain, of whom 100 were screened in a 45-day home trial to determine suitability for surgical SCS implantation during a 26-month period (December 1996–January 1999). Psychological prescreening was conducted by a clinical psychologist with an interest in chronic pain; patients with significant unresolved issues of secondary gain were rejected for the home trial. Candidates gave informed consent, and demographic and medical history data were collected. Patients received a neurological assessment (clinical evaluation, electromyography, clinical testing for thermal-tactile pain, and telethermography) to determine which pain types affected the areas under consideration. The pain types were defined as neuropathic or mixed neuropathic-nociceptive pain.

PAIN ASSESSMENT

The survey instrument was composed of five selected items of the Italian version of the Brief Pain Inventory (BPI) (Caraceni 1996): (1) pain intensity on a 0–10 visual analogue scale (pain VAS), (2) daily activity (function VAS), (3) improvement in life enjoyment (± 50% of basal level), (4) treatment satisfaction, assessed by yes/no questions about satisfaction with spinal cord stimulation, and (5) number of drugs used daily. The BPI (Cleeland 1994) is a powerful tool that has demonstrated its reliability and validity across cultures and languages; it is being adopted in many countries for clinical pain assessment, epidemiological studies, and studies of the effectiveness of pain treatment. Study patients were asked to assess the five parts of the survey before onset of treatment and 1 year after pulse generator implantation. An investigator not involved in the treatment was responsible for the outcome assessment. Data were collected at clinic visits and by telephone. Patients were also asked about the degree (incomplete, complete) of paresthesia coverage of the painful area.

We evaluated "success" in the screening trial by determining the fraction of those screened who were accepted for surgical implantation of the SCS pulse generator (a 50% reduction in pain VAS was necessary for pulse generator implant; see Technical Details below). "Efficacy" represents the percentage of patients implanted who showed an improvement at follow-up in at least three items surveyed.

TECHNICAL DETAILS

General inclusion-exclusion criteria and percutaneous implant protocol were similar to those later described in the Consensus Statement prepared in Brussels in 1998 (Gybels 1998). In all 100 patients, Pisces-Quad Model electrodes (Medtronic, Inc., Minneapolis, MN) were percutaneously inserted to determine the best possible paresthesia coverage. After a home trial stimulation period of 45 days, pulse generators (Itrel II and III) were subcutaneously placed in the patients who demonstrated improvement of at least 50% on the pain VAS. Stimulation parameters were adjusted to obtain the best patient satisfaction and consequently the best clinical result with the lowest possible level of energy consumption.

Statistical analysis was performed with both paired t test and nonparametric Wilcoxon test.

RESULTS

SUCCESS RATES IN INITIAL STIMULATION PERIOD

For analysis of success rates, we divided the initial 100 patients in two groups: the neuropathic pain (NP) group (n = 62 patients), in which the success rate was 53.3%; and the mixed pain (neuropathic-nociceptive) (MP) group (n = 38), in which the success rate was 63%. Thus, 33 NP patients and 24 MP patients underwent surgery for stimulator implant, for a total of 57.

Failure to obtain 50% reduction in pain VAS in the screening trial period was seen in the NP group in all seven patients with deafferentation pain, in four patients in whom it was not possible to obtain paresthesia in the painful area, and in two patients with poor motivation for the therapy. In the

MP group, patients with nociceptive back pain (n = 4) or nociceptive ischemic pain of the skin and deep tissues (n = 3) did not respond to SCS. Two patients had failures related to sudden development of vascular disease. The remaining 16 NP patients and 5 MP patients failed to obtain 50% reduction in pain VAS in the screening trial for reasons that were not obvious.

EFFICACY OF SCS AT 1-YEAR FOLLOW-UP

As noted above, we defined efficacious neurostimulation as significant improvement on at least three parameters of the assessment tool. In 57 patients at 1-year follow-up, the efficacy was 75.8% as the sum of 42.4% (success in 5 parameters), of 15.2% (4 parameters), and of 18.2% (3 parameters). Significant changes in these parameters are shown in Table I.

For efficacy assessment, we divided the patients in two groups according to paresthesia coverage of the painful area (complete or incomplete coverage). We noticed significant improvement at follow-up in both groups. The two groups showed differences in parameter values that were not statistically significant, but interesting in terms of patient satisfaction (Table II).

DISCUSSION

Neuropathic, rather than nociceptive, pain represents the main indication for SCS, according to the literature. Consistent with this conclusion, our data show many positive results in the NP group, which included patients

Table I
Efficacy of spinal cord stimulation, showing ratings in five categories of the five items of the Italian version of the Brief Pain Inventory at baseline and 1-year follow-up

	Pain VAS	Function VAS	Life Enjoyment	Treatment Satisfaction	Drug Amount
Neuropathic Pain					
Baseline	9.70	9.50	NA	NA	2.9
1 year	4.69	3.83	75.0	67.5	1.7
Mixed Pain					
Baseline	9.39	9.76	NA	NA	3.2
1 year	4.53	5.96	67.5	67.5	2

Note: Pain and function VAS are on a scale of 1–10; life enjoyment = percentage of patients showing at least 50% improvement; treatment satisfaction = percentage of patients satisfied; drug amount = number of drugs used daily; NA = not applicable.

Table II
Efficacy of spinal cord stimulation in patients with complete or incomplete paresthesia coverage of the painful area at baseline and 1-year follow-up

	Pain VAS	Function VAS	Life Enjoyment	Treatment Satisfaction	Drug Amount
Complete Coverage					
Baseline	9.55	9.78	NA	NA	2.9
1 year	4.20	4.68	82.0	77	1.8
Incomplete Coverage					
Baseline	9.69	9.41	NA	NA	3.1
1 year	5.46	5.58	78.5	58	1.8

Note: Details as in Table I.

with first-order neuron lesions (of the peripheral nerve or at nerve root levels) without deafferentation of the second-order neurons. However, results were poor in patients (n = 7) with first-order neuron lesions (five with plexus avulsion, two with postherpetic neuralgia) in whom there was marked neurophysiological evidence of deafferentation. In the MP group , the nociceptive component of pain, particularly in failed back surgery syndromes (n = 21) and in vascular patients (n = 17), was poorly controlled by SCS. Back pain and pain due to deep and cutaneous (ulcers) tissue ischemia were negative predictive factors. The high success rate in patients with peripheral vascular disease was related to a strict selection of patients in Fontaine third and fourth stages but with few finger ulcers. One such patient was dropped from the study after subcutaneous pocket infection.

In both NP and MP groups, lack of motivation for treatment and depression were negative predictive factors. The prolonged trial stimulation of 45 days was useful for the physician and patient to better predict the results in terms of pain relief, patient daily activity, and overall patient satisfaction. Patients who initially reported poor results during the prolonged screening period were unlikely to experience any subsequent improvement in pain relief.

If we consider the different degree of paresthesia coverage, the data show that incomplete coverage is not necessarily associated with failure (Table II). Even if complete paresthesia coverage is more important for patient satisfaction than for pain relief, it is beneficial to look for the best coverage of the painful area during electrode implant.

Despite clinical trial data demonstrating successful pain relief with several pharmacological and surgical treatment choices, the management of chronic neuropathic pain is difficult. As different mechanisms may coexist in the same clinical picture in different patients (or even in the same individual), a combination of different treatments may be the best approach in the management of chronic pain. Only careful clinical trials will clarify the role of SCS in a complex, mechanisms-based treatment.

REFERENCES

Caraceni A, Mendoza TR, et al. A validation study of an Italian version of the Brief Pain Inventory (Breve Questionario Per la Valutazione Del Dolore). *Pain* 1996; 65:87–92.

Cleeland CS, Ryan KM. Pain assessment: global use of the Brief Pain Inventory. *Ann Acad Med Singapore* 1994; 23:129–138.

De la Porte C, Van De Kelft E. Spinal cord stimulation in failed back surgery syndrome. *Pain* 1993; 61:52–55.

Fields HL, Rowbotham MC. Multiple mechanisms of neuropathic pain: a clinical perspective. In: Gebhart GF, Hammond DL, Jensen TS (Eds). *Proceedings of the 7th World Congress on Pain*, Progress in Pain Research and Management, Vol. 2. Seattle, IASP Press, 1994, pp 173–183.

Galer BS. Neuropathic pain of peripheral origin: advances in pharmacologic treatment. *Neurology* 1995; 45(Suppl 9):S17–S25.

Gybels J, et al. Neuromodulation of pain: a consensus statement prepared in Brussels 16-18 January 1988. *Eur J Pain* 1998; 2:203–209.

Portenoy RK. Neuropathic pain. In: Portenoy RK, Kanner RK (Eds). *Pain Management: Theory and Practice.* Philadelphia: F.A. Davis Company, 1996, pp 83–125.

Correspondence to: Cesare Bonezzi, MD, Pain Management Unit, Fondazione Salvatore Maugeri, I.R.C.C.S., Pavia, Italy. email: cbonezzi@fsm.it.

Proceedings of the 9th World Congress on Pain,
Progress in Pain Research and Management,
Vol. 16, edited by M. Devor, M.C. Rowbotham, and
Z. Wiesenfeld-Hallin, IASP Press, Seattle, © 2000.

94

Coronary Artery Bypass Grafting Versus Spinal Cord Stimulation in Severe Angina Pectoris: Further Results from the ESBY Study

Henrik Norrsell,[a] Martin Pilhall,[b] Tore Eliasson,[a] and Clas Mannheimer[a]

[a]Multidisciplinary Pain Center, Department of Medicine, and [b]Department of Clinical Physiology, Sahlgren's University Hospital, Östra, Göteborg, Sweden

Spinal cord stimulation (SCS) has been used since 1985 to treat therapy-resistant angina pectoris, with good clinical results. Several studies have consistently reported a reduction of myocardial ischemia as measured by exercise tests (Mannheimer et al. 1988; Sanderson et al. 1992; Eliasson et al. 1993; de Jongste et al. 1994a), long-term electrocardiographic (ECG) monitoring (de Jongste et al. 1994b), lactate metabolism tests (Mannheimer et al. 1993), or stress echocardiography (Kujacic et al. 1993). The ESBY (electrical stimulation versus bypass surgery) study (Mannheimer et al. 1998) investigated spinal cord stimulation (SCS) as an alternative to coronary artery bypass grafting (CABG) in patients with no prognostic benefit from CABG and increased surgical risk. The study included 104 patients, who were enrolled between January 1992 and March 1995; 51 patients were randomized to CABG and 53 to SCS.

Both groups had similar symptom relief, reflected in decreased frequency of anginal attacks and decreased consumption of short-acting nitrate. The CABG group performed better and had fewer ischemic changes in the S-T segment in the ECG compared to the SCS group when SCS was inactivated during exercise tests. However, the CABG group had a higher mortality and cerebrovascular morbidity compared to the SCS group. The report concluded that SCS might be an alternative to CABG in selected patient groups.

To further evaluate the effects of spinal cord stimulation versus CABG on ischemia symptoms, we subjected ESBY study patients to 24-hour Holter monitoring preoperatively and at 6-month follow up.

METHODS

We designed our study as a randomized, prospective, open comparison between CABG and SCS in patients with no proven prognostic benefit from CABG and with an increased risk for surgical complications. Patient characteristics, inclusion criteria, and the technique for implantation of the stimulation equipment have been described thoroughly (Mannheimer et al. 1998).

All patients included in the study underwent a 24-hour ambulatory ECG at inclusion, and 6 months later. For patients treated with SCS we discontinued the stimulation 24 hours before and during ECG monitoring. Patients were excluded from analyses if they were not able to participate in a follow-up test. Patients recorded anginal attacks in a diary during the 24 hours of monitoring. In the ST analyses, we excluded patients with left bundle branch block, left ventricular hypertrophy, digitalis medication, atrial fibrillation, and pacemakers.

Holter ischemia indices included: number of ischemia episodes (negative ST segment shifts of at least 1 mm lasting for at least 1 minute and separated from the previous episode by at least 1 minute), total ischemia duration (total time of negative ST segment shifts >1 mm), and total ischemia burden (the time-voltage area under the 1-mm cut-off value).

Heart rate variability (HRV) was analyzed by the triangular method. This time domain index has been documented as a reliable index of prognostic information regarding arrhythmic events after myocardial infarction (Malik et al. 1989). In the HRV analyses we excluded patients with atrial fibrillation and pacemakers.

We used repeated-measures analysis of variance (ANOVA) to analyze data after due normalization of variables. We used contingency tables and Fisher's exact probabilities test to analyze categorical data. In all instances, $P < 0.05$ was considered significant.

The study was performed according to the Helsinki declaration and was approved by the local ethics committee. All subjects provided informed consent.

RESULTS

Study results are summarized in Table I. The number and duration of ischemic episodes decreased in the CABG group, but remained unchanged

Table I
Results of comparison of CABG and SCS

	CABG (n = 30)		SCS (n = 39)		P	
Variable	Pre-op	Follow-up	Pre-op	Follow-up	Pre/Post	Treatment
Ischemic duration (min)	426.5 (495.3)	212.8 (420.8)	392.5 (511.4)	419.9 (506.9)	–	0.02
No. ischemic episodes	35.2 (39.9)	17.8 (21.4)	28.4 (32.1)	29.1 (30.8)	n.s.	<0.05
Ischemic burden (mm^2)	47.6 (124.6)	23.8 (78.5)	22.7 (39.3)	44.2 (124.2)	n.s.	n.s.
Anginal attacks (no./24 h)	2.1 (2.2) (n = 36)	0.5 (1.3) (n = 36)	1.5 (2.1) (n = 49)	0.7 (1.3) (n = 49)	0.0001	n.s.
Heart rate variability (ms)	542.6 (125.7)	464.3 (176.7)	545.0 (184.0)	540.6 (192.5)	0.053 (n.s.)	0.08 (n.s.)

Note: Values are given as means, with SD in parentheses. CABG = coronary artery bypass surgery; SCS = spinal cord stimulation; P values are for pre-treatment versus follow-up (Pre/Post) and for CABG versus SCS (Treatment). For Pre/Post the values shown are the outcome of the repeated-measures ANOVA of the corresponding variable and hence refer to the two types of treatment together. For Treatment, the values shown are the ANOVA interaction term Pre/Post × Treatment and hence refer to a comparison of the responses to CABG versus SCS treatment. n.s. = not significant.

in the SCS group (CABG vs. SCS; both $P < 0.05$). The groups also showed a nonsignificant trend toward differences in ischemic burden ($P = 0.1$). The number of reported anginal attacks decreased significantly at follow-up ($P < 0.0001$), without a significant difference between the treatment modalities. Even if the decrease appeared slightly greater in the CABG group, symptoms still decreased significantly in the SCS group when analyzed separately ($P < 0.02$). Three patients in the CABG group did not fill out their diaries and were excluded from this analysis. We observed a trend toward a decrease in heart rate variability at follow-up in the CABG group ($P = 0.08$).

DISCUSSION

The difference in effect on objective ischemic parameters as measured in this study favoring CABG is not surprising. These results are in accordance with the earlier results presented from this study population where CABG had a significant positive effect on ischemic variables at exercise test, whereas SCS had no effect on ischemic variables, even though both treatments had good and equal effects on anginal symptoms (Mannheimer et al. 1998). In both studies, SCS was discontinued during ischemia and HRV monitoring, which could explain the lack of effect on these parameters. The reason for discontinuing SCS was to assess the possible independent long-term effects of this treatment. The lack of effect of SCS on ischemic parameters contrasts with findings on acute effects of electrostimulation of earlier studies that monitored ischemia during ongoing stimulation. These studies have shown a consistent and reproducible anti-ischemic effect (Mannheimer 1984; Emanuelsson et al. 1991; de Landsherre et al. 1992; Sanderson et al. 1992; Eliasson et al. 1993; Kujacic et al. 1993; Mannheimer et al. 1993; de Jongste et al. 1994b; Haustvat et al. 1996). The lack of any long-term anti-ischemic effects has clinical implications, as it is considered essential to continue daily treatment, even when the frequency of anginal pain diminishes.

The number of anginal attacks significantly decreased in both groups without significant differences between the groups. The decrease in the CABG group was expected due to the decreased ischemia. The decrease in anginal symptoms in the SCS group, in the absence of a decrease in myocardial ischemia, can be explained by the two symptomatic effects of SCS: an acute anti-ischemic effect and a primary analgesic effect of longer duration.

Clinicians have observed that to alleviate persistent ischemic pain, patients must use high-intensity stimulation, which usually gives total pain relief in 30–120 seconds. Experience with SCS worldwide is largely based on use in patients with nonischemic pain conditions such as neuropathic pain, where clinical results have been quite good (Gybels and Kupers 1987; Lazorthes et al. 1995). In these conditions a partial pain-relieving effect usually begins in 1–15 minutes. This experience indicates that SCS has a different mechanism of action in neuropathic pain as compared to ischemic pain conditions, and this mechanism could theoretically be responsible for a long-term primary analgesic effect in ischemic pain conditions. This finding and these interpretations are somewhat in contrast to data presented earlier and should of course be treated with caution. However, the long-term mechanisms of SCS in angina pectoris have not been investigated thoroughly, and the present observation warrants further research.

In accordance with previous investigations, we found no significant change in HRV after SCS (Andersen 1998; Haustvat et al. 1998), but our study did not incorporate ongoing stimulation. The results indicate that SCS has no long-term or acute effects on cardiac autonomic activity as measured by HRV.

ACKNOWLEDGMENTS

This chapter was written on behalf of the ESBY study group. We would like to acknowledge the skillful work of laboratory technician Margareta Leijon at the Department of Clinical Physiology, Sahlgren's University Hospital/ Östra. This work was supported by the Faculty of Medicine, University of Göteborg, the Swedish Heart-Lung Foundation, and the Swedish Medical Research Council (projects B-93-19x-10404-01 and B96-19x-11239-02B).

REFERENCES

Andersen C. Does heart rate variability change in angina pectoris patients treated with spinal cord stimulation? *Cardiology* 1998; 89:14–18.

de Jongste M, Haustvat R, Hillege H, Lie K. Efficacy of spinal cord stimulation as adjuvant therapy for intractable angina pectoris: a prospective, randomized clinical study. *J Am Coll Cardiol* 1994a; 23:1592–1597.

de Jongste MJ, Haaksma J, Hautvast RW, et al. Effects of spinal cord stimulation on myocardial ischaemia during daily life in patients with severe coronary artery disease. A prospective ambulatory electrocardiographic study. *Br Heart J* 1994b; 71:413–418.

de Landsherre C, Mannheimer C, Habets A. et al. Effect of spinal cord stimulation on regional myocardial perfusion assessed by positron emission tomography. *Am J Cardiol* 1992; 69:1143–1149.

Eliasson T, Albertsson P, Hårdhammar P, et al. Spinal cord stimulation in angina pectoris with normal coronary arteriograms. *Coron Artery Dis* 1993; 4:819–827.

Emanuelsson H, Mannheimer C, Waagstein F. Changes in arterial levels and myocardial metabolism of catecholamines during pacing-induced angina pectoris. *Clin Cardiol* 1991; 14:567–572.

Gybels J, Kupers R. Central and peripheral electrical stimulation of the nervous system in the treatment of chronic pain. *Acta Neurochir* 1987; 38(Suppl):64–75.

Haustvat R, Blanksma P, DeJongste M, et al. Effect of spinal cord stimulation on myocardial blood flow assessed by positron emission tomography in patients with refractory angina pectoris. *Am J Card* 1996; 77:462–467.

Haustvat RW, Brouwer J, DeJongste MJ, Lie KI. Effect of spinal cord stimulation on heart rate variability and myocardial ischemia in patients with chronic intractable angina pectoris—a prospective ambulatory electrocardiographic study. *Clin Cardiol* 1998; 21:33–38.

Kujacic V, Eliasson T, Mannheimer C, et al. Assessment of the influence of spinal cord stimulation (SCS) on left ventricular function in patients with severe angina pectoris: an echocardiographic study. *Eur Heart J* 1993; 14:1238–1244.

Lazorthes Y, Siegfried J, Verdie JC, Casaux J. [Chronic spinal cord stimulation in the treatment of neurogenic pain. Cooperative and retrospective study on 20 years of follow-up]. *Neurochirurgie* 1995; 41:73–86.

Malik M, Farrell T, Cripps T, Camm AJ. Heart rate variability in relation to prognosis after myocardial infarction: selection of optimal processing techniques. *Eur Heart J* 1989; 10:1060–1074.

Mannheimer C. Transcutaneous electrical nerve stimulation (TENS) in angina pectoris. Göteborg, 1984.

Mannheimer C, Augustinsson L-E, Carlsson C-A, et al. Epidural spinal electrical stimulation in severe angina pectoris. *Br Heart J* 1988; 59:56–61.

Mannheimer C, Eliasson T, Andersson B, et al. Effects of spinal cord stimulation in angina pectoris induced by pacing and possible mechanisms of action. *BMJ* 1993; 307:477–480.

Mannheimer C, Eliasson T, Augustinsson L-E, et al. Electrical stimulation versus coronary artery bypass surgery in sever angina pectoris: the ESBY study. *Circulation* 1998; 97:1157–1163.

Sanderson JE, Brooksby P, Waterhouse D, et al. Epidural spinal electrical stimulation for severe angina: a study of its effects on symptoms, exercise tolerance and degree of ischaemia. *Eur Heart J* 1992; 13:628–633.

Correspondence to: Henrik Norsell, MD, PhD, Multidisciplinary Pain Center, Department of Medicine, Sahlgren's University Hospital, Östra, 416 85 Göteborg, Sweden. Fax: 46-31-3435933; email: henrik.norrsell@invmed.gu.se.

Proceedings of the 9th World Congress on Pain,
Progress in Pain Research and Management,
Vol. 16, edited by M. Devor, M.C. Rowbotham, and
Z. Wiesenfeld-Hallin, IASP Press, Seattle, © 2000.

95

Motor Cortex Stimulation for Chronic Neuropathic Pain

Dawn Carroll,[a] Carole Joint,[b] Tipu Aziz,[b] and Henry McQuay[a]

[a]*Pain Research Unit, University of Oxford, Oxford, United Kingdom;*
[b]*Department Of Neurological Surgery,*
Radcliffe Infirmary, Oxford, United Kingdom

Growing evidence from published case reports and case series supports the analgesic effectiveness of motor cortex stimulation in chronic neuropathic pain (Tsubokawa et al. 1990, 1991a,b, 1993; Hosobuchi 1993; Meyerson et al. 1993; Katayama et al. 1994, 1998; Canavero et al. 1995, 1998; Herregodts et al. 1995; Peyron et al. 1995; Ebel et al. 1996; Dario et al. 1997; Fujii et al. 1997; Nguyen et al. 1997, 1998, 1999; Rainov et al. 1997; Yamamoto et al. 1997; Saitoh et al. 1999). Although the possible mechanisms for motor cortex stimulation remain uncertain, some evidence from animal studies suggests that cortical stimulation activates thalamic nucleus relay systems (Namba and Nishimoto 1988). Positron emission tomography studies demonstrate changes in cerebral blood flow in patients reporting pain relief from motor cortex stimulation (Canavero et al. 1995; Peyron et al. 1995; Garcia-Larrea et al. 1997). Unlike other forms of neurostimulation, motor cortex stimulation can be tested for effectiveness by using double-blind techniques because the level of stimulation used to achieve pain relief is below the level that is capable of producing a motor response, and patients do not experience paresthesia or other sensations of any kind with stimulation. The only cue is the presence or absence of pain. This paper reports our experience of motor cortex stimulation together with the preliminary findings of a within-patient, "*n* of 1," multiple crossover, randomized, controlled trial.

PROSPECTIVE AUDIT OF 12 PATIENTS TREATED WITH MOTOR CORTEX STIMULATION

Patients and methods. Details of the 12 patients treated with motor cortex stimulation between 1995 and 1999 are summarized in Table I. Twelve patients with chronic neuropathic pain, who had failed to respond to all previous analgesic interventions, were treated with motor cortex stimulation. Patients received implants during a two-stage surgical procedure. The surgical technique has been reported elsewhere (Carroll et al. 2000). All 12 patients had intraoperative test stimulation. With the patients fully awake it was possible to confirm a reproducible motor response (muscle spasm or paresthesia) in the area of pain. A positive motor response was elicited in all 12 patients, who then received general anesthesia for the surgical implantation of the full motor cortex stimulation system, which was a fully programmable internal pulse generator device (Medtronic Itrel 2 or 3). Test stimulation was repeated after wound closure and again in the immediate postoperative period. Patients were discharged after surgery with the stimulator switched off. Four to six weeks later, when patients had fully recovered from the effects of their surgery, they were readmitted to hospital for programming and titration of the stimulator. Further retitration of the stimulator parameters is always needed, and is done as an inpatient. This method not only produces better analgesia results, but is more acceptable to patients.

Assessment and outcomes. All patients were assessed before and after surgery by at least one member of the multidisciplinary team. Pain outcomes, including measures of pain intensity and pain relief, were repeated whenever patients visited the department for any routine follow-up or retitration. All assessments were repeated before, during, and after any titration of the stimulator parameters. A summary of the main patient assessments and outcomes is shown below:

- Pain intensity: 4-point verbal rating scale (severe = 3, moderate = 2, mild = 1, none = 0).
- Pain intensity: 10-point numerical scale (0–10).
- McGill Pain Questionnaire (20 groups of 78 descriptors).
- Pain relief: 5-point scale (none = 0, slight = 1, moderate = 2, good = 3, complete = 4).
- Percentage pain relief.
- Volunteered and observed adverse effects attributable to motor cortex stimulation.
- Record of stimulator parameters (amplitude, pulse width, pulse rate, electrode settings, frequency of stimulation per day).
- Use of other analgesic interventions.

Results. The results for the analgesic outcomes are summarized in Table I. Six of the 12 patients treated responded positively (at least 50% relief) to intermittent motor cortex stimulation. Most patients received 15 minutes of active stimulation every 3–4 hours each day. Continuous stimulation was not necessary to produce pain relief. No epileptic seizures occurred in the patients who gained pain relief from stimulation. A seizure was induced in two patients who did not achieve any reproducible motor response or pain relief during the postoperative test stimulation despite the presence of a positive motor response during intra-operative test stimulation (Table I).

RANDOMIZED, DOUBLE-BLIND, ("*N* OF 1") WITHIN-PATIENT CROSSOVER TRIAL

Patients and methods. Three of six patients reporting at least 50% relief from long-term (>6 months), intermittent motor cortex stimulation participated in this randomized, double-blind, within-patient, repeated crossover study. Two patients died before the study began. The remaining patient has agreed to participate in the future. The study was approved by the local hospital ethics committee.

Patients were allocated to receive up to 10 sequential treatment periods of both: (a) active stimulation (5 treatments) and (b) no stimulation (5 treatments). For practical reasons, all three patients were admitted to hospital for the duration of the study. The 10 study treatments were given in a random order (by tossing a coin), and the randomization schedule was concealed by using sealed envelopes for each treatment, identified by patient name and treatment number (1–10). All study treatments followed double-blind protocol. Neither the patient nor the nurse observer knew whether the stimulator was switched on or off at any time during the study period. The person operating the internal programmer (on/off) was not involved with study assessments and had no other contact with patients. Each study treatment was administered for a minimum of one hour and lasted long enough for the patients to judge whether the stimulator was switched on or off during each treatment based on subjective changes in pain.

Assessment and outcomes. Outcomes were measured using the assessments listed above. They were evaluated immediately before each study treatment (baseline), and then immediately after patients requested to be switched over to the next treatment (post-treatment), according to the randomization schedule. At the end of each treatment period patients rated the overall treatment (poor = 0, fair = 1, good = 2, very good = 3, excellent = 4) before receiving the next study treatment. They were also asked whether the

Table I

Results for patients treated with motor cortex stimulation (MCS)

Patient No	Diagnosis, Year of Onset	Site and Characteristics of Pain	Age (y)/ Sex	Date of 1st stage MCS (2nd stage)	Adverse Effects/ Complications	Optimum Stimulator Settings	Amount and Duration of Relief	Comment
1 (DB)	*Post-stroke (thalamic infarct), 1991*	*Hemi-body; constant severe*	*62/m*	*Nov. 95 (Nov. 95)*	*Subdural hematoma, secondary wound infection. Explant Apr. 96.*	*Not documented*	*>50%, 2–3 weeks*	*Initial pain relief (>50%) lasted 2–3 weeks. Patient died of unrelated cause June 96.*
2 (SB)	*Post-traumatic neuralgia (brainstem gunshot injury), 1993*	*Face, neck, arm, shoulder; constant severe*	*54/f*	*Jul. 96 (Jul. 96)*	*Tender over implant. Secondary wound infection. High-amplitude stimulation gave sensation of tightness in area of pain, impaired speech.*	*Amp 2.1 V, PW 450 μs, PR 20 Hz*	*50–60%, 36 months*	*>50% relief overall. Titration limited by tightness and other symptoms.*
3 (TB)	Post-stroke (thalamic infarct), 1985	Facial; constant severe	80/m	Mar. 96 (Mar. 98)		None found	None	No relief. No clear postop. motor response
4 (RN)	*Post-stroke (occipital infarct), 1990*	*Hemi-body; constant severe*	*70/m*	*Jul. 96 (Dec. 96)*	*Itrel 2 affected by exposure to external magnetic field.*	*Amp 5.0 V, PW 450 μs, PR 15 Hz*	*100%, 31 months*	*No pain since Oct. 98. Stimulator switched off Feb. 99 with no recurrence of pain. Patient died of unrelated cause July 99.*
5 (CW)	*Phantom and stump, 1992*	*Leg; constant severe*	*48/m*	*Jan. 97 (Jan. 97)*	*Higher amplitudes gave tightness in area of pain.*	*amp 7.0 V, PW 450 μs, PR 25 Hz*	*70% phantom, 0% stump, 30 months*	*Good relief of phantom pain; no relief of stump pain.*
6 (ME)	Neuro-fibromatosis, 1990	Arm; constant severe	55/f	Jan. 97 (Jan. 97)	No postop. motor response.	None found	None	No pain relief; no postop. motor response. Stimulation discontinued.

7 (JC)	Post-stroke (thalamic infarct)	Hemi-body; constant severe	63/f	Mar. 97 (Mar. 97)		None found	None	No clear reproducible postop. motor response. No pain relief. Stimulation discontinued
8 (AG)	*Phantom limb, 1975*	*Arm and hand; constant severe*	*56/f*	*Apr. 97 (Apr. 97)*	*Secondary wound infection. Pain over implant site.*	*Amp 2.5 V, PW 450 μs, PR 75 Hz*	*Arm 75%, hand 5%, 27 months*	*Good long-term relief of phantom pain.*
9 (MP)	Phantom limb, 1979	Arm; constant severe	39/m	Oct. 97 (Oct. 97)	No evidence of any post-op. motor response. Possible contact with external magnetic field.	None found	None	Technical failure. Stimulation discontinued
10 (DT)	Post-stroke (brainstem) and trigeminal neuralgia, 1992	Facial; burning, constant, severe, episodic	80/f	Feb. 98 (Mar. 98)	Fit induced during postop. titration (9.6 V). No pain relief, despite clear motor response during post-op titration.	None found	None	Clear reproducible postop. motor response (8 V). No pain relief. Stimulation discontinued.
11 (EM)	Brachial plexus avulsion, 1976	Hand and arm; constant, but of variable intensity	36/f	Nov. 99 (Jan. 99)	Strong motor response elicited during intra-op. test stimulation. Fit during intra-op. test stimulation and postop. titration.	None found	None	Evidence for motor response postop.; no pain relief. Stimulation discontinued
12 (RD)	*Post-stroke, 1997*	*Hemi-body; constant, moderate to severe*	*68/m*	*Mar. 99 (Mar. 99)*	*Strong motor response elicited during intra-op. test stimulation.*	*Awaiting retitration*	*2 weeks relief from initial postop. titration; awaiting further titration*	*Complete relief of pain from propofol. Initial postop. titration produced 70% relief of pain in arm and hand, lasting 2–3 weeks.*

Note: PW = pulse width (microseconds); PR = stimulation pulse rate (pulses/second); Amp = stimulation amplitude (Volts). *Italic type designates patients reporting pain relief;* roman type indicates patients reporting no pain relief.

treatment they were receiving was active stimulation or not, based on changes in their pain during that treatment period.

Summary of main findings. Of the three participating patients, two were able to judge correctly when they had received the active and no stimulation treatments on 8 of 10 occasions, based on clinically relevant changes (decrease/increase) in their pain. Each cross over treatment lasted for 1 hour and treatments were given across two consecutive days. One patient could only guess correctly which treatment she had received on 4 of 10 occasions. She reported that the study treatment periods (1–2 hours) were not long enough for her to make a reliable judgment. For this patient we may repeat the "*n* of 1" trial with longer treatment periods.

CONCLUSIONS

Half of the patients in our case series have responded positively to intermittent motor cortex stimulation (>50% pain relief). Some of these patients benefited from long-term analgesia with motor cortex stimulation, but other patients may need repeated titration to achieve this effect. Any sudden increase in pain reported by patients was attributable to technical problems. The specific cause of technical problems was not always easy to identify, and surgical exploration was usually needed to find the source of the problem. Lead fractures or extension leads that required replacement were the most common problems in our current case series.

A positive analgesic response occurred in patients with phantom pain ($n = 2$), post-stroke pain ($n = 3$), and post-traumatic neuralgia ($n = 1$). However, we do not yet have any reliable way of predicting which patients are likely to respond to motor cortex stimulation, and the analgesic responsiveness does not seem to be specific to any one chronic pain condition.

The preliminary findings from our randomized, double-blind "*n* of 1" trial of three patients provides further supportive evidence for the analgesic effectiveness of motor cortex stimulation. Two of three patients were able to distinguish between active stimulation and no stimulation treatments (8 of 10 correct judgments), based on a clinically significant change in pain. A third patient failed to distinguish between the study treatments because the treatment periods were not of sufficient duration. We recommend that future "*n* of 1" studies be designed so that the treatment periods are long enough for patients to detect any clinically relevant changes in their pain.

Although this work provides further supportive data on the analgesic effectiveness of motor cortex stimulation, more randomized, placebo-controlled, double-blind studies of motor cortex stimulation are urgently needed if it is to become widely recognized as a useful intervention in the treatment of chronic neuropathic pain. Until more evidence is available the skeptics will simply dismiss motor cortex stimulation as an invasive, expensive, experimental, and unproven intervention. More research is also needed to identify possible mechanisms of pain relief by motor cortex stimulation. These studies may help us to predict which patients are likely to benefit from this technique.

ACKNOWLEDGMENTS

This work was done in collaboration between the Department of Neurological Surgery, Oxford Radcliffe Hospital NHS Trust, and the Pain Research Unit, University of Oxford. No external funding was provided. Technical and travel support was provided by Medtronic UK, Ltd.

REFERENCES

Canavero S, Bonicalzi V. Cortical stimulation for central pain. *J Neurosurg* 1995; 83(6):1117.

Canavero S, Bonicalzi V, Pagni CA, et al. Cortical stimulation for pain. *Abstracts: 4th IMS Conference Lucerne,* 1998, Free Poster 36.

Carroll D, Joint C, Maartens N, et al. Motor cortex stimulation for chronic neuropathic pain: a preliminary study of 10 cases. *Pain* 2000; 84:431–437.

Dario A, Marra A, Ramponi G, et al. A new approach to chronic central pain: the motor cortex stimulation. *Riv Neurobiol* 1997; 43(6):625–629.

Ebel H, Rust D, Tronnier V, Boker D, Kunze S. Chronic pre-central stimulation in trigeminal neuropathic pain. *Acta Neurochir* 1996; 138(11):1300–1306.

Fujii M, Ohmoto Y, Kitahara T, et al. Motor cortex stimulation therapy in patients with thalamic pain. *Neurol Surg* 1997; 25(4):315–319.

Garcia-Larrea L, Peyron R, Mertens P, et al. Positron emission tomography during motor cortex stimulation for pain control. *Stereotact Funct Neurosurg* 1997; 88(1-4):141–148.

Herregodts P, Stadnik T, De Ridder F, D'Haens J. Cortical stimulation for central neuropathic pain: 3-d surface MRI for easy determination of the motor cortex. *Acta Neurochir Suppl (Wien)* 1995; 64:132–135.

Hosobuchi Y. Motor cortical stimulation for control of central deafferentation pain. *Adv Neurol* 1993; 63:215–217.

Katayama Y, Tsubokawa T, Yamamoto T. Chronic motor cortex stimulation for central deafferentation pain: experience with bulbar pain secondary to Wallenberg Syndrome. *Stereotact Funct Neurosurg* 1994; 62(1–4):295–299.

Katayama Y, Fukaya C, Yamamoto T. Post stroke pain control by chronic motor cortex stimulation: neurological characteristics predicting a favourable response. *J Neurosurg* 1998; 89:585–591.

Meyerson BA, Lindblom U, Linderoth B, Lind G; Herregodts P. Motor cortex stimulation as a treatment of trigeminal neuropathic pain. *Acta Neurochir Suppl (Wien)* 1993; 58:150–153.

Namba S, Nishimoto A. Stimulation of internal capsule, thalamic sensory nucleus (VPM) and cerebral cortex inhibited deafferentiation hyperactivity provoked after gasserian ganglionectomy in cat. *Acta Neurochir Suppl (Wien)* 1988; 43:243–247.

Nguyen JP, Keravel Y, Feve A, et al. Treatment of deafferentation pain by chronic stimulation of the motor cortex: report of a series of 20 cases. *Acta Neurochir* 1997; Suppl 68:54–60.

Nguyen JP, Lefaucheur JP, Kondo S, et al. Chronic motor cortex stimulation in the treatment of central and neuropathic pain: correlations between clinical electrophysiological and anatomical datas. *Abstracts: 4th IMS Conference Lucerne,* 1998, Free Poster 32, p 180.

Nguyen JP, Lefaucheur JP, Decq P, et al. Chronic motor cortex stimulation in the treatment of central and neuropathic pain. Correlations between clinical, electrophysiological and anatomical data. *Pain* 1999; 82:245–141.

Peyron R, Garcia-Larrea L, Deiber MP, et al. Electrical stimulation of pre-central cortical area in the treatment of central pain: electrophysiological and PET study. *Pain* 1995; 62(3):275–286.

Rainov NG, Fels C, Heidecke V, Burkert W. Epidural stimulation of the motor cortex in patients with facial neuralgia. *Clin Neurol Neurosurg* 1997; 99(3):205–209.

Saitoh Y, Shibata Y, Mashimo T. Motor cortex stimulation for phantom limb pain. *Lancet* 1999; 353(9148):212.

Tsubokawa T, Katayama Y, Yamamoto T, Hirayama T, Koyama S. Motor cortex stimulation for control of thalamic pain. *Abstracts: VIth World Pain Congress,* Adelaide, 1990, p S491.

Tsubokawa T, Katayama Y, Yamamoto T, Hirayama T, Koyama S. Chronic motor cortex stimulation for the treatment of central pain. *Acta Neurochir Suppl (Wien)* 1991a; 52:137–139.

Tsubokawa T, Katayama Y, Yamamoto T, Hirayama T, Koyama S. Treatment of thalamic pain by chronic motor cortex stimulation. *Pacing Clin Electrophysiol* 1991b; 14(1):131–134.

Tsubokawa T. Katayama Y. Yamamoto T. Hirayama T. Koyama S. Chronic motor cortex stimulation in patients with thalamic pain. *J Neurosurg* 1993; 78(3):393–401.

Yamamoto T, Katayama Y, Hirayama T, Tsubokawa T. Pharmacological classification of central post-stroke pain: comparison with the results of chronic motor cortex stimulation therapy. *Pain* 1977; 72:5–12.

Correspondence to: Dawn Carroll, Pain Research Unit, The Churchill, Headington, Oxford, OX3 7LJ, United Kingdom. Tel: 44-1865-225775; Fax: 44-1865-226160; email: dawn.carroll@pru.ox.ac.uk.

Proceedings of the 9th World Congress on Pain, Progress in Pain Research and Management, Vol. 16, edited by M. Devor, M.C. Rowbotham, and Z. Wiesenfeld-Hallin, IASP Press, Seattle, © 2000.

96

Physical Therapy Assessment: Expanding the Model[1]

Maureen J. Simmonds,[a] Vicki Harding,[b] Paul J. Watson,[c] and Yvette Claveau[d]

[a]*School of Physical Therapy, Texas Woman's University, Houston, Texas, USA;* [b]*INPUT Pain Management, St Thomas' Hospital, London United Kingdom;* [c]*Rheumatic Diseases Centre, University of Manchester, Hope Hospital, Salford, United Kingdom;* [d]*Heritage MacCleod Physical Therapy, Calgary, Alberta, Canada*

Musculoskeletal pain (MSP) is a pervasive and diverse problem that is costly in both human and economic terms. MSP may be sudden or insidious in onset, and can result from major trauma or multiple episodes of micro-trauma. It may involve muscular, articular, nociceptive and/or neuropathic components and single or multiple sites of pain, and can persist for weeks, months, or a lifetime.

The presentation of MSP is diverse. Some persons with MSP continue an active and productive life and never seek professional health care. Others with apparently similar symptoms enter the health care system temporarily during symptom exacerbation. A small percentage enter the health care system and begin a downward spiral of distress, disability, and despair. It is apparent that individuals at risk for chronic disability are identifiable through psychosocial rather than biological factors. Unfortunately, most practitioners (physical therapists [PTs] or physicians) use a narrow assessment model that focuses on biological/physiological factors. MSP is clearly a complex biopsychosocial problem, and practitioners need to expand the way they conceptualize and assess the problems of patients with MSP. A suggested approach is to incorporate psychosocial measures into standard clinical assessment, and further explore the validity of biological assessment measures.

[1] Mini-review based on a congress workshop.

Given that optimal treatment is based on optimal assessment, it is imperative that assessment measures used in primary care be conceptually and psychometrically sound and be interpreted appropriately. It is beyond the scope of this chapter to review the myriad tests in clinical use (some of which are more credible than others). Rather, discussion will focus on a few tests that exemplify the construct. This chapter will briefly review and examine the psychometric and conceptual adequacy of some commonly used assessment measures. It also uses the biopsychosocial model as a framework for considering factors that may influence the assessment results and their interpretation. Finally, this chapter will discuss the use of screening assessments to identify patients who are at risk for chronic disability.

DEFINITIONS

Impairment, disability, and *handicap* are key terms that were defined by the World Health Organization (WHO) in 1980. Although not ideal, the following definitions encapsulate the differences between these commonly used terms: *Impairment*: any loss or abnormality of psychological, physiological, or anatomical structure or function. *Disability*: any restriction or lack (resulting from an impairment) of the ability to perform an activity in the manner or within the range considered normal. *Handicap*: a disadvantage for a given individual, resulting from an impairment or a disability, that limits or prevents the fulfillment of a role that is normal (depending on age, sex, and social and cultural factors) for that individual.

Nagi (1991) recognized the need for a concept that bridged impairment and disability, and proposed the term *functional limitation.* He constructed a model (Fig. 1) that illustrates the linkage from pathology through impairment and functional limitation to disability. His disablement model provides a conceptual framework for assessment and treatment. For example, *pathology* is defined as a change in the basic structure due to disease or injury. The diagnosis may be made through blood tests or imaging, e.g., a diagnosis of arthritis. *Impairment* is defined as in the WHO model. Impairment measures are familiar to most health care practitioners because they are so commonly used. They include measures of range of motion, muscle strength, pain intensity, or depression. *Functional limitation* is defined as compromised ability to perform tasks of daily life. Tasks include household tasks,

Pathology → Impairment → Functional Limitation → Disability

Fig. 1. Nagi (1991) model of functional limitation.

work, and recreational activities. Functional assessments include patient self-report and clinician-measured task performance. *Disability* is defined as an inability to perform an expected role in society. A person who is unable to return to work because of MSP is considered disabled.

Thus, impairment measures assess a part of a person, functional measures assess a person's abilities, and disability measures assess how the person functions in society. Assessment (and treatment) based on this model can encourage expansion in understanding and managing the problems of patients with MSP.

A limitation of Nagi's model is the implication of a linear progression from pathology to disability. Each of the constructs is complex and is influenced by many factors. Depending on when and how the different constructs are measured, and on the influence of mediating factors, the relations among the key constructs (pathology, impairment, functional limitation, and disability) and their relevance may be trivial. For example, degenerative changes noted on a plain X-ray in a 55-year-old person (pathology) may be surprisingly poor at predicting range of motion and are unlikely to predict pain (impairment). They are even less likely to predict the person's ability to climb stairs (functional ability) or work as a teacher (disability). A better predictor of work may be the unemployment rate or a flexible, satisfying work environment. These factors are external to the person, and the arthritic changes seen on X-ray are incidental. However, if the same person now breaks a leg (pathology), the X-ray becomes a much stronger predictor of work status.

MUSCULOSKELETAL PAIN: A COMPLEX BIOPSYCHOSOCIAL WEB

Low back pain (LBP) is one of the most prevalent and potentially disabling MSP conditions. LBP is typically a chronic recurrent problem that is frequently managed by the patient (Von Korff 1994). However, approximately 25% of those affected will seek health care (Von Korff et al. 1988) and about 3% of those absent from work or seeking health care will develop chronic disability (Waddell 1998). Although a relatively small percentage of persons with MSP become severely disabled, the economic costs (medical and social) are staggering, and the human costs are simply unacceptable. Clearly a priority of health care management of MSP is to prevent chronic disability.

LBP is the primary reason that adults seek outpatient physical therapy (Cats-Baril and Frymoyer 1991; Battie et al. 1994; Jette et al. 1994). A recent survey revealed that 80% of North American physicians from a variety of specialties identified physical therapy as the preferred management strategy for patients with LBP (Cherkin et al. 1995). Physical therapy is an accepted treatment option by most insurance companies and other third-party payers. Cats-Baril and Frymoyer (1991) estimated the costs of physical therapy for LBP in the United States to be $104 million a year.

PTs in primary care can spend substantial time with patients and are in an excellent position to identify those at risk for disability, provided the risk factors are known. To date, the strongest risk factors for chronic disability are psychosocial (see below), which is not surprising given that disability is a *social* construct. Unfortunately many PTs tend to ignore psychosocial factors, perhaps seeing them as "inconvenient baggage." PTs generally prefer to focus on factors that their education has best prepared them to handle, namely anatomical and biomechanical factors.

Psychological factors predictive of chronic disability include depressed mood, negative or passive coping, fear of pain and reinjury with consequent avoidance of activity (fear/avoidance beliefs), preoccupation with bodily symptoms or somatic anxiety, high self-report of stress or anxiety, and misunderstandings about the nature of the condition (Main and Watson 1995; Turk 1997). Social and economic factors predictive of chronic disability include dissatisfaction with current work, worries about safety at work, solicitous behavior of family, participation in medicolegal compensation claims, high level of wage replacement benefits, low educational level, and substance abuse (Main and Watson 1995; Turk 1997; Watson, in press).

Physical, psychological, and sociological factors thus are intricate, interwoven, and integral to the person. Although these factors can be conveniently compartmentalized for discussion, such compartmentalization is contrived. Psychosocial factors may predict physical dysfunction and disability, but psychosocial distress is also often a correlate and consequence of physical dysfunction rather than a cause. As such, this distress can be reversed by improvement in physical function (Simmonds et al. 1996), especially when physical dysfunction is the source of the distress (Main and Watson 1999). Thus, although studies provide support for the view that some patients are too distressed, depressed, or somatically focused to respond to physical therapy alone (Williams et al. 1995), measurable improvements in physical function may reduce distress.

MEASUREMENT OF IMPAIRMENT

Despite the frequent use of physical therapy, and clinicians' assertions of efficacy, reports from several task forces and research groups assert that the efficacy and effectiveness of many specific techniques or treatment regimens have not been adequately tested (Spitzer et al. 1987; Koes et al. 1991, 1992; Deyo 1993; Bigos et al. 1994; Fordyce et al. 1995; Feine and Lund 1997). Problems with measurements used in physical therapy account in part for some of the problems related to lack of evidence associated with this treatment approach (Campbell 1981; Rothstein 1985).

Clinical assessments used in physical therapy are traditionally limited to measures of impairment, which then guide treatment. Although restoration of function is one of the most common aims of treatment, function is not always directly assessed, but is inferred from the level of impairment. In the last two decades it has become increasingly obvious that impairment does not have a strong or stable relationship with functional limitation, disability, or rehabilitation outcome (e.g., Waddell 1987; Gatchel et al. 1995; Simmonds et al. 1998a), partly due to the complexity of the constructs and partly due to the difficulties in measuring them.

Although functional assessments may complement impairment-based assessments, the latter tests still predominate in primary care and are used to guide treatment. For example, in a recent survey on treatment goals for patients with LBP, Jette and colleagues (1994) reported that 87% (n = 895) of respondents cited reduction of pain as the primary treatment goal, 61% cited increase in range of motion, and 43% cited increase in muscle strength.

THE ORTHOPEDIC ASSESSMENT SCAN

The impairment-based orthopedic assessment scan typifies the clinical approach that focuses on the assessment of the part rather than on the person. Originally developed and described by Cyriax (1970), it has been the standard for physical therapy assessment for more than 20 years. The orthopedic assessment is described in its original form or with minor modifications in standard orthopedic texts (e.g., Cyriax 1983; Grieve 1984; Magee 1992; Lee and Walsh 1996). Briefly, the scan consists of observation of posture, measurement of active and passive joint range of motion, tests of muscle strength, and the presence and location of pain at rest, during muscle contraction, and during palpatory or provocative tests.

The scan was accepted untested and became entrenched in current practice and education. Only recently has it been subject to scientific scrutiny. The scan is primarily based on anatomy and joint biomechanics. It was (and still is) seductive because it promises simple solutions to complex problems. Cyriax (1970) originally promised that "diagnosis is only a matter of applying one's anatomy," a simplistic promise commonly reiterated in popular textbooks (Magee 1992; Lee and Walsh 1996; Tortensen 1997). The scan is technique driven and apparently logical. However, it is based on a mechanistic model of injury and acute pain (as it was understood 30 years ago), so the interpretation of the results is based on classical (hard-wired and stable) neurology and is frequently simplistic. Moreover, significant problems with the reliability and validity of the test components are apparent. The few studies that have tested reliability or validity are contradictory at best (Hayes et al. 1994; Pellecchia et al. 1996; Fritz et al. 1998).

For example, active and passive joint motions are key components of a spinal scan. But, except in extreme cases, the magnitude of spinal range of motion has limited clinical value because of the high level of individual variability and the trivial relations to disability. Mellin (1987) found lumbar spine mobility to have few significant correlations (none higher than r = 0.19) with the modified Oswestry questionnaire for LBP. It appears that standard tests of range of motion and muscle strength are not useful alone because they lack sensitivity, specificity, and responsiveness, and do not account for a patient's functional ability (Frese et al. 1987; Levack et al. 1988; Mooney et al. 1992; Pope 1992).

Not surprisingly, reliability studies have demonstrated visual estimation of range (probably the most common clinical method used) to be the least reliable method of measurement. Although instrumented measures of range are more reliable, agreement between instruments is still poor. Regardless of method, flexion and extension measurements are more reliable than side bend or rotation measures of the cervical or lumbar spine (Boline et al. 1992; Rondinelli et al. 1992; Breum et al. 1995; Saur et al. 1996; Moreland et al. 1997; Williams et al. 1998; Nitschke et al. 1999). This point is noteworthy and unfortunate, because the least reliable range of motion measure appears to be the best predictor of physical dysfunction (Mellin 1987).

Passive tests of joint motion are also part of a scan and do not fare well either. For example, postero-anterior (PA) passive intervertebral movement testing (PIVMS) is perhaps the most frequently practiced and investigated assessment and treatment technique (Maher et al. 1998). It requires that the therapist use the thumbs or the heel of the hand to apply a PA force to the patient's spine to put the joints through a range of motion while the patient remains relaxed. The therapist judges the relative stiffness and mobility of the resultant spinal motion and notes any provocation of the patient's pain or symptoms. Although the PA PIVMS test has acceptable reliability when a patient's report of pain is the goal of the test, therapists' judgments of stiffness and mobility are generally unreliable (Matyas and Bach 1985; Maher and Latimer 1992; Maher and Adams 1994; Binkley et al. 1995). A variety of factors account for poor reliability, but therapists' idiosyncrasies in technique and perceptual inaccuracy are certainly part of the problem.

For example, therapists may first have difficulty locating specific bony landmarks (Simmonds and Kumar 1993). Second, once the structure is found they may have difficulty applying an "ideal magnitude" of force to test joint stiffness/mobility. Simmonds and colleagues (1995) found that even under the same condition of joint stiffness, the magnitude of force applied by therapists varies by a factor of 3. Furthermore, other investigators have established and reported that tissue stiffness increases differentially in response to the magnitude and rate of applied force (Lee et al. 1996). So, although clinical authorities assert that tissue stiffness and the "end-feel" of movement are important for diagnosis and treatment progression, it is not clear how this information is obtained in the absence of a standardized, quantified test technique. Maybe this situation is not surprising when other clinical authorities in physical therapy assert that they can "release the liver" and palpate a "craniosacral rhythm."

MEASUREMENT OF FUNCTION

Traditional assessments based on impairment measures are now often complemented with functionally based measures. Functional measures assess at the level of the person rather than the "part." They assess the impact of any impairment and in that respect they are more meaningful to the patient. The assessment methods include patient self-report questionnaires and clinician-measured tasks.

PATIENT SELF-REPORT

The most commonly used self-report questionnaires in physical therapy are the Oswestry Disability Questionnaire (Fairbank et al. 1980), Roland and Morris Questionnaire (Roland and Morris 1983), and the SF-36 (Ware et al. 1993). The SF-36 is a multidimensional measure of general health status, whereas the Oswestry and Roland and Morris questionnaires are specific to patients with LBP. An advantage of questionnaires is that they sample a range of different activities, including self-care, mobility, the performance of household chores, and other work-related activity. They can be relatively quick, simple, and practical to administer and score. They have been widely used and have accepted norms, and clearly they have superior face validity when compared to health professionals' estimates of function. Ideally, objective outcome measures are employed in conjunction with self-report instruments to provide a multimethod assessment of clinical outcome (Klapow et al. 1993).

Self-report of function, however, may not be a valid reflection of a patient's actual functional status if an external reference is unavailable. Deyo and Centor (1986) found the Sickness Impact Profile (SIP) and the Roland and Morris scales to be more closely associated with other self-report measures of functioning than with physical capabilities observed by clinicians. Also, despite its usefulness, self-report of physical function at best assesses only what the patient is conscious or aware of. Persons have reporting biases, are likely to react to situational demands, and vary in their memory and verbal ability (Craig et al. 1992).

A person's perception and report of activity may not match actual activity. For example, Fordyce and colleagues (1981) demonstrated in 150 chronic pain patients that self-reported pain level was significantly related to self-reported activity limitation, but did not correlate strongly with the level of activity recorded in a patient diary. Sanders (1983) demonstrated a poor correlation of self-report measures of "uptime" (nonreclining) with more objective monitoring of activity using mechanical recording devices. However, this inaccuracy of reporting is not purposeful exaggeration of the problem. It has been shown that health care practitioners as well as patients also have difficulties with judgments of distance and time, as is reported in the following studies.

Sharrack and Hughes (1997) asked 100 physicians and 100 patients to estimate the dimensions of a hospital ward and the distances between five familiar sites. These estimates differed up to 14.6-fold from the measured distance, and the maximum estimates were up to 62.5 times greater than the minimum estimates. Time also is not easily estimated, and people find it difficult to say how long it took them to perform an activity or to predict how long it will take them. These findings have implications for concurrent validity of self-report measures of function.

PHYSICAL MEASUREMENT

A useful approach to determining function in general clinical practice involves the use of a range of standardized tests of physical function that essentially sample the construct. The tests must be simple, everyday tasks that are easy for the patient to perform so that motor learning is minimized. They must be easy to teach to patients, and easy to measure and interpret. In the absence of validated physical function measures, researchers have used other apparently related measures such as pain behavior observation (Romano et al. 1992).

Useful clinical tests should require minimal equipment and include tasks that are fundamental to day-to-day activity and are compromised by the patient's problem. Myriad activities can be sampled (e.g., lifting, bending, reaching, walking, rising from sitting, and picking up small or large objects). The tests can be measured using the time taken to complete the set task, or the distance walked or reached in the set time; both measures provide quantitative interval data. Depending on the patient's problem and on the research or clinical question, patients can be tested on one key task or on a battery of tasks.

Common sense and scientific sense are fundamental to the process. Collin and colleagues (1992) found a 10-meter walk useful for assessing function in lower limb amputees. Ringsberg and colleagues (1993) used a 30-m speed walk test to assess women with Colles wrist fractures, but not surprisingly, found this walk test unable to distinguish between those with and without fractures. From their results, we could conclude that the patients have no significant functional limitation (because they do not walk on their hands), that the affect of a Colles fracture is specific to the upper limb, or that the test is insufficiently sensitive to identify reasons for falling.

Nevertheless, walking is fundamental to function and so is a useful indicator of function in many (but not all) patient groups. The 12-minute walk was used first as a measure of function in subjects with obstructive respiratory disease (McGavin et al. 1976). However, Butland et al. (1982) found the 6-minute walk to be equally discriminative and time saving. Price and colleagues (1988) used a 5-minute walking test to evaluate patients with arthritis. Simmonds and colleagues have used a 5-minute distance walk to assess function in patients with LBP and those with cancer (Simmonds et al. 1998b; Simmonds et al. in press).

Some investigators have employed quite challenging tests of function. For example, Fan et al. (1998) used the Canada Fitness Award 50-m run to test patients with juvenile rheumatoid arthritis (Fan et al. 1998). Goh and Boyle (1997) used the 6-m and 12-m timed hop, crossover hop, and stairs hop tests to evaluating function at long-term follow-up on patients following reconstruction of the anterior cruciate ligament of the knee (Goh and Boyle 1997).

Less challenging tasks are used for testing function in the elderly and in populations of patients with rheumatoid arthritis, osteoarthritis, cancer, LBP, and chronic pain. The tasks have included distance walks, sit-to-stand, timed up-and-go, reaching, hand grip, fastening buttons, tying belts, and putting on socks. All the examples listed have demonstrated good reliability (Spiegel et al. 1987; Podsiadlo and Richardson 1991; Pincus and Callahan 1992; Harding et al. 1994a; Simmonds et al. 1998b, in press). The simplicity of the tests with respect to patient performance and clinician measurement obviously contribute to the consistently high levels of reliability.

For example, Harding and colleagues (1994) tested a battery of simple physical tests in 451 patients with heterogeneous pain problems attending a multidisciplinary pain management center. They established inter-rater and test-retest reliability and some validity, including a 10-minute walk test, a 2-minute stair climb, and a 2-minute sit-to-stand task. Reliability coefficients were $r = 0.9$, 0.9 and 0.8, respectively.

Simmonds and colleagues (1998) developed, tested, and refined a comprehensive but simple battery of performance tests to complement the assessment of patients with LBP. It is known that most persons with LBP have difficulty withstanding spinal loads (compressive and shear), and velocity and acceleration of motion are generally slower compared to persons who are pain free (Marras et al. 1995; Rudy et al. 1995; Simmonds and Claveau 1997). Therefore, performance on the task battery is generally measured by how quickly a task can be performed or how far a subject can reach forward (an indirect measure of spinal load). The timed tasks include repeated trunk bending, sit-to-stand, and 50-foot (~15-m) speed walk; the distance tasks include a 5-minute walk and distance in reaching forward while holding a 10-lb (4.6-kg) weight.

All measures have excellent inter-rater reliability. Intraclass correlation coefficients ($ICC_{1,1}$) were all equal to or greater than 0.95. Face validity, convergent, discriminant, and predictive validity have also been established (Simmonds et al. 1997, 1998a,b). In 66 patients with LBP, physical performance measures were excellent predictors of disability ($R^2 = 0.61$) compared to psychosocial factors ($R^2 = 0.59$) and impairment factors ($R^2 = 0.47$) (Simmonds et al. 1998a).

A person's performance on this or any task battery will be influenced by numerous factors. Studies have examined the influence of gender and pain location. Novy et al. (1999) compared the performance of men and women with and without LBP. Using a discriminant function analysis, she found that four groups of subjects performed differently in two major ways. The first difference, irrespective of gender, was that the healthy control subjects outperformed the patients with LBP on tasks that involved trunk control under heavy or quickly changing loads on the spine (sit-to-stand, repeated trunk flexion, Sorenson fatigue test, 50-foot speed walk). Healthy men outperformed healthy women, LBP men, and LBP women, respectively. The second difference, irrespective of patient or nonpatient status, was that men outperformed women on tasks involving anthropometric features of limb length (distance walk and loaded reach). Healthy men outperformed LBP men, healthy women, and LBP women, in that order.

In regard to pain location, subjects with radiating or referred leg pain were outperformed by subjects with back pain on the 50-foot speed walk, repeated trunk flexion, 360° rollover, and the loaded reach. The study found no performance difference between groups on the 5-minute walk, sit-to-stand, or Sorenson test. Subjects with leg pain appear to have much greater difficulties with tasks that involved high-compressive spinal loads or high-velocity movements.

Responsiveness of the task battery is moderate (Simmonds et al. 1999). Twenty-eight patients attending physical therapy were assessed initially and after 4–6 weeks of therapy. Standardized response means (SRM) of the 5-minute distance walk, loaded reach, and timed repeated flexion task were 0.81, 0.73, and 0.73, respectively. The SRM of the Roland and Morris Questionnaire was 0.81.

Finally, examination of the associations among patient self-report questionnaire items and the performance of similar tasks reveals moderate correlations (r = 0.28–0.5) (Lee et al. 1998). This finding suggests that function should be assessed using both patient self-report of ability and clinician-measured ability. These methods are complementary, and each taps a slightly different aspect of physical performance.

REINTERPRETATION OF THE MEANING OF THE MEASURES

Although chronic disabling MSP has been recognized and managed as a biopsychosocial problem for many years in tertiary care facilities, this is a relatively new concept for primary care practitioners who are not pain specialists. Therapists in outpatient clinics do not generally use operant or cognitive-behavioral approaches to pain management, do not assess psychosocial factors, and acknowledge having limited knowledge and interest in dealing with patients with chronic pain (Woolf et al. 1991).

Clinical assessments based on the biopsychosocial model have been recommended for use in primary care, but it is not clear what constitutes such an assessment. Neither is it clear whether a new assessment measure, a reinterpretation of an impairment measure, or a combination of both is required.

For example, although a standard impairment measurement such as range of motion appears to emphasize the "bio" aspect of the model, the measure is not free from the influence of psychological factors such as depressed mood or anxiety. Also, given that impairment measures are not performed in a vacuum, free of social context and social meaning, these social factors are likely to influence the results. Similarly, measures of depressed mood or anxiety may emphasize psychological aspects of the model, but again, the verbalization of those beliefs in a social (e.g., therapeutic) context means that the psychological assessment is susceptible to shaping by that context.

Any component of a physical therapy assessment taps into this complex biopsychosocial web of inter-related and multiple dimensions.

Although traditional diagnostic measures in fact have minimal diagnostic value, they can nevertheless provide different information. For example, measures of active range of motion provide little information about the patient's ability to function, but they do test the patient's willingness to move, and perhaps their fears or their self-efficacy beliefs about moving. For example, Estlander et al. (1994) investigated the role of self-efficacy in isokinetic performance in patients with LBP. They found that task performance was predicted by general self-efficacy beliefs about their ability to endure physical activity. Council et al. (1988) looked at a task-specific self-efficacy measure to assess its role in predicting range of lumbar flexion in LBP subjects. They demonstrated that LBP subjects' perceptions of their range of motion, rated on a cartoon representing increasing ranges of lumbar flexion, correlated highly with the measured range of motion. Of course, this finding may simply imply that patients are fairly accurate in their estimations of their ability. Lackner et al. (1996) found that subjects were able to accurately rate their ability to perform a wide variety of work-oriented tasks. In a group of subjects with LBP, they found that subjects' assessment of their physical capacity for specific tasks was highly predictive of their subsequent physical performance.

Repeatability of physical performance has been used as a measure of patients' sincerity of effort (Lechner et al. 1998). Sincerity of effort is a clinical question that stems from mistrust. Some investigators have suggested that variability in performance implies that the patients exert a submaximal effort or are "faking." Initial speculations about variability in performance were based on a study of movement in pain-free normal subjects, but recent work does not support this notion (Newton et al. 1993). Nevertheless, the search for a physical performance "lie detector" remains a popular quest. Simmonds and colleagues (1998b) have found that when compared to pain-free subjects, patients consistently have more performance variability in any task that requires repeated movements (e.g., repeated lumbar flexion and repeated sit-to-stand). This result may be due to physiological warm-up, increasing confidence that the movement will not cause injury, alteration in pain expectation when prediction does not match experience (Murphy et al. 1997), or a change in pain perception that may be due to a change in afferent (kinesthetic) input. What is significant is that variability in performance during a repeated movement is a characteristic of the task itself and not an indication of questionable patient motivation.

Letham et al. (1983) posited a "fear avoidance" model of exaggerated pain perception to explain the development of chronic pain syndrome and prolonged disability. In this quite simple model, the patients' responses to pain can be classified as confrontation or avoidance. This model implies that patients who avoid activity for fear of increased pain not only report more pain, but are much more likely to develop chronic incapacity. In contrast, patients who confront the pain "work through" the pain to maintain function and reduce disability. This model has been expanded to incorporate a fear of movement/(re)injury model (Vlaeyen et al. 1995) in which the pain patient develops a fear of movement, or kinesiophobia, partly arising from a mistaken fear of vulnerability to injury or reinjury (Kori et al. 1990). In extreme cases this can develop into a phobic response to physically challenging activities.

PSYCHOSOCIAL SCREENING MEASURES

The last decade and a half has seen increasing health care, litigation, and social costs associated with MSP such as low back pain, whiplash injury, and repetitive strain injuries. The increase in health care and social care costs due to disability has led to major reviews of the problem and the publication of clinical guidelines (Spitzer et al. 1987, 1995; Bigos et al. 1994; CSAG 1994; Fordyce 1995; Kendall et al. 1997).

Key guidelines in these reports include the identification of persons who require prompt medical attention (those with so-called "Red Flags") and those at risk for chronic incapacity (so-called "Yellow Flags") (Kendall et al. 1997). Recommendations with regard to the latter include conducting a psychosocial assessment between 4 and 12 weeks after onset in patients who fail to respond to routine therapy and reassurance. An assessment that reveals the presence of specific psychosocial factors (e.g., depressed mood, fear of pain and reinjury, somatic anxiety, misunderstandings about the pain, work dissatisfaction, medicolegal compensation, and low educational level) is an indication that recovery may be prolonged or outcome poor if steps are not taken to address these issues. An important point is that at no time have these reports ever suggested that the presence of psychosocial factors implies a question about the veracity of a patient's condition. The Clinical Standards Advisory Group (1994, p. 61) in the United Kingdom suggests that a biopsychosocial assessment may "be carried out by the patient's doctor or therapist." As noted earlier, numerous psychosocial factors potentially influence disability, and a plethora of questionnaires and screening tools are available. After a review of the evidence, Watson and Kendall (in press) have proposed guidelines for the use of "Yellow Flag" screening and offer suggestions for further research and development in this area. They advocate a combined approach using both simple screening tools and a clinical interview. Although the relative predictive value of psychosocial factors on outcome varies according to health care setting, duration of conditions, and treatment intervention, they suggest that the literature provides ample evidence to demonstrate the need to integrate psychosocial assessment into physical therapy practice.

SUMMARY AND RECOMMENDATIONS

MSP is a complex multidimensional (biopsychosocial) problem. Appropriate and effective management is predicated on an adequate conceptualization of the problem and adequate assessment of the person with the problem. Therefore, assessment of the patient with MSP must be expanded to encompass the biomedical, psychological, and sociological components of the problem. Assessment tests must be psychometrically sound, well understood, and meaningful to patient and practitioner. The biomedical component of the assessment should identify and guide the physical therapeutic focus of treatment. The psychosocial assessment should be complementary and inform the therapist of the *framework* in which treatment should be set so as to lead to more rational, individually focused treatment. Common sense suggests that poor physical performance due primarily to a patient's fear of activity should be managed quite differently than poor physical performance due to restricted range of motion.

ACKNOWLEDGMENTS

This work was supported by a NIH EARDA Pilot Project grant and a Texas Physical Therapy Education and Research Foundation grant to M.J. Simmonds.

REFERENCES

Battie MC, Cherkin DC, Dunn R, et al. Managing low back pain: attitudes and treatment preferences of physical therapists. *Phys Ther* 1994; 74:219–226.

Bigos S, Bowyer O, Braen G, et al. *Acute Low Back Problems in Adults.* Clinical Practice Guideline No. 14. AHCPR Publication No. 95-0642. Rockville, MD: Agency for Health Care Policy and Research, Public Health Service, U.S. Department of Health and Human Services, December 1994.

Binkley J, Stratford P, Gill C. Inter-rater reliability of lumbar accessory motion mobility testing. *Phys Ther* 1995; 75:786–795.

Boline PD, Keating JC, Haas M, et al. Interexaminer reliability and discriminant validity of inclinometric measurement of lumbar rotation in chronic low-back pain patients and subjects without low-back pain. *Spine* 1992; 17:335–338.

Breum J, Wiberg J, Bolton JE. Reliability and concurrent validity of the BROM 11 for measuring lumbar mobility. *J Manipulative Physiol Ther* 1995; 18:497–502.

Butland RJA, Pang J, Gross ER, Woodcock AA, Geddes DM. Two-, six-, and 12-minute walking tests in respiratory disease. *BMJ* 1982; 284:1607–1608.

Campbell SK. Measurement and technical skills-neglected aspects of research education. *Phys Ther* 1981; 61:523.

Cats-Baril WL, Frymoyer JW. In: Frymoyer JW (Ed), *The Economics of Spinal Disorders*. New York: Raven Press, 1991, pp 85–105.

Cherkin DC, Deyo RA, Wheeler K, et al. Physician views about treating low back pain. The results of a national survey. *Spine* 1995; 20:1–10.

Collin C, Wade DT, Cochrane GM. Functional outcome of lower limb amputees with peripheral vascular disease. *Clin Rehabil* 1992; 6:13–21.

CSAG (Clinical Standards Advisory Group). *Back Pain: Report of a CSAG Committee on Back Pain*. London: HMSO, 1994.

Council JR, Ahern DK, Follick MJ, Kline CL. Expectancies and functional impairment in chronic low back pain. *Pain* 1988; 33:323–331.

Craig KD, Prkachin KM, Grunau RVE. The facial expression of pain. In: Turk DC, Melzack R (Eds). *Handbook of Pain Assessment*. Guilford Press, 1992, pp 257–276.

Cyriax J. *Textbook of Orthopaedic Medicine, Diagnosis of Soft Tissue Lesions,* 8th ed. London: Bailliere Tindall, 1983.

Deyo RA. Practice variations, treatment fads, rising disability. Do we need a new clinical research paradigm? *Spine* 1993; 18:2153–2162.

Deyo RA, Centor RM. Assessing the responsiveness of functional scales to clinical change: an analogy to diagnostic test performance. *J Chron Dis* 1986; 39(11):897–906.

Estlander AM, Vanharanta H, Moneta GB, Kaivanto K. Anthropometric variables, self-efficacy beliefs and pain and disability ratings on he isokinetic performance of low back pain patients. *Spine* 1994; 19:941–947.

Fairbank JCT, Couper J, Davies JB, O'Brien JP. The Oswestry low back pain disability questionnaire. *Physiotherapy* 1980; 66:271–273.

Fan JS-W. Wessel J. Ellsworth J. The relationship between strength and function in females with juvenile rheumatoid arthritis. *J Rheumatol* 1998; 25:1399–1405.

Feine JS, Lund JP. An assessment of the efficacy of physical therapy and physical modalities for the control of chronic musculoskeletal pain. *Pain* 1997; 71:5–23.

Fordyce WE (Ed). *Back Pain in the Workplace: Management of Disability in Nonspecific Conditions*. Report of the IASP Task Force on Pain in the Workplace. Seattle: IASP Press, 1995.

Fordyce W, McMahon R, Rainwater G, et al. Pain complaints—exercise performance relationship in chronic pain. *Pain* 1981; 10:311–321.

Frese E, Brown M, Norton BJ. Clinical reliability of manual muscle testing: middle trapezius and gluteus medius muscles. *Phys Ther* 1987; 67:1072–1076.

Fritz JM, Delitto A, Erhard RE, et al. An examination of the selective tissue tension scheme, with evidence for the concept of a capsular pattern of the knee. *Phys Ther* 1998; 78:1046–1056.

Gatchel RJ, Polatin PB, Mayer TG. The dominant role of psychosocial risk factors in the development of chronic low back pain disability. *Spine* 1995, 20:2702–2709.

Goh S, Boyle J. Self evaluation and functional testing two to four years post ACL reconstruction. *Aust J Physiother* 1997; 43:255–262.

Grieve GP. *Mobilization of the Spine,* 4th ed. New York: Churchill Livingstone, 1984.

Harding VR, Williams ACdeC, Richardson PH, et al. The development of a battery of measures for assessing physical functioning of chronic pain patients. *Pain* 1994; 58:367–375.

Hayes KW, Petersen C, Falconer J. An examination of Cyriax's Passive Motion Tests with patients having osteoarthritis of the knee. *Phys Ther* 1994; 74:697–707.

Jette AM, Smith K, Haley SM, Davis KD. Physical therapy episodes of care for patients with low back pain. *Phys Ther* 1994; 74:101–115.

Kendall NAS, Linton SJ, Main CJ. *Guide to Assessing Psychosocial Yellow Flags in Acute Low Back Pain: Risk Factors for Long-Term Disability and Work Loss.* Wellington, New Zealand: Accident Rehabilitation and Compensation Insurance Corporation of New Zealand, and the National Health Committee, Ministry of Health, 1997.

Klapow JC, Slater MA, Patterson TL, et al. An empirical evaluation of multidimensional clinical outcome in chronic low back pain patients. *Pain* 1993; 55:107–118.

Koes BW, Bouter LM, Beckerman H, van der Heijden GJMG, Knipschild PG. Physiotherapy exercises and back pain: a blinded review. *BMJ* 1991; 302:1572–1576.

Koes BW, Bouter LM, van Mameren H, et al. Randomized clinical trial of manipulative therapy and physiotherapy for persistent back and neck complaints: results of one year follow-up. *BMJ* 1992; 304:601–605.

Kori SH, Miller RP, Todd DD. Kinesiophobia: a new view of chronic pain behavior. *Pain Manage* 1990; Jan/Feb:35–43.

Lackner JM, Carosella AM, Feuerstein M. Pain expectancies, pain and functional self-efficacy expectancies as determinants of disability in patients with chronic low back disorders. *J Consult Clin Psychol* 1996; 64,1:212–220.

Lechner DE, Bradbury SF, Bradley LA. Detecting sincerity of effort: a summary of methods and approaches. *Phys Ther* 1998; 78:867–888.

Lee DG, Walsh MC. *A Workbook of Manual Therapy Techniques for the Vertebral Column and Pelvic Girdle,* 2nd ed. Altona, Manitoba: Friesen, 1996.

Lee M, Steven G, Crosbie J, Feggs J. Towards a theory of lumbar mobilisation—the relationship between applied force and movements of the spine. *Manual Ther* 1996; 2:67–75.

Lee CE, Simmonds MJ, Novy DM, Jones S. Functional performance among patients with low back pain—a comparison of self-report and objective measures. *Physiother Canada* 1998; 50:30.

Letham J, Slade PD, Troup JDG, Bentley G. Outline of a fear-avoidance model of exaggerated pain perception. *Behav Res Ther* 1983; 21:401–408.

Levack B, Rassmussen L, Day S, Freeman MAR. Range of movement poor index of hip function. *Acta Orthop Scand* 1988; 59:14–15.

Magee DM. *Orthopedic Physical Assessment,* 2nd ed. Philadelphia: WB Saunders, 1992.

Maher CG, Adams R. Reliability of pain and stiffness assessments in clinical manual lumbar spine examination. *Phys Ther* 1994; 74:801–811.

Maher CG, Latimer J. Pain or resistance—the manual therapists' dilemma. *Aust J Physiother* 1992; 38:257–260.

Maher CG, Simmonds M, Adams R. Therapists' conceptualization and characterization of the clinical concert of spinal stiffness. *Phys Ther* 1998; 78:289–300.

Main CJ, Watson PJ. Screening for patients at risk of developing chronic incapacity. *J Occup Rehab* 1995; 5:207–217.

Main CJ. Watson PJ. Psychological aspects of pain. *Manual Ther* 1999; 4:203–215.

Marras WS, Parnianpour M, Ferguson SA, et al. The classification of anatomic- and symptom-based low back disorders using motion measure models. *Spine* 1995; 20:2531–2546.

Matyas T, Bach T. The reliability of selected techniques in clinical arthrometrics. *Aust J Physiother* 1985; 31:175–199.

McGavin CR, Gupta SP, McHardy GJR. Twelve-minute walking test for assessing disability in chronic bronchitis. *BMJ* 1976; 1:822–823.

Mellin GL. Correlations of spinal mobility with degree of chronic low back pain after correction for age and anthropometric factors. *Spine* 1987; 12:464–468.

Moreland J, Finch E, Stratford P, et al. Interrater reliability of six tests of trunk muscle function and endurance. *J Orthop Sports Phys Ther* 1997; 26:200–208.

Mooney V, Andersson GBJ, Pope MH. Discussion of quantitative functional muscle testing. In: Weinstein JN (Ed). *Clinical Efficacy and Outcome in the Diagnosis and Treatment of Low Back Pain.* New York: Raven Press, 1992, pp 115–116.

Murphy D, Lindsay S, Williams ACdeC. Chronic low back pain: predictions of pain and relationship to anxiety and avoidance. *Behav Res Ther* 1997; 35:231–238.

Nagi SZ. Disability concepts revisited: implications for prevention. In: Pope AM, Tarlov AR (Eds). *Disability in America: Toward a National Agenda for Prevention.* Washington, DC: Division of Health Promotion and Disease Prevention, Institute of Medicine, National Academy Press, 1991, pp 309–327.

Newton M, Thow M, Somerville D, Henderson I, Waddell G. Trunk testing with iso-machines: Part 2. Experimental evaluation of the Cybex II back testing system in normal subjects and patients with chronic back pain. *Spine* 1993; 18:812–824.

Nitschke JE, Nattrass CL, Disler PB, et al. Reliability of the American Medical Association Guides' Model for measuring spinal range of motion. *Spine* 1999; 24:262–268.

Novy DM, Simmonds MJ, Olson SL, Lee CE, Jones SC. Physical performance: differences in men and women with and without low back pain. *Arch Phys Med Rehabil* 1999; 80:195–198.

Pellecchia GL, Paolino J, Connell J. Intertester reliability of the Cyriax Evaluation in assessing patients with shoulder pain. *J Orthop Sports Phys Ther* 1996; 23:34–38.

Pincus T. Callahan LF. Rheumatology function tests: grip strength, walking time, button test and questionnaires document and predict long term morbidity and mortality in rheumatoid arthritis. *J Rheumatol* 1992; 19:1051–1057.

Podsiadlo D, Richardson S. The timed "up and go": a test of basic functional mobility for frail elderly persons. *J Am Ger Soc* 1991; 39:142–148.

Pope MH. A critical evaluation of functional muscle testing. In: Weinstein JN (Ed). *Clinical Efficacy and Outcome in the Diagnosis and Treatment of Low Back Pain.* New York: Raven Press, 1992, pp 101–113.

Price LG, Hewett JE, Kay DR, Minor MA. Five-minute walking test of aerobic fitness for people with arthritis. *Arthritis Care Res* 1988; 1:33–37.

Ringsberg K, Johnell O, Obrant K. Balance and speed of walking of women with Colles' fractures. *Physiotherapy* 1993; 79:689–692.

Roland M, Morris R. A study of the natural history of back pain. Part 1: development of a reliable and sensitive measure of disability in low-back pain. *Spine* 1983; 8:141–144.

Romano JM, Turner JA, Jensen MP. The chronic illness problem inventory as a measure of dysfunction in chronic pain patients. *Pain* 1992; 49:71–75.

Rondinelli R, Murphy J, Esler A, et al. Estimation of normal lumbar flexion with surface inclinometry: a comparison of three methods. *Am J Phys Med Rehabil* 1992; 71:219–224.

Rothstein JM. Measurement and clinical practice: theory and application. In: Rothstein JM (Ed). *Measurement in Physical Therapy.* New York: Churchill Livingstone, 1985, pp 1–46.

Rudy TE, Boston R, Lieber SJ, Kubinski JA, Delitto A. Body motion patterns during a novel repetitive wheel-rotation task. A comparative study of healthy subjects and patients with low back pain. *Spine* 1995; 20:2547–2554.

Sanders SH. Automated versus self-monitoring of up-time in chronic low-back pain patients: a comparative study. *Pain* 1983; 15:399–405.

Saur PM, Ensink FM, Frese K, et al. Lumbar range of motion: reliability and validity of the inclinometer technique in the clinical measurement of trunk flexibility. *Spine* 1996; 21:1332–1328.

Sharrack B, Hughes RAC. Reliability of distance estimation by doctors and patients: cross sectional study. BMJ 1997; 315:1652–1654.

Simmonds MJ, Claveau Y. Measures of pain and physical function in patients with low back pain. *Physiother Theory Pract* 1997; 13:53–65.

Simmonds MJ, Kumar S. Location of body structures by palpation: a reliability study. *Int J Ind Ergonomics* 1993; 11:145–151.

Simmonds M, Kumar S, Lechelt E. Use of a spinal model to quantify the forces and motion that occur during therapists' tests of spinal motion. *Phys Ther* 1995; 75:212–222.

Simmonds MJ, Kumar S, Lechelt E. Psychosocial factors in disabling low back pain: causes or consequences? *Disabil Rehabil* 1996; 18(4):161–168.

Simmonds MJ, Olson SL, Novy DM, et al. Classification of subjects with and without low back pain using novel tasks of physical performance. 16th Annual Scientific Meeting of the American Pain Society, New Orleans, LA, October 23–26, 1997.

Simmonds MJ, Olson S, Novy DM, Jones SC. *Disability Prediction in Patients with Back Pain Using Performance Based Models.* North American Spine Society/American Pain Society Meeting, Charlston, SC, April 1998.

Simmonds MJ, Olson SL, Jones SC, et al. Psychometric characteristics and clinical usefulness of physical performance tests in patients with low back pain. *Spine* 1998; 23:2412–2421.

Simmonds MJ, Lee CE, Jones S. *Pain Distribution and Physical Function in Patients with Low Back Pain.* 13th International Congress of the World Confederation for Physical Therapy, Yokohama, Japan, May 23–28, 1999.

Simmonds MJ, Felderman J, Massey PR, et al. Reliability and validity of physical performance tests for patients with cancer. *Phys Ther Abstract;* in press.

Speigel JS, Paulus HE, Ward NB, et al. What are we measuring? An examination of walk time and grip strength. *J Rheumatol* 1987; 14:80–86.

Spitzer WO, LeBlanc FE, Dupuis M, et al. Scientific approach to the assessment and management of activity-related spinal disorders: a monograph for clinicians. Report of the Quebec Task Force on Spinal Disorders. *Spine* 1987; 12:S4–S59.

Spitzer WO, Skovron ML, Salmi LR, et al. Scientific monograph of the Quebec Task Force on Whiplash-Associated Disorders: redefining "whiplash" and its management. *Spine* 1995; 20:S1–S73.

Tortensen TA. The physical therapy approach. In: J.W. Frymoyer (Ed), *The Adult Spine: Principles and Practice,* 2nd ed. Philadelphia: Lippencott-Raven, 1997, pp 1797–1804.

Turk DC. The role of demographic and psychosocial factors in transition from acute to chronic pain. In: Jensen TS, Turner JA, Wiesenfeld-Hallin Z. (Eds). *Proceedings of the 8th World Congress on Pain,* Progress in Pain Research and Management, Vol. 8. IASP Press, Seattle, 1997, pp 185–213.

Vlaeyen JWS, Kole-Snijders AMJ, Schuerman JA, Goenman NH, van Eek H. Fear of movement/(re)injury in chronic low back pain and its relation to behavioural performance. *Pain* 1995; 62:363–372.

Von Korff M. Perspectives on management of back pain in primary care. In: Gebhart GF, Hammond DL, Jensen TS (Eds). *Proceedings of the 7th World Congress on Pain,* Progress in Pain Research and Management, Vol. 2. Seattle: IASP Press, 1994, pp 97–110.

Von Korff M, Dworkin SF, LeResche L, Kluger A. An epidemiologic comparison of pain complaints. *Pain* 1988; 32:173–183.

Waddell G. A new clinical model for the treatment of low back pain. *Spine* 1987; 12:632–644.

Waddell G. The clinical course of back pain. In: *The Back Pain Revolution.* Edinburgh: Churchill Livingstone, 1998, pp 103–117.

Watson PJ. Psychosocial predictors of outcome from low back pain. In: Gifford L (Ed). *Topical Issues in Pain,* Vol. 2. Falmouth: NOI Press, in press.

Watson PJ, Kendall NAS. The assessment of psychosocial Yellow Flags in physiotherapy practice. In: Grifford L (Ed). *Topics in Pain,* Vol. 1. Falmouth: NOI Press, in press.

Ware J, Snow K, Kosinski M, Gandek B. *SF-36 Health Survey. Manual and Interpretation Guide.* Boston, MA: The Health Institute, New England Medical Center, 1993.

Williams MM, Grant RN, Main CJ. The Distress Risk *Assessment Method (DRAM) as a Predictor of Outcome in Chronically Disabled Workers Attending a Physical Rehabilitation Programme.* Abstracts, International Society for the Study of the Lumbar Spine, Helsinki, Finland, 1995, p 46.

Williams R, Goldsmith GH, Minuk T. Validity of the Double Inclinometer Method for measuring lumbar flexion. *Physiother Can* 1998; 50:147–152.

Woolf M S, Michel T, Krebs DE, Watts NT. Chronic pain-assessment of orthopedic physical therapists' knowledge and attitudes. *Phys Ther* 1991; 71:207–213.

World Health Organization. *World Health Organization International Classification of Impairments, Disabilities and Handicaps.* Geneva: World Health Organization, 1980.

Correspondence to: Maureen J. Simmonds, PT, PhD, Associate Professor, School of Physical Therapy, Texas Woman's University, 1130 MD Anderson Boulevard, Houston, TX 77478, USA. Tel: 713-794-2088; Fax: 713-794-2; email: HF_Simmonds@twu.edu.

Proceedings of the 9th World Congress on Pain,
Progress in Pain Research and Management,
Vol. 16, edited by M. Devor, M.C. Rowbotham, and
Z. Wiesenfeld-Hallin, IASP Press, Seattle, © 2000.

97

Differences between Patients with Fibromyalgia and Patients with Chronic Musculoskeletal Pain

Giancarlo Carli,[a] Anna Lisa Suman,[a] Flavio Badii,[b]
Valeria Bachiocco,[d] Gianpaolo Di Piazza,[c]
Giovanni Biasi,[b] Paolo Castrogiovanni,[c]
and Roberto Marcolongo[b]

Institutes of [a]Human Physiology and [b]Rheumatology, and [c]Division of Psychiatry, University of Siena, Siena, Italy; and [d]Institute of Anesthesiology, University of Bologna, Bologna, Italy

The 1990 American College of Rheumatology (ACR) classification criteria for fibromyalgia specify (Wolfe et al. 1990) the presence of widespread pain for more than 3 months and pain that can be elicited by manual pressure of approximately 4 kg/cm^2 at 11 or more defined tender points. The most characteristic symptoms of fibromyalgia are fatigue, sleep disturbance, and morning stiffness. Many patients also display diffuse hyperalgesia to mechanical, thermal, and chemical stimuli applied to skin or muscles and psychological and psychiatric disturbances (Winfield 1999). More recently, however, it has emerged (Croft et al. 1996; Wolfe 1997) that not only tender points but also other clinical aspects of musculoskeletal pain syndromes represent a continuum, with fibromyalgia producing the most severe clinical manifestations.

Our study investigated the possible differences in both sensitivity to experimental nociceptive stimuli and psychological factors between the patients with diffuse musculoskeletal pain who comply with the ACR tender point criteria for fibromyalgia (FS) and the patients who do not (nFS).

METHODS

Patients (n = 75; 3 males and 72 females) were recruited from the rheumatology clinic based on the presence of widespread pain for at least 3 months (Wolfe et al. 1990) after clinical examinations that excluded other rheumatic or pathological disorders. The protocol consisted in a single session during which the patients completed self-administered questionnaires and submitted to psychophysical tests. The session started with a detailed epidemiological-anamnestic questionnaire that also provided information about pain: pain intensity was expressed by a visual analogue scale (VAS) of 0–100, both at the onset of the disorder and presently; pain localization and extension were indicated by the pain drawings made by the patient (Margolis et al. 1986). Two additional questionnaires were administered: the SCL-90R (Symptom Check List; Derogatis 1977) and STAI-Y1 and STAI-Y2 (State Trait Anxiety Inventory; Spielberger 1983).

Superficial mechanoceptive function was assessed on the glabrous skin of the third phalanx of the second finger of the dominant hand using von Frey filaments (Aesthesiometer; Stolting Co.) according to the method of limits (Weinstein 1962). Electrocutaneous sensitivity was assessed by percutaneous stimulation (two silver electrodes, each 1 cm^2, applied to the skin 2 cm apart, over the external retromalleolar pathway of the sural nerve). Stimulation involved a volley of 10-ms rectangular pulses, delivered at 30–60 second intervals, at a strength varying from 0 to 20 mA. To determine pain threshold and tolerance, we applied stimuli in an ascending and descending order of magnitude in steps of 0.4 mA.

Pressure pain thresholds were assessed with a pressure algometer (foot plate surface 1.57 cm^2, scale range 0–5 kg) applied to the 18 defining tender points of Wolfe et al. (1990) and to 10 control sites (five pairs): mid-point of biceps brachii, distal third of the ventral forearm, thenar eminence, lower outer quadrants of buttocks, and upper third of the lateral aspect of quadriceps femoris. The pressure gauge was advanced at a rate of approximately 1 kg of pressure per second and arrested when the patient declared that the pressure pain level had been reached.

To produce ischemic pain we used both the cold pressor test (Wolf and Hardy 1941) and the submaximal effort tourniquet (Smith et al. 1966). In both instances the patients indicated the occurrence of pain threshold and pain tolerance. Heat and cold pain thresholds were determined with a thermal stimulator (TSA 2001 Thermal Sensory Analyzer). Four cold and four heat stimuli were delivered at 1.5°C/second starting from 32°C, and the patient was asked to press a button to interrupt the stimulus.

Table I
Outcome of epidemiological, Symptom Check List (SCL-90), and State Trait Anxiety Inventory (STAI) questionnaires and psychophysical measures in fibromyalgia (FS) and nonfibromyalgia (nFS) patients (mean ± SD)

	FS	nFS	*P* (*t* test)
Age (years)	41.64 ± 9.78	49.66 ± 12.61	–
Fatigue (0–100)	63.36 ± 33.92	59.56 ± 34.67	–
Stiffness (0–100)	57.40 ± 30.94	56.56 ± 29.83	–
Patients with sleep disturbance (%)	75.00	43.50	0.02 (χ^2)
Pain duration (months)	104.21 ± 96.95	144.0 ± 116.56	–
Pain area (%)	47.72 ± 19.38	41.61 ± 18.96	–
Vas 0–100 (onset)	53.36 ± 27.77	56.30 ± 25.01	–
Vas 0–100 (present)	69.42 ± 22.44	59.13 ± 30.06	–
von Frey (g/mm^2)	403.61 ± 212.92	386.79 ± 214.7	–
No. positive tender points	15.57 ± 2.15	6.47 ± 3.05	0.001
Threshold positive tender points (kg/cm^2)	2.06 ± 0.57	2.76 ± 0.38	0.001
Threshold positive controls (kg/cm^2)	2.24 ± 0.62	2.70 ± 0.62	0.004
Electrocutaneous threshold (μA)	5.75 ± 3.33	6.59 ± 3.09	–
Electrocutaneous tolerance (μA)	7.91 ± 4.41	9.30 ± 3.79	–
Cold pressure threshold (s)	10.57 ± 5.71	11.48 ± 4.73	–
Cold pressure tolerance (s)	24.41 ±17.71	23.33 ± 10.58	–
Tourniquet threshold (s)	84.50 ± 185.73	83.83 ± 174.97	–
Tourniquet tolerance (s)	216.29 ± 270.26	239.83 ± 260.51	–
Heat pain threshold (°C)	42.90 ± 3.76	43.68 ± 2.93	–
Cold pain threshold (°C)	4.44 ± 8.09	3.96 ± 4.99	–
SCL-90 depression	1.29 ± 0.73	0.82 ± 0.56	0.01
SCL-90 somatization	1.77 ± 0.79	1.25 ± 0.52	0.007
SCL-90 obsession	1.35 ± 0.76	0.95 ± 0.63	0.04
STAI-Y1	43.05 ± 9.38	36.9 ± 8.82	0.01
STAI-Y2	47.36 ± 9.42	42.19 ± 9.48	0.03

RESULTS

All patients referred diffuse musculoskeletal pain that was present at the time of the examination. However only 52/75 patients reached the tender point criteria for fibromyalgia (Wolfe et al. 1990). Table I shows the similarities and differences between the fibromyalgia (FS) and nonfibromyalgia (nFS) patients. The two patient populations did not differ for age, fatigue and morning stiffness, pain duration and extension, and pain intensity at onset. Pearson correlation coefficient showed a negative relationship (N =

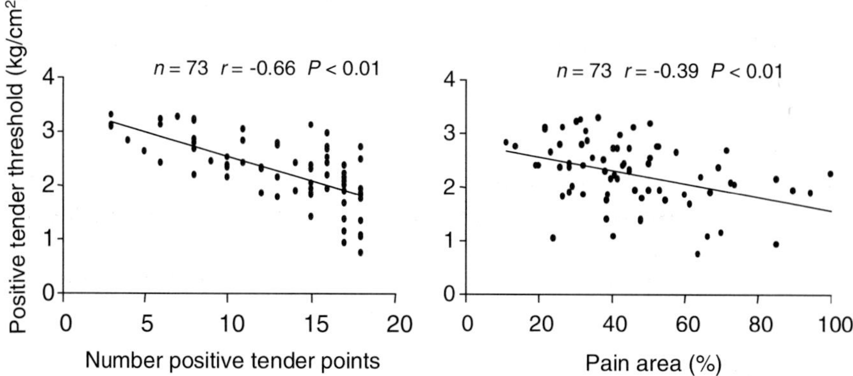

Fig. 1. Relationship between the threshold of positive tender points and the number of tender points (left) and the percentage of body area with pain (right) in fibromyalgia (FS) and nonfibromyalgia (nFS) patients. Positive tender point: a tender point in which the pain threshold to pressure stimuli applied at 1 kg/second is below 4 kg/cm^2. Statistical analysis was the Pearson correlation coefficient.

75, $r = -0.36$, $P < 0.005$) between present pain intensity (VAS) and electrocutaneous pain threshold. Although the difference in present pain intensity (VAS) did not reach significance (Table I), there was a strong trend ($P < 0.075$) toward higher values in FS than in nFS patients. The patients displayed similar sensitivity to punctate pressure (von Frey), electrocutaneous and thermal stimuli, and to the cold pressure test and the submaximum tourniquet technique. By definition (ACR criteria), FS had more positive tender points than did nFS. In addition, FS patients displayed a lower pain threshold than did nFS patients, both at positive tender and positive control points (Table I). In FS patients the pain threshold at positive tender points was lower than at positive control points (Student's *t* test, $P < 0.006$). The analy-

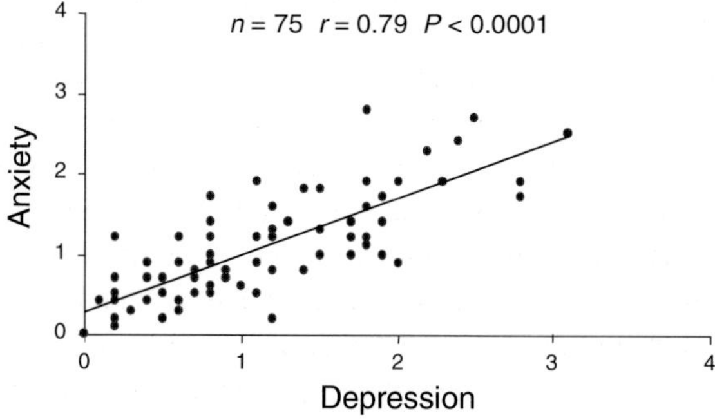

Fig. 2. Relationship between anxiety and depression scores obtained from the SCL-90R questionnaire in FS and nFS patients.

sis of the whole patient population revealed that the pain threshold at the tender points was negatively correlated both with the number of positive tender points (Fig. 1, left) and with the extension of the body pain area (Fig. 1, right).

Analysis of the questionnaires showed a positive relationship between depression and anxiety in the whole patient population (Fig. 2). Depression, somatization, obsession, and anxiety reached higher values in FS than in nFS patients (Table I). In addition, the percentage of patients with sleep disturbance was higher in FS than in nFS patients (Table I).

DISCUSSION

Our study shows that FS patients display higher sensitivity to pressure stimuli at both tender and control points and higher scores in some psychological aspects than do nFS patients.

It has often been reported (Arroyo and Cohen 1993; Lautenbacher et al. 1994; Vecchiet et al. 1994; Kosek et al. 1996) that FS patients display exaggerated responsiveness to somatosensory stimuli. In our patients with diffuse musculoskeletal pain the sensitivity to electrical, thermal, and ischemic stimuli was independent of the number of positive tender points. However, for pressure stimuli, our results confirm the findings that FS patients have a reduced pressure threshold for pain perception at tender and control points (Granges and Littlejohn 1993; Bedsen et al. 1997).In patients with diffuse musculoskeletal pain, their pressure-pain threshold is negatively correlated with the number of positive tender points and the extension of their pain area, and the parameters vary widely. These findings indicate that the tender-point pain threshold is a critical parameter that varies continuously.

Cognitive-behavioral parameters in the pain experience play a central role in the development and maintenance of persistent pain (Violon 1982; Linton 1994). In a recent review Walter et al. (1998) compared FS patients with rheumatoid arthritis (RA) patients. Their findings suggest that in FS patients the severity of the disease, and not the disease itself, results in affective distress: FS patients display higher pain levels, higher depression, and higher anxiety than do RA patients. In addition, Wolfe and Hawley (1999) have reported that fibromyalgia patients appraise medical symptoms and their importance more seriously than do RA patients. We have shown that anxiety and depression are positively related in both FS and nFS patients. In addition, FS patients display higher levels of anxiety, depression, somatization, sleep disturbance and, to a lesser extent, pain intensity than do nFS patients. These findings support the suggestion that fibromyalgia is a clinical syndrome at the severe end of a continuum rather than a well-defined disease syndrome (Croft et al. 1996; Wolfe 1997; Forseth et al. 1999).

In conclusion, our results suggest that the number of tender points and their reactivity to pressure in patients with diffuse musculoskeletal pain provide a good indication of the severity of the disease; maximum values of these parameters are observed in patients complying with the ACR criteria for fibromyalgia.

ACKNOWLEDGMENTS

This research was supported by Università degli Studi di Siena grants "Progetto di Ricerca 60% 1998" and "Piano di Ateneo per la Ricerca 1999." Dr. Anna Lisa Suman was the recipient of a contract "Fondi di Qualita 1996," University of Siena, Italy.

REFERENCES

Arroyo JF, Cohen ML. Abnormal responses to electrocutaneous stimulation in fibromyalgia. *J Rheumatol* 1993; 20:1925–1931.

Bedsen L, Norregaard J, Jensen R, Olesen J. Evidence of qualitatively altered nociception in patients with fibromyalgia. *Arthritis Rheum* 1997; 40:98–102.

Croft P, Burt J, Schollum J, et al. More pain, more tender points: is fibromyalgia just one end of a continuous spectrum? *Ann Rheum Dis* 1996; 55:482–485.

Derogatis LR. *Manual for SCL-90R*. Clinical Psychometric Research. Baltimore, MD: Johns Hopkins University School of Medicine, 1977.

Forseth KO, Forre O, Gran JT. A 5.5 year prospective study of self-reported musculoskeletal pain and fibromyalgia in a female population: significance and natural history. *Clin Rheumatol* 1999; 18:114–121.

Granges G, Littlejohn G. Pressure pain threshold in pain-free subjects, in patients with chronic regional pain syndromes, and in patients with fibromyalgia syndrome. *Arthritis Rheum* 1993; 36:642–646.

Kosek E, Ekholm J, Hanson P. Sensory dysfunction in fibromyalgia patients with implications for pathogenetic mechanisms. *Pain* 1996; 68:375–383.

Lautenbacher S, Rollman GB, McCain GA. Multi-method assessment of experimental and clinical pain in patients with fibromyalgia. *Pain* 1994; 59:45–53.

Linton SJ. The challenge of preventing chronic musculoskeletal pain. In: Gebhart GF, Hammond DL, Jensen TS (Eds). *Proceedings of the 7th World Congress on Pain*, Progress in Pain Research and Management, Vol. 2. Seattle: IASP Press, 1994, pp 149–166.

Margolis RB, Tait RC, Krause SJ. A rating system for use with patient pain drawings. *Pain* 1986; 24:57–65.

Smith GM, Egbert LD, Markowitz RA, Mosteller F, Beeker HK. An experimental pain method sensitive to morphine in man: the submaximal effort tourniquet technique. *J Pharmacol Exp Ther* 1966; 154:324–332.

Spielberger CD (Ed). *Manual for the State-Trait Anxiety Inventory* (Form Y) ("Self-evaluation questionnaire"). Palo Alto, CA: Consulting Psychologists Press, 1983.

Vecchiet L, Giamberardino MA, de Bigontina P, Dragani L. Comparative sensory evaluation of parietal tissues in painful and nonpainful areas in fibromyalgia and myofascial pain syndrome. In: Gebhart GF, Hammond DL, Jensen TS (Eds). *Proceedings of the 7th World Congress on Pain*. Progress in Pain Research and Management, Vol. 2, Seattle: IASP Press, 1994, pp 177–185.

Violon A. The process of becoming a chronic pain patient. In: Roy R, Tunks E (Eds). *Psychosocial Factors in Rehabilitation*. London: William and Wilkins, 1982, pp 20–35.

Walter B, Vaitl D, Frank R. Affective distress in fibromyalgia syndrome is associated with pain severity. *Z Rheumatol* 1998; 57:101–104.

Weinstein S. Tactile sensitivity of the phalanges. *Percept Motor Skills* 1962; 14:351–354.

Winfield JB. Pain in fibromyalgia. *Rheum Dis Clin North Am* 1999; 25:55–79.

Wolf S, Hardy JD. Studies on pain. Observations on pain due to local cooling and on factors involved in the "cold pressor" effect. *J Clin Invest* 1941; 20:521–533.

Wolfe F. The relation between tender points and symptom variables: evidence that fibromyalgia is not a discrete disorder in the clinic. *Ann Rheum Dis* 1997; 56:268–272.

Wolfe F, Hawley DJ. Evidence of disordered symptom appraisal in fibromyalgia: increased rates of reported comorbidity and comorbidity severity. *Clin Exper Rheumatol* 1999; 17:297–303.

Wolfe F, Smithe HA, Yunus MB, et al. The American College of Rheumatology 1990 criteria for the classification of fibromyalgia. Report of a multicenter criteria committee. *Arthritis Rheum* 1990; 33:160–172.

Correspondence to: Giancarlo Carli, MD, Istituto di Fisiologia Umana, Università di Siena, Via A Moro, 3100 Siena, Italy. Tel: 0039-0577-234038; Fax: 0039-0577-234037; email: carlig@unisi.it.

Proceedings of the 9th World Congress on Pain,
Progress in Pain Research and Management,
Vol. 16, edited by M. Devor, M.C. Rowbotham, and
Z. Wiesenfeld-Hallin, IASP Press, Seattle, © 2000.

98

No Influence of Naloxone on the Initial Hypoalgesic Effect of Spinal Manual Therapy

Bill Vicenzino,[a] James O'Callaghan,[b]
Felicity Kermode,[a] and Anthony Wright[c]

[a]Department of Physiotherapy, The University of Queensland, Queensland, Australia; [b]Multidisciplinary Pain Clinic, The Royal Brisbane Hospital, Queensland, Australia; [c]Division of Physical Therapy, School of Medical Rehabilitation, University of Manitoba, Manitoba, Canada

Manual therapy presents a striking paradox. Despite widespread use for millennia and emerging evidence from clinical trials that substantiates its clinical efficacy (Gross et al. 1996; Koes et al. 1996), little is known about the mechanisms by which it produces pain relief (Zusman 1994; Wright 1995).

Recently, a new approach to investigating the effects and mechanisms of manual therapy has revealed that a lateral glide treatment technique of the cervical spine produces a rapid onset hypoalgesia and a sympathoexcitatory response in patients suffering from chronic lateral epicondylalgia (Vicenzino et al. 1996, 1998). Interestingly, from a mechanistic point of view, the initial hypoalgesia and sympathoexcitation were significantly correlated (Vicenzino et al. 1998). This finding combined with the finding that the technique produces a selective mechanical hypoalgesia (Vicenzino et al. 1995, 1998) without influencing thermal pain perception suggests that the response has features in common with the coordinated response of the autonomic and sensory nervous systems to stimulation of the lateral periaqueductal gray (lPAG) region (Bandler and Keay 1996). A proposed model suggests that manual therapy may activate midbrain endogenous pain control centers and that such mechanisms may be responsible for a significant component of the initial pain-relieving effects of the therapy (Wright 1995).

The analgesia elicited following lPAG stimulation is not antagonized by the administration of naloxone and does not demonstrate tolerance following repeated stimulation or cross-tolerance to opioid-induced antinociception (Cannon et al. 1982; Morgan and Liebeskind 1987; Morgan 1991). Consequently, it had been classified as a nonopioid form of endogenous analgesia (Morgan 1991; Behbehani 1995). This form differs from the opioid-mediated analgesia that is evoked following stimulation of the ventrolateral periaqueductal gray (vlPAG) (Bandler and Keay 1996).

Several investigators have studied the role of endogenous opioids in manual therapy-induced hypoalgesia and found mixed results (Richardson et al. 1984; Vernon et al. 1986; Christian et al. 1988; Zusman et al. 1989). Zusman et al. (1989) reported no effect of naloxone on manual therapy-induced hypoalgesia but noted the relatively small doses (0.4 mg) of naloxone used and its post-treatment administration as possible reasons for the lack of effect. Christian et al. (1988) and Richardson et al. (1984) demonstrated no change in circulating β-endorphin levels, whereas Vernon et al. (1986) demonstrated a small but significant increase in this opioid peptide following manipulation. Several methodological issues may account for the disparate outcomes of these studies of manipulation. First and foremost, these studies used no measures to evaluate hypoalgesia, so it is difficult to ascertain whether the treatment techniques produced a therapeutic effect. Second, levels of circulating opioid peptides do not validly reflect the levels within the central nervous system and cerebrospinal fluid, the most likely site of action. In summary, the role of endogenous opioids in manual therapy-induced hypoalgesia awaits full evaluation. Such endeavors should attend to the methodological issues raised herein.

To further evaluate parallels between manual therapy-induced hypoalgesia and lPAG analgesia, we conducted a study that evaluated the effect of naloxone on the initial hypoalgesic effect of the lateral glide treatment technique.

METHODS

Twenty-four subjects (mean age 45.3 years) with chronic unilateral lateral epicondylalgia were recruited from medical and physiotherapy practices in the Brisbane metropolitan region. A screening test prior to the study ensured that the subjects had unilateral lateral epicondylalgia as diagnosed by well-established clinical tests (Haker 1993; Vicenzino and Wright 1996) and that no exclusion criteria were met (e.g., no coexisting neck or upper limb pain apart from pain in the lateral elbow and proximal forearm region). Details of the inclusion and exclusion criteria have been reported previously (Vicenzino and Wright 1996; Vicenzino et al. 1998). Since all subjects were to receive manual therapy of the cervical spine, an important exclusion criterion was any contraindication to manual therapy. All subjects signed consent forms indicating they were fully informed of their role in the study. The Medical Research Ethics Committee of the University of Queensland approved the study.

OUTCOME MEASURES (INDEPENDENT VARIABLES)

This study used outcome measures similar to those used in previous studies of the lateral glide treatment technique of the cervical spine in patients with lateral epicondylalgia (Vicenzino and Wright 1996; Vicenzino et al. 1998). These measures were pain-free grip strength, pressure-pain threshold, and thermal pain threshold. Pain-free grip strength was defined as the amount of force the subject was capable of producing at pain threshold (i.e., the first onset of elbow pain; Stratford et al. 1993). An isometric, digital grip dynamometer (MIE Medical Research, Ltd.) was used for this purpose. Pressure-pain threshold was the amount of pressure required to elicit the onset of pain. A digital algometer (Somedic AB) measured pressure-pain threshold over the most sensitive point of the lateral elbow as previously determined by digital palpation in the clinical examination. Thermal pain thresholds over the same site were measured with a contact thermode system (Somedic AB). Thermal pain threshold was defined as the temperature at which the subject perceived the onset of pain. Both the pressure and thermal pain threshold tests involved a graduated increase in the stimulus at a predetermined rate until the subject signaled pain onset by pressing a control switch. All measures were repeated three times, and measures were obtained on the asymptomatic side first. This approach facilitated familiarization with the test procedure because data from the asymptomatic side were not included in the analysis.

DEPENDENT VARIABLE (INTERVENTION)

The dependent variable had three levels: naloxone (0.8 mg in 2 mL saline i.v.), saline (2 mL i.v.), and control (no drug). An anesthetist administered these conditions in a randomized sequence. All other participants in the study were blind to the sequence of drug and control conditions.

DESIGN AND PROCEDURE

This study used a randomized, double-blind, placebo-controlled, repeated measures design. For the within-subjects component of the study, each subject experienced all three conditions in a randomized sequence over their 3-

day involvement in the experiment. Typically, on each day, the subject entered the laboratory, disrobed to expose the upper limbs, neck, and upper thoracic spine, and was positioned supine on a manual therapy treatment table. An i.v. line was inserted, and the pain threshold measurements were then made, followed by administration of either the naloxone, saline, or control conditions. To facilitate blinding of the subjects all conditions involved intravenous cannulation and the drawing up of a syringe. Immediately after the injection or sham procedure, an experienced manual therapist applied the treatment technique, which consisted of three sets of 30 seconds of lateral glide treatment separated by 60-second rest periods as used in previously published studies (Vicenzino et al. 1996, 1998, 1999). The therapist was blind to whether naloxone, saline, or control had been administered, as were the researchers responsible for obtaining pain threshold measures. The measures were then repeated immediately after the application of the treatment. Subjects received the lateral glide treatment procedure on each of the three days that they participated in the experiment.

The triplicate data were averaged and then expressed as a percentage change from preapplication to postapplication. We used a one-way within-subjects analysis of variance to analyze this change score.

RESULTS AND DISCUSSION

Data for pain-free grip strength, pressure-pain threshold, and thermal pain threshold are shown in Fig. 1. Statistical analysis of the data revealed no significant differences between naloxone, saline, and control conditions (Table I).

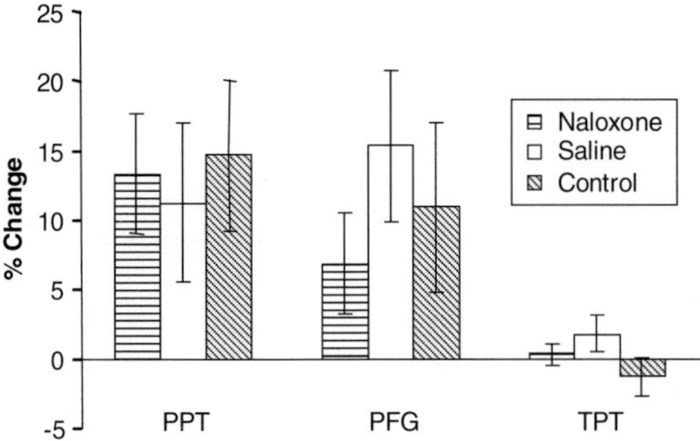

Fig. 1. The mean ± SEM percentage change in pressure-pain threshold (PPT), pain-free grip strength (PFG), and thermal pain threshold (TPT) under the naloxone, saline, and control conditions. A standardized dose of the manual therapy treatment procedure was administered on each occasion.

Table I
One-way ANOVA results (three levels: naloxone, saline, and control) for each dependent variable

Dependent Variable	$F_{2,46}$	P
Pain-free grip strength	0.86	0.43
Pressure pain threshold	0.11	0.89
Thermal pain threshold	1.59	0.22

The results of this study show that naloxone did not significantly alter the initial hypoalgesic effect of the manual therapy treatment when compared to a placebo saline injection or no intervention. This finding is similar to that of Zusman et al. (1989), who found no effect of naloxone on manual therapy-induced hypoalgesia, and suggests that the treatment may induce a non-opioid form of analgesia. This finding provides a further parallel with lPAG-mediated analgesia and supplies additional indirect evidence to support the postulated model that posited the involvement of a supraspinal control center in manual therapy-induced hypoalgesia. Nevertheless, naloxone reversal is only one of the suggested characteristics of opioid analgesia (Souvlis and Wright 1997). Other criteria include tolerance and cross-tolerance with morphine. Some additional evidence suggests that the hypoalgesic effect of manual therapy does not exhibit tolerance with six repeated administrations (Souvlis et al. 1999). To date no studies have considered whether subjects exhibiting tolerance to morphine can still show a hypoalgesic response to manual therapy. Further research is required to investigate in detail the phenomenon of manipulation-induced analgesia.

ACKNOWLEDGMENTS

This study was supported by funding from NHMRC grant No. 961219 and a grant from the Physiotherapy Research Foundation of Australia. We are grateful for the assistance of Dr. Bronwyn Williams.

REFERENCES

Bandler R, Keay KA. Columnar organization in the midbrain periaqueductal gray and the integration of emotional expression. *Prog Brain Res* 1996; 107:285–300.

Behbehani MM. Functional characteristics of the midbrain periaqueductal gray. *Prog Neurobiol* 1995: 46:575–605.

Cannon J, Prieto G, Lee A, Liebeskind J. Evidence for opioid and non-opioid forms of stimulation-produced analgesia in the rat. *Brain Res* 1982; 243:315–321.

Christian G, Stanton G, Sissons, D, et al. Immunoreactive ACTH, β-endorphin, and cortisol levels in plasma following spinal manipulative therapy. *Spine* 1988; 13:1411–1417.

Gross AR, Aker PD, Quartly C. Manual therapy in the treatment of neck pain. *Rheum Dis Clin North Am* 1996; 22:579–598.

Haker E. Lateral epicondylalgia: diagnosis, treatment and evaluation. *Crit Rev Phys Rehabil Med* 1993; 5:129–154.

Koes B, Assendelft W, van der Heijden G, Bouter L. Spinal manipulation for low back pain. An updated systematic review of randomized clinical trials. *Spine* 1996; 21:2860–2871.

Morgan M. Differences in antinociception evoked from dorsal and ventral regions of the caudal periaqueductal gray matter. In: Depaulis A, Bandler R (Eds). *The Midbrain Periaqueductal Gray Matter,* Vol. 213. New York: Plenum Press, 1991, pp 139–150.

Morgan M, Liebeskind J. Site specificity in the development of tolerance to stimulation-produced analgesia from the periaqueductal gray matter of the rat. *Brain Res* 1987; 425:356–359.

Richardson D, Kappler R, Klatz R, et al. The effect of osteopathic manipulative treatment on endogenous opiate concentration. *J Am Osteopath Assoc* 1984; 84:127.

Souvlis T, Wright A. The tolerance effect: its relevance to analgesia produced by physiotherapy interventions. *Phys Ther Rev* 1997; 2:227–37.

Souvlis T, Kermode F, Williams E, Collins D, Wright A. Does the initial analgesic effect of spinal manual therapy exhibit tolerance? *Abstracts: 9th World Congress on Pain.* Seattle: IASP Press, 1999, pp 454–455.

Stratford P, Levy D, Gowland C. Evaluative properties of measures used to assess patients with lateral epicondylitis at the elbow. *Physiother Canada* 1993; 45:160–164.

Vernon HT, Dhami MS, Howley TP, Annett R. Spinal manipulation and beta-endorphin: a controlled study of the effect of a spinal manipulation on plasma beta-endorphin levels in normal males. *J Manipulative Physiol Ther* 1986; 9:115–123.

Vicenzino B, Wright A. Lateral epicondylalgia I: a review of epidemiology, pathophysiology, aetiology and natural history. *Phys Ther Rev* 1996; 1:23–34.

Vicenzino B, Gutschlag F, Collins D, Wright A. An investigation of the effects of spinal manual therapy on forequarter pressure and thermal pain thresholds and sympathetic nervous system activity in asymptomatic subjects: a preliminary report. In: Shacklock M (Ed). *Moving In On Pain.* Adelaide: Butterworth-Heinemann Australia, 1995, pp 185–193.

Vicenzino B, Collins D, Wright A. The initial effects of a cervical spine manipulative physiotherapy treatment on the pain and dysfunction of lateral epicondylalgia. *Pain* 1996; 68:69–74.

Vicenzino B, Collins D, Benson H, Wright A. An investigation of the interrelationship between manipulative therapy induced hypoalgesia and sympathoexcitation. *J Manipulative Physiol Ther* 1998; 21:448–453.

Vicenzino B, Neal R, Collins D, Wright A. The displacement, velocity and frequency profile of the frontal plane motion produced by the cervical lateral glide treatment technique. *Clin Biomechanics* 1999; 14:515–521.

Wright A. Hypoalgesia post manipulative therapy: a review of a potential neurophysiological mechanism. *Manual Ther* 1995: 1:11–16.

Zusman M. What does manipulation do? The need for basic research. In: Boyling J, Palastanga N (Eds). *Grieve's Modern Manual Therapy: The Vertebral Column.* Edinburgh: Churchill Livingstone, 1994, pp 651–659.

Zusman M, Edwards B, Donaghy A. Investigation of a proposed mechanism for the relief of spinal pain with passive joint movement. *J Manual Med* 1989; 4:58–61.

Correspondence to: Anthony Wright, PhD, School of Medical Rehabilitation, University of Manitoba, 770 Bannatyne Avenue, Winnipeg, MB, Canada R3E 0W3. Tel: 204-787-1099; Fax: 204-787-1227; email: twright@ms.umanitoba.ca.

Proceedings of the 9th World Congress on Pain,
Progress in Pain Research and Management,
Vol. 16, edited by M. Devor, M.C. Rowbotham, and
Z. Wiesenfeld-Hallin, IASP Press, Seattle, © 2000.

99

Charisma and the Art of Healing: Can Nonspecific Factors Be Enough?

Richard H. Gracely

Clinical Measurement and Mechanisms Unit, Pain and Neurosensory Mechanisms Branch, National Institute of Craniofacial and Dental Research, National Institutes of Health, Bethesda, Maryland, USA

Until the time of Pasteur, individuals who assumed the role of health care provider dispensed health with a meager tool kit that included herbal remedies, physical interventions, and extensive ritual. These practices may be quite mystical (shamanic practices and the chants of a witch doctor are still associated with healing and magical cures) or more in line with contemporary Western medicine. For example, the method of audio analgesia enjoyed a brief popularity. Music and white noise were used to provide pain control during dental and other acute procedures until it became clear that the efficacy of the technique depended on factors such as anxiety and the charisma of the operator (Rosenberg 1964; Howitt 1967; Melzack 1973).

Charisma has been defined as a divinely inspired gift that bestows the power to elicit a response from others. This chapter will consider the broad array of clinician factors in treatment efficacy. Charisma in this context is a metaphor for general actions that the clinician can take to improve the power of a treatment. It is only one of many clinician factors that can evoke nonspecific mechanisms that can positively influence treatments for any disorder. Evidence indicates that these factors can be quite specific and provide therapeutic benefit by directly influencing a pathological process. In addition, nonspecific factors in one classification scheme, such as a biomedical model, may be specific factors in another scheme, for example a psychosocial model. Thus, the title of this chapter is potentially misleading. Noncharismatic clinicians may engage in purposeful behaviors that have specific therapeutic effects. The title should perhaps be rephrased: Can the behavior of the clinician alone evoke specific or nonspecific responses that are sufficient to result in a therapeutic success?

A review of the evidence indicates that the answer is yes. But first, it is useful to consider the recognized need for double-blind controls in clinical trials. There is no doubt that it is extremely important to blind the patient in the assessment of therapeutic agents. It is also universally understood that the clinician must be blinded as well. The person administering a treatment cannot be aware of the content of the treatment lest this knowledge influence the outcome. Early laboratory studies of morphine analgesia provide one of the first examples of this effect in pain research. Half a century ago, Hardy and colleagues at Yale were demonstrating experimental analgesia for several analgesics, including morphine (Hardy and Cattell 1950; Hardy et al. 1952). These studies lacked blind controls, and the investigators served as subjects. However, the Beecher group at Harvard could not duplicate their results, and so requested the aid of the Hardy group. An investigator from the Hardy group visited the Beecher laboratory and demonstrated experimental morphine analgesia in an open manner without experimental controls. When the Harvard group instituted such controls without the visitor's knowledge, they were unable to demonstrate morphine analgesia (Denton and Beecher 1949; Beecher 1959). This result is notable in that the controls used have become a standard for clinical trials of analgesics. This study is only one of many that show the necessity of controlling the influence of the person administering the treatments. It indicates that yes, the influence of the clinician can be sufficient. Those who doubt this statement must also doubt the need for double-blind controls. If the clinician has no influence, single blinding of the patient should be sufficient.

IATROPLACEBOGENESIS

The example of placebo-controlled trials raises the question of how clinician influence differs from the placebo effect. Overlap is considerable, and placebo data will be used as evidence for clinician factors. However, by focusing on the behavior of the clinician, not the behavior of the patient, we can address the contribution of clinician behavior to both placebo and active treatments, and the factors that modify this contribution. These factors may be treatments in their own right, not just a sham of some other treatment. Thus, the term placebo or placebo effect does not adequately describe the topic. Suggestion may be a factor (Lipkin 1984). However, this chapter will follow the proposal of Shapiro (1964, 1971), who recognized both the need for a new term and the similarity to placebo phenomena. He introduced the term *iatroplacebogenesis* (IPG) to describe the effects of the clinician on treatment efficacy.

Iatroplacebogenesis is not a single construct. Shapiro described two types of IPG. Direct IPG results from a conscious action of the clinician, intent on treating the patient; actions can range from carefully explaining the procedure to performing surgery. Indirect IPG results from unconscious behavior of the clinician and can include knowledge about the efficacy of the treatment or about the difficulty of treating the particular disease. The clinician's behavior may also reflect personality variables such as charisma. Direct and indirect IPG are not mutually exclusive and may overlap; a charismatic clinician may be aware of his or her power and use it purposefully to enhance treatment.

The evidence for IPG factors must be considered in the context of delivery of health care interventions for specific diseases. The evidence supporting the existence and efficacy of IPG will be divided into retrospective and prospective, with a consideration of future experimental designs. This chapter will conclude with the larger historical context of medical technology and political trends, and a brief summary of the implications for both research and clinical practice.

CLASSIFICATION OF INTERVENTIONS

ACTIVE AND PLACEBO INTERVENTIONS

It is quite clear that the placebo effect is not limited to the deliberate use of placebos. Placebo effects are present in all treatments; the power of the placebo effect is influenced by the power of the treatment. Clinician factors not only have influenced the efficacy of analgesics (Evans 1985), but also have affected treatments outside the pain field such as chemotherapy (Gallimore and Turner 1977) and the treatment of anxiety (Wheatley 1967) and depression (Kirsch and Saperstein 1998). As noted above, IPG factors operate in both placebo and active treatments. One issue is whether IPG modulation of the efficacy of an active treatment represents a simple placebo effect or an active treatment with specific effects.

PERCEIVED POWER OF INTERVENTIONS

Interventions may be classified by their perceived power. Surgery probably tops the list, followed by injections, and then pills. Within the pill domain there is evidence that size and color can have an influence. Words fall at the end of this continuum, but provide a baseline component to all treatments.

NCCAM CLASSIFICATION OF FIELDS OF PRACTICE

A review of existing classifications of pain interventions reveals a useful scheme from The National Center for Complementary and Alternative Medicine in the United States. The NCCAM has classified fields of practice into six categories. Of special interest is the category, "Mind-Body Control." Most of the procedures in this class do not involve any physical interaction with the patient. Some involve active movement or physical contact, but methods such as psychotherapy, relaxation, and hypnosis share the common features of verbal patient-clinician interaction without physical intervention. The NCCAM has concluded that these procedures are both effective and safe. Clearly, we must gain a thorough understanding of what these methods can do before we make statements about the efficacy of other alternative treatments and other conventional therapies. The underlying mechanisms of this group are undoubtedly present in all treatments, both conventional and alternative. These "nonphysical" therapies provide the therapeutic baseline against which all other treatments should be compared.

THERAPEUTIC MECHANISMS OF NONPHYSICAL THERAPIES

Curiosity naturally turns to the mechanisms by which non-physical therapies produce therapeutic benefit. Can such techniques improve normal functioning? Evidence is scant for improvement above normal. To the contrary, we have considerable evidence that nonphysical procedures can be harmful. Practices such as "Voodoo death" or the "giving-up-given-up" complex suggest that "beliefs can sicken and kill" (Engel 1968). Anecdotal evidence of primitive practices and present evidence of negative placebo (nocebo) effects (Hahn 1997) support the concept that cognitions can aversely impact health. The perceived connection between behavior and illness spawned the field of psychosomatic medicine in the 1940s and more recently, the new field of psychoneuroimmunology. The influence of psychological processes on the immune system has evoked increasing interest, especially with the recognition that the biomedical model has not been as successful in the treatment of chronic diseases as it has been in treating infectious diseases (Zachariae 1996). A review of this literature provides additional support for psychological processes that degrade immune function. In this context, treatments appear to be restorative—they improve health that has been adversely affected. It is well recognized that habitual behaviors can lead to stress-related and psychosomatic illnesses: "Thus it should not be surprising when the patient's decision to behave differently results in a reversal or alleviation of that condition" (Plotkin 1985, p. 247).

HEALTH DISINHIBITION AND THE PSYCHOLOGICAL U-TURN

The principle of reversing self-harm appears to be firmly established. We could use the term *health disinhibition* when patients stop specific behaviors that degrade health and thus allow health to return to normal. Improved health also can be referred to as a psychological U-turn; people first do things that make them sick, and then institute different behaviors that actively restore normal, healthy functioning. We may use the term *disinhibition* to refer to reversal of a specific health dimension and *psychological U-turn* to describe a general, beneficial change in behavior. Disinhibition may be similar to stopping cigarette smoking, while a psychological U-turn might be similar to an exercise program that leads to a cessation of smoking and other factors such as improved diet.

Disinhibition or U-turn mechanisms have at least two implications. First, these mechanisms suggest that IPG factors may heal disease primarily by restoring function, and thus may not improve function beyond a normal level. Second, these mechanisms may be particularly effective for conditions with a common etiology, with functional diseases that are caused or exacerbated by behavior. These factors may be less effective with "organic" injuries or diseases. However, this distinction becomes blurred because functional factors are also present in organic diseases. For example, morbidity and mortality in coronary artery disease are strongly related to psychosocial factors (Rozanski et al. 1999; Weidner and Mueller, in press).

CLASSIFICATION OF DISEASES

The influence of IPG factors most likely varies over disease categories. The limits of IPG factors need to be specified and efficacy must be established within these limits. The evidence suggests that ailments such as hypertension, angina, ulcers, esophageal-related chest pain, asthma, disorders of the skin, and psychological disturbances are particularly open to the influence of IPG factors (Abbot et al. 1952; Hass et al. 1959; Graham et al. 1962; Ikemi and Nakagawa 1962; Maslach et al. 1972; Bush 1974; Winters et al. 1984). Studies of the influence of these factors on immune function have produced mixed results, partly due to the complexity of immune response, to the many dependent variables that can be evaluated, and to lack of control of other important variables. In general, this literature indicates that positive effects on immune response occur, but without a consistent pattern. Positive effects vary across individuals, immune parameter measured, and type of psychological intervention technique (Zachariae 1996).

In addition to cataloging disorders sensitive to IPG factors, we can also divide diseases into those that are measured by subjective or objective dependent variables. This division implicitly suggests that subjective dependent variables such as self-report of pain, anxiety, or depression could represent a change predominantly in labeling behavior, while changes in physical parameters are more real and credible. Those in the pain field who have fought successfully for disease status for clinical pain syndromes may approach such a classification with ambivalence. As champions of the credibility of a "subjective disorder," pain researchers might eschew such a distinction, and yet seek the comfort of functional measures outside pain such as respiratory function in asthmatics, or exercise function in congestive heart failure (Chow et al. 1983; Fung et al. 1986; Archer and Leier 1992). They may be most firmly convinced by objective proof that can be measured on a physical dimension such as healing ulcers, reducing blood pressure, reducing postoperative swelling, changes in gastric secretions or skin temperature, or improvement of hypertension, dermatitis, or immune function (Abbot et al. 1952; Hass et al. 1959; Graham et al. 1962; Ikemi and Nakagawa 1962; Maslach et al. 1972; Bush 1974; Winters et al. 1984; Zachariae 1996). The evidence presented below will consider both subjective and objective dependent variables.

LINES OF EXPERIMENTAL EVIDENCE

Considerable evidence supports the concept that the clinician can powerfully influence treatment regardless of what treatment technique is used. Both retrospective evidence and prospective studies support the validity and efficacy of IPG. The following sections briefly describe the types of evidence and conclude with an experimental design synthesized from these studies.

RETROSPECTIVE EVIDENCE

Anecdotal evidence and folklore describe the power of the clinician to influence treatment success. In reviewing retrospective studies it is important to distinguish between the results of clinical trials and the occasional sensational case report. A successful case study can represent factors such as spontaneous remission, while a significant group effect provides credible evidence. However, evidence must be evaluated case by case. For example, although the results of clinical trials are more credible, case reports represent the results of a full clinical treatment in which many IPG factors can fully influence the outcome. In contrast, many clinical trials usually are conducted in an atmosphere in which these factors are deliberately suppressed. However, in other trials, patients may experience many more personally significant social interactions with more people than they would experience in a modern clinical setting (D.J. Clauw, personal communication). With these caveats in mind it is possible to distinguish two general lines of retrospective evidence: (1) therapies that become worthless over time after initial success, and (2) variation in the success rates of active and placebo treatments, over different active drugs and over definable clinician-patient relationships.

Efficacious therapies become worthless. Often new therapies are initially efficacious but eventually lose their effectiveness as clinician enthusiasm wanes. Examples include audio analgesia for dental and other acute procedures, the Vineberg procedure for angina, glomectomy for bronchial asthma, gastric freezing for duodenal ulcer, and treatment of herpes simplex virus infection with levamisole, organic solvents, or photodynamic inactivation (Benson and McCallie 1979; Roberts 1993; Turner et al. 1994). As Marchettini points out in this volume, therapies may become not only worthless, but harmful. The results of medical interventions can be much worse than doing nothing at all.

This line of evidence focuses on the natural history of a therapy. Why does the efficacy of many therapies begin at 70–90% and then decline to placebo, neutral, or even harmful levels? While the role of the patient's expectation cannot be ignored, it seems reasonable that the brunt of this effect can be attributed to the attitude of the treating clinicians. Disappointed in the lackluster performance of available tools, clinicians are naturally receptive to a new technological advance that promises dramatic improvements in treating problematic diseases. This enthusiasm and confidence are likely communicated to the patient through both direct and indirect IPG mechanisms, setting the stage for maximum treatment efficacy. Over time, it becomes obvious that the new treatment does not live up to its expectations; subsequent changes in clinician attitudes further reduce efficacy. Ultimately, the treatment is relegated to the pool of partially effective tools, and the stage is set for the excitement associated with the next promising novel therapy. Apart from suggesting that a patient use new treatments while they are still effective, this decline in treatment efficacy provides an important line of evidence for IPG. Most of the difference from initial high treatment rates to subsequent modest rates can be attributed to IPG factors in the clinician that are overtly and covertly communicated to the patient.

Variance of placebo and active treatment rates over medications, countries, cities, hospitals, and clinicians. The second line of retrospective evidence is the variance of effectiveness rates of placebo and active treatments.

Following Beecher's (1955) early classification of placebo efficacy, Evans (1985) took a slightly different tack and compared the power of placebo to the power of the active treatment substituted by the placebo. In the clinical analgesic trials reviewed he found that the mean placebo efficacy was 56% of the efficacy of the active treatment. Remarkably, this percentage was found over a number of analgesics ranging from high (morphine, 56%) to low (aspirin, 54%) potency. Thus, placebo aspirin is quite weak, while placebo morphine is much stronger. This percentage can be expected to vary, depending on how efficacy is defined and quantified, but there is little argument that these and other studies show that the power of placebo is always about half that of an active analgesic treatment.

In analgesic trials, knowledge of the power of the active drug provides a context that modulates placebo efficacy. The power of the active treatment is not the only contextual influence; the influence of additional factors is evident in studies that deliver the same treatment. In meta-analyses of treatments for anxiolytics and ulcers, the efficacy of the placebo is influenced by the fluctuating efficacy of the active treatment, with a correlation between active and placebo treatment of about 0.4 (Moerman 1999). As in the pain studies reviewed by Evans (1985), the mean placebo rate for the ulcer treatments was close to half of that of the active treatments. These observed fluctuations could represent the relative influence of several contextual variables or fluctuations in the effect of specific variables. Such factors could also explain geographical differences in placebo rates. In the literature on pharmacological trials of treatments for ulcers, the placebo rate varies dramatically between countries from a low of 7% in Brazil to a high of 59% in Germany. Neighboring Denmark and The Netherlands only demonstrate about half the rate found in Germany (Moerman 1999). The rate also can vary systematically between cities in the same nation; MacDonald et al. (1980) reported an ulcer placebo rate of 73% in Dundee and only 44% in London.

Geographic variation is also found for active treatments. A meta-analysis of anti-acid treatment for ulcers in the United States found that the effectiveness varied by hospital and ranged from 17% to 79% (Littman et al. 1977).

What is responsible for variation of identical active or placebo treatments? IPG factors likely play an important role in these variations, although other factors cannot be ruled out. Patient expectation and regional differences in the culture of health care delivery also must be considered. IPG factors may be implicated more strongly by differences within the same region and culture. One example is a study of ulcer treatment in France in which different physicians in the same trial had different placebo rates, expressed as mean pain duration and ranging from 3.55 to 12 days. One clinician who participated in a subsequent trial provided evidence that these rates were stable characteristics of the clinicians. The mean pain duration of the patients he treated by placebo was 12 (SEM = 0.73) days for the first trial and 12.04 days for the second; with no treatment, mean pain duration was 19.53 days (Sarles et al. 1977).

In summary, this line of evidence suggests that the context in which placebo and active treatments are delivered modulate efficacy. The studies by Sarles et al. (1977) strongly implicate the influence of the clinician but need to be replicated with repeat testing of more than one clinician. In other studies the context may result from the attitudes of the patients, independent of the influence of the clinician. The role of patient conditioning, desires, beliefs, expectation, and attitude has received much interest in the literature. However, patient factors represent part of an equation that includes clinician factors and the "doctor-patient relationship." Evans (1985, p. 224) emphasized the role of the clinician in placebo analgesia: "The conviction of the therapist about the drug's potency ... seems to be a powerful mediator of therapeutic effectiveness. This power may be due to direct clinician factors, and also to the clinician's control of the "doctor-patient relationship."

Rapport. It is likely that one significant variable modulating IPG factors is the degree of rapport between doctor and patient. In this view it is not a specific behavior of the doctor or patient, but the interaction between them, that critically determines treatment success (Benson and McCallie 1979). The positive influence of indirect IPG factors such as charisma may be due in part to behaviors that establish and increase rapport. While considerable anecdotal evidence supports the importance of the interaction between the individuals in a therapeutic setting, rapport is difficult to define or measure. A comment by Zachariae (1996, p. 195) about the influence of psychological interventions on immune function applies equally well to treatment of most diseases and emphasizes the difficulty in evaluating rapport:

> The personality traits and training of the therapist may also influence the results of psychological intervention trials. These factors influence the degree of rapport with the participating subjects, which is extremely difficult to assess. An operator may easily be able to influence certain subjects and be unable to influence others. This may depend on such factors such as gender, age, personality and other sociocultural variables. ... Future investigations would benefit if they include and develop indicators and measurements of the characteristics of the therapist or operator and his or her influence on the subjects.

Rapport, though ill defined, is an important if not critical independent variable in studies of IPG. The importance of rapport gains support from the extensive literature on persuasion and attitude change in the fields of social and counseling psychology. This literature strongly suggests that a clinician's ability to establish rapport, rather than specific clinician attributes such attractiveness or behavioral style, is the critical variable in effecting lasting beneficial changes in patient behavior (Strong 1995). Further studies of this elusive but important construct are needed.

PROSPECTIVE EVIDENCE

Prospective studies of IPG include therapies shown to be worthless, studies that manipulate the clinician's social or physical interaction or manipulate the clinician, and studies that attempt to remove the influence of the clinician.

Therapies shown to be worthless. In contrast to retrospective studies in which therapies become worthless, several studies have used appropriate sham controls to assess the efficacy of invasive procedures ranging from experimental pain studies of audio analgesia to clinical surgery (Turner et al. 1994). One of the most famous is the use of sham controls for mammary artery ligation, which was assumed to treat angina-related myocardial ischemia by increasing collateral circulation to the heart. Fig. 1 shows the result of two placebo-controlled studies using sham surgery (Cobb et al.

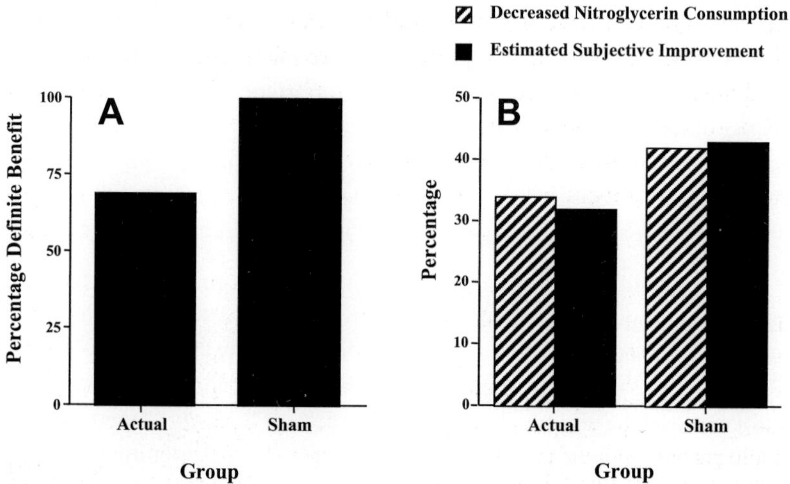

Fig. 1. Results of controlled trials of actual mammary artery ligation versus sham ligation for relief of angina pain. (A) Results of a study by Dimond et al. (1960) in which patients' subjective benefit was based on reduced nitroglycerin consumption and increased exercise tolerance. (B) Results of a study by Cobb et al. (1959) in which subjective improvement and nitroglycerin consumption were evaluated as separate variables. In all cases improvement was greater in the sham condition.

1959; Dimond et al. 1960). These studies demonstrated that sham surgery can even be superior to the actual surgery. Following their publication, the ligation procedure was abandoned (Benson and McCallie 1979).

Manipulation of the clinician's social interaction with the patient. This line of prospective evidence directly assesses IPG factors. In some cases the interventions fall under the NCCAM "Mind-Body" classification because the treatment does not involve a physical intervention. In other cases IPG factors are manipulated as a component of a treatment that also includes a physical intervention.

Manipulation of direct IPG factors improved treatment efficacy in several studies. Gryll and Katahn (1978) varied several factors in a study of the pain of mandibular block for dental procedures, including whether a dentist or technician delivered the message, whether their attitude was warm or neutral, and whether they employed message oversell or undersell. Message oversell had the most pronounced effect of reducing the pain of this procedure. In a simple study in a general practice, Thomas (1987) randomly gave one of two messages to 200 patients with undiagnosed symptoms. They were told either that the doctor knew what they had and they would get better in a few days, or that the doctor did not know what was wrong with them. Fig. 2 shows that the group that had received the positive consultation had a significantly greater number of patients with improved symptoms.

Simple, short preoperative communications and subsequent postoperative interactions can have a profound effect. Fig. 3 shows the result of purposeful communications in which morphine requirements were significantly reduced during the first 5 postoperative days. Patients in the treatment group required 70% of the opiates needed by the untreated patients, and this difference increased to only a 39% requirement by 5 days postsurgery. In addition, the postoperative inpatient recovery was significantly shortened

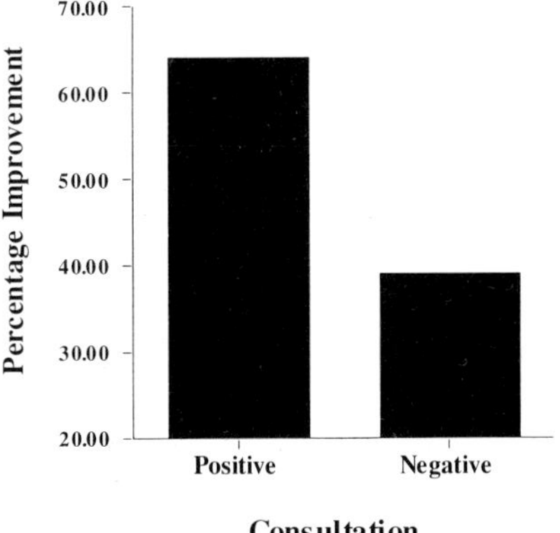

Fig. 2. Influence of brief verbal communication of undiagnosed physical complaints. Two hundred consecutive patients in a general medical practice were either told that they would get better in a few days or that the doctor did not know what was wrong with them. Sixty-four percent of the 100 patients with the positive message reported improvement in symptoms while only 39% of the 100 patients receiving the negative message reported improved symptoms.

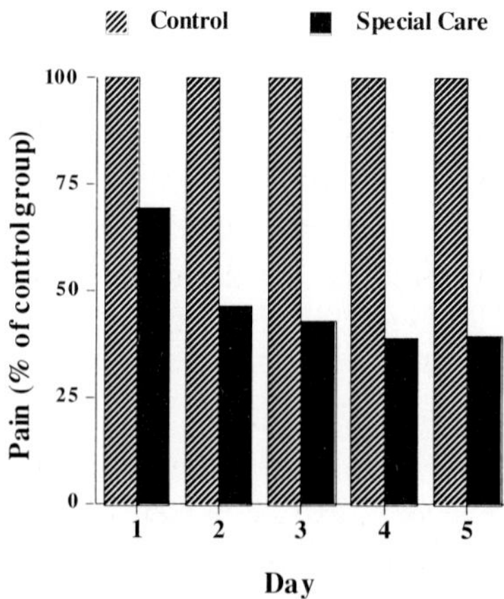

Fig. 3. Influence of preoperative instructions and specialized postoperative care on postoperative morphine requirements. In comparison to 51 patients in the control group, 46 patients in the special care group required less than 75% of the morphine on Day 1 and less than 50% on subsequent days. Blind observers rated specialized care patients as appearing to be more comfortable.

by 2.7 days (Egbert et al. 1964). Notably, the physicians performing the surgery, administering the medications, and discharging the patients from the hospital were blind to the treatments.

Even simple communications, such as the use of a brand name instead of a generic name, can have an effect (Fig. 4). In this study the use of a brand-name aspirin produced a small but significant increase in efficacy in both the active and placebo groups (Branthwaite and Cooper 1981).

One of the most elaborate studies of clinician behavior evaluated the effect of an antidepressant in three hospitals in two cities. Clinicians were chosen and trained for a warm, therapeutic role or for a more reserved, uncertain, or experimental role (Uhlenhuth et al. 1966). The results showed an overall beneficial effect for enthusiasm, but it varied by location. It was greatest in an inner-city hospital where both the patients and clinicians were predominantly of lower socioeconomic status, and less or absent in teaching hospitals with patients of greater socioeconomic status. Thus, the positive

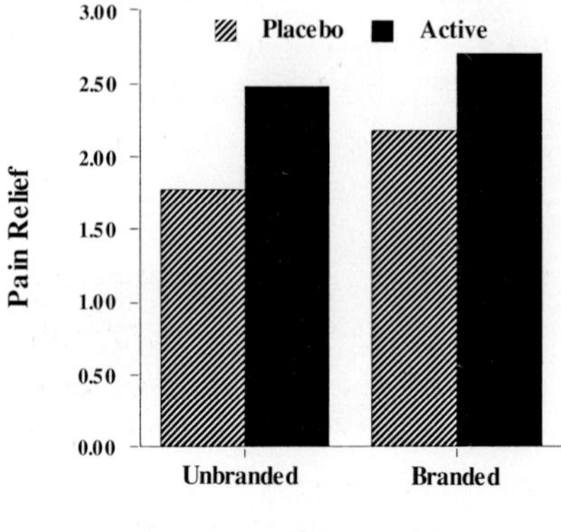

Fig. 4. Influence of brand name on the influence of active and placebo aspirin. In comparison to the use of a generic aspirin, use of a brand name produced a significant increase in analgesic efficacy in both the active and placebo groups.

effect of enthusiasm was not related to the specific role per se, but to how appropriate the role was for a given patient. This prospective study provided additional evidence for the importance of rapport. The effect of the treatment was enhanced with a specific behavioral style congruent with characteristics of both the clinician and patient. Good clinicians are not characterized by specific attributes, but more by their ability to see the world as the patient sees it, to understand the patient from within his or her frame of reference, and to communicate within this model.

Manipulation of the clinician's physical interaction with the patient. In addition to what doctors *say,* considerable evidence suggests that what doctors *do* can exert specific or nonspecific effects (Beecher 1961). Medical treatments have symbolic value, and clearly the most potent of all is surgery. It is the ultimate treatment, with the drama of preparation, contact with a surgical team, anesthesia, and invasion of the body. Surgery carries strong implications of success, and almost no clinical trials have interfered with this perception. The studies of mammary artery ligation described above probably highlight one of many procedures in which surgical success may be unrelated to the procedure performed. Other examples include the effects of sham surgery for arthroscopic treatment of the knee (Moseley et al. 1996) and relief of sciatica and back pain in at least one-third of back surgery patients who proved to have no disk herniation (Spangfort 1972; Turner et al. 1994).

The treatment of trigeminal neuralgia offers several examples in which surgical exploration alone has brought significant relief (Adams 1989; Gybels and Sweet 1989; Sweet 1990). These and other examples may indicate the powerful psychological effects of surgery, but also may indicate the effect of other mechanisms. Interpretations of these results cannot exclude a physiological mechanism evoked by the anesthesia or by minimal surgical tissue damage (Adams 1989; Gybens and Sweet 1989; Sweet 1990; Eliav and Gracely 1999; J. Gybels, personal communication). Studies that distinguish between IPG and physiological mechanisms may be difficult to perform. Most surgical techniques have not been subject to the scrutiny of controlled trials that is required for analgesic agents. However, the U.S. Food and Drug Administration recently reversed this trend by requesting controlled proof of efficacy for new surgical techniques. One popularized example is the brain implantation of fetal tissue for treatment of Parkinson's disease. Trials of this procedure include a sham surgery in which a burr hole is drilled but no implantation is performed. The adverse consequences are minimal for the patient because the burr hole is used in a subsequent surgery. The act of drilling a burr hole, however, supplies a potent psychological and physiological stimulus. In this study both actual and sham surgery produced positive subjective reports that did not significantly differ (Freed et al. 1999). It would be informative to compare the results of this procedure to those of other sham conditions with less trauma, such as minor scalp incision. Evaluation of the therapeutic response to a range of physiological insults might distinguish between physiological and psychological mechanisms of sham improvement. Such studies are unlikely because the adverse effects would have to be weighed against this minor goal versus the clinically significant goal of demonstrating surgical efficacy.

Sham controls have been used in conjunction with implantation of stimulating electrodes for control of intractable pain. Our own laboratory has produced some evidence that simply implanting electrodes reduces pain responses. Twenty years ago we performed an extensive inpatient analysis of the mechanisms and efficacy of deep brain stimulation of paraventricular gray for treatment of intractable pain disorders. We observed a trend ($P <$ 0.07–0.09) for a reduction in baseline pain responses after the surgical procedure (Wolskee et al. 1982). We also assessed the effects of deep brain stimulation. We observed significant morphine analgesia in comparison to placebo before the surgery, which was antagonized by the narcotic antagonist naloxone. After surgery we observed that sham brain stimulation was just as effective as real brain stimulation, and that naloxone did not influence the putative opioid-mediated effect of real stimulation. This negative result is consistent with the natural history of this technique. The use of paraventricular gray stimulation has declined in the intervening 20 years, replaced to some extent by stimulation of other brain regions such as the lateral thalamus.

Surgery is the most extreme example of physical interventions for pain control. Surgical procedures define the top of a continuum that includes invasive treatments, manipulation such as transcutaneous electrical nerve stimulation or acupuncture, and delivery of medications by injection or the oral route (Beecher 1961). Treatments such as sham tooth grinding have produced 64% relief in patients with chronic orofacial pain (Goodman et al. 1976), while sham ultrasound treatments have reduced postoperative swelling after oral surgical procedures (Hasish et al. 1986; Ho et al. 1988). Spiro (1986, p. 41) posits that physicians perceive the placebo effects of an injection to be greater than that of oral medications. Within the realm of oral medications, greater effects have been found with specific colors, bigger pills, and with capsules instead of tablets (Buckalew and Ross 1981; Buckalew and Coffield 1982a,b). A hierarchy of placebo power, if verified by further studies, could result from attitudes related to the efficacy of the actual treatments. The hierarchy of placebo potency could reflect the relative efficacy of these genuine interventions. Efficacy also may be related to general factors such as invasiveness and treatment-evoked sensation or side effects.

The reader can appreciate that these factors may be convoluted. Greater perceived efficacy of an invasive procedure could directly result in a greater placebo effect, or indirectly contribute to the perceived power of such active treatments, which in turn increases the placebo effect. The relation between these variables can only be evaluated by studies that independently manipulate physical invasiveness and attitudes toward treatment efficacy.

All these treatments represent clear cases of direct IPG, actions that a clinician can take within ethical bounds to increase treatment efficacy. Indirect IPG factors also play a role because the clinician possesses ingrained attitudes of treatment efficacy. Indirect factors have been addressed in prospective studies that manipulate clinicians' knowledge and attitudes.

Manipulation of the clinician's knowledge and attitude. One of the most interesting lines of evidence is provided by a few "triple-blind" studies that not only blind the patient and clinician but also further manipulate the clinician's knowledge (Hoffer and Osmond 1961; Paul et al. 1972; Henker et al. 1979). Beecher's (Beecher 1959; Denton and Beecher 1949) use of double-blind controls, described at the beginning of this chapter, can be viewed as an example in which an operator was unaware that he was part of the experiment. Another classic example is the study by McGlashan and colleagues (1969), in which the physician believed he was administering either an analgesic or placebo, when in fact all of the treatments were placebo. These studies used deception to manipulate the knowledge of the clinician, with attendant ethical issues of informed consent (see Galer and Turner [1997] for a study of clinicians' knowledge that does not involve deception).

In our laboratory we performed an experiment similar in concept to that of McGlashan et al. (1969) but with a different manipulation (Gracely et al. 1985). We administered placebo under a condition in which the powerful opiate fentanyl was a random possibility, or in a condition in which fentanyl was not a random possibility. We instructed the clinicians to inform the patients that fentanyl could always be a possibility, and this was also stated in the informed consent. Thus, while the clinicians and patients in the McGlashan et al. (1969) study thought that an active drug could be delivered, the clinicians in our study knew this was not the case in one condition. Fig. 5 shows the result of fentanyl and placebo when fentanyl was a possibility in a traditional double-blind design. Fentanyl significantly reduced the postoperative pain of third-molar extractions, and a robust placebo effect was about half that of fentanyl. This figure also shows the result when the clinician knew that fentanyl was not a randomized possibility, but the patient still believed that fentanyl could be delivered. The effect of the placebo was significantly reduced. The only difference was the clinician's knowledge, which was somehow communicated to the patient.

Disguised or hidden administration. The last category of prospective evidence comes from studies that disguise the administered drug or hide its delivery. The influence of the clinician in an active drug treatment can be assessed by comparing the effect observed when the clinician delivers the drug to the effect when the drug is delivered without the patient's knowledge. The difference can represent the influence of the doctor-patient relationship, and differences in this effect with different clinician behaviors would provide a direct measure of the IPG factors. In our studies of pain mechanisms we introduced the use of a hidden infusion to isolate the pharmacological action of a drug from the psychological effect related to the patient's knowledge that a drug has been delivered (Gracely et al. 1983). The introduction of this method in pain studies was preceded by studies of Ross et al. (1962) and Lyerly et al. (1964), who examined the effects of stimulants and sedatives on mood and psychomotor performance in healthy volunteers. They used the term "disguised" in a manner similar to the use of "hidden." However, "disguised" or a similar term might be better used to describe the condition of a masqueraded administration in which the identity of a drug is paired with the action of another. These types of manipulations possess the experimental power to evaluate IPG effects and the factors that modulate these effects.

Fig. 6 shows a 12-cell research design that focuses on the role of the

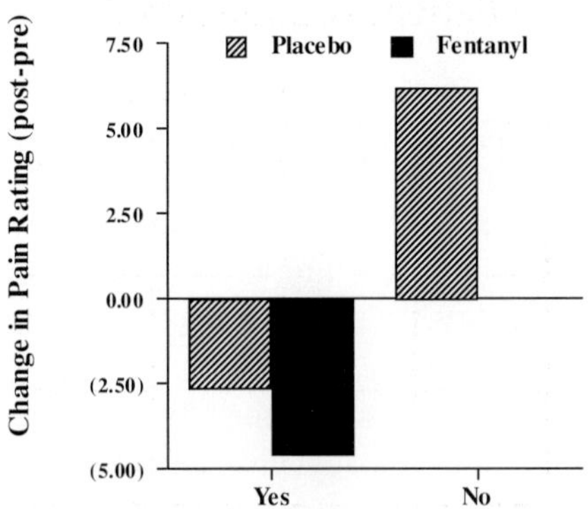

Fig. 5. Influence of clinician's knowledge on magnitude of placebo analgesia. Following extraction of a lower third molar tooth, two groups of patients received blinded intravenous infusions. Both groups read a consent form and received verbal information that indicated that opiate analgesia was a random possibility but the clinician administering the drugs knew that fentanyl was only a possibility in the group shown on the left. Placebo in this group resulted in significantly greater analgesia than that produced by placebo administered to the group in which fentanyl was not a possibility, shown on the right. From Gracely et al. (1985).

clinician and incorporates hidden infusions and disguised administrations. It contains a clinician factor of three levels. In the first two conditions, the clinician believes that either an active or placebo treatment is delivered, and in the third, common in a clinical trial, either active or placebo treatment is a random possibility. The design specifies either open or hidden administration, and a treatment identity factor for delivery of the actual treatment or the placebo treatment. In this design, IPG can be assessed by several comparisons. In the condition in which the clinician believes an active drug has been delivered, the comparison of the active drug delivered by hidden or open administration assesses IPG, as does the comparison of placebo-delivered hidden or open administration. The same comparisons can be performed under double-blind conditions (last row) with an expected decrement in IPG. The range of IPG influence can also be assessed by comparing cells in the first row with those directly below. These disguised conditions test the effect of contrary clinician beliefs, and the hidden infusions provide a baseline against which to test the relative increases or decreases in the putative effect of the treatment.

The design in Fig. 6 presents only a static comparison, and fails to include a temporal factor to assess effects such as altered expectation. It also presents theoretical possibilities unhampered by current trends of informed consent. It involves both delivery of treatments without the knowledge of

Patient Administered:

Clinician Believes ↓	Active		Placebo	
	Open	Hidden	Open	Hidden
Active				
Placebo				
Either				

Fig. 6. A design to assess influence of the clinician during administration of an analgesic or other medication. This design crosses three factors: what the clinician believes is being administered, shown on the left; whether the patient is administered an active or placebo treatment; and whether the patient is aware of the treatment administration. The influence of the clinician can be assessed by comparisons such as those between the open and hidden conditions on the top row, for example, comparing the effect of openly giving a placebo or active treatment versus administering the same treatment hidden when the clinician believes that an active treatment is being administered. Comparisons between rows evaluate the manipulation of clinicians' beliefs during open treatment administration.

the subject and misrepresentation of the treatment identity to the clinician. These ethical issues lead to a tension between quality data and reservations about the temporary need for deception until a post-study debriefing. Resolution of the opposing needs for scientific rigor and ethical treatment of subjects depends on an evolving ethical and political climate and is one of three historical trends that influence the investigation and clinical efficacy of IPG.

TRENDS IN IPG RESEARCH

IPG research involves three themes that are not mutually exclusive: medicine before technology, the decline of paternalism and deception, and the influence of technology and practice of medicine on treatment efficacy and patient satisfaction. These themes are three aspects of the continued scientific progression in medical treatment in an informed society. If this trend continues, patients might someday choose their own treatments through an Internet browser with passive tacit physician approval. In this scenario, evidence-based medicine would dominate decision-making. Patients would be protected from worthless treatments, but the art of medicine would be lost.

Medicine before Pasteur. Prior to the advent of biomedical approaches, doctors had to depend on IPG factors and were aware of the importance of their own attitudes and behavior. The literature of the past two decades essentially repeats statements made throughout the history of medicine. In 1628 Burton observed that the physician must "be confident he can cure or at least make the patient believe so, otherwise his Physick will not be effectual. ... confidence and hope do more good than Physick" (Burton 1951).

In 1938 Houston presented an address to the American College of Physicians entitled, "The Doctor Himself as a Therapeutic Agent," in which he argued that physicians at the time of Hippocrates were exceptionally skillful at dealing with the emotional dimensions of therapy and that they were the therapeutic agents by which cures were effected (Houston 1938; Spiro 1986).

In Beecher's (1961) classic paper, "Surgery as Placebo," he states what he erroneously claimed to be a new principle of therapeutic action: "Certain drugs are effective only if a required mental state is present. My material indicates that is also true for surgery, and that success depends in certain situations upon an appropriate mental state of the patient and surgeon."

Decline of paternalism and deception. The classic figure of the all-knowing, kind, and caring doctor is firmly entrenched in literature and folklore. The physician was the ultimate authority, respected and trusted. The doctor-patient relationship was sacred, and patients shared a greater personal and physical intimacy with their doctors than they would permit with spouses or parents. A physician's treatment was augmented by potent IPG factors related to his confidence, the patient's trust and admiration, and the relationship established between them. This relationship was not hampered by present standards of informed consent, as Holmes aptly stated: "Your patient has no more right to all the truth you know than he has for all your medicine in your saddle bags ... he should get only as much as is good for him" (Holmes 1883). The ethics of deception were heavily influenced by Percival's 1803 publication of *Medical Ethics*, which supported the use of benevolent deception (King 1971; Rawlinson 1985). Informed consent had not yet dictated doctor behavior, and physicians were free to engage in the "benevolent lie" in caring for their patients. During this time, toxic effects of drugs could be avoided by delivering a weaker or inert substance in combination with both direct IPG behavior and indirect IPG factors fostered in part by the paternalistic doctor-patient relationship.

Times changed. The public attitude of "doctor knows best" has been steadily replaced by a demand to know everything about every treatment. The use of deception met with strong moral objections for its negative consequences to society, the clinician, and the patient. Deception has become incompatible with modern principles of informed consent, and has long been criticized for weakening the patient's already damaged autonomy (Kant 1949; Augustine 1961; Bok 1974, 1978; Rawlinson 1985).

Presently, the delivery of deception can be considered by the same criteria used to assess any treatment, that of weighing the benefit with the cost. In some cases deception might be justified, such as delivery of a placebo opiate to a patient with compromised respiratory function. Rawlinson (1985) described criteria for the use of placebo therapy that include benefit for the patient rather than the physician, use only when justifiably necessary, and attention to the negative medical and psychological consequences.

Treatment environments: managed scientific care and the increasing popularity of alternative medicine. Many practicing clinicians express the concern that the managed care environment does not allow them to practice their "magic" anymore, and that doctors would be much more effective if they had a clinical rotation in witch doctor school. This complaint is not new. Benson and Epstein (1975) sounded the alarm 25 years ago: "The placebo effect is a neglected and berated asset of patient care. Any health care system that minimizes and fragments the relationship between the physician and the patient will lessen the effects of this asset." The present climate of managed care in many countries has further exacerbated this trend. Patients are becoming dissatisfied with conventional medicine and are increasingly drawn toward alternative therapies that provide the elements of personal relationship and time that are missing from modern medical practice. The influence of IPG factors in the therapeutic success of the various fields of alternative practice has yet to be determined. Studies of these methods (and of conventional therapies as well) should include the necessary controls to assess IPG effects and also the influence of patient-specific variables that operate independently of IPG effects. As noted above, the results of such studies on mind-body therapies are of particular relevance because they indicate a therapeutic baseline from which to compare all other therapies.

IMPLICATIONS

Research. The questions are obvious. Are physical or pharmacological interventions, with potential adverse effects, more efficacious than baseline therapies devoid of physical contact or interventions? Or do they provide some other benefit such as a more consistent response over a diverse group of subjects? Do physical interventions and IPG-mediated effects differ in their mechanisms? How much of an active effect is due to IPG factors? In a recent study of pharmacological treatment for depression, Kirsch and Saperstein (1998) concluded that only one-quarter of the therapeutic effect was due to the drug, while twice as much effect, or fully half, was due to IPG and patient-related factors.

Clinical practice. The implications are also clear, and not new. Clinicians should strive to understand how their patients view the world and should provide a rational explanation for their disease and its treatment within this framework. The social graces of deception may be needed occasionally and used sparingly, but the ethics of deception are a minor issue. The evidence indicates that, regardless of the natural gifts of charisma and related traits, treatment will be most effective if time is spent searching for the best possible treatment and then administering it with the utmost confidence.

ACKNOWLEDGMENTS

The author thanks Michael J. Farrell and Masilo A.B. Grant for their technical assistance and comments on the manuscript.

REFERENCES

Abbot FK, Mack M, Wolf S. The action of Banthine on the stomach and duodenum of man with observations on the effects of placebos. *Gastroenterology* 1952; 20:249-261.

Adams CBT. Microvascular compression: an alternative review and hypothesis. *J Neurosurg* 1989; 57:1–12.

Archer TP, Leier CV. Placebo treatment in congestive heart failure. *Cardiology* 1992; 81:125–133.

Augustine. *Enchiridion*. Paolucci H (Ed). Chicago: Henry Regnery, 1961.

Beecher HK. The powerful placebo. *JAMA* 1955; 159:1602–1606.

Beecher HK. *Measurement of Subjective Responses*. New York: Oxford University Press, 1959.

Beecher HK. Surgery as placebo. *JAMA* 1961; 156:1102–1107.

Benson H, Epstein MD. The placebo effect: a neglected asset in the care of patients. *JAMA* 1975; 232:1225–1227.

Benson H. McCallie DP. Angina pectoris and the placebo effect. *N Engl J Med* 1979; 300:1424–1429.

Bok S. The ethics of giving placebos. *Sci Am* 1974; 231:17–22.

Bok S. *Lying*. New York: Pantheon, 1978.

Branthwaite A, Cooper P. Analgesic effects of branding in treatment of headaches. *BMJ (Clin Res Ed)* 1981; 282:1576–1578.

Buckalew LW, Coffield KE. Drug expectations associated with perceptual characteristics: ethnic factory. *Percept Motor Skills* 1982a; 55:915–918.

Buckalew LW, Coffield KE. An investigation of drug expectancy as a function of capsule color and size and preparation form. *J Clin Psychopharmacol* 1982b; 2:245–248.

Buckalew LW, Ross S. Relationship of perceptual characteristics to placebo efficacy. *Psychol Rep* 1981; 49:955–961.

Burton R. *The Anatomy of Melancholy*. Dell F, Smith PJ (Eds). New York: Tudor, 1955, originally published 1628.

Bush PJ. The placebo effect. *J Am Pharmaceutical Assoc* 1974; NS14:671–652.

Chow OK, Qo SY, Lam WK, Yu DY, Yeung CY. Effect of acupuncture on exercise-induced asthma. *Lung* 1983; 161:321–326.

Cobb LA, Thomas GI, Dillard DH, Merendinio KA, Bruce RA. An evaluation of internal-mammary-artery ligation by a double-blind technique. *N Engl J Med* 1959; 2608:1115–1118.

Denton JE, Beecher HK. New analgesics I. Methods in the clinical evaluation of new analgesics. *JAMA* 1949; 141:1051–1057.

Dimond EG, Kittle CF, Crockett JE. Comparison of internal mammary ligation and sham operation for angina pectoris. *Am J Cardiol* 1960; 5:483–486.

Egbert LD, Battit GE, Welch CE, Bartlett MK. Reduction in postoperative pain by encouragement and instruction of patients. *N Engl J Med* 1964; 270:825–827.

Eliav E, Gracely RH. Trigeminal neuralgia. In: Block AR, Kremer E, Fernandez E (Eds). *Handbook of Chronic Pain Syndromes*. Mahwah, NJ: Erlbaum and Associates, 1999, pp 435–453.

Engel G. A life setting conducive to illness: the giving-up-given-up complex. *Ann Intern Med* 1968; 69:292–300.

Engel G. The need for a new medical model: a challenge for biomedicine. *Science* 1977; 196:129–136.

Evans FJ. Expectancy, Therapeutic instructions, and the placebo response. In: White L, Tursky B, Schwartz GE (Eds). *Placebo: Therapy, Research and Treatment*. New York: Guilford Press, 1985, pp 235–228.

Freed CR, Breeze RE, Greene PE, et al. Double-blind placebo-controlled human fetal dopamine cell transplants in advanced Parkinson's disease. *Soc Neurosci Abstr* 1999; 27:212.

Fung KP, Chow OK, So SY. Attenuation of exercise-induced asthma by acupuncture. *Lancet* 1986; 2:1419–1422.

Galer BS, Schwartz L, Turner JA. Do patient and physician expectations predict response to pain-relieving procedures? *Clin J Pain* 1997; 13:148–351.

Gallimore RG, Turner JL. Contemporary studies of placebo phenomena. In: Jarvik ME (Ed). *Psychopharmacology in the Practice of Medicine*. New York: Appleton-Century Crofts, 1977.

Goodman P, Green CS, Laskin. Response of patients with myofascial pain-dysfunction syndrome to mock equilibration. *J Am Dental Assoc* 1976; 92:755–758.
Gracely RH, Dubner R, Deeter WR, Wolskee P. Naloxone and placebo alter postsurgical pain by separate mechanisms. *Nature* 1983; 306:264–265.
Gracely RH, Dubner R, Deeter WR, Wolskee P. Clinician's expectations influence placebo analgesia. *Lancet* 1985; 1:8419–8443.
Graham DT, Kabler JD, Graham FK. Physiological response to the suggestion of attitudes specific for hives and hypertension. *Psychosom Med* 1962; 24:159–167.
Gybels J, Sweet WH. *Neurosurgical Treatment of Persistent Pain*. Basel: Karger, 1989, pp 10–69.
Gryll SL, Katahn M. Situational factors contributing to the placebo effect. *Psychopharmacology* 1978; 57:253–261.
Hahn RA. The nocebo phenomenon: concept, evidence, and implications for public health. *Prev Med* 1997; 26:607–611.
Hashish I, Harvey W, Harris M. Anti-inflammatory effects of ultrasound therapy: evidence for a major placebo effect. *Br J Rheumatol* 1986; 25:77–81.
Hardy JD, Cattel McK. Measurement of pain threshold-raising action of aspirin, codeine, and meperidine (Demerol). *Fed Proc* 1950; 9:280.
Hardy JD, Wolff HG, Goodell H. *Pain Sensation and Reactions*. Baltimore: Williams and Wilkins, 1952.
Hass H, Fink H, Hartfelder G. Das Placeboproblem. *Prog Drug Res* 1959; 1:279–454.
Henker B, Whalen CK, Collins BE. Double-blind and triple-blind assessments of medication and placebo responses in hyperactive children. *J Abnorm Child Psychol* 1979; 7:1–13.
Ho KH, Hashish I, Salmon P, Freeman R, Harvey W. Reduction of post-operative swelling by a placebo effect. *J Psychosom Res* 32:197–205, 1988.
Hoffer A, Osmond H. Double blind clinical trials. *J Neuropsychol* 1961, 2:221–227.
Holmes OW. *Medical Essays*. Boston: Houghton Mifflin, 1883.
Houston WR. The doctor himself as a therapeutic agent. *Ann Intern Med* 1938; 11:1416–1425.
Howitt JW. An evaluation of audio-analgesia effects. *J Dent Children* 1967; 5:406–411.
Ikemi Y, Nakagawa S. A psychosomatic study of contagious dermatitis. *Kyudhu J Med Sci* 1962; 13:335–350.
Kant I. On a supposed right to lie from benevolent motives. In: Beck LW (Ed). (edited and translated). *Critique of Practical Reason and Other Writings in Moral Philosophy*. Chicago: University of Chicago Press, 1949 (originally published 1797).
King LS. *The Medical World of the Eighteenth Century*. New York: Huntington, Robert E. Krieger, 1971.
Kirsch I, Sapirstein G. Listening to Prozac but hearing placebo: a meta-analysis of antidepressant medication. *Prev Treat* 1998; 1:article 0002a.
Lipkin M. Suggestion and healing. *Perspect Biol Med* 1984; 28:121–126.
Lyerly SB, Ross S, Krugman AD, Clyde DJ. Drugs and placebos: the effects of instructions upon performance and mood under amphetamine sulphate and chloral hydrate. *J Abnorm Soc Psychol* 1964; 68:321–327.
Littman A, Welch R, Fruin RC, et al. Controlled trials of aluminum hydroxide gels for peptic ulcer. *Gastroenterology* 1977; 73:6–10.
MacDonald AJ, Peden NR, Hayton R, et al. Symptom relief and the placebo effect in the trial of an antipeptic drug. *Gut* 1980; 21:323–326.
Maslach D, Marshall G, Zimbardo P. Hypnotic control of peripheral skin temperature. *Psychophysiology* 1972; 9:600–605.
McGlashan TH, Evans FJ, Orne MT. The nature of hypnotic analgesia and placebo response to experimental pain. *Psychosom Med* 1969; 31:227–246.
Melzack R. *The Puzzle of Pain*. New York: Basic, 1973.
Moerman DE. Cultural variations in the placebo effect: ulcers, anxiety and blood pressure. *Med Anthropol Q*; 1999: in press.
Moseley JB Jr, Wray NP, Kuykendall D, Willis K, Landon G. Arthroscopic treatment of

osteoarthritis of the knee: a prospective, randomized placebo-controlled trial. Results of a pilot study. *Am J Sports Med* 1966; 24:28–34.

Paul GL, Tobias LL, Holly BL. Maintenance psychotropic drugs in the presence of active treatment programs: a triple-blind withdrawal study with long term mental patients. *Arch Gen Psychiatry* 1972; 27:106–115.

Plotkin WB. A psychological approach to placebo: the role of faith in therapy and treatment. In: White L, Tursky B, Schwartz GE (Eds). *Placebo: Theory, Research and Treatment.* New York: Guilford Press, 1985, pp 237–254.

Rawlinson MC. Truth-telling and paternalism in the clinic: philosophical reflections on the use of placebos in medical practice. In: White L, Tursky B, Schwartz GE (Eds). *Placebo: Theory, Research and Treatment.* New York: Guilford Press, 1985, pp 403–41.

Roberts A, Kewman DB, Mercier L, Hovell M. The power of nonspecific effects in healing: implications for psychosocial and biological treatments. *Clin Psychol Rev* 1993; 13:375-391.

Rosenberg JL. A re-evaluation of audio analgesia. *Oral Surg Oral Med Oral Pathol* 1964; 17:319–324.

Ross S, Krugman AD, Lyerly SB, Clyde BJ. Drugs and placebos: a model design. *Psychol Rep* 1962; 10:383–392.

Rozanski A, Blumenthal J, Kaplan J. Impact of psychological factors on the pathogenesis of cardiovascular disease and implications for therapy. *Circulation* 1999; 99:2192–2217.

Sarles H, Camatte R, Sachel J. A study of the variations in the response regarding duodenal ulcers when treated with placebo by different investigators. *Digestion* 1977; 16:289–292.

Shapiro AK. A contribution to a history of the placebo effect. *Behav Sci* 1960; 5:109–135.

Shapiro AK. Etiological factors in the placebo effect. *JAMA* 1964; 187:712–714.

Shapiro AK. Placebo effects in medicine, psychotherapy, and psychoanalysis. In: Nergina AE, Garfield SL (Eds). *Handbook of Psychotherapy and Behavior Change: an Empirical Analysis.* New York: John Wiley and Sons, 1971.

Spangfort EV. The lumbar disc herniation: a computer-aided analysis of 2504 operations. *Acta Orthop Scand* 1972; 342(Suppl):1–95.

Spiro HM. *Doctors, Patients, and Placebos.* New Haven: Yale University Press, 1986.

Strong SR. From social psychology: what? *Counsel Psychol* 1995; 23:686–690.

Sweet WH. Complications of treating trigeminal neuralgia: an analysis of the literature and response to a questionnaire. In: Rovit RL, Murali A, Jannetta PJ (Eds). *Trigeminal Neuralgia.* Baltimore: Williams & Wilkins, 1990, pp 251–279.

Thomas KB. General practice consultations: is there any point in being positive? *BMJ* 1987; 294:1200–1202.

Turner JA, Deyo RA, Loeser JD, Von Korff M, Fordyce WE. The importance of placebo effects in pail treatment and research. *JAMA* 1994; 271:1609–1614.

Uhlenhuth EH, Rickels K, Fisher S, et al. Drug, doctor's verbal attitude and clinic setting in symptomatic response to pharmacotherapy. *Psychopharmacology* 1966; 9:392–418.

Weidner G, Mueller H. Emotions and coronary heart disease. In: Goldman MB, Hatch MC (Eds). *Women and Health.* San Diego: Academic Press, in press.

Wheatley D. Influence of doctors' and patients' attitudes in the treatment of neurotic illness. *Lancet* 1967; 2:1133–1135.

Winters C, Artnak EJ, Benjamin SB, et al. Esophageal bouginage in symptomatic patients with nutcracker esophagus. *JAMA* 1984; 252:363–366.

Wolskee PJ, Gracely RH, Greenberg RP, Dubner R, Lees D. Comparison of effects of morphine and deep brain stimulation on chronic pain. *Am Pain Soc Abstr* 1982, p 36.

Zachariae R. *Mind and Immunity: Psychological Modulation of Immunological and Inflammatory Parameters.* Munksgaard: Rosinante, 1996.

Correspondence to: Richard H. Gracely, PhD, CMMU/PNMB/NIDCR, NIH-10/1N-103D, Bethesda, MD 20892, USA. Tel: 301-496-5238; Fax: 301-496-1005; email: richard.gracely@nih.gov.

Proceedings of the 9th World Congress on Pain,
Progress in Pain Research and Management,
Vol. 16, edited by M. Devor, M.C. Rowbotham, and
Z. Wiesenfeld-Hallin, IASP Press, Seattle, © 2000.

100

Can Cognitive-Behavioral Therapies Succeed Where Medical Treatments Fail?

Francis J. Keefe

Duke University Medical Center, Durham, North Carolina, USA

Individuals whose pain has failed to respond to medical and surgical treatments are increasingly being referred for specialized programs in cognitive-behavioral therapy (CBT). This trend raises the important question of how helpful such therapy is in treating patients who have persistent and disabling pain. The purpose of this chapter is to provide an overview of recent studies examining the efficacy of CBT. In the first section I describe and analyze the conceptual background and basic components of CBT treatment programs. In the next section I critically review outcome studies that have examined the efficacy of CBT. To illustrate the nature, strengths, and limitations of these studies, I will examine data on the outcome of CBT in various chronic pain conditions including arthritis pain, cancer pain, sickle cell disease pain, and back pain. In the final section of the chapter, I highlight important future directions for CBT outcome research, such as early intervention to prevent pain and disability and the integration of CBT into medical and surgical pain management approaches.

CONCEPTUAL BACKGROUND

Historically, pain has been conceptualized as the direct result of underlying tissue damage or injury. This model assumes that pain is proportional to the degree of tissue damage or injury, such that patients with extensive disease activity or serious injury would be expected to have high levels of pain, while those with little or no evidence of disease or injury would be expected to have low levels of pain. This conceptual model has served as the basis for many conventional approaches to pain, whose goal was first to identify the source of underlying tissue damage and then to eliminate its effects through medical or surgical treatment. Consistent with this model is the notion that pain relief is the primary outcome by which treatment efficacy is evaluated.

Clinical observations and research studies have revealed several problems with the model of pain described above. First, in many cases, the pain reported by a patient is not proportional to the evidence of underlying tissue damage. Studies of battlefield casualties (Beecher 1959) and emergency department patients (Melzack et al. 1982) have shown that some individuals with obvious injuries report little or no pain, while others with minimal injuries may report severe or excruciating pain. Second, patients who have the same tissue pathology basis for their pain often show quite varied responses to the same surgical or medical treatment. For example, in clinical settings we have observed that patients with very similar levels of osteoarthritis of the knees often respond quite differently to knee replacement surgery (Keefe and Caldwell 1997). Following surgical treatment, many of these patients experience little or no pain, become involved in a much wider range of daily activities, and are optimistic about their abilities to cope with pain, while other patients are overwhelmed by their pain, may be confined to a wheelchair, and are pessimistic about the future. Finally, the model fails to acknowledge the important role that behavioral and psychological factors play in influencing the pain experience (Melzack and Wall 1996).

Dissatisfaction with this traditional model of pain was a major factor in the emergence of the field of pain research and practice, stimulating pain researchers to develop new experimental approaches that have increased our understanding of basic pain processes and leading to the development of new theoretical models of pain. The cognitive-behavioral model of pain is one of these models (Turk et al. 1983).

The hallmark of the cognitive-behavioral model is its insistence that in order to understand pain, we must not only consider underlying tissue damage, but also take into account cognitive factors (e.g., expectations, beliefs, and memories) and behavioral factors (e.g., activity level, home or work environment) that can influence the pain experience. Because this perspective views pain as a complex phenomenon, it not only considers pain relief as a key index of therapeutic improvement, but also emphasizes the importance of improvements in psychological functioning (e.g., coping, self-efficacy, and amelioration of depression and anxiety) and social functioning (e.g., marital satisfaction, family environment, and social support).

The cognitive-behavioral model of pain is based on two research traditions. The first is the behavioral and social learning theory and research tradition. Social learning theory maintains that behavioral factors, such as an overly sedentary and restricted lifestyle, and social factors, such as a supportive work environment, can be influential in determining whether pain develops or persists (Fordyce 1976; Keefe and Lefebvre 1994). Research shows that behavioral interventions based on social learning principles can reduce pain and improve function (Turner and Clancy 1988). Behavioral intervention is an important component of CBT protocols, which often include self-monitoring, goal setting, activity pacing, and graded activation. Interestingly, these interventions not only are commonly employed in CBT, but also are increasingly utilized in many multidisciplinary pain management programs.

The second theoretical and research tradition that served as a foundation for CBT is that of cognitive theory and research (Turk et al. 1983). This tradition holds that cognitive processes such as thoughts, expectations, beliefs, and memories are important not only because they can influence the pain experience, but also because they can lead to problematic changes in feelings (e.g., increased depression) and behaviors (e.g., overdependence on family members or friends) that contribute to pain-related disability.

In many ways, the gate control theory (Melzack and Wall 1965) set the stage for the emergence of a cognitive perspective on pain. This theory proposed that brain activity in areas responsible for cognition and affect can influence the pain experience by activating descending neural pathways that serve to block pain at the level of the spinal cord. Research studies, both at the basic and clinical levels, have provided considerable support for the gate control theory (Melzack 1999; Wall 1999). This theory and the research it generated led to heightened recognition of the role that cognitive processes can play in chronic pain and increased interest in the use of psychological and behavioral pain management methods.

The emergence of the cognitive-behavioral perspective on pain has also been heavily influenced by numerous research studies documenting the importance of cognitive variables such as pain coping, self-efficacy, and fear-avoidance beliefs (Lester and Keefe 1997). Studies of coping strategies, for example, have found that patients who rely on passive and ineffective strategies (such as catastrophizing) are much more likely to experience high levels of pain and psychological distress and to develop maladaptive pain behavior patterns (Keefe et al. 1992). Other research has demonstrated that patients who rate their self-efficacy for pain as high not only report lower levels of clinical pain, but also have higher thresholds and greater tolerance for controlled experimental pain stimulation (Keefe et al. 1997). Recent investigations also have shown that the beliefs of chronic pain patients about the need to avoid pain are closely associated with excessive pain and disability (Vlaeyen et al. 1995). The results of such studies have enabled cognitive-behavioral researchers to develop treatment protocols designed to enhance coping strategies and alter patients' appraisals of pain.

Cognitive-behavioral protocols for managing pain have several basic elements (Keefe and Caldwell 1997). First, they provide patients with a rationale that helps them view pain in a different way. The gate control theory, for example, might be used to help a patient understand the influence that thoughts and feelings can have on pain. Alternatively, an adaptational model might be used that emphasizes the role that learning can play in the development and maintenance of problematic ways of responding to pain (Keefe et al. 1996b). Patients in chronic pain may be skeptical about the utility of CBT, and it is very important that they be provided a compelling rationale and an opportunity to discuss their own thoughts, attitudes, and beliefs about pain before treatment techniques are introduced. A second important element of CBT is training in multiple pain coping skills. Most protocols train patients in a variety of behavioral skills (e.g., pacing one's activities, relaxation training, and communication skills) and cognitive skills (e.g., imagery, distraction, and calming self-statements). These skills are often presented as a menu from which patients can select, modify, and combine. A third element of CBT is practice and rehearsal of learned skills. During training sessions, patients have the opportunity to practice their skills while being given feedback from a therapist. Home practice sessions are also important in developing a sense of mastery of pain control skills. Finally, CBT emphasizes training in relapse prevention techniques (Keefe and Van Horn 1993). Patients learn how to attend to early warning signs of setbacks, develop strategies for handling pain flares and challenging situations, and re-institute their pain coping efforts after a relapse.

THE EFFICACY OF COGNITIVE-BEHAVIORAL THERAPY

Several randomized controlled studies have tested the efficacy of CBT for chronic pain. Many of these studies are methodologically sophisticated and have positive design features, including random assignment to CBT or one or more control conditions, comprehensive assessments of outcome, and long-term follow-up evaluations. Therapy might include multiple sessions of training in a variety of pain coping skills (e.g., relaxation, activity pacing, imagery, and problem solving) and the use of treatment manuals. Randomized studies of CBT have been conducted in a wide variety of pain populations such as arthritis pain, cancer pain, sickle cell disease pain, back pain, and mixed chronic pain patients.

COGNITIVE-BEHAVIORAL THERAPY FOR ARTHRITIS PAIN

Pain is major problem for patients who have rheumatic diseases such as osteoarthritis and rheumatoid arthritis. Medical approaches (e.g., nonsteroidal anti-inflammatory drugs [NSAIDs]) are helpful in managing the pain, but side effects limit their long-term use. There is increasing interest in educational and cognitive-behavioral pain management approaches for patients with rheumatic diseases (Superio-Cabuslay et al. 1996).

We conducted a controlled study to test the effects of a CBT protocol for osteoarthritis patients with persistent knee pain (Keefe et al. 1990a). In this study, 99 such patients were randomly assigned to one of three groups. Patients in the CBT group attended 10 weekly, 2-hour group sessions of training in a wide variety of behavioral and cognitive pain coping skills. Patients in the arthritis education group attended 10 weekly, 2-hour group sessions that provided them with detailed information about osteoarthritis and its medical and surgical treatment, but no training in pain coping skills. Patients in the standard care control condition continued with the routine care provided to patients with osteoarthritis. The use of two comparison conditions in this study is noteworthy. The arthritis education comparison condition provided a control for nonspecific effects of CBT, such as contact with a caring therapist, whereas the standard care control condition enabled us to compare the effects of CBT to those obtained with routine medical care alone. Note that all patients assigned to control conditions in this study, as in most studies of CBT, were allowed to continue their regular medical care. Thus, these studies enable us to determine what CBT contributes over and above routine medical care.

The CBT and arthritis education protocols used in the Keefe et al. (1990a) study were carefully standardized. For each of these interventions, therapists followed a manual that provided a very detailed outline of each session. Treatment sessions were also audiotaped, and therapists met with a supervisor weekly to review the tapes. Records of attendance at group sessions showed high levels of attendance (over 90%) for both the CBT and arthritis education sessions. Finally, patients were asked to provide ratings of the credibility of treatment to ensure that differences in outcome were not due to variations in how credible or logical the treatment seemed. Interestingly, mean ratings of credibility were high (over 8 on a 10-point scale) for both CBT and arthritis education conditions.

Data analysis performed to evaluate treatment outcome revealed that, at the completion of treatment, patients in the CBT group had significantly lower levels of pain and psychological disability than did patients in the arthritis education and standard care control groups (Keefe et al. 1990a). A subsequent long-term follow-up study showed that patients in the CBT group were able to maintain their gains in psychological functioning and that they began to show improvements in physical disability when compared to patients in the arthritis education group (Keefe et al. 1990b). Patients in the CBT group, however, did not maintain their gains in pain relief over the long term. This finding led us in subsequent studies to explore other strategies for maintaining treatment effects, such as spouse-assisted CBT training (Keefe et al. 1996c) or systematic training in relapse prevention methods (Keefe and Van Horn 1993).

The effects of CBT have also been tested in rheumatoid arthritis patients. Bradley et al. (1987), for example, found that CBT led to significant reductions in pain behavior, anxiety, and disease activity in such patients. Parker et al. (1995) found that a comprehensive CBT protocol focusing on pain and stress management was also effective.

Over the past few years, several systematic reviews have evaluated the effects of CBT in arthritis patients (Keefe and Caldwell 1997; Compas et al. 1998; Bradley and Alberts 1999). The only meta-analysis of this literature, to our knowledge, is that of Superio-Cabuslay et al. (1996), who examined data from 19 education trials in rheumatoid arthritis patients. This meta-analysis was more broadly focused on patient education trials, only some of which used CBT methods, but its results are interesting. Although the average effect size for pain in these education trials was modest (0.17), the effect sizes for pain obtained in studies that used the type of comprehensive CBT intervention we have discussed were generally much higher (range = 0.27–0.60). The authors also calculated the added benefits of providing the educational intervention to arthritis patients who may be taking NSAIDs. These benefits were 20–30% as great as the effects of NSAIDs for pain relief in osteoarthritis and rheumatoid arthritis, 40% as great as the effects of NSAIDs for improvements in functional disability in rheumatoid arthritis, and 60–80% as great as the effects of NSAIDs for improvements in tender joint counts in rheumatoid arthritis.

COGNITIVE-BEHAVIORAL THERAPY FOR SICKLE CELL DISEASE PAIN

Episodes of severe and disabling pain afflict many patients suffering from sickle cell disease. This pain, due to vaso-occlusion secondary to sickling of cells, often occurs unpredictably and may last for days or weeks. Patients vary considerably in their use of health care resources during sickle cell pain episodes, and evidence indicates that patients' coping efforts are related to health care utilization (Gil et al. 1989).

In the past few years, several well-controlled randomized studies have examined the effects of CBT for sickle cell disease pain. In one study (Gil et al. 1996), 64 African Americans with sickle cell disease were randomly assigned to either a CBT condition or an education control condition. The CBT protocol involved a series of three 45-minute sessions. During each session, patients were taught two new coping skills (e.g., relaxation, imagery) and were then given an opportunity to practice applying these skills during exposure to a laboratory pain stimulus (Forgione-Barber pressure pain stimulator). Patients receiving CBT had significant improvements in coping (increased coping attempts, decreased negative thinking) and a decrease in their ratings of laboratory pain stimuli. A subsequent follow-up report (Gil et al., in press) revealed that on days when CBT participants practiced learned coping strategies for pain they were much less likely to contact their health care providers.

Another recent study by Gil et al. (1997) examined the effects of CBT in children with sickle cell disease pain. In this study, 49 children (mean age = 11.9 years) were randomly assigned to either a CBT coping skills training group or to a standard care control group. The CBT protocol involved only a single session of training and focused on three coping skills (deep breathing/counting relaxation, pleasant imagery, and calming self-statements). Data analysis revealed that CBT produced a significant decrease in negative thinking and a reduction in ratings of a low-intensity laboratory pain stimulus.

Taken together, these studies suggest that CBT may be effective altering pain coping and pain perception in sickle cell patients. These studies, however, have failed to show that CBT can result in measurable improvements in clinical pain or health care use. Given the severity and disabling nature of sickle cell disease pain, more intensive and comprehensive CBT interventions may need to be developed for this patient population.

COGNITIVE-BEHAVIORAL THERAPY FOR CANCER PAIN

Pain is a major concern of cancer patients and their health professionals. Studies have shown that up to 80% of cancer patients with advanced disease have significant pain (Bonica et al. 1990). Medical interventions for managing cancer pain have been developed, but many patients with advanced disease do not experience adequate pain relief (Zelman et al. 1987).

Syrjala and her colleagues at the University of Washington have carried out several controlled studies to test the effectiveness of CBT in managing cancer pain in patients having bone marrow transplantation. There are several reasons why this procedure provides a good model in which to test the effects of CBT (Syrjala et al. 1992). First, the medical treatment (chemotherapy and radiation) is well standardized and is delivered in a controlled environment. Second, patients undergoing this treatment regimen experience significant oral mucositis pain that interferes with their ability to eat and speak. Third, opioid treatments often fail to eliminate or significantly reduce mucositis pain. Thus, there is a need to explore alternative approaches to pain control in such patients.

Syrjala et al. (1992) randomly assigned such patients to one of four groups: (1) training in cognitive-behavioral pain coping skills, (2) hypnosis, (3) attention control, or (4) standard care control. Therapists met with patients twice prior to admission to the clinic and then followed the patients during their 3-week inpatient stay. While hypnosis was effective in reducing mucositis pain, the CBT intervention had no effect on pain relief.

A subsequent study by Syrjala and her colleagues (1995) tested the effects of a more comprehensive CBT protocol in managing pain during bone marrow transplantation treatment. In this study, 94 patients were randomly assigned to (1) a comprehensive CBT protocol that included training in relaxation, imagery, coping self-statements, distraction, goal setting, and problem solving; (2) a more limited CBT protocol that focused on relaxation and imagery training only; (3) a control condition of therapist attention; or (4) a control condition of standard care only. Patients receiving either the comprehensive or the more limited CBT protocol had significant reductions in pain when compared to the two control conditions. Patients receiving either of the CBT interventions also reported significant improvements in their ability to manage the pain and nausea associated with their treatment.

Three recent meta-analytic reviews have examined the effects of psychoeducational interventions (many of which include training in CBT techniques) in controlling cancer pain and other symptoms (Smith et al. 1994; Devine and Westlake 1995; Meyer and Mark 1995). These reviews have found support for the efficacy of such interventions in cancer pain control. Devine and Westlake (1995), for example, noted a positive treatment effect in 92% of the studies they reviewed. Studies using relaxation-based interventions were particularly effective and had a large and homogeneous overall effect size (0.91).

COGNITIVE-BEHAVIORAL THERAPY FOR BACK PAIN

Back pain is the most common chronic pain disorder, and in many countries it is the leading cause of disability and work loss (Waddell 1998). Over the past decade, several systematic reviews and meta-analyses have examined the efficacy of cognitive-behavioral interventions for back pain. In this section, we highlight two of the most recent reviews.

Flor (in press) conducted a meta-analysis of 80 studies involving over 3000 patients with back pain or mixed chronic pain symptoms. This review compared patients receiving psychological interventions (most of which were based on CBT) to those receiving medical treatment only. Data analysis revealed that, at the completion of treatment, patients who had received a psychological intervention had 54% greater improvement than those receiving medical treatment alone. Interestingly, these benefits were maintained at the 1-year follow-up, with patients receiving psychological intervention showing an average of 48% improvement relative to medical care alone.

Linton (in press) conducted an evidence-based review of the literature on CBT for neck and back pain. He concluded that "multidimensional programs that include CBT are statistically and clinically superior to control groups," and that CBT programs produce moderate to large improvement on the key outcome variables as compared to waiting-list controls. Linton's review, in particular, found that CBT was likely to produce improvements in pain, psychological function, and medication intake. Linton also noted that CBT was superior to control conditions at long-term follow-up.

Taken together, the results of recent systematic reviews provide strong support for the efficacy of CBT in the treatment of back pain.

MIXED CHRONIC PAIN SAMPLES

Morley et al. (1999) conducted the most systematic and comprehensive meta-analysis of the efficacy of CBT for chronic pain. The authors compiled data from 25 controlled studies that examined a wide range of chronic pain conditions including low back pain, arthritis, and mixed chronic pain syndromes. The patients in these studies had long histories of pain (mean = 12.27 years).

Morley et al.'s meta-analysis had two important methodological advantages. First, it included explicit information on the methods for estimating effect sizes and the reliability of the coding schemes used in categorizing the studies. Second, the authors identified and operationally defined a variety of key outcome domains that must considered in evaluating CBT studies. Consistent with the cognitive-behavioral perspective, these domains included not only measures of pain experience, but also measures of mood/affect, cognitive coping and appraisal, pain behavior, social role functioning, biological/physical fitness, use of health care resources, and miscellaneous outcomes. The delineation of these domains provides a framework for conceptualizing outcomes that may be used in future systematic reviews and meta-analyses of the CBT literature on pain.

Morley et al. calculated effect sizes for two comparisons. The first evaluated the effects of CBT versus other active treatments such as physical therapy, occupational therapy, and education, and revealed that CBT had significant effects on three outcomes: pain experience, pain behavior, and coping and appraisal. The second comparison evaluated the effects of CBT versus waiting-list control conditions, during which patients most likely continued with their usual or standard medical care. This comparison revealed that CBT had significant effects on all outcome domains, with a median effect size of 0.5. Based on these data, these authors concluded that "active psychological treatments based on the principle of cognitive-behavioral therapy are effective."

Morley et al. (1999) also highlighted several methodological and clinical issues that must be considered in evaluating the literature on CBT. First, the subjects in these studies are volunteers who met strict inclusion and exclusion criteria. The findings of these studies thus may not generalize to patients seen in clinical practice, who often have severe pain and high levels of disability and may be unwilling to participate in research studies. Second, controlled studies of CBT are often conducted in specialized research centers located in tertiary care medical centers. The results achieved may differ from those obtained in more typical clinical settings such as the primary care setting. Interestingly, a recent study by Von Korff et al. (1998) evaluated the effects of a self-management program based on cognitive-behavioral principles in the management of back pain in a primary care setting. When compared to patients randomly assigned to usual care, patients who were trained in self-management had significant reductions in activity limitations, lower levels of worry about back pain, and more positive attitudes toward self-care.

A third limitation of controlled studies of CBT for pain management is that the sample sizes are typically small (Morley et al. 1999). Many studies use samples of 20–30 patients per treatment condition. Although this number provides sufficient power to detect differences between CBT and usual care or waiting-list conditions, it is often not large enough to detect differences between different CBT protocols. A final limitation of these studies is that the mechanisms underlying the effects of CBT are unknown. Findings from many studies suggest that improvements in cognitive variables, in particular in self-efficacy and the use of coping strategies, are related to the short- and long-term improvements following CBT (Keefe and Caldwell 1997). Careful experimental studies are needed to isolate the active components of CBT. Such research is important because it may identify key processes responsible for change and lead to a streamlining of treatment interventions.

FUTURE DIRECTIONS

The evidence reviewed above indicates that CBT is effective in treating chronic pain. Future research on cognitive-behavioral interventions for chronic pain may follow several important directions. In this section we evaluate three of these directions: CBT as an early intervention, the integration of CBT into ongoing medical treatment, and tailoring CBT to meet the needs of individual patients.

COGNITIVE-BEHAVIORAL THERAPY AS AN EARLY INTERVENTION

All too often, CBT is held out as a last resort for patients who have had poor results from all other medical or surgical options. After years of pain, patients may have developed entrenched pain-related behavioral problems that are difficult to modify (e.g., an overly sedentary lifestyle or excessive reliance on pain medications). Early intervention with CBT is useful, not only because it can prevent the development of persistent pain, but also because it can reduce the likelihood of pain-related behavioral problems.

S.J. Linton and T. Andersson recently conducted a randomized controlled study evaluating the effects of CBT in preventing pain and disability in patients with acute back or neck pain (unpublished manuscript). Participants, 243 individuals having acute or spinal pain, were considered at risk for the development of chronic pain. All subjects were randomly assigned to one of three conditions: (1) a six-session CBT protocol that provided training in problem solving, relaxation techniques, communication skills, and activity pacing; (2) a six-session educational program that used a "back school" approach to teach patients about back care; or (3) an information-only condition where patients received a pamphlet of basic information on spinal pain and its management. Patients were evaluated prior to treatment and at 1-year follow-up. Data analysis revealed that, at follow-up, all three groups showed significant improvement on measures of pain and that there were no differences among the three groups in pain relief. However, patients in the CBT group made significantly fewer visits to doctors and physical therapists than did patients in the other groups. In addition, while patients in the educational program and information-only groups showed increases in their average number of sick days at 1-year follow-up, patients in the CBT group decreased their sick days to an average of 0.5 days per month. In fact, the risk for long-term sick leave was nine times lower in patients receiving CBT than in patients in the educational and information-only groups.

Linton and Andersson's study is noteworthy for several reasons. First, in contrast to the studies reviewed earlier, the patients had much shorter histories of pain and thus were more similar to back pain patients seen in primary care settings. Second, the CBT intervention was conducted in groups, thereby reducing the costs. Finally, the magnitude of reduction in risk for absenteeism was not only statistically significant, but also clinically meaningful. Taken together, these findings suggest that CBT is a promising technique for reducing the risk of long-term disability in back pain patients.

INTEGRATING COGNITIVE-BEHAVIORAL THERAPY INTO ONGOING MEDICAL OR SURGICAL PAIN TREATMENT

Cognitive-behavioral therapy is often seen as an alternative to conventional medical or surgical treatment. There are many opportunities, however, to integrate CBT into ongoing conventional pain management. For example, it could be a very useful adjunct for patients undergoing a physical therapy regimen that might temporarily increase their pain. In this context, CBT may help patients deal with exercise-related pain and may enhance their compliance with home-based exercise. CBT also could be helpful in patients who are receiving long-term opioid medications for pain by providing them with alternative strategies for managing periodic flares and setbacks. Finally, CBT may be useful in patients who are at high risk for postsurgical pain.

A good example of how CBT can be integrated into surgical treatment is provided by a recent, unpublished study conducted by D.A. Williams (1997). This study, conducted in the context of a busy surgical practice, was focused on patients who were candidates for implantable spinal cord stimulators or morphine pumps. Using pre-implant screening procedures, Williams identified a group of patients who were considered "candidates with reservations"(the implant team considered them candidates for the surgery but had some concerns about them). Prior to undergoing implantation, these patients were given a psychotherapy protocol that used several CBT methods. Outcome evaluations were conducted prior to treatment and at long-term follow-up. Interestingly, 60% of the patients who received the psychotherapy protocol were judged to have long-term success following their implants. This success rate contrasts with a much lower long-term success rate (19%) reported in a comparable sample of patients from another treatment center who had not received such a psychotherapy program. These results must be interpreted with caution, since Williams' study used a single-group design and did not randomly assign patients to a control group. Nevertheless, this study demonstrates how CBT can be integrated into surgical treatment for pain and illustrates the potential benefits of this approach.

TAILORING COGNITIVE-BEHAVIORAL THERAPY INTERVENTIONS

Research suggests that patients in chronic pain vary in their response to CBT (Keefe and Van Horn 1993; Compas et al. 1998). Some patients are more active in their coping efforts, find that CBT fits with their coping style, and respond well to training in pain coping skills. Other patients, however, are much more passive in coping, view medical approaches such as drugs or surgery as the best solution for their pain, and are skeptical about trying to learn coping skills.

Prochaska and his colleagues have developed a transtheoretical model that can be used to understand whether or not a patient is ready to initiate a self-management approach to his or her pain (Prochaska and DiClemente 1998). This model has identified five stages in terms of readiness to change. Individuals at the *precontemplation* stage are not intending to change their behavior. Those at the *contemplation* stage intend to change but are not certain about when they will begin. Individuals at the *preparation* stage are actively planning to make changes in the near future, but have not yet begun. Individuals at the *action* stage are currently taking action, and those at the *maintenance* stage are working on methods to sustain change and overcome setbacks and relapses.

Kerns et al. (1997) recently developed a Pain Stages of Change Questionnaire that is based on Prochaska and DiClemente's model. This questionnaire, designed for use with chronic pain populations, has four scales (precontemplation, contemplation, action, and maintenance) that assess a patient's readiness to adopt a self-management approach. These scales were reliable, both in terms of internal consistency and stability (Kerns et al. 1997). In a recent unpublished study, R.D. Kerns and R. Rosenberg found that scores on these scales were related to participation in a cognitive-behavioral pain management program. Patients who scored lower on the precontemplation scale and higher on the contemplation scale were much more likely to complete treatment. Furthermore, patients who completed treatment had significantly higher scores on the action and maintenance scales, and improvements in these scales were related to better outcomes.

Using a slightly different stages of change measure, the University of Rhode Island Change Assessment Questionnaire (URICA; McConnaughy et al. 1989), we recently conducted a study of arthritis patients' readiness to adopt a self-management approach to managing their pain and other arthritis symptoms (Keefe et. al. 1999). This study sought to determine whether, within a heterogeneous sample of arthritis patients, we could identify homogeneous subgroups of patients who were similar in terms of their responses to a stages of change questionnaire. The subjects in this study included 103 patients with rheumatoid arthritis and 74 patients with osteoarthritis. Consistent with the transtheoretical model, a cluster analysis of questionnaire responses revealed five distinct subgroups: (1) precontemplation, 44% of the sample; (2) contemplation, 11% of the sample; (3) preparation, 22% of the sample; (4) unprepared action, 6% of the sample; and (5) prepared maintenance, 17% of the sample. The fact that the largest subgroup was made up of patients at the precontemplation stage suggests that many arthritis patients may deny they have problems in self-management of their symptoms, and thus may have difficulty in becoming involved in formal programs to learn coping skills.

Although the transtheoretical model has only recently been applied to chronic pain patients, the results already obtained suggest that a patient's stage of change may be important in understanding variations in participation and response to treatment and that treatment must be based on the patient's stage. Thus, to engage patients who are at the precontemplation stage, health care professionals may need to use tailored educational messages or support group formats. Such interventions improved recruitment rates, reduced attrition, and improved outcome in studies of CBT in the treatment of smoking, obesity, and other health conditions (Prochaska et al. 1994).

CONCLUSIONS

In sum, cognitive-behavioral therapy interventions are based on behavioral and cognitive-behavioral theory and research. Recent meta-analyses and systematic reviews indicate that CBT is effective in reducing pain and disability and in improving pain coping and mood in a wide variety of disease-related and other chronic pain conditions. By focusing more on early intervention, on integrating CBT protocols into medical treatment, and on developing tailored interventions, pain clinicians may be much better able to prevent pain and improve the quality of life of patients suffering from persistent pain.

REFERENCES

Beecher HK. *The Measurement of Subjective Responses*. New York: Oxford University Press, 1959.

Bonica JJ, Ventafridda V, Twycross RG. Cancer pain. In: Bonica JJ (Ed). *The Management of Pain*, 2nd ed. Philadelphia: Lea & Febiger, 1990.

Bradley LA, Alberts KR. Psychological and behavioral approaches to pain management for patients with rheumatic disease. *Med Clin N Am* 1999; 25:215–232.

Bradley LA, Young LD, Anderson KO, et al. Effects of psychological therapy on pain behavior of rheumatoid arthritis patients: treatment outcome and six-month follow-up. *Arthritis Rheum* 1987; 30:1105–1114.

Compas BE, Haaga DAF, Keefe FJ, Leitenberg H, Williams DA. A sampling of empirically supported psychological treatments from health psychology: smoking, chronic pain, cancer, and bulimia nervosa. *J Consult Clin Psychol* 1998; 66:89–112.

Devine EC, Westlake SK. The effects of psychoeducational care provided to adults with cancer: meta-analysis of 116 studies. *Oncol Nurs Forum* 1995; 22(9):1369–1381.

Flor H. Der Stellenwert verhaltenstherapeutischer Ansätze bei der Behandlung chronischer Schmerzen [The value of behavior therapy in the treatment of chronic pain]. *Der Kassernatz;* in press.

Fordyce WE. *Behavioral Methods for Chronic Pain and Illness*. St. Louis: CV Mosby, 1976.

Gil KM, Abrams MR, Phillips G, Keefe FJ. Sickle cell disease pain: the relationship of coping strategies to adjustment. *J Consult Clin Psychol* 1989; 57:725–731.

Gil KM, Wilson JJ, Edens JL, et al. Effects of cognitive coping skills training on coping strategies and experimental pain sensitivity in African American adults with sickle cell disease. *Health Psychol* 1996; 15(1):3–10.

Gil KM, Wilson JJ, Edens JL, et al. Cogntive coping skills training in children with sickle cell disease pain. *Int J Behav Med* 1997; 4(4):364–377.

Gil KM, Carson JW, Sedway JA, et al. Follow-up of coping skills training in adults with sickle cell disease: analysis of daily pain and coping practice diaries. *Health Psychol,* in press.

Keefe FJ, Bonk V. Psychosocial assessment of pain in patients having rheumatic diseases. *Rheum Dis Clin North Am* 1999; 25(1):81–103.

Keefe FJ, Caldwell DS. Cognitive behavioral control of arthritis pain. *Med Clin North Am* 1997; 81:277–290.

Keefe FJ, Lefebvre JC. Behaviour therapy. In: Melzack R, Wall P (Eds). *Textbook of Pain*. London: Churchill Livingstone, 1994, pp 1367–1380.

Keefe FJ, VanHorn Y. Cognitive-behavioral treatment of rheumatoid arthritis pain: maintaining treatment gains. *Arthritis Care Res* 1993; 6(4):213–222.

Keefe FJ, Caldwell DS, Williams DA, et al. Pain coping skills training in the management of osteoarthritic knee pain: a comparative study. *Behav Ther* 1990a; 21:49–62.

Keefe FJ, Caldwell DS, Williams DA, et al. Pain coping skills training in the management of osteoarthritic knee pain: follow-up results. *Behav Ther* 1990b; 21:435–448.

Keefe FJ, Salley AN, Lefebvre JC. Coping with pain: conceptual concerns and future directions. *Pain* 1992; 51:131–134.

Keefe FJ, Kashikar-Zuck S, Opiteck J, et al. Pain in arthritis and musculoskeletal disorders: the role of coping skills training and exercise interventions. *J Orthop Sports Phys Ther* 1996a; 24(4):279–290.

Keefe FJ, Beaupre PM, Gil KM. Group therapy for patients with chronic pain. In: Turk DC, Gatchel RJ (Eds). *Psychological Treatments for Pain: A Practitioner's Handbook*. New York: Guilford Press, 1996b.

Keefe FJ, Caldwell DS, Baucom D, et al. Spouse-assisted coping skills training in the management of osteoarthritic knee pain. *Arthritis Care Res* 1996c; 9(4):279–291.

Keefe FJ, Lefebvre JC, Kerns RD, et al. *Understanding the Adoption of Arthritis Self-Management: Stages of Change Profiles among Arthritis Patients*. Paper presented at the American Pain Society Annual Meeting, Ft. Lauderdale, Florida, 1999.

Kerns RD, Rosenberg R, Jamison RN, Caudill MA, Haythornthwaite J. Readiness to adopt a self-management approach to chronic pain: the Pain Stages of Change Questionnaire (PSOCQ). *Pain* 1997; 72:227–234.

Lester N, Keefe FJ. Coping with chronic pain. In: Baum A, McManus C, Newman S, Weinman J, West R (Eds). *Cambridge Handbook of Psychology, Health and Medicine*. Cambridge: Cambridge University Press, 1997.

Lorig KR, Mazonson PD, Holman HR. Evidence suggesting that health education for self-management in patients with chronic arthritis has sustained health benefits while reducing health care costs. *Arthritis Rheum* 1993; 36(4):439–446.

McConnaughy EA, DiClemente CC, Prochaska JO, Velicer WF. Stages of change in psychotherapy: a follow-up report. *Psychotherapy* 1989; 26(4):494–503.

Melzack R. From the gate to the neuromatrix. *Pain* 1999(Suppl 6):S127–S132.
Melzack R, Wall PD. Pain mechanisms: a new theory. *Science* 1965; 150:971–979.
Melzack R, Wall PD. *The Challenge of Pain*. London: Penguin Books, 1996.
Melzack R, Wall PD, Weisz TC. Acute pain in an emergency clinic: latency of onset and descriptor patterns. *Pain* 1982; 14:33–43.
Meyer TJ, Mark MM. Effects of psychosocial interventions with adult cancer patients: a meta-analysis of randomized experiments. *Health Psychol* 1995; 4:101–108.
Morley S, Eccleston C, Williams A. Systematic review and meta-analysis of randomized controlled trials of cognitive behaviour therapy and behaviour therapy for chronic pain in adults, excluding headache. *Pain* 1999; 80:1–13.
Parker JC, Smarr KL, Buckelew SP, et al. Effects of stress management on clinical outcomes in rheumatoid arthritis. *Arthritis Rheum* 1995, 38:1807–1818.
Prochaska JO, DiClemente CC. Towards a comprehensive, transtheoretical model of change: stages of change and addictive behaviors. In: Miller WR, Heather N (Eds). *Treating Addictive Behaviors,* 2nd ed. New York: Plenum Press, 1998, pp 3–24.
Prochaska JO, Norcross JC, DiClemente JC. *Changing for Good*. New York: William Morrow & Co., 1994.
Smith MC, Holcombe JK, Stullenbarger E. A meta-analysis of intervention effectiveness for symptom management in oncology nursing research. *Oncol Nurs Forum* 1994; 21(7):1201–1209.
Superio-Cabuslay E, Ward MM, Lorig KR. Patient education interventions in osteoarthritis and rheumatoid arthritis: a meta-analytic comparison with nonsteroidal antiinflammatory drug treatment. *Arthritis Care Res* 1996; 9(4):292–301.
Syrjala KL, Cummings C, Donaldson GW. Hypnosis or cognitive-behavioral training for the reduction of pain and nausea during cancer treatment: a controlled clinical trail. *Pain* 1992; 63:137–146.
Syrjala KL, Donaldson GW, Davis MW, Kippes ME, Carr JE. Relaxation and imagery and cognitive-behavioral training reduce pain during cancer treatment: a controlled clinical trial. *Pain* 1995; 63:189–198.
Turner JA. Educational and behavioral interventions for back pain in primary care. *Spine* 1996; 21(24):2851–2859.
Turner JA, Clancy S. Comparison of operant behavioral and cognitive-behavioral treatment for chronic low back pain. *J Consult Clin Psychol* 1988; 50:757–765.
Turner JA, LeResche L, Von Korff M, Ehrlich K. Back pain in primary care. *Spine* 1998; 23(4):463–469.
Vlaeyen JWS, Kole-Snijders AMJ, Boeren RGB, van Eek HF. Fear of movement/(re)injury in chronic low back pain and its relation to behavioral performance. *Pain* 1995; 62:363–372.
Von Korff M, Moore JE, Lorig K, et al. A randomized trial of a lay person-led self-management group intervention for back pain patients in primary care. *Spine* 1998; 23(23):2608–2615.
Waddell G. *The Back Pain Revolution*. New York: Churchill Livingston, 1998.
Wagner EH, Austin BT, Von Korff M. Organizing care for patients with chronic illness. *Milbank Q* 1996; 74(4):511–544.
Wall PD. *Pain: The Science of Suffering*. London: Weidenfeld & Nicolson, 1999.
Williams ACdeC, Richardson PH, Nicholas MK, et al. Inpatient vs. outpatient pain management: results of a randomized controlled trial. *Pain* 1996; 6:13–22.
Williams DA. Psychosocial considerations for implantable pain management devices. Paper presented at the 16th Annual Meeting of the American Pain Society, New Orleans, LA, 1997.
Zelman DC, Cleeland CS, Howland EW. Factors in appropriate pharmacologic management of cancer pain: a cross-institutional investigation. *Pain* 1987; (Suppl):S136.

Correspondence to: Francis J. Keefe, PhD, Box 3159, Duke University Medical Center, Durham, NC 27710, USA. Tel: 919-416-2363; email: keefe003@mc.duke.edu.

Proceedings of the 9th World Congress on Pain,
Progress in Pain Research and Management,
Vol. 16, edited by M. Devor, M.C. Rowbotham, and
Z. Wiesenfeld-Hallin, IASP Press, Seattle, © 2000.

101

Factors That Determine the Magnitude and Presence of Placebo Analgesia[1]

Donald D. Price

*Departments of Oral and Maxillofacial Surgery and Neuroscience,
Brain Institute, University of Florida, Gainesville, Florida, USA*

The potentially powerful influence of placebo effects in studies of analgesia was emphasized by Beecher (1955, 1959), whose studies have led to the commonly held view that placebo analgesic effects are, in general, both powerful and prevalent and that we would all be fools to ignore them. The assertion that approximately 33% of patients have significant responses to placebo treatments is commonly quoted in papers and textbooks; the origin of this percentage is Beecher's (1955) figure of 35.2%. However, he based this value on an average of 11 of his own studies, most of which varied considerably from the average. The placebo analgesia literature from Beecher's era to the present identifies fractions of placebo responders that vary between 0% and 100% (see Jospe 1978; Turner et al. 1994; Wall 1994, for reviews). Clinical pains are claimed to be associated with larger numbers of placebo responders than are experimental pains, and some types of placebo treatments are supposed to generate larger placebo effects than others (see Jospe 1978 and Wall 1994 for reviews).

All of these claims are unsubstantiated because they are founded on erroneous assumptions from studies whose considerable methodological problems and difficulties of interpretation have only recently been acknowledged. The aims of this chapter will be to explain why these claims are not valid, to briefly review some factors that may co-determine the magnitude of placebo effects, and to suggest a new strategy for measuring these factors and assessing placebo effects in analgesic studies.

---

[1] Mini-review based on a congress workshop.

PROBLEMS OF MEASURING PLACEBO EFFECTS AND PLACEBO RESPONSES

The placebo analgesic effect is the measured mean reduction in pain for a group of individuals given a placebo treatment, and the placebo analgesic response is the reduction in pain that occurs in an individual as a result of placebo administration (Fields and Price 1997). Measurement of both placebo analgesic effects and responses requires estimates of pain intensity under both untreated baseline and placebo treatment conditions. The difference in pain intensity between these two conditions provides a measure of the placebo effect for groups and a measure of the placebo response for individuals. The untreated baseline pain in experimental studies usually results from presentation of a controlled pain stimulus. This gives experimental studies an enormous advantage in that the stimulus that produces pain can be repeated at different times in relationship to the placebo manipulation. Using multiple trials of baseline stimuli and multiple trials of stimuli after placebo administration, researchers can identify and measure a placebo response in an individual participant.

The measurement of a placebo response in one person is not nearly as feasible in the case of clinical pain. Unlike experimental pain, whose intensity can be controlled to some extent by stimulus parameters, in clinical studies investigators must rely on the "natural history" of pain intensity, that is, the temporal profile of pain intensity that occurs without any treatment whatsoever (Fields and Price 1997). Natural histories of pain vary according to type of clinical pain and circumstances. For example, the natural history of most postoperative pains is an initial slow increase in intensity over time, whereas that of migraine headaches is often a gradual rise in pain intensity to a severe level followed by a decline to no pain at all. Natural histories of pain also vary considerably across patients. As a result of both of these sources of variation, any treatment may be followed by a reduction in pain level as a result of the natural history rather than as a result of the treatment itself. To attribute a reduction in pain to any antecedent treatment, including placebo, is therefore an inference. Without a natural history control condition, this attribution is not valid because we do not know what change in pain intensity would have occurred without the treatment. The mean magnitude of a placebo analgesic effect in a group of patients can only be assessed by comparing a no-treatment condition with the placebo treatment condition. *For this reason, nearly all studies of clinical analgesia fail to measure the placebo effect.* They measure the *difference* between the placebo condition and the active treatment condition. Having a placebo group in a study does not provide a measure of the placebo effect. Since both pharmacological and nonpharmacological studies of analgesia rarely include an untreated comparison group or condition (in crossover studies), little knowledge exists with regard to the magnitude and time course of placebo effects or frequency of occurrence of placebo responses among individuals. Indeed, in the absence of a no-treatment group or condition, it is difficult to know whether a placebo treatment has produced any effect at all.

To obtain a general assessment of the prevalence of consideration of placebo effects and natural history in analgesic studies, I conducted PubMed key word searches from 1966 to the present, using words relevant to this issue. The words "placebo analgesic effect" yielded 3397 references, which suggests that many analgesia studies may have acknowledged the importance of the placebo analgesic effect or its potential influence in their results. However, when the words "natural history" were added, only 11 references were found. Apparently, the natural history of pain is only very rarely given consideration in clinical studies that have placebo control groups. Even among the 11 studies, most did not use a natural history group to help assess the placebo effect. Rare exceptions include studies by Gracely et al. (1983) and Levine and Gordon (1984). The latter demonstrates a strong placebo effect, approximately equivalent to the effect of 8 mg of intravenous morphine but less than that of 12 mg of morphine.

One might assume that measuring baseline pain in clinical studies helps to provide a way to estimate the magnitude of a placebo effect. This could be true in the case of a well-controlled stimulus-evoked pain or a baseline pain intensity that remains very stable over time; these conditions are often satisfied in studies of experimental pain. Thus, placebo effects are more commonly ascertained in experimental than in clinical studies. However, baseline pain in clinical studies is the level of pain prior to treatment. Since the natural history of most clinical pains shows changes in pain intensity over time, assessment of baseline pain in clinical studies usually does not allow an evaluation of the placebo effect. For this reason, nearly all postsurgical analgesia studies have failed to assess the magnitude of placebo effects, although most of them include an evaluation of baseline pain as well as a placebo control condition.

Lack of consideration of the influences of multiple psychological factors and the necessity of taking into account the natural history of the pain condition have resulted in the frequently unwarranted conclusion that a placebo response has occurred if a patient's pain is observed to decrease following placebo treatment. Overlooking the importance of an untreated comparison group remains a major source of confusion in current literature on placebo (Wickramasekera 1985; Wall 1994). Without a natural history control comparison, we can neither exclude the possibility that a placebo response is absent nor confirm that it has occurred. The two types of pain mentioned above can serve as examples. Giving a placebo treatment at the peak of a migraine headache would most likely be followed by a reduction in pain, regardless of whether the placebo had any effect. The reduction, however, does not establish the presence of a placebo response. Likewise, a postoperative pain that has steadily increased in intensity may continue to increase in intensity despite any small reduction in pain produced by the placebo treatment. The absence of an overall reduction in pain does not mean that a placebo response did not occur. In both examples, the placebo response of individual patients is the measured difference between the level of pain with and without the presence of the placebo treatment. In a situation where there is a strong placebo response, it may be difficult or impossible to determine anything about the effects of the test agent.

An example of a study that infers a strong placebo effect without sufficient evidence is one in which headache patients admitted to the emergency department were assigned to one of three treatment groups: ketorolac, meperidine, and saline placebo (Harden et al. 1996). Approximately equally large reductions in headache pain were found in all three groups. The authors interpret these results as reflecting a strong placebo effect in this clinical situation. They state: "Thus, the present study suggests that the treatment of acute headache in an emergency department setting provides an excellent demonstration of the placebo effect, but provides a poor model for the evaluation of analgesic interventions." A reasonable alternative explanation is that the headache patients sought relief at or near the peak intensity of their headache pain. Given the natural history of headache pain, it is very possible that their headache pain would have decreased without any treatment whatsoever. The authors readily acknowledged that a natural history comparison would have been ideal, yet persisted in inferring the presence of a strong placebo effect.

However, it is also important to emphasize that the lack of natural history comparison groups in clinical studies is not just a matter of oversight or negligence on the part of clinical investigators. There are humane reasons to be reluctant *not* to treat patients, such as headache patients entering the emergency room. It may be possible to find other ways to assess the presence and magnitude of placebo analgesia under these circumstances.

FACTORS THAT CO-DETERMINE THE MAGNITUDE OF PLACEBO EFFECTS

Given the problems that have obscured knowledge about the magnitudes and prevalence of placebo responses and effects in analgesic studies, we need to know more about factors that mediate the presence and magnitude of placebo analgesia as well as about psychological and neural mechanisms of placebo analgesia. In this section, I briefly consider the potential roles of classical conditioning, expectancy, desire for relief, and distortions in memory as factors that may mediate placebo analgesia.

CONDITIONING AND EXPECTANCY

Current explanations of mechanisms of placebo analgesia propose that multiple factors co-determine its magnitude and prevalence (Fields and Price 1997; Price and Fields 1997). These factors include classical conditioning, desire for relief, and expectancy. Repeated exposure to effective analgesics (i.e., conditioning) can produce large placebo effects by increasing expectation of relief. Furthermore, the degree of threat that is present in the context in which placebo treatments are administered would contribute to desire for pain relief. The combination of these factors could co-determine the magnitude of placebo analgesia. Both classic studies and recent studies of placebo effects confirm the roles of expectancy and conditioning in producing placebo analgesia (Montgomery and Kirsch 1996, 1997; Price et al. 1999). Consistent with the classical conditioning hypothesis, a landmark study of patients clearly showed that prior treatments with effective analgesic drugs enhanced the analgesic effectiveness of a subsequent placebo (Laska and Sunshine 1973). In this study, a second medication, always placebo, followed graded doses of propoxyphene HCl (three dose levels), propoxyphene napsylate (three dose levels), or placebo. There were seven groups of patients with 14–20 patients in each group. The results showed convincing evidence of a dose-response relationship between the dose of the first medication and the analgesic response to the subsequent placebo, although the magnitudes of placebo effects were lower than effects of corresponding doses of the active drug. Placebo given as a second treatment was more effective when it followed a more potent analgesic, whereas placebo following a placebo continued to have the same slight analgesic effect as did the first placebo administration. These results support learning, even classical conditioning, as a major factor in placebo analgesia. However, the results do not distinguish the contributions of conditioning versus expectation in producing placebo analgesia.

The roles of expectation and conditioning in placebo analgesia are complementary and not mutually exclusive. Modern interpretations of conditioning emphasize that it depends on expectations of effects (Rescorla 1988). Recent work by Montgomery and Kirsch (1997) demonstrated that placebo analgesia can be produced by repeated pairings of placebo cream with surreptitious lowering of stimulus strength, i.e., conditioning, but that the effect is mediated by participants' expectations. Benedetti and colleagues likewise have shown that placebo analgesia can be produced by conditioning with repeated morphine treatments or by simple expectancy manipulations consisting of verbal instructions (Amanzio and Benedetti 1999). Both types of experimental manipulations produced placebo analgesia that was naloxone reversible, which provides further evidence for endogenous opioid mechanisms (see Gracely et al. 1983 and Levine and Gordon 1984 for prior literature on this issue). Interestingly, conditioning with a non-opioid drug, ketorolac, produced placebo analgesia that was *not* naloxone reversible. Benedetti et al. (1999) followed up this elegant study by testing the hypothesis that placebo analgesia develops as a result of a highly specific response expectancy and is mediated by endogenous opioid mechanisms. The authors produced pain simultaneously in four limbs by intradermal capsaicin injections and applied placebo cream to only one or two of the four sites. Placebo analgesia developed only in the limb(s) that were treated, an effect that is consistent with a highly specific response expectancy. This result rules out the possibility that placebo analgesia consists of nothing more than a reduction in anxiety or some other global mechanism that would affect the entire body. Although specific to only one part of the body, the effect could be eliminated by prior intravenous injection of naloxone, suggesting mediation by somatotopically organized opioid mechanisms.

A study by Price et al. (1999) corroborated and extended the results of both Benedetti et al. (1999) and Montgomery and Kirsch (1997). We applied two "strengths" of placebo creams (A and B) and a control agent (C) to three adjacent areas on the forearms, and conditioned the participants by combining these treatments with varying degrees of surreptitious lowering of the strength of painful skin temperature stimuli. In comparison to the pretreatment baseline condition, participants experienced no reduction, a small reduction, and a large reduction in areas C, B, and A, respectively. When stimulus strength was returned to equal levels in all three areas, the assessed placebo effects were graded in proportion to the extent to which stimulus strength had been secretly lowered during manipulation trials. Since these three areas were immediately adjacent, the results provide even more evidence for somatotopic specificity of the placebo effect than was demonstrated by Benedetti et al. (1999). Second, these effects were strongly associated with participants' *expected* levels of pain within each area, expectations that were assessed just prior to trials for which placebo effects were assessed. The combination of these results demonstrates that expectations directed toward highly specific body locations can mediate placebo analgesia under at least some circumstances. Under clinical circumstances, specific expectations of patients can be potently influenced by clinicians' expectations (Gracely et al. 1985). Thus, a double-blind study format is necessary to assess placebo analgesia in clinical studies.

DESIRE FOR PAIN RELIEF

A second likely factor in placebo analgesia is the desire for pain relief (Price and Fields 1997). Placebo effects occur in clinical contexts wherein patients not only expect pain reduction but also have a strong need or desire for relief. Unfortunately, there have been very few explicit attempts to assess this factor in studies of placebo effects. A role of desire for relief is indirectly supported by the fact that placebo effects are larger in experimental pain studies that create threatening circumstances (Jospe 1978).

Contrary to what was hypothesized, however, ratings of desire for pain relief were not significantly associated with the magnitudes of placebo analgesia in the study by Price et al. (1999) described above. Although this result casts some doubt on the possible contribution of desire for pain relief on placebo analgesia, the hypothesis should not be completely dismissed for several reasons. First, nearly all participants of the study had some degree of desire for pain relief, as determined by their ratings of this factor. Second, as discussed above, desire for pain relief may be a much more critical factor in placebo effects during clinical pain. This factor needs to be assessed in clinical pain studies.

A third reason for not completely rejecting the hypothesis that desire or motivation contribute to placebo analgesia is based on a study by Jensen and Karoly (1991). Although the study was not about pain relief, the authors explicitly assessed the contribution of a desire for symptom change in a study of placebo manipulations designed to suggest sedative or stimulant effects. Jensen and Karoly (1991) assessed separate contributions of *motivation* and *expectancy* to placebo responses. According to the authors, *motivation* referred to "the degree to which subjects desire to experience a symptom change" and *expectancy* was considered the subjects' expectation of symptom change. They manipulated both of these factors by separate instructions and then later checked (by subject self-ratings) whether either or both factors had been influenced. Thus, the study was a two by two factorial design containing four groups (high motivation + high expectancy, etc.).

The authors found that motivation accounted for a significant amount of variance in placebo responses that included perceived sedation in the case of placebo tranquilizers or perceived arousal in the case of placebo stimulants.

MEMORY DISTORTION OF BASELINE PAIN AS A MEDIATOR OF PLACEBO ANALGESIA

A factor that has recently been demonstrated to make a major contribution to the magnitude of placebo analgesia is the method used to assess pain relief. In a study in which placebo analgesia was produced by applying a placebo cream in the guise of a local analgesic, placebo effects were modest when assessed concurrently with placebo trials (0.5–1.3 visual analogue scale [VAS] units on a 10-unit scale) (Price et al. 1999). However, when the same participants rated pain and pain reduction based on *remembered* pain intensities, placebo effects were 3–4 times larger than those assessed *during* placebo trials- (2.0–4.3 VAS units). The main reason for these differences was that participants remembered the untreated pain as being much more intense and unpleasant than it actually was. Finally, ratings of expected pain levels prior to placebo trials were similar to participants' ratings of remembered pain intensities, and in fact were strongly associated with them (r = 0.5–0.6). Expectations and memory distortions mediate large placebo effects based on retrospective ratings of pain or pain relief. Large placebo effects based on memory distortion may demonstrate potent psychological influences, rather than potent antinociceptive effects.

The selective exaggeration of remembered pain intensity and the consequent enhancement of apparent placebo analgesia are consistent with a previous study showing that memory distortion of pretreatment pain contributes to an exaggeration of self-reports of pain relief (Feine et al. 1998). The authors found that pain relief scores based on memory were over three times higher than those based on pretreatment minus present pain VAS ratings, consistent with the results of Price et al.'s (1999) study of placebo analgesia.

As pointed out by Feine and colleagues (1998), patients' reports of relief following treatment are often used to establish the effectiveness of treatments. To the extent that such measures are used in clinical studies of pain treatments, estimates of magnitudes of analgesic effects from both placebo and active treatments are likely to be significantly enhanced when reports are made retrospectively. We can only speculate about the extent to which commonly quoted magnitudes of placebo analgesia (Beecher 1955, 1959; Turner et al. 1994) as well as reported magnitudes of analgesia from active treatments have been based on retrospective judgments of pain relief.

AN ALTERNATIVE STRATEGY FOR ASSESSING PLACEBO RESPONSES AND EFFECTS IN ANALGESIA STUDIES

Given the problems inherent in assessing the magnitude of placebo analgesia and the multiple factors that contribute to it, including memory distortion, we cannot conclude that powerful placebo effects take place in most clinical analgesia studies. Placebo analgesic effects in experimental pain studies are negligible to modest. However, among clinical studies, for which the pain is more threatening or severe, we cannot rule out the possibility of potent analgesic effects of placebo, particularly since we know that such effects can result from other psychological interventions, such as hypnosis. However, past and current studies of analgesia do not allow definitive conclusions concerning the potency or prevalence of placebo effects because placebo effects and responses are not really characterized in the vast majority of analgesia studies.

However, a strategy could be developed whereby it is possible to assess most or all of the relevant mediating factors that contribute to placebo effects. The proposed strategy would be based on two considerations. The first is that expectancy and desire for pain relief could be measured and integrated within the designs of analgesia studies. If, as shown by several studies of experimental pain, one or both of these parameters can account for most of the variance in placebo effects, then they could be incorporated into clinical analgesia studies. Their measurement could provide an important adjunct, if not a substitute means of assessing the contribution of placebo effects. A secondary purpose of their inclusion would be to assess the "blindness" of the studies. After all, if pain patients in double-blind analgesia studies cannot subjectively distinguish active from placebo treatments, then their levels of expectation and desire for relief should be the same across both types of treatment. And if they *can* subjectively distinguish the two treatments, it would be *really* important to understand the contribution of desire for relief and expectation to the resultant analgesia.

The second consideration would be to design the pain measurements in a manner that takes into account the confounding influences of memory distortion and natural history in assessment of the placebo effect. Thus, it would be far better to assess analgesia concurrently than retrospectively, and it would be extremely important to take into consideration all that is known about the natural history of the pain.

The possibility of a refined analysis of placebo effects within studies has far-reaching scientific and medical implications (Price and Fields 1997; Wall 1994). Our present limited capacity to ascertain, measure, and control for placebo effects is at the heart of complex and difficult questions about pharmacological therapies for pain as well as many nonpharmacological therapies, particularly those related to surgery, hypnosis, electrical stimulation, and "alternative" medical treatments. If the magnitudes of desire for and expectation of a specific therapeutic effect account for most of the variance in placebo effect, then measures of such factors could be incorporated into studies in which it is extremely difficult to provide a flawless placebo control treatment condition. Measurement of desire and expectation factors in analgesia studies could serve as an additional or substitute method for analyzing placebo effects and make it unnecessary to rely on questionable control treatment conditions. This possible improvement could be applied not only to studies of "alternative" treatments such as acupuncture, but also to any study in which the active analgesic treatment can be subjectively distinguished from its placebo control. This improvement may apply to the vast majority of analgesic studies.

REFERENCES

Amanzio M, Benedetti F. Neuropharmacological dissection of placebo analgesia: expectation-activated opioid systems versus conditioning-activated specific subsystems. *J Neurosci* 1999; 19:484–494.

Beecher HK. The powerful placebo. *JAMA* 1955; 159:1602–1606.

Beecher HK. *Measurement of Subjective Responses: Quantitative Effects of Drugs.* New York: Oxford University Press, 1959.

Benedetti F, Arduino C, Amanzio M. Somatotopic activation of opioid systems by target-directed expectations of analgesia. *J Neurosci* 1999; 19(9):3639–3648.

Fields HL, Price DD. Toward a neurobiology of placebo analgesia. In: Ann Harrington (Ed). *Placebo: Probing the Self-Healing Brain.* Boston: Harvard University Press, 1997.

Feine JS, Lavigne GJ, Dao TTT, et al. Memories of chronic pain and perceptions of relief. *Pain* 1998; 77:137–141.

Gracely RH. Psychophysical assessment of human pain. In: Bonica JJ, Liebeskind JC, Albe-Fessard DG (Eds). *Advances in Pain Research and Therapy,* Vol. 3, New York: Raven Press, 1979.

Gracely RH, Dubner R, Deeter WR, et al. Naloxone and placebo alter postsurgical pain by separate mechanisms. *Nature* 1983; 306:264–265.

Gracely RH, Dubner R, Deeter WR, et al. Clinician's expectations influence placebo analgesia. *Lancet* 1985; 1:8419–8423.

Harden RN, Gracely RH, Carter T, et al. The placebo effect in acute headache management: ketorolac, meperidine, and saline in the emergency department. *Headache* 1996; 36(6):352–356.

Jensen MP, Karoly P. Motivation and expectancy factors in symptom perception: a laboratory study of the placebo effect. *Psychosom Med* 1991; 53:144–152.

Jospe M. *The Placebo Effect in Healing.* Lexington, Massachusetts: Lexington Books, 1978.

Laska E, Sunshine A. Anticipation of analgesia: a placebo effect. *Headache* 1973; 1:1–11.

Levine JD, Gordon NC. Influence of the method of drug administration on analgesic response. *Nature* 1984; 312(5996):755–756.

Montgomery GH, Kirsch I. Mechanisms of placebo pain reduction: an empirical investigation. *Psychol Sci* 1996; 7:174–176.

Montgomery GH, Kirsch I. Classical conditioning and the placebo effect. *Pain* 1997; 72:103–113.

Price DD, Fields HL. Where are the causes of placebo analgesia? An experiential behavioral analysis. *Pain Forum* 1997; 6(1):44–52.

Price DD, Milling LS, Kirsch I, et al. An analysis of factors that contribute to the magnitude of placebo analgesia. *Pain* 1999; 83(2):147–156.

Rescorla RA. Pavlovian conditioning: it's not what you think it is. *Am Psychol* 1988; 43:151–160.

Turner JA, Deyo RA, Loeser JD, et al. The importance of placebo effects in pain treatment and research. *JAMA* 1994; 271(20):1609–1614.

Wall PD. The placebo and the placebo response. In: Wall PD, Melzack R (Eds). *Textbook of Pain*. New York: Churchill Livingstone, 1994.

Wickramasekera I. A conditioned response model of the placebo effect: predictions from the model. In: White L, Turskey B, Schwartz GE (Eds). *Placebo: Theory, Research, and Mechanisms*. New York: Guilford Press, 1985.

Correspondence to: Donald D. Price, PhD, Department of Oral and Maxillofacial Surgery, Claude Denson Pepper Center for Research on Oral Health in Aging, University of Florida, 1600 Southwest Archer Road, JHMHC, Box 100416, Gainesville, FL 32610, USA. Tel: 352-846-2718; Fax: 352-846-0588; email: dprice@dental.ufl.edu.

Proceedings of the 9th World Congress on Pain,
Progress in Pain Research and Management,
Vol. 16, edited by M. Devor, M.C. Rowbotham, and
Z. Wiesenfeld-Hallin, IASP Press, Seattle, © 2000.

102

Attitudinal Barriers to Effective Pain Management in the Nursing Home

Debra K. Weiner[a,b,e] and Thomas E. Rudy[b,c,d,e]

[a]Department of Medicine, Division of Geriatric Medicine, [b]Department of Psychiatry, [c]Department of Anesthesiology, [d]Department of Biostatistics, and [e]Pain Evaluation and Treatment Institute, University of Pittsburgh, Pittsburgh, Pennsylvania, USA

Unrelieved pain may plague at least 80% of older adults who live in nursing homes (NH) (Roy and Thomas 1986; Ferrell et al. 1990; Sengstaken and King 1994; Parmelee 1994; Weiner et al. 1999); most such pain is persistent (Weiner et al. 1998, 1999). The result is unnecessary suffering, often exacerbated by depression, compromised cognitive function, sleep disturbance, functional disability, and compromised quality of life. Perhaps the most serious consequence of persistent pain is functional disability, which fosters learned helplessness, social isolation, and greater health care costs due to greater dependency in activities of daily living and thus a greater need for nursing care. With the anticipated future steady increase in NH utilization (Kemper and Murtaugh 1991) combined with older and more disabled residents inhabiting these facilities, persistent pain in the NH is likely to become an increasingly prevalent problem for our society.

Attitudes held by residents and staff may contribute significantly to the underdiagnosis and undertreatment of NH pain. Residents, having lived for many years with chronically painful stimuli, may accept their pain as an expected companion of old age and be reticent to complain or seek treatment (Harkins et al. 1984; Yates et al. 1995). Fears of not being heard, being labeled a "bad patient," or becoming overly dependent may also drive some NH residents' apparent pain-related stoicism (Fagerhaugh and Strauss 1977; Harkins et al. 1984; Hofland 1992; Yates et al. 1995).

NH staff prioritize maximizing function and tend to devalue management of persistent pain (Fagerhaugh and Strauss 1977; Haley 1983). Other attitudes and beliefs that may impede effective detection and management of persistent pain include lack of time (Schnelle and Reuben 1999), belief that pain is a normal part of aging and is unresponsive to treatment (McCaffery and Ferrell 1991), fears of addiction to analgesics (Charap 1978; Cohen 1980; Degner et al. 1982), and disbelief in the validity of pain complaints without physical deformity (Jacox 1979). The purpose of this investigation was to systematically explore NH resident and staff attitudes that serve as barriers to detection and management of persistent pain.

METHODS

SUBJECTS

The participants were 35 NH nurses and 38 communicative NH residents without acute illness, acute pain, receptive aphasia, severe hearing impairment, or severe dementia, who had persistent pain as defined by an affirmative response to the question "Do you have some pain or discomfort every day or almost every day?" This question has demonstrated reliability based on previous research (Weiner et al. 1999). Demographic data for residents and staff were collected on age, gender, ethnicity, highest level of education, marital status, and for staff only, length of time in the field of nursing and in long-term care.

PROCEDURES

We performed a comprehensive literature review to identify potential attitudes among NH residents and staff that might serve to perpetuate persistent pain by interfering with its detection and treatment. Based on this review, we identified 12 pain constructs common to residents and staff: (1) lack of time, (2) lack of prioritization of persistent pain treatment in the NH, (3) the belief that persistent pain treatment is unnecessary in the face of adequate function, (4) belief that persistent pain is a normal part of aging, (5) the belief that persistent pain has little potential for change, (6) disbelief in the validity of pain complaints without physical deformity or well-defined pathology, (7) fear of addiction, (8) fear of functional dependence, (9) desensitization, (10) fear of the "bad patient" label, (11) ageism, and (12) fear of pain complaints being ignored or unheard. We created separate resident and staff questionnaires to explore these 12 constructs as well as persistent pain-related knowledge deficits among staff. There were two to four questions per construct. Attitudinal responses were collected on a 5-point scale: strongly disagree (–2), disagree (–1), uncertain (0), agree (1), strongly agree (2). For example, for the construct, "complaints unheard," the attitudes and beliefs of residents were: (1) I feel that complaining about pain is a waste of my energy, because no one will listen anyway; and (2) I am reluctant to let nursing staff know when I have pain because I fear that my complaints will not be taken seriously. The staff attitudes about this construct were: (1) Some nurses tend not to listen to residents who have a lot of pain complaints; and (2) sometimes nurses are so busy with other, more important problems (e.g., aggressive behavior, wandering) that when residents voice their chronic pain complaints, nurses may not act on them. For the construct, "desensitization," the attitudes and beliefs of the residents were: (1) When you live with pain every day, eventually you start not to feel it; and (2) I am so used to living with pain that I don't even notice it. The staff attitudes for this construct were: (1) Over time, with repeated exposure, some nurses may become desensitized to residents in chronic pain; (2) if a resident complains of pain every day it is difficult to take him or her seriously; (3) if the resident has the same pain complaints day after day, after a while I stop listening; and (4) so many nursing home residents act as though they are in pain (e.g., they walk slowly, appear stiff, and often have a pained expression on their faces), much of the time I don't even notice it. Resident questionnaires were administered by a trained research assistant. Staff questionnaires were self-administered in the setting of a nursing in-service meeting. Twenty-five residents and 15 nurses were asked to repeat the questionnaire 1 week later.

Scale scores were created for each pain construct by computing the mean of the items used to measure that construct. One-week test-retest reliability was calculated using the intraclass correlation coefficient (ICC). Attitudinal differences between the two groups were evaluated with *t* tests.

RESULTS

NH resident age ranged from 40 to 94 years (mean ± SD, 81.2 ± 9.6); 13% of residents were male, 68% high school graduates, 89.5% Caucasian, and 7.9% married. Nurse age ranged from 23 to 66 years (45 ± 10.3); 8.6% of nurses were male, and 82.9% Caucasian; 54.3% were registered nurses (RNs), 40% licensed practical nurses (LPNs), and 5.7% held a bachelor's degree in nursing (BSN). The mean number of years in nursing was 16.8 ± 11.4 (range, 1.5–43.6), and number of years in long-term care was 7.5 ± 6.3 (0.5–30.0). Reliability coefficients for each of the 12 constructs are shown in Table I. Ten of the 12 constructs demonstrated good to excellent test-retest reliability. Constructs that demonstrated insufficient reliability included lack of prioritization of persistent pain treatment in the NH and fear of the

Table I
Pain construct test-retest reliability indices

Construct	Intraclass R Nurses ($n = 15$)	Intraclass R Residents ($n = 25$)
Lack of time	0.524	0.796
Prioritization	0.189	0.449
Emphasis on function	0.813	0.656
Pain part of old age	0.711	0.716
Chronic pain doesn't change	0.679	0.728
Belief in pathology	0.699	0.676
Fear of addiction	0.760	0.685
Fear of dependence	0.667	0.460
Desensitization	0.737	0.614
Fear of "bad patient"	0.873	0.206
Ageism	0.678	0.736
Complaints unheard	0.658	0.565

"bad patient" label. Attitudinal differences between NH residents and staff for the 10 reliable constructs are shown in Fig. 1. Constructs for which significant attitudinal differences were demonstrated between NH residents and staff included the beliefs that (1) persistent pain treatment is unnecessary in the face of adequate function, (2) persistent pain is a normal part of aging, (3) persistent pain has little potential for change, and (4) pain complaints are invalid without physical deformity or well-defined pathology, as well as (5) fear of functional dependence and (6) fear that pain complaints will be ignored or unheard. For the construct, "complaints unheard," nurses tended to agree that residents' pain complaints would fall on deaf ears, but residents did not. For the other five constructs in which residents and nurses demonstrated significant differences, residents tended to remain neutral while nurses tended to disagree with these constructs.

DISCUSSION

Our questionnaires on persistent pain attitudes among NH residents and nurses are reliable and highlight significant differences between these two groups. The results of this survey suggest that undertreatment of persistent pain in NH residents may not be related to staff attitudes. However, the degree to which nurses' responses on this attitude survey were influenced by social desirability cannot be determined from the results of this study. Since pain is undertreated in NH residents, our results suggest that "correct"

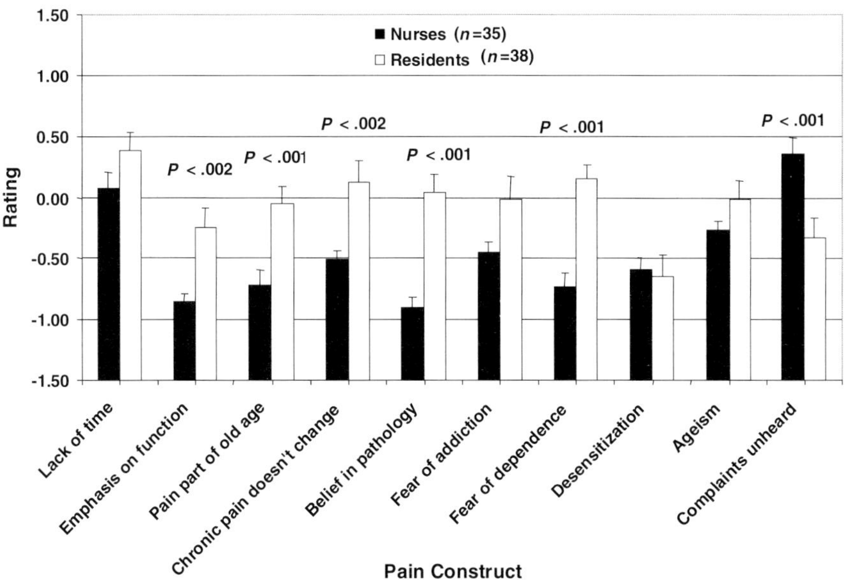

Fig. 1. Pain construct ratings by group. Mean (± SEM) ratings are shown ranging from strongly disagree (–2) to strongly agree (+2).

staff attitudes are not being translated into behaviors that promote pain management, perhaps because of nurses' already burdensome workload or other factors such as inadequate persistent pain management skills or lack of knowledge regarding appropriate pain assessment tools.

The tendency of NH residents to remain neutral about the idea that persistent pain need not be treated in the face of adequate function, that pain is a normal part of aging, that persistent pain is unlikely to respond to treatment, that they should not ask for help when they are in pain, and that nurses will not believe that they hurt if they are without physical deformity, suggests that staff are not communicating to NH residents the therapeutic optimism that they themselves expressed on the nurse attitude survey. Alternatively, residents, having lived for many years with pain, may have become grounded in perceptions that have become immutable. While staff may, in fact, be encouraging residents to seek treatment for their persistent pain, residents may be unwilling to do so.

Certified nursing assistants (CNAs), as the primary caregivers in nursing homes, are a critical part of the pain management team. Because behavioral manifestations of pain (e.g., grimacing, guarding, sighing) are often manifested when individuals move from one position to another (e.g., turning in bed, moving from a supine to a sitting position), CNAs are in an ideal position to determine when NH residents experience pain. The attitudes of

CNAs toward persistent pain and its management and thus the degree to which CNAs' pain behavior observations are communicated to nursing staff may strongly influence whether or not pain is treated in NH residents. We are currently investigating the attitudes of CNAs toward persistent pain in NH residents.

Finally, while CNAs and nurses are the hands-on caregivers of nursing homes, physicians remain responsible for prescribing treatment. In both NH and elderly non-NH populations, physicians may underprescribe pain medications, even for those with metastatic cancer (Cleeland et al. 1994; Bernabei et al. 1998; Weiner et al. 1999). Age and cognitive impairment may be risk factors for inadequate pain management (Feldt et al. 1998). This study did not explore the degree to which physician attitudes lead to inadequate pain relief among NH residents.

Effective pain management in the NH requires that all members of the primary caregiving team (CNAs, nurses, and physicians) have the necessary knowledge, attitudes, and skills to carry out this important agenda. Open communication between residents and CNAs, CNAs and nurses, residents and nurses, and nurses and physicians is also critical. A breakdown in communication of any one of these dyads fosters suboptimal pain management. Clearly, additional research is warranted to enhance the management of persistent pain in NH residents and thus improve the quality of life of this increasingly prevalent segment of our population.

ACKNOWLEDGMENTS

This work was supported by grants from the National Institutes of Health, K08 AG00643 and P01 HD33989.

REFERENCES

Bernabei R, Gambassi G, Lapane K, et al. Management of pain in elderly patients with cancer. *JAMA* 1998; 279:1877–1882.

Charap AD. The knowledge, attitudes, and experience of medical personnel treating pain in the terminally ill. *Mt Sinai J Med* 1978; 45:561–580.

Cleeland CS, Gronin R, Hatfield AK, et al. Pain and its treatment in outpatients with metastatic cancer. *New Engl J Med* 1994; 330:592–596.

Cohen FA. Postsurgical pain relief: patients' status and nurses' medication choices. *Pain* 1980; 9:265–274.

Degner LF, Fujii SH, Levitt M. Implementing a program to control chronic pain of malignant disease for patients in an extended care facility. *Cancer Nursing* 1982; 5:263–268.

Fagerhaugh SY, Strauss A. Inattentiveness to chronic pain: geriatric wards. In: Fagerhaugh SY, Strauss A (Eds). *Politics of Pain Management*. Menlo Park: Addison-Wesley Publishing Company, 1977, pp 181–192.

Feldt KS, Ryden MB, Miles S. Treatment of pain in cognitively impaired compared with cognitively intact older patients with hip-fracture. *J Am Geriatr Soc* 1998; 46:1079–1085.
Ferrell BA, Ferrell BR, Osterweil D. Pain in the nursing home. *J Am Geriatr Soc* 1990; 38:409–414.
Fordyce WE. Evaluating and managing chronic pain. *Geriatrics* 1978; 33:59–62.
Haley WE. Priorities for behavioral intervention with nursing home residents: nursing staff's perspective. *Int J Behav Geriatr* 1983; 1:47–51.
Harkins SW, Kwentus J, Price DD. Pain and the elderly. In: Benedetti C, Chapman CR, Moricca G (Eds). *Advances in Pain Research and Therapy,* Vol. 7. New York: Raven Press, 1984, pp 103–121.
Hofland SL. Elder beliefs: blocks to pain management. *J Gerontol Nursing* 1992; 18:19–24.
Jacox AK. Assessing pain. *Am J Nursing* 1979; 79:895–900.
Kemper P, Murtaugh CM. Lifetime use of nursing home care. *New Engl J Med* 1991; 324:595–600.
McCaffery M, Ferrell BR. Patient age—does it affect your pain-control decisions? *Nursing* 1991; 21:44–48.
Parmelee PA. Assessment of pain in the elderly. In: Lawton MP, Teresi J (Eds). *Annual Review of Gerontology and Geriatrics.* New York: Springer, 1994, pp 281–301.
Roy R, Thomas M. A survey of chronic pain in an elderly population. *Can Fam Physician* 1986; 32:513–516.
Schnelle JF, Reuben DB. Long-term care in the nursing home. In: Calkins, Boult C, Wagner EH, Pacala JT (Eds). *New Ways to Care for Older People—Building Systems Based on Evidence.* New York: Springer, 1999, pp 168–181.
Sengstaken EA, King SA. The problem of pain and its detection among geriatric nursing home residents. *J Am Geriatr Soc* 1994; 41:541–544.
Weiner DK, Peterson B, Logue P, Keefe FJ. Predictors of pain self-report in nursing home residents. *Aging Clin Exp Res* 1998; 10:411–420.
Weiner D, Peterson B, Ladd K, McConnell E, Keefe F. Pain in nursing home residents: an exploration of prevalence, staff perspectives and practical aspects of measurement. *Clin J Pain* 1999; 15:92–101.
Yates P, Dewar A, Fentiman B. Pain: the views of elderly people living in long-term residential care settings. *J Adv Nursing* 1995; 21:667–674.

Correspondence to: Debra K. Weiner, MD, University of Pittsburgh, Keystone Building, 3520 Fifth Avenue, Suite 300, Pittsburgh, PA 15213-3313, USA. Tel: 412-624-4018; Fax: 412-383-1972; email: dweiner+@pitt.edu.

Proceedings of the 9th World Congress on Pain, Progress in Pain Research and Management, Vol. 16, edited by M. Devor, M.C. Rowbotham, and Z. Wiesenfeld-Hallin, IASP Press, Seattle, © 2000.

103

Self-Efficacy as a Mediator of Depression and Pain-Related Disability in Chronic Pain

Paul Arnstein,[a,b,c] Margaret Caudill,[c] and Carol Wells-Federman[b,c]

[a]*School of Nursing, Boston College, Chestnut Hill, Massachusetts, USA;* [b]*Beth Israel Deaconess Medical Center, Boston, Massachusetts, USA;* [c]*Dartmouth-Hitchcock Pain Clinic, Manchester, New Hampshire, USA*

Self-efficacy refers to personal judgments about one's ability to perform specific behaviors in particular situations (Bandura 1977). Studies have demonstrated the significance of self-efficacy for the ability to manage chronic pain (Jensen et al. 1991; Lorig et al. 1993). A growing base of research indicates that a low level of self-efficacy (self-doubt regarding the ability to manage pain or to function or cope) is a significant contributor to the extent to which a person is disabled by chronic pain (Dolce et al. 1986; Council et al. 1988; Kores et al. 1990; Estlander et al. 1994; Arnstein et al. 1999; Keefe et al. 1999) and the degree of depression experienced when pain persists (Wright et al. 1996; Arnstein et al. 1999). To provide further evidence that self-efficacy acts as a mediator and acts as an intrinsic mechanism explaining how or why the disability and depression associated with chronic pain occurs (Baron and Kenny 1986), we tested two path analytic models in three samples of chronic pain patients.

METHODS

Sample. We obtained data from convenience samples of consecutive chronic pain patients from three clinics in the northeastern United States. One sample represented patients evaluated at a major referral center and a second sample represented patients at a community-based primary care and specialty clinic in a nonurban center. We obtained a third combined sample from both those settings and an additional outpatient setting, but screened these patients to exclude those with a history of depression prior to the onset of pain. All patients completed questionnaires prior to an initial consultative visit with a pain specialist at one of the three outpatient pain clinics in New England. A total of 515 participants (tertiary, n = 248; community-based, n = 141; and combined setting, no prior depression, n = 126) provided data on model variables, met the eligibility criteria, and consented to be included in the study. Most subjects were Caucasian (95%), female (70%), married or living in a committed relationship (61%), and had at least some college education (70%). On average, patients were 44 years old with a mean duration of pain of 4.5 years.

Instruments. The primary instruments used were a visual analogue scale to measure pain intensity, the Center for Epidemiological Studies Depression scale to measure the frequency and intensity of depressive symptoms, the Pain Disability Index to determine the extent that pain interferes with daily living, and the Chronic Pain Self-Efficacy Scale to measure subjects' beliefs about their own ability to manage pain and to cope and function despite the persistence of pain. The validity and reliability of these instruments have been reported in the literature and are supported in these samples (Cronbach's alpha range; α = 0.85–0.95). The Chronic Pain Self-Efficacy Scale is a 22-item questionnaire that reveals the patient's perceived ability to manage pain in specific circumstances, to cope with pain and related symptoms, and to perform specific tasks (e.g., walk half a mile or lift 10 pounds). The scale was developed from a widely used Arthritis Self-Efficacy Scale and through extensive research (on self-efficacy beliefs and effective pain control behaviors) and was refined based on rigorous testing among different samples of chronic pain patients (Anderson et al. 1995).

Data analysis. Preliminary statistics (e.g., means, medians, standard deviations, correlations) were computed for all study variables and examined for the assumptions required for path analysis. We conducted a series of regression analyses with a $P < 0.05$ level of significance to test for mediation effects of the proposed model. The standardized coefficients and their statistical significance were calculated and are reported as beta (β) for each path in the model. We examined the adjusted R^2 values to determine the amount of variance in the variable of interest (disability or depression) that is explained by each step of the equation. An F statistic for the regression model was calculated to test the statistical significance of the improved ability to explain variance in the outcome variable of each model. Additional statistical tests identified potential sources of error in interpreting these models.

RESULTS

Results from regression analysis supported self-efficacy as a mediator of the relationship between pain intensity and disability. Note (Table I) that the coefficient for the relationship between pain and disability decreased (β = 0.42–0.21) when the influence of self-efficacy (step 2) was added. Entering depression into the model added 2% (R^2 = 0.34–0.36) to the explained variance in disability (step 3), so we added depression to the model in the combined sample. All paths remained statistically significant ($P <$ 0.001) in the final step, fulfilling the requirements for a mediation model (Baron and Kenny 1986) and supporting a partial mediation effect exerted by self-efficacy. Data supported the model drawn in Fig. 1 ($F_{3,476} = 84$; $P <$ 0.001), which accounted for 36% of the explained variance in disability.

Table I
Mediators of pain-related disability (combined sample, standardized β coefficients)

Model	Step 1	Step 2	Step 3
Pain intensity	0.42***	0.21***	0.17***
Self-efficacy		–0.45***	–0.38***
Depression			0.18***
Adjusted R^2	0.18	0.34	0.36

*** $P \leq 0.001$.

Results also supported lower self-efficacy as a mediator of the relationship between pain intensity and depression. Note (Table II) that the coefficient for the relationship between pain and depression decreased (β = 0.41–0.23) when the influence of self-efficacy (step 2) was added. The addition of disability into the model added 2% (R^2 = 0.28–0.30) to the explained variance in depression (step 3), and thus we added disability to the model in the

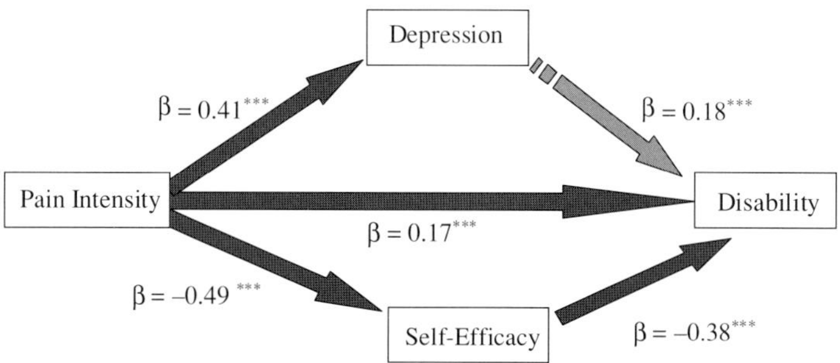

Fig. 1. Self-efficacy mediates pain-related disability. The broken arrow indicates a pathway that is not significant in all samples.

Table II
Mediators of depression in chronic pain (combined sample, standardized β coefficients)

Model	Step 1	Step 2	Step 3
Pain intensity	0.41***	0.23***	0.19***
Self-efficacy		–0.38***	–0.29***
Disability			0.20***
Adjusted R^2	0.17	0.28	0.30

*** $P \leq 0.001$.

combined sample. All paths remained statistically significant ($P < 0.001$), fulfilling the requirements for the mediation model drawn in Fig. 2 ($F_{3,449}$ = 87; $P < 0.001$), which accounted for 30% of the explained variance in depression.

Separate examinations of the three samples supported the disability model with slight differences (Fig. 3). In the group with no history of depression, the greatest amount of variance in disability (a total of 47%) was explained by pain (33%) and self-efficacy (14%). Although in the tertiary sample these accounted for less of the explained variance (37%), self-efficacy completely mediated the effect of pain on disability, meaning that it was low self-efficacy, not high pain intensity that accounted for the extent of disability reported. Both samples that included patients with prior depression found that depression contributed only 2–3% of the explained variance, which could be attributed to pain intensity and self-efficacy alone.

Fig. 4 shows a similar testing of the depression model in different samples. In all three groups, self-efficacy mediated the relationship between pain intensity and depression ($P < 0.001$). The model explained the most variance in depression (17% pain plus 19% self-efficacy plus 3% disability for a total of 39%) for the tertiary center sample. Low self-efficacy beliefs accounted for more of the explained variance in depression than did pain

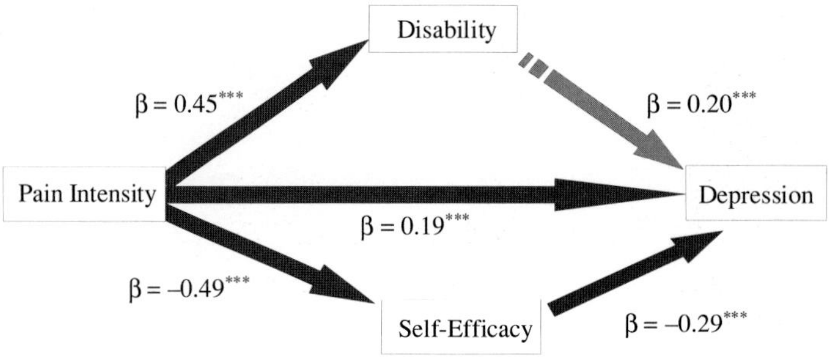

Fig. 2. Self-efficacy mediates depression. (Broken arrow as in Fig. 1.)

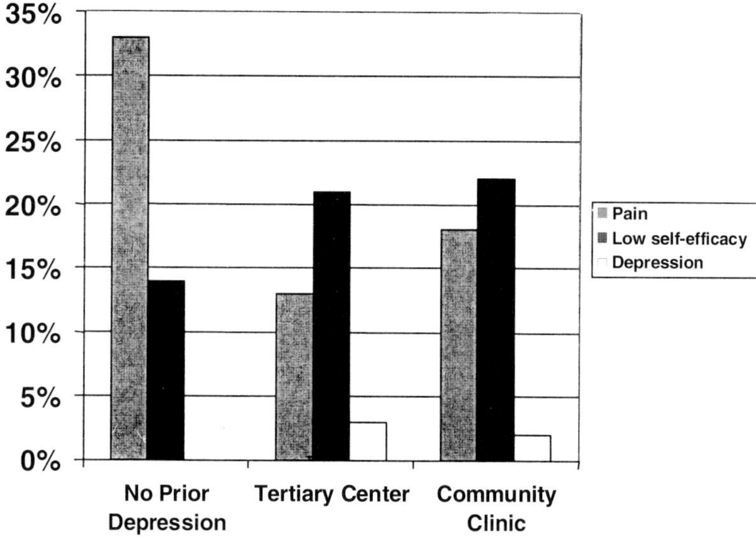

Fig. 3. Explained variance of pain-related disability: comparison of predictors of disability in different samples.

intensity in both samples that included patients with a history of depression. In the sample that excluded patients with a history of prior depression, pain intensity accounted for twice as much explained variance as did low self-efficacy (23% versus 11%, respectively).

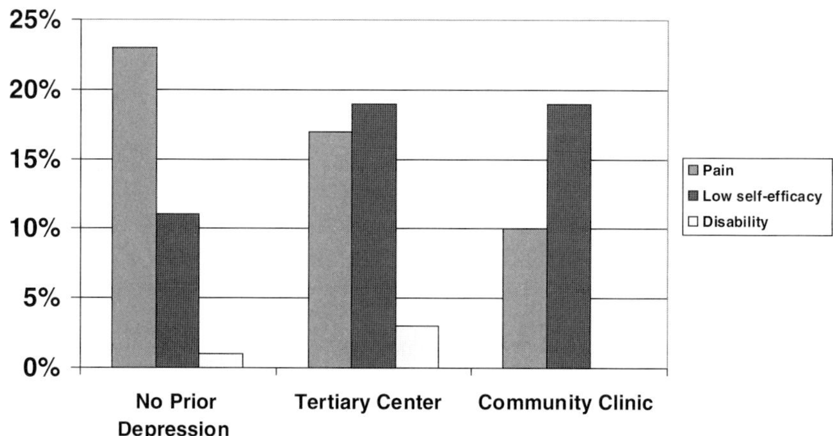

Fig. 4. Explained variance of depression: comparison of predictors of depression in different samples.

CONCLUSIONS

Pain intensity directly and indirectly contributes to disability by lowering self-efficacy beliefs. In a similar fashion both pain intensity and low self-efficacy contribute to a depressed mood. This study is consistent with others that support the influence of self-efficacy beliefs on mood (Wright et al. 1996; Arnstein et al. 1999) and physical functioning (Dolce et al. 1986; Council et al. 1988; Kores et al. 1990; Estlander et al. 1994; Jensen et al. 1994; Anderson et al. 1995; Levin et al. 1996). The combination of high pain intensity and low self-efficacy beliefs accounted for nearly half the explained variance in disability and nearly a third of the variance in depression. Differences noted between samples imply the need for research to determine whether patients who have a history of depression prior to the onset of chronic pain are more vulnerable to the effects of low self-efficacy.

Our results confirm that the lack of belief in one's ability to manage pain and to cope and function despite the persistence of pain (low self-efficacy) is an important contributor to the disability and depression of chronic pain patients. Therefore, evaluating and bolstering the patient's belief in personal abilities may be an important component of therapy. According to Bandura (1997), self-efficacy beliefs can be enhanced through skill mastery, sharing vicarious experiences, verbal persuasion, and providing information about the patient's physiological and affective state. An enhancement of self-efficacy beliefs may protect patients from the disability and despair that often results from chronic pain.

REFERENCES

Anderson KO, Dowds BN, Pelletz RE, Edwards WT. Development and initial validation of a scale to measure self efficacy beliefs in patients with chronic pain. *Pain* 1995; 63:77–84.

Arnstein PM, Caudill M, Mandle CL, Norris A, Beasley R. Self efficacy as a mediator of the relationship between pain intensity, disability and depression in chronic pain patients. *Pain* 1999; 80(3):483–491.

Bandura A. *Social Learning Theory*. Englewood Cliffs, NJ: Prentice-Hall, 1977, pp 58–93.

Bandura A. Self efficacy: the exercise of control. New York: W.H. Freeman, 1997.

Baron RM, Kenny DA. The moderator-mediator variable distinction in social psychological research: conceptual, strategic and statistical considerations. *J Pers Soc Psychol* 1986; 51:1173–1182.

Council JR, Ahern DK, Follick MJ, Kline CL. Expectancies and functional impairment in chronic low back pain. *Pain* 1988; 33:323–331.

Dolce JJ, Crocker MF, Moletteire C, Doleys DM. Exercise quotas, anticipatory concern and self efficacy expectancies in chronic pain: a preliminary report. *Pain* 1986; 24:365–372.

Estlander AM, Vanharanta H, Moneta G, Kaivanto K. Anthropometric variables, self efficacy beliefs and pain and disability ratings on the isokinetic performance of low back pain patients. *Spine* 1994; 19(8):941–947.

Jensen MP, Turner JA, Romano JM. Self efficacy and outcome expectancies: relationship to chronic pain coping strategies and adjustment. *Pain* 1991; 44:263–269.

Jensen MP, Turner JA, Romano JM, Lawler BK. Relationship of pain-specific beliefs to chronic pain adjustment. *Pain* 1994; 57:301–309.

Keefe FJ, Bradley LA, Main CJ. Psychological assessment of the pain patient for the general clinician. In: Max M (Ed). *Pain 1999—An Updated Review.* Seattle: IASP Press, 1999, pp 219–230.

Kores RC, Murphy WD, Rosenthal TL, Elias DB, North WC. Predicting outcomes of chronic pain treatment via a modified self efficacy scale. *Behav Res Ther* 1990; 28:165–169.

Levin JB, Lofland KR, Cassisi JE, Poreh AM, Blonsky ER. The relationship between self efficacy and disability in chronic low back pain patients. *Int J Rehabil Health* 1996; 2(1):19–28.

Lorig KR, Mazonson PD, Holman HR. Evidence suggesting that health education for self management in patients with chronic arthritis has sustained health benefits while reducing health care costs. *Arthritis Rheum* 1993; 36(4):439–446.

Wright GE, Parker JC, Smarr KL, et al. Risk factors for depression in rheumatoid arthritis. *Arthritis Care Res* 1996; 9(4):264–272.

Correspondence to: Paul Arnstein, RN, CS, PhD, 140 Commonwealth Avenue, Chestnut Hill, MA 02467, USA. Tel: 617-552-1605; email: arnstein@bc.edu.

Proceedings of the 9th World Congress on Pain,
Progress in Pain Research and Management,
Vol. 16, edited by M. Devor, M.C. Rowbotham, and
Z. Wiesenfeld-Hallin, IASP Press, Seattle, © 2000.

104

Solicitousness Revisited: A Qualitative Analysis of Spouse Responses to Pain Behaviors

Toby R.O. Newton-John
and Amanda C. de C. Williams

Department of Pain Management, National Hospital for Neurology and Neurosurgery, London, United Kingdom; and Guy's, King's and St. Thomas' Medical School, London, United Kingdom

The operant behavioral formulation of chronic pain (Fordyce et al. 1968; Fordyce 1976) drew attention to the importance of social factors in the development and maintenance of chronic pain problems. Since the introduction of this model, evidence has accumulated that the social responsiveness of others, and the patient's spouse in particular, can be important in these processes (Block et al. 1980; Turk et al. 1985; Schwartz et al. 1994). For example, an early study by Block et al. (1980) demonstrated that patient pain reports may be influenced by the presence or absence of the spouse—a finding confirmed in several other contexts (e.g., Gil et al. 1987; Lousberg et al. 1992).

In attempting to quantify patient-spouse interactions in chronic pain, researchers have developed measures for categorizing spouse responses to patient expressions of pain and suffering (i.e., pain behaviors; Keefe and Block 1982). These spouse responses have been examined for their effect upon the physical and emotional functioning of patients. The Spouse Response Scale of the Multidimensional Pain Inventory (MPI: Kerns et al. 1985) is the most widely used self-report instrument, and may be completed by either the patient or the spouse. It identifies three kinds of spouse behavioral response to expressions of pain behavior: solicitous responses (e.g., "I get him medications"), punishing or negative responses ("I express my anger"), and distracting responses ("I turn on the TV to take his mind off the pain"). Other scales for categorizing spouse responses include observer rating scales (Romano et al. 1992) and diary recording methods (Flor et al. 1987); however, these scales have also categorized spouse responses within similar three-response formats.

By contrast, perusal of the marital interaction literature suggests that spouses are capable of responding to each other's behaviors in more varied ways than noted by these chronic pain data. Fincham (1994, 1997) has emphasized the importance of spouse cognitions in determining behavioral responses. As attributions and appraisals of behavior within relationships vary according to context, mood, and a host of other factors (Cheung 1996), spouse responses may also vary widely. To reflect this variability, the assessment of spouse behaviors in the marital interaction literature supports a much broader range of categories. For example, the Category System for Partnership Interaction (Hahlweg et al. 1984) contains 26 categories for coding verbal and nonverbal behaviors during within-couple interactions. The Couples Interaction Scoring System (Gottman 1979) contains eight codes to reflect just the verbal responses of the speaker in a dyadic interaction. Admittedly, the response of a spouse to the expression of pain behavior by a patient is a specific form of dyadic interaction, as opposed to these more general evaluations of couple interaction. Nevertheless, the wide range of responses that the marital literature acknowledges as being important in marital interactions suggests the behavioral view of spouse response that dominates the chronic pain literature may be excessively narrow.

We designed a study to investigate whether spouse responses to patient pain behaviors are more varied when this interchange is viewed from a marital interaction perspective rather than a purely behavioral perspective. A second but related issue was the effect of the spouse responses upon the patients. More particularly, what affective response does spouse solicitousness generate in chronic pain patients? Throughout the study, the term "spouse" indicates a primary adult relationship, but not necessarily legal matrimonial status.

METHOD

STUDY POPULATION

Eighty heterogeneous chronic pain patients and their spouses (see Table I for demographics) participated in the study. Subjects were recruited from consecutive patient referrals to an inpatient, multidisciplinary pain management program (Williams and Erskine 1995). To participate, pain patients had to be in a primary relationship and cohabiting with their partner for at least 12 months. Of the eligible couples that were approached, 59% agreed

Table I
Patient and spouse demographics

Demographic	Patients ($N = 95$)	Spouses ($N = 95$)
Age (years)		
Mean (SD)	48.2 (10.4)	49.1 (11.5)
Range	25–68	28–71
Sex		
Male	38	57
Female	57	38
Ethnicity (%)		
White	93	94
Black/Afrocaribbean	2	2
Asian	4	4
Other	1	—
Pain Site (%)		
Low back	64	
Upper limb	17	
Head/neck	12	
Other	7	
Pain Duration (years)		
Mean (SD)	9.7 (9.2)	
Range	1–50	

to join the study. Eighty-nine percent of the sample were married, with a mean relationship duration of 20.9 years (SD = 12.8 years). There were no same-sex couples. Inspection of scores on standardized assessment measures indicated that the couples were reporting mild levels of psychological distress. Mean scores on the Beck Depression Inventory (Beck et al. 1961) were 18.2 (SD = 8.0) for the patient sample, well below the cut-off recommended by Eisser et al. (1999) to indicate significant depressive symptoms in chronic pain patients. Compared to norms for the general population, the spouse sample also reported little depressive symptomatology (mean = 8.4, SD = 5.2). Scores on the Dyadic Adjustment Scale (Spanier 1976), a commonly used measure of marital satisfaction, were also well above the cut-off indicating marital distress (patients' mean = 114.2, SD = 19.4; spouses' mean = 111.9, SD = 19.2). Neither measure showed significant gender differences between the patient and spouse groups.

PATIENT AND SPOUSE ASSESSMENT

To explore the two research questions stated above, we conducted semistructured, separate interviews with patients and their spouses. Spouses were first shown a series of 14 written vignettes depicting various everyday situations (e.g., socializing, watching television, doing household chores). Each vignette describes the patient as exhibiting pain behavior of some kind (e.g., grimacing, talking about pain, refusing to continue with an activity because of pain). Spouses were asked to identify which of the 14 vignettes they had personally experienced. Then they were asked: "In this situation, how would you respond? What would you normally do?" Their responses to these questions were recorded verbatim on protocol sheets.

The patients independently read the same vignettes and identified those they had experienced personally. For consistency, only those vignettes previously identified by the spouse were included. Patients were asked: "In this situation, how would your spouse respond? What would he/she do?" After replying, patients were asked the supplementary question, "When your spouse responds in that way, how does it make you feel?" If patients had difficulty identifying their affective reaction to the spouse response, they were given one prompt: "Does that kind of response make you feel good, bad, or neutral?" This question concluded the semistructured interviews.

DATA ANALYSIS

All data were transcribed verbatim onto recording sheets, and then onto a word processor for analysis. Content analysis (Krippendorff 1980; Weber 1990) was the qualitative method chosen to analyze the data. Content analysis, which has been used with a variety of clinical populations including those with chronic illness (Viney 1983; King et al. 1999), involves transforming a data set into groups or categories of homogeneous responses. Once "saturation" is reached (Glaser and Strauss 1967) and no further categories can be generated from the data, the existing categories are reviewed for any duplication or overlap. They are finally reduced further until a core set of response categories has emerged (Weber 1990). Categories are then analyzed according to the frequency of their occurrence, either within the text or from subject report. All categories are mutually exclusive in that a particular response may not be coded into more than one category. An integral part of the content analytic method is the examination of intercoder reliability to ensure that the categories are generalizable to other populations.

RESULTS

The 80 spouses produced 540 responses to the 14 vignettes (mean = 6.6 responses, range 3–13 responses). Saturation was reached in the initial coding run after 36 categories had been generated; however, subsequent cross-comparison of the categories reduced this total to a final set of 12 core responses. The first author tested the intercoder reliability of the 12 categories with the assistance of three other clinical psychologists with at least three years' experience working with chronic pain patients. Twenty percent of the data (120 responses) was randomly selected from the entire data set and coded by all experimenters after standardized training. Kappa coefficients ranged from $\kappa = 0.84$ to $\kappa = 0.89$, which indicates high intercoder reliability (Everitt 1996).

A brief description of each spouse response category, in descending order of the frequency of reported use, follows:

1) Providing Help (35% of all responses): This set of responses encompasses the traditional conceptualization of solicitousness. The behaviors represented by this category are specifically aimed at either relieving pain (e.g., giving a massage, getting pain medications, taking over patient's activity) or decreasing pain-related distress (e.g., expressing sympathy). Spouses most frequently reported this category of response.

2) Observe Only (15% of all responses): The spouses reported that they do not respond with an overt helping behavior when witnessing patient expressions of pain. Instead, spouses prefer to observe and monitor the patient. A variety of different reasons were given for the observe only response: "You can't always be jumping up to help them," "I like to see how he gets on himself," "She doesn't like me fussing, but I want to know what's happening." This category therefore represents a cognitive rather than a behavioral response to pain behavior, and was the second most frequently reported response cited by spouses.

3) Offer Help (11% of all responses): This response represents a verbal offer of assistance (e.g., "Would you like me to take over?"; "Do you need any help?") as opposed to the first category, in which the spouse simply performs the pain-relieving action. A distinction was drawn between these two responses, as the offer help category allows the patient to reject the offer.

4) Discouraging Pain Talk (8% of all responses): We were particularly interested in the spouse response to patient verbal expressions of pain. This category refers to attempts by the spouse to interrupt, change the topic, or otherwise inhibit patient discussion of his or her pain problem.

5) Encouraging Pain Talk (7% of all responses): In this response, the opposite of the above category, the spouse attempts to engage the patient in a discussion of his or her pain. This category was reported only slightly less frequently than discouraging pain talk.

6) Physical Assurance (6% of all responses): This somewhat broader category of response refers to the spouse's attempt to reassure the patient

that he or she is physically capable of managing a current task—despite the acknowledgment of pain behavior. Physical assurance responses may relate to specific activities such as socializing (e.g., “We don’t need to go back home right now—you’ll be OK in a short while”) and domestic chores (e.g., “You look like you can cope with that”) or represent more general examples of encouragement (e.g., “Come on, you can do it”).

7) Shielding (6% of all responses): The spouse tries to avoid emotionally upsetting the patient by either protecting him or her from further stress (e.g., not relating bad news) or by terminating an argument or disagreement when pain behavior becomes apparent.

8) Express Frustration (4% of all responses): This is equivalent to the MPI category of Punishing/Negative responses. The spouse directly expresses anger or irritation with the patient (e.g., “For goodness sake, stop complaining!”).

9) Ignoring (4% of all responses): The spouse pretends that the pain behavior had not occurred, and intentionally disregards the patient’s action. This response contrasts with that of observing only, where the spouse does not intend to ignore or disregard the patient, but to defer making any behavioral response at that time. Spouses seldom reported the Ignoring response.

10) Problem-Solving (3% of all responses): The spouse makes specific efforts to assist the patient to maintain a given activity or achieve a particular goal, despite the patient’s expression of pain behavior. Examples include suggesting that the patient still prepare the evening meal, but prepare the vegetables sitting down rather than standing; or discussing how the patient might attend a social event by pacing of walking and sitting tolerances.

11) Hostile-Solicitous (2% of all responses): This response conforms to the traditionally accepted notion of solicitousness in that the spouse is attempting to relieve pain or distress, but the response is underpinned by an aggressive or irritated affect (e.g., “I’ll get him the tablets, but only when I am good and ready”; “I’ll shout at her, ‘How many times have I told you not to carry those bags—put them down now’”).

12) Distraction (1% of all responses): This response is also equivalent to the MPI category of distracting—the spouse’s response is intended to divert the patient’s attention from the pain and onto some other task (e.g., “I start talking to her about anything I can think of, anything other than her back”).

The patient sample generated 353 responses to the 14 vignettes (mean = 3.45 responses, range 1–8 responses); the lower mean reflects the inclusion in the analysis of only those vignettes that the spouse also had previously chosen. We coded the patient data according to the 12 categories generated above, and again obtained very high intercoder reliabilities ($\kappa = 0.85$ to $\kappa = 0.87$).

The responses to the patient question, "When your spouse responds in that way, how does it make you feel?" were then coded into three categories of affect: positive, negative, or neutral. However, unlike the 12 response categories, these affective categories were not mutually exclusive. For example, the patient may report feeling "cared for" by a providing help response but also "guilty" for receiving the assistance; or feeling "upset" by the expressing frustration response but also "relieved" that the spouse had noticed that the patient was in pain. On these occasions, the response was coded as having both a positive and a negative affective value.

Fig. 1 presents the affective reactions to the 12 response categories. The responses most often rated positively by patients were physical assurance, observe only, and problem-solving. Providing help, the category that encompasses the traditional view of solicitousness, was rated the third least favorable response. The most common affective consequences for this response included feeling "guilty," "useless," and "burdensome." None of the patients reported any instances of distraction.

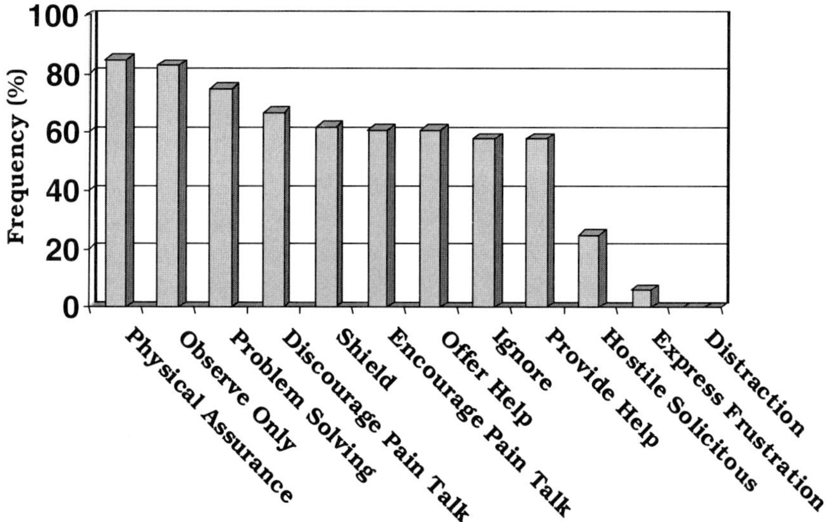

Fig. 1. Patient affective reactions to spouse responses. The graph shows the frequency of each spouse response being rated as "Positive" by patients.

CONCLUSIONS

Our study had two principal aims: First, to determine whether spouse responses to the pain behaviors of chronic pain patients showed greater variability than the behavioral model has hitherto acknowledged; and second, to evaluate the immediate affective influence of spouse responses upon patients. We used a qualitative data analytic technique to answer these questions and better capture the phenomenological aspects of the interaction.

In contrast to the prevailing notion of just three spouse responses to pain behaviors, our content analysis generated 12 forms of response. Intercoder reliability checks indicated that these categories were highly reliable and were not generated according to idiosyncratic coding rules that could not be applied to another data set. Hence, it appears that spouses do exhibit a greater variety of responses than has been recognized. Of note was the generation of two new categories of response: observe only, a primarily cognitive reaction to pain behavior, and hostile-solicitous, which combines elements of helping behaviors with frustration or annoyance.

We found that the spouse responses reported by patients as the most positive are among the least frequently used. Physical assurance and problem-solving responses, which are wholly consistent with cognitive behavioral principles of pain management (Williams and Erskine 1995), were rarely reported by spouses although highly valued by patients. Alternatively, the solicitous response categories of providing help and offering help were rated much less favorably by patients—and yet they are the most common forms of spouse response by a considerable margin.

Several limitations pertaining to the nature of the sample need to be considered when interpreting these results. The patients were predominantly white, lower back pain sufferers with lengthy pain histories but without the high levels of depressive symptomatology often seen in this patient group (Rudy et al. 1988). Equally important, the marital satisfaction scores for both patients and spouses fell above the norms set for healthy populations. Given that the mean length of relationship was slightly above 20 years for the sample as a whole, these data suggest that this group of pain couples may not be as representative of the population of chronic pain couples as might be wished. It is an empirical question whether a similar set of results would be obtained with a less maritally satisfied, more distressed, more culturally diverse patient-spouse sample.

Finally, these results offer some suggestions for the inclusion of spouses in pain management interventions (Moore and Chaney 1985; Keefe et al. 1996). It seems that spouses are capable of a wider repertoire of responses than has been acknowledged, but may rely on solicitous behaviors such as providing help because they lack awareness of the acceptability of other responses. The patient data indicate that the most desirable responses are being given minimal assistance, providing encouragement, or just acknowledging the pain—without any instrumental response. These results thus offer an empirical basis for the development of a couples-based, cognitive behavioral pain management program.

REFERENCES

Beck AT, Ward CH, Mendelson M, Mock N, Erbaugh J. An inventory for measuring depression. *Arch Gen Psychiatry* 1961; 4:561–571.

Block AR, Kremer EF, Gaylor M. Behavioral treatment of chronic pain: the spouse as a discriminative cue for pain behavior. *Pain* 1980; 9:243–252.

Cheung S. Cognitive-behaviour therapy for marital conflict: refining the concept of attribution. *J Family Ther* 1996; 18:183–203.

Fincham FD. Cognition in marriage: current status and future challenges. *Appl Preventative Psychol* 1994; 3:185–198.

Fincham FD. Understanding marriage: from fish scales to milliseconds. *Psychologist* 1997; 10:543–547.

Flor H, Kerns RD, Turk DC. The role of spouse reinforcement, perceived pain, and activity levels of chronic pain patients. *J Psychosom Res* 1987; 31:251–259.

Fordyce WE. *Behavioral Methods in Chronic Pain and Illness*. St. Louis: Mosby, 1976.

Fordyce WE, Fowler RS, DeLateur B. An application of behavior modification technique to a problem of chronic pain. *Behav Res Ther* 1968; 6:105–107.

Gil KM, Keefe FJ, Crisson JE, Van Dalfsen PJ. Social support and pain behavior. *Pain* 1987; 29:209–217.

Glaser BG, Strauss AL. *The Discovery of Grounded Theory: Strategies for Qualitative Research*. Chicago: Aldine, 1967.

Gottman JM. *Marital Interaction: Experimental Investigations*. New York: Academic Press, 1979.

Hahlweg K, Reisner L, Kohli J, et al. KPI category system for partnership interaction. In: Hahlweg K, Jacobson N (Eds). *Marital Interaction: Analysis and Modification*. New York: Guilford Press, 1984.

Keefe FJ, Block AR. Development of an observation method of assessing pain behavior in chronic low back pain patients. *Behav Ther* 1982; 13:363–375.

Keefe FJ, Caldwell DS, Baucom DH, et al. Spouse-assisted coping skills training in the management of osteoarthritic knee pain. *Arthritis Care Res* 1996; 9:279–291.

Kerns RD, Turk DC, Rudy TE. The West Haven-Yale Multidimensional Pain Inventory (WHYMPI). *Pain* 1985; 23:345–356.

King C, Kennedy P. Coping effectiveness training for people with spinal cord injury: preliminary results of a controlled trial. *Br J Clin Psychol* 1999; 38:5–14.

Krippendorff K. Analytical techniques. In: Krippendorff K. *Content Analysis: An Introduction to its Methodology*. Beverly Hills, California: Sage, 1980, pp 109–118.

Lousberg R, Schmidt AJM, Groenman NH. The relationship between spouse solicitousness and pain behavior: searching for more experimental evidence. *Pain* 1992; 51:75–79.

Moore JE, Chaney EF. Outpatient group treatment of chronic pain: effects of spouse involvement. *J Consult Clin Psychol* 1985; 53:326–334.

Romano JM, Turner JA, Friedman LS, et al. Sequential analysis of chronic pain behaviors and spouse responses. *J Consult Clin Psychol* 1992; 60:777–782.

Rudy TE, Kerns RD, Turk DC. Chronic pain and depression: towards a cognitive-behavioral mediation model. *Pain* 1988; 35:129–140.

Schwartz L, Slater MA, Birchler GR. Interpersonal stress and pain behaviors in patients with chronic pain. *J Consult Clin Psychol* 1994; 62:861–864.

Spanier GB. Measuring dyadic adjustment: new scales for assessing the quality of marriage and similar dyads. *J Marriage Family* 1976; 38:15–28.

Turk DC, Rudy TE, Flor H. Why a family perspective for pain? *Int J Family Ther* 1985; 7:223–234.

Viney LL. The assessment of psychological states through content analysis of verbal communications. *Psychol Bull* 1983; 94:542–563.

Weber RP. Content classification and interpretation. In: Weber RP. *Basic Content Analysis.* Newbury Park, California: Sage Publications, 1990, pp 15–40.

Williams AC de C, Erskine A. Chronic pain. In: Broome A, Llewelyn S (Eds). *Health Psychology: Processes and Applications.* London: Chapman and Hall, 1995; pp 353–376.

Correspondence to: Toby R.O. Newton-John, PhD, Department of Pain Management, National Hospital for Neurology and Neurosurgery, Queens Square, London WC1N 3BG, United Kingdom. Tel: 44-171-837-3611; Fax: 44-171-419-1714.

Proceedings of the 9th World Congress on Pain,
Progress in Pain Research and Management,
Vol. 16, edited by M. Devor, M.C. Rowbotham, and
Z. Wiesenfeld-Hallin, IASP Press, Seattle, © 2000.

105

Talking to Others about Pain: Suffering in Silence

Stephen Morley, Katharine Doyle, and Angela Beese

Division of Psychiatry and Behavioural Sciences, School of Medicine, University of Leeds, Leeds, United Kingdom

Contemporary analysis of communication in chronic pain patients is dominated by two schools that rely on an observer's account of behavior, often in the context of marital interactions, via operant behavioral analysis (Sanders 1996) and the analysis of facial expression (Craig et al. 1992). Little is known about the circumstances in which chronic pain sufferers choose to communicate information about their pain to members of their social network. Our work was stimulated by clinical observations of pain patients who reported problems in social settings. How should they manage the conflicting demands engendered by the need to maintain social interaction when they are experiencing pain? Disclosing their pain state might enable others to understand and accommodate to the pain sufferer's behavioral limitations, but this advantage may have unacceptable costs, such as not being believed and social withdrawal (Osborn and Smith 1998). One feature that may facilitate disclosure is whether the sufferer has a socially plausible "story" to tell the recipient. We speculated that sufferers with a known cause for their illness (postherpetic neuralgia) would be more able to disclose their pain than sufferers without a known cause (chronic low back pain).

METHODS

PARTICIPANTS

We recruited 25 patients with chronic low back pain and 20 patients with postherpetic neuralgia from two neighboring pain clinics. The gender ratio within each group was identical (male:female = 3:2) but the chronic low back pain patients were significantly younger (51.1 years, SD = 11.8) than the postherpetic pain patients (71.8 years, SD = 7.9, $t_{(43)} = 6.68$, $P < 0.001$). The mean duration of pain was 8.86 years (SD = 7.9) for the low back pain group and 6.03 years (SD = 4.3) for the postherpetic neuralgia group: these means were not significantly different. Few patients were employed: 17 low back pain patients had retired due to ill health, while 11 postherpetic patients were retired because of their age. Relationship status was 78% married, 16% widowed, 4% divorced, and 2% single. A significant proportion (48%) had comorbid chronic physical illness (diabetes, cardiovascular disorders), and the postherpetic pain patients were more likely to report respiratory problems ($P < 0.05$).

MEASURES

Participants completed several self-report measures to assess aspects of pain and psychological distress: (1) McGill Pain Questionnaire-Short Form (MPQ; Melzack, 1987); (2) Pain Perceptions and Beliefs Inventory (PBPI; Williams and Thorn, 1989); (3) Hospital Anxiety and Depression Scale (HAD; Zigmond and Snaith, 1983); and (4) Back Pain Locus of Control Scale (BPLC; Härkäpää et al. 1996; Vakkari 1990). We slightly modified this scale for use in both groups by replacing the phrase "back pain" with "pain."

We developed a structured interview to systematically explore participants' accounts of their interpersonal communication. The content of the interview was based on ideas from current theories of communication and social cognition research. We pilot tested the interview over three development cycles on chronic pain patients who were not participants in the main study. The general questionnaire format posed open questions to encourage participants to talk freely about an issue. Then followed specific closed questions that required participants to provide a rated response on a Likert scale. This strategy has been used successfully in other research to map personal accounts of epilepsy (Kemp et al. 1999) and the development of chronicity in pain (Royle 1997). The interview consisted of three sections. Section A comprised a series of questions designed to assess in general terms how, and under what circumstances, participants communicate their pain to others. Section B required participants to recall in as much detail as possible the last time they spoke to four specific individuals about their pain; their "closest other" (usually spouse or family member), an acquaintance, their family doctor, and their pain clinic doctor. This section used the cognitive interview technique to elicit memories (Bekerian and Dennett 1993). Section C comprised a series of questions designed to assess illness representations.

PROCEDURE

Suitable participants were identified through the clinic database and contacted by letter. All participants signed consent forms prior to the interview; 18 participants chose to be interviewed at home and 27 at the clinic. After we collected demographic data, participants completed the structured interview followed by the standardized questionnaires. Interviews lasted up to 2 hours. The interviewer recorded participants responses verbatim and made additional memo notes at the end of each interview.

RESULTS

The mean scores for the two groups on the standardized questionnaires are shown in Table I. The groups showed no differences in their reports of

Table I
Summary of mean group characteristics (SD) on the standardized questionnaires; the groups did not differ on any of these measures

	Group	
Measure	Low Back Pain	Postherpetic Neuralgia
McGill Pain Questionnaire		
Sensory	15.7 (8.4)	13.8 (7.3)
Affect	7.0 (3.7)	4.8 (3.3)
Present pain intensity	4.3 (1.3)	3.6 (1.4)
HAD		
Anxiety	9.8 (4.5)	8.2 (4.5)
Depression	8.0 (4.9)	6.0 (4.3)
*PBPI**		
Constancy	8.1 (1.7)	9.0 (1.2)
Permanence	11.9 (1.2)	12.3 (1.1)
Self-blame	9.0 (2.2)	9.3 (1.7)
Mysteriousness	10.4 (2.3)	11.2 (1.4)
BPLC		
Internal control	3.3 (1.1)	3.4 (1.1)
Control by others	3.9 (1.0)	3.2 (1.3)
Chance	3.9 (0.9)	4.2 (0.9)

Note: HAD = Hospital Anxiety and Depression Scale; PBPI = Pain Beliefs and Perceptions Inventory; BPLC = Back Pain Locus of Control Questionnaire.
* The scoring for the PBPI items was changed to 1, 2, 3, 4 from –1, –2, +1, +2.

pain intensity, but the low back pain group reported slightly higher pain affect on the MPQ. The groups did not differ in their self-reported depression or anxiety, or on measures of locus of control or on the subscales of the PBPI.

The data from the structured interview were subjected to content analysis. We developed a list of provisional codes and categories (Bogdan and Biklen 1992) and took a sample of 70 statements from 15 randomly selected participants. Each statement was pasted onto an index card for presentation to three independent raters. After initial orientation and discussion, pairs of raters achieved inter-rater agreement on category allocation of 90%, 94%, and 88%. Reliability checks for repeated coding (1-week interval) yielded 100% agreement. We tabulated the frequency of observation for each code and examined the proportional differences between the two groups by using confidence interval analysis (Gardner et al. 1989). The following section reports analysis of the data from sections A and B of the interview.

HOW DO PATIENTS COMMUNICATE TO OTHERS?

The two groups of patients showed few differences in their self-reports of how they communicate their pain to others. Only 7% of patients said that they did not talk to anyone about their pain. Most patients (78%) said that verbal disclosure was the main mode, but a significant subgroup (22%) reported that "others just know" because of nonverbal cues (posture, facial expression, and para-vocalizations). Over 50% of patients in both groups said that they only talked about their pain when asked, and 22% felt it was inappropriate to talk when their pain was very severe. When pain is disclosed it appears that most patients say little about its intensity and quality, and back pain patients (32%) were more likely to try and "play down" their pain and distress compared with postherpetic neuralgia patients (0%, $P < 0.01$). Not surprisingly, most communication (70%) is within the family, but 13% of patients said they talk to friends and 11% said they talk only to their doctor about their pain.

More than one-third of participants (38%) identified certain aspects of their pain experience they would not talk about even in their most confiding relationship (pain severity, sexual difficulties consequent on pain, and new health threats); reported concealment was more likely in low back pain ($P < 0.05$). Notably, most sufferers (90%) said they tried to hide their pain from others, an approach most likely in public places, with new people, and with non-family members and when pain was severe, and 64% identified a particular person they would not talk to about their pain (this included medical staff).

We identified several reasons pain patients gave for concealment. More than 60% of sufferers said that they had experienced, and therefore expected, negative consequences (others' inability to sympathize, expectation of being judged negatively, distrusting others, expectation of others' disbelief). Sufferers also reported that not disclosing was a strategy for maintaining a relationship; they were concerned about being perceived as a social burden and preferred to maintain a public view of their competence in a given role. Finally, over half of the participants reported that hiding their pain was important in preserving a sense of self-competence and self-esteem.

COMMUNICATING IN GIVEN ROLES

Our study revealed marked differences in how participants described their communication to others in given social roles. A few participants (7%) could not name a *closest other* because their partner had died. The mode of disclosure of pain was almost equally divided between verbal (40%) and nonverbal (37%: "They can see it in my face—I don't need to talk"). The remaining participants reported using a mixture of both modes. While 75% reported they received a positive response from their partner, 13% reported that the response had been negative. This was more likely in the low back pain group ($P < 0.05$). Most participants (55%) had disclosed information about the "physical" component of pain (intensity, symptoms). The next most frequent category of communication was an excuse or reason why they could not carry out a particular domestic task. In contrast to the report of universal disclosure to a closest other, more than half (53%) of participants said that they would never disclose their pain to an *acquaintance*. If they do disclose to another it is most likely to be to a fellow sufferer (22%), whom they expect to be less likely to respond negatively.

Most participants reported verbal disclosure (84%) to their *family doctor,* but a few relied on either the doctor's sensitivity to their nonverbal expression or direct questioning before they would disclose their pain. Most participants (70%) reported that they felt able to disclose information on any matter to their doctor, and only 9% reported difficulties in talking to the doctor because the relationship was poor. In contrast, the report of disclosure to a *pain clinic doctor* was more circumscribed. While 58% reported disclosure about the physical aspects of their pain, only 2.2% reported having talked about psychological concerns, although the vast majority (90%) said that they would talk about their psychological and social concerns were they to be asked. However, 30% made statements suggesting that they felt the pain clinic doctor might be unsympathetic.

DISCUSSION

The subjective experience of pain is loosely coupled with behavioral indices, e.g., facial expression, that indicate its presence. For chronic pain patients the choice about whether to express or suppress their experience of pain is difficult and marked by conflicting elements: wishing to disclose, the fear of not being understood or believed, and the need to present themselves as positive contributors to a relationship and as a competent person. Participants reported exercising caution about how and when they disclosed the presence of pain, and showed marked differences in both the frequency and content of disclosure that corresponded to the function of the relationship and the need to maintain it. While most participants described their closest other as supportive, they also described frequent attempts to conceal pain in an effort to maintain the relationship. Concealment of pain was even more marked in the presence of non-pain-suffering acquaintances. In contrast, disclosure of pain and distress to doctors and other pain sufferers is more marked because of their roles. While the focus of the doctor's role is to attend to the symptom of pain, disclosure to fellow pain sufferers was characterized by the experience of safety, of being believed, and having one's experience validated. It is thus not surprising that patients use pain management groups to express their pain. What professionals may see as unhelpful "pain talk" may serve a critical function in maintaining the sufferer's self-esteem. Elsewhere suffering in silence may be socially necessary.

ACKNOWLEDGMENT

We thank the Northern and Yorkshire NHSE for funding Katharine Doyle.

REFERENCES

Bekerian DA, Dennett JL. The cognitive interview technique: reviving the issues. *Applied Cognitive Psychol* 1993; 7:275–297.

Bogdan R, Biklen SK. *Qualitative Research for Education: An Introduction to Theory and Methods,* 2nd ed. Boston: Allyn and Bacon, 1992.

Craig KD, Prkachin KM, Grunau RVE. The facial expression of pain. In: Turk DC, Melzack R (Eds). *Handbook of Pain Assessment*. New York: Guilford Press, 1992, pp 257–276.

Gardner SB, Winter PD, Gardner MJ. *Confidence Interval Analysis: Software Package*. London: British Medical Association, 1989.

Härkäpää K, Järvikoski A, Vakkari T. Associations of locus of control beliefs with pain coping strategies and other pain-related cognitions in back pain patients. *Br J Health Psychol* 1996; 1:51–63.

Kemp S, Morley S, Wilkinson E. Coping with epilepsy: do illness representations play a role? *Br J Clin Psychol* 1999; 38:43–58.

Melzack R. The short form McGill Pain Questionnaire. *Pain* 1987; 30:191–197.
Osborn M, Smith JA. The personal experience of chronic benign lower back pain: and interpretative phenomenological analysis. *Br J Health Psychol* 1998; 3:65–83.
Royle J. Illness representations of pain states. University of Leeds, doctoral thesis, 1997.
Sanders SH. Operant conditioning with chronic pain: back to basics. In: Gatchel RJ, Turk DC (Eds). *Psychological Approaches to Pain Management*. New York: Guilford Press, 1996, pp 112–130.
Vakkari T. Chronic low back pain and health locus of control. University of Helsinki, master's thesis, 1990.
Williams DA, Thorn BE. An empirical assessment of pain beliefs. *Pain* 1989; 36:351–358.
Zigmond AS, Snaith RP. The Hospital Anxiety and Depression Scale. *Acta Scand Psychiat* 1983; 67:361–370.

Correspondence to: Stephen Morley, PhD, Division of Psychiatry and Behavioural Sciences, School of Medicine, University of Leeds, Leeds, LS2 9JT, United Kingdom. Tel: 44-113-233-2733; Fax: 44-113-243-3719; email: s.j.morley@leeds.ac.uk.

Index

Locators in *italic* refer to figures.
Locators followed by t refer to tables.

O

P